PART IV
Health Patterns: Psychosocial Funtions

Restoration and Rehabilitation: Special Populations

Rehabilitation Nursing

PREVENTION, INTERVENTION, AND OUTCOMES

FOURTH EDITION

Shirley P. Hoeman, PhD, MPH, RN, CS

Health Systems Consultations, International
Naples, Maine

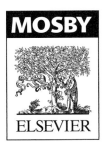

MOSBY

ELSEVIER

MOSBY
ELSEVIER

11830 Westline Industrial Drive
St. Louis, Missouri 63146

Notice

Knowledge and best practice in this field are constantly changing. As new research and experience broaden our knowledge, changes in practice, treatment and drug therapy may become necessary or appropriate. Readers are advised to check the most current information provided (i) on procedures featured or (ii) by the manufacturer of each product to be administered, to verify the recommended dose or formula, the method and duration of administration, and contraindications. It is the responsibility of the practitioner, relying on their own experience and knowledge of the patient, to make diagnoses, to determine dosages and the best treatment for each individual patient, and to take all appropriate safety precautions. To the fullest extent of the law, neither the Publisher nor the Author assumes any liability for any injury and/or damage to persons or property arising out or related to any use of the material contained in this book.

The Publisher

Previous editions copyrighted 2002, 1996, 1989

ISBN: 978-0-323-04555-1

Executive Editor: Susan R. Epstein
Senior Developmental Editor: Jean Sims Fornango
Publishing Services Manager: John Rogers
Senior Project Manager: Beth Hayes
Design Direction: Julia Dummit

Printed in the United States of America

Last digit is the print number: 9   8   7   6   5   4   3   2   1

To my grandchildren

Isaiah 40:31   "But those that wait upon the Lord
                    Shall renew their strength;
                    They shall mount up with wings like eagles,
                    They shall run and not be weary,
                    They shall walk and not faint."

Unit Managers

Barbara J. Boss, PhD, RN, CFNP, CANP
School of Nursing
University of Mississippi Medical Center
Jackson, Mississippi

Pamela M. Duchene, DNSc, RN, CRRN
St. Joseph Hospital
Nashua, New Hampshire

Aloma R. Gender, MSN, RN, CRRN
Administrator/Director of Nursing
Christus St. Michael Rehabilitation Hospital
Texarkana, Texas

Patricia L. McCollom, MS, RN, CRRN, CDMS, CCM, CLC
President and Nurse Consultant
LifeCare Economics, Management, Consulting, and Rehabilitation Services, Inc.
Ankeny, Iowa

Contributors

Joan Alverzo, PhD, MSN, CRRN
Chief Clinical Officer
Kessler Institute for Rehabilitation
West Orange, New Jersey

Angela L. Boleware, RN, MSN, FNP-C
Department of Orthopedic Surgery
University of Mississippi Medical Center
Jackson, Mississippi

Barbara J. Boss, PhD, RN, CFNP, CANP
School of Nursing
University of Mississippi Medical Center
Jackson, Mississippi

Leslie Neal Boylan, PhD, RN, CRRN, FNP-C
Associate Professor of Nursing
University of Southern Maine
Portland, Maine

Joyce Brewer, PhD, CNM, CFNP
Assistant Professor
University of Mississippi, School of Nursing
Jackson, Mississippi

Linda Brewer, RN, MSN, CFNP, CACNP
Pelahatchie Clinic
Pelahatchie, Mississippi

Lisa Cyr Buchanan, MS, RN, CRRN
Rehabilitation Clinical Nurse Specialist
The Maine Rehabilitation Center
Eastern Maine Medical Center
Bangor, Maine

Theresa Perfetta Cappello, PhD, RN
Dean and Professor
School of Health Professions
Marymount University
Arlington, Virginia

Lenore Coover, RN, MSN, AE-C
Owner–Consultant
Pediatric Case Management Services
Highland, Indiana

Sally M. Davis, MSc, RN, PGEA, DipMan
Program Lead Rehabilitation
School of Health and Social Care
Oxford Brookes University
Oxford, United Kingdom

Pamela M. Duchene, DNSc, RN, CRRN
St. Joseph Hospital
Nashua, New Hampshire

Darlene N. Finocchiaro, MSN, RN, CRRN, PN
Lecturer/Clinical Instructor
California State University–Los Angeles
Los Angeles, California

Cindy Gatens, MN, RN, CRRN-A
Clinical Nurse Specialist
Dodd Rehabilitation Center
Ohio State University
Columbus, Ohio

Aloma R. Gender, MSN, RN, CRRN
Administrator/Director of Nursing
Christus St. Michael Rehabilitation Hospital
Texarkana, Texas

Nancy H. Glenn-Molali, MSN, RN, CRRN
Rehabilitation Nurse Specialist
Private Practice
Havre de Grace, Maryland

Cynthia Gronkiewicz, RN, MS, APRN, AE-C
Pulmonary Nurse Consultant
Adjunct Faculty
University of Illinois College of Nursing
Chicago, Illinois

Maureen L. Habel, MA, RN, CRRN
Nurse Writer, Consultant
Long Beach, California

Dalice L. Hertzberg, RN, MSN, APRN, BC
Instructor, JFK Partners and School of Nursing
University of Colorado at Denver and Health Sciences Center
Denver, Colorado

Dierdre F. Jackson, MSN, APRN, CRRN
Director, Continuing Educations and Staff Development
Children's Specialized Hospital
Mountainside, New Jersey

Kelly M.M. Johnson, RN, MSN, CRRN, CNAA
Vice President Patient Care Services
Craig Hospital
Englewood, Colorado

Margaret Kelly-Hayes, EdD, RN, CRRN, FAAN
Clinical Professor of Neurological Nursing
Boston University School of Medicine
Boston, Massachusetts

Deborah J Konkle-Parker, PhD, FNP
Assistant Professor, Nurse Practitioner
University of Mississippi Medical Center
Jackson, Mississippi

Karen Liszner, BSN, MHA, CRRN
Director of Nursing and Ancillary Services
Kessler Institute for Rehabilitation
West Orange, New Jersey

Fleetwood Lostalot, RN, NP C
Nurse Practitioner/Instructor
University of Mississippi Medical Center
Jackson, Mississippi

Barbara J. Lutz, PhD, RN, CRRN
Assistant Professor
College of Nursing
University of Florida
Gainesville, Florida

**Patricia L. McCollom, MS, RN, CRRN, CDMS,
    CCM, CLC**
President and Nurse Consultant
LifeCare Economics, Management Consulting,
    and Rehabilitation Services, Inc.
Ankeny, Iowa

Jill Milner, RN, MSN, CRRN, CNS, CHTP, HTSM-HTP
Health Care Consultant
Health ReCreation
Chicago, Illinois

Christina M. Mumma, PhD, RN, CRRN
Professor Emerita, School of Nursing
University of Alaska
Anchorage, Alaska

Maureen Musto, RN, BNS, CRRN
Dodd Rehabilitation Center
Ohio State University Medical Center
Columbus, Ohio

Audrey Nelson, PhD, RN, FAAN
Director, Patient Safety Center of Inquiry
James A. Haley Veterans Affairs Medical Center
Tampa, Florida

Rhonda S. Olson, MS, RN, CRRN
Rehabilitation Nurse Consultant
RS Consulting
Houston, Texas

Marion A. Phipps, RN, MS, CRRN, FAAN
Clinical Nurse Specialist
Massachusetts General Hospital
Boston, Massachusetts

Linda L. Pierce, PhD, RN, CNS, CRRN, FAHA
Professor
Medical University of Ohio at Toledo College
    of Nursing
Toledo, Ohio

Elizabeth Predeger, PhD, RN
Associate Professor
School of Nursing
University of Alaska
Anchorage, Alaska

**Maureen Preston, MSN, APRN, BC, CRRN,
    CWOCN**
Adult Nurse Practitioner
Craig Hospital
Englewood, Colorado

Christy A. Price-Rabetroy, MSN, RN, NP
Nephrology Nurse Practitioner
Nephrology Associates
Salt Lake City, Utah

Julie Pryor, RN, RM, BA, MN, PhD
Associate Director, Rehabilitation Nursing Research
    and Development Unit
Royal Rehabilitation Center
Sydney, Australia

Maria L. Radwanski, RN, MSN, CRRN
Administrator
Health Calls Home Health Agency
Wyomissing, Pennsylvania

Kathleen A. Stevens, PhD, RN, CRRN
QI Coordinator
Rehabilitation Institute of Chicago
Chicago, Illinois

Cherisse Tebben, BSN, MSN, CWOCN, CFNP
Nurse Practitioner
Craig Hospital
Englewood, Colorado

Lewis Vierling, JD
Attorney-at-law
Ankeny, Iowa

Robin Wilkerson, PhD, RN
Associate Professor, School of Nursing
University of Mississippi
Jackson, Mississippi

Contributors to the Third Edition

Judith C. Allen, EdD, RN, CRRN
Nursing Education Coordinator
Kessler Institute for Rehabilitation
West Orange, New Jersey

Joan P. Alverzo, PhD(c), MSN, CRRN
Vice President, Clinical Support Services
Kessler Institute for Rehabilitation
West Orange, New Jersey

Jean M. Benjamin, MSN, RN, CRRN
Senior Consultant
Gill/Balsano Consulting
Atlanta, Georgia

Jean K. Berry, PhD, RN, CS
Clinical Assistant Professor, College of Nursing
University of Illinois at Chicago
Chicago, Illinois

Barbara J. Boss, PhD, RN, CFNP, CANP
Professor of Nursing
University of Mississippi
Jackson, Mississippi

Nicole Brandt, PharmD, CGP
Assistant Professor, Geriatric Pharmacotherapy
Deputy Director, Lamy Center on Drug Therapy and Aging
University of Maryland School of Pharmacy
Baltimore, Maryland

Linda Brewer, MSN, RN, CFNP, CACNP
Acute Care, Family Nurse Practitioner
Scott Regional Hospital
Morton, Mississippi

Lisa Cyr Buchanan, MS, RN, CRRN
Rehabilitation Clinical Nurse Specialist
The Maine Rehabilitation Center
Eastern Maine Medical Center
Bangor, Maine

Theresa Perfetta Cappello, PhD, RN, CtHy
Associate Professor, School of Health Professions
Marymount University
Arlington, Virginia

Gloria T. Aubut Craven, MS, RN
Partner
Craven & Ober Policy Strategists, LLC
Boston, Massachusetts

Pamela M. Duchene, DNSc, RN, CRRN
Vice President, Patient Care Services
St. Joseph Hospital
Nashua, New Hampshire

Cindy Gatens, MN, RN, CRRN-A
Clinical Nurse Specialist
Dodd Hall/Rehabilitation
The Ohio State University Medical Center
Columbus, Ohio

Aloma R. Gender, MSN, RN, CRRN
Senior Vice President, Clinical Services
Good Shepherd Rehabilitation Hospital
Allentown, Pennsylvania

Carol A. Gleason, MM, RN, CRRN, CCM, LRC
Director of Resource Management
Shaughnessy Kaplan Rehabilitation Hospital
Salem, Massachusetts

Nancy H. Glenn-Molali, MSN, RN, CRRN
Rehabilitation Clinical Nurse Specialist
Private Practice
Havre de Grace, Maryland

Susan B. Greco, MSN, RN, CRRN
Director of Nursing
Touro Rehabilitation Center
New Orleans, Louisiana

A. René Hébert, MS, RN, CRRN-A
Clinical Instructor
Adult Health and Illness
The Ohio State University College of Nursing
Columbus, Ohio

Diane Huber, PhD, RN, FAAN, CNAA
Associate Professor, College of Nursing
The University of Iowa
Iowa City, Iowa

Deirdre F. Jackson, MSN, APRN, CRRN
Director, Continuing Education and Staff Development
Children's Specialized Hospital
Mountainside, New Jersey

Joyce H. Johnson, PhD, MS, RN
Associate Professor, College of Nursing
University of Illinois at Chicago
Chicago, Illinois

Kelly M. M. Johnson, MSN, RN, CFNP, CRRN
Vice President, Patient Care Services
Craig Hospital
Englewood, Colorado

Margaret Kelly-Hayes, EdD, RN, CRRN, FAAN
Clinical Professor of Neurological Nursing
Boston University School of Medicine
Boston, Massachusetts

Deborah J. Konkle-Parker, MSN, FNP, ACRN
Nurse Practitioner, Division of Infectious Diseases
University of Mississippi Medical Center
Jackson, Mississippi

Patricia L. McCollom, MS, RN, CRRN, CDMS, CCM, CLCP
President and Nurse Consultant
LifeCare Economics and Management Consulting
    and Rehabilitation Services, Inc.
Ankeny, Iowa

Christina M. Mumma, PhD, RN, CRRN
Professor, School of Nursing
University of Alaska
Anchorage, Alaska

Leslie J. Neal, PhD, RNC, CRRN
Assistant Professor, School of Health Professions
Marymount University
Arlington, Virginia

Audrey Nelson, PhD, RN, FAAN
Associate Chief, Nursing Service for Research
James A. Haley Veterans Affairs Medical Center
Tampa, Florida

Grace Nolde-Lopez, MSN, RN, CWOCN, CRRN
Clinical Nurse Specialist
Craig Hospital
Englewood, Colorado

Rhonda S. Olson, MS, RN, CRRN
Rehabilitation Nurse Consultant
RS Consulting
Houston, Texas

Billie R. Phillips, PhD, RN, CDFS
Assistant Professor
Tennessee Wesleyan College
Fort Sanders School of Nursing
Athens, Tennessee

Marion A. Phipps, MS, RN, CRRN, FAAN
Rehabilitation Nurse Specialist
Beth Israel Deaconess Medical Center
Boston, Massachusetts

Marilyn Pires, MS, RN, CRRN-A
Rehabilitation Clinical Nurse Specialist
Rancho Los Amigos National Rehabilitation Center
Downey, California

Christy A. Price, MSN, RN, NP
Nephrology Nurse Practitioner
Nephrology Associates
Salt Lake City, Utah

Julie Pryor, CM, BA, MN, RN
Senior Lecturer in Rehabilitation Nursing
University of Western Sydney
Associate Director, Rehabilitation Nursing Research
    and Development Unit
Royal Rehabilitation Centre
Sydney, Australia

Maria B. Radwanski, MSN, RN, CS, CRRN
Gerontological Clinical Nurse Specialist
Private Practice
Reading, Pennsylvania

Gail Lynn Sims, MSN, RN, CRRN
Nurse Manager
TIRR Systems
Houston, Texas

Mary Ann Solimine, MLS, RN
Research Consultant
Westfield, New Jersey

Kim Vander Ploeg, MS, RN
Clinical Nurse Specialist
Pediatrics and Pediatric Intensive Care
Lutheran General Children's Hospital
Park Ridge, Illinois

Contributors to the First and Second Editions

Kay Lewis Abney, PhD, RN, CPNP
Denise B. Angst, DNSc, RN
Mila A. Aroskar, EdD, RN
Judith A. Behm, MSN, RN, CRRN
Rita J. Boucher, EdD, RN
Dorothy P. Byers, MS, RN
Marci Catanzaro, PhD, RN, CS
Sandra Chenelly, MS, RN
Susan L. Dean-Baar, PhD, RN, CRRN, FAAN
Sharon S. Dittmar, PhD, RN
Theresa P. Dulski, MS, RN,C
Susan M. Evans, MS, RN
Elizabeth Forbes, MSN, EdD, RN, FAAN
Mary Frances Gainer, EdD, RN
Kathy M. Graham, MS, RN
Cheryl Graham-Eason, MS, RN, CRRN
Margaret J. Griffiths, MSN, RN
Maureen Habel, MA, RN, CRRN
Denise Hanlon, MS, RN
Brenda P. Haughey, PhD, RN
Margaret M. Hens, MS, RN

Linda M. Janelli, EdD, MS, RN,C
Janet G. LaMantia, MA, RN, CRRN
Janet L. Larson, PhD, RN
Judith A. Laughlin, PhD, RN
Martha F. Markarian, MS, RN
Elizabeth A. Moody-Szymanski, MS, RN
Angela Moy, MSN, RN, CRRN
Mary Sue Niederpruem, MS, RN
Elizabeth C. Phelps, MS, RN
Josephine Ricci-Balich, MSN, RNC, CRRN
Dorothy Sager, RN, CRRN, CIRS, CCM
Joyce Santora, MS, RN
Yvonne Krall Scherer, EdD, RN
Jill A. Scott, MS, RN
Margie L. Scott, EdD, RN
Elizabeth L. Sharkey, MS, RN
Anaise Theuerkauf, BS, MEd, RN, CRRN, CCM
Margaret A. Umhauer, MS, RN
Barbara H. Warner, MS, RN
Barbara G. White, EdD, RN
Barbara Wisnom, MS, RN

Reviewers for this Edition

Elizabeth R. A. Beattie, PhD, RN, FGSA
Adjunct Associate Professor
University of Iowa College of Nursing
Research Compliance Associate
Office of Human Research Compliance Review
Office of the Vice President for Research
University of Michigan
Ann Arbor, Michigan

Pamela M. Beley, RN, BS, CCM, QRP, LHRM, ABQUARP Diplomat
Qualified Rehabilitation Provider
Sunrise, Florida

Ann S. Bines, RN, MS, CCRN
Nurse Manager, Brain Injury
The Rehabilitation Institute of Chicago
Chicago, Illinois

Maryann Brigante, RNC, MSN, CRRN
Director of Nursing and Ancillary Services
Kessler Institute for Rehabilitation
East Orange, New Jersey

Barbara Brillhart, RN PhD CRRN FNP-C
Associate Professor
Arizona State University
College of Nursing and Healthcare Innovation
Phoenix, Arizona

Evelyn Calvillo, DNSc, RN
Professor
School of Nursing
California State University–Los Angeles
Los Angeles, California

Christie Campbell-Grossman RN, PhD
University of Nebraska Medical Center
College of Nursing–Lincoln
Lincoln, Nebraska

Cheryl Crisp, MSN, RN, APRN, BC, CDDN, CRRN
Pediatric Clinical Nurse Specialist
Riley Child Development Center
Indianapolis, Indiana

Doreen Casuto, RN, BSN, MRA, CRRN, CCM
Rehabilitation Nurse Case Manager
Rehabilitation Care Coordination
San Diego, California

Shelby L. Corman, PharmD, BCPS
Assistant Professor of Pharmacy and Therapeutics/Drug
   Information Specialist
University of Pittsburgh School of Pharmacy
Pittsburgh, Pennsylvania

Anne Deutsch, RN, PhD, CRRN
Clinical Scientist
Rehabilitation Institute of Chicago
Research Assistant Professor/Northwestern University
Feinberg School of Medicine
Chicago, Illinois

Merry E. Dreier, RN, BSN, CRRN, ONC
Nurse Clinician
Marianjoy Rehabilitation Hospital
Wheaton, Illinois

Karen Dunn, PhD, RN
Assistant Professor
Oakland University School of Nursing
Rochester, Michigan

Charles D. Fricks, RRT, RPSGT
Clinical Coordinator Sleep Disorder Center
Christus St. Michael Rehabilitation Hospital
Texarkana, Texas

Jeanne Gant, RN, CCM
Board Member and Past President
Virginia Association of Rehabilitation Nurses
State Farm Insurance Companies
Fairfax, Virginia

Jane M. Georges, Ph.D., RN
Associate Professor
University of San Diego School of Nursing
San Diego, California

Mary A. Gollinger, MS, BSN, CRRN
Director, Patient Care Services
Instructor, College of Nursing
University of Illinois Medical Center
Chicago, Illinois

Joan Earle Hahn, PhD, APRN, BC, CDDN
Adjunct Associate Professor
School of Nursing
Tarjan Center at UCLA
University of California Los Angeles
Los Angeles, California

Elizabeth H. Hall, RN, BS
Wound Care Specialist
University of Washington
Harborview Medical Center
Seattle, Washington

Barbara Harrison, PhD, APRN, BC
Assistant Professor
Oakland University School of Nursing
Rochester, Michigan

Kathleen J. Haydon, MS, RN, BC, CRRN
Education Program Manager
St. Mary's Hospital and Medical Center
Grand Junction, Colorado

Dalice Hertzberg, RN, MSN, APRN, BC
Instructor, JFK Partners and School of Nursing
University of Colorado at Denver and Health Sciences
   Center
Denver, Colorado

Donna P. Jernigan, RN, BSN, MS, CRRN
Patient Services Manager III
University of North Carolina Hospitals Rehabilitation
   Center
Chapel Hill, North Carolina

Steven D. Johns, MS, CRC, CCM, CLCP
Rehabilitation Consultant
RNS Healthcare Consultants
Sacramento, California

Kathleen J. Kalemba, RN, MA, CRRN
Education Coordinator, Nursing
Kessler Institute for Rehabilitation
East Orange, New Jersey

Cathleen M. King, RN, BS, MHA, CRRN
Director of Operations, Rehabilitation Program
Veterans Affairs North Texas Health Care System
Dallas, Texas

Maria Knikou, PT, PhD
Associate Professor
City University of New York
New York, New York
Northwestern University
Chicago, Illinois

Marilyn Long, MSN, RN, CRRN
Clinical Education Specialist/Stroke Program
Harris Methodist Fort Worth Hospital
Fort Worth, Texas

Barbara J. Lutz, PhD, RN, CRRN
Assistant Professor
College of Nursing
University of Florida
Gainesville, Florida

Linda Marler, RN, BSN, CRRN
Education Coordinator
Baylor Institute for Rehabilitation
Dallas, Texas

Michelle Z. Matthews, RN, BSN, BS, MSN
Director of Nursing
Kessler Institute for Rehabilitation
West Orange, New Jersey

Bobbie McCarty, RN, CCM, CRP, LNC
Clinical Liaison
Lakeview Neuro-Rehabilitation Center
Richmond, Virginia

**Jill Milner, RN, MSN, CRRN, CNS,
   CHTP, HTSM-HTP**
Health Care Consultant
Health ReCreation
Chicago, Illinois

Anne Oakley, RN, MSN, APNC
Nurse Practitioner
Kessler Institute for Rehabilitation
West Orange, New Jersey

Patrice R. Oliver, RN, BSN, CRRN
Rehabilitation Nurse Manager
Medical Center of Arlington
Arlington, Texas

Lorraine J. Phillips, MSN, RN, FNP
Graduate Research Assistant
The University of Texas at Austin School of Nursing
Family Nurse Practitioner, SunStar Geriatrics
Austin, Texas

Linda L. Pierce, PhD, RN, CNS, CRRN, FAHA
Professor
The University of Toledo College of Nursing
Toledo, Ohio

Marie Povey, BSN, MSN, ARNP-BC, CRRN
Past President West Coast District FSARN
Florida State Association of Rehabilitation Nurses
    SIG Chair
Clearwater, Florida

Gail M. Powell-Cope, PhD, ARNP, FAAN
Associate Chief Nursing Service Research
James V. Haley Veterans Affairs Medical Center
Tampa, Florida

Karen Preston, PHN, MS, CRRN, FIALCP
Nurse Consultant
RNS Healthcare Consultants
Sacramento, California

Judith P. Salter, MSN, CRRN
Clinical Nurse Specialist
Metropolitan Medical Center
Cleveland, Ohio

Mary Scherbring, MS, RN, OCN
Clinical Nurse Specialist
Cancer Adaptation Team
Mayo Clinic
Rochester, Minnesota

Linda M. Schultz, PhD, CRRN-A
Clinical Instructor
Washington University School of Medicine
St. Louis, Missouri

Janet M. Simpson, RN, BSN, CRRN
Pediatric Outpatient Nurse/Clinical Instructor
Rehabilitation Institute of Chicago
Chicago, Illinois

Matthew Sorenson, PhD, RN
Assistant Professor
DePaul University
Chicago, Illinois

Carole Stolte-Upman, RN, MA, CRC, CDMS, CCM
President
Chesapeake Disability Management, Inc.
Baldwin, Massachusetts

Alexa M. Stuifbergen, PhD, RN, FAAN
Professor, Dolores Sand Chair in Nursing Research
Associate Dean of Research, School of Nursing
The University of Texas at Austin
Austin, Texas

Stephanie Vaughn, Ph.D., RN, CRRN
Assistant Professor
Department of Nursing
California State University–Fullerton
Fullerton, California

Donna M. Vittorio, RN, CRRN
Rehabilitation/Restorative Care Consultant
Senior Disability Analyst and Diplomat
Adjunct Faculty
Waubonnsee Community College
Sugar Grove, Illinois

Lori Watkins, RN, MSN
Nurse Manager
Infectious Diseases Division
Washington University School of Medicine
St. Louis, Missouri

Reviewers for the Third Edition

Jane H. Backer, DNS, RN
Associate Professor, School of Nursing
Indiana University
Indianapolis, Indiana

Barbara J. Boss, PhD, RN, CFNP, CANP
Professor of Nursing
University of Mississippi
Jackson, Mississippi

Carol Boswell, EdD, RN
Assistant Professor, School of Nursing
Texas Tech University Health Sciences Center
Odessa, Texas

Barbara Brillhart, PhD, RN, CRRN
Associate Professor, College of Nursing
Arizona State University
Tempe, Arizona

Teresa A. Bryan, BSN, MSN, RN, CRRN
Nurse Manager
Craig Hospital
Englewood, Colorado

Lisa Cyr Buchanan, MS, RN, CRRN
Rehabilitation Clinical Nurse Specialist
The Maine Rehabilitation Center
Bangor, Maine

Joanne Bullard, MN, APRN
Assistant Professor of Nursing
Our Lady of Holy Cross College
New Orleans, Louisiana

Nancy E. Dayhoff, EdD, RN
Clinical Nurse Specialist
CEO, Clinical Solutions, LLC
Columbus, Indiana

Paula DiBenedetto, MSN, RN
Instructor, Clinical Nursing
Texas Tech University Health Sciences Center
Lubbock, Texas

Pamela M. Duchene, DNSc, RN, CRRN
Vice President, Patient Care Services
St. Joseph Hospital
Nashua, New Hampshire

Kristen L. Easton, PhD(c), MS, RN, CRRN-A, CS
Assistant Professor of Nursing
Valparaiso University
Valparaiso, Indiana

Janet M. Farahmand, EdD, RN
Adjunct Professor of Nursing
Neumann College
Aston, Pennsylvania
Immaculata College
Immaculata, Pennsylvania

Mitzi A. Forbes, PhD, RN
Assistant Professor
School of Nursing
University of Wisconsin–Milwaukee
Milwaukee, Wisconsin

Judith K. Glann, MSN, RN, CCRN
Clinical Nurse Specialist, Cardiovascular/Critical Care
Lovelace Health Systems
Albuquerque, New Mexico

Nancy H. Glenn-Molali, MSN, RN, CRRN
Rehabilitation Clinical Nurse Specialist
Havre de Grace, Maryland

Cheryl Graham-Eason, PhD(c), MEd, MS, RN
Professor
Community College of Allegheny County
Adjunct Faculty, Carlow College
Pittsburgh, Pennsylvania

Philip A. Greiner, DNSc, RN
Associate Professor and Director
Health Promotion Center, Fairfield University
Fairfield, Connecticut

Amy E. Guilfoil-Dumont, MSN, RN, CCRN
Clinical Nurse Specialist
Holy Family Hospital and Medical Center
Methuen, Massachusetts

Mary E. Hanson-Zalot, MSN, RN, OCN
Clinical Resource Coordinator
University of Pennsylvania Hospital
Philadelphia, Pennsylvania

Susanne R. Hays, MS, RN, CRRN
Advanced Practice Nurse
Albuquerque, New Mexico

Dalice L. Hertzberg, MSN, RN, CRRN
Instructor
University of Colorado Health Sciences Center
Denver, Colorado

Cynthia S. Jacelon, PhD(c), RN, CRRN
Clinical Assistant Professor, School of Nursing
University of Massachusetts
Amherst, Massachusetts

Mary Ann Jacobs, MSN, RN, CRRN
Nurse Practitioner, Spinal Cord Injury
Jefferson Barracks Veterans Administration Hospital
St. Louis, Missouri

Linda L. Kerby, BA, BSN, MA
Registered Nurse Consultant
Leawood, Kansas

Christina M. Mumma, PhD, RN, CRRN
Professor, School of Nursing
University of Alaska
Anchorage, Alaska

Sarah E. Newton, PhD, RN
Assistant Professor, School of Nursing
Oakland University
Rochester, Michigan

Maria E. Nowicki, PhD, RN
Director of Nursing
Mercy College of Northwest Ohio
Toledo, Ohio

Rhonda S. Olson, MS, RN, CRRN
Rehabilitation Nurse Consultant
RS Consulting
Houston, Texas

Phyllis Peterson, MN, RN
Assistant Professor, Division of Nursing
Our Lady of Holy Cross College
New Orleans, Louisiana

Mary L. Pickerell, BA, RN, CCM, CPUR
Nurse Review Specialist, Marriott International, Inc.
Washington, District of Columbia

Janet Johnson Prince, BSN, RN, CWOCN, CGRN
Clinical Nurse Manager, Endoscopy Unit Wound
    and Ostomy Management Services
St. Joseph Hospital
Nashua, New Hampshire

Patricia A. Quigley, PhD, ARNP, CRRN
Rehabilitation Clinical Nurse Specialist
James A. Haley Veterans Affairs Hospital
Faculty, University of Phoenix
St. Petersburg, Florida

Terry Savan, BSN, MA, RN, CRNP, PA-C
Assistant Professor, PA Program
DeSales University
Center Valley, Pennsylvania

Mary R. Stange, MS, RN, CRRN
Clinical Nurse Specialist, Neurological Rehabilitation
Drake Center
Cincinnati, Ohio

Teresa L. Cervantez Thompson, PhD, CRRN-A
Assistant Professor, School of Nursing
Oakland University
Rochester, Michigan

Karen L. Tomajan, MS, RNC, CRRN
Director, Clinical Education
Integris Health
Oklahoma City, Oklahoma

Mary Joe White, PhD, RN
Associate Professor of Nursing
University of Texas Health Sciences Center
Houston, Texas

Preface

When I entered the emerging specialty of medical rehabilitation, I was fortunate to be in the company of the forerunners of the field, including nurses such as Ruth Stryker and Nancy Holt, who wrote the first rehabilitation nursing textbooks. These landmark classics were foundations upon which nurses built their practice using rehabilitation principles. In addition to specialized rehabilitation nursing skills and techniques, they stressed intensive patient and family education, attention to the processes of coping and adaptation, and practice within the team approach. Over time I envisioned a book for rehabilitation nurses that would become a comprehensive standard for education and excellence in practice and administration for the specialty, as well as an inspiration for conducting research. The vision was to advance the specialty practice of professional rehabilitation nursing and ensure the best practices to bring about improved outcomes for patients, families, and communities. I wanted to instill qualities of commitment, competence, caring, and compassion as fundamental to rehabilitation nursing.

This edition of the book continues to incorporate the philosophy of the interdisciplinary team and to bridge levels of intervention and prevention with all settings for rehabilitation nursing practice, that is, primary care and acute care through community living. Ideal rehabilitation nursing practice employs high-level assessments of functional health patterns, establishes mutual patient and nursing goals targeting optimal levels of function, implements evidence-based interventions that lead to realistic outcomes, and incorporates evaluation as an essential component of practice. Nursing measures for early intervention and those that prevent further impairment or complications encourage patient satisfaction and quality of life and promote higher levels of functional outcomes. As people live longer and survive formerly fatal illnesses, few escape the experiences of acute or chronic conditions, comorbidity, or impairment. While changes in health care delivery and advances in medical science have been rapid and monumental, being able to provide care that makes a difference in a patient's life never goes out of style.

The content of this fourth edition has matured and developed in complexity to reflect the comprehensive scope of the specialty. During this process, I have been privileged to work with contributors and reviewers who are among the foremost rehabilitation nursing experts in the world. The fourth edition grew beyond the range of a single editor, and four exceptional colleagues joined me as Unit Managers—Barbara Boss, Pam Duchene, Aloma Gender, and Patricia McCollom. Together we have shaped the content and direction of the book. We retained the conceptual frameworks that reflect a systems approach using health patterns rather than a medical model. The organization creates a smoother flow of content in each chapter from the nursing process and evaluation into case studies that are tied to critical thinking questions and concept maps. While keeping to the framework, several chapters were moved within the table of contents to create a more logical order and a few chapters were combined, such as legislative and ethics. Chapter 14 is a combination of three former chapters, with new content to illustrate how synthesis of a concept, that of immobility, with the nursing process can set new directions and outcomes. The new chapters, such as the chapter on developmental disabilities, are in response to changes in the scope of practice or, as with patient safety, demonstrate the growing relationship among research findings, education, and practice. We have maintained our commitment to producing a timely and scholarly work that serves as a reliable text for educators and students and offers a key reference with guidelines for practicing nurses.

Practical applications are based on evidence from research findings and written for all levels and settings of nursing practice across the continuum of care. This edition makes a strong bid for increased use in the community and restorative care with emphasis on patients' independent functioning. Demographics of an aging population and a new surge of wounded veterans, reduced hospital stays, increased costs for health services, and patient preferences place the future of rehabilitation nursing practice in the community, as well as with traditional practice in institutions. The decision to retain foundational content, illustrations for correct positioning, transfer techniques, or range-of-motion exercises, for instance, was intended to benefit nurses who are new to rehabilitation or who are responsible for teaching others, such as health workers or families. The scope of the book chapters is comprehensive and current for rehabilitation nursing and sets future directions for the specialty. However, the content is not exhaustive; entire books may be written about topics such as research, ethics, or specific neuromuscular problems.

Features in the fourth edition include: A change in the subtitle to include *prevention*. A more comprehensive edition, it covers rehabilitation care across the life span and the continuum of care. It provides current guidelines, such as for a rehabilitation nursing research agenda, and for practice, such as the new pressure ulcer staging guidelines. New chapters and chapters with new combinations or configurations enhance the scope of practice. Chapters are organized around the nursing process, including evaluation with updated NANDA-I and NIC/NOC tables, and case studies that are accompanied by related critical thinking questions. Clinical chapters contain a new feature of concept maps (described later). Contributors include key content experts in the specialty and several international contributors. The book is scholarly but practical, with classic and current references, updated and usable illustrations, and peer-reviewed chapter content and lists World Wide Web resources throughout. Chapter 7 contains relevant pharmacology content for ready reference. Important illustrations of rehabilitation procedures, such as range-of-motion exercises, transfers, and management of the neurogenic bladder, are placed strategically throughout the book.

This fourth edition places a focus on the whole person, as a person who has an existence and worth apart from whatever experience of the chronic, disabling, or developmental condition. In this life, some aspect of rehabilitation or restorative care will touch all of us, at some time, whether personally or through family and friends. We all will need and can hope to encounter a rehabilitation nurse who has understood and embraced our conceptual philosophy, and who practices in accordance with our efforts in this book. It is written for all of us.

Acknowledgments

A highly functioning interdisciplinary team is a hallmark of rehabilitation and designed to improve outcomes. In a similar approach, a team of editorial, production, and management professionals joined with rehabilitation nurse experts to produce this fourth edition of *Rehabilitation Nursing*. Jean Fornango has been an epicenter of the publication process. An experienced senior developmental editor, she deserves our gratitude for her proficient guidance, unwavering assistance, and masterful coordination in all aspects of the project. We thank our Executive editor Suzi Epstein for sponsoring and maintaining support for the project, Beth Hayes for a diligent tattoo on the production process, Julia Dummitt for creative inspirations as our designer, and Mary Jo Adams for steady assistance in the editorial process. Whether sharing expertise and resources, collaborating to resolve problems, injecting great ideas, offering support, or providing a spot of humor, we modeled the team approach. The outcome of our efforts is reflected in the quality and integrity of this book.

Once again, I credit my husband, family, and friends and thank them for their encouragement, patience, and prayers. I am honored and humbled to have had the opportunity to edit another edition of this book. I hope it will contribute toward making a positive difference for rehabilitation nurses and patients throughout the world.

S.P.H.

CLASSIC FEATURES.

- **Functional health patterns** form conceptual framework.
- **Clinical chapters** follow the **nursing process.**
- The most current **Nursing Interventions Classifications and Nursing Outcomes Classifications** are included for many key diagnoses.
- **Exceptional reference sections** presents foundational references as well as the most recently published, evidence-based practice references for each chapter.

- **Case Study** feature has been expanded.
- **Comprehensive coverage** continues to reflect the broad scope of rehabilitation nursing practice, including chapters on *Legal and Ethical Issues in Rehabilitation* (3), *Cultural and Medical Systems: Conventional, Alternative, and Complementary Health Patterns* (6), and *Quality: Indicators and Management* (9)

NEW TO THIS EDITION

- *New Chapter!* **Patient Safety for Persons With Disabilities** focuses on specific patient safety issues in the rehabilitation setting.
- *New Chapter!* **Functional Mobility With Activities of Daily Living** provides *a completely* new treatment of mobility impairment including a comprehensive section on spinal cord injury.
- *Groundbreaking New Chapter!* **Rehabilitation Nursing Care of People With Intellectual/Developmental Disabilities** covers this challenging topic including issues of community integration, consent and guardianship, aging issues for those with developmental disabilities, and more.
- *New Chapter!* **Pharmacology** coverage has been expanded from an end-of-book appendix to a full chapter.
- **Critical thinking** questions have been added to each case study to provide a method of integrating chapter topics with real-life patient situations.
- **Concept maps** have been added to the case studies in the clinical chapters (Chapters 14 through 29) as a method of demonstrating the evaluation process critical to managing complicated patient needs in a rehabilitation setting.

A Word About Concept Maps

Concept maps are a method of graphic organization that provides a system for heuristic problem solving through the use of schematic diagrams. They present key concepts in a pictorial arrangement that builds upon existing knowledge to create new meaning for an event or object—or, in this case, a patient's problem. Business has used such tools for many years, such as the fishbone or cause-and-effect diagram, the organizational chart and, of course, the spider diagram. In developing the concept map, the nurse begins with knowledge of the patient that is available and adds to the map in a way that makes sense to the user.

Through concept mapping, diagrams illustrate the interrelationship of concepts and situations. Such maps promote a way of retaining new information or understanding. In nursing, we often rely on rote memory for formulas, calculations, complications, and other scientific facts. The concept map enables us to move away from rote memorization and draw upon spatial learning strategies. When developing a concept map, the nurse: (1) develops a basic skeleton drawing; (2) analyzes and categorizes data; (3) identifies nursing diagnoses relationships; (4) identifies goals, outcomes, and interventions; and (5) evaluates patient's responses.

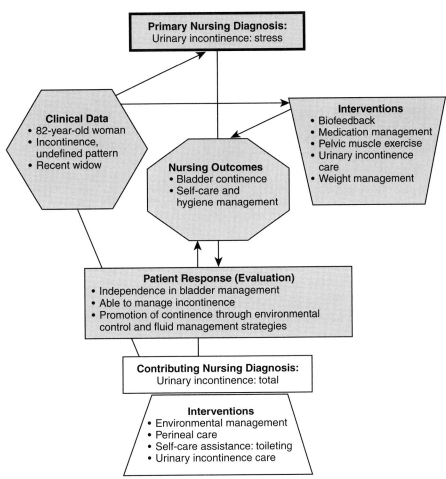

Concept Map. Mrs. Jones' problem with urinary incontinence has not been assessed. It is likely a problem with stress incontinence, but could be more complex, as a total incontinence pattern. Interventions should be directed at assessment with identification of strategies that match the cause and pattern of incontinence. The rehabilitation nurse will focus on coordinating interventions to achieve the outcomes of incontinence management.

The following figure illustrates the principles of a basic concept map.

Throughout this edition of *Rehabilitation Nursing*, concept maps are presented to promote comprehension of the interrelationship of rehabilitation concepts and situations. Each of the case studies is followed by a concept map that provides a graphic organization of the rehabilitation nursing care.

The case study concept maps in this edition of *Rehabilitation Nursing* were created by Pamela M. Duchene, DNSc, ARNP, CNAA, and John B. Muhm, PhD.

Contents

PART V
Restoration and Rehabilitation: Special Populations

1

History, Issues, and Trends

Shirley P. Hoeman, PhD, MPH, RN, CS

EVOLUTION OF REHABILITATION NURSING

Most nurses reading this book have never seen the polio wards; those who have will never forget them (Figure 1-1). Nurses who worked there often had served in World War II and knew about battle wounds; they found polio to be an uneven fight against a fearful disease with an unknown cause. Maneuvering the cumbersome equipment was backbreaking as nurses extended their arms into the sleeve openings of the iron lung respirators and straddled hoses and tubing to reach their patients. So many were children hospitalized for lengthy periods with unpredictable, often heartrending, outcomes. Then in 1954 Salk developed the polio vaccine that led to global eradication of polio.

During this era other advances in medicine and technology dramatically changed health care. Patients survived formerly fatal diseases, and the general population, not only war veterans, began to receive rehabilitation services for conditions such as paraplegia, stroke, or multiple injuries. Rehabilitation nursing was poised for these challenges. From inception as a specialty practice in 1964, it resonated with the teachings of Nightingale (1859/1992); its principles were foundations for excellent nursing practice and respect for each individual's potential. Rehabilitation nursing is "a creative process that begins with immediate preventive care in the first stage of accident or illness. It is continued through the restorative stage of care and involves adaptation of the whole being to a new life" (Stryker, 1977, p. 15).

Defining a Specialty

Formally, rehabilitation nursing is "A specialty practice area of professional nursing. Rehabilitation nursing is the diagnosis and treatment of human responses of individuals and groups to actual or potential health problems relative to altered functional ability and lifestyle" (ARN, 2000, p. 4).

The core principles and practices of rehabilitation nursing are applicable at all levels of intervention, essential to quality care in all sectors of health, and foundational to other nursing specialties. In a world of aging populations, advances in biomedical technology, and global health concerns, rehabilitation nurses are experts in preventing complications and averting further disability for their patients. They coordinate and manage increasingly complex systems of care. Chronic conditions, associated with reduced life satisfaction and limited functional abilities, are often precursors to disability. Rehabilitation nurses assist persons with disabilities or chronic conditions with attaining or maintaining maximum functional abilities, optimal health and well-being, and effective coping with changes or alterations in their lives.

Rehabilitation nurses cannot rely on specific care plans standardized to medical diagnoses if they intend to practice on a level that will enable patients to achieve optimal outcomes. Individualized assessment and interventions based on functional health patterns and systems are essential for the multiple conditions that are not only chronic and disabling, but also complex, involving comorbidity or secondary stages of diseases. To further this level of practice, rehabilitation nurses require unique expertise in educating patients and their families and in enabling them to become authorities on their own condition and situation. They assist patients with negotiating mutually acceptable, lifelong goals, including patients who have developmental disabilities or unique and persistent problems not defined by medical diagnosis and those who have different cultural perceptions.

Rehabilitation is an active intervention to achieve maximum function and to improve quality of life; it is not a third stage of health care, a kind of final resort. When epidemiological principles and levels of prevention for chronic, disabling conditions are integrated, prevention and health promotion are shown to be as critical to outcomes in tertiary levels of intervention as in primary or secondary levels. Thus early preventive interventions, whether primary care or proper positioning, apply within all care levels (Table 1-1). Rehabilitation nurses are involved in assessment and innovations from prevention to incident or onset and provide coordination and continuity through optimal health restoration. The goals and objectives of *Healthy People 2010* (U.S. Department of Health and Human Services [USDHHS], 2000b) include reducing disparities in access to health care and enabling persons to live healthy and functioning, as well as longer, lives. Rehabilitation nurses are well suited to examine ways health institutions, community services, and components of health systems can participate in meeting these goals. They are responsible for ensuring patient participation, comprehensive care, continuity, and support for rehabilitation goals.

Conceptual Basis

To date, no one unified model or combination of theories has proven adequate to serve as the sole paradigm for the practice of rehabilitation nursing. Content from core theories, models, and concepts from a variety of disciplines have enriched and

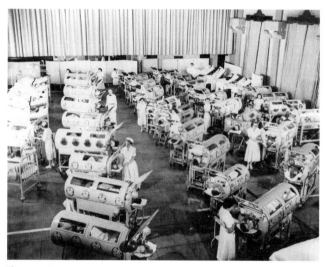

Figure 1-1 A polio ward during the epidemics of the 1950s. (Reproduced with permission of Rancho Los Amigos National Rehabilitation Center, Downey, CA.)

broadened the scope of rehabilitation nursing. Along with findings from research, relevant concepts have furthered the scientific knowledge base, influenced education and practice, offered efficacious options, and improved outcomes for the multiple and complex problems that beset patients and their families. The development of theories, models, and concepts important to rehabilitation nursing is discussed in detail in Chapter 2.

Professional Education

The tradition of nursing by women at home or in religious settings changed with Nightingale in the Crimean War and Barton in the U.S. Civil War. These leaders recognized that many soldiers died needlessly because of lack of basic care, unhygienic conditions, and inadequate distribution of medical goods in the field (Oates, 1994). Convinced of the need for trained nurses, in 1862 Nightingale founded St. Thomas School for Nurses in London; 11 years later her model was replicated in the United States: Massachusetts General Nurses' Training School in Boston, Bellevue Training School in New York City (Morrissey, 1951), and the Connecticut Training School in New Haven. Nursing studies in 1892 featured massage and muscle treatments and therapy with water and electricity, and nursing topics including anatomy and physiology (Young, 1989). The earliest textbook (1879) described care for paralysis and bedsores (Box 1-1). The first *American Journal of Nursing* (1900) encompassed occupational and physical therapy treatments into nursing practice but did not mention paraplegia. Nursing practice with "nervous system diseases" began at the New York Neurological Institute during the first polio epidemic in 1909. Standards improved after findings from the 1910 Flexner Report forced medical education to align with universities, although professional

TABLE 1-1   Levels of Prevention as Interventions Over the Natural Course of a Chronic Disease or Disability

Level of Prevention	Types of Interventions	Applications
Primary	Interventions: health promotion, education, and specific protections	Conducted before a condition or problem is clinically evident or at any stage to improve the situation and prevent further disability or complications
Secondary	Interventions for early diagnosis and treatment and to limit disability and impairments or control the disease processes	Screening or surveys, curative actions or treatments, halting of the disease process, and prevention of spread or complications after the disease has shown early signs or advanced
Tertiary	Interventions for restoration and rehabilitation toward optimal independence and function with quality of life, convalescence from acute or injury problems, and adaptation to impairments	Community, education, or vocation planning; self-care and ADL education; minimizing disability; primary prevention for whole persons, not a focus on disease or disablement

This modification from the original model is retained because it depicts the relationships between any level of prevention and a level of intervention more clearly than current versions. Modified from Leavell, H. R., & Clark, E. G. (Eds.). (1965). *Preventive medicine for the doctor in his community* (3rd ed.). New York: McGraw-Hill.
ADL, Activity of daily living.

roles and control of programs became issues (Braddom, 1988). The National League for Nursing Education issued a standard curriculum for schools of nursing in 1915.

POLITICAL AND SOCIOCULTURAL CONTEXT

Function and Vocation

Wars, disasters, medical/technological advances, social movements, cultural and political philosophies, and religion all influence ways of thinking in any era. The ability to work was a consistent theme. After the Civil War, the federal government set aside a sum of $15,000 for "limb makers" to fashion prostheses for disabled veterans so they could find work (Davis, 1973). Likewise, during the great European immigration (1820 to 1910) when 30 million persons passed through Ellis Island, only those whose functional abilities and health status indicated they could work entered the United States. Function was a priority in 1887 for the new American Orthopedic Association and the Children's Aid Society in New York City, operating a School for Crippled Children with limb and brace care (Young, 1989).

The events of World War I drew attention to the vocational needs of disabled veterans. Patterned after the Belgian-French Ecole Joffre and funded by the Millbank family, the Red Cross Institute for Crippled and Disabled Men opened in New York

---

BOX 1-1 Nursing Guidelines in the Late Nineteenth Century

Regarding Paralysis

"Paralysis is a symptom of other diseases that can occur gradually or suddenly. Generally, a first and partial attack is successfully treated. Friction, healthful living, digestible food, and electricity are common ways of domestic treatment. A physician is responsible for treating the cause. When long continued, great care must be taken that bedsores do not develop" (p. 96).

Regarding Bedsores

"When any part of the body is compressed for a long time, it loses its vitality; this would be the case even in health, but when a person is debilitated by disease, is paralyzed or wounded, and is obliged to remain in one position, the skin covering the points of the body that are pressed upon becomes congested and inflamed, and sometimes excoriated without any pain being felt so far by the patient, the lowered vitality of the part having to a certain extent deprived it of feeling" (p. 141). "The nurse intervened by daily examining the patient for herself all the parts upon which pressure comes: the hip, the seat, the shoulders, elbows, heels, and so forth. It is not so much the severity, but the continuance that concerns. The patient is to be kept clean and dry, placed on a waterbed, and bathed 3-4 times daily with spirits of wine or 2 grains of bi-chloride of mercury dissolved in wine" (p. 141).

Modified from *A handbook of nursing.* (1879). New Haven, CT: U.S. Surgeon General's Office under direction of the Connecticut Training School for Nurses, State Hospital, New Haven.

City in 1917. The director, Douglas McMurtrie, coined the term *rehabilitation*, replacing *physical reconstruction of the disabled.* Army hospitals adopted the term, and the 1918 Senate bill for vocational rehabilitation of servicemen legitimized the term. Soon there emerged large charitable foundations, such as Rockefeller and Carnegie; private and religious organizations, such as Jewish Vocational Services; and sheltered workshops, such as Goodwill and the Rehabilitation Center for the Disabled. In the 1920s local chapters of national organizations, such as the National Society for Crippled Children and Adults, promoted rehabilitation centers in cities across the country (Morrissey, 1951). Residential specialized hospitals were established for children; The Children's Country Home in Westfield, New Jersey (Children's Specialized Hospital), Blythesdale Children's Hospital in Valhalla, New York, and Elizabethtown Hospital and Rehabilitation Center in Pennsylvania remain.

A new social consciousness led influential women to sponsor charitable organizations and protest the harsh, hazardous labor conditions for children. Bertha Wright and Mabel Weed established the Baby Hospital in Oakland, California, in 1907. Although challenged by male paternalism, their work fostered the Federal Children's Bureau (later part of the U.S. Public Health Service [USPHS]), where preventive health was a priority, and eventually the Shepherd-Towner Act, which provided maternal and child health services (Nichols & Hammer, 1998). Efforts of the social reformers also contributed to the Workmen's Compensation Laws drafted in 1911 in response to increased occupational injuries (Cioschi, 1993). In 1920 the Civilian Rehabilitation Act addressed persons with industrially acquired disabilities, and the same year the Vocational Rehabilitation Act transferred vocational rehabilitation from the Surgeon General to a nonphysician-led federal department. Despite multiple amendments, the Vocational Rehabilitation Board retained control over civilian rehabilitation, and physical therapists established interdependent relationships with physicians.

Negotiating Professional Roles

During World War II, physicians who used therapy methods (*physical therapy physicians*) and physical therapy technicians (some were nurses) worked closely; at the war's end, the situation changed. In 1918 the American Medical Association used its leadership in the USPHS to effectively lobby the Surgeon General for control of both medical and functional restoration. As a result, physical therapists were supervised by physicians for diagnosis and treatment, while retaining authority over their modalities. The physical therapy physicians struggled within their own profession, joining physical therapists in 1921 to form the American College of Physical Therapy (changed to the American *Congress* of Physical Therapy in 1930). This was a contentious but mutually beneficial association. Initially tied with the radiology groups, the physical therapists formed their own organization, the American Physical Therapy Association, in 1929, 3 years after a physical therapy school began at Northwestern University Medical

School in Chicago (Young, 1989). At first, occupational therapists moved into mental institutions and tuberculosis sanitariums. They organized in 1923 and applied their skills in sensory and cognitive areas as complements to physical therapy and vocational rehabilitation.

The USPHS gained control over programs to assist the 123,000 disabled veterans and established the first spinal treatment centers in the United States, modeled after those in Europe; one was Massachusetts General Hospital. They recruited nurses, especially wartime physical therapy technicians, for veterans affairs (VA) hospitals to work with orthopedic physicians or to assist physicians with hydrotherapy, massage, and exercises. Initially the nurses sought to manage therapy departments. Not wanting to lower standards of nursing training to do so, they concentrated instead on acute care (Young, 1989) and abandoned their heritage in the community.

With Roosevelt's New Deal (1933 to 1938), the government concentrated on social reform to combat domestic issues and considered the health and education needs of children as a national interest. Nurses were active in programs for early detection and treatment for children with potentially handicapping conditions and led health promotion, education, and prevention programs in schools, precursors of fitness programs. In 1935 Social Security granted civilians access to rehabilitation services formerly reserved for the military and veterans, creating market competition between physical therapy physicians and others. The physical therapy physicians wanted supervision of therapists and thus to control the fee-for-service benefits. Physicians wanted to head physical therapy departments in hospitals to gain referrals, especially from orthopedic physicians. Although physical therapy schools were approved in 1934 and 1936, therapists struggled for years to define their role and functions (Gritzer & Arluke, 1985).

Physical therapy, radiology, and physician organizations then changed names. The American College of Physical Therapy became the American Congress of Physical Therapy until reorganized in 1945 as the American Congress of Rehabilitation Medicine (ACRM) (Cole, 1993). The American Medical Association endorsed the medical specialty of physical therapy physicians, establishing the American Academy of Physical Medicine and Rehabilitation (AAPM&R) in 1938. Their publication evolved to the *Archives of Physical Medicine and Rehabilitation* (Kottke & Knapp, 1988).

Legitimizing Rehabilitation

World War II manpower needs highlighted the health and fitness of the population. Despite perceptions of the United States as a young, healthy, and strong nation, 40% of military draftees were rejected, or classified as 4F, because they did not meet the standard physical requirements for service. Once enlisted, the most common reason for discharge was for neuropsychiatric problems (Kessler, 1970). The question of disability versus capability became more complex and critical to the national interest. The military demanded quantifiable explanations about what recruits were able to do under what circumstances and began to classify impairments and name

the condition, as well as to state whether a disability was permanent, continuous, or temporary. These data eventually applied to vocational evaluations.

Dr. Henry Kessler's (1968) descriptions of his experiences in the field operating theater during World War II are illuminating in their rendering of the human destruction of war. He questions how, as an orthopedic physician dedicated to rehabilitation, he can be laboring to sever limbs from young soldiers, even to save their lives. But save their lives for what kind of life, he struggles to understand. At what point is an individual to be declared "unhealthy or unfit" and for what activities? How can negative labels be avoided, prejudicial social attitudes be contained, emotional factors associated with disability be managed, and the person reach peace in the situation and achieve productivity?

The tragedies of World War II created a forum for a rehabilitation model that combined care and cure. Antibiotics, improved trauma care, and other advances increased the survivors who returned home with injuries and functional limitations; many still young men, they demanded to be accommodated into society. One response was for the Veterans' Bureau to create the VA hospitals and assistance programs under General Omar Bradley, which solidified the Army Physical Medicine Consultants Division's control over military rehabilitation. Initially overwhelmed with the numbers of patients, the VA instituted programs of education, research, and clinical advances that legitimized rehabilitation medicine in federal regulation and funding opportunities (Gritzer & Arluke, 1985).

When the value of early mobility prevailed over traditional bed rest recuperation, rehabilitation gained another foothold in medical science, although therapy methods still were considered unconventional. "The physically handicapped person must be retrained to walk and to travel, to care for his daily needs, to use normal methods of transportation, to use ordinary toilet facilities, to apply and remove his own prosthetic appliances, and to communicate either orally or in writing. Too frequently these basic skills are overlooked" (Rusk, 1957). In 1938 Dr. Frank Krusen continued to promote the Society of Physical Therapy Physicians, in opposition to Dr. Howard Rusk, who wanted therapy within rehabilitation teams of the Army Air Corps Medical Corps (Cioschi, 1993). Rusk and Taylor (1965) presented the notion of "rehabilitation as the third or last phase of health care" to appease medical and surgical colleagues so they would include rehabilitation in the overall plan of care. This phrase was to haunt the specialty for years.

Private philanthropy funded the Baruch Committee to study the utility of physical modalities, to identify the medical education programs to best foster the specialty, and to assist veterans. The committee recommended university teaching and research centers with fellowship and residency programs (Cole, 1993). With Donald Covalt and George Deaver, Rusk joined the medical faculty at New York University Bellevue Hospital in 1945 and created the Department of Rehabilitation Medicine, precursor to the Rusk Institute.

The Vocational Rehabilitation Act of 1943 included vocational evaluation in rehabilitation services (Cioschi, 1993), and the Social Security Act amendments provided vocational rehabilitation and maintenance funds for persons with emotional problems or mental retardation. The Rusk Institute provided treatment for civilians, and parents became involved, promoting study of "mental deficiency," brain diseases, and retardation in children. Stroke, spinal cord injuries, back pain, spastic problems, and sequelae to traumatic injuries created new rehabilitation markets. The Stoke Mandeville Center for Spinal Cord Injury Research in England used a team approach and vocational rehabilitation and community integration programs, which were replicated in the United States by 1944.

Poliomyelitis Years

Reports of polio in the United States began in 1894; a major epidemic occurred in 1909 to 1916. During 1952, reported cases of acute polio numbered 21,269 with 1,200 dead and many with residual problems (Martin, 1988). For every hospital admission, another 100 persons presented with subclinical polio. The mortality rate for high levels of spinal or bulbar polio was nearly 40%; many were children (McCourt & Novak, 1994). In 1943, the National Foundation for Infantile Paralysis (1943) began the national March of Dimes campaign. Citizens and schoolchildren contributed to a cure, depositing dimes into cardboard replicas of "iron lungs" placed on the countertop of every business place. Children in mechanical ventilators were displayed on the new medium of television (Figure 1-2), and the nation was fearful.

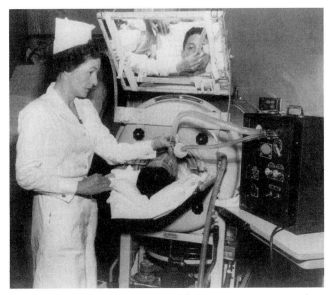

Figure 1-2 Until the mirror was added, a person in an iron lung could not see beyond its rim. When a film crew wanted to show the face of a young man in the ventilator, they realized this environmental barrier. The film crew supplied all those in the polio ward with mirrors. (Reproduced with permission of Rancho Los Amigos National Rehabilitation Center, Downey, CA.)

Polio care centers included the Alfred I. duPont Institute for Pediatric Rehabilitation in Wilmington, Delaware; Rancho Los Amigos in California; and Sister Kenny Rehabilitation Institute in Minneapolis. Sr. Kenny argued with physicians over methods but convinced many at the Mayo Clinic, Rochester, Minnesota, that applying her special hot packs relieved muscle pain that produced acute muscle spasms. With less pain, the patient could perform range-of-motion exercises and improve or retain strength and mobility; that in turn would prevent paralysis, contractures, deformity, loss of function, and pain. Classic rehabilitation nursing courses taught her principles.

Research triumphed in 1954, when Jonas Salk administered polio serum, and Enders and Weiler won the Nobel Prize for study of the poliomyelitis virus. Widespread vaccinations reduced cases; 988 were reported in 1961; then, combined with the Sabin oral vaccine, less than 100 cases were reported in 1967, and between 1979 and 1983, only 12 cases annually (Martin, 1988). The March of Dimes continued to support treatment and rehabilitation and educate health professionals. Infectious disease control, including eradication of polio and smallpox, and clean water and nutrition for children became global concerns.

Government Involvement

Federal legislative involvement in rehabilitation became evident in 1946 with the Hill-Burton Act (Hospital Survey and Construction Act) and the Vocational Rehabilitation Act amendments of 1954 authorizing federal funds for research, training, and building of rehabilitation facilities. The National Mental Health Act and the Federal Security Agency (the Department of Health, Education, and Welfare in 1953) also began. The Office of Vocational Rehabilitation supported development of rehabilitation centers staffed by physicians trained in physical medicine and rehabilitation under the 1958 Vocational Rehabilitation Act. In the 1950s federal funds supported diverse health, transportation, and communications programs for the stated purpose of building and protecting the nation's defense. Leaders emerged, such as Mary Switzer, Director of the Federal Office of Vocational Rehabilitation (1950 to 1970). Heralded as the champion of government-funded programs of research and training in rehabilitation, she initiated inclusion of persons with disabilities at all levels of planning and laid the groundwork for the Independent Living Movement (Affeldt, 1988), ideas that would influence rehabilitation profoundly over the next decades.

REHABILITATION CENTERS AND THE TEAM

The Team Concept

Multidisciplinary and interdisciplinary teams are the hallmark of rehabilitation medicine (see Chapter 2). The early concept of the team was highly regarded, but hierarchical in practice. Rusk claimed the physician as "captain of the team," who is aided by other professionals (Davis, 1973). Health professionals traditionally retained control of information and set goals; the patient was not a member of the team. Although the team existed for the patient, patients must assist to the fullest extent of their capacity to achieve the goals established for them (Lance & Landes, 1957). Team members were to have mutual respect and confidence in one another because "long education in a profession" often leads to the conscious or unconscious assumption that treatment is centered in their particular specialty. Innovators such as Karl and Berta Bobath (who in 1958 founded the neurodevelopmental approach for treatment of persons with cerebral palsy or stroke) had conflicts with physician roles. Their experience was difficult, like that of Sr. Kenny and others who had differences with the medical establishment model or suggested a team leader other than a physician.

Despite conflicts, the team remained foundational to rehabilitation medicine in the first regional rehabilitation research and training centers: the New York University Medical Center and the Sister Kenny Institute in Minneapolis (University of Minnesota Medical School affiliate), home of The American Rehabilitation Foundation. The multidisciplinary team and activities of daily living (ADLs) were included in Krusen's *Physical Medicine and Rehabilitation Handbook*. Hirschberg, Lewis, and Thomas (1964) described the team and functional health patterns and stressed efficiency, economy, and continuity of care.

Other teams contributed to rehabilitation outcomes, such as early interventions by the mobile army support hospital staff (MASH units) and air rescue teams employed in combat situations. Veterans injured during the wars in Korea and Vietnam, workers with occupational injuries, and young adults with injuries resulting from automobile or diving accidents needed rehabilitation services. Disabilities were classified as primary—those resulting from congenital disorders, disease processes, or injury—and secondary, those arising from misuse or disuse syndromes. The community and environment were considered in the plan of care with attention to individual differences.

Introducing Rehabilitation Nursing

Alice Morrissey, nursing supervisor at Rusk Institute and Bellevue Medical Center, authored the first textbook on rehabilitation nursing in 1951. Nurses who performed the dual roles of provider and coordinator of care for persons with chronic or disabling conditions became *rehabilitation nurses*. Use of the term *activities of daily living* (ADLs), referring to self-care, ambulation, and hand activities, began at Rusk Institute (Young, 1989). In Boston, Liberty Mutual Insurance Company hired Harriet Lane as a rehabilitation insurance nurse and Lena Plaisted, a nurse trained in physical therapy. Lane developed a program in geriatric rehabilitation education in the early 1960s at Boston University, where Plaisted, directing the first graduate program in rehabilitation nursing, wrote *The Clinical Specialist in Rehabilitation*, published in 1969 (Cioschi, 1993).

Rehabilitation nursing fared well as Barbara Madden (who established regional respiratory centers for the National Foundation for Infantile Paralysis) became director of nursing at Rancho Los Amigos Medical Center and inaugurated a graduate residency program for rehabilitation nursing specialization in 1965 (Fliedner & Rodgers, 1990). Nurses were so active in rehabilitation services that the American Nurses Association (ANA) published *Guidelines for Practice of Nursing on the Rehabilitation Team: An Answer to a Growing Need*. The National League for Nursing (NLN) published a series of programmed instruction on the "rehabilitative aspects of nursing" (NLN, 1966). The Sister Kenny Institute published manuals on techniques and for ADLs, patient teaching materials (Ellwood, 1964); and Stryker and colleagues offered specialty courses in rehabilitation nursing. The Association of Rehabilitation Nurses (ARN), founded in 1964, and the Rehabilitation Nursing Institute (RNI), founded in 1976, offered national rehabilitation nursing courses. Mary Ann Mikulic edited the *ARN Journal*, and Ruth Stryker revised her rehabilitation nursing text (1977).

During the decades of 1960 to 1980 nurses coordinated patient care, as well as activities of other team members with patients and families. A key role function was preventing complications following a medical event, such as stroke, or due to a chronic condition, such as arthritis. Family and patient education was documented as a modality, much as any medical or therapy procedure. Nurses taught techniques for ADLs, positioning, and exercises for joint range of motion; they prescribed wheelchairs and adaptive equipment and initiated and managed bowel and bladder programs to prepare the patient to return home to live in the community. Patients and families practiced procedures and then "returned demonstrations" to ensure their understanding. Not only did they have access to a special apartment within the rehabilitation facility where they could work with family members or attendants to practice what life would be like on their return home, they also spent several trial weekends at home before discharge from the unit (Hoeman, 1998).

Accountability and Community Integration

An emphasis on vocational training and independent living or community placement underscored coordination efforts between the rehabilitation program and resources from the person's community. What was clear then was that restoration of the person for effective living was a responsibility of the community (Spier, 1957). "Our greatest need is for a rehabilitation program for every community. Most of the rehabilitation problems of a community can be handled at that level if the philosophy of rehabilitation is present, and the resources of the community are utilized" (Covalt, 1957).

> Rehabilitation embodies the democratic ideals that each individual is unique, that each person has the right to participate in all aspects of life, and that each member of the community should contribute to society to the fullest extent of which he is capable. It (rehabilitation) is concerned with the physically disabled person as a human being who requires specialized help to realize his physical, social, emotional, and vocational potentials. It assumes an ideal goal—full development and

utilization of abilities and maximum reduction of the effects of disabilities (Roberts, 1957).

Legislation, injury, and morbidity statistics contributed to the growth of rehabilitation programs and disciplines. By the 1970s medical advances led everyone to expect more from a longer life. Reduced mortality from infectious diseases or infection increased opportunities for people to develop chronic diseases and experience disabling conditions. Automobile accidents, sports injuries, and occupational hazards soon replaced armed conflict as major causes of disabilities. The incidence of head trauma, spinal cord injury, and multiple traumas was increasing in the general population. Questions arose about the role of rehabilitation as a specialty. Who would reimburse for services to patients following a stroke or for children with special needs? What was the role of the insurance industry and the government in paying for services? What were the limits of technology? Who would decide ethical and moral issues? Rehabilitation was at another crossroads (Hoeman, 1998).

In the community, rehabilitation nurses became central to holistic and comprehensive care across levels of care, especially to patients who survived infectious disease and trauma, once fatal conditions, only to develop chronic, disabling conditions. And they advocated for persons to attain optimal levels of function and independence with dignity. They educated families and caregivers along with patients about managing their daily care and about special programs or procedures, and they made referrals to appropriate services or care (Hoeman, 1998).

Rehabilitation nurses joined campaigns to prevent spinal cord injury from diving accidents and for legislation requiring seatbelts and infant car seats. These types of measures saved lives and sent survivors to rehabilitation. Social concerns about the environment and quality of goods were fueled by events such as birth defects after use of thalidomide during pregnancy. Food additives were scrutinized; DDT was banned; and the federal government strengthened warranties on goods and services, began licensing and reviews, wrote more regulations, and began quality control through agencies. Demands for accountability flooded businesses and corporations, products for the consumer, and government agencies; health care was not immune. The rehabilitation team noticed that adherence to new criteria, computer data recording, and government reporting allowed less time for direct care and productivity. Dr. Carl Granger called on the AAPM&R to conduct outcome-based research. Private programs developed to satisfy budding insurance programs led to special interest groups in the AAPM&R (Granger, 1988).

Legislative Provisions Across the Life Span

The government accepted more responsibility for citizens' health as Congress passed Medicare and Medicaid legislation, the Workmen's Compensation and Rehabilitation Law, and Public Law (PL) 89-333, the Vocational Rehabilitation Act amendments of 1965. Within government the Social and Rehabilitation Service (SRS) became a federal administrative

department headed by experienced Mary Switzer. The Commission on Accreditation of Rehabilitation Facilities (CARF) formed in 1967 (Johnson, 1988).

Social change was visible with passage of PL 90-391, the Vocational Rehabilitation Act amendments of 1968. Persons deprived of environmental, social, or cultural factors were considered handicapped and eligible for services. National activities, such as the President's Committee on Employment of the Handicapped, attended to rehabilitation (Figure 1-3). Mental retardation and handicaps became civil rights issues, and the Independent Living Movement was launched (De Jong, 1983).

Issues and programs related to children with mental retardation, formerly assigned to various bureaus, moved to the Division of Maternal Child Health, Title V of the Social Security Act amendments. In 1962 President Kennedy created the National Institute of Child Health and Human Development and the President's Committee on Mental Retardation. This launched the University-Affiliated Facilities (UAFs), and in 1967 the Mental Retardation amendments (PL 91-170) extended UAF programs to research, training, physical education, and recreation. Beginning in 1970 the Developmental Disabilities Services and Construction Act defined mental, developmental, congenital, and related conditions.

The Developmental Disability Assistance and Bill of Rights Act (PL 94-103) provided persons with developmental disabilities the right to treatment, services, and habilitation according to each state plan. Earlier, developmental disabilities

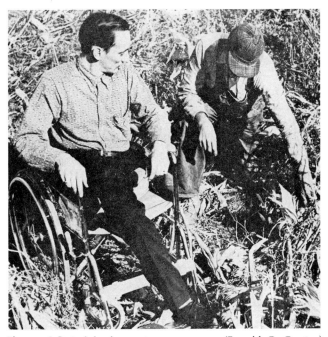

Figure 1-3 A federal crop insurance agent (Ronald C. Cutting) worked his wheelchair into cornfields as part of the President's Committee on Employment of the Handicapped in 1964. (From the President's Committee on Employment of the Handicapped. [1964]. *Performance: The story of the handicapped* [Vol. XIV, No. 8, February]. Washington, DC: U.S. Government Printing Office.)

legislation included mental retardation, cerebral palsy, and epilepsy and related problems, and now autism. All were defined functionally and categorically. The idea of writing individualized care plans and goals bolstered accountability and advocacy (Eberly, Eklund, & Simon, 1986).

The rehabilitation team discovered roles in the community when PL 94-142, the Education for All Handicapped Children Act, passed in 1975. All children were to receive appropriate free education, regardless of disability in the least restrictive environment and with medically necessary services in school and preschool settings, the concept of mainstreaming. Although overall treatment of persons with disabilities was better in the United States than in many places, the social construction of disability and the language describing disability remained negative and derisive for decades. Researchers traced legislation dealing with children who had special needs from 1903 to 1990. They found changes in the language to refer to the children coincided with changes in the social construction and in turn became evident in legislation. No longer are words like *imbecile* or *cripple* used, nor are children classified as *trainable, educable,* or *minimally brain damaged* (Repetto & Hoeman, 1991).

In 1972 Medicare incorporated services for disabilities, and the federal government issued a host of specific guidelines for conducting inpatient rehabilitation services suitable for Medicare reimbursement. Initial regulatory concerns were quality control; issues of fraudulent billing and proper services arose later. The Rehabilitation Act of 1973 provided protection against discrimination in the workplace and addressed barriers in the community. Persons severely injured and those with multiple or complex disabilities needed coordinated expert team care, which eventually resulted in the creation of the Model Systems programs. Team roles in the community were bolstered by Medicare amendments authorizing care in Comprehensive Outpatient Rehabilitation Facilities (CORFs) (Ditunno, 1988). Community-based agencies, including visiting nurse associations (VNAs), sought to capitalize on rehabilitation and restorative nursing. Physical therapists and speech-language pathologists flourished under Medicare reimbursement and contractual agreements with VNAs. Occupational therapists had contracts but did not gain independent reimbursement function until the mid-1980s, when the Health Care Financing Administration (HCFA) studied cost controls.

The Rehabilitation Act amendments of 1978 (PL 95-602) created the National Institute of Handicapped Research, provided comprehensive services for independent living, and promoted research (Verville, 1988). New methods and approaches to managing and understanding disability and chronic conditions were introduced in the mid-to-late 1970s. Dr. John Basmajian pioneered research in electromyograms (EMGs) and education. Biofeedback interventions for paralysis, "psychosocial considerations in spinal cord injury, medical record keeping and team care, neuromuscular physiology, transcutaneous electrical nerve stimulation (TENS), and traditional clinical examination expertise" were significant advances (Granger, 1988).

Negotiating Rehabilitation's Identity

Martin, Holt, and Hicks (1981) published *Comprehensive Rehabilitation Nursing,* and the ARN offered a core curriculum in rehabilitation nursing with a second edition in 1987 (Mumma). ARN conducted the first national certification examination in rehabilitation nursing in 1984, followed by the *Rehabilitation Nursing Standards and Scope of Practice* (1988/2000). By its thirtieth anniversary the ARN had published *Rehabilitation Nursing* and *Rehabilitation Nursing Research* journals, numerous specialized publications and videos, a third and a fourth core curriculum (Edwards, 2000; McCourt, 1993), and an advanced practice core curriculum (Johnson, 1997) and had new editions in process. The ARN established the Rehabilitation Nursing Foundation (RNF), which funded rehabilitation nursing research by 1988. Dittmar (1989) edited *Rehabilitation Nursing,* and Hoeman (1996, 2002) edited the second and third editions.

Initially, rehabilitation nurses practiced insurance nursing or in rehabilitation facilities. By the mid-1980s rehabilitation nurse entrepreneurs founded consulting companies for assessment, case management, legal expertise, and related contracts. Between 1980 and 1983 legislation such as PL 96-374 and PL 98-199, the Carl D. Perkins Vocational and Technical Education Act, and PL 98-524 ensured funding and other access to vocational educational services for persons with a wide range of disabilities and for those considered disadvantaged. Congress proclaimed 1981 as The International Year of Disabled Persons. The Hastings Institute examined the ethics of medical rehabilitation; their publications stirred public debate and challenged the moral beliefs of health professionals and the society.

Rehabilitation resources were tested by the needs of an aging population with increased prevalence of chronic, disabling conditions, aggregates of survivors, entitlements for children with disabilities, and poorly developed injury and disease prevention programs. The Rehabilitation Act amendments of 1986 (PL 99-506), the Technology-Related Assistance for Individuals With Disabilities Act of 1988 (related provisions were included in the 1975 Education for All Handicapped Children Act), and an amendment in 1992 (PL 102-569) each provided for some assisted technology. The Catastrophic Health Bill for the Elderly, designed to prevent poverty resulting from catastrophic illness or trauma, and PL 99-457 for children at risk were enacted. In 1986 the National Council on Disability recommended the Centers for Disease Control and Prevention (CDC) develop a program using public health expertise and systems to prevent disabilities. The Disabilities Prevention Program launched in 1988. Accessible, affordable, appropriate, available, and acceptable care available for persons with disabilities from sources that are accountable was (and is) needed.

The U.S. Senate proposed a National Center for Medical Rehabilitation Research (NCMRR) within the National Institutes of Health (NIH) in 1988 (Title V of S.2222) (Verville, 1988). Rehabilitation nurses participated, Dorothy Gordon served on the panel, and Hoeman (1989) provided testimony for ARN. Within the decade NCMRR claimed institute status and engaged in collaborative activities with other institutes. In the mid-1980s the National Institute on Disability and Rehabilitation Research (NIDRR) funded the nationwide Model Systems for Spinal Cord Injury (16 centers) and for Traumatic Brain Injury (17 centers) to demonstrate the efficacy of coordinated systems of rehabilitation care and research. The years between 1970 and 1990, while active in legislation for persons with disabilities, polarized relationships between rehabilitation and the federal government. Many in rehabilitation wanted decentralized federal services and proposed expanding both private and public sectors. They gained recognition of unmet needs for rehabilitation in the community, increased international collaboration and service, and initiated funded research precisely for rehabilitation and outcomes.

Capstones for the Twentieth Century

Disability rights became visible during the 1990s, as the grassroots social actions and community planning of the 1950s sprouted. The Americans With Disabilities Act (ADA) solidified social responses to needs of persons with disabilities (see Chapter 3). Not only were new populations of persons with chronic, disabling, or developmental disorders surviving, they were entering the community in daily life and vocational pursuits. Nursing manpower was short, and HCFA pressured Medicare funds to reduce costs, services, and lengths of stay in institutions. In an effort to advance a role for the "rehabilitationist," in 1993 the ACRM separated (as in 1968 to 1969) from the physicians of the AAPM&R.

Awareness of the hazards, injuries, and social effects of environment and occupation and the impact of culture and community grew. The interplay of medical advances and technology with public expectations for life satisfaction and quality influenced policy and practice. The Rehabilitation Act amendment of 1992 (PL 102-569) extended rehabilitation to those who were most severely disabled. Patients gained rights to participate in planning with the interdisciplinary team, and persons from minority aggregates had priority funding. The Family Leave Act of 1993 was to ease the challenges of caregiver and family roles.

Exposed to the goals of *Healthy People 2000*, the public vaguely began to appreciate a national agenda for preventive actions, including preventing disabilities, but cure remained the desired outcome. People had expectations to live longer, better, and with more functional abilities and with disparities reduced. Public interest in alternative treatments fostered the Office of Alternative Medicine (OAM) in 1992, and its research centers for holistic approaches were established in 1995 (see Chapter 6). The World Health Organization (WHO) Collaborative Centers in Traditional Medicine Research began in 1996. Some rehabilitation professionals were concerned about quality and found ways to negotiate and participate with governmental agencies in matters of policy, research involvement, and funding. Others identified private resources as means to proceed without federal funding or to exercise research options apart from priorities set by the government.

INTERNATIONAL REHABILITATION

International programs emerged following World War I. The Red Cross Institute for the Crippled and Disabled began in 1917 (the International Center for the Disabled) and the International Society of Crippled Children in 1922 (Rehabilitation International). The National Rehabilitation Organization originated in 1923 with a heavy emphasis on vocational rehabilitation. World War II slowed international rehabilitation activities for a time. The United Nations formed the Council of World Organizations Interested in the Handicapped (International Council on Disability) in 1953 (Groce, 1992) in an attempt to stimulate governments to recognize the needs and take some responsibility for poor and disabled citizens. Governments predictably reserved resources for "worthy" persons, especially those with potential to be "productive." International models influenced rehabilitation programs and thinking in the United States for many years. Facilities and schools were organized in the European manner (i.e., based on specific disabilities [schools for the deaf or blind] and isolating patients from society). The medical model and socially devalued persons superseded concerns for the individual's environment or empowerment (Groce, 1992).

Switzer (Federal Office of Vocational Rehabilitation) was in a position to carry progressive program and social ideas forward. She enabled international rehabilitation funding for more than 500 researchers conducting projects in 14 countries under the International Rehabilitation Research and Demonstration Program (PL 83-840 and PL 86-610). By 1978 the NIDRR funded two projects to foster international linkages of persons and professionals with expertise in rehabilitation or disability studies by participating in short-term fellowships for study abroad. The International Exchange of Experts and Information in Rehabilitation (IEEIR) was administered on the East Coast by the World Rehabilitation Fund, and the International Disability Exchanges and Studies Project (IDEAS) was administered on the West Coast by the World Disability Institute (WDI).

Rehabilitation physicians were interested in learning about the technology and equipment developed in Europe and the Soviet Socialist Union, where political differences had impeded sharing scientific progress. Rusk, Kessler, and Basmajian (Basmajian, 1993) traveled worldwide to collaborate with colleagues. Differing social and cultural definitions of disability affected how persons with disabilities were treated, but interest in international training and collaboration grew in centers such as the Rusk Institute of Physical Medicine and Rehabilitation and the Kessler Rehabilitation Institute. These activities synchronized with the new medical specialty of physical medicine and rehabilitation in 1947. Soon international exchanges flourished with conferences attended by academic faculty and education or service programs sponsored by nongovernmental and voluntary organizations.

International Rehabilitation Nursing

Although eligible, rehabilitation nurses have not sought funding through NIDRR projects. They have participated in international conferences, and Hertzberg and Hoeman (1991) worked with an interdisciplinary team (Project Hope) to develop pediatric rehabilitation and education programs in Armenia. Hoeman (1992, 1999) served as a Fulbright Senior Scholar in Greece and in Jordan and has collaborated on research and projects in multiple countries. International delegations, volunteer mission programs, or nongovernmental organizations (NGOs) offer opportunities for global collaboration and service according to their mission statements, funding, and the needs of specific countries. The second edition of *Rehabilitation Nursing* was translated into Portuguese. The global scene is changing with more nurses becoming involved.

In the United Kingdom (UK) rehabilitation nursing is organized within the National Health Service (NHS) policy. The National Service Frameworks for Older People (DOH, 2001) and Long-Term Conditions (DOH, 2005) are charged with the goal of intermediate care to raise quality standards in health care, and rehabilitation is a key component. The Rehabilitation and Intermediate Care Nursing Forum (formed as the Rehabilitation Nurses' Forum in 1990) is linked with the Royal College of Nursing and creates an arena for sharing ideas and raising the profile of rehabilitation nursing. Members participated in a survey on the International Classification of Functioning, Disability, and Health (ICFHI) (see chapter 2) have developed rehabilitation skills workbooks, and conduct research. Davis and O'Connor (1999) wrote *Rehabilitation Nursing: Foundations for Practice*, and Davis' *Rehabilitation Models and Theories* is due in 2006. The Forum convenes annual conferences and a biannual international rehabilitation nursing conference.

Australia's first postgraduate rehabilitation nursing programs were offered in 1997, and Australia's first Chair of Rehabilitation Nursing was established in 2001. The Australasian Rehabilitation Nurses Association holds annual conferences, as well as research programs, and publishes a journal. They published the *Rehabilitation Nursing Competency Standards for Registered Nurses* in 2003, a *Scope of Practice and Curricula*, a *Position Statement*, and *Scope of Practice* in 2002. Pryor (1999) edited a textbook for rehabilitation nursing. The goals are as follows: to promote rehabilitation nursing as a specialist field, to service as a forum for the exchange of ideas related to rehabilitation nursing, to strive to update rehabilitation services in line with current advances in the field of rehabilitation, and to create opportunities to advance knowledge and skill in rehabilitation nursing through continuing education.

The World Health Organization and Disability

Community-based rehabilitation and primary health care programs became international priorities for WHO in 1978. The WHO definitions include multiple determinants of health status that differ from the predominant views in the United States. WHO and the World Bank sponsored a study in 1992 to identify and quantify health problems and to make projections about the cause and extent of mortality and disability through 2020. The idea was to direct public health policy using evidence from data about health outcomes of disease and injury that resulted in chronic, morbid, or disabling situations. Problematically, data were not measured or collected in many parts of the world. Although the impact of chronicity, disability, and related morbidity on the social, economic, and overall fiber of a society was tremendous, without data, the health areas were not included in planning or objectives for improving health outcomes (*Lancet* Editor, 1997).

Thus the Global Burden of Disease (GBD), developed in 1993, updated in 2000, offered a means for measuring the gap between current health status and an ideal situation of longevity free from disease or disability. The GBD measures severity, incidence, duration, and prevalence of 107 diseases and injury conditions with corrections for regional differences. A standard unit of measurement, the disability-adjusted life year (DALY), compared risk factors that influenced the problems. Prevention, control, and injury management were considered along with socioeconomic, cultural, educational, and technological factors in a society (Murray & Lopez, 1997a, 1997b). Without DALY, depression, ischemic heart disease, osteoarthritis, and alcohol abuse would have been omitted from health planning (Ezzati et al., 2002; Schopper et al., 2000). Then in 2000 WHO introduced the disability-adjusted life expectancy summary measure (DALE), changed to health-adjusted life expectancy (HALE) in 2002, to include all states of health in the calculations. The measures are intended to assist in predicting needs, setting priorities for distribution of resources and services, and allocating funds.

In 1980, the WHO prepared a supplement to the *International Classification of Diseases* (ICD) (1977) after much debate among countries about internal consistencies, word connotations, and use of frameworks, such as Pope and Tarlov (1991) and use of Nagi (1965). In 2001 the *International Classification for Functioning, Disability and Health* (ICF) became a new standard for classifying health conditions/status of people with disabilities. One premise important for rehabilitation is that a disabling condition is not a total health status measure. ICF is discussed further in Chapter 2.

NIDRR Collaboration and Priorities

In the United States the NIDRR collaborates with the ICF initiative. NIDRR has been a key player in the development, dissemination, and adoption of the shift to conceptualize disability from a medical to a sociomedical model. NIDRR sponsors comprehensive and coordinated programs of research and related activities that assist people with disabilities with achieving full inclusion, social integration, employment, and independent living. The long-range plan emphasizes "five 'domains' as areas for expanded research efforts in the next five years (2005-2009) in support of people with disabilities: employment; participation and community living; health and function; technology for access and function; and disability demographic" (NIDRR, 2005). The total proposed fiscal year 2001 budget was $141 million ($100 million for research; $41 million for technology requirements), which supports 344 projects (NIDRR, 2005). Clearly, chronic, disabling conditions have come to attention as major factors in the future of any country or region and have earned rehabilitation programs and research a place in the world of global health.

Disability Prevalence in the United States

Based on self-reports and using definitions from national surveys, an estimated 54 million individuals have disabilities in the United States. Disability status is determined in various ways, such as qualification for civil rights claims, work disability compensation, or public-funded programs, including childhood early intervention programs, special education, and Medicaid or supplemental income. Although such claims or programs are important, not everyone considered to have a disability uses them. Some people with disabilities remain unrecognized despite improved data collection, analysis, and tracking systems for managing information about the incidence and prevalence of chronic, disabling conditions. In 1982 NIDRR convened member agencies to form the Interagency Subcommittee on Disability Statistics (ISDS). The goal was to coordinate and generate improved statistics about disability populations and eventually to enlarge the scope and capabilities in order to interface data systems in multiple directions.

One U.S. household survey, the National Health Interview Survey (NHIS), is used to gather data about health conditions and impairments related to disability (i.e., "a limitation in social or other activity that is caused by a chronic mental or physical disorder, injury, or impairment"). Congenital, acquired, or secondary deficits of psychical structure or function, sensory impairments, loss of limb, or problems in orthopedic or neuromuscular function all are defined as impairments and coded in a classification developed by the National Center for Health Statistics, CDC. Diseases and injuries are coded per the WHO ICD and in collaboration with the ICF network. Although some respond with more than one condition, analysis of the data reveals an extensive problem (National Center for Health Statistics, 2000). One in 8 to 10 persons worldwide has limitation severe enough to prohibit activity.

The 10 most common conditions that cause U.S. citizens to have limitations in activity are conditions within the domain of rehabilitation nursing practice. Thirty-eight million persons in the United States report 61 million disabling conditions encompassing 42 million chronic conditions, 16.3 million impairments, 2 million mental health disorders, and 1 million other injuries. Injuries cause 13.4% of all disabling conditions, highlighting the need for increased preventive actions in rehabilitation nursing interventions. Heart disease leads at 13% of all conditions, combined orthopedic and arthritis-like conditions near 25%, and sensory impairments exceed 5% (LaPlante, 1996).

Despite progress, rehabilitation services are not universally available or affordable. Confusion persists about the proper introduction and institution of rehabilitation practices for a patient, differences between levels of prevention and levels of

intervention, and interrelationships among body, mind, and spirit. A business mentality promotes narrow medical models without incorporating the social and cultural situation. Life satisfaction is compromised further when a person must add a classifiable, named disability or chronic condition to the cultural load.

REHABILITATION NURSING ROLES

Rehabilitation nurses recognize the impact of context and social and physical environment. Understanding concepts from role theory is central to professional rehabilitation nursing practice. Role expectations, clarity, and boundaries must be understood, but more importantly the rehabilitation nurse must be able to communicate these to others on the team and in the community. Decision making, conflict resolution, team building among professional colleagues, and collaboration among various organizational departments or community providers are essential skills.

Rehabilitation nurses have clarified their roles on the team, frequently coordinating expanded teams in the community. Appropriate roles are coordinator, educator, researcher, consultant, case manager, advocate, enabler/facilitator, expert practitioner, and team member. Rehabilitation nurses may be certified for both rehabilitation nursing (CRRN) and advanced practice (CRRN-A) and practice in emerging roles. For example, chapters in this book specify roles with special populations who require cardiac, pulmonary, renal, human immunodeficiency virus (HIV), cancer, or burn care and roles that attend to pediatric, adult, or geriatric age-groups. With advanced practice (APRN), roles are added: administrator, international consultant, expert witness or legal consultant, advanced researcher, and advanced practice functions. Advanced practice occurs in a growing variety of programs, agencies, residences, and centers.

A rehabilitation nurse's role as an advocate and agent of change is to equalize power and reduce disparities while building partnerships with patients, families, and communities. Thus enabled, patients can know, envision, and evaluate options; plan mutual strategies and solutions; and identify the behaviors or actions to achieve the outcomes. Not only agents of change but also adaptable to change, rehabilitation nurses historically have solid experiences in setting new directions for practice.

Key role functions for rehabilitation nurses are managing complex health situations, intervening throughout the life span, perfecting advanced skills to improve patient outcomes, forging partnerships with patients and communities, coordinating interdisciplinary plans of care, and meeting global health challenges.

As rehabilitation nurses form partnership with patients, community agencies, and other professionals, their goals remain consistent. Prevention of chronic, disabling, or developmental disorders; prevention of further disability or complications; promotion of optimal levels of freedom and independent function; reinforcement of effective coping and adaptation; and formation of therapeutic relationships never go out of style for rehabilitation nurses. Ideally the future holds more community and patient involvement, improved clarity on ethical dilemmas, more international collaboration, improved outcomes, and stronger role clarity.

As the point of service has expanded to the community and beyond the institution, the team configuration necessarily has become fluid and more diverse and patients have become more interactive. Rehabilitation goals fit well with those to enable persons to live longer and better and to reduce disparities or inequality (USDHHS, 1990, 2000a). Stating goals and actualizing them are not the same process. Services organized according to population-based or aggregate needs with community involvement have been discussed for half a century. Changes in service needs, that is, for transportation, housing (independent and assisted living), shopping patterns, foods, pharmaceuticals, services, communication, and safety needs, are growing, especially for aging populations in most countries.

Trends predicted to be important for rehabilitation nurses and their patients are listed in Box 1-2. Some trends that will emerge and affect rehabilitation nursing are visible only as possibilities, and their outcomes remain to be evidenced. As Stryker (1977) observed, "the impact of rehabilitation programs is just beginning" (p. 11).

REFERENCES

Affeldt, J. E. (1988). The 1987 Mary E. Switzer Lecture: The tapestry of rehabilitation, its weavers and threads. *Journal of Allied Health, February*, 53-59.

Association of Rehabilitation Nurses. (1988). *Standards and scope of rehabilitation practice.* Glenview, IL: Author.

Association of Rehabilitation Nurses. (2000). *Standards and scope of rehabilitation practice.* Glenview, IL: Author.

Australian Rehabilitation Nurses' Association. (2002). Position statement: Rehabilitation nursing—Scope of practice (2nd ed.). Putney, NSW, Australia: Author.

Australian Rehabilitation Nurses' Association. (2003). *Rehabilitation nursing: Competency standards for registered nurses.* Putney, NSW, Australia: Author.

Basmajian, J. V. (1993). *I.O.U.: Adventures of a medical scientist.* Hamilton, Ontario, Canada: J&D Books.

Braddom, R. L. (1988). Medical education in the academy: Past, present, and a glimpse of the future. *Archives of Physical Medicine and Rehabilitation, 69,* 53-58.

Cioschi, H. (1993). The history of rehabilitation and rehabilitation nursing in the 20th century. In A. E. McCourt (Ed.), *The specialty practice of rehabilitation nursing: A core curriculum* (3rd ed., pp. 6-12). Glenview, IL: The Rehabilitation Nursing Foundation of the Association of Rehabilitation Nurses.

Cole, T. M. (1993). The greening of physiatry in a golden era of rehabilitation. The 25th Walter J. Zeiter Lecture. *Archives of Physical Medicine and Rehabilitation, 74,* 231-237.

Covalt, D. (1957, February-March). Rehabilitation in war and peace. In *Rehabilitation Service Series No. 420. The planning of rehabilitation centers. Proceedings of the Institute on Rehabilitation Center Planning* (pp. 26-32). Washington, DC: U.S. Department of Health, Education, and Welfare.

Davis, A. B. (1973). *Triumph over disability: The development of rehabilitation medicine in the U.S.A.* Washington, DC: National Museum of History and Technology, Smithsonian Institution.

Davis, S., & O'Connor, S. (Eds.). (1999). *Rehabilitation nursing: Foundations for practice.* London: Bailliere Tindall.

De Jong, G. (1983). Defining and implementing the independent living concept. In N.M. Crewe & I. K. Zola (Eds.), *Independent living for physically disabled people.* San Francisco: Jossey-Bass.

Department of Health. (2005). *Long-term conditions.* Norwich, U.K.: HMSO.

Dittmar, S. (1989). *Rehabilitation nursing.* St. Louis, MO: Mosby.

Ditunno, J. F. (1988). Maturation of a specialty: The early 1980s. *Archives of Physical Medicine and Rehabilitation, 69,* 35-40.

Eberly, S., Eklund, E., & Simon, R. (Eds.). (1986). *Profiles in excellence: Twenty-five years of UAF accomplishment.* Silver Spring, MD: American Association of University Affiliated Programs for Persons With Developmental Disabilities.

Edwards, P. A. (Ed.). (2000). *The specialty practice of rehabilitation nursing: A core curriculum* (4th ed.). Glenview, IL: Association of Rehabilitation Nurses.

Ellwood, P. (1964). *A handbook of rehabilitative nursing techniques in hemiplegia.* Kenny Rehabilitation Institute. Minneapolis, MN: Sister Elizabeth Kenny Foundation.

Ezzati, Mi., Vander Hoorn, S., Rogers, A., Lopez, A., Estimates of global and regional potential health gains. Mathers, C., & Murray, C. (2003). From reducing multiple major risk factors. *The Lancet, 362*(9380), 271-280.

Fliedner, C., & Rodgers, M. (1990). *Centennial Rancho Los Amigos Medical Center 1888-1988.* Downey, CA: Rancho Los Amigos Medical Center.

Granger, C. V. (1988). Breaking new ground: Academy growth from 1975 to 1979. *Archives of Physical Medicine and Rehabilitation, 69,* 30-34.

Gritzer, G., & Arluke, A. (1985). *The making of rehabilitation: A political economy of medical specialization, 1890-1980.* Berkeley and Los Angeles: University of California Press.

Groce, N. (1992). *The U.S. role in international disability activities: A history and a look toward the future.* Washington, DC: Rehabilitation International, World Institute on Disability, and World Rehabilitation Fund.

Hertzberg, D., & Hoeman, S. P. (1991, October). *Pediatric rehabilitation nursing in Armenia: An opportunity for change.* Presented at the 17th Annual Association of Rehabilitation Nurses Educational Conference, Kansas City, MO.

Hirschberg, G. G., Lewis, L., & Thomas, D. (1964). *Rehabilitation: A manual for the care of the disabled and elderly.* Philadelphia: J. B. Lippincott.

Hoeman, S. P. (1972). *Memories of Sister Kenny Rehabilitation Institute.* Personal files: unpublished notes.

Hoeman, S. P. (1989). *Testimony for a Rehabilitation Research Institute in the National Institutes of Health.* Representing the Association of Rehabilitation Nurses to the NIH Panel on Physical Medicine and Rehabilitation Research. Report of the Panel C-83-86 (November 20). Bethesda, MD: NIH.

Hoeman, S. P. (1992). *Community and rehabilitation nursing in Greece.* Fulbright Senior Scholar award. Washington, DC: International Exchange of Scholars.

Hoeman, S. P. (Ed.). (1996). *Rehabilitation nursing* (2nd ed.). St. Louis, MO: Mosby.

Hoeman, S. P. (1998). Dynamics of rehabilitation nursing. In G. Goldstein & S. R. Beers (Eds.), *Rehabilitation* (pp. 71-87). New York: Plenum Press.

Hoeman, S. P. (1999). *Community and rehabilitation nursing in Jordan. Fulbright Senior Scholar award.* Washington, DC: International Exchange of Scholars.

Hoeman, S. P. (Ed.) (2002). Rehabilitation nursing (3rd ed.). St. Louis, MO: Mosby.

Institute on Rehabilitation Center Planning. (1957, February-March). In *Rehabilitation Service Series No. 420. The planning of rehabilitation centers. Proceedings of the Institute on Rehabilitation Center Planning.* Washington, DC: U.S. Department of Health, Education, and Welfare.

Johnson, E. W. (1988). Struggle for identity: The turbulent 1960s. *Archives of Physical Medicine and Rehabilitation, 69,* 20-25.

Johnson, K. M. M. (Ed.). (1997). *Advanced practice nursing in rehabilitation: A core curriculum.* Glenview, IL: Association of Rehabilitation Nurses.

Kessler, H. H. (1968). *The knife is not enough.* New York: W. W. Norton.

Kessler, H. H. (1970). *Disability—Determination and evaluation.* Philadelphia: Lea & Febiger.

Kottke, F. J., & Knapp, M. E. (1988). The development of physiatry before 1950. *Archives of Physical Medicine and Rehabilitation, 69,* 4-14.

Lance, H. E., & Landes, R. H. (1957, February-March). Personnel recruitment, selection, and retention. In *Rehabilitation Service Series No. 420. The planning of rehabilitation centers. Proceedings of the Institute on Rehabilitation Center Planning* (pp. 205-216). Washington, DC: U.S. Department of Health, Education, and Welfare.

Lancet Editor. (1997). Editorial: From what will we die in 2020? *Lancet, 349*(9061), 1263.

LaPlante, M. P. (1996). Health conditions and impairments causing disability. *Disability Statistics Abstracts* (No. 16). San Francisco, CA: Disability Statistics Rehabilitation Research and Training Center, University of California, San Francisco, U.S. Department of Education, National Institute on Disability and Rehabilitation Research.

Leavell, H. R., & Clark, E. G. (Eds.). (1965). *Preventive medicine for the doctor in his community* (3rd ed.). New York: McGraw-Hill.

Martin, G. M. (1988). Building on the framework: The Academy in the 1950s. *Archives of Physical Medicine and Rehabilitation, 69,* 15-19.

Martin, N., Holt, N. B., & Hicks, D. (1981). *Comprehensive rehabilitation nursing.* New York: McGraw-Hill.

Maslow, A. H. (1968). *Toward a psychology of being* (2nd ed.). Princeton, NJ: Van Nostrand Reinhold.

McCourt, A. (Ed.). (1993). *The specialty practice of rehabilitation nursing: A core curriculum* (3rd ed.). Glenview, IL: Rehabilitation Nursing Foundation.

McCourt, A. E., & Novak, S. (1994, September). *A history of the Association of Rehabilitation Nurses Association.* Presented at the Annual Educational Conference; Orlando, FL.

Morrissey, A. B. (1951). *Rehabilitation nursing.* New York: G. P. Putnam's Sons.

Mumma, C. M. (Ed.). (1987). *Rehabilitation nursing: Concepts for practice—A core curriculum* (2nd ed.). Evanston, IL: Rehabilitation Nursing Foundation.

Murray, C. J. L., & Lopez, A. D. (1997a). Regional patterns of disability-free life expectancy and disability-adjusted life expectancy: Global Burden of Disease study. *Lancet, 349,* 1347-1352.

Murray, C. J. L., & Lopez, A. D. (1997b). Global mortality, disability, and the contribution of risk factors: Global Burden of Disease study. *Lancet, 349,* 1436-1442.

Nagi, S. Z. (1965). Some conceptual issues in disability and rehabilitation. In M. B. Sussman (Ed.), *Sociology and rehabilitation.* Washington, DC: American Sociological Association.

National Center for Health Statistics. (accessed 2000). The national health interview survey. http://www.cdc.gov/nchs/. Atlanta: Centers for Disease Control and Prevention.

National Institute on Disability and Rehabilitation Research. (2005). Retrieved 2006, from http://www.ed.gov/osers/nidrr.

The National Service Frameworkers for Older People. (2001). Norwich, U.K.: HMSO.

National League for Nursing. (1966). *Rehabilitative aspects of nursing.* New York: Author.

Nichols, D. J., & Hammer, M. S. (1998). Case study of institution-building by Nurse Bertha Wright and colleagues. *Image—The Journal of Nursing Scholarship, 30*(4), 385-389.

Nightingale, F. (1859/1992). *Notes on nursing: What it is, and what it is not* (Commemorative edition). Philadelphia: J. B. Lippincott.

Oates, S. B. (1994). *A woman of valor: Clara Barton and the Civil War.* New York: Free Press.

Pope, A. M., & Tarlov, A. R. (Eds.). (1991). *Disability in America: Toward a national agenda for prevention.* Washington, DC: Institute of Medicine, National Academy Press.

Pryor, J. (Ed.) (1999). *Rehabilitation: A vital nursing function.* Deakin, ACT, Australia: Royal College of Nursing.

Repetto, M. A., & Hoeman, S. P. (1991). A legislative perspective on the school nurse and education for children with disabilities in New Jersey. *Journal of School Health, 61*(9), 388-391.

Roberts, D. W. (1957, February-March). Evolution of the rehabilitation center concept. In *Rehabilitation Service Series No. 420. The planning of rehabilitation centers. Proceedings of the Institute on Rehabilitation Center Planning* (pp. 1-17). Washington, DC: U.S. Department of Health, Education, and Welfare.

Roper, N., Logan, W. W., & Tierney, A. J. (1996). *The elements of nursing: A model for nursing based on a model of living* (4th ed.). Edinburgh: Churchill Livingstone.

Rusk, H. A. (1957, February-March). International aspects of the rehabilitation center movement. In *Rehabilitation Service Series No. 420. The planning of rehabilitation centers. Proceedings of the Institute on Rehabilitation Center Planning* (pp. 11-25). Washington, DC: U.S. Department of Health, Education, and Welfare.

Rusk, H. A., & Taylor, E. (1965). Rehabilitation as a phase of preventive medicine. In H. R. Leavell & E. G. Clark (Eds.), *Preventive medicine for the doctor in his community* (3rd ed., pp. 474-494). New York: McGraw-Hill.

Schopper, D., Pereira, J., Torres, A., Cuende, N., Alonso, M., Baylin, A., et al. (2000). Estimating the burden of disease in one Swiss canton: What do disability adjusted life years (DALY) tell us? *International Journal of Epidemiology, 29*(5), 871-877.

Stryker, R. (1977). *Rehabilitative aspects of acute and chronic nursing care* (2nd ed.). Philadelphia: W. B. Saunders.

Switzer, M. E. (1957, February-March). Foreword. In *Rehabilitation Service Series No. 420. The planning of rehabilitation centers. Proceedings of the Institute on Rehabilitation Center Planning* (p. v). Washington, DC: U.S. Department of Health, Education, and Welfare.

U.S. Department of Health and Human Services. (1990). *Healthy People 2000.* Retrieved 2006 from http://web.health.gov/healthypeople.

U.S. Department of Health and Human Services. (2000a). *Healthy People 2010.* Retrieved 2006 from http://web.health.gov/healthypeople.

U.S. Department of Health and Human Services. (2000b). *Healthy People 2010: Conference edition.* Retrieved 2000 from http://web.health.gov/healthypeople/document.

Verville, R. E. (1988). Fifty years of federal legislation and programs affecting the PM&R. *Archives of Physical Medicine and Rehabilitation, 69,* 64-68.

World Health Organization. (1980). International classification of impairments, disabilites, and handicaps. Geneva, Switzerland: Author.

Young, M. (1989). *A history of rehabilitation nursing: Fifteen years of making the difference.* Skokie, IL: Association of Rehabilitation Nurses.

2

Theory and Practice Models for Rehabilitation Nursing

Barbara J. Lutz, PhD, RN, CRRN
Sally M. Davis, MSc, RN, PGCEA, DipMan

A number of uniprofessional models and theories from nursing, rehabilitation, and the social sciences offer discipline-specific foundations for rehabilitation nurses and other professionals to use when conducting research, providing care, and developing programs of service. The use of theoretical models often is explicit in rehabilitation research; however, rehabilitation nurses integrate theories more implicitly in practice. In-depth discussions with rehabilitation nurses about their nursing practice revealed rich theoretical underpinnings and principles that were highly consistent with major nursing and other discipline-specific theories and models. However, these same nurses had difficulty articulating the theoretical foundations of their practice (Mumma, 2000).

Rehabilitation is a complex process that necessitates a multidisciplinary or interdisciplinary theoretically based approach to care. However, there were no interprofessional theories or models available to guide rehabilitation research and practice until the World Health Organization (WHO) (2001) introduced an integrated model for the interdisciplinary approach so critical to rehabilitation research and practice.

This chapter provides a basic overview of selected theories and models from nursing and other disciplines that are highly relevant for rehabilitation nursing research and practice. Building on the works of Hoeman (1993, 1996, 2001) and Edwards (2000), the chapter begins by describing the overarching frameworks of disability. The discussion compares and contrasts the individual and social models of disability and provides an overview of the newer integrated WHO model, the International Classification of Functioning, Disability, and Health (ICF) (WHO, 2001). The second part of the chapter presents selected theories from nursing and other disciplines important to rehabilitation nursing practice and concludes with descriptions of relevant practice models and settings.

CONCEPTUAL MODELS OF DISABILITY

The early overarching frameworks of disability supported either the individual model or the social model and had a goal to improve the health and quality of life for individuals with physical disabilities (Nagi, 1991; Swain, Finkelstein, French, & Oliver, 1993). How this goal is achieved is dictated by each model's focus or implicit set of assumptions. One way to better understand rehabilitation is to explore the contexts through which these models evolved.

Individual Model of Disability

The individual model of disability was first introduced by Nagi (1965). The model, referred to as the Nagi Scheme is based on the conventional biomedical model (Figure 2-1) and on Parsons' theory of functionalism (1951). The goal of the individual model of disability is to return the patient to normal functioning and expected social roles. In the individual model the problems associated with disability arise from an individual's disabling illness or injury. In the late 1970s the World Health Organization developed a model, the International Classification of Impairments, Disabilities, and Handicaps (ICIDH) (WHO, 1980), which has important similarities to the Nagi Scheme; both are linear, arise from the biomedical model, and focus on the functioning individual. The Nagi Scheme, prominent in the United States, and the WHO/ICIDH model, prevalent in international studies, were the most commonly referenced models in rehabilitation until the early 2000s. Figure 2-2 illustrates the models and definitions of the concepts. Important conceptual differences, which are beyond the scope of this chapter, are described in the literature (Jette, 1994; Nagi, 1991).

In an attempt to further delineate the dimensions and clarify the concept of "disability," several researchers revised the Nagi and ICIDH models. They added societal limitations (Jette, 1994); environmental, individual, and risk factors

(Verbrugge & Jette, 1994); and quality of life and health status (Ebrahim, 1995; Pope & Tarlov, 1991). The revisions incorporated three distinguishable broad areas: (1) physiological function, (2) ability to perform activities of daily living, and (3) ability to function as a member of society (Whiteneck, 1994). However, the models remained linear with a focus on the disease process and resulting functional limitations.

Social Models of Disability

Like the individual models, the goal of the social models was to improve quality of life for persons with disabilities. Unlike individual models, social models identify the locus of the problem of disability as barriers in the physical/social environments, owing to societal/environmental discrimination, prejudice, and stigmatization (Hahn, 1993) and forced dependence on health care/other professionals (DeJong, 1979).

The social model is based in earlier sociological and psychological theories of disability, including stigma theory (Goffman, 1963); spread theory (Dembo, 1969); social consciousness and disability (Wright, 1960); and the three levels of disability (personal, social, and cultural) (Safilios-Rothschild, 1970). These theorists proposed a view of disability that was alternative to the prevailing functionalist medical perspective proposed by Parsons. In this alternative construction, disability is defined as a product of societal attitudes, rather than specific attributes of an individual. These theories highlight the influence of the nondisabled observers' views in the construction of disability, perceptions that often make disability central, "overriding everything else about the person" (Wright, 1980, p. 275).

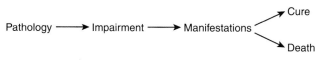

Figure 2-1 The Biomedical Model.

The most widely used and referenced social models of disability are the Independent Living (IL) model in the United States and the *Fundamental Principles of Disability* by the Union of the Physically Impaired Against Segregation (UPIAS) (1976) in the United Kingdom. Similar in nature, they were developed as a response to the perceived inadequacy of the medically focused individual models. During the 1960s and 1970s disability was defined as a problem of *individual* functioning, which promoted dependency and further disabled persons with impairments. Advocates of the social model proposed that persons with disabilities trade the dependent role of patient for the independent role of consumer (DeJong, 1979). Proposed solutions to problems deriving from disability included empowerment, self-determination, advocacy, consumer control, and environmental modifications such as curb cuts, ramps, and widened doorways and halls (Barnes, 2003; DeJong, 1979; Swain et al., 1993).

Integrated Model—The International Classification of Functioning, Disability, and Health

The WHO (2001) designed the ICF as a universal model intended to integrate the individual and social models of disability for all people, irrespective of age and health condition. The ICF defines a health condition as a "disease (acute or chronic), disorder, injury, or trauma . . . [which] may also include other circumstances such as pregnancy, aging, stress, congenital anomaly, or genetic predisposition" (WHO, 2001, p. 212).

The ICF uses categories within health and health-related domains to classify health and health-related conditions. There are two component parts, each with codes that reflect the different aspects. Part 1, Functioning and Disability, contains codes for body functions and structures and activities and participation, and Part 2, Contextual Factors, addresses environmental factors and personal factors. In the ICF, disability exists when there is dysfunctioning at one or more of these levels.

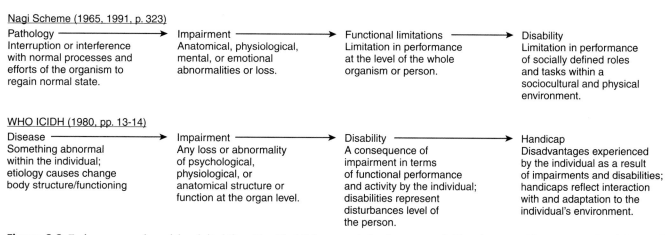

Figure 2-2 Early conceptual models of disability—The Nagi Scheme and the International Classification of Impairment, Disability, and Handicap (ICIDH).

The ICF provides rehabilitation nurses and other professionals with a framework to move away from a discipline-specific focus on illness and impairment toward a multidisciplinary focus on health and quality of life. The ICF is available on the World Health Organization website (http://www.WHO.int). Box 2-1 represents a range of literature, including research studies, that evaluates use of the ICF.

The ICF is not without critique. A reclassification of the earlier International Classification of Impairments, Disabilities and Handicaps (ICIDH), the ICF carries with it the functionalist and medically focused underpinnings of that model. Although a goal of the ICF is to integrate the individual and social models of disability, the guiding concept is the health condition or disease of the individual and its impact on body structures and functions. Therefore the resulting classification system remains grounded in the concepts of functionalism and the practices of Western medicine and science. However, with the inclusion of environmental and personal factors, the ICF is an improvement over its predecessor, the ICIDH (Barnes, 2003; Hurst 2003; Lutz & Bowers, 2003).

Kearney and Pryor (2004) describe the ICF as a useful conceptual framework with potential to expand nursing practice by increasing nurses' awareness of the social, political, and cultural dimensions of disability. As the ICF continues to be used and developed internationally, and across disciplines and contexts, rehabilitation nurses have opportunities to collaborate with other professionals to continue to evaluate and refine the ICF to better integrate the concepts from the social model.

THEORIES AND CONCEPTUAL MODELS FOR REHABILITATION

A number of discipline-specific theories and conceptual models useful to rehabilitation nursing center on life processes, well-being, and/or optimum functioning. They address ways individuals interact with their environments and function during health and illness. This section discusses the relevance of selected theories from nursing and other disciplines to rehabilitation nursing.

Relevant Nursing Theories and Models

Orem's Self-Care Deficit Theory. Orem first introduced her theories related to self-care in 1959 and has continued to refine and develop them (Orem, 1971, 2001). The Orem Self-Care Deficit Theory for nursing is composed of three subtheories: the theory of self-care, the theory of self-care deficit, and the theory of the nursing system. In Orem's theory one goal of nursing is to assist patients with their self-care needs and to return the patient to self-care. Therefore nursing interventions related to self-care may be wholly compensatory, partly compensatory, and supportive-educative (Orem, 1995, 2001). For example, a patient recovering from an acute illness can be expected to transition over time, moving from wholly compensatory through partly compensatory to supportive-educative interventions.

According to Davis and O'Connor (1999), deliberate nonintervention is oftentimes an effective strategy for rehabilitation nurses. The nurses' expertise cues them when to intervene and when to stand back, an aspect lacking in Orem's theory. Burks (1999) described a nursing practice model based on the concept of intentional action, using the Orem Self-Care Deficit Theory as the conceptual framework. In this model, rehabilitation nurses relinquish control of a patient and support the patient's management skills, thus reconceptualizing the meaning of "self-care." That is, patients with severe disabilities or chronic illnesses, who are wholly dependent in areas of self-care, can become responsible for self-directing care and ultimately become able to direct others in how to provide care that meets their self-defined needs and preferences. In this situation all three of Orem's nursing interventions for self-care would operate simultaneously.

Roy's Adaptation Model. The Roy Adaptation Model (RAM) (Roy & Andrews, 1991, 1999) considers human beings as "adaptive systems." Adaptation occurs within four adaptive modes: physiological, self-concept, interdependence, and role-function. When the need for adaptation exceeds the individual's current ability to adapt, the rehabilitation nurse intervenes by working within the patient's adaptive modes to increase adaptation or by changing environmental stimuli to

---

BOX 2-1   Literature Citing the ICF as the Theoretical Framework

Bornman (2004): This description of the ICF illustrates how the ICF can determine whether a particular intervention program has been effective at the levels of body function and structure, activity and participation.

Ogonowski, Kronk, Rice, and Feldman (2004): This study looks at the interreliability in assigning ICF codes to children with disabilities in the United States.

Heerkens, van der Brug, Napel, and van Ravensberg (2003): These researchers concluded that the ICF is too general to be used to describe functioning of an individual on the level of detail needed by health care professionals.

Jette and Keysor (2003): This U.S. survey identifies distinct concepts within physical functioning that fit with specific activities and participation levels.

Rentsch et al. (2003): The focus on improved quality of life can be achieved by identifying goals for participation, involving the family, and taking into account contextual factors.

Wade and Halligan (2003): These researchers suggest an expanded ICF model to include a description of quality of life and other concepts such as happiness and role satisfaction.

decrease the demands. This model focuses on the functioning individual and is consistent with the individual models of disability. The Roy Adaptation Model has been used as the framework for research exploring mobility and environmental barriers (Shyu, Liang, Lu, & Wu, 2004), chronic pain (Tsai, Tak, Moore, & Palencia, 2003), and issues related to multiple sclerosis (Gagliardi, 2003; Gagliardi, Frederickson, & Shanley, 2002).

Rogers' Model of the Science of Unitary Human Beings.

Rogers' Science of Unitary Human Beings (1990) is a framework for holistic nursing care that involves recognition of patterns that emerge from person-environment interactions. Human beings are energy fields in constant interaction with environmental energy fields, both of which are infinite and irreducible. Rogers' principles of homeodynamics (resonancy, helicy, and integrality) are useful when assessing patterns that emerge from interactions between patients and their environments. Parses' Theory of Human Becoming and Newman's Theory of Health as Expanding Consciousness are both based on Rogers' model. Several studies have applied Rogers' model through the use of therapeutic touch and energy fields as a nursing intervention (Biley, 1996; Herdtner, 2000; Turner, Clark, Gauthier, & Williams, 1998).

King's Open Systems Framework and Theory of Goal Attainment.

King's theory of goal attainment is an open systems framework containing three interacting systems: individual or personal systems, group or interpersonal systems, and society or social systems (Figure 2-3). Individuals are in constant interaction with their environments and one another. They bring a set of values, ideas, attitudes, and perceptions to those interactions. The goal of nursing is "to help individuals to maintain their health so they can function in their roles" (King, 1981). As nurses and patients interact, "each perceives the other in the situation and, through communication, they set goals, explore means, and agree on means to achieve goals." Mutually set goals among nurses, patients, and their families is a key component of rehabilitation nursing practice that is consistent with King's theory of goal attainment.

Neuman's Systems Theory.

Neuman Systems Model is another open systems framework that combines constructs from several theories, including general systems, ecological, epidemiological, and stress and coping. Focusing on the whole person in interaction with his or her environment, concepts such as adaptation, stressors, whole person, and preventive intervention are woven throughout the model (Hoeman, 1996; Neuman, 1989).

This complex model proposes a holistic, wellness and prevention orientation that is particularly useful for rehabilitation nursing interventions with community-living persons with disabilities. It also has the capacity to be used by transdisciplinary teams for lifelong care planning and continuity

across the continuum of the health care from acute care to home.

Omaha System.

Developed with the goal of coordinating and documenting the efforts of a multidisciplinary health team, Omaha System provides a standardized framework for problem solving that focuses on three key components: problem classification, intervention, and a rating scale for outcomes. When taken as a whole, the system is reflective of the nursing process and is recognized by the American Nurses Association. Box 2-2 summarizes the process.

Roper's Model for Living.

Concepts from the Roper Model for Living (Roper, Logan, & Tierney, 1996) constitute part of the framework for this book. Roper et al. developed a Model for Living and a corresponding Model for Nursing. The major components of both models are the activities of daily living (ADLs) (Table 2-1), which characterize the person. These ADLs represent all of the things persons do on a daily basis, and each is placed on a dependence-independence continuum. The multiple factors that have potential to influence ADLs are categorized as biological, psychological, sociocultural, environmental, or politicoeconomic. Adding to the complexity of the model is that all of the ADLs are interrelated and affect functioning of the whole person. For example, one patient with impaired mobility of the lower extremities may experience significant loss of interpersonal

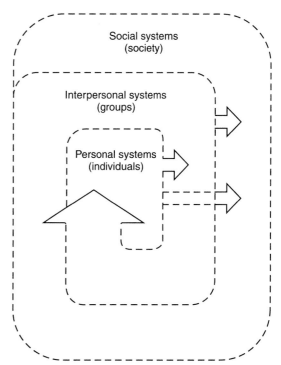

Figure 2-3 King's conceptual framework for nursing. (Reprinted with permission of Sage Publications, from Frey, M. A., & Sieloff, C. L. [Eds.]. [1995]. *Advancing King's systems framework and theory of nursing* [p. 19]. Thousand Oaks, CA: Sage.)

BOX 2-2 Omaha System

Problem Classification Scheme

Domain I—Environmental
01. Income
02. Sanitation
03. Residence
04. Neighborhood/workplace safety

Domain II—Psychosocial
06. Communication with community resources
07. Social contact
08. Role change
09. Interpersonal relationship
10. Spirituality
11. Grief
12. Mental health
13. Sexuality
14. Caretaking/parenting
15. Neglect
16. Abuse
17. Growth and development

Domain III—Physiological
19. Hearing
20. Vision
21. Speech and language
45. Oral health
23. Cognition
24. Pain
25. Consciousness
26. Integument
27. Neuro-musculo-skeletal function
28. Respiration
29. Circulation
30. Digestion-hydration
31. Bowel function
46. Urinary function
47. Reproductive function
48. Pregnancy
49. Postpartum
50. Communicable/infectious condition

Domain IV—Health Related Behaviors
35. Nutrition
36. Sleep and rest patterns
37. Physical activity
38. Personal care
39. Substance use
40. Family planning
41. Health care supervision
42. Medication

Intervention Scheme Categories
I. Teaching, Guidance, and Counseling
II. Techniques and Procedures
III. Case Management
IV. Surveillance

Intervention Scheme Targets
01. Anatomy/physiology
64. Anger management
02. Behavioral modification
03. Bladder care
04. Bonding/attachment
05. Bowel care
07. Cardiac care
08. Caretaking/parenting skills
09. Cast care
10. Communication
65. Community outreach worker services
66. Continuity of care
11. Coping skills
12. Day care/respite
67. Dietary management
13. Discipline
14. Dressing change/wound care
15. Durable medical equipment
16. Education
17. Employment
68. End-of-life care
18. Environment
19. Exercises
20. Family planning care
21. Feeding procedures
22. Finances

24. Gait training
69. Genetics
25. Growth and development care
27. Home
70. Homemaking/housekeeping
71. Infection precautions
28. Interaction
72. Interpreter/translator services
29. Laboratory findings
30. Legal system
31. Medical/dental care
32. Medication actions/side effects
33. Medication administration
73. Medication coordination/ordering
74. Medication prescription
34. Medication setup
35. Mobility/transfers
75. Nursing care
38. Nutritionist care
39. Ostomy care
40. Other community resources
77. Paraprofessional/aide care
41. Personal hygiene
78. Physical therapy care
42. Positioning

44. Relaxation/breathing techniques
80. Respiratory care
81. Respiratory therapy care
45. Rest/sleep
46. Safety
47. Screening procedures
48. Sickness/injury care
49. Sign/symptoms—mental/emotional
50. Signs/symptoms—physical
51. Skin care
52. Social work/counseling care
53. Specimen collection
82. Speech and language pathology care
54. Spiritual care
55. Stimulation/nurturance
56. Stress management
83. Substance use cessation
58. Supplies
59. Support group
60. Support system
61. Transportation
62. Wellness
63. Other (specify)

Rating Scales for Outcomes

Knowledge—Level of

1	2	3	4	5
None	Minimal	Basic	Adequate	Superior

Behavior—Appropriateness of

1	2	3	4	5
Never	Rarely	Inconsistently	Usually	Consistently

Modified from Martin, K. S. (2005). *The Omaha System: A key to practice, documentation, and information management.* St. Louis, MO: Elsevier Saunders.

TABLE 2-1 Roper's Activities of Living Model (1996) and Gordon's Functional Health Patterns (2000)

Activities of Living	Functional Health Patterns
Maintaining a safe environment	Health perception–health management pattern
Communicating	Cognitive-perceptual pattern Coping-stress-tolerance pattern Value-belief pattern
Breathing	Activity-exercise pattern
Eating and drinking	Nutritional-metabolic pattern
Eliminating	Elimination pattern
Personal cleansing and dressing	Activity-exercise pattern
Controlling body temperature	Nutritional-metabolic pattern
Mobilizing	Activity-exercise pattern
Working and playing	Activity-exercise pattern Self-perception–self-concept pattern Role-relationship pattern
Expressing sexuality	Sexuality-reproductive pattern Role-relationship pattern
Sleeping	Sleep-rest pattern
Dying	Self-perception–self-concept pattern

Data from Gordon, M. (2000). *Manual of nursing diagnosis* (9th ed.). St. Louis, MO: Mosby; and Roper, N., Logan, W., & Tierney, A. (1996). *The elements of nursing: A model for nursing based on a model of living* (4th ed.). Edinburgh: Churchill Livingstone.

relationships, inability to dress independently, and difficulty accessing toilet facilities. Another patient, with a similar impairment, using a wheelchair for mobility, may be independent in those same ADLs.

Roper's Model for Nursing combines the steps of the nursing process (assessing, diagnosing, planning, implementing, and evaluating) with the Model for Living to achieve desired patient outcomes. Rehabilitation nurses use the nursing process when working with patients to prevent potential problems, alleviate actual problems, and cope effectively with problems that cannot be cured or solved. Health teaching, individuality, and active patient participation are explicit in the model, an attractive feature for rehabilitation nurses.

Gordon's Functional Health Patterns. Gordon (2000) developed the typology of Functional Health Patterns (FHPs) primarily as a system for organizing assessment data. The FHPs are used in the care of individuals, families, and communities and evolve from patient-environment interactions. Patterns are highly interrelated and are fully understood only within the context of the whole person. Because the FHPs can be used to effectively organize assessment data from patients with disabilities and chronic illnesses, they have been

integrated with the Roper Model for Living in the organizing framework for this book.

Other Relevant Theories

The following section includes descriptions of selected theories from other disciplines that are particularly relevant to rehabilitation nursing. Other theories and constructs (Table 2-2) are discussed throughout this book when they are applicable to the specific chapter content.

Social Cognitive Theory. In 1962 Bandura pioneered social learning theory, which later evolved into social cognitive theory (1977, 1986). The theory proposes that human behavior is based on an interaction between personal factors (including cognition), behavior, and environment. When deciding on or learning a particular behavior, the person attends to the situation, retains the observation, has a certain capacity to perform the action, and identifies rewards or punishments associated with performing the action. According to this theory, behavior change is based on the interaction between expectations about the outcomes of a behavior and expectations about the ability to carry out the behavior. The most important factor in behavior change, according to Bandura (1986) and others is the degree of self-efficacy or confidence a person has in his or her ability to performing an activity or behavior. Rehabilitation nurses frequently apply the tenets of social cognitive theory and self-efficacy by breaking desired tasks or behaviors into small sequential steps to facilitate a patient's confidence in performing them, and then transferring those new behaviors to a variety of situations.

Social cognitive theory and self-efficacy provide the theoretical basis for many research studies and interventions in rehabilitation. Resnick developed a program of research based on the theory of self-efficacy in which several interventions, tools, and models focusing on rehabilitation of older adults were tested. Examples include the Self-Efficacy for Functional Activities Scale (Resnick, 1999), the Exercise Plus Program (Resnick, Magaziner, Orwig, & Zimmerman, 2002), and the Restorative Care Intervention for nurses and nursing assistants working in nursing homes (Resnick et al., 2000).

Social and Cultural Models. Social and cultural diversity have implications for rehabilitation because outcomes, interactions, and responses to rehabilitation services are influenced by social and cultural factors. Based in nursing and anthropology, Leininger's Culture Care Theory (Leininger, 1976; Reynolds & Leininger, 1993) proposes that health and illness experiences can be fully understood only within the context of culture. Culture is not based solely on ethnicity. When groups of people have similar experiences over a period of time, a "culture" develops based on those similar experiences. In inpatient rehabilitation, for example, a unique culture linking patients, families, and staff often emerges.

A goal of Culture Care Theory is to provide nursing care that is congruent with the values, health beliefs, and

TABLE 2-2 Selected Theories, Models, and Concepts Relevant to Rehabilitation Nursing

Type of Theory	Contributor	Theories, Models, and Concepts
Behavioral Theories		
Change theories	Lewin (1947)	Theories of planned change and reducing barriers to change
	Lippitt, Watson, and Westley (1958)	Change agent, advocacy, and informed decision making
Stress and coping	Lazarus and Folkman (1984)	Theories of stress and coping (see Chapter 22)
	Selye (1956)	First of the modern stress theorists
Health beliefs	Becker (1974)	Health Belief Model—combines stimulus-response theory and social cognitive theory
Resilience	Antonovsky (1979, 1996)	Salutogenesis—resilience; sense of coherence
Health and Wellness		
	Dunn (1959)	High-level wellness based on holistic balance and maximum potential
	Leavell and Clark (1965)	Epidemiology integrated with levels of prevention (see Chapter 1)
	Erbst (1984)	Multidimensional model of wellness; wellness is relative and governed by an ecological model, balance and synergy
Alternative Constructions of Disability		
	Wright (1960, 1983)	Identified the link between environment and disability; eschewed the individual (medical) models of disability in favor of a social/environmental approach
	Goffman (1963)	Theories related to stigma, spoiled identity, passing for normal
	Dembo (1969)	Spread theory—person devalued by attributes or altered body status
	Safilios-Rothschild (1970)	Three levels of disability—personal, social, and cultural; integrates stigma and spread theory; perceptions of disability; self-concept and body image
	Union of the Physically Impaired Against Segregation (1976)	*Fundamental Principles of Disability*—the first social model of disability
	DeJong (1979)	Independent Living model—the U.S. version of the social model
	NIDRR (2005)	Universal design, focusing on the built environment with a goal of creating an environment that is all-inclusive
Chronic Illness Management		
	Corbin and Strauss (1992)	Chronic Illness Trajectory model
	Charmaz (1991)	The Self in Chronic Illness and Time
	Lubkin (1995)	Complexities in the concepts of chronicity and disability

lifestyles of different cultures. Within rehabilitation, nurses can bridge cultural barriers to facilitate care and improve access, while being sensitive and competent in cultural matters. Chapter 6 discusses cultural care within the context of conventional, complementary, and alternative care.

Chronic Illness Theories. Several theories focusing on chronic illness are applicable to rehabilitation nursing. For example, the Chronic Illness Trajectory framework developed by Corbin and Strauss (1992) proposes that disabling and chronic conditions have a predictable course over time that can be influenced or managed. Providers or patients

themselves can attempt to produce outcomes that differ from the trajectory when they understand the nature of their condition. As a result, persons with disabilities or chronic disease can learn ways of managing limitations to participate as fully as possible in everyday activities.

Charmaz's theory (1991) of The Self in Chronic Illness and Time illustrates the influence of chronic illness on self and how persons with chronic illnesses manage their disease process over time. She addresses issues such as living with chronic illness, disclosing illness, the intrusion of illness into one's life, and lessons learned from the illness experience. Charmaz's work provides in-depth insight for rehabilitation nurses and other health professionals into the everyday lives of persons with chronic illness.

Environmental and Ecological Models. Ecological models take into account the multifaceted social and environmental context in which individuals experience health and illness. These include the natural environment, such as climate, topography, flora, and fauna; the built environment, such as community buildings and accessible housing; the social environment, such as attitudes, social norms, and support systems; and cultural factors and norms. Ecological models operate at five levels: individual, interpersonal, organizational, community, and public policy (Sallis & Owen, 2002). These factors are prominent in theories and models such as those of Reynolds and Leininger (1993), Rogers (1990), Neuman (1995), and Wright (1980). Ideally, patients experience rehabilitation in a setting that best prepares them to deal with their critical life situation so they may return successfully to community living. Rehabilitation nurses consider all of the contextual factors of the ecological model in order to help patients accomplish this goal.

Family Systems Theories. Many theories address family systems. Bowen (1966), Satir (1967), and Minuchin (1974) are familiar to nurses because they presented ways to facilitate counseling and psychotherapy with families. Friedemann (1995) and Anderson (2000) developed theories for nurses to use for promoting comprehensive family health. For example, Anderson's Family Health System theory (FHS) (2000) is a process-oriented, holistic approach to health and illness that combines elements of the ecological model with those of family systems and life span developmental theories, change theory, and illness beliefs. The FHS proposes that the patient is integrally linked to the family system, as well as the larger social system. In FHS "family health is systemic and . . . includes an interaction of biopsychosocial and contextual phenomena" (p. 106). Therefore competent care must include assessment and care of the family, as well as the patient. The FHS suggests five interrelated processes—interactive, developmental, coping, integrity, and health—that constitute family health. This approach to care recognizes the complexity of variables that converge when family members of different sexes, generations, and developmental stages, as well as differing life experiences, interact with environmental structures and social systems.

For example, the challenges are evident with a 50-year-old woman who experienced a left hemisphere stroke, resulting in right body paresis, sensory loss, aphasia, and dysphagia. Following inpatient rehabilitation in an urban center, she returned to a geographically remote area. She lives in a small home with her husband, three children, and one grandchild. Her successful reintegration into the community and continued rehabilitation depend to a large extent on the involvement and capabilities of her family and the community resources.

REHABILITATION NURSING PRACTICE—MODELS AND SETTINGS

Models of practice that guide care and settings where rehabilitation nurses provide care are discussed in this section.

Specialty Practice

The design of rehabilitation specialty programs was shaped in part, by the criteria set by the Commission on Accreditation of Rehabilitation Facilities (CARF). Although most rehabilitation care models attempt to address the unique needs of their patients, the heterogeneity of the patient population can make this difficult. Specialization is one way to address unique consumer needs by targeting services to particular patient groups. Rehabilitation services are frequently specialized by age or developmental level (e.g., pediatric or geriatric), setting, or by diagnosis (e.g., stroke, traumatic brain injury, or spinal cord injury). CARF has research-based diagnosis- and age-specific standards for spinal cord injury, stroke, burns, brain injury, and pediatric specialty units. These standards help to ensure high-quality specialized care for patients in need of rehabilitation services.

Specializing by Age or Developmental Level. Rehabilitation programs may be specialized according to the age or developmental level of the patient. For example, pediatric rehabilitation nursing goals related to comprehensive and holistic care blend with creative strategies to address the unique developmental needs of children. Children need a program environment appropriate for their age and stage where their parents can spend extended time with them. The plan of care for infants and children with chronic illness and disability must emphasize collaboration and partnership with parents. Rehabilitation services for adolescents address their critical development needs of independence, socialization, and sexuality education. Chapter 31 discusses pediatric rehabilitation in detail.

Evaluation and promotion of restorative function is important in planning care with the older adult. Functionally impaired elderly patients are at greater risk for secondary sequelae such as falls, adverse reactions to medications, and complications from comorbid conditions. Specialized units, such as inpatient geriatric assessment units or transitional care centers, provide evaluation and rehabilitation specifically designed for older adults. These programs focus on promoting self-care activities and improved function to decrease nursing home placement and reduce mortality. Chapter 32 discusses gerontological rehabilitation nursing in more detail.

Specializing by Type of Disability. Rehabilitation units may be designated to provide comprehensive, coordinated care for homogeneous groups based on a specific disability or chronic condition. These specialized units are designed using standardized guidelines from CARF or model systems programs from the National Institute on Disability and Rehabilitation Research (NIDRR). For example, NIDRR has model systems programs specializing in spinal cord injury and traumatic brain injury including services for acute care, rehabilitation, community reintegration, and long-term follow-up. Outcome data and detailed information on research projects are available on the NIDRR website (http://www.ed.gov/about/offices/list/osers/nidrr/index.html). In 2005 CARF added new practice guidelines for inpatient rehabilitation for persons recovering from stroke (CARF, 2006).

National Rehabilitation Information Center (n.d.).

Acute care hospitals are also beginning to have specialized units focusing on specific disabilities or conditions. For example, The Joint Commission (TJC) in conjunction with the American Stroke Association (ASA) has developed evidence-based standards for primary stroke centers to improve outcomes for stroke patients in acute care (JCAHCO & ASA, 2005). These interdisciplinary centers may be physically based on a particular floor within the hospital or they may consist of mobile teams that go to the floor or department where the patient in located. In either case, teams that include physicians, nurses, and therapists who specialize in stroke care and rehabilitation follow patients from admission to acute care through discharge back to the community.

One disadvantage of disability-specific programs is that their centralized locations, often in urban areas, require patients to undergo treatment at a distance from family and community. Program protocols that are dedicated to detailed care of a particular problem or disease may overlook comorbidity or fail to consider the complexity of multiple chronic conditions for a patient. However, a community of caring or peer support often emerges when patients and families are exposed to others dealing with the same condition and similar challenges. Viewing the whole patient necessitates early recognition and control of complications, reconditioning, attention to retraining in ADLs, and prevention of secondary conditions.

Patient/Family-Centered Practice

In rehabilitation nursing, working with patients and their families to develop and achieve goals for restoring function and living as independently as possible is paramount to practice. Patient/family-centered models of care (PCC) provide an overarching framework for all rehabilitation nursing care.

PCC, a critical rehabilitation element, has two working definitions. In the first, care is designed based on the specific needs of a patient; however, those needs are measured by the provider's system. Secondly, PCC is an approach that consciously adopts the perspective of the patients and their families, with careful consideration of what is important to each and how care is likely to affect them (Box 2-2) (Lutz & Bowers, 2000). PCC embraces a philosophy of respect and partnership between patients and providers that is essential to effective rehabilitation care. This model also is referred to as patient driven because it emphasizes the needs, thoughts, feelings, and expectations of the patient (Gerteis, Edgman-Levitan,

---

> **BOX 2-3** **Patient-Centered Practice**
>
> **Dimensions of Patient-Centered Care**
> - Respect for patient's values, preferences, and expressed needs
> - Coordination and integration of care
> - Information, communication, and education
> - Physical comfort
> - Emotional support, alleviation of fear and anxiety
> - Involvement of family and friends
> - Transition and continuity (Gerteis, Edgman-Levitan, Daley, & Delbanco, 1993)
>
> **Key Concepts**
> - Individual autonomy and choice
> - Partnership
> - Nurse and patient responsibility
> - Enablement
> - Contextual congruence
> - Accessibility
> - Respect for diversity

Daley, & Delbanco, 1993). Family systems theories, discussed earlier, offer useful concepts for patient and family-centered practice.

Full cooperation and commitment from the family, as well as the patient, in the rehabilitation process are crucial for the patient's recovery and reintegration into community living. Therefore the rehabilitation team often must also consider the family's needs and preferences. Ideally, long-term rehabilitation is a joint team-family-patient partnership that addresses the physical and emotional impact of disabling illness or chronic condition. The rehabilitation nurse has an important role in identifying family, as well as patient, concerns with issues such as caregiving and helping to secure the resources for continued recovery at home. Identifying family and patient needs and instituting short-term interventions at known crisis points in the rehabilitation process when family members are occupied with specific concerns are likely to be effective strategies because their attention is focused.

Ideally, patients and families are comanagers in the rehabilitation process, participating as fully as possible in planning, implementing, and evaluating care. Family systems theories help rehabilitation nurses in understanding family dynamics, including patterns of communication, interaction, power, and economics (Anderson, 2000), while maintaining a PCC approach to care. Chapter 22 discusses coping and family in rehabilitation.

Practice Settings in Rehabilitation Nursing

Acute Inpatient Rehabilitation Care. Many rehabilitation nurses practice in acute inpatient rehabilitation settings. Acute inpatient rehabilitation units were developed after World War II to provide intensive rehabilitation for patients with disabling conditions. Units can be part of a larger tertiary hospital system or can be freestanding hospitals. Patients admitted to these units must be able to tolerate several hours of therapy each day, and families are encouraged to participate in the patient's care and therapy sessions. Care is usually designed and provided through a team-based approach. Teams include rehabilitation nurses; speech, occupational, physical, and recreational therapists; rehabilitation counselors; physiatrists; social workers; case managers; and patients and their families.

Recent focus on cost containment, including prospective payment systems in the United States, has caused shorter lengths of stay and lower reimbursement for acute inpatient rehabilitation facilities. Facilities have responded to these changes with strategies including utilization management and specialty care. Given the continued focus on cost containment and shifting care to less costly settings (e.g., subacute and home health care), the configuration of acute inpatient rehabilitation programs will continue to change for years to come.

Subacute and Long-Term Care.
Subacute rehabilitation units emerged in the 1990s as a potentially lower-cost option for rehabilitation care, serving patients who required skilled medical and nursing care but not diagnostic or invasive procedures. Many subacute units admit persons whose medical treatment makes their participation in an acute rehabilitation program difficult or for those who cannot tolerate the intensive therapy provided in acute rehabilitation programs. The overall rehabilitation goals are congruent with those in other settings—maximum independent functioning and quality of life.

These facilities generally provide a variety of rehabilitation services to patients with disabilities, including nursing and speech, physical, and occupational therapies. The scheduled number of hours of therapy per week compared with that in acute inpatient rehabilitation facilities is reduced. Within subacute settings, nurses serve as primarily planners, coordinators, and evaluators of patient outcomes, as well as direct care providers. Nursing assistants and licensed practical nurses provide much of the direct care in these settings.

Accurate statistics on the total numbers of persons with chronic disability residing in long-term care facilities are not readily accessible. In the United States an estimated 5% of Medicare beneficiaries live in long-term care institutions. Approximately half of these are 65 to 85 years, and a third are over 85 years old (National Center for Health Statistics, 2005). The number of younger persons with chronic disabilities who reside in long-term care facilities is more difficult to determine. Certainly many residents in long-term care facilities could live in the community if adequate services, such as personal care and housekeeping, home-delivered meals, and transportation, were available.

Subacute and long-term inpatient rehabilitation settings may be viewed in a number of different ways. For some patients these facilities are an appropriate, cost-effective alternative to rehabilitation in a more acute setting. For others

these settings may be only one of several stops along their rehabilitation continuum of care. Others will be discharged to home from acute rehabilitation and later admitted to a subacute or long-term care facility.

Community Settings.
The community, rather than the hospital or inpatient setting, has become a primary treatment setting in which many persons with disabilities manage their care and daily activities. The term *community-based rehabilitation* (CBR) has been broadly defined and applied to a variety of programs and settings within which patients receive rehabilitation services. CBR services may include outpatient care, home health care, independent living centers, senior citizen centers, community reentry programs, rural outreach, and mobile rehabilitation teams (Quigley, 2000). Community-based rehabilitation is discussed in detail in Chapter 12.

Residents in rural areas, in particular, have more difficulty accessing rehabilitation services. Problems central to rural rehabilitation include limited access to the variety of services for individuals with disabilities, the number of persons who are elderly or have limited income, and time and money burdens of travel to centralized rehabilitation. In addition, there is a scarcity of health care providers, including nurses, who make up the majority of direct-care providers in rural areas, and they often lack specialized expertise in rehabilitation.

The rehabilitation literature includes a number of reports of rural communities that have successfully met the challenge of providing rehabilitation care in areas where resources are scarce. The entire community can learn to participate in the plan of care. One strategy is through a mobile interdisciplinary rehabilitation team. These teams have increased patients' access to rehabilitation services and improved outcomes in both rural and urban areas internationally (Geddes & Chamberlain, 2003; Lavallee & Crupi, 1992). For example, patients discharged early from an acute care stroke unit received services from a mobile rehabilitation team. They experienced improved quality of life and better functional status 1 year post discharge (Fjaertoft, Indredavik, Johnsen, & Lydersen, 2004; Fjaertoft, Indredavik, & Lydersen, 2003).

Home Health Care.
Rehabilitation in home health care settings has increased dramatically in the last decade, along with community awareness of the availability and effectiveness of home health care (Moffa-Trotter & Anemaet, 1999). Home rehabilitation is generally viewed as a continuation of rehabilitation programs initiated in other settings, such as acute inpatient rehabilitation facilities, outpatient programs, and long-term care settings. Returning home is often one of the strongest desires for patients involved in inpatient rehabilitation programs. A measure of successful rehabilitation is the generalization or translation of skills to the natural setting—home. Home rehabilitation promotes patient autonomy, independence, and community reintegration (Mayo, Wood-Dauphinee, & Cote, 2000; Neal, 1998). Community awareness of the availability and effectiveness of home health

care is growing dramatically. There are essential differences between home health care and hospital or rehabilitation facility care. Regardless of how "patient friendly" inpatient units are designed to be, patients will quickly remind anyone listening that these settings are not home.

Several models applicable to rehabilitation nursing are cited in the literature, including the Albrecht (1990) nursing model for home health care, which supports the congruence between rehabilitation principles and home health nursing practice; a model integrating case management and home health care (Aliotta & Andre, 1997); the Rice (1994) model for dynamic self-determination; and the Neal (1998) model of home health nursing practice.

Telerehabilitation. Technology is changing the way outpatient rehabilitation services are delivered, especially in remote areas of the country. With videoconferencing and data acquisition technologies, telerehabilitation has been used in rehabilitation nursing, physical and occupational therapy, pediatric and geriatric rehabilitation services (Garrett & Shapcott, 1998; Levine, 1996), and computer-based support groups (Pierce et al., 2004). Applications of telerehabilitation include providing the following: (1) comprehensive rehabilitation services to patients for whom transportation and disability limit access, (2) alternatives to on-site home evaluations, (3) a link between providers at remote sites and real-time consultation at a specialty hub, (4) support for patients and families transitioning to home by contact with rehabilitation staff, and (5) education programs among clinicians and rehabilitation experts (Cudney & Weinert, 2000). For example, a spinal cord injury rehabilitation team at one Veterans Administration (VA) hospital implemented a telerehabilitation intervention with community-living patients with spinal cord injuries (SCIs). These patients and their caregivers communicate weekly with the team via videophone to address issues related to their post-SCI recovery. Although the number of enrolled patients thus far is small (14), these patients have fewer rehospitalizations and reduced lengths of stay when they are admitted to the hospital (Galea, Tumminia, & Garback, 2006). With the rapid advance of telerehabilitation technologies, these types of programs will continue to increase.

MODELS OF CARE

In addition to the variety of settings described above, there are two models of care that guide rehabilitation nursing practice: provider-based and team-based models, which are described in the following section.

Provider-Based Models

The number and type of health care providers is integrally linked to the practice models used in the different rehabilitation settings. Staffing needs in rural settings differ from those in suburban or urban areas. Reimbursement systems and third-party payers also shape the type of providers and thus the type of rehabilitation. Provider-based models of care

include primary nursing, case management, and advanced practice/consultation.

Primary Nursing. Primary nursing as a care delivery system emerged more than 30 years ago as a response to fragmentation and depersonalization of team nursing. Under the team nursing model, a team leader (usually a registered nurse) supervises a variety of team members in the total care for assigned patients. Members of the nursing team perform different care functions composing the patients' total care. A drawback of team nursing is that each patient has multiple caregivers with no individual nurse clearly accountable for coordination of all care given.

An essential feature of primary nursing is the professional nurse's 24-hour responsibility for care provided to patients to whom that nurse is assigned. A successful primary nursing system requires considerable communication and collaboration with the patient and family, as well as with others involved in the care. Thus primary nursing continues to prove useful in settings where patients have chronic conditions (Jonsdottir, 1999).

Within acute inpatient rehabilitation settings, primary nursing has been modified in keeping with the interdisciplinary team approach to care. Acute rehabilitation settings that successfully use a primary nursing model have sufficient staff so that each primary nurse is accountable for a maximum number of patients at a time. Financial constraints and decreased availability of registered nurses may alter primary nursing.

Case Management. The goal of case management is comprehensive, patient-centered, continuous care provided by a multidisciplinary team (Coile & Matthews, 1999). A rehabilitation nurse case manager who receives a referral for initial assessment while the patient is in an acute inpatient rehabilitation setting may continue to provide follow-up for the patient through outpatient and home settings. The concept and purposes of case management, including patient- and family-centered care, are highly congruent with rehabilitation philosophies and purposes. Individual patient goals related to maximizing functional ability and quality of life are integral to both rehabilitation and case management.

Case management is a care delivery model whose popularity and usefulness will continue to grow. Naylor et al. (1999) have demonstrated the effectiveness of an advanced practice nursing case management model for frail elders. Advanced practice nurses provided comprehensive discharge planning and in-home follow-up for elderly patients who were at risk for rehospitalizations. Total Medicare costs for the intervention group were 50% lower than the control group at 24 weeks.

For many rehabilitation patients with complex health care needs, the most appropriate case management system may be a well-organized interdisciplinary team. The VA Care Coordination Home Tele-Health Program is an example of an interdisciplinary case management model (Chumbler, Mann, Wu, Schmid, & Kobb, 2004). Although it is important to recognize the benefits of case management, it is important to conduct additional research focusing on its effectiveness. Case management is discussed in detail in Chapter 13.

Advanced Practice. Opportunities abound for nurses prepared for advanced practice. In an increasingly complex health system with mandates for the highest quality care at the lowest cost, nurse practitioners and clinical specialists are in demand. Some advanced practice nurses specialize in the care of patients with chronic illness and disability. Collaborative practice between nurse practitioners and clinical nurse specialists can be the basis for excellent, cost-effective care, using the expertise of both roles for the benefit of patients (Conger & Craig, 1998).

Nurse-to-nurse referral and consultations benefit provider and patient alike. For example, an advanced practice rehabilitation nurse specialist can provide consultation throughout an acute care hospital and assist primary nurses in making patient care decisions. When patients with severe limitations are admitted to a medical-surgical floor, the advanced practice nurse can provide expert advice, helping the primary nurse to assess the patient for potential problems, such as skin breakdown, mobility issues, and incontinence, and devise the appropriate interventions to address these problems. By working collaboratively with the medical-surgical nurses, rehabilitation nurse specialists are able to help improve the quality of patient care (Phipps, 1990).

Opportunities for advanced practice nurses are expected to expand considerably. Rehabilitation nurses in advanced practice roles can have an impact on care in acute settings by ensuring that patients receive care to prevent complications that would disrupt or prohibit their performing well in rehabilitation.

Team-Based Models of Care

Treatment teams traditionally have been considered the best way to work with patients who have multiple complex rehabilitation needs. Coordinated, concurrent care from the onset of the disability through all phases of rehabilitation is critical to achieving the best results.

Teams vary in their structure, composition, configuration, and functions, all of which influence outcomes. The traditional rehabilitation team is composed of representatives from various disciplines united in purpose to improve rehabilitation outcomes for a patient. Although the combination varies according to patient needs and goals, team members typically include specialists in nursing; medicine; physical, occupational, recreational, and speech therapies; psychology; social work; dietetics; and orthotics. In rehabilitation the patient and family are critical members of the team. Multidisciplinary, interdisciplinary, and transdisciplinary teams differ in philosophy, structure, leadership, goal-setting practices, and goal-attainment strategies.

Multidisciplinary Teams. Multidisciplinary teams include members from various disciplines. Each discipline within a multidisciplinary team submits findings and recommendations, sets its own discipline-specific goals, and works within the discipline boundaries to achieve these goals independently. Discipline-specific progress in goal attainment is communicated directly or indirectly to the rest of the team. Thus the team's outcomes are the sum of each discipline's efforts (Dean & Geiringer, 1990). Effective communication between team members is viewed as the key to success (Figure 2-4).

Many rehabilitation professionals believe that the whole is greater than the sum of its parts, emphasizing the need for integrating the efforts of team members in a holistic manner. Physical, psychological, social, and spiritual goals for each individual cannot be fully met by isolating the goals and assigning responsibility to a specific discipline. Holistic care requires that each patient be viewed as a whole, with the entire team working toward the attainment of all goals. Interdisciplinary and transdisciplinary teams are more likely to strive to achieve comprehensive holistic care than are multidisciplinary teams. These methods of team interaction (interdisciplinary and transdisciplinary) have been described as synergistic in that more comprehensive outcomes are produced than any one discipline alone would be able to accomplish (Norrefalk, 2003).

Interdisciplinary Teams. Collaboration replaces communication as the key to successful interdisciplinary teams. Although membership on an interdisciplinary team is quite similar to that on a multidisciplinary team, the way the disciplines function is different (Figure 2-5). Rather than each discipline identifying treatment goals, the team identifies goals and strives to avoid duplication or conflict in goals. Team members are involved in problem solving beyond the confines of their discipline. Once the team goals are identified, each discipline sets out to work toward goal attainment within the parameters of the discipline, collaborating when goals overlap discipline boundaries.

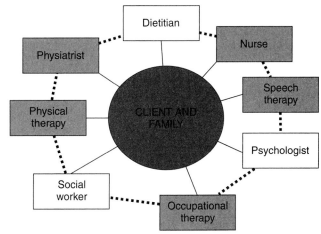

Figure 2-4 Multidisciplinary rehabilitation team, characterized by discipline-specific goals, clear boundaries between disciplines, and outcomes that are the sum of each discipline's efforts. Effective communication is the key to success for this type of team.

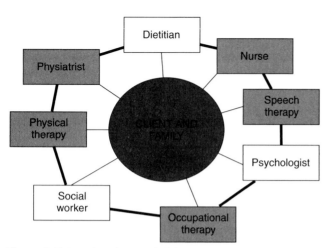

Figure 2-5 Interdisciplinary rehabilitation team. This type of team collaborates to identify patient goals and is characterized by a combination of expanded problem solving beyond discipline boundaries and discipline-specific work toward goal attainment.

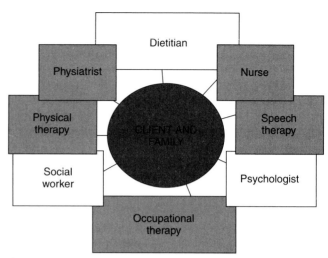

Figure 2-6 Transdisciplinary rehabilitation team, characterized by blurring of boundaries between disciplines, as well as implied cross-training and flexibility to minimize duplication of effort toward patient goal attainment.

One obstacle to interdisciplinary efforts is that although each discipline is programmatically dedicated to the interdisciplinary team, organizationally they are aligned to their own discipline. To promote interdisciplinary team collaboration, some rehabilitation models have endorsed organizational changes to include a program director responsible for organizational leadership of several disciplines. Babicki and Miller-McIntyre (1992) described such a rehabilitation program model.

Transdisciplinary Teams. As resources shrink and patient care demands grow, health care providers are looking for ways to accomplish goals efficiently without jeopardizing quality. Transdisciplinary teams maximize the strengths of team members and minimize duplication in effort (Figure 2-6). One member of the team is selected to be the primary therapist, depending on the specific patient needs (Diller, 1990), while the other team members contribute information and advice through that team member. Transdisciplinary teamwork involves a certain amount of boundary blurring between disciplines in that team members are cross-trained to accomplish duties and tasks that are usually discipline specific in situations when one team member can effectively accomplish the task, regardless of discipline. However, all standards of care and professional practice guidelines are observed as team members collaborate to effectively and efficiently implement the patient's plan of care. Determining the range of capability of various team members is essential, and team members must be receptive and learn to cope with a wider domain of functioning. Hoeman (1993) described a transdisciplinary team model for the care of infants with special needs.

Future of Teams in Rehabilitation. The future use of teams in rehabilitation must begin with a critical analysis of the strengths and weaknesses of this approach to care delivery.

Major strengths of teams are that they are well established, promote good communication and collaboration among disciplines, address comprehensive aspects of care, energizes staff, and view the patient holistically (Gibbon, 1999; Wagner, 2000). Weaknesses of the team approach may include increased cost, inefficiency, and reduction in time for direct patient care. Rothberg (1981) stated that the team approach places psychological strain on staff from having to deal with problems related to role diffusion, ambiguity, status concerns, interpersonal conflicts, lack of commitment of some team members, and concerns regarding competency. From an operational standpoint, coordinated, cooperative, goal-directed teamwork that includes the patient and family as integral members is often is difficult to achieve.

Although the comprehensive treatment team has been viewed as the foundation of rehabilitation, Schofield and Amodeo (1999) questioned whether the team approach will erode in the face of economic constraints and health care reform. Accounts of third-party payers opting for a limited number of specific services, rather than paying for comprehensive care, are becoming more common. Others have questioned the effectiveness of comprehensive treatment teams in rehabilitation, citing cost, inefficiency, and lack of research documenting the value of teams, advocating instead for the development of alternate treatment models, for example, making teams smaller, increasing consultations from other specialties, and even using rehabilitation technicians to address the shortage of health care professionals (Keith, 1991).

However, comprehensive specialized teams focusing on specific populations demonstrated improved outcomes. For example, a systematic review of the research on stroke-specific inpatient care indicates that stroke patients should receive "coordinated and organized" rehabilitation by multidisciplinary teams specializing in stroke care as soon as the patient is medically stable (Rodin, Saliba, & Brummel-Smith,

2006, p. 159). This approach to care has been found to improve mortality, functional status, and ability to live independent (Stroke Unit Trialists Collaboration, 2006), resulting in evidence-based practice guidelines and certification requirements from TJC, CARF, and the VA for stroke-specific rehabilitation. Another systematic review concluded rehabilitation for geriatric patients should be conducted by an interdisciplinary team (Wells, Seabrook, Stolee, Borrie, & Knoefel, 2003). The evidence from these systematic reviews would suggest that a comprehensive, specialized team approach for specific populations improves outcomes and may be the future of rehabilitation care.

SUMMARY

Models and theories from nursing and other relevant disciplines described in this chapter provide a theoretical basis for rehabilitation nursing care. The ICF (WHO integrated model), provides a way for all rehabilitation professionals to collaborate within one interdisciplinary, unified model. However, because this model is new, nurses and other rehabilitation professionals need to evaluate its usefulness for research and practice. Whichever models or theories underpin research and care delivery in particular settings, services need to be integrated, comprehensive, appropriate, and patient/family-centered, incorporating patient-defined goals. The expertise required of rehabilitation nurses in their multiple roles and diverse work settings with challenging and complex patient situations requires them to understand and know how to make effective use of models and theories relevant for rehabilitation.

CRITICAL THINKING

1. Compare and contrast the nurse's role within multidisciplinary, interdisciplinary, and transdisciplinary rehabilitation teams.
2. Describe several strategies that can facilitate active involvement of the patient and family in the rehabilitation program.
3. How might the ICF enhance the interprofessional working in a rehabilitation team?

REFERENCES

Albrecht, M. N. (1990). The Albrecht nursing model for home health care: Implications for research, practice, and education. *Public Health Nursing, 7*, 118-126.

Aliotta, S., & Andre, J. (1997). Case management and home healthcare: An integrated model. *Home Healthcare Management & Practice, 9*(2), 1-2.

Anderson, K. H. (2000). The family health system approach to family systems nursing. *Journal of Family Nursing, 6*(2), 103-117.

Antonovsky, A. (1979). *Health, stress, and coping.* San Francisco: Jossey-Bass.

Antonovsky, A. (1996). The salutogenic models as a theory to guide health promotion. *Health Promotion International, 11*(1), 11-18.

Babicki, C., & Miller-McIntyre, K. (1992). A rehabilitation programmatic model: The clinical nurse specialist perspective. *Rehabilitation Nursing, 17*, 84-86.

Bandura, A. (1977). *Social learning theory.* Englewood Cliffs, NJ: Prentice-Hall.

Bandura, A. (1986). *Social foundations of thought and action: Social cognitive theory.* Englewood Cliffs, NJ: Prentice-Hall.

Barnes, C. (2003). Rehabilitation for disabled people: A 'sick' joke? *Scandinavian Journal of Disability Research, 5*(1), 7-24.

Becker, M. H. (Ed.). (1974). *The health belief model and personal health behavior.* Thorofare, NJL Slack.

Biley, F. C. (1996). Rogerian science, phantoms, and therapeutic touch: Exploring potentials. *Nursing Science Quarterly, 9*(4), 165-169.

Bornman, J. (2004). The World Health Organisation's terminology and classification: Application to severe disability. *Disability and Rehabilitation, 26*(3), 182-188.

Bowen, M. (1966). The use of family therapy in clinical practice. *Comprehensive Psychiatry, 7*, 345-374.

Burks, K. (1999). A nursing practice model for chronic illness. *Rehabilitation Nursing, 24*(5), 197-200.

Charmaz, K. (1991). *Good days, bad days: The self in chronic illness and time.* New Brunswick, NJ: Rutgers University Press.

Chumbler, N. R., Mann, W. C., Wu, S., Schmid, A., & Kobb, R. (2004). The association of home-telehealth use and care coordination with improvement of functional and cognitive functioning in frail elderly men. *Telemedicine Journal and E-Health, 10*(2), 129-137.

Coile, R. C., & Matthews, P. (1999). Nursing case management in the millennium: Two perspectives. *Nursing Case Management, 4*(6), 244-254.

Commission on Accreditation of Rehabilitation Facilities. (n.d.). *Medical Rehabilitation program descriptions.* Retrieved May 28, 2006, from http://www.carf.org/Providers.aspx?content=content/Accreditation/Opportunities/MED/What.htm.

Conger, M., & Craig, C. (1998). Advanced nurse practice: A model for collaboration. *Nursing Case Management, 3*(3), 120-127.

Corbin, J. M., & Strauss, A. (1992). A nursing model for chronic illness management based on the trajectory framework. In P. Woog (Ed.), *The chronic illness trajectory framework: The Corbin and Strauss nursing model* (pp. 9-28). New York: Springer.

Cudney, S. A., & Weinert, C. (2000). Computer-based support groups: Nursing in cyberspace. *Computers in Nursing, 18*(1), 35-43.

Davis, S., & O'Connor, S. (Eds.). (1999). *Rehabilitation nursing: Foundations for practice.* London: Harcourt Brace.

Dean, B. Z., & Geiringer, S. R. (1990). Physiatric therapeutics. The rehabilitation team: Behavioral management Part 6. *Archives of Physical Medicine and Rehabilitation, 71*(Suppl. 4), 275-277.

DeJong, G. (1979). Independent living: From social movement to analytic paradigm. *Archives of Physical Medicine and Rehabilitation, 60*, 435-446.

Dembo, T. (1969). Rehabilitation psychology and its immediate future: A problem of utilization of psychological knowledge. *Rehabilitation Psychology 16*, 63-72.

Diller, L. (1990). Fostering the interdisciplinary team: Fostering research in a society in transition. *Archives of Physical Medicine and Rehabilitation, 71*, 275-278.

Dunn, H. L. (1959). High level wellness for man and society. *American Journal of Public Health, 49*, 786-792.

Ebrahim, S. (1995). Clinical and public health perspectives and applications of health-related quality of life measurement. *Social Science and Medicine, 41*(10), 1383-1394.

Edwards, P. A. (Ed.). (2000). *The specialty practice of rehabilitation nursing: A core curriculum* (4th ed.). Glenview, IL: Association of Rehabilitation Nurses.

Erbst, R. M. (1984). Defining health: A multidimensional model. *Journal of School Health, 54*(3), 99-104.

Fjaertoft, H., Indredavik, B., Johnsen, R., & Lydersen, S. (2004). Acute stroke unit care combined with early supported discharge: Long-term effects on quality of life—A randomized controlled trial. *Clinical Rehabilitation 18*, 580-586.

Fjaertoft, H., Indredavik, B., & Lydersen, S. (2003). Stroke unit care combined with early supported discharge: Long-term follow-up of a randomized controlled trail. *Stroke 34*, 2687-2692.

Friedemann, M. L. (1995). *The framework of systemic organization: A conceptual approach to practice and research with families and family members.* Thousand Oaks, CA: Sage.

Gagliardi, B. A. (2003). The experience of sexuality for individuals living with multiple sclerosis. *Journal of Clinical Nursing, 12*(4), 571-578.

Gagliardi, B. A., Frederickson, K., & Shanley, D. A. (2002). Living with multiple sclerosis: A Roy adaptation model-based study. *Nursing Science Quarterly, 15*(3), 230-236.

Galea, M., Tumminia, J., & Garback, L. M. (2006). Telerehabilitation in spinal cord injury persons: A novel approach. *Telemedicine Journal and E-Health, 12*(2), 160-162.

Garrett, R., & Shapcott, N. (1998, November 26). *Applications of videoconferencing in rehabilitation.* Presented at the First South Australian Seminar on Technology for People With Disabilities (ARATA).

Geddes, J., & Chamberlain, M. A. (2003). Stroke community rehabilitation: A classification of four different types of services. *International Journal of Therapy and Rehabilitation (10)*7, 299-304.

Gerteis, M., Edgman-Levitan, S., Daley, J., & Delbanco, T. (Eds.). (1993). *Through the patient's eyes.* San Francisco: Jossey-Bass Publisher.

Gibbon, B. (1999). An investigation of interprofessional collaboration in stroke rehabilitation team conferences. *Journal of Clinical Nursing, 8*(3), 246-252.

Goffman, E. (1963). *Stigma: Notes on the management of spoiled identity.* New York: Simon & Schuster.

Gordon, M. (2000). *Manual of nursing diagnosis* (9th ed.). St. Louis, MO: Mosby.

Hahn, H. (1993). The political implications of disability definitions and data. *Journal of Disability Policy Studies, 4*(2), 41-51.

Heerkens, Y., van der Brug, Y., Napel, H. T., & van Ravensberg, D. (2003). Past and future use of the ICF (former ICIDH) by nursing and allied health professionals. *Disability and Rehabilitation, 25*(11-12), 620-627.

Herdtner, S. (2000). Using therapeutic touch in nursing practice. *Orthopedic Nursing, 19*(5), 77-82.

Hoeman, S. (1993). A research-based transdisciplinary team model for infants with special needs and their families. *Holistic Nursing Practice, 7,* 63-72.

Hoeman, S. P. (1996). Conceptual basis for rehabilitation nursing. In S. P. Hoeman (Ed.), *Rehabilitation nursing: Process and applications* (2nd ed., pp. 3-20). St. Louis, MO: Mosby.

Hurst, R. (2003). The international disability rights movement and the ICF. *Disability and Rehabilitation, 25*(11-12), 572-576.

Jette, A. M. (1994). Physical disablement concepts for physical therapy research and practice. *Physical Therapy, 74*(5), 380-386.

Jette, A. M., & Keysor, J. J. (2003). Disability models: Implications for arthritis exercise and physical activity interventions. *Arthritis and Rheumatology, 49*(1), 114-120.

Joint Commission on Accreditation of Healthcare Organizations & American Stroke Association. (2005). *The Joint Commission Certificate of Distinction for Primary Stroke Centers.* Retrieved June 8, 2006, from http://www.jointcommission.org/NR/rdonlyres/D795E85D-DE78-4A9F-A070-0E8ECE0DE3D8/0/Mktg_PStroke_brochure.pdf.

Jonsdottir, H. (1999). Outcomes of implementing primary nursing in the care of people with chronic lung diseases: The nurses' experience. *Journal of Nursing Management, 7*(4), 235-242.

Kearney, P. M., & Pryor, J. (2004). The International Classification of Functioning, Disability and Health (ICF) and nursing. *Journal of Advanced Nursing, 46*(2), 162-170.

Keith, R. A. (1991). The comprehensive treatment team in rehabilitation. *Archives of Physical Medicine and Rehabilitation, 72,* 269-274.

King, I. M. (1981). *A theory for nursing: Systems, concepts, process.* Albany, NY: Delmar Publishers.

Lavallee, D. J., & Crupi, C. D. (1992). Rehabilitation takes to the road. *Holistic Nursing Practice, 6,* 60-66.

Lazarus, R. S., & Folkman, S. (1984). *Stress, appraisal, and coping.* New York: Springer.

Leavell, H. R., & Clark, E. G. (Eds.). (1965). *Preventive medicine for the doctor in his community* (3rd ed.). New York: McGraw-Hill.

Leininger, M. (Ed.) (1976). *Health care dimensions (Vol. 3): Transcultural health care issues and conditions.* Philadelphia: F. A. Davis.

Levine, K. (1996). Internet update. *OT Update, 1*(18), 14-15.

Lewin, K. (1947). Frontiers in group dynamics: Concepts, methods, and reality in social sciences. *Human Relations, 1,* 5-41.

Lippitt, R., Watson, J., & Westley, B. (1958). *The dynamics of planned change.* New York: Harcourt, Brace, & World.

Lubkin, I. M. (1995). *Chronic illness: Impact and interventions* (3rd ed.). Boston: Jones and Bartlett.

Lutz, B. J., & Bowers, B. J. (2000). Patient-centered care: Understanding its interpretation and implementation in health care. *Scholarly Inquiry for Nursing Practice 14*(2), 165-183.

Lutz, B. J., & Bowers, B. J. (2003). Understanding how disability is defined and conceptualized in the literature. *Rehabilitation Nursing, 28*(2), 74-78.

Mayo, N. E., Wood-Dauphinee, S., & Cote, R. (2000). Prompt hospital discharge and home rehab is more beneficial for stroke patients. *Geriatrics, 55*(8), 60-61.

Minaire, P. (1992). Disease, illness and health: Theoretical models of the disablement process. *Bulletin of the World Health Organization, 70*(3), 373-379.

Minuchin, S. (1974). *Families and family therapy.* Cambridge, MA: Harvard University Press.

Moffa-Trotter, M. E., & Anemaet, W. K. (1999). Cost effectiveness of home rehabilitation: A literature review. *Topics in Geriatric Rehabilitation, 14*(4), 1-33.

Mumma, C. (2000). *Lecture notes on theory based practice.* Anchorage, AK: University of Alaska.

Mumma, C. M., & Nelson, A. (2002). Theory and practice models for rehabilitation nursing. In S. P. Hoeman (Ed.), *Rehabilitation nursing: Process, applications, and outcomes* (3rd ed., pp. 20-36). St. Louis, MO: Mosby.

Nagi, S. Z. (1965). Some conceptual issues in disability and rehabilitation. In M. B. Sussman (Ed.), *Sociology and rehabilitation* (pp. 100-113). Washington, DC: American Sociological Association.

Nagi, S. Z. (1991). Disability concepts revisited: Implications for prevention. In A. M. Pope & A. R. Tarlov (Eds.), *Disability in America: Toward a national agenda for prevention* (pp. 309-327). Washington, DC: National Academy Press.

National Institute on Disability and Rehabilitation Research. (2005). Retrieved 2006, from http://www.ed.gov/osers/nidrr.

National Center for Health Statistics. (2005). *Health, United States, 2005 with chartbook on trends in the health of Americans.* U.S. Department of Health and Human Services (No. 2005-1232). Washington, DC: U.S. Government Printing Office.

National Rehabilitation Information Center. (n.d.). *NIDRR project database.* Retrieved May 28, 2006, from http://www.naric.com/research/.

Naylor, M. D., Brooten, D., Campbell, R., Jacobsen, B. S., Mezey, M. D., Pauly, M. V., et al. (1999). Comprehensive discharge planning and home follow-up of hospitalized elders: A randomized clinical trial. *Journal of the American Medical Association (JAMA), 281*(7), 613-620.

Neal, L. (1998). The Neal model of home health nursing practice. In L. J. Neal (Ed.), *Rehabilitation nursing in the home health setting* (pp. 263-279). Glenview, IL: Association of Rehabilitation Nurses.

Neuman, B. (1989). *The Neuman Systems Model* (2nd ed.). East Norwalk, CT: Appleton & Lange.

Neuman, B. (1995). *The Neuman systems model* (3rd ed.). Norwalk, CT: Appleton & Lange.

Newman, M. A. (1986). *Health as expanding consciousness.* St. Louis, MO: Mosby.

Norrefalk, J. R. (2003). How do we define multidisciplinary rehabilitation? *Journal of Rehabilitation Medicine, 35*(2), 100-101.

Ogonowski, J., Kronk, R., Rice, C., & Feldman, H. (2004). Inter-rater reliability in assigning ICF codes to children with disabilities. *Disability and Rehabilitation, 26*(6), 353-361.

Orem, D. (1971). *Nursing: Concepts of practice.* New York: McGraw-Hill.

Orem, D. (2001). *Nursing: Concepts of practice* (6th ed.). St. Louis, MO: Mosby.

Parse, R. R. (1981). *Man-living-health: A theory of nursing.* New York: Wiley.

Parsons, T. (1951). *The social system.* Glencoe, IL: The Free Press.

Phipps, M. (1990). Rehabilitation nursing specialist practice in an acute care setting. *Nursing Administration Quarterly 14,* 12-16.

Pierce, L. L., Steiner, V., Govoni, A. L., Hicks, B., Thompson, T. L. C., & Friedemann, M. L. (2004). Internet-based support for rural caregivers of persons with stroke shows promise. *Rehabilitation Nursing, 29*(3), 95-99, 103.

Pope, A. M., & Tarlov, A. R. (Eds.). (1991). *Disability in America: Toward a national agenda for prevention.* Washington, DC: National Academy Press.

Quigley, P. (2000). Environment of care and service delivery. In P. A. Edwards (Ed.), *The specialty practice of rehabilitation nursing: A core curriculum* (4th ed., pp. 342-349). Glenview, IL: Rehabilitation Nursing Foundation.

Rentsch, H. P., Bucher, P., Nyffeler, I. D., Wolf, C., Hefti, H., Fluri, E., et al. (2003). The implementation of the 'International Classification of Functioning, Disability and Health' (ICF) in daily practice of neurorehabilitation: An interdisciplinary project at the Kantonsspital of Lucerne, Switzerland. *Disability and Rehabilitation, 25*(8), 411-421.

Resnick, B. (1999). Reliability and validity testing of the Self-Efficacy for Functional Activities Scale. *Journal of Nursing Measurement, 7*(1), 5-20.

Resnick, B. (2002). Geriatric rehabilitation: The influence of efficacy beliefs and motivation. *Rehabilitation Nursing, 27*(4), 152-159.

Resnick, B., Magaziner, J., Orwig, D., & Zimmerman, S. (2002). Evaluating the components of the Exercise Plus Program: Rationale, theory, and implementation. *Health Education Research, 17*(5), 648-658.

Resnick, B., Simpson, M., Bercovitz, A., Galik, E., Gruber-Baldini, A., Zimmerman, S., et al. (2006). Related articles, links, and pilot testing of the Restorative Care Intervention: Impact on residents. *Journal of Gerontological Nursing, 32*(3), 39-47.

Reynolds, C. L., & Leininger, M. M. (1993). *Madeleine Leininger: Cultural care diversity and universality theory.* Newbury Park, CA: Sage.

Rice, R. (1994). Procedures in home care conceptual framework for nursing practice in the home: The Rice model for dynamic self-examination. *Home Healthcare Nurse, 12*(2), 51-53.

Rodin, M, Saliba, D., & Brummel-Smith, K. (2006). Guidelines abstracted from the Department of Veterans Affairs/Department of Defense Clinical Practice Guideline for the management of stroke rehabilitation. *Journal of the American Geriatrics Society 54*, 158-162.

Rogers, M. E. (1990). Nursing: Science of unitary, irreducible human beings: Update 1990. In E. Barrett (Ed.), *Patterns of nursing theories in practice* (pp. 83-92). New York: National League for Nursing.

Roper, N., Logan, W., & Tierney, A. (1996). *The elements of nursing: A model for nursing based on a model of living* (4th ed.). Edinburgh: Churchill-Livingstone.

Rothberg, J. (1981). The rehabilitation team: Future directions. *Archives of Physical Medicine and Rehabilitation, 62*, 407-410.

Roy, C., Sr., & Andrews, H. A. (1991). *The Roy adaptation model: The definitive statement.* Norwalk, CT: Appleton & Lange.

Roy, C., Sr., & Andrews, H. A. (1999). *The Roy adaptation model: The definitive statement* (2nd ed.). Stamford, CT: Appleton & Lange.

Safilios-Rothschild, C. (1970). *The sociology and social psychology of disability and rehabilitation.* New York: Random House.

Sallis, J. F., & Owen, N. (2002). Ecological models of health behavior. In K. Glanz, B. K. Rimmer, & F. M. Lewis (Eds.), *Health behavior and health education: Theory, research, and practice* (3rd ed.) (pp. 462-484). San Francisco: Jossey-Bass.

Satir, V. (1967). *Conjoint family therapy.* Palo Alto, CA: Science & Behavior Books.

Schoenhofer, S. O. (1995). Rethinking primary care: Connections to nursing. *Advances in Nursing Science, 17*(4), 12-21.

Schofield, R. F., & Amodeo, M. (1999). Interdisciplinary teams in health care and human services settings: Are they effective? *Health and Social Work, 24*(3), 210-219.

Selye, H. (1978). *The stress of life.* New York: McGraw-Hill.

Shyu, Y. I., Liang, J., Lu, J. F., & Wu, C. C. (2004). Environmental barriers and mobility in Taiwan: Is the Roy adaptation model applicable? *Nursing Science Quarterly, 17*(2), 165-170.

Stroke Unit Trialists' Collaboration. (2006). Organized inpatient (stroke unit) care for stroke. *Cochrane Library, 2006*(1).

Swain, J., Finkelstein, V., French, S., & Oliver, M. (Eds.). (1993). *Disabling barriers: Enabling environments.* London: Sage Publications.

Tsai, P. F., Tak, S., Moore, C., & Palencia, I. (2003). Testing a theory of chronic pain. *Journal of Advanced Nursing, 43*(2), 158-169.

Turner, J. G., Clark, A. J., Gauthier, D. K., & Williams, M. (1998). The effect of therapeutic touch on pain and anxiety in burn patients. *Journal of Advanced Nursing, 28*(1), 10-20.

Union of the Physically Impaired Against Segregation. (1976). *Fundamental principles of disability.* London: Author.

Verbrugge, L. M., & Jette, A. M. (1994). The disablement process. *Social Science and Medicine, 38*(1), 1-14.

Wade, D. T., & Halligan, P. (2003). New wine in old bottles: The WHO ICF as an explanatory model of human behaviour. *Clinical Rehabilitation, 17*(4), 349-354.

Wagner, E. (2000). The role of patient care teams in chronic illness management. *British Medical Journal, 320*(7234), 569-572.

Wells, J. L., Seabrook, J. A., Stolee, P., Borrie, M. J., & Knoefel, F. (2003). State of the art in geriatric rehabilitation. Part I: Review of frailty and comprehensive geriatric assessment. *Archives of Physical Medicine and Rehabilitation, 84*, 890-897.

Whiteneck, G. G. (1994). Measuring what matters: Key rehabilitation outcomes. *Archives of Physical Medicine and Rehabilitation, 75*, 1073-1076.

World Health Organization. (1980). *International classification of impairments, disabilities, and handicaps.* Geneva, Switzerland: Author.

World Health Organization. (2001). *ICF: International classification of functioning, disability, and health.* Geneva, Switzerland: Author.

Wright, B. (1960). *Physical disability: A psychological approach.* New York: Harper & Row.

Wright, B. (1980). Developing constructive views of life with a disability. *Rehabilitation Literature, 41*(11-12), 273-279.

3

Ethical and Legal Issues in Rehabilitation Nursing

Shirley P. Hoeman, PhD, MPH, RN, CS
Pamela M. Duchene, DNSc, RN, CRRN
Lewis Vierling, JD

Ethics involves the study of morals (Online Ethics Center for Engineering and Science, 2005) and moral evaluation, distinguishing right from wrong, beneficial from harmful, and virtuous from vicious. Ethics evolves from beliefs and values and thus has religious and cultural bases. Ethical behavior requires moral reasoning, problem solving, and decision making; in research studies ethics includes informed consent and analysis of risk benefits. Professional codes or standards, such as the American Nurses Association (ANA) *Code of Ethics for Nurses With Interpretive Statements* (ANA, 2001), guide expected ethical behavior for nurses. The Association of Rehabilitation Nurses (2003) supports the ANA Code of Ethics and adds specific ethical expectations for rehabilitation nurses. Ethical issues or *dilemmas* result when *answers are not evident* in the codes or expectations.

FOUNDATIONS OF ETHICS

Hippocrates recognized the need for ethics when he created the first code, the Hippocratic Oath (Dupont, 2005), in which he set the foundation for concepts of nonmaleficence, beneficence, veracity, and the sanctity of life. Nightingale's writings and practice emphasized advocacy and privacy (Hunt, 2001). Although Hippocrates' and Nightingale's basic ethical tenets have been endorsed in nursing practices throughout decades, they could not have envisioned the ethical dilemmas today resulting from advances in science, technology, and genetics. For example, a 90-year-old man was admitted to an acute care hospital. He lived independently, and his granddaughters were very involved in his care. He had not been feeling well, and the physician suspected diverticulitis. A work-up with computerized tomography revealed a large intestinal mass. Unfortunately, while he was hospitalized, he fell, developed pneumonia, and experienced delirium. The surgeons evaluated

him and thought that his only chance of survival was removal of the tumor, although they explained to the granddaughters that he might never be weaned from the ventilator. The granddaughters felt their grandfather would want to try surgery if there was a chance of his recovery. The surgeons operated, and the patient remained on the ventilator. At the end of a month, the granddaughters met with the health care team and requested that their grandfather be allowed to die in dignity and without the ventilator. The ventilator was disconnected, and the patient surprised all involved by breathing without support. He was transferred to a medical unit for recovery and, after almost 100 days of hospitalization, was admitted to rehabilitation for strengthening and a return to independence. The bill exceeds $200,000 and will continue to grow with the expense of rehabilitation, home health care, and outpatient therapy. The outcome is a happy one and certainly seems right for all concerned. Ethical dilemmas occurred throughout the case, beginning with the decision to do surgery although the status of the patient's pneumonia was known. Termination of ventilatory support was another ethical quandary. Admission to acute rehabilitation was also an ethical question—should the patient have gone to long-term care, skilled care, or acute rehabilitation? Hippocrates and Nightingale could not have imagined such questions.

Eckenhoff (1981) noted that rehabilitation developed to ease the uneasy situation created by advances in science. Because it is morally and ethically questionable to place a value on a life with a disability, rehabilitation provides a solution: achieving the biopsychosocial potential possible. In the illustration of the 90-year-old receiving extensive surgery, rehabilitation made return to independence conceivable. Scientific advances never come without a price. The costs of implementing new advances in efforts to save lives and to promote quality care are staggering; rehabilitation can be expensive. In the United States the direct cost of treating stroke, for example, exceeds 33 billion dollars; 41% is for acute hospital and rehabilitation expenses (Sharma et al., 2005).

Conversely, for every $1 spent on rehabilitative care, an estimated $11 are saved on long-term disability costs (Stoolman, 2005). The value of a productive life, or even a life with decreased burden on the health care system, outweighs the expense of acute, subacute, and outpatient rehabilitation. Although rehabilitation may provide added value, it cannot be assumed to be indispensable. The full impact of the Balanced Budget Act of 1997 and revised 75% rule that set limits on rehabilitation services provided to Medicare beneficiaries is yet to be determined. What is known is that there will be fewer individuals eligible for acute rehabilitation services and limitations on rehabilitation provided in subacute settings and home health care (Esselman, 2004).

Uncharted Waters

Increasingly, people are surviving formerly fatal conditions and are living longer lives due to medical advances and technological assistance. Society has never been without individuals afflicted by chronic illness or disability. Ways of managing such situations have varied, and although technology has advanced the ability to provide care, little has been done to decrease the burdens faced by caregivers. Funding for assistance, transportation, medical needs, and respite care is often unavailable or insufficient for caregivers, resulting in an ever escalating load of caregiver responsibilities. The ethical concerns with care persevere long after the acute episode has resolved.

Rehabilitation nurses need to have a clear understanding of their own values and a premise for logical, critical thinking because personal ethics often differ from patient beliefs, public rules, or professional codes. Compliance with regulations is complex when outcomes are uncertain and engender ethical debates. As an example, a 35-year-old patient recovering from a traumatic brain injury was admitted to an acute rehabilitation program. He was violent and verbally abusive to staff members and to family members. He demanded to leave the facility. A psychiatric consultation was completed, and although decision-making capacity was impaired, the psychiatrist could not state that the patient was incapable of making decisions. Guardianship could be sought but would take days. In the meantime, the patient demanded to leave, and the rehabilitation staff members were required to allow him to do so or be guilty of restraining him against his will. The family members pleaded with the staff to do something to keep him hospitalized, but all strategies were unsuccessful. Staff members explained to the family that if the patient was violent after leaving the facility, the police should be contacted and the patient could be arrested and taken to a mental health facility for an involuntary emergency admission. All of these actions were in compliance with legal regulations, yet a quandary existed for all involved. The patient had rights, which were not violated, yet the family and rehabilitation staff felt it would be

a greater good to complete rehabilitation. However, rehabilitation could not be completed without restraining the patient against his will.

SCOPE OF REHABILITATION CONCERNS

Throughout this book, rehabilitation and the specialty practice in nursing are shown as integral and essential across the levels of the health system. It follows that ethical principles emerge that are of concern to rehabilitation nursing regarding care throughout the health care continuum. Ethical principles in and of themselves cannot resolve many of the complexities, quandaries, and dilemmas found in the scope of rehabilitation. Values and expectations include ideas about what constitutes care. Examples are presented in the following section.

Levels of Intervention

Prevention is a key intervention level for rehabilitation nurses. For example, rehabilitation nurses spearheaded campaigns for prevention of spinal cord injury from diving accidents, for helmet laws to prevent head injury during bicycle and motorcycle accidents, and for education of elderly persons about home safety to prevent falls. Education programs such as the ThinkFirst National Injury Prevention Foundation have reached over 8 million young people (ThinkFirst, 2005). Such efforts are resulting in changes. However, encouraging people to alter unhealthy lifestyle choices and noncompliance (e.g., substance abuse or failure to monitor high blood pressure), all preventable, is more taxing for health care providers.

The case for prevention and intervention within rehabilitation nursing is clear in secondary level interventions. Calculate the cost and devastation that result when proper skin care, positioning, and nutrition are omitted in acute care. Interventions can prevent contractures, skin breakdown, and problems of immobility, as well as maximize functioning following total joint-replacement surgery, a cerebrovascular accident, or head injury. Rehabilitation nursing interventions have improved outcomes in specialty areas, such as cardiac, renal, burn, and cancer rehabilitation, and improved length of stay and function in many settings.

Selection Criteria

Not all who become disabled or impaired have access to rehabilitation services. Many fail to consider rehabilitation because they or their provider have no understanding or experience in the specialty, and no one requests a referral. Others simply may not have confidence in rehabilitation outcomes, or they consider the person too old, severely disabled, or unmotivated. The ability to finance rehabilitation has become a screening mechanism in itself; the uninsured live outside the system, vulnerable, invisible, and marginal. Third-party reimbursement and criteria for coverage vary greatly, and now with the advent of prospective payment for rehabilitation and the enforcement of the updated 75% rule, access to acute rehabilitation is more restrictive than in prior times. A patient who might benefit from rehabilitation may not receive services because of changes in reimbursement or because programs are at capacity. Under the new regulations regarding the 75% rule, the number of admissions for acute rehabilitation declined by 34,000 the first year (American Hospital Association [AHA], 2005).

Those who do receive rehabilitation must continue to demonstrate their potential, meet the system requirements, and participate in the individually designed program. What truly is unique is the process the rehabilitation team uses, evaluating persons before selecting those who will be candidates for rehabilitation and the setting where they will receive services.

Rehabilitation is oriented strongly toward care, easily accomplished while expectations for cure remain low. Conflict and dissonance can occur when patients and family hold hope for cure while providers promote rehabilitative themes, challenging advocacy. Certain themes are inherent in a rehabilitation world view including self-care, maximum independence, potential for education or vocation, caregiver involvement, and participation in the plan for care, especially when setting goals. Rehabilitation requires involvement of the person served, while asserting that pushing just a little harder for independence today makes a difference in the level of function possible tomorrow.

THEORETICAL BASES FOR ETHICAL PRACTICE

Although individuals may have defined values and beliefs, an understanding of ethical theories and principles is necessary to understand the society in which we live and practice. Four ethical theories (Table 3-1) encompass principles important for rehabilitation nurses to understand in making decisions. Table 3-2 illustrates how ethical principles relate to situations encountered in rehabilitation nursing practice or sphere of concern. The theories and principles reflect centuries of thought and hypothesis. If one doubts that theories written more than 250 years ago can influence the way we think today, the works of Jeremy Bentham, founder of the utilitarian (happiness) theory, should be reviewed. Bentham (1748-1832), a nonpracticing attorney, campaigned for social reform by proposing that actions be evaluated against the yardstick of happiness. Actions that yielded the greatest happiness for the most people were the best actions (Hinman, 2004).

Access

Access is a multidimensional word; it functions as both a verb and a noun, with the noun having extended connotations. Thus we refer to access to facilities or structure, access to goods and services, and access to the World Wide Web, and then we debate the accessibility of the same for all individuals, regardless

TABLE 3-1 Ethical Theories for Practice

Theory	Description	Examples Within Rehabilitation Nursing
Ethics of divine commands	Religious moralities: Right and wrong defined through divine commands (e.g., the Bible).	Many nurses believe that they have a calling to practice nursing. As such, their practice will be in line with their religious beliefs concerning right and wrong.
Ethics of selfishness	Egoism: Individuals define what is the ethical right for them. This is acceptable as long as the ethical right for oneself does not interfere with the ethical right for another.	Rehabilitation nurses have a responsibility to complete patient education on the importance of pressure releases for position changes for the prevention of pressure ulcers. Patients choose whether to comply with the instructions. It is their right to choose, as long as the consequences of such actions (pressure ulcer) do not interfere with the rights of others (which could occur through preventable consumption of health care resources).
Ethics of duty and respect	Deontological theory: The science of "right." The theory specifies that there are definable principles of natural right associated with jurisprudence.	In rehabilitation nursing, the nurse has a responsibility to provide competent care in accordance with the nursing practice act. For example, it is right for nurses to administer medications and treatments in synchronization with physician orders. To violate this would be to fail the patient in delivery of nursing care and to violate the ethic of duty.
Ethics of consequences	Utilitarian theory: Stipulates that principles or actions can be proved to be good. The best principles or actions are those resulting in good feelings. Also known as the happiness theory.	Rehabilitation leads to increased independence. This is good as long as independence is known to be good. For example, for many years rehabilitation specialists encouraged individuals with significant disabilities to walk without considering energy-conservation principles. Is walking "good" if the individual expends an excessive amount of energy in walking?

From Hinman, L. (2002). *Ethics: A pluralistic approach to moral theory* (3rd ed.). Belmont, CA: Thomson-Wadsworth.

TABLE 3-2 Relationship of Ethical Principles to Situations Encountered in Rehabilitation Nursing Practice or Sphere of Concern

Ethical Principle	Description	Examples
Autonomy	An individual's actions are independent from the actions and the will of others. Individuals have the ability to form their own perspectives on right, wrong, and values.	Rehabilitation nurses must acknowledge that individuals for whom they care have freedom regarding their bodies and actions. Nurses may provide education on wellness and health promotion, but compliance with programs cannot be forced. Patients have autonomy in their health care programs.
Nonmaleficence	The concept of doing no harm.	Rehabilitation nurses, like all health care practitioners, have a duty to do no harm to a patient. To intentionally administer a lethal dose of medication to a patient is an example of violation of the ethical principle of nonmaleficence. It is unthinkable for a nurse to intentionally harm a patient.
Beneficence	The concept of doing good for another.	Nursing care is based on the concept of beneficence. Rehabilitation nurses intend to do good for others. The motivation that drives rehabilitation nurses to go the extra distance in care of their patients is an example of beneficence.
Advocacy	Loyalty: Championing the needs and interests of another.	Rehabilitation nurses are in an ideal position to advocate for their patients. Nurses often see patients on a 24-hour basis and have an awareness for and appreciation of patient's abilities and energy levels that other disciplines may not. It is critical that such information be shared with team members in a way to advocate for the best plan for patients.
Veracity	Responsibility to speak the truth.	Nurses have an obligation to speak truthfully in all aspects of their role.
Financial responsibility (cost-benefit analysis)	Stewardship: Ensuring that there is sufficient benefit for the expense provided.	There is an ethical responsibility to meet the patient's needs as well as possible while using as few resources as possible. For example, extending lengths of stay in hospitals, home health care, and subacute programs, when a patient is capable of being discharged to a lesser level of care, is not in line with the nurse's financial responsibility for care.
Care	Providing for and meeting the needs of others for compassion, empathy, and good.	Care is a component of the rehabilitation nurse's role, regardless of the setting.
Sanctity of life	Value of life, right to life.	Rehabilitation nurses have an obligation to care for all patients, regardless of the extent of disability or potential for recovery, because all life is of value.
Quality of life	Condition of one's life, based on assessment of correlation between life and participation in valued activities and interests.	Quality of life is a frequent question for individuals with devastating disabilities and chronic illnesses. Rehabilitation nurses can assist individuals and families in reframing situations to find quality of life in remaining abilities.
Consent	Voluntary agreement with a procedure, process, or treatment.	The role of the rehabilitation nurse in informed consent is key. Because patients often confide in nurses, the rehabilitation nurse is in a position to validate understanding of a procedure, treatment, or course of therapy. As an advocate, the rehabilitation nurse supports the patients' abilities to make decisions and participate in their plans of care.
Confidentiality	Responsibility to keep information private.	Rehabilitation nurses are entrusted with substantial amounts of private information. Such information must be kept confidential, to be shared only as related to the nursing care and needs of the patient.
Competence	The ability or legal right to make appropriate decisions.	The need for rehabilitation sometimes follows a disability or illness that affects the clarity the patient's decision-making ability. This should not be confused with legal competence.
Values	Worthwhile or positive qualities held by an object or outcome. These should be chosen carefully but freely.	The question of the value of a life after a disability or chronic illness is sometimes placed in question. Rehabilitation nurses recognize the value of independence and of reframing prior values to achieve higher levels of life satisfaction.

From Ursery, D. (2005). *Principles of normative ethics.* Austin, TX: St. Edwards University.

of functional status. The idea of access has become associated with the ability to obtain a goal or a right.

Persons with chronic, disabling conditions have made gains in the social construction of what "ought to" constitute proper accesses for them. The Americans With Disabilities Act (ADA) and inclusion of children in education (discussed later in this chapter), and the patient Bill of Rights Act of 1998 are examples of access-promoting legislation. *Healthy People 2010* lists priority areas for reducing disparities in access to health goods and services (U.S. Department of Health and Human Services, 2000). *Healthy People 2010* targets access as a national priority, based on the evidence that strong predictors for quality health care are access to health insurance, access to a regular primary care provider, and decreased financial, structural, and personal barriers to care.

Mass media regularly feature positive images of people with disabilities and highlight Special Olympics games. Certainly the open discussions of their chronic, disabling conditions by prominent individuals such as Christopher Reeve (spinal cord injury), Michael J. Fox (Parkinson's disease), and Annette Funicello (multiple sclerosis) have dented the wall of silence and invisibility. Options, such as assisted living homes or group caregiver living arrangements, have served some needs. Activists for disability rights would argue that access to "homes" is not needed as much as access to "their own homes." Figure 3-1 features a campaign poster for accessible housing within one's own home, rather than institutional types of housing.

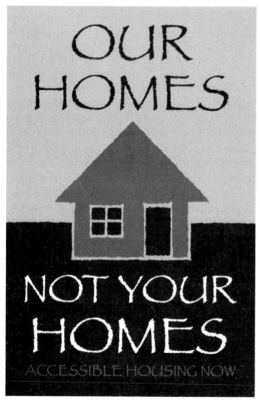

Figure 3-1 (Courtesy The Nth Degree, Luckey, OH.)

At all levels of care and stages of life diminishing funds, services, manpower, and durable goods supplies compete with escalating needs and demands. Early intervention programs for infants have no openings. Young adults with disabilities have few choices for community and independent living and sparse attendant care. Restricted benefits and reduced services, coupled with strict criteria for assistance in the home, limit older persons attempting to maintain their independent living. Inaccessibility reduces visibility, as with the example of voting. Of the 33.7 million disabled adults eligible to vote, 10% are less likely to register and 20% less apt to vote than able-bodied voters; furthermore, the voting areas and booths in more than 20,000 polling sites are inaccessible for persons with disabilities (Schriner & Ochs, 2000). Table 3-2 illustrates more about ethical theories applied to practice.

Family Responsibilities. As families have more responsibility to care for their members, the stress and burden on caregivers rises. Despite love and dedication, caregiving is a difficult, exhausting, and isolating role (Tsai, 2003). (See details in Chapter 22.) The Family and Medical Leave Act, company benefits with elder care programs, and lenient family care leave policies for workers are helpful, but more government-funded programs will not be the answer. At some point programs and bureaucracies break down, they set limits and restrictions for care, and they take away individual rights because they give according to their own rules. Many states are seeking waivers from the federal government to allow significant changes in Medicaid that would limit access to care and increase the load on family members. Examples of state actions are to restrict medical treatment to the least costly, but clinically effective option available; a limited funds approach where beneficiaries can determine how they will spend the dollars available to them; and requiring family members (regardless of the state or location of residence) to pay for long-term and postacute care (Rowland, 2005).

Ultimately, the community has the foremost role and responsibility for rehabilitation of its members. Ethically, efforts to remove barriers and obstacles must be purposeful to the targeted population. Family and patient access to the community is a key, whether through churches, voluntary organizations, specialty associations, support groups, or others.

Advocacy

Advocacy is an acknowledged role for rehabilitation nurses. A nurse advocate can and has made enormous differences in outcomes for patients with chronic, disabling disorders. Rehabilitation nurses educate patients and families to ensure that they know their rights, are fully informed and able to consent, and gain all benefits they are entitled to for their needs.

Advocacy is a role that attempts to clarify the situation and broker the gap that may exist between ethics and the law. Patients in rehabilitation typically have complex, multidimensional, and lengthy problems. It is essential to clarify whether the problem involves ethics, regulations, or other factors before moving to advocate. Unnecessary dilemmas and complications may be avoided by identifying the exact problem. Ethics are of broader scope than laws, but standards of practice and licensure are legal processes. Other advocacy actions important to the rehabilitation nurse are assisting patients in clarifying their values, resolving conflicts, solving problems effectively, and making decisions that leave them with satisfaction as well as quality of life.

Clarifying Values. Values are rooted in a person's culture, family, and beliefs and are moderated by experiences. Actions reflect values, but individuals are not always aware of the connections, especially when under duress from competing values. Identifying and clarifying values is a sequential process that involves a person's freely choosing from alternatives, willingly accepting the choice, and acting (Edge & Groves, 2005).

Kohlberg's theory of moral development (Burkhart & Nathaniel, 2002) has three levels of development. Level I, or preconventional level, is when rules are recognized and obeyed out of fear of punishment, such as levying significant fines for traffic violations. This is a primarily egocentric level philosophy that a fear of fines will cause individuals to obey the rules. Level II, or conventional level, is when people desire good relationships. Moral reasoning is employed, and there is a sense that duty and respect are important. For example, an individual is not fined or punished for "pushing the limit" on an organization's dress code—however, it is a sign of disrespect for the organization, and in some instances the individual may be asked to change or leave the premises. This differs from failure of duty by neglecting to wash the hands between patient contacts. Level III is postconventional and principled. Individuals are able to assess the relativity of social values and exercise moral decision making based on principles, internalized rules, and conscience. Decisions are based on impartial universal moral principles, even when the outcome may conflict with societal standards. An example of the Level III concept would be to choose the generic medication over a brand medication to conserve expense—even though the insurance company might pay for the more expensive drug. Through choosing a low-cost option, the individual shows an awareness of an impartial universal moral principle of stewardship of resources.

Autonomy

One ethical value proffered in rehabilitation is autonomy for the patient. Persons with chronic, disabling conditions often must deal with the health care system for extended periods. Invasive, intensive, highly technological treatments may or may not be a patient's choice. Regardless, if cures and treatments fail, they may be forced into a model of care. If obtaining needed care is one concern, finding life satisfaction in daily living is another. Consider how difficult it is for a patient to achieve intimacy in relationships apart from clinical discussions, shared rooms, and caregiver scrutiny or how important it is to be included, not just mainstreamed, into schools. Consider the difficulty of living in managed housing or group homes with strangers, or being segregated in residential areas,

or to be without transportation. Ethical dilemmas about a patient's autonomy are predictable when a nurse serves as advocate, as well as regulator or keeper of the system.

Patient-centered, rather than system-driven, advocacy might include ensuring a patient's right to autonomy in refusing a treatment, or offering assertiveness training to patients who must deal with the system, or ensuring that patients are involved in their care plan and rehabilitation processes. Nurses are attuned to issues of confidentiality, anonymity, fully informed consent, and prevention of all aspects or threats of abuse and neglect. Likewise, they are exposed to applications of the Omnibus Budget Reconciliation Act (OBRA) Self-Determination Act of 1990, including advance directives, physical and chemical restraint policies, or guardianship and durable power of attorney issues. Many of these are compounded when a patient is not able to function with autonomy or when decision making is impaired.

Life Satisfaction and Quality. Perhaps life satisfaction and quality of life issues arise from within the varying belief systems and world views of individuals. Safeguarding cultural or religious beliefs is an increasingly important advocacy action. Rehabilitation is complicated by competing values, ethical dilemmas, cultural experiences, health problem expression, and the conventional medical system. These are difficult issues for the most dedicated advocate.

When catastrophic or progressive conditions occur, gathering information about a patient's wishes, desires, and beliefs may become an ethical assessment. It may follow that a person's behaviors in life and stated beliefs or values are expressions or inferences of their intended meaning and thus become useful in making choices when the person cannot do so. In addition to the cultural assessment (see Chapter 6) and the steps in clarifying values, an advocate learns the patient's wishes about personal suffering or use of technology and medical interventions. Patients may talk about what constitutes quality and satisfaction in their lives and express opinions about decisions and who else should make them. They will have differing perceptions about how their conditions place economic, emotional, or physical burdens on others. For example, some older adults invest in long-term care insurance to avoid placing their care needs on their children—often without involving their children in the decision.

Power in Relationships. Attaining and maintaining a therapeutic relationship grounded in trust is important for patients and nurses. Honesty, active listening, cooperation, and shared responsibility for decisions and outcomes are effective actions in relationship building. One of the tripping stones in a relationship is power, especially when unevenly distributed. Nurses are well acquainted with roles that offer responsibility without sufficient authority and uneven power in team settings. The medical model maintains a dominant role in the social construction of disability; that is, medical diagnoses determine by definition who has what problem, whether something is to be done about it, how much will be done, by whom, and for what expense.

However, power imbalance in the patient-provider relationship is extensive and symbiotic. Without persons with chronic or disabling disorders, there would be no need for rehabilitation, providers, equipment manufacturers, or all of the others who interface with patients and families. As it stands, patients or their payment sources reimburse rehabilitation providers who are expected to attend educational conferences, obtain funding to conduct research, or provide patient care in clinics and centers. Providers have social prestige and good incomes. Patients spend time and money in hope of improving their condition, although many times they are not fully included in the decision-making process regarding their case. In spite of this, however, most find time to thank their providers—even though they may not have agreed with or understood the approach taken by the provider regarding their care (Tan, 2002).

Changes in Practice Environment. Decisions about care of the patient have always been a chief concern of nurses. For rehabilitation nurses the implications are serious. Twenty years ago autonomy in rehabilitation meant giving patients and their families sufficient time and alternatives so they could deal with treatment decisions, such as stopping services due to a patient's a lack of progress or lack of physical or cognitive function. The team made decisions, and ideally the process involved the patient or the family (Caplan, Callahan, & Haas, 1987). Today, although the patient may be closely involved in the rehabilitation process, the length and intensity of treatment is dictated by the setting and by progress made. Twenty years ago individuals who were possible candidates for rehabilitation could be given a "brief" 10-day trial of acute rehabilitation; today the average length of stay for acute rehabilitation is 16 days or less.

Rehabilitation nurses must learn to consider the context of the social system (i.e., the political, legal, economic, educational, and microhealth situation) in understanding ethical situations, defining true dilemmas, and making judgments or decisions. In an environment constrained by business ventures, managed care may become incompatible with autonomy and advocacy roles of nurses. Conflicted values about offering optimal levels of care as opposed to efficiency or cost measures quickly erode a therapeutic relationship.

VALUE OF THE PERSON

Few employees missed the 1980 to 1990 management mantra of the "paradigm shift." Whether the shift meant moving into the new economy, postmodernism, or another realm, most agree that some things once believed to be permanently in place did, indeed, shift. However, when proposed legislation shifts health care providers away from the original tenet of "do no harm," it may constitute a landslide. Concerns about risk versus benefits of a treatment or conflicts between conventional or alternative health practices became overshadowed in comparison. Managed care shifts led to conflicts among members of the team as the need to "do more with less" called principles into question for some, but not all, team members.

Self-determination, once deemed important for informed consent, is subject to legislative dictates that stretch the ethical principle taut.

Self-determination legally permits patients to refuse unwanted treatment or to have full disclosure and information before consent. Suicide is not illegal. However, movement toward legislation that targets persons for approaches to suicide (legal ones) on the basis of their health status, age, or other attributes refutes the ethical principles upon which self-determination was based. As of this writing, euthanasia and assisted suicide are legal in Oregon, the Netherlands, Switzerland, and Belgium (Canadian Broadcasting Corporation, 2004).

If social values dictate beliefs about self-determination and life satisfaction, persons with chronic, disabling disorders are at risk for socially promoted suicide even if they are not terminally ill. Consider the Danish arguments for the legislation of voluntary euthanasia (Hartling, 2006). Patients who feel they are a burden on their family may perceive euthanasia as a way out of the situation. The notion of dying as a life stage and a process is lost as they reject nursing hospice and palliative care programs in favor of aids to rapid death. Eventually, resources used for pain management, palliative care, family cohesiveness, and other support are open to challenge and they may no longer be justified.

Not Dead Yet is a grassroots national disability rights group formed in 1996 to oppose legal motions for assisted suicide and euthanasia. They hold that movements supporting assisted suicide and euthanasia actually promote legislation that would target persons with severe disabilities, whether their condition is terminal or not, and create a double standard for treatment and survival. According to Diane Coleman, the founder and president of Not Dead Yet, "If the values of liberty really dictate that society legalizes assisted suicide, then legalize it for everyone who asks for it, not just the devalued old, ill and disabled. Otherwise, what looks like freedom is really only discrimination" (Not Dead Yet, 2005). Highly public debates sparked by court cases involving patients in persistent vegetative states have elicited comments such as, "I would not want to live like that." Others have thought, "I would not want to die under circumstances like that."

The ANA (1994) statement on assisted suicide does not support assisted suicide in any of its forms. Suicide, euthanasia, managed death, self-deliverance, or whatever name it is called—these are not nursing words. Assisted suicide in any variation for persons with disabilities is not a dilemma; it is a plan for earmarking devalued persons.

Moral Decision Making and Conflict Resolution

The ethical debates influencing rehabilitation nursing are significant and have the potential to affect all levels of practice. Rehabilitation nurses have influence in determining the outcomes of ethical questions through moral decision making and conflict resolution. Moral decision making is the use of ethical principles to guide decision making through a rational

---

BOX 3-1 Process of Moral Decision Making

A. Recognizing the Moral Dimension
The first step is recognizing the decision as one that has moral importance. Important clues include conflicts between two or more values or ideals.

B. Who Are the Interested Parties? What Are Their Relationships?
Carefully identify who has a stake in the decision. In this regard, be imaginative and sympathetic. Often there are more parties whose interests should be taken into consideration than is immediately obvious.

Look at the relationships between the parties. Look at their relationships with yourself and with each other, and with relevant institutions.

C. What Values Are Involved?
Think through the shared values that are at stake in making this decision. Is there a question of trust? Is personal autonomy a consideration? Is there a question of fairness? Is anyone to be harmed or helped?

D. Weigh the Benefits and the Burdens
Benefits—broadly defined—might include such things as the production of goods (physical, emotional, financial, social, etc.) for various parties, the satisfaction of preferences, and acting in accordance with various relevant values (such as fairness).

Burdens might include causing physical or emotional pain to various parties, imposing financial costs, and ignoring relevant values.

E. Look for Analogous Cases
Can you think of other similar decisions? What course of action was taken? Was it a good decision? How is the present case like that one? How is it different?

F. Discuss With Relevant Others
The merits of discussion should not be underestimated. Time permitting, discuss your decision with as many persons as have a stake in it. Gather opinions, and ask for the reasons behind those opinions. Remember that your ability to discuss topics with others may be limited by the other people's expectations of confidentiality.

G. Does This Decision Accord With Legal and Organizational Rules?
Some decisions are appropriately made based on legal considerations. If one option is illegal, we should at least think very seriously before taking that option.

Decisions may also be affected by rules set by organizations of which we are members. For example, most professional organizations have Codes of Ethics which are intended to guide individual decision making. Institutions (hospitals, banks, corporations) may also have policies which limit the options available to us.

Sometimes there are bad laws, or bad rules, and sometimes those should be broken. But usually it is ethically important to pay attention to laws and rules.

H. Am I Comfortable With This Decision?
Sometimes your "gut reaction" will tell you if you've missed something.

Questions to be asked in this regard might include:
1. If I carry out this decision, would I be comfortable telling my family about it? My clergyman? My mentors?
2. Would I want children to take my behavior as an example?
3. Is this decision one which a wise, informed, virtuous person would make?
4. Can I live with this decision?

From *Guide to moral decision making*, © by Chris MacDonald, http://www.ethicsweb.ca/guide/1.

---

course (McDonald, 2002). A guide for moral decision making is included in Box 3-1.

PROFESSIONAL ADVOCACY

Rehabilitation nurses also have rights that must be protected. Recent practice issues range from unsafe staffing ratios to protections for whistle-blowers to preventing violence against nurses in the workplace. No one should be forced or threatened to perform duties or actions that are against their moral beliefs. However, rehabilitation nurses also have a moral responsibility to professional standards, legal regulations, their employer, and their fellow team members. Many problems in the health care system lend themselves to corrective action when reasonable efforts are undertaken to demonstrate solutions.

The so-called "organizational culture," the underlying currents of how the mission statement and goals of the organization are handed down in daily practice, determines an ethical path or climate that affects professionals. Ethical paths are evident in the way problems are handled, such as professional misconduct or errors, the perceived ability for staff to express opinions openly, and a sense of continuity in values from the top to the lower levels of the employee hierarchy. The organizational culture influences how providers make decisions or conduct moral reasoning during situations in which ethics are in question (Crosby & Croskerry, 2004).

Nurse leaders must work within the structure of the organization and the regulations of their state's nurse practice act to ensure that standards and guidelines for nursing practice are met (Burkhart & Nathaniel, 2002). This ethical responsibility includes ensuring appropriate staffing ratios for patient acuity, work conditions that are conducive to optimal nursing practice, and stewardship of community and organizational resources. Only 2% of the nation's hospitals have achieved Magnet designation, which is awarded to organizations based on their ability to attract and retain nurses. The American Nurses Credentialing Center recognizes Magnet status as one way that nurse leaders can advocate for the nurses on staff and ensure the best care practices for their patients (American Nurses Credentialing Center, 2005).

Ethics Committees

Every health care organization benefits from an ethics committee composed of interdisciplinary professionals and consumer representatives. Accreditation organizations, such as the Joint Commission on Accreditation of Healthcare Organizations and the Commission on Accreditation of Rehabilitation Facilities (CARF), mandate organizations to establish an ethics committee that reviews questions and investigates allegations that arise within the organization (CARF, 2005). Potential ethical questions include, "Can program evaluation and monitoring of patient outcomes realistically (read, ethically) serve as the basis for making decisions about allocating services to patients?" Leadership in establishing an ethics committee and ensuring proper representation is an example of an organizational advocacy role for rehabilitation nurses.

Research. Two landmark events in human subject research have forever changed the way in which medical research is conducted. The Nuremberg Code was developed to prevent a reoccurrence of the medical experiments that occurred in Nazi Germany during World War II. The Nuremberg Code specifies 10 basic requirements for all medical experimentation (Box 3-2). The National Institutes of Health specifies the guidelines for clinical research involving human subjects, codified in Title 45, Code of Federal Regulations, Part 46 (Protection of Human Subjects, 1995). Any rehabilitation nurse participating in a clinical trial or research initiative must be familiar with the basic requirements for research involving human subjects.

Ethical considerations with rehabilitation research deal primarily with informed consent. Nurses often participate in obtaining informed consent and collecting data for research conducted on patient populations. An institutional review board evaluation with full informed consent materials must be in place before any data collection, treatment interventions, or new product tests occur.

BOX 3-2 Nuremberg Code (Paraphrased)

1. Informed, voluntary consent of the subject is essential.
2. The study must be expected to have a result that will be of benefit to others.
3. The study must be based on an understanding of pathophysiology of the disease or problem or on prior animal studies.
4. Suffering of subjects will be prevented during the study.
5. Death or disability are not expected or predicted as a result of the study.
6. The degree of risk does not outweigh the potential good to be gained.
7. Subjects will be protected and safeguarded against problems that may occur during the study.
8. Researchers will have the appropriate credentials to complete the research.
9. Subjects may withdraw from studies if they cannot continue.
10. Researchers will stop the study if at any time they deem it in the best interests of the subjects to discontinue the study.

Codes of Ethics. Patients may express interest in euthanasia, assisted suicide, suicide, and related topics. Be clear that in these situations they are not presenting the rehabilitation nurse with an ethical dilemma. Rather, these topics are legal issues and subject to the professional codes of practice.

Each professional discipline on the team, nursing, physical therapy, occupational therapy, medicine, and speech pathology has a code of ethics. However, no single code of ethics applies to rehabilitation as a specialty, despite the prevalence of chronic and disabling disorders treated at the tertiary level of care. Many conflicts arise regarding the balance between the needs of patients with complex, severe disabilities and managing costs. Statements related to ethics are found in standards for practice, state nursing practice acts, institution or agency policies and procedures, research ethics, and reviews of research involving human subjects, vulnerable populations, and others. Table 3-3 contains a listing of disciplines with websites documenting their codes of ethics.

The National Academy of Science (2005) issued the first guidelines for researchers using stem cells in the United States. More than 50 recommendations are intended to help academic and private institutions and states govern projects and control unregulated research. For example, institutions with stem cell research should establish an oversight committee, researchers should not pay donors for eggs or sperm, and some research should be avoided altogether (e.g., injecting human stem cells into monkeys). Using eggs for cloning procedures is highly discouraged. Federal funding for projects is closely regulated and seldom involves human embryos, but research funded by private and charitable sources is less restricted. The research has created complex ethical dilemmas because it is viewed by some as akin to murder/abortion and by others as potentially life saving. Clarity and guidelines are imperative.

TABLE 3-3 Websites for Codes of Ethics Prepared by Professional Specialty Organizations Relevant to Rehabilitation

Organization	Website for Code of Ethics
American Physical Therapy Association	http://www.apta.org/PT_Practice/ethics_pt/code_ethics
American Occupational Therapy Association	http://www.aota.org/members/area2/links/LINK03.asp
American Speech-Language-Hearing Association	http://www.asha.org/library/code_of_ethics.htm
American Therapeutic Recreation Association	http://www.recreationtherapy.com/rt.htm
American Academy of Physical Medicine and Rehabilitation	http://www.aapmr.org/about/codea.htm
American Nurses Association	http://www.nursingworld.org/ethics/ecode.htm
International Council of Nurses	http://www.icn.ch/icncode.pdf

ETHICAL ISSUES IN REHABILITATION NURSING

Rehabilitation nurses are confronted with issues that need resolution in areas where answers are not readily found and few responses are satisfactory. Important examples of ethical areas likely to create conflict are listed below. Although not an all-inclusive list, most of these pose concerns for persons with impairments.

- Care of potentially vulnerable populations, including the elderly, prisoners, children, cognitively impaired individuals, or people who are economically or educationally disadvantaged (Trials of war criminals, 1949)
- Application of genetic engineering research (Clayton, 2003)
- Changes in death certification decisions based on technological advances in delaying death
- Use of transplant technology, stem cell research, and other organ research
- Proposed legislation for assisted suicide and related movements
- Controversies over an individual's "right to live" and "right to die"
- Judicial decisions involving the state's rights versus federalism or families in moral judgments
- Regulatory decisions concerning approval for "promising" investigational drugs for persons with terminal illnesses

The ANA Code of Ethics (2001) clearly comes down on the side of patients and against assisted suicide. Rehabilitation nurses advocating for patients not only keep themselves knowledgeable but also ensure that other members of the team are aware of covert, as well as publicized issues. They also advocate for ethical decision-making processes, including ethics committees with patient representation, to be in place and for authority to operate with documented ethical quality standards.

LEGAL ISSUES IN REHABILITATION NURSING

No area of health care or professional nursing practice is unaffected by law or regulation. Laws govern the scope of nursing practice and delivery of care; protect licensure; define specifics of provision, access to services, and reimbursement; and finance education and research. Laws also create the forum to test ethical issues related to health care dilemmas. Rehabilitation nursing practice is uniquely tied to law and regulation owing to its affiliation with medical rehabilitation and the federal legislation written after both world wars, chiefly for veterans. Disability definitions and laws have broadened to support adaptation to chronic, disabling conditions, including education, entitlements, and access to the public arena. Significant changes in legislation nearly always have some relationship with economic factors in health care. The federal government is responsible for funding many programs of interest to rehabilitation, making the plans proposed by the National Institute on Disability and Rehabilitation Research (NIDRR) relevant to rehabilitation nurses and patients. (See Chapter 1 for more information about NIDRR.) At this writing, NIDRR has proposed a long-range plan for disability-related funding for fiscal years 2005 to 2009.

Whenever NIDRR offers a new proposal, the Institute publishes its intent, as for this 5-year plan (2005 to 2009). It invites review and comments from people with disabilities, their families and advocates, and service providers, as well as organizations and professionals seeking funds for research. All relevant information is available on the NIDRR website and in published government documents. The current proposal emphasizes five domains that will be recognized over the next 5 years in support of people with disabilities. Those designing programs and research should direct their efforts toward the priorities of (1) employment, (2) participation and community living, (3) health and function, (4) technology for access and function, and (5) disability demographics for persons with disabilities. Once the comments are received and reviewed, the final guidelines, including deadlines and fiscal boundaries, are published. Grants and proposals are subject to peer review for acceptance or approval, and ideally for allocation of funds.

Government agencies important to rehabilitation are housed within the U.S. Department of Education, notably the Rehabilitation Services Administration (RSA). The No Child Left Behind Program and New Freedom Initiative are important legislation for patients. The office of Special Education Programs (OSEP) offers support to parents, individuals, school systems, and state programs concerning special education, vocational rehabilitation, and research. OSEP funds programs to offer technical assistance to individuals of all ages. The Center for National Rehabilitation Research Information and Exchange (CIRRIE) is another relevant program. Until recently, rehabilitation nurses have not participated in these programs and research opportunities. The scope of pertinent information on the website is comprehensive, directly related to practice, and should be required reading for action by all rehabilitation nurses.

Americans With Disabilities Act Definition of Disability

Disability, as defined in the ADA (1990), is a physical or mental impairment that substantially limits one or more major life activities, a record of such an impairment, or being regarded as having an impairment. The Equal Employment Opportunity Commission (EEOC) issued guidelines for complying with the ADA law. Within the EEOC's regulations was an expansion of the ADA legislative definition. The ADA took effect on July 26, 1992, 2 years after President George Bush signed the act.

Supreme Court Decisions and Legal Summaries

All eight Supreme Court cases relative to this chapter and a summary of the opinions rendered are presented in Box 3-3. Summaries of disability laws are presented in Box 3-4.

NURSING PROCESS

Assessment

Ask the patient and family about values and beliefs important to them. In a trust relationship, this process will be easier and responses more reliable than when a patient senses conflict or coercion. The person who decides not to participate has made a choice; however, the nurse advocate must ensure that the patient has made a fully informed choice and no penalties are assigned.

Assessment of children's values is a unique category that includes assessment of a child's development of moral reasoning; the child's ability to understand the illness or disability; the severity, extent, and type of disability or condition; family or guardian involvement; and other subtle, complex factors.

Value/belief questions are about the following:
• Patient and family self-ratings of life satisfaction and perceptions of quality of life

---

BOX 3-3 Supreme Court Decisions

Title of Case	Opinion of the Court
Bragdon v. Abbott (1998)	Abbott's HIV is a disability under ADA and reproduction is a major life activity, but no "per se disabilities" under ADA.
	A risk assessment must be based on medical or other objective evidence.
Cleveland v. Policy Management Systems (1999)	The application for or receipt of Social Security benefits does not preclude an ADA claim. A claim for Social Security and an ADA claim can exist "side-by-side." (Court listed five specific examples.)
Sutton v. United Airlines (1999)	Determination of disability under the ADA must take into account corrective or mitigation measures.
	The inability to perform a single job does not constitute a substantial limitation in the major life activity of work.
Murphy v. United Parcel Services (1999)	Medication is a corrective or mitigation measure.
	Inability to perform a single, particular job does not constitute a substantial limitation in the major life activity of working.
	"Regarded as" unable to perform a single, particular job does not constitute discrimination under the ADA "third prong."
Albertson's Inc. v. Kirkingburg (1999)	Monocular vision is not a "per se disability."
	The body's own ability to compensate is considered a mitigating measure.
Toyota Motors v. Williams (2002)	In determining a substantial limitation in the major life activity of performing manual tasks, must assess whether or not the impairment prevents or severely restricts tasks that are of central importance to most people's daily lives.
	Impairments must have a permanent or at least a long-term effect.
Chevron v. Echazabal (2002)	Employers do not have to hire individuals who are unable to carry out the essential function of the job without incurring risk to their own health.
	The ADA does not entitle individuals to jobs that might jeopardize their health.
Clackamas Gastroenterology v. Wells (2003)	A covered entity is an employer who is "engaged in an industry affecting commerce who has 15 or more employees for each working day in each of 20 or more calendar weeks in the current or preceding calendar year."
	An employee is defined as "an individual employed by an employer."

ADA, Americans With Disabilities Act; *HIV*, human immunodeficiency virus.

BOX 3-4 Summaries of Disability Laws

Employment	*Americans With Disabilities Act, Title I:* Prohibits discrimination in the workplace against people with disabilities. *Section 501, Rehabilitation Act (1973):* Requires affirmative action and nondiscrimination in employment by federal agencies of the executive branch. *Section 503, Rehabilitation Act:* Requires affirmative action and prohibits employment discrimination by federal government contractors and subcontractors with contracts of more than $10,000. *Section 188, the Workforce Investment Act:* Prohibits discrimination against people with disabilities in employment service centers funded by the federal government.
State and local government programs and services	*Americans With Disabilities Act, Title II:* Prohibits discrimination in the provision of public benefits and services (e.g., public education, employment, transportation, recreation, health care, social services, courts, voting, and town meetings). *Section 504, Rehabilitation Act:* Requires that buildings and facilities that are designed, constructed, or altered with federal funds, or leased by a federal agency, comply with federal standards for physical accessibility.
Housing	*Fair Housing Act:* Prohibits discrimination in any aspect of selling, renting, or denying housing on the basis of disability. Owners are further required to make reasonable accommodations in their housing policies to afford equal housing opportunities to those with disabilities. *Americans With Disabilities Act, Title II:* Prohibits discrimination by public housing authorities and other state and local government housing. *Americans With Disabilities Act, Title III:* Does not apply to regular privately owned residential dwelling units. However, it does apply to residences that are also public accommodations, such as nursing homes and school dorms. In addition, parts of residential facilities that serve a group of people or the public might be considered public accommodations, such as a swimming pool or a sales and leasing office. *Section 504, Rehabilitation Act:* Prohibits discrimination by public housing authorities that receive federal funds, cities and towns that receive Community Development Block Grants (CDBGs) or other federal funds, private for-profit or nonprofit housing developers that receive federal funds, and colleges and universities that receive federal funds (student housing). *Architectural Barriers Act:* Applies accessibility standards to housing constructed with federal funding.
Education	*Individuals With Disabilities Education Act (IDEA):* Requires public primary and secondary schools to make available to all eligible children with disabilities a free appropriate public education in the least restrictive environment appropriate to their individual needs. *Section 504, Rehabilitation Act:* Prohibits discrimination against students with disabilities in primary, secondary, or postsecondary schools receiving federal funds. *Americans With Disabilities Act, Title II:* Prohibits discrimination against students with disabilities in all educational institutions that receive funds from state or local government. *Americans With Disabilities Act, Title III:* Prohibits discrimination against students with disabilities in private schools.
Travel and transportation	*Americans With Disabilities Act, Title II:* Prohibits discrimination in transportation provided by state and local governmental entities such as bus, railway, subway, and other forms of ground transportation. *Section 504, Rehabilitation Act:* Prohibits discrimination in privately operated transportation services that receive federal funds. *Americans With Disabilities Act, Title III:* Prohibits discrimination in privately operated transportation services such as limousines and hotel shuttle services. *Air Carrier Access Act:* Prohibits discrimination on the basis of disability in air travel. It applies only to air carriers that provided regularly scheduled services for hire to the public. Requirements address a wide range of issues, including boarding assistance and certain accessibility features in newly built aircraft and new or altered airport facilities.
Technology and telecommunications	*Section 508, Rehabilitation Act:* Requires federal agencies to make their electronic and information technology accessible to people with disabilities. *Americans With Disabilities Act, Title IV:* Requires telephone companies to establish telecommunications relay services for callers with hearing and speech disabilities. Title VI also requires closed captioning of federally funded public service announcements. *Section 255, Telecommunications Act:* Requires manufacturers of telecommunications equipment and providers of telecommunications services to ensure that such equipment and services are accessible to and usable by persons with disabilities; that people with disabilities will have access to a broad range of products and services such as telephones, cell phones, pagers, call waiting, and operator services.

- Future goals or plans and awareness of bias for those who are not future oriented
- Involvement in community or other activities outside of self and self-care
- Support mechanisms, especially religious or spiritual
- Things that are considered important to do, such as rituals or family traditions

Nurse's Self-Assessment. Nurses bring their own values into a conflict or paradoxical situation. Clarifying personal values and identifying biases, as well as cultural differences, are preliminary to advocacy about values. Weis and Schank (2000) developed an instrument, the Nurses Professional Value Scale, intended for use in measuring professional nursing values and enhancing professional socialization. They found caregiving and activism to be the major factors. Caregiving included "providing care without prejudice" and "establishing standards as guides for daily nursing practice" (Weis & Schank, 2000, p. 203).

Nursing Diagnoses

Decisional conflict: There is uncertainty about the optimal course among competing actions, and the course involves risk, loss, or challenge to personal life values (Dochterman & Bulechek, 2004, p. 805).

Related Factors. Social construction or beliefs about health, illness, and disability; knowledge of the natural history of the disability; and full information concerning regimens and interventions are related factors. The person's coping and

adaptation patterns and supports influence acceptance of the situation, and previous experiences with the system may alter acceptance. Difficulties arise when the person is not fully oriented, wavers among options, or breaks down in the process. Cultural differences are complex and make value clarification or mutual goal setting tenuous (see Chapter 6).

Nursing Interventions

- Invoke codes of ethics and patient rights and *Nursing's Agenda for Healthcare Reform* (ANA, 1992).
- Educate patient and family about the disease or disability, treatment options, and full disclosure.
- Refer to community and other resources for assistance and support.
- Offer therapeutic support or effective coping mechanisms, such as companion pets, humor, stress reduction and relaxation, music or art therapy, guided imagery, and so forth.
- Use cognitive or behavioral therapy to improve thinking and communication.
- Institute culture broker activities when indicated.
- Refer for genetic counseling.
- Help patient to locate legal aid or assistance.
- Encourage spiritual resources.
- Use touch (if appropriate), time, and support from self as professional nurse.

Nursing Outcomes

- Knowledge, fully informed, values clear
- Consistent, logical information processing
- Participation in health care decisions
- Acceptance of health or disability status

Case Study

Frank is dying of advanced prostate cancer. His wife manages his care at home with the assistance of hospice care nurses and assistants. His care is complicated by a gangrenous foot ulcer. The only corrective treatment for the wound is amputation, yet the surgeons are wary of performing the amputation on Frank because his cancer is nearing end stage. They are concerned that he may not withstand the surgery and that the surgery may hasten his demise. His pain, however, is intractable. While fully alert and oriented, Frank cries throughout the day and night and is unable to move from his bed due to the pain of the wound. His wife appeals to the ethics committee at the hospital to request the amputation for her husband, stating that his quality of life with the pain is not worth continuing.

Members of the ethics team meet with Frank's wife and discuss the case and possible options. The chairperson of the committee meets with Frank to validate that Frank understands the risks of the surgery, in addition to benefits and alternatives. He explains that he loves his wife and wishes that the circumstances were different, yet he cannot bear to continue living if living means experiencing such extreme pain. Medications have not been sufficient to relieve the

pain, and he spends all day, every day, in bed, a constant burden to his wife. He comprehends the risks of surgery, recognizes that he may die during or following the surgery.

The burden of the caregiver, his wife, is an ethical problem. In his current situation, Frank requires complete care, 24/7, for his condition. He is never pain free, and his wife is on a family medical leave of absence from her job to provide care for him. There are no adult children or other family members to assist with Frank's care. Although hospice nurses and assistants are available, they are limited by Medicare guidelines in the number of visits made and the time available.

Frank's wife has requested that he receive an amputation of his gangrenous limb, which is likely to cause his demise. Ethical questions for consideration are the following:

- What is the cost of his current care? This analysis should include his wife's current leave of absence from work, in addition to the physical and emotional demands of caregiving.
- What is the efficacy of his current care regimen? Currently Frank is completely dependent for all physical care needs, with the exception of feeding and washing his face. His pain is ineffectively managed, and he is confined to bed.

Case Study—cont'd

- *What is the rationale for the amputation? Removal of his diseased limb is the immediate goal. However, if his pain is decreased, he could become more independent and perhaps participate in rehabilitation.*
- *Do the benefits of the surgery outweigh the risks? Only Frank and his wife can make this decision. The burden on the physicians is to ensure that their decision is informed. The burden on the nurses is to ensure that strong advocacy exists to allow Frank and his wife to make a decision, independent of pressures from the busy health care system. Such pressures may include attempts to reduce pain through additional pharmacological interventions rather than provide costly surgery and interdisciplinary rehabilitation.*

In Frank's situation in the case study, although he and his wife admitted to significant and disruptive levels of pain and their options were quite limited, they opted for amputation of his limb. At this point in time, they had no expectations for the future—whether he died, or if the surgery was successful, in either situation his pain would end or decrease.

Nurses advocated for Frank and his wife in relaying information to the surgeon and assuring him that the family was fully aware of the possible negative outcome of the surgery.

The family is devoutly Catholic, and the nurses contacted the family priest, who visited and remained with Frank's wife during the morning of surgery.

Given Frank's situation, the nurses might have been biased toward doing only hospice-level care, yet they were first and foremost to advocate for his chance at surgery. The nurses did not display a prejudice toward Frank relative to his late stage of cancer.

Nursing Diagnoses

Acute pain: related to metastatic prostate cancer and gangrene of the left foot

Grieving: related to anticipating end of life and managing advanced prostate cancer

Decisional conflict: related to question of surgical appropriateness and possible adverse outcome

Outcome

Frank did very well through surgery. His pain level was easily managed with 5 mg of oxycodone IR every 4 hours. Following surgery, he experienced increased energy and was able to transfer in and out of the chair with assistance.

His diet increased, his participation in his care improved, and he was referred for acute inpatient rehabilitation. Following a 2-week course of acute rehabilitation, Frank was independent in wheelchair mobility and was able to return home with his wife. They regained involvement in their home church and in community activities. They were able to go out for dinner and occasionally to the movies.

Six months following surgery, Frank experienced a significant setback, with a new tumor of the left lower lobe of his lung. He deteriorated quickly and succumbed to lung cancer.

His widow continues to visit the nurses on rehabilitation and states that she will be forever grateful for the 6 months she had with Frank when he was pain free.

CRITICAL THINKING

1. Given that rehabilitation care can be expensive and consumes limited resources, is there a time when promotion of rehabilitation is unethical?
2. There are many different approaches to rehabilitation care, and patients with chronic illness and disabilities are susceptible to the latest promise for cure and return to normal. What are key ways of assessing that claims made by rehabilitation programs or approaches are valid?

INTERNET RESOURCES

American Academy of Pediatrics: http://www.aap.org
Institute on Independent Living: http://www.independentliving.org
Justice for All: http://www.jfanow.org
National Council on Disability: http://www.ncd.gov/index.html
National Council on Independent Living: http://www.ncil.org
National Spinal Cord Injury Association: http://www.spinalcord.org
New Mobility: http://www.newmobility.com/index.cfm
Not Dead Yet: http://www.notdeadyet.org
TASH-Disability Advocacy Worldwide: http://www.tash.org
World Institute on Disability (WID): http://www.wid.org

REFERENCES

American Hospital Association. (2005). *AHA comment letter on Medicare inpatient rehab facility PPS for FY 2006 proposed rule.* Retrieved October 15, 2005, from http://www.hospitalconnect.com/aha/key_issues/rehab/content/20050718comment.pdf.

American Nurses Association. (1994). *Position statement: Assisted suicide.* Washington, DC: Author.

American Nurses Association. (2001). *Code of ethics for nurses with intepretive statements.* Washington, DC: Author.

American Nurses Association. (2002). *Nursing's agenda for the future: A call to the nation.* Washington, DC: Author.

American Nurses Credentialing Center. (2005). *ANCC Magnet Recognition Program®–Recognizing excellence in nursing services.* Washington, DC: Author. Available from http://www.nursingworld.org/ancc/magnet/index.html.

Americans With Disabilities Act of 1990, 42 U.S.C.A. § 12101 *et seq.* (West 1993). Available from http://www.usdoj.gov/crt/ada/publicat.htm.

Association of Rehabilitation Nurses. (2003). *ARN position statement on ethical issues.* Glenview, IL: Author. Available from http://www.rehabnurse.org/profresources/pethical.html.

Burkhart, M., & Nathaniel, A. (2002). *Ethics and issues in contemporary nursing* (pp. 83-84). Clifton Park, NY: Delmar,.

Canadian Broadcasting Corporation. (2004, September 27). Indepth: Assisted suicide. The fight for the right to die. *CBC News Online,* September 27, 2004. Retrieved May 17, 2006, from http://www.cbc.ca/news/background/assistedsuicide/.

Caplan, A. L., Callahan, D., & Haas, J. (1987). *Ethical and policy issues in rehabilitation medicine* (Special supplement, August, pp. 1-19). Briarcliff Manor, NY: Hastings Center.

Clayton, E. (2003). Ethical, legal, and social implications of genomic medicine. *New England Journal of Medicine, 349*(6), 562-569.

Commission on Accreditation of Rehabilitation Facilities. (2005). *Standards manual: Medical rehabilitation, July 2005-June 2006.* Tucson, AZ: Author.

Crosby, K., & Croskerry, P. (2004). Profiles in patient safety: Authority gradients in medical error. *Academy of Emergency Medicine, 11*(12), 1341-1345.

Dochterman, J. M., & Bulechek, G. M. (2004). *Nursing interventions classification (NIC)* (4th ed.). St. Louis, MO: Mosby.

Dupont, E. (2005). Hippocrates, father of semiology and medical deontology. *Revue Medicale de Bruxelles, 26*(3), 193-197.

Eckenhoff, E. (1981). The value of the disabled life. In N. Martin, N. Holt, & D. Hicks (Eds.), *Comprehensive rehabilitation nursing.* New York: McGraw-Hill.

Edge, R. S., & Groves, J. R. (2005). *Ethics of health care: A guide for clinical practice.* Boston: Thomson Delmar Learning.

Esselman, P. (2004). Inpatient rehabilitation outcome trends: Implications for the future. *JAMA 292*(14), 1746-1748.

Flax, H. J. (2000). The future of physical medicine and rehabilitation. *Archives of Physical Medicine and Rehabilitation, 79,* 79-86.

Greene, J., Haidt, J. (2002). How (and where) does moral judgment work? *Trends in Cognitive Sciences, 6*(12), 517-523

Hartling, O. (2006). Euthanasia—The illusion of autonomy. *Medical Law, 25*(1), 189-199.

Hinman, L. (2002). *Ethics: A pluralistic approach to moral theory* (3rd ed.). Belmont, CA: Thomson-Wadsworth.

Hinman, T. (2004). *Utilitarianism.* Available from http://ethics.sandiego.edu/theories/Utilitarianism/.

Hunt, G. (2001). Human rights or responsibilities? Remembering Florence Nightingale. *Nursing Ethics, 8*(3), 179-180.

McDonald, C. (2002). Physical activity, health impairments, and disability in neuromuscular diseases. *American Journal of Medical Rehabilitation, 81*(11 Suppl.), S108-S120.

National Academy of Science. (2005). *Guidelines released for embryonic stem cell research.* Washington, DC: Author. Available from http://www4.national academies.org/news.nsf/isbn/0309096537?OpenDocument.

Not Dead Yet. (2005). *Disability rights groups to rally against assisted suicide.* Forest Park, IL: Author. Available from http://www.notdeadyet.org/docs/gonzalesorals1005pr.html.

Online Ethics Center for Engineering and Science. (2005). *The Online Ethics Center for Engineering and Science.* Retrieved August 18, 2005, from http://onlineethics.org/cite-link.html.

Protection of Human Subjects, 45 C.F.R. Part 46. (1995).

Rowland, D. (2005). Medicaid: Implications for the health safety net. *New England Journal of Medicine, 353*(14), 1439-1441.

Schriner, K., & Ochs, L. (2000). "No right is more precious": Voting rights and people with intellectual and developmental disabilities. *Policy Research Brief* (University of Minnesota, Minneapolis, Institute on Community Integration), *11* (1).

Sharma, M., Clark, H., Armour, T., Stotts, G., CotÈ, R., Hill, M. D., et al. (2005, July). *Acute stroke: Evaluation and treatment.* Evidence Report/Technology Assessment No. 127 (Prepared by the University of Ottawa Evidence-based Practice Center under Contract No. 290-02-0021). AHRQ Publication No. 05-E023-2. Rockville, MD: Agency for Healthcare Research and Quality.

Stoolman, R. (2005). *A second chance: Helping people return to work after a disabling injury or illness.* Philadelphia: Cigna. Available from http://www.nraf-rehabnet.org/images/rehabweek2005FINALfor distribution.pdf.

Tan, S. (2002). Deconstructing paternalism—What serves the patient best? *Singapore Medical Journal, 43*(3), 148-151.

ThinkFirst. (2005). *Mission.* Rolling Meadows, IL: Author. Available from http://www.thinkfirst.org/About/.

Trials of war criminals before the Nuremberg Military Tribunals under Control Council Law No.10, Vol. 2 (pp. 181-182). (1949) Washington, DC: U.S. Government Printing Office.

Tsai, P. (2003) A middle-range theory of caregiver stress. *Nursing Science Quarterly, 16*(2), 137-145.

U.S. Department of Health and Human Services. (2000). *Tracking Healthy People 2010.* Washington, DC: U.S. Government Printing Office.

Weis, D., & Schank, M. J. (2000). An instrument to measure professional nursing values. *Journal of Nursing Scholarship, 32*(2), 201-204.

4

Research-Based Rehabilitation Nursing Practice

Linda L. Pierce, PhD, RN, CNS, CRRN, FAHA
Elizabeth J. Predeger, PhD, RN
Christina M. Mumma, PhD, RN, CRRN

Nursing has a rich research history of building the art and science. In the 1850s Florence Nightingale's research on epidemiology and the detection of the contagion began the process of discovery in nursing (Nightingale, 1859/1946). Rehabilitation nursing research has a short chronology, rooted in the twentieth century, specifically following World Wars I and II when many veterans survived and aged with disabilities (see Chapter 1). The first issue of *Nursing Research* published an article about the adjustment of chronically ill older adults who were receiving home health care (Mack, 1952); however, it was nearly 10 years later before the journal published a research article specific to rehabilitation nursing, development of an objective measure for decubitus ulcers (Verhonick, 1961). Table 4-1 lists research progress relevant to rehabilitation nursing for each decade.

RESEARCH PRIORITIES FOR REHABILITATION NURSES

This chapter demonstrates the importance of building programs of nursing research and offers examples of rehabilitation nurse scientists and their funded work. Another highlight is funding opportunities for beginning and experienced researchers. Several sources with established research priorities of particular interest to rehabilitation nurses are discussed below.

The National Institute of Nursing Research

For several decades the National Institute of Nursing Research (NINR) has set research priorities (NINR, 2006b), which are redirected in light of new discoveries (National Institutes of Health [NIH], 2005). One NINR program priority is the integration of biological and behavioral research. Three dimensions, promoting health and preventing disease, managing the symptoms and disability of illness, and improving the

environments in which care is delivered, provide broad areas of opportunities for nurse researchers (NINR, 2006b).

The Rehabilitation Nursing Foundation

The purpose of the Rehabilitation Nursing Foundation (RNF) is to advance practice by promoting, supporting, conducting, and disseminating research that has the potential to improve the quality of health care to individuals with disability or chronic illness. The RNF makes funding available to novice and seasoned researchers totaling nearly $50,000 each year. The inaugural research grant was awarded to Kathleen Sawin and June Marshall in 1988 for their study, *Developmental Competence in Adolescents With an Acquired Disability*. RNF has funded a total 41 research projects to 39 researchers (ARN, 2006).

Since the mid 1990s RNF research grant recipients' studies have reflected the identified priorities of the Rehabilitation Nursing Research Agenda (RNRA) (Association of Rehabilitation Nurses, 2006). In 1993 the Association of Rehabilitation Nurses (ARN) directed the RNF to develop a research agenda over the next 2 years. Findings from combined quantitative (survey) and qualitative (focus group) methods yielded the critical issues needed for research to advance practice in rehabilitation nursing. Thus the RNRA covered a broad range of issues, described by 25 clinical priorities and 20 contextual statements and synthesized into five categories or areas. The areas were (1) nursing interventions, including management of symptoms, to promote function in people with chronic illness and physical disability; (2) health promotion and prevention strategies to facilitate self-care and independence for people with or at risk for physical disability and chronic illness; (3) rehabilitation practices in the changing health care system; (4) community context of care for people with or at risk for physical disability or chronic illness and for their quality of life; and (5) outcomes and costs influenced by

TABLE 4-1 Changing Focus of Rehabilitation Nursing Research

Decade	Nursing Research Focus	Noteworthy Events
Early 1900s	Nursing education	Basic guidelines, few textbooks written.
1940s	Nursing manpower, supply and demand of nurses explored	Walter Reed Army Institute of Nursing research established.
1950s	Self-study of nurses, nursing actions, and functions	*Nursing Research* journal published in 1952.
1960s	Theoretical bases, conceptual frameworks, and the nursing process	University graduate level education established in clinical areas.
1970s	Clinical problems, improving patient care	Professional specialty organizations set research priorities (e.g., the American Association of Critical-Care Nurses [AACN] and the Oncology Nursing Society [AACN, 2004; Berry, 2003]). Association of Rehabilitation Nurses (ARN) founded in 1974. First research article (Steels, 1976) published in the *ARN Journal* (now *Rehabilitation Nursing*).
1980s	Setting research priorities at federal and national levels	Rehabilitation Nursing Foundation (RNF) of the ARN established research grant award program in 1988 (ARN, 2006). The National Center for Nursing Research (now National Institute of Nursing Research [NINR]) established in 1986; elevated to institute status at National Institutes of Health in 1993 (NINR, 2006a).
1990s	Outcomes research, research utilization	*Rehabilitation Nursing Research* published (1992 to 1997). The Expert Panel on Quality Health Care established the Agency for Healthcare Policy and Research (AHCPR) (now known as the Agency for Healthcare Research and Quality [AHRQ] [2006a]). Publication of *Qualitative Health Research and Clinical Nursing Research*.
2000s	Evidence-based practice, outcomes research; research initiatives to address global health	International Council of Nurses; Sigma Theta Tau International Honor Society of Nursing (2005); National Institutes of Health road map (2005).

rehabilitation nurses in multidisciplinary settings and across the continuum of care (Gordon, Sawin, & Basta, 1996).

In 2005 RNF evaluated and revised the RNRA, as described in detail elsewhere (Jacelon, Pierce, & Buhrer, 2006, 2007). A search of the Cumulative Index to Nursing and Allied Health Literature (CINAHL) database between 1995 and December 2004 identified publications cited as research in *Rehabilitation Nursing* and *Rehabilitation Nursing Research* journals. Two hundred three of these publications resulted from some relationship with the RNRA. RNF grant recipients also published studies in a variety of nursing and interdisciplinary journals: *Cancer, Cancer Practice: A Multidisciplinary Journal of Cancer Care, Cancer Nursing, Journal of Christian Nursing, Journal of Cultural Diversity, Journal of Neuroscience Nursing, Journal of Nursing Scholarship, Nursing Research, Oncology Nursing Forum, Qualitative Health Research, Research in Nursing & Health, Topics in Stroke Rehabilitation,* and *Western Journal of Nursing Research* (Jacelon et al., 2006).

The revised RNRA of 2005 (Box 4-1) consists of 18 statements of research priorities grouped into four categories (ARN, 2006). The categories are (1) nursing and nursing-led interdisciplinary interventions to promote function in people of all ages with disability and/or chronic health problems, (2) experience of disability and/or chronic health problems for individuals and families across the life span, (3) rehabilitation in the changing health care system, and (4) the rehabilitation nursing profession (ARN, 2005). This agenda has the potential to direct and promote rehabilitation nursing research for the next 10 years and is widely disseminated both within the ARN and throughout the nursing and rehabilitation professions (Jacelon et al., 2007).

NURSES' INVOLVEMENT IN RESEARCH

Rehabilitation nurses are becoming recognized as researchers, as nurses involved in all aspects of a research study, and as nurse scientists, that is, nurses who develop and lead programs of research. The work of these researchers and scientists is focused on identified research priorities spread across clinical, educational, and administrative dimensions of practice. The actual involvement of rehabilitation nurses in research has been reported and has grown in numbers. In 1993 only 186 (2%) of the 8,000 ARN members responded to a newsletter survey about their involvement in research. Forty-one per cent of respondents reported that they had no involvement in research (Hoeman, Dayhoff, & Thompson, 1993). In contrast, when 0.2845% of the 6,000 members of ARN (n = 1701) were contacted by e-mail in 2005 and invited to evaluate and comment

---

BOX 4-1 *The Rehabilitation Nursing Research Agenda,* Second Edition, 2005

The agenda, developed by the Rehabilitation Nursing Foundation (RNF), addresses four areas and includes brief descriptions of the high-priority research issues for each area:

1. **Nursing and nursing-led interdisciplinary interventions to promote function in people of all ages with disability and/or chronic health problems**
   1.1. Interventions to promote management of physiologic processes including, but not limited to, bowel, bladder, and skin care
   1.2. Interventions, including behavior management, to promote health, increase independence, and/or improve quality of life in individuals and their families
   1.3. Interventions to promote management of sexuality based on the individual's values, beliefs, and developmental stage
   1.4. Interventions to improve assessment and management of chronic pain
   1.5. Interventions to promote access and safety
   1.6. Interventions and programs for individual education to enhance independence and wellness
   1.7. Interventions using technology to improve lives
2. **Experience of disability and/or chronic health problems for individuals and families across the lifespan**
   2.1. Experience and meaning of disability and/or chronic health problems as it relates to diverse individuals and their families
   2.2. Experience and meaning of independence of individuals with disabilities and/or chronic health problems
   2.3. Response of individuals and families to alterations in independence and caregiving in relation to disability and/or chronic health problems
   2.4. Experience and meaning of accessibility as it relates to diverse individuals, families, and communities
3. **Rehabilitation in the changing healthcare system**
   3.1. Relationships between and among individual characteristics such as behavior and functional status, and caregiver staffing within rehabilitation settings
   3.2. Individuals' functional outcomes in relation to the type, intensity, and duration of rehabilitation nursing services received
   3.3. Effectiveness of rehabilitation programs with respect to individual and/or family outcomes across the continuum of care
4. **The rehabilitation nursing profession**
   4.1. Ethical issues related to the practice of rehabilitation nursing
   4.2. The effect of changing healthcare priorities on the practice of rehabilitation nursing
   4.3. The contributions and the cost of rehabilitation nurses as components of the rehabilitation process
   4.4. The effects of rehabilitation nursing practice models, advanced practice nursing, and nurses' competency levels on individual outcomes in various service settings

From Association of Rehabilitation Nurses. (2005). *The rehabilitation nursing research agenda.* Retrieved May 14, 2006, from http://www.rehabnurse.org/research/researchagenda.html.

on the proposed items for the revised RNRA (Jacelon et al., 2007), 286 members (17% of those queried) responded to the survey. Of the respondents, 20% identified themselves as researchers (Jacelon et al., 2007).

Involvement in some aspect of research is recommended for any nurse intent on providing optimum rehabilitation care for persons with disability and chronic illness. Reading research reports and attending research conferences, and then discussing the relevance of the findings for clinical practice with colleagues, are ways of engaging in rehabilitation nursing research. Reviewing and analyzing published research studies to determine best practices can also provide a basis for using this evidence to improve patient care. Learning more about the research process and collaborating with members of a research team to study human responses to rehabilitation will advance the discipline and provide a scientific foundation for nursing practice. Participation can range from generating research questions based on observations in clinical practice to designing and implementing complex studies.

Rehabilitation nurses assume various roles in research activities dependent, in part, upon their educational preparation. Nurses with associate degrees in nursing and nursing diplomas contribute value in research when they raise questions

about the effectiveness of nursing interventions and participate in data collection to answer these questions. Nurses with baccalaureate, master's, and doctoral degrees receive more research education and can be involved in interpreting and evaluating research for practice, assisting with and conducting investigations, and disseminating research findings. Simply put, nurses in practice identify relevant clinical problems for investigation; nurse scientists design studies to address these problems (American Nurses Association [ANA], 1994; Bartels, 2005). Pierce (2005) takes this one step further in describing the importance of collaborative research relationships between nurse clinicians and researchers, both intradisciplinary (one discipline) and interdisciplinary (many disciplines). Collaborative research teams cultivate liaisons that can move beyond academic degrees and practice roles to make important contributions toward improving health outcomes. Research teams provide an opportunity for mentoring and support among members (Pierce, 2005). The RNF also provides research mentorship opportunities for conference attendees at the ARN annual education meeting. One-to-one sessions can be scheduled with seasoned researchers to discuss potential research ideas, as well as RNF research grant mechanisms.

The roles just described are supported by the ARN scope of practice statement for the rehabilitation nurse researcher (ARN, 2001). Accordingly, rehabilitation nurse researchers (a) identify health care issues in collaboration with patients and others; (b) develop, coordinate, and conduct investigative studies to solve problems within established research guidelines; and (c) disseminate findings. They also analyze and synthesize evidence for best practice, serve as research reviewers, are educators and mentors for beginning researchers, and act as change agents to promote research use in practice (ARN, 2001).

BUILDING A PROGRAM OF RESEARCH

During doctoral study, nurses begin to develop a research trajectory to promote the science. Postdoctoral study provides extended time with mentors when nurses acquire skills to refine and/or redirect their research productivity (Conn, 2004). The National Institutes of Health (NIH) research training offers opportunities for persons with doctoral degrees or those in a research training program (NIH, 2006). Collaboration is essential in the research enterprise starting with small, preliminary studies that lead to larger projects and a program of research. Dissemination of findings in scientific journals, presentations at professional meetings, and competing for sessions at national and international scientific conferences is crucial in the journey to become a nurse scientist (Conn, 2004, 2005; Pierce, 2005).

Rehabilitation nurse scientists are growing in numbers. The following funded programs of inquiry by rehabilitation nurses are representative of their work.

1. Health promotion in adults with chronic disabling conditions, such as multiple sclerosis, postpolio syndrome, and fibromyalgia by Stuifbergen at the University of Texas (http://www.nur.utexas.edu/)
2. Health, adaptation, self-management, and quality of life outcomes in individuals with disabilities and their families (e.g., spina bifida, spinal cord injury, and cerebral palsy), as well as the risk and protective factors that are associated with these outcomes by Sawin at the University of Wisconsin (http://cfprod.imt.uwm.edu/)
3. Persons with stroke and caregivers, a joint project by Bakas at the University of Indiana, King at Northwestern University, Lutz at the University of Florida, Ostwald at the University of Texas, and Pierce at the University of Toledo (http://nursing.iupui.edu/; http://www.northwestern.edu/; http://www.nursing.ufl.edu/; http://son.uth.tmc.edu/; http://hsc.utoledo.edu/)
4. Safe patient care by designing and testing safety defenses for the patient, provider, technology, and organization by Nelson at the Tampa Veterans Administration, VISN 8 Patient Safety Center of Inquiry (http://www.visn8.med.va.gov/patientsafetycenter/)

These nurse scientists have funded research with a combined total of millions of dollars in grants awarded by private organizations, university, and/or government agencies.

FUNDING OPPORTUNITIES

Grants are helpful, even essential, for building a continuous research program, whether a novice investigator or seasoned nurse scientist. In addition to the RNF, national professional and nursing organizations make monies available for conducting research. For example, the American Heart Association (http://www.americanheart.org), the American Stroke Association (http://www.strokeassociation.org), the American Cancer Society (http://www.cancer.org), Sigma Theta Tau International (http://www.nursingsociety.org), the Oncology Nursing Society (http://www.ons.org), and the American Association of Neuroscience Nurses (http://www.aann.org) have research funds. University incentive and/or foundation grants are resources for pilot studies and projects. Numerous federal programs provide funding for a broad range of research priorities. The following are a few exemplars of government funding sources.

The NINR has a budget of nearly $138 million to support clinical and basic research to establish a scientific basis for the care of individuals across the life span. This includes managing persons during illness and recovery, reducing risks for disease and disability, promoting healthy lifestyles, promoting quality of life with chronic illness, and caring for individuals at the end of life (NINR, 2006b). The Agency for Healthcare Research and Quality (AHRQ) supports a broad program of health services research and works with partners, such as NINR, to promote improvements in clinical and health systems practices, including the prevention of diseases and other health conditions. The AHRQ mission is to improve U.S. health care, including quality, safety, efficiency, and effectiveness (AHRQ, 2006a). These areas of interest provide appropriate avenues for rehabilitation nurses to conduct research.

The National Center for Medical Rehabilitation Research (NCMRR) has been a component of the National Institute of Child Health and Human Development (NICHD) since 1990. The primary interest of NCMRR is rehabilitation research. Research initiatives and opportunities are offered in seven crosscutting areas identified as needing increased research effort. Those areas are the following:

1. Improving functional mobility.
2. Promoting behavioral adaptation to functional losses.
3. Assessing the efficacy and outcomes to medical rehabilitation therapies and practices.
4. Developing improved assistive technology.
5. Understanding whole body system responses to physical impairments and functional changes.
6. Developing more precise methods of measuring impairments, disabilities, and societal and functional limitations.
7. Training research scientists in the field of rehabilitation (NCMRR, 2005). The NCMRR has a budget request for 2007 of $1.25 billion with 54% of that money designated for research project grants (NCMRR, 2006).

The National Institute on Disability and Rehabilitation Research (NIDRR) is a component of the Office of Special Education and Rehabilitative Services (OSERS) in the United States Department of Education. NIDRR is specific to and funds rehabilitation research (NIDRR, 2006). This institute, created in 1978, is a legacy of Mary Switzer and Dr. Howard Rusk that originated with the rehabilitation research program begun with the 1954 amendments to the Vocational Rehabilitation Act. The NIDRR is probably among the first federal funding agencies for rehabilitation researchers and leads in support of research that is responsive to basic changes in the lives of individuals with disabilities. The NIDRR's largest program is the Rehabilitation Research and Training Centers (RRTCs). Each center focuses on a particular aspect of the behavioral, medical, or vocational rehabilitation of people with disabilities. Investigators should also be aware of the Field Initiated Research (FIR) program and Switzer Research Fellowships. The FIR is a 36-month program, $150,000 per year, and the Switzer Research Fellowship is an award of $45,000 to 55,000 per year (NIDRR, 2006).

The Centers for Disease Control and Prevention (CDC) also funds rehabilitation-related research and works through local health departments, advocacy groups, and other partners (e.g., nonprofit and voluntary organizations; schools and universities; community, professional, and philanthropic organizations) to accomplish their goals. From 2001 to 2004, the CDC convened three workgroups charged with recommending an agency-wide research agenda to serve as a blueprint for the next decade. The proposed *Research Guide* contains themes focused on early identification of developmental disabilities, health among persons with disabilities, and care for children with chronic conditions, to name a few (CDC, 2006).

A final example of potential funding is the U.S. Department of Veterans Affairs (2006). In the Veterans Affairs (VA) Office of Research and Development, the Rehabilitation Research and Development Service is charged with discovering knowledge, developing VA researchers and health care leaders, and creating innovations that advance health care for veterans and the nation. Rehabilitation Research and Development Centers of Excellence are sites of rehabilitation research throughout the country. Grants for research are available to VA employees. For instance, a rehabilitation nurse scientist directs the Rehabilitation Outcomes Research Center in Gainesville, Florida, where scientists enhance access, quality, and efficiency of rehabilitation services through interdisciplinary research and dissemination activities. The center is affiliated with the University of Florida and Brooks Center for Rehabilitation Studies, where nurse faculty and employees have opportunities to apply for funds and engage in rehabilitation nursing research (U.S. Department of Veterans Affairs, 2006).

RELATIONSHIPS AMONG PRACTICE, RESEARCH, AND THEORY

The value of rehabilitation nursing in the care of persons with disability and chronic illness is maximized through strong connections, which require communication and collaboration, among practice, research endeavors, and theory development.

The research process depends upon researchers posing an important, answerable question derived from practice and collecting and analyzing data to answer the question. Many excellent research textbooks describe the steps in the research process, as well as how to read and critically analyze research reports.

It is conventional to refer to the steps in research, suggesting a linear sequence, whereas the actual process is more likely to involve moving back and forth among these steps. For instance, a researcher may identify a problem for study, formulate hypotheses, design the research, and then need to reformulate the problem as more information about what is known and the realities of the clinical situation are better understood.

One perspective on ways to organize and improve the research endeavor is to view research in terms of levels that build to develop theory, which in turn, guides nursing practice. The purpose of theory is to describe, explain, and predict phenomena. Before any proposed theory can guide practice, an understanding of the concepts involved in the theory is necessary. For example, practice based on a theory of helping individuals cope with disability is possible only if there is a clear understanding of the concepts of coping, patient teaching, and outcome variables, such as independence.

Research based on rehabilitation nurses' experiences in clinical practice ensures that the outcome of the research will be relevant to the very essence of rehabilitation nursing: caring for individuals and groups with actual or potential health problems due to disability and chronic illness. Understanding which nursing actions under which conditions produce which patient outcomes will allow rehabilitation nurses to provide care that can predictably accomplish desired results.

Levels of Research for Theory Development

Describing Phenomena: What Is This? In the first stage of theory development, little is known about the topic or concept and the researcher must ask the question, "What is this?" This question can be answered in a number of ways, using either qualitative or quantitative research methods. Qualitative methods are characterized by the collection of narrative information, conducted in naturalistic rather than controlled research conditions, and inductive or thematic analyses. In contrast, quantitative methods are characterized by the collection of numerical data, relatively controlled research conditions, and statistical analyses. Research at this level relies on literature review, open-ended questions, unstructured observations, interviews and field notes, and exploration of the phenomenon of interest in various settings.

Typically reports of level one research (i.e., "What is it?") fully identify and describe the phenomenon of interest. Data might include a verbal description of a phenomenon, graphs, and/or descriptive statistics. The nursing and social science literatures are replete with descriptions of phenomena and studies that examine coping, adaptation, and the meaning of various disabilities and illnesses for the individual and for family members. Pilkington's work (1999) describing quality of life from the perspective of the person with stroke is representative. Another example is a qualitative study by Rittman et al. (2004) that explored the transition from hospital to home during the first month after an acute stroke and found changes in the temporal aspect of daily order were related to functional impairments.

Mixed methods (qualitative and quantitative data collected and analyzed) have also been used to more fully describe and validate phenomena of interest to rehabilitation nursing. As an illustration, Lucke, Coccia, Goode, and Lucke (2004) completed a mixed-method descriptive, longitudinal, feasibility study to describe and compare perceptions of health-related quality of life in a small group of spinal cord injured persons and their family caregivers during the initial 6 months following rehabilitation. Health-related quality of life instruments (quantitative surveys) and in-depth interviews (qualitative narrative) were undertaken at 1, 3, and 6 months following inpatient rehabilitation. Differences among perceptions of perceived disability suggested that further work was needed to identify critical interventions to improve quality of life during this transition period (Lucke et al., 2004). Regardless of the methods, the ultimate goal is to maximize the complementary strength of multiple methods in exploring phenomena about which little is known (Kroll, Neri, & Miller, 2005).

Secondary analysis of previously collected data is another approach useful to achieve a full description of phenomena. Predeger and Mumma (2004) analyzed narrative data gathered from multiple qualitative studies over a 13-year period to describe the experiences of women living with chronic illness in exploring the notion of connectedness. Connections considered important and sustaining for women were fully described with implications for nursing roles in supporting and facilitating connectedness in chronic illness (Predeger & Mumma, 2004). In another study, Pierce, Steiner, Hicks, and Dawson-Weiss (2007) presented a case report of a 55-year-old husband's perceived experience as a new caregiver while caring for his wife with stroke, as learned from his 1-year of participation in a web-based support intervention. Additional analysis of data previously collected for another project revealed that the spousal caregiver was (1) providing support, (2) offering solutions, and (3) taking control. He spent a significant amount of his energy in creating order and stability within his environment in order to maintain balance in his life. These findings may be useful to identifying and designing interventions for male spousal caregivers new to the role of caring.

Concept analysis is another approach to answering the question "What is this?" Concept analysis is a process of examining written and unwritten sources of information on phenomena to clarify their uses and meaning. An exemplar (Box 4-2) demonstrates a concept analysis that describes human dignity (Jacelon, Connelly, Brown, Proulx, & Vo, 2004). Other examples of concept analyses appropriate to rehabilitation practice include imagery used by athletes in sport injury (Driediger, Hall, & Callow, 2006), self-organization in chronic

---

BOX 4-2 Research Example 1: Describing Phenomena

Jacelon, C., Connelly, T. W., Brown, R., Proulx, K., & Vo, T. (2004). A concept analysis of dignity for older adults. *Journal of Advanced Nursing, 48*(1), 76-83.

The aim of this study was to develop a definition of dignity in older adults. Data were collected concurrently using literature review and focus groups composed of older adults. About 400 abstracts were reviewed, and of these, 130 were read with 80 being included in this review. The literature provided data about professionals' ideas of dignity. Five focus groups were composed of individuals who ranged in age from 65 to 92 years and provided qualitative data about the nature of dignity in older people. Data were synthesized, and the findings revealed that dignity is an inherent, but learned, characteristic of being human. Dignity can be subjectively felt as an attribute of the self and is made manifest through behavior that demonstrates respect for self and others. An individual's dignity is affected by the treatment received from others. Nurses need to develop interventions that foster dignity for older people.

---

pain (Monsivais, 2005), quality of life of orthopedic patients (Mandzuk & McMillan, 2005), and aloneness in elderly women (Pierce, Wilkerson, & Anderson, 2003). Each of these rather abstract ideas was defined and described to more fully explain or examine the concept.

Determining Relationships: What Is Happening Here? Once concepts have been described and analyzed through research, the next step in making these studies applicable to practice is to determine how the concepts are related to one another. The researcher asks, "What is happening here?" Much of rehabilitation nursing research has explored the relationship between concepts. For example, marital status, education, employment, perceived social support, perceived economic adequacy, and their relationship to functional limitation were studied in a large sample of adult women with multiple sclerosis (Clingerman, Stuifbergen, & Becker, 2004). Results showed that unmarried women with less than 12 years of education, who reported disability-related unemployment, and had the least amount of social support and the least economic adequacy, displayed relationships with greater functional limitations.

Other studies examined gender. Heid and Schmelzer (2004) found that gender played a role in women's participation in a cardiac rehabilitation program at a midsize urban hospital in the southwest United States (Box 4-3). Through extensive chart review and follow-up interviews, they determined that women and men were referred equally to the programs, but women were significantly less likely to actually enroll in cardiac rehabilitation programs (Heid & Schmelzer, 2004). In another view of gender, Stiller and Holt (2004) examined variables influencing referrals to cardiac rehabilitation for men and women. They found significant evidence that male physicians were more likely to refer patients to

---

BOX 4-3 **Research Example 2: Determining Relationships**

Heid, H. G., & Schmelzer, M. (2004). Influences on women's participation in cardiac rehabilitation. *Rehabilitation Nursing, 29*(4), 116-121.
This study answered the question, What factors influenced women's decisions to enroll or not enroll in a cardiac rehabilitation program? Two hundred and two hospital charts were reviewed. The mean age of the men (62 years) and women (65 years) was not significantly different (t 1.646 = 0.793, p = <0.05). The researchers found that eligible men and women were equally likely to be referred to the program (chi-square (1) = 0.115, p = 0.734), but women were significantly less likely to enroll (chi-square (1) = 8.756, p = 0.003). The 20 women who did enroll and the 10 women who did not enroll were interviewed to determine factors that influenced their participation in the program. Major factors to enroll included a desire for better health and strength of health care provider's recommendation. Barriers to enrollment were uncovered (e.g., transportation problems, physical limitations, expenses, and concern of family member). All the women who did not enroll showed interest when contacted after hospitalization. Based on these findings, the researchers recommend that staff telephone women after discharge to answer questions, clarify misconceptions, solicit family support, and encourage participation in a cardiac rehabilitation program.

---

cardiac rehabilitation than were their female counterparts. These findings have important implications for practice, especially with the growing awareness of the impact of cardiovascular disease on women's morbidity and mortality.

Qualitative and quantitative studies have been conducted to examine relationships among other variables relevant to rehabilitation nursing practice. For instance, in viewing quality of life after a stroke, Robinson-Smith (2002) studied 63 stroke survivors from an inpatient rehabilitation facility. The researcher found that quality of life and recovery for stroke survivors were enhanced when self-care efficacy was high (Robinson-Smith, 2002). In a study of perceived health and life satisfaction among older adults, the variable of worry was related to lower life satisfaction, negative emotions, physical discomforts, and decreased functional ability (Fakouri & Lyon, 2005). These researchers found that assessment of worry is significant in planning nursing care in the rehabilitation setting (Fakouri & Lyon, 2005). Another exemplar is a longitudinal analysis of illness, coping hopefulness, and mood for 52 persons participating in a 2-year clinical drug trial (Wineman, Schwetz, Zeller, & Cyphert, 2003). Results revealed that participants with higher levels of hopefulness were more effective in coping and had more positive moods, while those individuals with more uncertainty about their disease were likely to be less hopeful with more negative moods (Wineman et al., 2003). Information such as this provides needed insight to guide nursing interventions.

Research designed to determine the relationships among concepts uses more structured observations, asks more precise questions, and uses descriptive statistics to explain the connection among the concepts. Exploring the relationship among concepts is one step further along the continuum of establishing a theoretical base for rehabilitation nursing practice. Research at this level explains how one factor might be manipulated to influence another factor. Descriptive statistics including correlation statistics, *t* tests of group differences, and chi-square tests of independence are useful analytical strategies.

Testing Relationships: What Will Happen If? After phenomena are named and described and research findings have demonstrated that various phenomena are related, the next question that researchers ask is, "What will happen if...?" This stage of theory development is important because it permits testing of relationships that were identified in the previous level of theory development. Factors thought to predict the relationships among the variables are stated and tested. Murrock (2002) conducted a study to examine the effects of music on the rate of perceived exertion and general mood among people with a coronary artery bypass graft enrolled in a cardiac rehabilitation program. The researcher used random assignment to group A (exercise with music, n = 15) or group B (exercise without music, n = 15). The hypothesis that listening to music during exercise would result in a greater decrease in rate of perceived exertion than exercising without music was not supported. The hypothesis that listening to music during exercise would result in a greater increase in general mood than exercising without music was supported (Murrock, 2002). Despite the limitations of a small sample size and a convenience sample, this study contributed to the developing body of knowledge regarding the therapeutic effects of music within rehabilitation settings.

Hiltunen et al. (2005) tested a set of efficacy-enhancing interventions based on social cognitive theory in a sample of individuals 65 years of age and older who had experienced either myocardial infarction or coronary artery bypass graft surgery (n = 248). Participants were randomly assigned to either the treatment group or to usual care. The results of the study supported the use of efficacy-enhancing interventions to promote recovery of elders with cardiac illness (Hiltunen et al., 2005). Another example of testing relationships with caregivers of persons with multiple sclerosis by Stuifbergen, Seraphine, and Roberts (2000) is described in Box 4-4.

Studies that test relationships are more challenging than studies at lower levels of theory development, because they require the specification of necessary and sufficient conditions that will produce a desired effect. The research designs used in studies that test relationships among concepts are similar to the designs used in the studies described in the following category, producing situations. In both of these categories of research, designs are used that exert as much control as is feasible over extraneous variables. Control of extraneous variables allows the researcher to say that the results are due to manipulation of the variables and not to chance interference.

BOX 4-4 Research Example 3: Testing Relationships

Stuifbergen, A. K., Seraphine, A., & Roberts, G. (2000). An explanatory model of health promotion and quality of life in chronic disabling conditions. *Nursing Research, 49*(3), 122-129.

The aim of this study was to test an explanatory model of variables influencing health promotion and quality of life in persons living with the chronic disabling condition of multiple sclerosis (MS). The sample, 786 persons with MS, completed instruments measuring severity of illness-related impairment, barriers to health-promoting behaviors, resources, self-efficacy, acceptance, and perceived quality of life. Antecedent variables accounted for 58% of the variance in the frequency of health-promoting behaviors and 66% of the variance in perceived quality of life. The model supports the hypothesis that quality of life is based on complex interactions among contextual factors, antecedent variables, and health-promoting behaviors. The authors suggest the need for interventions to enhance social support, decrease barriers, and increase self-efficacy with the goal of improving health-promoting behaviors and quality of life.

BOX 4-5 Research Example 4: Producing Situations

Janelli, L. M., Kanski, G. W., & Wu, Y. B. (2005). The influence of individualized music on patients in physical restraints: A pilot study. *Journal of the New York State Nurses Association, 35*(2), 22-27.

This study examined the relationship between listening to preferred music and the behavioral responses of 30 patients, age 65 to 93 years, who were physically restrained. There were three groups. Group 1 patients were out of the restraining devices while listening to music, group 2 patients were out of restraining devices and not listening to music, and group 3 patients were in restraining devices while listening to music. There was no significant effect on decreasing the patients' negative behavior or on increasing positive behavior while listening to preferred music. However, the researchers reported that group 1 patients had higher mean scores for positive behaviors and lower mean scores for negative behaviors. Nurses need to be aware of these findings, because this may suggest some benefits for patients who are out of restraint devices and listening to preferred music.

Producing Situations: How Can X Be Made to Happen? The last stage in theory development is goal oriented and situation producing and has been referred to as prescriptive theory. A prescriptive theory gives directions or rules as to how something should work or be carried out. The question researchers ask is, "How can X be made to happen?" Studies at this level often are referred to as clinical trials, in which researchers test the feasibility of a new treatment, determine the optimal use of a regimen or procedure, or compare the efficacy of two treatments or programs in achieving a desired outcome (Burns & Grove, 2005). An example is an experimental study conducted to determine the effects of music as an alternative to physical restraints in a sample of 40 middle-age and elderly hospitalized patients (Janelli, Kanski, & Wu, 2002). The study was conducted in an acute medical-surgical setting but has relevance for any setting where physical restraints are used. The results of the study supported the use of music as an alternative to physical restraints (Janelli et al., 2002). The researchers were appropriately cautious in the interpretation of their results, based on the small size of the sample and the need for more research in this area. A similar study to extend this work by Janelli, Kanski, and Wu (2005) is presented in Box 4-5.

Another example is the research of Stuifbergen, Becker, Blozis, Timmerman, and Kullberg (2003), who reported the results of a clinical trial conducted to test the effectiveness of a wellness intervention for women with multiple sclerosis. They found a statistically significant effect of the intervention on self-efficacy for health-promoting behaviors and some aspects of quality of life, particularly pain and mental health (Stuifbergen et al., 2003). The researchers were appropriately prudently optimistic in interpreting the findings due to the limitations of a convenience sample and possible selection bias.

Despite these limitations, this study makes important contributions to the knowledge base for providing rehabilitative care to women with chronic illness.

Rehabilitation nursing is building the knowledge basis for understanding the underlying mechanisms for nursing interventions, which precludes the conduct of situation-producing studies related to most rehabilitation nursing phenomena at this time. Testing prescriptive theory requires that the findings be generalized beyond the specific situation. Studies that test theoretical relationships among concepts must be done first.

Application of Research Findings to Practice

The opportunity to explore phenomena related to rehabilitation and to examine how various phenomena are related provides a basis for understanding practice. Further exploration ultimately can lead to confidence that prescriptions for nursing interventions will influence patient outcomes in the expected direction. Unlike the laboratory, where circumstances can be tightly controlled, the clinical arena provides additional challenges related to its complexity.

Research findings are intended to be applied in ways that enhance practice and ultimately improve outcomes. Outcomes research evaluates the impact of care on the outcomes of patients and populations.

Research Utilization and Evidence-Based Practice. Not every nurse needs to be involved in generating research findings, but every nurse is expected to use credible research findings appropriately to improve care. Research utilization processes occur when scientific research is reviewed and critiqued with the findings applied to clinical practice. Evidence-based practice (EBP) represents a broader concept. Evidence-based practice is a systematic process for using research findings to improve practice. The most effective evidence base combines clinical expertise with critical analysis of research results.

Rosswurm and Larrabee's Model (1999). Rosswurm and Larrabee (1999) placed research utilization as a major component of their model for change to EBP. Their model is based in part on earlier research utilization models (Stetler, 1994; White, Leske, & Pearcy, 1995). The steps are (1) assess the need for change in practice, (2) link problem with interventions and outcomes, (3) synthesize best evidence, (4) design practice change, (5) implement and evaluate change in practice, and (6) integrate and maintain change in practice.

The model offers specific guides for each step that can be used by nurses as they work through the changes necessary for incorporating EBP into their routine or setting. In step 1, internal data are collected and compared to external data to determine the need for change. When data indicate a problem with an aspect of practice, discipline-specific or multidiscipline teams come together to discuss and clearly delineate the problem using language of standardized classifications. The problem is linked in step 2 with classification of interventions and outcomes. Classification systems help to define concepts and facilitate communication. For example, Nursing Outcomes Classification (http://www.nursing.uiowa.edu/centers/cncce/noc/nocoverview.htm) and Nursing Interventions Classification (http://www.duke.edu/~goodw010/vocab/NIC.html), used throughout this book, facilitate linkages of outcomes and interventions appropriate for identified nursing diagnoses.

Within step 3 of the model (synthesis), results of both quantitative and qualitative research studies are critically analyzed. Numerous electronic databases are available for searching the literature (e.g., Medical Literature Analysis and Retrieval System Online [MEDLINE] and Cumulative Index to Nursing and Allied Health Literature [CINAHL]). Once the literature is found, a careful critique of the research is done that includes the problem studied, literature reviewed, setting and participants, design, instruments and measures, data analysis, and discussion and conclusions. The scientific and practice components of the research are analyzed at each phase of the critique (Rosswurm & Larrabee, 1999).

The idea that health care decisions should be based on best evidence is unassailably wise and not controversial. One prominent example of formalizing the process for synthesizing clinical evidence for use in health care decision making is the Cochrane Collaboration (CC). The CC is an international nonprofit and independent organization dedicated to making up-to-date, accurate information about the effects of health care readily available worldwide. It produces and disseminates systematic reviews of health care interventions and promotes the search for evidence in the form of clinical trials and other studies of interventions (see Chapter 6). In addition, the AHRQ evidenced-based practice guidelines are also available online to nurses. Their rigorous, evidenced-based approach has made AHRQ guidelines a gold standard in health care. These systematic reviews gather the existing

evidence that may be included in practice guidelines, but they do not create new evidence or knowledge. Additional research may be needed before making decisions to change policy or practice.

The model continues with the fourth, fifth, and sixth steps of its application (Rosswurm & Larrabee, 1999). In step 4 (design) a plan for pilot testing of the proposed change is developed for a particular clinical setting. Step 5 involves the implementation and evaluation of the change in practice, and in step 6 the change is integrated into practice, assuming the pilot study results support such integration. The decision to apply the research to practice may confirm existing practice or require modifying or changing existing practice (Rosswurm & Larrabee, 1999). Pipe, Wellik, Buchda, Hansen, and Martyn (2005) described the use of this model to answer the clinical question "Is there evidence to support the use of an early warning scoring system and communication triggers to guide nurses in clinical decision-making in the medical-surgical environment?" (p. 367).

The Rosswurm and Larrabee model (1999) could be used effectively to guide the process of evaluating evidence for many nursing interventions and professional practice activities of interest to rehabilitation nurses. Box 4-6 provides an example of application of the model to the care of patients with dysphagia.

Critiques of Research Utilization and EBP. One indication of the progress toward EBP is the publication of clinical protocols and guidelines based on systematically evaluated research evidence. Examples include the comprehensive work conducted by Nelson and Baptiste (2004) on safe moving and handling of patients and research-based protocols for the management of constipation (Hinrichs & Huseboe, 2001) and the prevention of pressure ulcers (Frantz, 2004). The National Guideline Clearinghouse (http://www.guideline.gov), an initiative of AHRQ, includes numerous evidence-based protocols of relevance to rehabilitation nursing practice on topics that include hydration management, fall prevention, promoting spirituality, and assessment of stroke complications (AHRQ, 2006b).

Many challenges to research utilization, and more recently to EBP, have been described in the nursing literature (Nicoll & Beyea, 1999; Retsas, 2000). These challenges can be categorized as intrapersonal, interpersonal, and organizational. Some intrapersonal challenges or barriers to research use that have been identified include lack of interest or motivation to use research results, lack of knowledge about the research process, and resistance to change (Estabrooks et al., 2003; Nicoll & Beyea, 1999; Retsas, 2000). Interpersonal barriers include lack of collaboration between researchers and clinicians, research articles not written for clinicians, and lack of availability of consultants to assist clinicians with critically analyzing research articles (Newhouse, Dearholt, Poe, Pugh, & White, 2005).

Factors within organizations or care systems have also been identified as barriers to research utilization and include lack of time and money allocated to research participation,

---

BOX 4-6 Application of Rosswurm and Larrabee's Evidence-Based Practice Model (1999) to Patients With Dysphagia

Step 1. Assess Need for a Change
- Discuss clinical problem of dysphagia with nurse managers, nurses, speech pathologists, and other rehabilitation team members.
- Review quality assurance and risk management data on associated adverse events (primarily choking and dehydration).
- Assess nursing knowledge about dysphagia in patients with neurological and neuromuscular impairment.
- Compare internal data with external data from similar rehabilitation settings.
- Identify from findings the need to improve nursing staff knowledge and care of patients with dysphagia.

Step 2. Link Problem With Interventions and Outcomes
- Link dysphagia with the appropriate Nursing Interventions Classification interventions.
- Include dysphagia management and aspiration prevention activities in nursing protocols.
- Identify outcomes such as fluid intake levels, indicators of nutritional balance, and choking events.

Step 3. Synthesize Best Evidence
- Review literature on dysphagia management.
- Include nurses in critiquing research literature using worksheets.
- Synthesize quantitative and qualitative research evidence.
- Combine research evidence with clinical judgment and contextual data.
- Assess system feasibility and benefits and risks of protocol to patients.

Step 4. Design a Change in Practice
- Include nurses from pilot study units in drafting the evidence-based protocol.
- Prepare forms for pilot study and its evaluation with input from unit nurses.
- Identify tools for measuring outcomes such as fluid intake levels, indicators of nutritional balance, and choking events.
- Educate all nurses on pilot study units in use of the evidence-based protocol.

Step 5. Implement and Evaluate the Practice Change
- Implement pilot study on selected clinical units.
- Monitor use of protocol throughout pilot study period.
- Collect and analyze data.
- Recommend adoption of protocol if indicated by pilot study results.

Step 6. Integrate and Maintain the Practice Change
- Meet with staff nurses on pilot study units to review any revisions.
- Present evidence-based protocol to hospital/agency-wide practice committees.
- Communicate information to administration and collaborating practitioners.
- Conduct in-service education for all nursing staff about the protocol.
- Plan ongoing monitoring of outcomes on all units.

Modified from Rosswurm, M. A., & Larrabee, J. H. (1999). A model for change to evidence-based practice. *Image: Journal of Nursing Scholarship, 31*(4), 317-322.

---

lack of expectation for involvement in the research process, and lack of reward or positive reinforcement for research and research utilization (Newhouse et al., 2005; Pravikoff, Tanner, & Pierce, 2005; Retsas, 2000). All of these challenges or barriers can be reframed as opportunities and, when present, can facilitate practice based on the best available evidence that achieves the best possible outcomes.

Outcomes Research. Outcomes research is concerned with the impact of care on the outcomes of patients and populations. It may also examine and evaluate the quality and/or economic impact linked to health outcomes, such as with quality compared to cost-effectiveness and cost utility. Outcomes research activities increased significantly from 1990

forward, partly in response to the high costs of health care (Kirchhoff & Rakel, 1999; Lutz, 2004). The primary goal of any nursing quality improvement program is the ongoing betterment of the delivery, quality, efficiency, and outcome of patient care and services. This is accomplished through a systematic examination of information provided through ongoing monitoring, evaluation, and improvement activities (see Chapter 9). All quality activities are done in accordance with standards of professional health care practices and regulatory and licensing agencies and support the overall mission and strategic plans of the organization.

The purpose of an outcome study is to measure the effects or impact of a particular clinical program or intervention. Specific documented indicators that serve as measures of patient outcome are selected depending on the purpose of the research. For instance, measures may be data about infection or injury rates, patient satisfaction with care, and number of nursing care hours provided per patient day; or scores documented on standardized tools, such as the functional independence measure (FIM). Additional outcome measures of particular interest for rehabilitation facilities include functional health status, discharge to the community, rates of employment after rehabilitation, postdischarge medical complications, hours of outpatient rehabilitation therapy, and social integration (Hart, Whyte, Polansky, Kersey-Matusiak, & Fidler-Sheppard, 2005; Kirchhoff & Rakel, 1999; Quigley, 1997; Yu & Richmond, 2005).

One ongoing program of rehabilitation outcomes research is located at the Center for Rehabilitation Outcomes Research at the Rehabilitation Institute of Chicago (http://www.ric.org/research/outcomes/). One study at the Center is focused on developing an instrument that would become a comprehensive assessment tool to identify supports and barriers to participation in lifestyle physical activity among person with arthritis; no other comprehensive tool is available (Mallinson, 2006). The knowledge gained from this study has potential to help patients with arthritis and their care providers to develop individualized treatment plans and interventions that would enhance patients' full participation in lifestyle physical activities.

Research Trends

There continue to be many questions about the effect of research on practice and research trends. Rehabilitation nursing research has concentrated on describing the concepts of interest identified by the RNF and others discussed earlier and on exploring how these factors are related. A goal is to establish clearly what the rehabilitation nurse does in practice to bring about specific outcomes for patients in rehabilitation. A proactive approach to developing knowledge based on scientific evidence will inform practice and evaluate rehabilitation outcomes.

What will the future bring for rehabilitation nursing research? Changing health care priorities that reflect ongoing concerns about spiraling health care costs, an emphasis on cost-effectiveness, and an outcome-oriented society will continue to change the landscape of rehabilitation nursing well into the twenty-first century. The integration of theory-guided research and practice will provide solid ground to ensure that rehabilitation nurses are included in whatever health care configuration evolves.

Rehabilitation nursing research will expand the qualitative description of living with chronic illness and disability from the perspective of persons living those experiences. An example is described by Warms, Marshall, Hoffman, and Tyler (2005) in a unique secondary analysis of comments written in the margins of a large pain survey. In addition to promoting dialogue with these researchers, the narrative, subjective experiences of pain offered in the margins provided insight and direction for ways to improve future pain research and

treatment for those who live with the condition (Warms et al., 2005). Studies such as this can encourage critical review, be compared with findings across other studies, and ideally, launch research to develop and test concepts. Studies that relate phenomena in such ways that allow predictions of the rehabilitation outcome for selected indicators or characteristics are critical to advancing the knowledge base for practice.

Single case studies and designs appropriate for small research samples allow inquiries to build on findings from one another. Nurse-led large, multisite studies, as well as emphasis on interdisciplinary/transdisciplinary rehabilitation research with nurses actively involved as members of the research team, will occur as the high-priority areas included in the 2005 RNF Rehabilitation Nursing Research Agenda (ARN, 2006) are addressed. Predictably, EBP guidelines for the care of persons in need of rehabilitation care, such as *Multiple Sclerosis: Best Practices in Nursing Care* (Harris & Halper, 2004), will be developed and implemented. Equally important, interdisciplinary efforts toward EBP, as well as research utilization and outcomes research, will produce guidelines and protocols for practice within rehabilitation settings; innovations in rehabilitation research and practice will follow.

Finally, the information explosion in a highly technological world will continue to expand rehabilitation nursing research beyond national borders; an international collaborative research effort with colleagues across the globe is already occurring. With the World Wide Web connection, opportunities to design and carry out collaborative studies working (virtually) side by side have become a reality. This potential to uncover universal responses to the human condition will strengthen the quality and use of nursing research and add to the body of scientific evidence that guides rehabilitation nursing practice.

CRITICAL THINKING

1. Give at least one example of a clinical problem within your rehabilitation nursing practice that would benefit from research.
   a. Give an example of a research study that answers the question, What is this?
   b. Give an example of a research study that answers the question, What is happening here?
   c. Give an example of a research study that answers the question, What will happen if?
   d. Give an example of a research study that answers the question, How can X be made to happen?
   e. Identify several sources of potential funding for a research study.
2. Describe the state of research utilization in your rehabilitation setting.
   a. What types of research utilization studies have been conducted?
   b. What were the barriers encountered in the application of the outcomes?

c. List some possible strategies that could be used to overcome barriers to research utilization within rehabilitation settings.

3. Discuss what is considered "evidence" for evidence-based practice in your rehabilitation agency or organization.

a. How does evidence-based practice differ from program evaluation and research utilization?

b. Estimate how much of the practice in your rehabilitation setting is actually based on research studies.

c. Are the barriers to research utilization also the same barriers in your setting for evidence-based practice?

d. Are regulatory bodies for your rehabilitation setting demanding evidence-based practice?

REFERENCES

Agency for Healthcare Research and Quality. (2006a). *AHRQ at a glance.* Retrieved August 15, 2006, from http://www.ahrq.gov/.

Agency for Healthcare Research and Quality. (2006b). *Evidence-based practice.* Retrieved August 15, 2006, from http://www.ahrq.gov/.

American Association of Critical-Care Nurses. (2004). *AACN's research priority areas.* Retrieved August 15, 2006, from http://www.aacn.org.

American Nurses Association. (1994). *Education for participation in nursing research.* Retrieved August 15, 2006, from http://www.nursingworld.org/readroom/position/research/rseducat.htm.

Association of Rehabilitation Nurses. (2001). *Role description: The rehabilitation nurse researcher.* Retrieved August 15, 2006, from http://www.rehabnurse.org/profresources/researcher.html.

Association of Rehabilitation Nurses. (2005). *The rehabilitation nursing research agenda.* Retrieved August 15, 2006, from http://www.rehabnurse.org/research/researchagenda.html.

Association of Rehabilitation Nurses. (2006). *Research.* Retrieved August 15, 2006, from www.rehabnurse.org.

Bartels, J. E. (2005). Educating nurses for the 21st century. *Nursing & Health Sciences, 7*(4), 221-225.

Berry, D. (2003). *Oncology Nursing Society research agenda 2003-2005.* Retrieved August 15, 2006, from www.ons.org.

Burns, N., & Grove, S. (2005). *The practice of nursing research: Conduct, critique and utilization* (5th ed.). St. Louis, MO: Elsevier Saunders.

Centers for Disease Control and Prevention. (2006). *Office of Public Health Research: Developing the CDC health protection research guide, 2006-2015.* Retrieved August 14, 2006, from www.cdc.gov.

Clingerman, E., Stuifbergen, A., & Becker, H. (2004). The influence of resources on perceived functional limitations among women with multiple sclerosis. *Journal of Neuroscience Nursing, 36*(6), 312-321.

Conn, V. S. (2004). Editorial: Building a research trajectory. *Western Journal of Nursing Research, 26*(6), 592-594.

Conn, V. S. (2005). Editorial: Postdoctoral research preparation. *Western Journal of Nursing Research, 27*(7), 799-801.

Driediger, M., Hall, C., & Callow, N. (2006). Imagery use by injured athletes: A qualitative analysis. *Journal of Sports Sciences, 24*(3), 261-271.

Estabrooks, C. A., Floyd, J. A., Scott-Findlay, S., O'Leary, K. A., & Gushta, M. (2003). Individual determinants of research utilization: A systematic review. *Journal of Advanced Nursing, 43*(5), 506-520.

Fakouri, C., & Lyon, B. (2005). Perceived health and life satisfaction among older adults: The effects of worry and personal variables. *Journal of Gerontological Nursing, 31*(10), 17-24.

Frantz, R. A. (2004). Evidence-based protocol treatment of pressure ulcers. *Journal of Gerontological Nursing, 30*(5), 4-10.

Gordon, D. L., Sawin, K. J., & Basta, S. M. (1996). Developing research priorities for rehabilitation nursing. *Rehabilitation Nursing Research, 5*(2), 60-66.

Harris, C., & Halper, J. (2004). *Multiple sclerosis: Best practices in nursing care.* Denmark: BioScience Communications. Retrieved August 15, 2006, from http://www.neura.net/channels/1.asp?id=370.

Hart, T., Whyte, J., Polansky, M., Kersey-Matusiak, G., & Fidler-Sheppard, R. (2005). Community outcomes following traumatic brain injury: Impact of race and preinjury status. *Journal of Head Trauma Rehabilitation, 20*(2), 158-172.

Heid, H. G., & Schmelzer, M. (2004). Influences on women's participation in cardiac rehabilitation. *Rehabilitation Nursing, 29*(4), 116-121.

Hiltunen, E. F., Winder, P. A., Rait, M. A., Buselli, E. F., Carroll, D. L., & Rankin, S. H. (2005). Implementation of efficacy enhancement nursing interventions with cardiac elders. *Rehabilitation Nursing, 30*(6), 221-229.

Hinrichs, M. D., & Huseboe, J. (2001). Research-based protocol: Management of constipation. *Journal of Gerontological Nursing, 27*(2), 17-28.

Hoeman, S. P., Dayhoff, N. E., & Thompson, T. C. (1993). The initial RNF research survey: Rehabilitation nursing research interests of ARN members. *Rehabilitation Nursing, 18*(1), 40-42.

Jacelon, C., Connelly, T. W., Brown, R., Proulx, K., & Vo, T. (2004). A concept analysis of dignity for older adults. *Journal of Advanced Nursing, 48*(1), 76-83.

Jacelon, C., Pierce, L., & Buhrer, R. (2006). Evaluation of the research agenda for rehabilitation nursing. *Rehabilitation Nursing, 31*(6), 242-248.

Jacelon, C., Pierce, L., & Buhrer, R. (2007). Revision of the research agenda for rehabilitation nursing. *Rehabilitation Nursing 32*(1), 23-30.

Janelli, L. M., Kanski, G. W., & Wu, Y. B. (2002). Individualized music—A different approach to the restraint issue. *Rehabilitation Nursing, 27*(6), 221-226.

Janelli, L. M., Kanski, G. W., & Wu, Y. B. (2005). The influence of individualized music on patients in physical restraints: A pilot study. *Journal of the New York State Nurses Association, 35*(2), 22-27.

Kirchhoff, K. T., & Rakel, B. A. (1999). Outcomes evaluation. In M. Mateo & K. Kirchhoff (Eds.), *Using and conducting nursing research in the clinical setting* (2nd ed., pp. 76-89). Philadelphia: W. B. Saunders.

Kroll, T., Neri, M. T., & Miller, K. (2005). Using mixed methods in disability and rehabilitation research. *Rehabilitation Nursing, 30*(3), 106-113.

Lucke, K. T., Coccia, H., Goode, J. S., & Lucke, J. F. (2004). Quality of life in spinal cord injured individuals and their caregivers during the initial 6 months following rehabilitation. *Quality of life research: An international journal of quality of life aspects of treatment, care and rehabilitation, 13*(1), 97-110.

Lutz, B. J. (2004). Determinants of discharge destination for stroke patients. *Rehabilitation Nursing, 29*(5), 154-163.

Mack, M. J. (1952). The personal adjustment of chronically ill old people under home care. *Nursing Research, 1*(1), 9-31.

Mallinson, T. (2006). *Development of an instrument to promote physical activity in persons with arthritis.* Retrieved August 15, 2006, from http://www.ric.org/research/outcomes/arth_phys.php.

Mandzuk, L. L., & McMillan, D. E. (2005). A concept analysis of quality of life. *Journal of Orthopaedic Nursing, 9*(1), 12-18.

Monsivais, D. (2005). Self-organization in chronic pain: A concept analysis. *Rehabilitation Nursing, 30*(4), 147-151.

Murrock, C. J. (2002). The effects of music on the rate of perceived exertion and general mood among coronary artery bypass graft patients enrolled in cardiac rehabilitation phase II. *Rehabilitation Nursing, 27*(6), 227-231.

National Center for Medical Rehabilitation Research. (2005). *Seven priority areas.* Retrieved August 14, 2006, from http://www.nichd.nih.gov/ncmrr/seven.htm.

National Center for Medical Rehabilitation Research. (2006). *Congressional budget justification FY 2007.* Retrieved August 14, 2006, from http://www.nichd.nih.gov/about/about.cfm.

National Institute of Nursing Research. (2006a). A brief history of the NINR. Retrieved August 14, 2006, from http://ninr.nih.gov/ninr/about/history.html.

National Institute of Nursing Research. (2006b). *Division of extramural activities.* Retrieved August 15, 2006, from http://ninr.nih.gov/ninr/index.html.

National Institute on Disability and Rehabilitation Research. (2006). *Welcome to NIDRR!* Retrieved August 15, 2006, from http://www.ed.gov/about/offices/list/osers/nidrr/index.html.

National Institutes of Health. (2005). *Setting research priorities at the National Institutes of Health.* Retrieved August 14, 2006, from http://www.nih.gov/about/researchpriorities.htm.

National Institutes of Health. (2006). *Research and training opportunities at the National Institutes of Health.* Retrieved August 15, 2006, from http://www.training.nih.gov/.

Nelson, A., & Baptiste, A. S. (2004). Evidence-based practices for safe patient handling and movement. *Online Journal of Issues in Nursing, 9*(3). Retrieved August 15, 2006, from http://www.nursingworld.org/ojin/topic25/tpc25_3.htm.

Newhouse, R., Dearholt, S., Poe, S., Pugh, L. C., & White, K. M. (2005). Evidence-based practice: A practical approach to implementation. *Journal of Nursing Administration, 35*(1), 35-40.

Nicoll, L. H., & Beyea, S. C. (1999). Research utilization. In J. A. Fain (Ed.), *Reading, understanding and applying nursing research* (pp. 261-280). Philadelphia: F. A. Davis.

Nightingale, F. (1859/1946). *Notes on nursing: What it is and what it is not.* Philadelphia: J. B. Lippincott.

Pierce, L. (2005). Rehabilitation nurses working as collaborative research teams. *Rehabilitation Nursing, 30*(4), 132-139.

Pierce, L., Steiner, V., Hicks, B., & Dawson-Weiss, J. (2007). Perceived experience of caring for a wife with stroke: A case report. *Rehabilitation Nursing, 32*(1), 35-40

Pierce, L., Wilkinson, L., & Anderson, J. (2003). Analysis of the concept of aloneness as applied to older women being treated for depression. *Journal of Gerontological Nursing, 29*(7), 20-25.

Pilkington, F. B. (1999). A qualitative study of life after stroke. *Journal of Neuroscience Nursing, 31*(6), 336-347.

Pipe, T. B., Wellik, K. E., Buchda, V. L., Hansen, C. M., & Martyn, D. R. (2005). Implementing evidence-based nursing practice. *Urologic Nursing, 25*(5), 365-370.

Pravikoff, D. S., Tanner, A. B., & Pierce, S. T. (2005). Readiness of U.S. nurses for evidence-based practice: Many don't understand or value research and have had little or no training to help them find evidence on which to base their practice. *American Journal of Nursing, 105*(9), 40-52.

Predeger, E., & Mumma, C. (2004). Connectedness in chronic illness: Women's journeys. *International Journal for Human Caring, 8*(1), 13-19.

Quigley, P. (1997). Program evaluation and measurement of outcomes. In K. Johnson (Ed.), *Advanced practice nursing in rehabilitation: A core curriculum* (pp. 277-285). Glenview, IL: Association of Rehabilitation Nurses.

Retsas, A. (2000). Barriers to using research evidence in nursing practice. *Journal of Advanced Nursing, 31*(3), 599-606.

Rittman, M., Faircloth, C., Boylstein, C., Gubrium, J. F., Williams, C., Van Puymbroeck, M., et al. (2004). The experience of time in the transition from hospital to home following stroke. *Journal of Rehabilitation Research & Development, 41*(3A), 259-268.

Robinson-Smith, G. (2002). Self-efficacy and quality of life after stroke. *Journal of Neuroscience Nursing, 34*(2), 91-98.

Rosswurm, M. A., & Larrabee, J. H. (1999). A model for change to evidence-based practice. *Image: Journal of Nursing Scholarship, 31*(4), 317-322.

Sigma Theta Tau International. (2005). *Global health and nursing research priorities resource paper.* Retrieved August 15, 2006, from http://www.nursingsociety.org/research/main.html.

Steels, M. M. (1976). Perceptual style and the adaptation of the aged to the hospital environment. *ARN Journal, 1*(6), 9-14.

Stetler, C. B. (1994). Refinement of the Stetler/Marram model for application of research findings to practice. *Nursing Outlook, 42*(1), 15-25.

Stiller, J. J., & Holt, M. M. (2004). Factors influencing referral of cardiac patients for cardiac rehabilitation. *Rehabilitation Nursing, 29*(1), 18-23.

Stuifbergen, A. K., Becker, H., Blozis, S., Timmerman, G., & Kullberg, V. (2003). A randomized clinical trial of a wellness intervention for women with multiple sclerosis. *Archives of Physical Medicine & Rehabilitation, 84*(4), 467-476.

Stuifbergen, A. K., Seraphine, A., & Roberts, G. (2000). An explanatory model of health promotion and quality of life in chronic disabling conditions. *Nursing Research, 49*(3), 122-129.

U.S. Department of Veterans Affairs. (2006). *Rehabilitation research and development service.* Retrieved August 15, 2006, from http://www1.va.gov/resdev/programs/rrd.cfm.

Verhonick, P. J. (1961). Decubitus ulcer observations measured objectively. *Nursing Research, 10,* 211-218.

Warms, C. A., Marshall, H. M., Hoffman, A. J., & Tyler, E. J. (2005). There are a few things you did not ask about my pain: Writing on the margins of a survey questionnaire. *Rehabilitation Nursing, 30*(6), 248-256.

White, J. M., Leske, J. S., & Pearcy, J. M. (1995). Models and processes of research utilization. *Nursing Clinics of North America, 30*(3), 409-420.

Wineman, N. M., Schwetz, K. M., Zeller, R., & Cyphert, J. (2003). Longitudinal analysis of illness uncertainty, coping, hopefulness, and mood during participation in a clinical drug trial. *Journal of Neuroscience Nursing, 35*(2), 100-106.

Yu, F., & Richmond, T. (2005). Factors affecting outpatient rehabilitation outcomes in elders. *Journal of Nursing Scholarship, 37*(3), 229-236.

5

Outcome-Directed Patient and Family Education

Maureen L. Habel, MA, RN, CRRN

Rehabilitation nurses have an essential duty to provide quality patient and family education. Effective education helps patients learn to live with a chronic or disabling condition in their own environment and as independently as possible. The education process promotes independence by helping patients acquire new information, develop self-care skills that they can competently apply to functional activities, develop adaptive behaviors to manage the illness or impairment, and prevent further disability. Outcomes are measured by the person's ability to incorporate new health behaviors into a preferred lifestyle. The following examples illustrate challenges that rehabilitation nurses face in teaching critical self-care skills and achieving desirable outcomes in a dynamic health and social environment. We will discuss four patients and their families whose unique learning needs are influenced by limited rehabilitation stays, cultural differences, limited English literacy, and the impact of the Internet. Henry and Sarah Wall own a small upholstery shop. Mr. Wall bids out work and supervises their small staff; Mrs. Wall does all the skilled finish sewing. Eight days ago, Mrs. Wall had a left hemisphere stroke, leaving her aphasic and with right extremity weakness. Mrs. Wall's insurance pays for a limited amount of inpatient rehabilitation. The entire family is concerned about how they will meet her care needs when she returns home. June Tang emigrated to the United States from Cambodia 8 years ago. Mrs. Tang has severe chronic obstructive pulmonary disease (COPD) and requires increasing assistance with activities of daily living (ADLs). Mrs. Tang does not speak English and is suspicious of Western medical practices. Her daughter has a full-time job and small children. As a result, she has little time to visit her mother or to participate in a rehabilitation education program. Mac Mowery, a maintenance man at an apartment complex, has had poorly controlled type 2 diabetes for 6 years and now has a diabetic foot ulcer. Mr. Mowery also has a history of seizures and has had several serious falls in the past. His wife, Susan, is a frequent visitor; however, she reads at a fifth-grade level, and her husband is illiterate. Sally Hirsch has had rheumatoid arthritis for 4 years. She is an avid Internet user and often seeks opinions about arthritis treatment she has found online.

FORMING PARTNERSHIPS: A CHANGING EDUCATION PARADIGM

Until the mid–twentieth century, acute disease was the primary health problem in the United States. Health care professionals dictated treatment, transmitted specific limited information to patients, and maintained control over health care. Following World War II, patient education became a priority as young adults with acquired disabilities spent weeks and months learning skills that enabled them to manage their needs in daily life. In the twenty-first century, chronic diseases are the major cause of disability, and the reason for the majority of health expenditures.

The prevalence and consequences of chronic, disabling conditions significantly alters the responsibilities and relationships between health care professionals and the patients for whom they provide care. The model of expert provider and passive recipient of information and care no longer apply. Persons with chronic conditions expect to have specific information about their disease, its implications, available treatments, and the impact of an altered health status on their lifestyle. Consumers demand that care be continuous and coordinated, including management of the physical and psychosocial consequences of their condition (Holman, 2004). Acknowledging that chronic conditions are not curable, a person's continuous participation in health practices that maximize health and prevent disability is essential. Ideally, a patient will become the knowledgeable expert about the consequences of the condition and apply that knowledge to its long-term management. Ultimately, patients and health professionals who share complementary knowledge achieve better outcomes in the health maintenance process.

The Arthritis Self-Management Program is a model that has decreased physician visits and reduced pain despite an increase in physical disability (Holman, 2004). Key elements of the program include solving disease-related problems, managing medications, using cognitive strategies to control symptoms, coping with emotional responses, practicing communication skills to build partnerships with health professionals, and learning how to access community resources (Holman, 2004). A group visit program developed by the Kaiser Health System in Denver is another example of the positive effects of developing collaborative partnerships. This program allows patients with chronic disease to meet regularly with a physician and nurse to discuss an agenda set by the patients. Over a period of time, the discussions address most of the information the patients seek (Holman, 2004). Improved health outcomes occurred in addition to benefits the patients participating in these programs received from their medical care (Holman, 2004). One of the most important outcomes of these learning experiences was growth in self-efficacy—the confidence that one can achieve a goal. Individuals participating in both programs reported that learning from and helping other patients solve problems was the most important part of their experiences (Holman, 2004).

Partnering with patients requires more than mutual agreement about treatment decisions. To work as partners, health care professionals must value the patient's role in health and wellness (Huffman, 2005). This shift parallels a growing consumer movement in health care in which the consumer has access to health information via television, print media, and the Internet and expects to participate in health care decisions (Allen, 2002).

Nurses and other rehabilitation team members have an obligation to provide patients with understandable information and to collaboratively develop learning goals. *It is essential for the nurse educator to remember that patients* **cannot** *follow health care instructions they do not understand and* **will not** *follow recommendations they do not agree with.*

PATIENT EDUCATION

Patient education empowers learners by giving them the knowledge and skills needed to manage their own care and to have control over their lives. A reduced length of stay is a significant barrier to providing effective learning experiences. Patients come to rehabilitation more acutely ill than in the past and have less education provided while in acute care. The need to teach about acute and comorbid conditions reduces the opportunity for learning about rehabilitation skills and coping (Allen, 2002). As a result, the rehabilitation team needs to concentrate on a few priority learning goals and design an education plan that can continue in the community. Time constraints require that each contact with the patient and family become a "teachable moment," and all interactions should be seen as an opportunity to help patients, their family members, or other caregivers learn new skills and incorporate adaptive behaviors into their lifestyles (Allen, 2002).

Renewed emphasis on patient and family education began in 1993 when The Joint Commission (TJC) incorporated patient education standards into its guidelines. TJC (2004) has continued to refine the standards addressing patient-family education with the stated goal of improving patient health care outcomes by promoting healthy behaviors and involving patients in care and care decisions. The Commission on Accreditation of Rehabilitation Facilities (CARF) (2004) also addresses education in its standards. Accreditation standards describe patient education as an interactive, outcome-oriented process that is a primary responsibility of hospitals. Continued emphasis placed on patient and family education by accreditation organizations has helped support patient education efforts that have previously struggled for resources and recognition. The rehabilitation nursing philosophy of helping patients, families, or communities learn to be as independent as possible also recognizes the central role of patient education in nursing practice (Allen, 2002).

CONCEPTUAL FOUNDATIONS OF PATIENT EDUCATION

An outcome-based approach to patient education requires learning about multiple factors that produce behavior change and tailoring teaching strategies to meet individual needs. Theories and models from the social sciences can help rehabilitation nurses learn about how behavior change occurs (Table 5-1).

Health Belief Model

The health belief model (HBM) (Becker, 1974) describes a sequence of stages necessary for behavior change. According to the HBM, people are more receptive to education when they believe (1) they are personally at risk of acquiring a health problem, (2) the risk is serious enough to affect their lives negatively, (3) the benefits of action outweigh the barriers to action, and (4) they are confident they can take action to that improve their health status. Rehabilitation nurses can use the HBM to assess an individual's readiness to participate in health behavior change and can customize strategies to encourage and reinforce change efforts. For example, the nurse can provide information about risks and consequences of inaction to the patient who is unaware of risk factors. In working with a person who acknowledges the risk but sees barriers to change as overwhelming, the nurse can develop strategies that focus on problem solving to minimize or overcome barriers.

Self-Efficacy Theory

Self-efficacy theory (Bandura, 1997), a social learning theory, considers an individual's self-efficacy or confidence in his or her ability to perform a specific behavior. A person with low self-efficacy is less likely to change behavior than a person with high self-efficacy. Educators can help increase self-efficacy by developing educational interventions that build confidence so that patients can accomplish the desired health care behavior (Robinson-Smith, Johnston, & Allen, 2000). Factors that help

TABLE 5-1 Education and Behavioral Models and Theories

Theory	Theorist	Summary	Application
Health belief model	Hochbaum	Framework developed to predict health behaviors and understand motivation and decision making.	Assess what is needed for behavioral change; select teaching strategies based on patient's stage of readiness for behavioral change.
Self-efficacy model	Bandura	A social learning theory that looks at the role of a person's confidence in learning a new health behavior.	Plan education to build a person's confidence; break tasks into small, achievable parts and give learner recognition and reinforcement.
Locus of control	Wallston	An individual's belief about whether personal behaviors results in outcomes; persons who believe they are in control of their health status are more likely to change behavior than those who believe forces outside themselves are in control.	Design strategies to assist those with an external locus of control to achieve goals.
Cognitive dissonance	Festinger, Lewin	Sense of discomfort (dissonance) occurs due to conflict between two beliefs, attitudes, or emotions.	Plan education to foster discomfort with present behavior; when change occurs, work to keep dissonance low.
Developmental theories	Erickson, Piaget, Duvall	The individual's developmental level influences learning.	Match teaching strategies to the person's developmental level.
Adult learning theory	Knowles	Adults are self-directed learners who are concerned with managing and solving their own problems. Adult learners bring life experiences to the learning situations; internal motivators are stronger than external motivators for change.	Educator is the facilitator of learning; learner takes active role in developing learning goals and objectives. Learning is problem centered with opportunity for application.

build self-efficacy include helping the person see that a task is achievable; breaking down complex tasks into small, sequential parts that are easier to perform; providing opportunities to repeat the task; and recognizing success.

Locus of Control

Locus of control (LOC) is a social psychology theory that describes individuals' beliefs about how much control they have over their own health and the relationship between behavior and outcomes. Those with an internal LOC believe their own actions influence outcomes; thus they are more likely to accept responsibility for personal health practices. Persons with an external LOC believe that external forces, fate, God, or authority figures are responsible for outcomes (Wallston, Wallston, & DeVellis, 1978). When an external LOC stems from a cultural belief, patients are unlikely to change behaviors. LOC can be evaluated during an educational needs assessment. In developing a teaching plan, patients with an internal LOC will be receptive; for those with external LOC, the educator can suggest actions to reach specific goals without focusing on patient responsibility.

Cognitive Dissonance Theory

This social theory (Festinger, 1957) is useful in identifying motivators that can influence behavior change through education. Cognitive dissonance is the sense of discomfort individuals

feel when what they do differs from what they believe. This difference produces a sense of discomfort that individuals strive to reduce. For instance, a woman may be overweight; she knows it is unhealthy and feels uncomfortable being overweight. The discomfort she feels may make her receptive to reading information on healthy eating and taking steps to change her eating habits. Educators can use any dissonance on the patient's part to motivate behavior change (Allen, 2002).

Developmental Theory

An individual's developmental level is an important factor to consider in designing an effective education plan. Developmental frameworks such as those described by Erickson, Piaget, and Duvall, which are taught in nursing education programs as a basis for assessment and intervention, are useful in preparing age-appropriate teaching plans.

Adult Learning Theory

Knowles (1984) developed the dominant theory about how adults learn. His model of adult learning is based on several key assumptions (Box 5-1). Because most rehabilitation patients are adult learners, teaching strategies are designed to be problem centered, and the learner helps develop objectives and evaluates learning. Full application of adult learning principles requires learners who are willing to take responsibility for directing their own learning and are comfortable in this role. This condition may not always exist because of patients' previous educational experiences, response to their illness or disability, or the presence of a cognitive or related impairment.

Pratt (1988) proposed a framework for examining teaching-learning situations based on the degree of direction and support needed by the learner. In the first phase, learners need both direction and support because they lack both content knowledge and confidence in their ability to learn unfamiliar information and skills. In the second phase, learners need direction in mastering content but need less direct support because they are becoming more confident about their learning potential. In the third phase, learners continue to need support but are increasingly self-directed in determining content needs and require less direction. In the last phase, learners provide their own direction and support. This framework uses the principles of adult learning but allows for the reality that in some situations learners may be unable or unwilling to assume responsibility for their own learning. It allows the rehabilitation nurse to assess individual learning needs and to develop a teaching plan that capitalizes on the nurse's content expertise in areas that the patient might be totally unfamiliar with, such as bowel and bladder management.

The Transtheoretical Model of Change

The Transtheoretical Model of Change (TMM) describes states that are associated with behavior change (Prochaska & Velicer, 1997). This model has been successfully applied to a variety of health behaviors, including smoking cessation, weight control, condom use for human immunodeficiency virus (HIV) protection, mammography screening, and the use of sunscreen to prevent skin cancer (University of Rhode Island, 2005). The TTM involves five change stages: precontemplation, contemplation, preparation, action, and maintenance. Precontemplation is the stage at which there is no intention to change behavior in the foreseeable future.

In the contemplation stage an individual is aware that a problem exists and is considering behavior change but has not yet made a commitment to act. In the third stage, preparation, the person expresses the intention to take action in the near future. In the action state the person modifies his or her behavior, experiences, or environment in order to confront the health care problem. The action stage involves the most overt behavior changes and requires a commitment of time and energy. During maintenance, the stage in which the individual strives to prevent a return to the previous unhealthy state, the focus is on consolidating gains achieved during the action state (University of Rhode Island, 2005). Traditional change interventions often assume that individuals are ready for an immediate and permanent behavior change. In contrast, the TMM makes no assumptions about how willing individuals are to participate in behavior change but recognizes that educational interventions must be personalized because individuals are in different stages.

THE NURSE AS EDUCATOR

Because patient education has always been an integral part of their practice, rehabilitation nurses need to develop knowledge and skill as educators. Although it often assumed that anyone with a health care background could provide patient education, helping patients and families to make behavior change is a complex process. In addition to teaching patients and families, rehabilitation nurses may participate in teaching other health care professionals and ancillary nursing staff. Some rehabilitation team members have received little or no formal training to prepare them to conduct patient education. As nurses work with other rehabilitation team members, they can help improve the team's overall educational expertise by coordinating, developing, and sharing patient education principles and strategies.

Benner's Model

In basic nursing education programs nurses learn the basics about learning theories and methods and have opportunities to develop teaching plans for individuals and groups. As with other aspects of professional development, nurses gain increasing expertise with continuing education and experience (Benner, 1985, 2001). Benner describes a model of nursing career development that progresses from advanced beginner to competent to proficient and eventually to expert practice. Her model is useful in acknowledging the educational developmental needs of rehabilitation nurses (Allen, 2002). Nurses new to rehabilitation may be more concerned with learning new information themselves than in meeting the unique teaching needs of patients and families. They may lack experience in adapting teaching to patients who have a wide range of impairments and chronic conditions. For example, the novice rehabilitation nurse may not recognize how to select appropriate teaching strategies for a person with sensory-perceptual deficits (Table 5-2). Academic and continuing education, in-service programs, self-study, and mentoring

TABLE 5-2 Teaching Strategies: Patients With Sensory-Perceptual Deficits

Deficit	Teaching Strategy
Deficit in one or more sensory areas (e.g., vision, hearing, touch)	Engage intact senses in learning.
Neglect/visual field cuts	Identify area of intact vision, and direct teaching methods to area where perception is unimpaired.
Short attention span/inability to focus or maintain attention	Break learning into small concepts, and use short teaching segments. Vary topics to hold interest and keep person engaged. Alternate using cognitive and psychomotor domains; stimulate all intact senses.
Impaired directional concepts	In teaching, use environmental cues rather than directional cues. For example, say, "Pull your slacks toward your waist" rather than "Pull your slacks up."
Altered perception of body part or position	Patient may respond better to gestures indicating the body part rather than words; touch the body part when teaching the person to dress or move a part.
Apraxia (inability to perform a previously learned action)	Give instructions that refer to a goal rather than to a specific action. For example, say, "Get dressed" rather than "Put your arm into your shift sleeve."
Agnosia (inability to recognize familiar objects and symbols by means of senses)	Use alternate senses to help the patient recognize an object. For example, if the person cannot recognize an object by sight, he or she may know it by touch.

are ways nurses can become expert patient and family educators.

The Effective Patient Educator

The effective patient educator knows what needs to be taught, thinks critically, communicates effectively, is aware of her or his attitudes and values, respects the learner, creates a caring environment, includes the patient as a participant, and monitors and evaluates the education process. Knowledge of and comfort with teaching content is vital for effective patient education. The insecure teacher may impart inadequate or inaccurate information or no information at all. Although no one can expect to be expert in all areas, it is a professional responsibility to keep abreast of research and practice changes in the rehabilitations population for which one provides care. Not everyone is comfortable teaching all topics. For example, learning about alterations in sexual functioning is important for many individuals with disabilities. A nurse who is both knowledgeable and comfortable with this topic should teach this important information.

Critical thinking skills are crucial for assessing learning needs, developing teaching plans, solving problems, and conducting and evaluating patient education. As an educator, the nurse must clearly identify what must be learned and initiate a timely, effective teaching plan.

All aspects of communication influence the teaching-learning process. The educator is an active listener who communicates not only with words but also with the eyes, gestures, body language, and voice inflection. Barriers to communication may be one's own attitudes and values, the language used to communicate, or environmental distractions. Simple, factual information that is to the point is most effective. An effective educator recognizes patient and family concerns; has empathy, patience, and sensitivity to the person's mood; and allows sufficient time to encourage questions and to address concerns. Effective educators also focus on avoiding common teaching errors (Box 5-2).

BOX 5-2 Common Teaching Errors

- Ignoring the restrictions of the patient's environment
- Not accepting that the patient has the right to change his or her mind
- Failing to negotiate goals
- Duplicating teaching the other team members have done
- Overloading the patient with information
- Choosing the wrong time for teaching
- Not evaluating what the patient has learned

From Habel, M. (2005). *Putting patient teaching into practice* (pp. 139-140). King of Prussia, PA: Nursing Spectrum Continuing Education.

THE LEARNING PROCESS IN REHABILITATION

The familiar steps of the nursing process apply to patient education. Documentation of education process is vital to ensure that learning is a continuous process (Figure 5-1).

Assessing Learning Needs

Assessment of the patient's educational needs, the first step in the educational process, should begin at admission and continue throughout the patient's stay. Assessment yields basic data for a teaching plan, including determining learner needs, evaluating what is already known and what the patient wants and needs to know, patient and family learning readiness and learning style, and factors that affect learning. Assessment also provides the opportunity to develop rapport with the patient and to start building a helping relationship (Pestonjee, 2000). Important assessment areas include the person's age, cognitive and developmental level, sex, occupation, culture, language proficiency, educational level, motivation, belief system, access to caregivers, and ability to teach others.

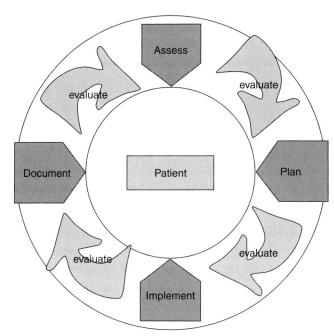

Figure 5-1 Model of patient education.

The patient's functional limitations, social needs, psychological needs, and vocational considerations influence learning needs. Asking questions such as "Which hand do you use to eat with?" "Do you use mobility aids?" or "Does your apartment building have an elevator?" will provide clues about functional limitations that affect mobility and self-care. Social needs are also an important consideration. How has the impairment compromised the patient's life roles? For example, if the patient was the sole financial support of the family before the disability, how will this role be fulfilled in the future? Other social factors include living arrangements, whether the patient owns or rents a home or apartment, who else will live with him or her or provide help, whether the patient is married, whether there are children in the home, and whether the environment is accessible and safe (Allen, 2002).

Anxiety and depression are powerful psychological emotions that can interfere with learning. Patients may feel overwhelmed by a sense of hopelessness. They may experience grief, despair, and discouragement as they realize the changes imposed on their lives by disease or disability. Instilling hope and dispelling hopelessness are an important part of patient education. A patient and family may use denial or rationalization to protect them from the reality of the situation. For example, a person with a spinal cord injury who has not acknowledged or accepted functional losses will be unlikely to learn about a bowel management program. Common reactions of those who are anxious or in denial are to "not hear" what they are told; they may even deny later that the information was ever presented. Incorporating strategies such as repetition and reinforcement into teaching when a patient has a great deal of anxiety or denial may help transmit the information (Allen, 2002).

Vocational counseling and training may be needed to address unemployment or loss of job-related skills. How patients understand the course of illnesses or disability, how they view relationships, and their lifestyle preferences are important factors in developing an effective educational plan. For example, does the patient with an amputation understand the relationship between peripheral vascular disease and smoking? Does the patient with a stroke see the relationship between heart disease and decreased endurance? An individual's knowledge level may not relate to the length of time he or she has experienced an impairment or illness because knowledge about the condition may be inaccurate, incomplete, or obsolete (Allen, 2002).

Assessing Learning Readiness

Learning readiness refers to how likely a person is to participate in behavioral change (Habel, 2005). Many factors influence learning readiness. The physiological capacity to learn depends on more than neuromuscular functioning; any previous or current physical or psychological limitations can significantly impair learning readiness. Immediate basic needs, such as pain relief or anxiety, or limitations, such as joint stiffness from arthritis, sensory deficits, or decreased cardiac reserve, take priority over learning. In addition, the physiological capacity for learning needed skills may not have been reestablished during shortened stays in rehabilitation. For example, a young man with paraplegia spends 5 days in acute care and then spends 2 weeks on the rehabilitation unit. This may not allow sufficient time before discharge to resolve the spinal shock resulting from the trauma to the spinal cord. His physiological capacity for any learning is poor. His bowel and bladder program will not be established and will need continued adjustment at home. As spinal shock resolves, he may experience new problems, such as spasticity. As a result, he, his family members, or other caregivers will need to know how to anticipate and solve potential problems.

Awareness of and sensitivity to family needs must be an ongoing focus. How well family members adapt and their readiness to participate actively in the learning process are significant factors in the patient's ability to achieve positive health outcomes. Families with close relationships before the onset of injury or disability are more likely to have positive attitudes and demonstrate supportive behaviors that enhance the patient's rehabilitation and successful community reentry. Conversely, in families where hostility, alienation, or other negative attitudes prevail, the support system is likely to be less effective.

Another important factor is how the learner feels toward the family member designated as the "backup" learner; compatibility between the patient and the designated family member facilitates carryover of learning. The family member should realize that he or she backs up the patient and provides assistance only with activities the patient is unable to perform. Providing information about the impairment and management options throughout the rehabilitation process enhances family participation. The perceptions and concerns of the family about the care required and its impact on family functioning are important considerations.

Assessing Learning Style

Learning style refers to the way in which an individual receives, processes, organizes, and comprehends information (Marcy, 2001). Taking time to answer the question "How does this person learn best?" helps the nurse to plan strategies that result in positive learning outcomes within the shortest time period. Assessing a patient's preferred learning style can be done by a formal method such as using a learning style questionnaire or by informally asking the patient to share details about the best learning experience he or she ever had. Learning style is influenced by previous learning experiences. For example, individuals with low literacy skills may recall very unpleasant experiences in school, especially with written or complex material.

Some individuals are visual learners; others learn by listening or by doing. Visual learners prefer pictures, posters, videos, and diagrams (Hamilton, 2005). When teaching someone who is a visual learner, the nurse should encourage the person to create a mental picture of the material being presented. Auditory learners learn best by listening to an explanation or an audiotape presentation. If possible, provide the person with a tape recording for future review (Hamilton, 2005). Those who are kinesthetic learners learn best by doing and respond to demonstration and return demonstration as teaching strategies. Using real-life examples or case studies before providing theory and practice may also help meet the needs of kinesthetic learners (Hamilton, 2005).

Meeting the Challenge of Low Health Literacy

Health literacy, the ability to read, understand, and use health information to make appropriate health care decisions and to follow treatment instructions needed to maintain health, is a significant problem in the United States (Brown et al., 2004). Twenty percent of Americans—those who read at the fifth-grade level or less—are functionally illiterate (Doak, Doak, & Root, 1996). People who are functionally illiterate are unable to follow directions on prescription bottles, read appointment slips, complete health insurance claims, follow instructions for diagnostic tests, or understand written self-care and discharge instructions (Kleinbeck, 2005). Another thirty percent of the U.S. population have marginal reading skills and are only able to read materials between a fifth- and ninth-grade level.

Multiple studies have shown that low literacy skills are associated with poorer health outcomes, decreased adherence with treatment instructions, more hospitalizations, and significantly increased health care costs (Mayer & Villaire, 2004). The Agency for Healthcare Research and Quality (AHRQ) has found that people who read at lower levels are $1\frac{1}{2}$ to 3 times more likely to have adverse outcomes than are those who read at higher levels (Dewalt, 2005). Illiteracy is an invisible impairment; those with limited literacy are not easily identified because they have learned to cope with and hide their limitations from others (Allen, 2002). Although persons who are

elderly or have limited education, those who are members of ethnic minority groups, and recent immigrants are at highest risk for low health literacy, the problem affects individuals in all segments of society (Institute of Medicine, 2004). Nursing interventions to improve literacy learning include the following:

- Using health literacy resources such as the National Library of Medicine (http://www.nlm.hih.gov/pubs/cbm/literacy)
- Teaching in a step-by-step process, presenting the most essential information first
- Keeping sessions as brief as possible without leaving out important information
- Asking the patient to restate information or to return demonstrate skills
- Repeating each step to reinforce the learning process
- Selecting materials written at the fifth-grade level and using visual aids that illustrate key points
- Using videotapes or audiotapes that use simple words and give clear instructions (Doak et al., 1996)

Learner Characteristics

Developmental Level. The learner's developmental level has a significant effect on the educational process.

Teaching Children. Teaching and learning programs for children take into account the child's growth and development, as well as the cognitive level and chronological age. Information from school reports and developmental assessments describe the child's learning potential and special needs. Children are included in decisions about learning as appropriate; however, the fact remains that the parents will oversee the child's care. Learning readiness and the quality of the parent-child relationship are important variables. Sensitivity to child-rearing practices and cultural issues also plays a role in planning effective education for the pediatric patient (Allen, 2002). Children have short attention spans, so material is best presented in limited amounts over short periods. Affection and praise nurture the child during the educational sessions. Children learn through play and active participation. Excellent play therapy and teaching programs are available; most involve the family and an interdisciplinary team approach.

Teaching Adolescents. Adolescents are in a time of transition, and their learning needs are wide and varied. Although education includes the family, the focus of teaching is on the adolescent because adolescents are independent and control the outcomes of education. Adolescents are capable of abstract thought and logical reasoning. An attitude of "it won't happen to me" often leads them into risk-taking behaviors. Peer groups are strong influences. Adolescents are in the process of adapting to a changing body and are concerned with body image and appearance. In teaching the adolescent patient, consider the following (Allen, 2002):

- Adolescents need to assert their independence; they may rebel against authority figures.
- A guidance approach to learning works better than lecturing.
- Honesty and trust are important when working with adolescents.

- Adolescents may have less knowledge about their bodies than is assumed.
- The importance of the peer group should be used through group learning.
- Body image is important to adolescents.

Teaching Older Adults. Learning by elderly persons may be affected by sensory impairments, altered cognitive processes, endurance, a need for frequent toileting, medication side effects, and impaired nutritional status. Using medical jargon or speaking too rapidly or too softly may become learning barriers. When teaching older adults, the nurse should be sensitive to their unique needs and should reinforce individual strengths (Williams, Kemper, & Hummert, 2004). Older patients learn effectively when educational programs are tailored to their unique needs; for instance, material written in large type helps those with diminished vision. Older persons may feel intimidated when faced with lengthy learning modules, tests, or quizzes. Teaching strategies for elderly patients include the following (Allen, 2002):

- Presenting the material at a slower pace and presenting small amounts of information at a time
- Speaking in a low tone of voice because elderly persons hear low tones better than high-pitched sounds
- Allowing time for integration and assimilation of conceptual material
- Repeating information frequently
- Reinforcing oral presentations with audiovisual materials
- Using written examples and analogies
- Decreasing outside distractions
- Using group experiences to improve problem-solving abilities
- Remembering that elderly patients are cautious and do not make changes easily

Culture and Language. Cultural factors have a profound effect on patient education. Providing culturally relevant patient education requires understanding and applying transcultural concepts, including considering cultural needs, appreciating the patient and family's cultural context, selecting culturally teaching sensitive strategies, and using resources from a variety of cultural subsystems in the community. A cultural component should be part of every patient assessment. Useful Internet links for learning about cultural diversity include Diversity Rx (http://www.diversity.org), Ethnomed (http://www.ethnomed.org), and the Transcultural Nursing Society (http://www.tcns.org.).

Language barriers can create frustration and misunderstanding for both patients and providers. Interpretive services are preferable to those of a translator because interpreters are trained to interpret the accurate meaning of words into the patient's language and to communicate the patient's questions and concerns to the health care team. An informal translator may not have fluency in both languages, may lose cultural meanings in the translation, or may be unaware of medical or health-related words. Family members are least desirable as translators because they may edit what the educator is telling the patient or filter what the patient is saying to the health

care professional. Most health care facilities have lists of language interpreters, and AT&T offers fee-based interpretive services. Written materials and videos about specific conditions and treatments are available in a variety of languages. Pharmaceutical and medical supply companies provide information about their products in several languages. For example, consumer product information about warfarin sodium (Coumadin) is published in 51 languages (Allen, 2002).

Planning and Implementation

Planning learning experiences involves developing goals and objectives, identifying learning activities, developing content, and identifying resources. After an initial assessment the nurse and patient work to set mutually agreed-on learning goals and objectives they both believe to be achievable. Goals direct the educator and the learner toward expected behavioral changes and are the basis for measuring learning outcomes. Learning objectives are specific behaviors that lead to goal accomplishment (Box 5-3). For example, a person with diabetes may identify keeping his blood glucose within specific parameters as a goal. Learning objectives related to this goal may include learning how to use insulin, how to balance diet and exercise, and how to use a blood glucose monitor.

Families have major roles in identifying goals and objectives, and the extent of their investment influences success or failure. Family involvement in planning the learning experiences enhances the patient's potential for rehabilitation and helps ensure that the goals are realistic. Common patient and family goals include acquiring care survival skills, recognizing and solving problems, adapting to disability, and integrating the limitations of the disability into a preferred lifestyle.

Much of the teaching that occurs in rehabilitation is focused specifically on accommodating the cognitive, sensory-perceptual, and motor impairments resulting from an impairment, disability, or chronic condition. Members of the rehabilitation team must collaborate to identify the specific strategies that will work best for each patient. In an ideal world seamless communication of the education plan moves from the inpatient setting to the community setting, whether the outpatient clinic, the home, the physician's office, or the support group. To promote continuity, teaching plans and projected outcomes can be sent along with discharge records to clinics or home health care agencies. Patients can be instructed to call help lines, where they can talk with familiar staff for advice and help (Allen, 2002).

In addition to goal development, a comprehensive teaching plan includes appropriate learning domains, instructional

---

BOX 5-3 Example of Goal and Objective

Goal: The desired outcome of learning (e.g., maintain intact skin)
Objective: Specific statement related to goal that describes in more detail the behavior that will be performed to meet the goal (e.g., weight shift every 30 minutes when seated in wheelchair)

methods, and resources (Tables 5-3 and 5-4). Learning activities should match the planned objectives and the learner's functional and cognitive abilities. The rehabilitation environment provides learners with opportunities to practice new behaviors with the support and encouragement of the staff. When feasible, an overnight or weekend home pass gives the patient and family a chance to try skills or behaviors and to review areas of perceived difficulty with the team. An independent-living center in the facility serves the same purpose as the patient and family try out behaviors, identify successes or problems, and overcome barriers with the staff on call.

TABLE 5-3 Behavior Domains and Learning Activities

Domain	Definition	Teaching-Learning Method
Cognitive	Knowledge, intellectual skills	Lecture, discussion, printed materials, independent study, demonstration, tests, simulation; learning facts, information
Psychomotor	Performing physical skills within limits of disability	Demonstration, practice, simulation, role-playing
Affective	Attitudes, values, feelings	Discussion, role-playing, simulation

Educators classify behaviors into three categories known as domains. The cognitive domain describes intellectual tasks. The affective domain consists of feelings, attitudes, and values. The psychomotor domain involves learning motor skills and tasks. Each domain is further divided into a ranked taxonomy—a sequence beginning with the least to the most complex learned behavior. Taxonomies guide the development of learning objectives and the selection of appropriate learning methods. Learning a new medication regimen is an example of a behavior in the cognitive domain. Behavioral objectives progress from naming medications to explaining primacy actions and side effects and avoiding potential drug-food interactions. In teaching a psychomotor skill, behaviors progress from observing the task to practicing with guidance, to practicing independently, and finally to task mastery (Allen, 2002). Rehabilitation needs often involve learning in all three domains. For example, to prevent skin breakdown, a person with paraplegia must learn new knowledge, skills, and attitudes.

Instructional Methods and Instructional Resources

Teaching can be conducted for individuals, groups, or a combination of these to accomplish learning objectives. In groups patients share information and experiences and provide support for one another. Families learn about the impairment and ways of providing care and form their own support groups to discuss adjustments or ask questions of those who have related problems. Although conducted by patients or families,

TABLE 5-4 Uses and Advantages of Selected Learning Activities

Learning Activity	Uses and Advantages
Lecture	Most often used in transmitting information. Effective in teaching cognitive information. Most effective when used with discussion. Enhanced by handouts and visual aids; presented at the level of the patient's understanding; should be limited in length.
Demonstration	Most useful for psychomotor learning. Can be presented in person or by video; return demonstration and repetition needed.
Group discussion	Actively involves learners; promotes understanding and application of knowledge and development of problem-solving skills.
Role-playing and return demonstration	Helps learner apply knowledge by practicing and obtaining feedback to improve skill performance. Helps patients recognize and solve problem situations.
Printed material (brochures, handouts)	Most common teaching tool; content must be appropriate for patient's language and literacy level. Review written information with the patient; provide a reference for community use.
Games and simulations	Involves the patient in teaching and learning. Introduce information, and provide practice in simulated situations; incorporate problem solving. Can take a course of action and look at consequences in a nonthreatening way.
Computer-assister learning and programmed instruction	Self-paced, self-directed learning. Many commercial products available; older adults may not be familiar with use. Nurse should introduce materials and follow-up with learning.
Slides and transparencies	Helps learner focus thoughts; pictures and diagrams can promote understanding.
Audiotapes	Small, inexpensive, and easy to use; particularly helpful for those with low literacy skills and visual impairments. Commercial tapes available on many topics; should be in short segments to maintain interest.
Videotapes	Present life situations that promote understanding and problem solving. Introduce and follow with discussion. Can be shown over in-house television systems with staff follow-up.

support groups may be sponsored by the health care facility, a local or national organization, or community agencies. These groups recognize the benefits of mutual support in adjustment to chronic disease and management of disabling conditions. One-on-one teaching is an effective strategy for teaching psychomotor skills such as self-catheterization. Individual teaching provides a means for sharing confidential information and problems and overcoming barriers such as cultural differences, anxiety, or low literacy.

Increasingly, patient education is incorporated into care maps and critical pathways that guide the sequence and timing of a patient's progress. Care maps and critical pathways with an education component have been developed for various diseases and conditions; they prescribe approaches and combine individual, group, and self-directed learning. Patients and families are taught from standardized content that is tailored for individual situations and to promote effective problem solving.

The Internet as a Resource in Patient Education

The Internet has changed the way we obtain information and documents and how we communicate. Although patients are increasingly seeking health information via the Internet, they may lack skills in understanding and evaluating the wealth of information at their fingertips (Jenkins & Dunn, 2004). Studies show that most consumers use a general search engine such as Google or Yahoo that may or may not provide accurate and timely information (Eysenback & Kohler, 2002). Medline Plus (http://www.medlineplus.gov) is a highly recommended portal for authoritative health information. Medline Plus is a consumer-focused website developed by librarians at the National Library of Medicine. It provides interactive tutorials on over 100 diseases, procedures, and health enhancement strategies that are presented in a user-friendly and easy-to-read format (Jenkins & Dunn, 2004).

Documentation of Education

Documenting the educational process informs all rehabilitation team members about individual patient and family progress and is also a major focus of accreditation review and health maintenance organization (HMO) standards. Effective documentation can help ensure continuity in the education process. Document what was taught, who was taught, when and where the teaching took place, what teaching methods were used, and how learning was evaluated. The teaching plan and the patient's progress in meeting the goals and objectives are part of the permanent patient record available to all members of the interdisciplinary team to track progress and to avoid duplication. It also provides a legal record of teaching and learning for reimbursement.

Evaluation in Patient Education

Evaluating what patients and families have learned is a vital part of the educational process that is often overlooked. Evaluation completes the loop back to assessment to determine

further education needs throughout each stage of the learning process. Feedback at each stage helps the educator adjust information, methods, and materials to make changes if needed to reach the agreed-upon goal. The nurse can refer to the information in the Nursing Interventions Classification (NIC) (Dochterman & Bulechek, 2004) and the Nursing Outcomes Classification (NOC) (Moorhead, Johnson, & Maas, 2004) for nursing interventions and outcomes related to patient education. Examples of NOC outcomes relevant to patient and family education include adherence behaviors, learning facilitation, learning readiness enhancement, and health education (Moorhead et al., 2004). A challenge for patient educators is to evaluate learning as behavior change. A patient and family may demonstrate understanding of information and perform associated skills successfully in the health care setting but may not transfer the new behaviors to the community. For example, how do we determine that patients with diabetes follow their diet at home? How do we know that patients will make changes to reduce stroke risk factors? In the past, individuals who failed to follow treatment instructions were termed *noncompliant*. Today, the terms *adherence* or *concordance* are more commonly used, and efforts are being made to determine why patients find adherence difficult. Box 5-4 outlines strategies that can help increase patient adherence (Habel, 2005).

BOX 5-4   Strategies to Improve Adherence

- Ask the patient why he or she is not able to follow treatment instructions. The patient's view of why adherence is a problem is the one that counts.
- Avoid proposing an immediate solution. Focusing efforts on helping the patient learn problem-solving skills will pay greater dividends.
- Determine whether or not the patient believes that adherence will solve the health care problems. If the answer is "no," assess the patient's beliefs about the problem.
- Does the patient understand what he or she is to do? It is difficult for adults to acknowledge they do not know how to do something. Verify that the person understands instructions, and ask for a return demonstration if appropriate.
- Determine that the person has the skills to adhere.
- Is adherence punishing? For example, some drugs have uncomfortable side effects, or an exercise program may produce pain and stiffness.
- Is the new health care behavior too complex? Simplify tasks and steps if needed.
- Does the patient have a memory problem that interferes with adherence? Using memory aids to recall when to take medications or linking the new behavior with an already learned activity can help.
- Does the person have the physical and/or mental capacity to learn the self-care skill? If physical limitations are a barrier, provide assistive devices or arrange caregiver support. If the patient has problems with mental capacity, enlist a spouse, family member, or friend to assist.

THE REHABILITATION NURSE AND COMMUNITY EDUCATION

Patients return to the community from acute care and rehabilitation facilities with unmet learning needs. The rehabilitation nurse can facilitate patients' integration into the community by connecting them with persons, groups, and services to provide support and assistance. Knowing the community services available is central to preparing patients for home and developing a teaching plan that can continue after discharge. Being aware of agencies and support groups in their community helps patients return home better prepared to resume independent living (Allen, 2002).

Nurses can develop reciprocal relationships with community groups. For example, volunteering to teach rehabilitation skills, such as safe transfers, through a church or community group introduces better care to the community. The result is safer care and helpful association with groups that could benefit others, including support for family caregivers. Other continuing education programs might deal with the prevention of chronic disease or care for persons with specific impairments. Resources for patient education in the community include national organizations for special disease conditions (e.g., the American Heart Association), local health departments, local churches, hospital websites, and Internet consumer health sites.

A national initiative to improve the health of the nation, *Healthy People 2010*, establishes priorities for health promotion, prevention, and health protection services. The goals of *Healthy People 2010* are to help individuals change negative health behaviors, equalize access to health care, and prevent chronic conditions that are costly in terms of lives and dollars.

CHALLENGES FOR PATIENT EDUCATION

Increased emphasis on cost containment and treatment outcomes is forcing rehabilitation facilities to critically assess the value of patient and family education. The introduction of the prospective payment system (PPS) for acute rehabilitation is expected to affect length of stay and, in turn, further streamline patient education using critical pathways and care maps. Educators will be challenged to demonstrate that patient education can improve health status, reduce complications, and reduce readmission to hospitals. The potential for producing educational outcomes for persons with disabling conditions and chronic illness that can be replicated in various health care settings is a formidable and exciting challenge for rehabilitation nurses.

CRITICAL THINKING

Refer to the four patients introduced in the opening of this chapter:

1. How do you plan to teach the Wall family what they need to know about Mrs. Wall's posthospital care? What are teaching priorities for this family?

2. What community resources would you consider to help Mrs. Tang and her daughter?

3. How would you plan to ensure that Mr. Mowery can follow his treatment plan if his wife becomes ill or must leave their home for a period of time?

4. How would you respond to Mrs. Hirsch if she asks your opinion about Internet claims for arthritis treatment that are scientifically unsubstantiated?

REFERENCES

Allen, J. C. (2002). Outcome-directed patient and family education. In S. P. Hoeman (Ed.), *Rehabilitation nursing: Process, application & outcomes* (3rd ed., pp. 144-161). St. Louis, MO: Mosby.

Bandura, A. (1997). *Self-efficacy.* New York: W. H. Freeman.

Becker, M. H. (Ed.). (1974). *The health belief model and personal health behavior.* Thorofare, NJ: Slack.

Benner, P. (1985). *From beginner to expert: Excellence and power in clinical nursing practice.* Reading, MA: Addison-Wesley.

Benner, P. (2001). *From novice to expert* (Commemorative 1st ed.). Upper Saddle River, NJ: Prentice Hall.

Brown, D. R., Ludwig, R., Buck, G. A., Durham, D., Shurard, R., & Graham, S. S. (2004). Health literacy: Universal precautions needed. *Journal of Allied Health, 33*(2), 150-155.

Commission on Accreditation of Rehabilitation Facilities. (2004). *The 2004 standards manual.* Tucson, AZ: Author.

Dewalt, D. A., Berkman, N. D., Sheridan, S., Lohr, K. N., & Pignone, M. P. (2005). Literacy and health outcomes: A systematic review of the literature. *Journal of General Internal Medicine, 19*, 1228-1239.

Doak, C., Doak, L., & Root, J. (1996). *Teaching patients with low literacy skills* (2nd ed.). Philadelphia: J. B. Lippincott.

Dochterman, J. M., & Bulechek, G. M. (2004). *Nursing interventions classification (NIC)* (4th ed., pp. 244, 301-309). St. Louis, MO: Mosby.

Eysenback, G., & Kohler, C. (2002). How do consumers search for and appraise health information on the World Wide Web: A qualitative study using focus groups, usability tests, and in-depth interviews. *British Medical Journal, 314*, 573-577.

Festinger, L. (1957). *Theory of cognitive dissonance.* Stanford, CA: Stanford University Press.

Habel, M. (2005). *Putting patient teaching into practice* (pp. 139-140). King of Prussia, PA: Nursing Spectrum Continuing Education.

Hamilton, S. (2005). How do we assess the learning style of our patients? *Rehabilitation Nursing, 33*(4), 129-131.

Hoffman, C., Rice, D., & Sung, H. Y. (1996). Persons with chronic conditions: Their prevalence and costs. *JAMA, 276*, 1473-1479.

Holman, H. (2004). Patient self-management: A key to effectiveness and efficiency in care of chronic disease (Viewpoint). *Public Health Reports,* May 1, 2004.

Huffman, M. H. (2005). Compliance, health outcomes & partnering in PPS: Acknowledging the patient's agenda. *Home Healthcare Nurse, 23*(1), 23-28.

Institute of Medicine of the National Academies. (2004, April). *Health literacy: A prescription to end confusion.* Report Brief. Washington, DC: National Academies Press.

Jenkins, M. L., & Dunn, D. (2004). Ask an expert: Enhancing web-based health information for consumer education. *Applied Nursing Research, 17*(1), 68-70.

Joint Commission on Accreditation of Healthcare Organizations. (2004). *Comprehensive accreditation manual for hospitals.* Oakbrook, IL: Author.

Kleinbeck, C. (2005). Reaching positive diabetes outcomes for patients with low literacy. *Home Healthcare Nurse, 23*(1), 17-22.

Knowles, M. (1984). *Andragogy in action.* San Francisco: Jossey-Bass.

Marcy, V. (2001). Adult learning style: How VARK learning style inventory can be used to improve student learning. *Perspectives on Physician Assistant Education, 12*, 117-120.

Mayer, G. G., & Villaire, M. (2004). Low health literacy and its effects on patient care. *Journal of Nursing Administration, 34*(10), 440-442.

Moorhead, S., Johnson, M., & Maas, M. (Eds.). (2004). *Nursing outcomes classification (NOC)* (3rd ed., pp. 140-142). St. Louis, MO: Mosby.

Pestonjee, S. (2000). *Nurse's handbook of patient education.* Springhouse, PA: Springhouse.

Pratt, D. D. (1988). Andragogy as a relational construct. *Adult Education Quarterly, 38*, 160-181.

Prochaska, J. O., & Velicer, W. F. (1997). The transtheoretical model of health behavior change. *American Journal of Health Promotion, 12*, 38-48.

Robinson-Smith, G., Johnston, M., & Allen, J. (2000). Self-care efficacy, quality of life and depression after stroke. *Archives of Physical Medicine and Rehabilitation, 81*, 460-464.

University of Rhode Island. (2005). *Transtheoretical model: Stages of change.* Available from www.uri/edu/research/cprc/TTM/StagesOfChange.htm.

Wallston, K., Wallston, B., & DeVellis, R. (1978). Development of the multi-dimensional health locus of control (MHLC) scales. *Health Education Monographs, 6*(2), 160-170.

Williams, K. W., Kemper, S., & Hummert, M. L. (2004). Enhancing communication with older adults: Overcoming elderspeak. *Journal of Gerontological Nursing, 39*(10), 17-24.

6

Culture and Medical Systems: Conventional, Alternative, and Complementary Health Patterns

Shirley P. Hoeman, PhD, MPH, RN, CS
Theresa Perfetta Cappello, PhD, RN

With traditional and complementary practices appearing in the mainstream of health care, it is inevitable that rehabilitation nurses will encounter practitioners of complementary therapies, and likely they personally will use them. At times the nursing assessment and plan for care will differ from a patient's or family's view of what is being done or what should be done; studies may yield conflicting evidence. Lifestyle preferences, religious beliefs, family system patterns, and traditions of healing may not match a nursing or team plan of care. Traditional healers may join the team or collaborate, or the patient may request a referral, use alternative therapeutics independent of the team, or rely on cultural practices in tandem with conventional rehabilitation practices.

Cultural competence includes sensitivity to patients' desires and preferences for use of integrated therapies. Care is provided in ways that are acceptable, respectful, and relevant to the patient's worldview. Critical thinking requires that nurses become aware of their own biases and gaps in their knowledge about a cultural group. Although no one can learn about all cultural beliefs and practices and individuals differ widely in their own adherence to cultural practices, nurses can focus on those groups with whom they come into contact more regularly. Continuous learning is part of gaining competence. Patients have a right to meet their culturally based health care needs as much as possible. However, this right does not require nurses to conform to situations or participate in practices that are illegal or unsafe or to violate and refute their own moral or religious beliefs. It does require that nurses be very clear about the rationale for decisions. The "emerging universe of disability" (National Institute on Disability and Rehabilitation Research [NIDRR], 2005) discussed later will have a notable impact on community-based rehabilitation nursing practice.

The purpose of this chapter is to acquaint the rehabilitation nurse with some of the ways that cultural factors influence health assessment, interventions, and outcomes. A goal is to explain the relevance of alternative medical systems and complementary therapeutics in rehabilitation nursing practice. Certainly this is not an exhaustive discussion. The view is toward holism in nursing offered from an anthropological approach; it is not intended to be a presentation of holistic nursing per se. A goal is to provide information and access to information that will enable rehabilitation nurses to make informed and critical decisions about cultural, alternative, and complementary beliefs and practices.

CULTURE AND WORLDVIEWS

Historical Development

From tribal times, healing was ascribed to selected persons who knew proper use of magic, herbs, and rituals and how to connect with a spiritual domain. Most enduring of primitive healer-spiritual roles is the shaman, whose interactions with the spiritual world empowered healing. Romans, Greeks, and Druids associated healers with their gods; Arab physicians emphasized mathematical and scientific approaches with a spiritual health component. The Indo-Asian concepts attribute Ayurvedic medicine to Dhanvantari, patron of physicians. Early Christian monks tended the sick as a spiritual calling and honed their herbal apothecary skills. Despite varying success with cure or even palliative care, all of these healers held holistic views supporting elementary concepts of prevention and health maintenance. They envisioned an individual life force, acknowledged a need to maintain balance or harmony, and attempted to align the natural world with spiritual forces. Certainly every culture had specific requirements, taboos, beliefs, and practices. However, body, mind, spirit, and their interaction with the natural and supernatural environments influenced health and healing.

Culture, Health, and Disability

The health system is an underlying system of society as are education, legislation, religion, family, and economics. The World Health Organization (WHO) promotes a system of community-based rehabilitation, a global definition of holistic health, and a system to classify disability. (See Chapter 2 for discussion of the International Classification for Functioning, Disability and Health [ICF].) Each culture assigns meaning to health or illness and teaches under what circumstances and symptoms a person becomes ill or disabled, a process referred to as "cultural modeling" (Micozzi,1996). The social construction of the situation defines roles and actions for persons who are well, ill, or impaired and sets expectations for the person and responsibilities of family and society. Thus, health or illness, modes of care and caring, and identities of practitioners are defined, understood, and communicated, and the behaviors are carried out, within the boundaries of the culture.

Culture and Symptoms

When Zborowski's landmark study (1958) found responses to pain differed among patients from three sociocultural groups, the implications launched research about culture and health. Parsons' classic study (1951) affirmed cultural prescriptions and definitions of illness behavior. Others attributed persons' descriptions of their condition and the cause, appropriate treatment, and expected outcomes to products of cultural "explanatory models" (Kleinman, Eisenberg, & Good, 1978). Symptoms and names of some diseases may be recognized and understood only within a particular culture. The fact that a disease or syndrome is not listed in the materia medica does not mean that it does not exist; it simply may not have diagnostic labeling for conventional medicine. For example, professionals in the People's Republic of China did not accept attention-deficit hyperactivity disorder (ADHD) as a diagnosis; they considered it a Western condition (Hoeman, 1992). Similarly, practitioners in Asian, Hispanic, and African cultures are astounded at the inability of Western medical practitioners to diagnose or treat based on a person's psychosocial or spiritual symptoms. Findings from bioethnographic research have been well received, so that "culture-bound" symptoms and syndromes, spiritual curses, and treatment theories, such as hot-cold theory, are documented in the literature.

Ethnocentrism, or the tendency to gauge situations and filter experiences through one's own cultural point of view, is a typical response. Not only do providers bring their own cultural backgrounds to the therapeutic encounter, but they also come with the extensive beliefs and practices of their medical culture system. Fadiman (1997) effectively illustrated how ethnocentric cultural dissonance prevailed in a Hmong family's encounter with conventional medicine despite highly competent, caring physicians. In this ethnographic account,

physicians and family desired the best outcome for the child. However, physicians misconstrued cultural cues as nonadherence or simply dismissed them as irrelevant information for the medical diagnostics. The family, mistrusting the physicians, continued their remedies and explained the situation through the spirit world. Both sides sincerely wanted to help the child, but, unable to attain real understanding, ultimately failed.

The importance of how language is used when describing symptoms or subjective experiences or reporting health status has been devalued and underrated in conventional medicine. Zola (1991), who had postpolio syndrome, emphasized language and insisted on being referred to as a person "using the wheelchair" and not one "confined to a wheelchair."

Culture-bound symptoms have been associated with modern living, such as problems arising from human activity in the environment or iatrogenic problems resulting from medical diagnostic procedures, especially medical errors or acquired infections. Other conditions may be born of responses to civilization and technological advances, such as stress, obesity, anorexia, repetitive motion injury, or sick building syndrome. Some cultural rituals may prescribe substances such as hallucinogens or tobacco to circumvent or ease symptoms, whereas other groups engage in violence as an acceptable means of problem solving.

Patients from other than Western cultures have two common complaints about conventional medicine: the short time allotted for the visit and the number of questions they are asked by the provider. A healer may use special skills, apply therapeutic techniques, provide herbal or other remedies, or form connections with the nonphysical world to identify the person's problem. Because alternative or traditional healers spend time with patients, more information emerges, which the healer incorporates into a statement of what the person needs to restore balance and regain health.

SOCIAL CONSTRUCTION OF DISABILITY

Persons with impairment or disability have been treated unequally and devalued for centuries, their conditions being considered as punishment for wrongdoing; the result of a curse; or less often, an insight, blessing, or call to a special role in the society. Deformity, often associated with being a fool, frequently was a target of cruel ridicule or debasement among adults, as well as children. Negative attributes were applied to those with deformities or disabilities, from Richard III to the Hunchback of Notre Dame. Only in the last 50 years have ideas about life satisfaction and quality in developed countries provoked legislation with protections for these persons.

In the professional culture of rehabilitation nursing, a holistic mind-body-spirit view extends beyond mere survival with intact physical abilities as outcome criteria. The love of family members and their role in a community is neither one-dimensional nor linear (Hoeman & Nordin, 2003). Holism takes into account what Sobel (1979) identified as nonmedical determinants of health, that is, genetic, behavioral, and physical and psychosocial environmental factors. He envisioned an integrated approach, a synthesis of conventional science and alternate systems of healing, and a mutual approach by healer and patient. Too often conventional medicine regards the mind and the body as if on separate planes to the point of providers' excluding subjective history and intuition born of experience.

Simply gathering information is not equal to understanding the cultural meaning. Haddad and Hoeman (2000) stress the significance of the nurse's learning about the history of a patient's culture and how events have shaped beliefs and practices within the context of the culture. Paul's classic anthology (1955) demonstrates repeatedly that culture is a system larger than the sum of its parts. In one encounter a Peruvian village woman confronts health workers who attempt to have her boil contaminated water. She reasons that any microbes, should these invisible organisms exist, would drown themselves; they must have become "stuck on" from other sources. She questions why she should worry about minuscule, invisible animals when cold, hunger, and poverty are real threats. Clearly, interpersonal trust and mutual faith in the intervention are essential because healer and patient "behold one another through different kinds of cultural glasses" and "sickness is as much a moral as a physical crisis" (Wellin, 1955).

Cultures construct definitions of chronic conditions, impairment, and disability and how the social system will manage the situation (Box 6-1). However, individuals can and do rise above social constructions of relativism and negative designations. Rehabilitation nurses are advocates to support patients' self-confidence and to forestall language and situations that devalue them.

DOMINANT ROLE OF CONVENTIONAL MEDICINE

The undisputed cultural model of health care in the United States is conventional medicine, that is, the Western or allopathic model. The 20 medicine system's ways of knowing are to determine whether something is scientific, as opposed

---

BOX 6-1   Social Construction of Illness

Social construction means that cultures or societies use their systems to define and prescribe the following:

- How and why illness or disability occurred
- What should be done about it
- Who should perform healing
- Which interventions should be used
- How the person and others are to respond to and perform roles
- What meaning is given to the illness or disability
- What is the cost (financial, social, and otherwise)
- What should be the outcome
  Members of the culture know these ways; although social meanings are powerful, it is essential to remember that they do not prevent individuals from constructing their own meanings

---

to unscientific. Practitioners are indoctrinated into the culture of the system and adhere to the professional roles and standards of practice. Initially they viewed the body mechanistically, as a machine, to be dealt with apart from the mind and spirit. Based on Cartesian concepts, positivism, objectivism, and reductionism (Micozzi, 1996), and augmented by advances in pharmaceutics, technology, and surgery, the dominant political and economic power of conventional medicine as a cultural system is unparalleled (Starr, 1982).

Practitioners of conventional medicine found it easy to disregard other health systems and interventions as illogical and unproven, effectively excluding them from legitimate status and, importantly, from the reimbursement process. Conventional medicine flourished and dominated, its blatant paternalism abetted by consumer expectations for cures and technological solutions. Initiatives for preventive care and self-care were discarded in lieu of fantastic and expensive procedures, equipment, and technology that promised more cures. Ironically, before World War II rehabilitation medicine itself was considered alternative and noncure and struggled to be accepted as a specialty by conventional medicine.

Erosion of Trust in Medical Diagnosis and Care

Reliance on treatments and technology interfered with the interpersonal relationship between health professionals and patients, dismantling the worth of the family physician, house calls, and bedside manner. Some patients blamed themselves when drugs or surgical interventions did not resolve their conditions. Ziporyn (1992) discusses the miserable status of the person who lives with multiple unexplained symptoms. Eventually an unwelcome diagnosis of multiple sclerosis assigns meaning and validates the person's suffering situation. Once symptoms and suffering had a name, the person could begin to deal with it. More importantly, both the person and others realized the symptoms were real and the feelings legitimate. On the other hand, diagnostic labeling with a chronic, disabling condition may become the definition of the person.

Functional Health Patterns as a Foundation

Rehabilitation nurses understand that chronic conditions and comorbidity cannot be fit into a single diagnostic label and that the responses and reserves of an individual cannot be cataloged. They recognize the exquisite fine-tuning needed to identify a person's optimal abilities, eke out every possibility, and then minimize problems. Rehabilitation nurses examine functional patterns to assess a patient's multiple strengths and unique deficits, such as those that might follow a stroke. Interventions are specific to each patient beyond the scope of the diagnosis and a more holistic approach. This is superior because no single medical diagnosis can encompass an individual's whole situation when the goal is to restore or maintain optimal levels of function on all fronts. The disease or disability does not exist on its own and is not representative of the person. Likewise, no one discipline or single approach is prepared to manage the complexity of chronic, disabling conditions. In part, this rationale justifies use of functional health patterns for the holistic conceptual framework throughout this book.

Self-Healing

Many of the complex problems encountered by patients with chronic, disabling, or developmental disorders remain out of reach of conventional medical cures. Patients and families learn about treatment options through sources such as the World Wide Web and choose to inform themselves and manage or design aspects of their own health care. They seek improved quality, not only cure, in their lives and no longer believe that medical science and technology alone will provide it. Complementary therapies, used in conjunction with conventional medicine, may enable patients to access a variety of modes of treatment and exercise their greatest potential for healing (Barnes, Powell-Griner, McFann, & Nahin, 2004).

In the realm of *psychoneuroimmunology* (PNI) (discussed later) (a term signifying a body of research that examines mind-body connections), cognitive, emotional, and psychological factors are found to influence the body's immune system, that is, these factors can effect self-healing. Eisenberg's landmark study (1997) found that 58% of alternative therapies in use were for health promotion or disease prevention. Among adults in the United States, 62% of those over age 18 had used complementary/alternative medicine (CAM) within the previous year, when prayer for health reasons was included in the definition (Barnes et al., 2004). This interest combined with an emphasis on the body's ability to heal itself and correct imbalance makes alternative therapies and remedies enticing options for patients with previously incurable chronic or disabling conditions.

Self-report measures of impairment and disability have some reliability and validity. However, patients' assessments of quality of care may be related to their satisfaction with social interaction with the health professional (Callahan, Bertakis, & Azari, 2000). Of equal concern is the lack of culturally relevant tools or ways to measure patient outcomes or satisfaction. The fact that a person is participating in a rehabilitation program indicates some degree of experience with the medical system (Hoeman, 1989). However, it remains unclear whether satisfaction or rating of quality of care is influenced by cultural factors, including values, perceptions, expectations, mode of expressing agreement or concerns, use of complementary therapies, or other reasons (Murray-Garcia, Selby, Schmittdiel, Grumbach, & Quesenberry, 2000). Skepticism about conventional medicine does not justify anyone's indulging in risky behavior or placing excessive trust in untested remedies.

Socioeconomic status and poor access to care may lead to early death with certain conditions (Frankset al., 2003). However, researchers found that homeless persons, including many with chronic disabling conditions, would seek care when referral mechanisms were in place and when they believed their situation was serious (Gelberg, Andersen, & Leake, 2000).

Diversity and Utilization

Diversity is a growing reality that extends beyond cultural lines to encompass persons who are disenfranchised, marginalized, refugees, immigrants, or in a low socioeconomic class (Hyde, 2004). Falling into stereotypical thinking about these categories is unwise. In particular, intraethnic diversity is often overlooked or underestimated by providers eager to become culturally sensitive (Hoeman, 1996).

Multiple factors, such as education, acculturation, and economic status, do influence how closely patients admit or adhere to their traditional beliefs and practices. When families with higher education and socioeconomic status were asked, they "perhaps" knew about folk or traditional healing practices and "some people who used them" but said they did not personally use them. They did use conventional medicine, pharmacologics, surgery, and technology (Hoeman, 1998). A national study found the use of CAM, defined as herbal medicine, acupuncture, chiropractic, traditional healer, and home remedy, was equally prevalent among white, African American, Latino, Asian, and Native American populations. Certain modalities were used by specific ethnic groups (e.g., Native Americans were more likely to use herbal medicine than acupuncture). In contrast to previous research, 28% of those using CAM in this study did so because they believed that conventional medicine would not help them (Mackenzie, Taylor, Bloom, Hufford, & Johnson, 2003). On the other hand, conventional medicine may be the last resort when other means fail. Some patients vacillate among a cadre of complementary and allopathic practitioners, or they may devise their own version and combinations, adding other interventions. Box 6-2 contains useful definitions for topics in this chapter.

Prevalence of Complementary or Integrative Therapies

Cyberspace provides a moratorium from reality and a forum for individuality (Kelly & Fitzsimons, 2000). Demographics changes and global travel and communications have created an awareness of options in selecting health care; practitioners from multiple cultures are evident in the social mainstream. The World Wide Web provides electronic mailing lists, chat rooms, and support groups in an electronic forum that allows individuals to ask questions and share interests or problem-solving information. Refer to Box 6-3 for online resources. Consumers not only have access to information and resources, they are willing to pay for them. The percentage of the U.S. population using alternative therapies has nearly doubled from 33.8% to 62% since the original study (Eisenberg et al., 1993).

Integrative therapy is the next goal level. The Centers for Disease Control and Prevention National Health Interview Study (2000) was administered to 31,000 adults in the United States. Fifty-five percent believed that a combination of CAM and conventional medicine treatments would help them. Half of the respondents thought it would be interesting to try, while 26% used CAM because their physicians suggested they try it (Barnes et al., 2004). It is logical that patients would turn to their physicians for guidance and information about

---

BOX 6-2 Medical System Definitions

Conventional (biomedical, traditional, contemporary, and allopathic) medicine: The dominant philosophical paradigm of medicine in the Western developed world. This scientific, reductionist method of medicine is taught in all U.S. medical schools. Rehabilitation is a specialty within conventional medicine.
Complementary/alternative medicine (CAM): A broad range of nonallopathic healing practices primarily stemming from Eastern medical philosophy and spiritual traditions of many cultures. Western conventional medicine does not commonly use, accept, study, understand, or make available CAM therapies. Until recently, CAM therapies were not found in U.S. medical school curricula and generally were not recognized by third-party payers in the United States. However, many medical schools have developed courses, and reimbursement for selected modalities has become more common. CAM therapies are considered holistic, considering the physical, mental, emotional, and spiritual aspects of each person.
   The terms *complementary* and *alternative* often are used interchangeably. However, *alternative medicine* refers to a system of treatments that replace conventional medical practices, whereas *complementary medicine* refers to a system of treatments that enhance, support, or supplement conventional medicine.
Integrated medicine or therapies: The next level goal based on evidence. It requires mutual patient and practitioner education and understanding, and acceptance.

BOX 6-3 Online Resources and Websites

- NCCAM website: http://nccam.nih.gov
- CAM Citation Index: http://nccam.nih.gov/nccam/resources/search.cgi
- Combined Health Information Database: http://chid,nih.gov
- Rosenthal Center: http://cpmcnet.columbia.edu/dept/rosenthal/
- Cochrane Collaboration: An essential resource—http://www.cochrane.dk.org
- Agency for Healthcare Research and Quality: http://www.ahrq.gov/
- The Office of Minority Health, Public Health Service has begun a project—Assuring Cultural Competence in Health Care: Recommendations for National Standards and an Outcomes-Focused Research Agenda: http://omhrc.gov/CLAS/po.html
- A federal and privately funded online registry of clinical trials, both those proposed with opportunities for participation and completed trials: http://www.clinicaltrials.gov/database
- American Holistic Nurse's Association (AHNA) website, which contains conference listings and message boards for those interested in holistic nursing: www.ahna.org/home/html
- A website devoted to exposing fraudulent practices and claims or to debunking commonly held misconceptions, as a consumer protection: http://www.quackwatch.com

CAM therapies; however, less than 40% of patients discuss their use of CAM with their primary care physicians (Wetzel, Kaptchuk, Haramati, & Eisenberg, 2003).

Too often providers neglect to ask patients about their use of alternative treatments or fail to understand what they hear. Certainly *Healthy People 2010* data document socioeconomic and ethnic disparities that exist in health care quality and access (U.S. Department of Health and Human Services, 2000). Inability to cure is the negative benchmark for conventional medicine, whereas care, prevention of further disability, and maintenance of function are left begging. Failure of conventional medicine to produce the now expected cure for many conditions has encouraged consumers to seek alternatives, especially in our aging global population. This is a major breakdown in the interpersonal and therapeutic relationship and the basis for erosion of trust.

Similarly, persons of all ages who have survived formerly fatal conditions only to continue to battle with multiple complex problems seek relief in any form. Hope is strong for finding cures for diseases such as cancer, multiple sclerosis, or Parkinson's disease and for progress toward relieving chronic back pain and other painful conditions. Restoring nerve function for spinal cord injury and other nerve-related conditions is a heady goal. As more complementary therapies are integrated into mainstream practices, critical thinking demands having an understanding of how their conceptual bases differ from those of conventional medicine. Nurses are familiar with patients who hold cultural health beliefs and practices and who rely on remedies from folk, family, or other lay sources or religious healing. Other persons call on specific practitioners from particular cultural origins.

Nurses as Healers

For centuries, nurses have employed healing practices that complemented mechanistic medical procedures, such as touch, hot/cold applications, pain management, or the relaxation response. CAM therapeutics are of particular interest to rehabilitation nurses because many of these techniques maximize patients' independence in terms of care and function and are practices within the standards and scope of professional rehabilitation nursing In the twenty-first century, nurses practice integrative care with an understanding of cellular and organic disease, movement theory, and pharmaceutical and technological advances. They integrate the patient's combined personal, familial, and cultural history into the therapeutic relationship so that physical and mechanical data explain only a portion of a person's health.

NATIONAL CENTER FOR COMPLEMENTARY AND ALTERNATIVE MEDICINE

The National Center for Complementary and Alternative Medicine (NCCAM), one of 27 institutes and centers within the National Institutes of Health (NIH) of the U.S. Public

Health Service, is part of the U.S. Department of Health and Human Services. The NCCAM was mandated by Congress in 1998 (Omnibus Appropriations Bill, Pub. L. No. 105-277, 11 Stat. 2681). Originating as the Office of Alternative Medicine (OAM) in 1991, it became established solidly under the NIH Revitalization Act of 1993 (Pub. L. No. 103-43). The complex and challenging mission of the NCCAM is to identify complementary and alternative healing practices, examine patterns of use, investigate efficacy and safety through rigorous science, disseminate information to the public and professionals, validate outcomes, and train practitioners to integrate tested therapies into mainstream health care practice and gain reimbursement. Today the NCCAM has established clinical research and project centers, an information clearinghouse, a system for organizing and conducting clinical trials, advisory panels for managing specific data such as for cancer treatment, and various transgovernmental agency and advisory groups.

NCCAM CLASSIFICATIONS

The following classifications are according to the NCCAM. Although other versions and groupings of categories, and some disagreements, exist, at this time the NCCAM is the major source of funding and research (NCCAM, 2005). Table 6-1 contains information about selected complementary/alternative modalities.

Whole or Traditional Medical Systems

Whole or traditional medical systems have been portrayed erroneously as a type of folk or lay healing. Traditional medical systems are complete systems that include conceptual frameworks, practice guidelines, standards for practitioners, and detailed pharmacopoeia. They have evolved parallel to conventional medicine, but from the viewpoint of conventional medicine the concepts are difficult to comprehend.

TABLE 6-1 Selected Complementary/Alternative Modalities

Selected Therapeutic Interventions	
Acupuncture	An ancient Chinese method in which fine needles which are inserted at specific points on the body to unblock energy that circulates throughout the body along pathways called meridians. *Acupressure* uses firm finger pressure instead of needles to exert pressure along the same points as acupuncture for relief of symptoms. It has proven effective to decrease pain and increase function with osteoarthritis of the knee (NCCAM, 12/20/04). Both methods are useful as adjuncts to conventional interventions.
Mind-body interventions	Interventions based on recognition that the mind and body are integrated and thus influence one another for healing. Examples are: *Biofeedback:* A technique for patients to listen to signals from their bodies and respond in ways that improve their condition; a means of training for control over involuntary body functions. It has been used to promote movement in paralyzed muscles following stroke, for stress reduction, and in pain management. *Hypnotherapy:* A hypnosis therapy that uses a state of heightened awareness that alters subjective feelings or creates expectancy so the patient is likely to follow suggestions posed by the therapist or via autosuggestion. Hypnosis has been successful for pain management (Cuellar, 2005).
Magnet therapy	Magnets are veritable energy interventions that generate a static unchanging magnetic field intended to accelerate healing by attracting and repelling charged particles in the blood. Patients seeking pain relief wear magnets in shoe soles, as bracelets, belts, or headbands and place them in mattresses. Although popular, magnets are not proven effective for muscle pain to date; some may benefit edema and ischemic conditions (NCCAM, 2/21/07). Electromagnets are medical diagnostic devices and have changing fields and may pulse with electrical current.
Manual therapy and massage therapy	Both therapies involve manipulating the musculoskeletal system. Manual therapy uses musculoskeletal adjustments involving pressure to relieve pathologic pressure on nerves or reduce blocked energy channels in the body. Massage therapy manipulates the soft tissues in a specified manner. Massage increases blood flow to muscles, promoting relaxation and relieving pain.
Nursing interventions for imagery/visualization, meditation, progressive relaxation, and prayer	These interventions are recognized in professional nursing practice and are discussed in detail in Chapter 29, Spirituality.
Qi gong	Often used with acupressure, this Chinese based intervention involves movement, meditation, and regulation of breathing in order to enhance the flow of *qi (chi)* and healthy balance. Benefits are increased blood circulation, improved immune functions, and possible help with asthma.
Reflexology	Reflexologists use their thumbs to apply pressure to "reflex zones" on the feet (sometimes hands) to produce a signal to the peripheral nervous system. The zones are mapped to correspond to different parts of the body. As with a reflex, the signal passes to the central nervous system and is processed by the brain before being relayed to the motor system for response. The purpose is to mitigate symptoms by adjusting the body's tone for reduced stress and improved well-being.

Continued

TABLE 6-1 Selected Complementary/Alternative Modalities—cont'd

Reiki	Reiki is a Japanese practice that involves placing the hands on or just above the patient. The practitioner senses and transmits the universal life energy, or *ki*, through specific body channels in order to promote healing and balance. A recognized therapy, it is known to reduce stress and blood pressure and promote relaxation. It has a strong spiritual component and is practiced by trained Reiki masters (NCCAM, 2/21/07).
Movement techniques and methods	During the 1950s a number of practitioners developed methods that relied on body positioning and movements to improve health. The *Alexander technique:* A technique promoting posture to facilitate health and prevent injury, such as from repetitive motion or stress. Treatment focus is on chronic conditions of the head, neck, or back, myalgias, and breathing problems. The F*eldenkrais Method* relies on awareness of movement and integrated movement as a means to improve functional abilities in daily life. With the *Trager method* a gentle bodywork of rocking and stretching loosens stiffness in joints and muscles. The pleasurable sensations and deep relaxation have been used with multiple sclerosis, muscular dystrophy, polio, asthma, and emphysema. *Rolfing* creates changes in a patient's posture and structure by manipulating the body's myofascial system. The more efficiently muscles operate, the more the body can conserve energy and develop more economical and refined patterns of movement for daily activities. Rolf's Structural Integration technique also is intended to reduce chronic pain and stress.
Therapeutic touch (TT) (noncontact)	TT is a putative energy method developed by Krieger (1979). The goal is to restore health of the body, mind, and spirit by bringing the patient into alignment with *qi (chi)*, the universal energy that sustains all life. Practitioners move their hands over the body without contact to restore harmony and balance qi.
Healing touch	A hand-mediated energy healing method certified by Healing Touch International.
Transcutaneous electrical nerve stimulation (TENS)	This battery-operated electronic device is attached to the skin with several electrodes; a conductive cream is used. The TENS unit generates electrical signals that stimulate local nerves intending to block pain. Although popular with physical therapists, no conclusive evidence of effectiveness was found for TENS.
Yoga and t'ai chi	These therapies are discussed in this chapter text.

Selected Botanicals

Use current data to evaluate all botanicals for effectiveness, adverse effects, and interactions with prescription drugs. Many cultural preparations are not listed.

Aloe	The gel of the aloe plant is used topically for minor burns and skin irritations. Evidence supports aloe may help heal pressure ulcers and wounds (NCCAM, 7/12/05) and prevent mouth ulcers following chemotherapy (NCCAM, 1/9/06). Strong caustic properties **prohibit** use as a laxative.
Asian ginseng	May lower blood glucose and aid immune function; use cautiously with diabetes. Increases effects of caffeine. Current studies include use with Alzheimer's disease and chronic lung infection (NCCAM, 8/18/05).
Assorted herbals	Chamomile and peppermint are examples of herbs in common use. Feverfew may relieve migraines and mild rheumatoid arthritis symptoms (NCCAM, 2/21/07).
Bismacine	The Federal Drug Administration (FDA) **banned** this bismuth preparation, including use with Lyme disease (FDA, 7/21/06).
Capsicum (cayenne)	Specific types and doses may relieve muscle and back pain and reduce gastric problems.
Chelation with ethylenediamine tetraacetic acid (EDTA)	Chelation has been used to treat high levels of lead in the blood. EDTA is a man-made amino acid administered intravenously (with oral vitamin supplements) during an international research study to determine whether chelation therapy is safe and effective for treating heart disease (NCCAM, 2/21/07).
Cranberry	A popular berry under review; it may prevent urinary tract infections and reduce dental plaque.
Echinacea	Echinacea was found ineffective against colds, but may treat upper respiratory infections (NCCAM, 2002/2003).
Ephedra	The FDA **banned** all supplements containing ephedrine alkaloids (NCCAM, 2/18/07).
European mistletoe	European variety found to kill cancer cells and stimulate the immune system. Any raw, unprocessed mistletoe and American mistletoe are **poisonous** (NCCAM, 6/30/05).
Evening primrose	Potentially effective with mild rheumatoid arthritis symptoms (NCCAM, 12/6/06).
Flaxseed and flaxseed oil	Evidence supports effective use as a laxative and potential to reduce cholesterol (NCCAM, 3/29/06).
Garlic	Potential but unclear benefits for arterial disease, lowering blood pressure, and against low-density lipoprotein cholesterol (The German E Commission) Difficult to establish effective dosage and preparations (NCCAM, 4/28/06). May be **harmful** used with certain human immunodeficiency virus (HIV) drugs (FDA).
Ginger root	Effective for nausea/vomiting (NCCAM, 8/3/03). Current studies are of ginger used with turmeric against arthritis and asthma.
Ginkgo biloba	NCCAM studies for use in multiple sclerosis, vascular and cognitive function, and preventing Alzheimer's disease. Potential benefits for certain macular degenerations and tinnitus; emerging evidence with cognitive impairments and dementias (Cochrane Library, 7/26/02) and with ischemic stroke. Interactions with anticoagulant drugs may increase bleeding risks.

TABLE 6-1 Selected Complementary/Alternative Modalities—cont'd

Hawthorne	Potentially effective and safe for mild heart failure (NCCAM, 12/5/06).
Kava	FDA **warning** links kava to severe liver damage; not recommended for use (NCCAM, 3/30/06).
Licorice root	May reduce symptoms with hepatitis C (NCCAM, 5/30/06). Role with stomach ulcers is unclear. High doses can elevate blood pressure and alter electrolyte balances.
Saw palmetto fruit	Moderate gains in urinary function associated with benign prostatic hypertrophy. Long term effects are unknown (NCCAM, 2/21/07).
St. John's wort	Popular in Europe; specific extracts/doses are helpful to treat mild-moderate depression (Cochrane Library, 2/25/05). **Alert:** Lowers blood levels of HIV drug indinavir.
Valerian root	Used for insomnia. Effectiveness with anxiety disorders being studied (NCCAM, 8/21/06).

Nutrition Plans and Dietary Supplements

Dietary supplements	Oral products labeled as dietary supplements, such as vitamins, minerals, herbal mixtures, and other substances that contain ingredients, for example, amino acids, enzymes, or glandulars, intended to supplement the diet. They are not a meal or conventional food. Studies concerning the safety and efficacy of supplements are available at http://www.ods.od.nih.gov. Megavitamin regimens remain a source of controversies; while some may help, others can be harmful and are under further study.
Specialty diets	Trade books present a large number and a wide variety of diet plans tailored to specific needs. Some diets, such as vegetarian, have cultural foundations and several variations. Popular diets use food regimens may target weight loss, cardiovascular benefits, and overall well-being, such as Pritikin's high fiber and low fat, Ornish's low fat vegetarian with calorie control, or Atkins' high protein foods; they also propose exercise and stress reduction measures. Macrobiotic diets are complex vegetarian and organic food regimens studied for cardiovascular benefits and lower cancer rates. The Zone diet targets weight loss and control of type 2 diabetes in that it stresses hormonal balance of low carbohydrates with protein and calorie control.
Diets targeting the immune system	Some untested diets are based on a theory of disease causation; they tend to require adherence to complicated therapy programs, but claim to counteract specific diseases. Most evidence is anecdotal or nonsupporting. The National Institutes of Health is investigating *Gerson* therapy, which views malignant growths as results of metabolic dysfunction within cells; for example, a cellular imbalance between sodium and potassium in each cell. Patients eat a highly specialized diet, including supplements and enzymes, and detoxify the body with certain agents that eventually eliminate abnormal substances, such as cancer cells. The *Kelly-Gonzales* diet also is under study. It consists of large amounts of natural and organic foods, especially raw fruits, juices, raw and steamed vegetables, cereals, and nuts. When combined with massive quantities of dietary supplements and freeze-dried pancreatic enzymes and practiced together with a "detoxification" process involving coffee enemas, it is said to slow the growth of cancerous tumors.

Data compiled from National Center for Complementary and Alternative Medicine, available at http://www.nccam.nih.gov; the Cochrane Library, available at www.cochrane.org; the U.S. Food and Drug Administration, available at www.fda.gov; and Blumenthal, M., Goldberg, A., & Brinckman, J. (Eds.). (2000). *Herbal medicine: Expanded Commission E monographs.* Newton, MA: Lippincott Williams & Wilkins.

Thinking of the body in terms of meridians or types, studying the flow of energy, or being concerned with restoring humeral balance are not conventional medicine concepts, nor is the belief that imbalance or restricted flow of energy (chi, *prahna*, and others) leads to illness. Nonetheless, traditional Chinese medicine has been practiced for more than 2000 years, and its practitioners engage in programs of study that are longer and more intensive than those of their Western physician counterparts. Usually traditional systems are best understood from worldviews of the particular cultures or regions where they have been practiced for centuries.

The major whole medical systems are listed briefly. Attempting to describe any one traditional system would be comparable to discussing the conventional medical system. Because rehabilitation nurses integrate CAM interventions with conventional practice, they have particular purposes in understanding more about the source, theoretical base, and context of the therapeutics.

Traditional Chinese medicine deals with balance and imbalance of the vital energy called qi (chi) and with yin and yang. It is a complex system that has ancient origins dating to 206 BC. Acupuncture is the intervention most familiar in the West; herbal preparations, *qi gong*, special types of massage, moxibustion, and proper attention to diet, exercise, and rest are important therapeutics. A great deal of rehabilitation research is centered on providing evidence for the benefits of traditional Chinese medicine. Acupuncture has been reported as effective in reducing pain due to osteoarthritis, rotator cuff disease, and fibromyalgia (Berman, Swyers, & Ezzo, 2000; Green, Buchbinder, & Hetdrick, 2005). Acupuncture is currently under review by the Cochrane Collaboration (CC) for efficacy in treating chemotherapy-induced nausea or vomiting among cancer patients and in reducing incidence and duration of seizures in patients with epilepsy (Cheuk & Wong, 2005; Richardson et al., 2004).

India's traditional medical system, Ayurveda, which literally means "science of life," has gained attention in the West. *Prahna* is an essential energy flow, and diet, massage, herbal preparations, fresh air, and sunshine are prescribed according to individual body types. Programs of exercise (yoga), meditation, and a form of controlled breathing place emphasis on maintaining or restoring harmony and connection among the body, mind, spirit, and environment. Traditional and *Maharishi* are two approaches to Ayurveda. In a randomized controlled trial to evaluate the efficacy of yoga for chronic low back pain, the outcome revealed significant improvement in functional ability, as well as reductions in pain intensity, and a decrease in pain medication in the yoga group (Williams, Petronis, Smith et al., 2005).

In Germany as early as 1776, Hahnemann hypothesized "the principle of similars," which holds that a condition could be cured by administering small doses of a substance of which large doses produce specific disease symptoms in health, persons to induce a mild form of a like condition. Small doses of potentially toxic remedies, often involving several preparations to be taken in a certain order, time, and dose, are used to stimulate the body's self-healing mechanisms against illness. Every illness is thought to have its own remedy within itself. Homeopathy became popular in the West during the mid-nineteenth century then diminished by the 1920s. Today it is practiced by those who place emphasis on the body's capacity for self-healing. A large pharmacopoeia includes many remedies prepared from herbal and plant sources, minerals, and some animal secretions and venom. Systematic reviews and meta-analysis of the effectiveness of homeopathic remedies have produced conflicting results (Cucherat, Haugh, Gooch, & Boissel, 2000; Jones, Kaptchuck, & Linde, 2003).

Naturopathic medicine, another system that focuses on prevention of disease and restoration of health, is less concerned with treatments. The rationale incorporates the philosophy that the body has potential for healing itself when one lives within the laws of nature. Thus it follows that naturopathic practitioners rely on noninvasive remedies of diet modification, nutritional supplements, herbal preparations, and counseling, especially about prevention and lifestyle. In addition, ultrasound, electric therapies, soft tissue and spinal manipulations, acupuncture, multiple types of hydrotherapy, and pharmacology are used. Practitioners study premedicine as a biological science and then study for 4 years incorporating conventional medicine curricula and naturopathic therapeutics. Naturopathic physicians are accredited and licensed under the Council on Naturopathic Medical Education (CNME).

Mind-Body Medicine

As discussed earlier, PNI is a framework for research of the body-mind connection using biological measures of outcome. Research supports the mind-body pathway's influence on the immune system. Simplistically the higher cognitive and limbic (emotional) centers of the brain affect health and healing via the autonomic nervous system and neuroendocrine body-mind pathways to the immune system (Waitkins in Micozzi, 1996). Complementary therapies activate brain-immune pathways to improve well-being. To this end, nurses incorporate interventions such as prayer, spirituality, relaxation, meditation, group sessions, guided imagery and visualization, hypnotherapy, t'ai chi, *qi gong*, reframing and cognitive or behavior modification, pet therapy, humor, and support groups into practice. Table 6-1 provides short descriptions of selected complementary alternative modalities of interest to nurses (see also Chapter 29).

Examples of studies in the mind-body category include effectiveness of movement therapies, such as yoga, t'ai chi, and dance therapy. T'ai chi has been found to promote physical function, including flexibility and strength, to reduce pain, and to enhance immune response (Klein & Adams, 2004). In seven recent studies, t'ai chi has been shown to improve strength and balance, thus helping prevent falls in elderly persons (Choi, Moon, & Song, 2005; Li, Harmer, Fisher, & Mcauley, 2004; Hart et al., 2004; Lin & Lane, 2005; Tsang & Hui-Chan, 2005; Wong, Chou, Tang, & Wong, 2001; Zwick, Rochell, Choksi, & Domwicz, 2000). These results indicate that dynamic exercise has improved muscle strength and aerobic capacity. Additional studies have demonstrated positive effects of t'ai chi in blood pressure control and in retarding bone loss in postmenopausal women (Chan et al., 2004; Klein & Adams, 2004).

The benefits of pet therapy and service dogs have been documented in several studies that report the positive results of increased social interaction and decreased agitated behaviors. (Modlin, 2000; Richeson, 2003). In rehabilitation, pets have provided assistance as well as companionship. Equine therapy is therapeutic horseback riding. The motion of the horse in movement helps patients to develop muscle strength, control, and balance. Children who have developmental disabilities or cerebral palsy have benefited from horseback therapy, although riders of all ages gain a sense of confidence, improved self-image, and access to the larger world viewed from the saddle.

Related therapies, such as music, art, and dance, influence the brain hemisphere responses and cognitive processes in positive ways. Used in conjunction with relaxation and visualization or guided imagery, these therapies have potential for improving outcomes for patients. Journal writing is a favorite technique used in conjunction with these therapies. Smith, Holcoft, Rebeck, Thompson, and Werkowitch (2000) found journal writing influential in helping chronically ill patients overcome situational depression. Nurses with special training do participate in other techniques complementary to mind-body concepts (e.g., hypnosis, psychotherapy, and biofeedback). Biofeedback training has been found effective in improving bed-wetting and improving recurring urinary track infections (Rutters, 2005). The literature is replete with studies chronicling the positive effects of hypnosis therapy for many conditions, including pain management in older adults who were depressed and complained of poor quality of life (Cuellar, 2005).

Biological-Based Practices

This category is popular in the community owing to use of nutritional programs, dietary supplements, herbal preparations, and therapies or products to treat special conditions or diseases. Sales of dietary supplements in the United States have reached an annual estimated cost of $18.7 billion (NCCAM, 2002). Examples are glucosamine supplements for arthritis; bee pollen supplements for autoimmune diseases; diet programs such as those by Drs. Atkins, Pritikin, and Ornish; megavitamin regimens; macrobiotic diets; antioxidant supplements; and melatonin supplements. The range of herbal medicine choices is huge. All are biological based.

Aromatherapy and hydrotherapy have entered the public domain in various products ranging from candles to body oils to massage kits. Aroma as therapy differs from simply selecting scents; choices for use as therapies are highly selective based on multiple factors and may be introduced complementary to other interventions. Allergies or sensitivities to aromas are not uncommon, but purveyors of essential oils claim that, unlike fragrances, they do not stimulate allergic attacks. Proper informed use of aromatherapy may bring soothing relief and relaxation.

Many herbal products are available over-the-counter at local health food stores or pharmacies; others must be prepared at ethnic apothecaries. Studies have shown that glucosamine and chondroitin supplements give moderate-to-large relief of symptoms due to osteoarthritis (Jordan et al., 2004; Manson & Rahman, 2004; Šimánek, Kren, Ulrichová, & Gallo, 2005; Thompson, 2004). Similarly, injectable gold has been shown to be effective for short-term treatment of swollen joints due to rheumatoid arthritis, although toxicity was a risk for some patients (Clark, Tugwell, Bennett et al., 2004). However, there is controversy regarding the popular herb echinacea. In clinical trials echinacea has been found ineffective in preventing colds or reducing cold symptoms (Sampson, 2005). Currently NCCAM has three more active randomized clinical trials of echinacea. Miller (2005) found echinacea to extend the life span of aging mice and leukemic mice and to abate leukemia. Given the 97% genetic similarity between mice and humans, the potential immuno-enhancing property of echinacea is of interest.

Interactions with food, conventional medicines, and herbal products occur, but as a body of knowledge the implications of consecutive or concurrent use are relatively unknown. For example, St. John's wort, used successfully for decades to treat depression and perimenopausal symptoms, was found to produce reduced blood levels of indinavir, a human immunodeficiency virus (HIV) protease inhibitor and to cause decreased anticoagulant effect in cardiac patients (Izzo, Di Carlo, Borelli, & Ernst, 2005; Linde & Knuppel, 2005; Piscitelli, Burstein, Chaitt, Alfaro, & Falloon, 2000). Nutrition and lifestyle changes are modalities of high interest to nurses.

Manipulative and Body-Based Practices

Physiatrists and therapists in rehabilitation, chiropractors, osteopathic physicians, massage therapists, and certain alternative practitioners manipulate the musculoskeletal system during treatments. Rehabilitation practitioners are interested in myofascial release as an adjunct to pain management. The diversity of practitioners ranges from licensed chiropractors to therapists performing massage, shiatsu, reflexology, Rolfing, *Tui Na*, and acupressure for soft tissues and deep muscle manipulation.

Nurses have some practice in this category; more often physical therapists use methods such as those originated as Feldenkrais, Alexander, Trager, and others. Although chiropractors and massage therapists receive standardized training and are licensed, the methods referred to as "bodywork" may be practiced under a vast array of labels by persons who have no regulation or formal training. The Cochrane Collaboration systematic reviews on manipulative and bodywork practices (2005) revealed that numerous clinical trials on the safety and effectiveness of many manipulative techniques have been inconclusive.

Energy Fields Medicine

These therapies deal with two types of energy fields. The first is from endogenous fields (also called putative or biofields) within the individual's body, and the other is from exogenous fields (external energy). Putative or biofield energy was described more than 2000 years ago, when practitioners in various cultures described a vital energy or life force (called qi, ki, *doshas*, *prana*, etheric energy, *fohat*, orgone, *odic forme*, or *mamna*) that is inherent in each individual. It is believed that the flow and balance of vital energy is required for optimal health. Therapists correct imbalances and restore energy flow by removing blockages in the body or by transmitting vital energy to restore health. *qi gong*, Reiki, healing touch, intercessory prayer, and therapeutic touch are examples of healing modalities during which the therapist accesses a healing energy force to facilitate healing for the individual.

The therapist must be able to enter into a centered state of consciousness and continually assess and evaluate the process while directing energy. Based on the research initiated by Krieger (1979) (a rehabilitation nurse later joined by Kunz), the principle of "undivided wholeness" is one that resonated with nurses. They have embraced therapeutic touch (TT) in research and practice, including a NANDA International (NANDA-I) diagnosis of *disturbed energy field* (NANDA-I, 2007) and Nursing Outcomes Classification of "Energy Field, Disturbed" (Moorhead, Johnson, & Maas, 2004, p. 599).

Also classified as a nursing intervention, TT is defined as "attuning to the universal healing field, seeking to act as an instrument for healing influence, and using the natural sensitivity of the hands to gently focus and direct the intervention process" (Dochterman & Bulechek, 2004, p. 734). Although many research findings support TT, results are mixed. Woods, Craven, and Whitney (2005) compared therapeutic touch with placebo on behavioral symptoms of persons with dementia and found significantly fewer adverse behaviors in those who received TT. The Nurse Healers Professional Associated International lists policies and procedures for health care professionals on their website (http://www. therapeutic-touch.org) along with a position statement on credentialing, standards of practice, and a code of ethics for practitioners of therapeutic touch.

Kwapien and Kulakowski (2005) found healing touch and Reiki treatments reduced pain, stress, and nausea and vomiting in cancer patients. Closely aligned with Krieger's therapeutic touch and Rogerian theory, healing touch is a hand-mediated energetic healing intervention. Healing Touch International (http://www.healingtouchinternational.org) is an organization that certifies nurses, other health professionals, and lay practitioners in healing touch. The organization has established international standards and a code of ethics, as well as sponsoring research and education programs.

The use of electromagnetic field energy relies on devices maneuvered by the individual or a therapist. Static and time-varying magnetic products have achieved popular use for pain relief, muscle spasms, osteoarthritis, and multiple sclerosis. Low-level laser therapy (classes I, II, and III) has been used as noninvasive treatment for reducing rheumatoid arthritis symptoms associated with morning stiffness, range of motion and function, and local swelling. Randomized controlled clinical trials (RCCTs) yielded some benefits for reduced pain and stiffness after treatment. Overall additional research is needed, especially regarding specific details such as dose, intensity, and site (McDonald, 2005; NCCAM, 2005).

There has long been an interest and belief in healing properties from electromagnetic fields. Multiple products, ranging from wrist or knee magnets to magnetic mattress pads, are available widely in the market. To date, studies find some hope for improving outcome in sleep and certain neurological disorders and pain management; further evidence is unclear (Eccles, 2005; Kroeling, Gross, Goldsmith & Cervical Overview Group, 2005).

Current Research at NCCAM

Clinical and basic scientific research, including formal clinical trials to determine the safety, clinical activity and efficacy, and potential problems of currently known and available therapies and substances, are NCCAM's highest priority. Initially five specialized research centers across the nation received funding to study the use of complementary and alternative medicine in areas of aging, arthritis, craniofacial disorders, neurological disorders, women's health, and cardiovascular disease in African Americans. Current areas of special interest important to rehabilitation include examining the safety and efficacy of the following:

- Anxiety and depression—basic and preclinical research on CAM approaches
- Cardiovascular diseases—preclinical and early-phase clinical studies of CAM approaches to secondary prevention and management of hypertension, atherosclerosis, and congestive heart failure
- Ethnomedicine—identification, description, and study of potentially valuable, vanishing traditional or indigenous health care practices in geographic areas where there is little preservation
- HIV/acquired immunodeficiency syndrome (AIDS)—use and effects of CAM therapies for HIV/AIDS and its complications
- Immune modulation/enhancement—basic and preclinical studies of CAM approaches that may enhance or inhibit immune response, including inflammation
- Insomnia—CAM approaches to primary and secondary insomnia
- Liver—CAM approaches to liver disease
- Obesity/metabolic syndrome—CAM modalities, particularly mind-body treatments, as adjuvant therapies, especially with respect to the metabolic syndrome and type 2 diabetes
- Respiratory diseases—CAM approaches to prevention and treatment of infectious respiratory disease and asthma

NATIONAL INSTITUTE ON DISABILITY AND REHABILITATION RESEARCH: EMERGING UNIVERSE OF DISABILITY

The National Institute on Disability and Rehabilitation Research (NIDRR) conducts ongoing monitoring of demographical characteristics of the U.S. population and notes changes in the distribution of disability. Over the last 4 years of the past long-range plan (1999 to 2003), certain indicators in the population changed, namely, age, income, education, ethnic composition, and immigrant status. Poverty, ethnic background, family structure, and social risks are known to negatively impact patients with disabilities who are from diverse groups. Key concerns revealed in the demographic data analysis were new impairments and consequences for existing disabilities that were associated with emergent health challenges such as those that arise from different socioeconomic, regional, and cultural causes. NIDRR refers to this phenomenon as an "emerging universe of disability." Researchers are called upon to study the impact of this universe on outcomes for citizens with disabilities and to do so in a comprehensive evaluation of complex variables. Community-based rehabilitation nurses may be positioned to have key roles in meeting this challenge (NIDRR, 2005).

Monitoring Claims for Cure

When cure is not forthcoming, persons with terminal, chronic, or disabling conditions may seek hope wherever promised, regardless of evidence. The Food and Drug Administration (FDA) is the government agency charged to protect consumers from danger, fraud, false expectations, and ineffective or unacceptable claims. The FDA requires pharmaceutical companies and manufacturers of dietary supplements and other health products to meet stringent standards, involving costly and lengthy procedures, whenever the label promises cure for a specific condition. However, products that are intended to improve health undergo less scrutiny.

Germany is the world leader in evaluating herbal safety and efficacy. Since 1978 the German Commission E, a panel of physicians, pharmacists, pharmacologists, and toxicologists, has evaluated data from studies, clinical trials, and case studies. Available in English, results from the German Commission E are regarded as the most accurate information on the safety and efficacy of herbal remedies (Freeman, 2004). Computer Access to Research on Dietary Supplements (CARDS) is a database of federally funded research projects on dietary supplements. The database is compiled as part of the Dietary Supplement Health and Education Act of 1994 with free access at the Office of Dietary Supplements (ODS) website (http://ods.nih.gov/Research/CARDS). Also available from ODS is the International Bibliographic Information on Dietary Supplements

(IBDS) database, which provides access to published international and scientific literature on dietary supplements.

Composition and standards for preparation of dietary supplements vary among companies and products. Nearly 70% of households use some type of vitamin, herbal product, or supplement. Some products are ineffective, and product sales prey on the hopes of desperate patients and families. One example is laetrile, although banned nearly 20 years ago by the FDA. A simple Internet search for laetrile will find it offered for sale on multiple websites as laetril, or B17, and as a treatment for cancer.

Evidence-Based Practice

Evidence-based practice has become a phrase for ensuring quality of service, therapeutic interventions, remedies, and preparations. The process examines the abilities of the practitioner, as well as the rigor of research to evaluate safety and effectiveness. At stake are reimbursement for effective products and therapies and eventual integration of proven therapies into mainstream conventional medicine and education. Gathering evidence and disseminating findings are lengthy processes that become longer when coupled with safeguards for research on human subjects and translations of foreign language publications. Clinical decisions rely on critique of the literature, then conclusions about what is safe, effective, and economically sound, often only to determine that more evidence is needed or to declare interventions as outright unsafe or ineffective. A scheme for rating evidence of research findings combines ranking of several medical groups. The tomes of information about potential therapeutics, research findings, and resources create a huge backlog of material for investigation. Answers about safety and efficacy have fallen far behind public demands, and consumers continue to use products based on sparse data.

The NCCAM collaborated with a group of national organizations to enhance the speed and improve the quality of research reports from clinical investigations. The gold standard for evaluating any intervention has been recognized as the RCCT. This method sits directly in the domain of scientific approaches of conventional medicine and will be fraught with problems that are methodological, philosophical, and concerned with feasibility (Margolin, Avants, & Kleber, 1998). Critical evaluation of research conducted worldwide and databases of information gathered with organizational collaboration will assist in providing data about the validity and reliability of findings.

In fact, the FDA has a program that encourages pharmaceutical companies to submit information from their clinical trials to a website as a contribution to a federal and private registry. Because Medicare reimbursement is tied to results of clinical trials, patients will have a vested interest in several ways. Some who have chronic conditions may choose to participate in trials with varying degrees of risk, others may seek payment for procedures or medications, and health providers may be bombarded with appropriate and inappropriate requests for services from patients (FDA on-line, 2005, www.clinicaltrials.gov).

The CC provides an international register of (RCCTs) in CAM-related research. A not-for-profit organization that prepares, maintains, and disseminates systematic, current reviews of RCCTs and/or controlled clinical trials, the CC issues reports of interest including those about CAMs to health care groups; some are specific treatments in rehabilitation. The CC uses a similar scheme to evaluate research findings suitable for clinical practice. Evidence must be accompanied by sufficient information about use of the therapeutic technique, instrument, or preparation, such as the dose response, strength, frequency, intensity, cautions, and adverse effects (www.cochrane.org).

Rehabilitation nurses are in positions to serve as advocates for patients on either hand: to protect them from improper participation in trials or use of products and services, or to assist them in gaining access to efficacious interventions. Becoming knowledgeable and staying current must be tempered with understanding the implications and evaluating the outcomes on individual patient bases. If not evidence based, then what does formulate medical decisions? (Dickersin, Straus, & Bero, 2007).

Organizational Collaboration

Once the NCCAM scientifically investigates the effectiveness of a treatment or procedure and determines the type of evidence needed, one or more of the following organizations conduct systematic reviews for evidence.

- Centers for Disease Control and Prevention (CDC) has direct access to providers and skill in survey research.
- Cancer Advisory Panel for Complementary and Alternative Medicine (CAPCAM) operates in collaboration with the National Cancer Institute (NCI) to target evaluation of cancer treatment proposals.
- Agency for Healthcare Research and Quality (AHRQ), formerly the Agency for Health Care Policy and Research (AHCPR), offers publications about best practices and guidelines for professionals and consumers.
- The Cochrane Collaboration reports can be used when deciding whether to use research findings in practice.
- Topics discussed at NIH Consensus Development Conferences sponsored by NCCAM are pertinent to practice and research.

Dissemination of Information

Not only are patients becoming active partners in their health care, in some instances they are researching and directing their care using information and resources from around the world, such as from the FDA-sponsored clinical trials database and registry mentioned earlier. Dissemination of information in reputable channels is important for providers. Alternative and complementary health care and related interventions have captured a great deal of attention in research, publications, conference proceedings, and practice settings, and dozens of schools of medicine, nursing, and allied health now include courses in these fields.

The Richard and Hinda Rosenthal Center for Complementary and Alternative Medicine at Columbia University is a resource on the World Wide Web for databases concerning complementary and alternative health care (www.rosenthal. hs.columbia.edu). This website lists many and varied websites related to CAM. In addition, the NCCAM has its own clearinghouse for dissemination of information about the program and research findings to providers and the public. The NCCAM maintains a citation index since 1963 available through the National Library of Medicine's (NLM's) MEDLINE database. Entrez PubMed is the NLM search service that provides access to citations on MEDLINE and PreMEDLINE. NCCAM and the NLM have partnered to create CAM on PubMed, a subset of NLM PubMed that provides free access to data limited to the CAM subset of PubMed. The Consortium of Academic Health Centers for Integrative Medicine (CAHCIM) is composed of a group of 32 medical centers in North America affiliated with academic institutions. They publish a journal, *Alternative Therapies in Health and Medicine.*

Referral to a CAM Practitioner

Collaboration with and referral to a practitioner of complementary or conventional health care can be problematic without criteria for evaluating the person and the practice. Box 6-4 offers guidelines for referrals. Practitioners, such as chiropractors and some therapists, may be licensed by the state, but practice laws and licensure requirements differ among states. To complicate the process, many CAM providers have no established education or training, no formal organization, and no standard name for their practice. For instance, more than 30 titles fall under the category of bodyworks. CAM practice is regulated by a variety of rules that may differ by state. Major areas of concern are licensure, scope of practice, ethics, and malpractice. Legal issues regarding CAM practice are evolving, and many health insurers are providing coverage for certain CAM practices or providers. However, when working in collaboration

with any provider or making a referral to an unknown practitioner, liability issues may emerge should the patient suffer injury due to negligence or inappropriate care (Cohen, 2003).

NURSING PROCESS

Assessment

Conceptual frameworks that may be useful include the Health Belief Model, Leininger's transcultural model, and Neuman's Systems Model (see Chapter 2).

Cultural Assessment. Recognize that the community and familial environments are part of the person's assessment. Elicit their explanatory model of the health condition or situation; ask for their own description of the condition.

- What does it mean to you or your family that you have this disease or disability?
- What do you think is the cause of the problem? Does it have a name? Why do you think it happened?
- Explain how you think this disease or disability will work. How long will it last? How sick or disabled do you think, or do others say, you are?
- What should be done to treat the condition? What have you or someone else done already? Did it work?
- Who could best treat this condition? What are problems or concerns that you have about the treatment? What support is available from your family, religious group, or community? Do you need help in contacting these groups?
- What do you plan to do? What can you expect as a result of treatment or lack of treatment?
- Are nontraditional, complementary, or alternative healers involved? What treatments are under consideration? What assistance is needed to accommodate this approach?
- Are there legal or ethical considerations? How best can these be addressed?
- What will not work or should not be done in the situation? Are there things you believe you should not talk about or say?
- What would you like the result or outcome to be?

   Learning and asking about specific areas will provide better understanding of the meaning of data collected during the assessment.

Learn About

- History of the culture
- Patient's perception of personal identification with the culture
- Patient/family degree of acculturation with the dominant society
- Where they place themselves regarding intraethnic diversity
- Language skills (assess oral and reading/writing separately)
- Education level and socioeconomic status
- Length of time they have lived in the United States

Ask About

- Lifestyle, preferences, and prohibitions
- Dietary habits or needs
- Religious practices, including restrictions, and spiritual values
- Traditional healing practices and the use of nutraceuticals, over-the-counter medications, and complementary and alternative medical practices

---

BOX 6-4   Suggestions When Making a Referral to a Practitioner of Complementary/ Alternative Medicine or of Conventional Medicine

Determine whether the practitioner:

- Holds membership in specialty organizations or associations
- Is certified or accredited by specialty area
- Has liability insurance for practice
- Honors (does not violate) professional practice acts of conventional medicine professionals
- Obtains reimbursement or coverage from insurance companies
- Attends continuing education or other workshops
- Is known to other providers (conventional and alternative) in the community
- Communicates with the team members about the plan for care
- Uses safe practices and ethical behaviors, as far as can be ascertained, and avoids practices known to be unsafe or ineffective per randomized controlled clinical trials (RCCTs)
- Provides treatment options and indicates length of the treatment
- Does not continue process or treatments indefinitely
- Has no public, professional, or patient complaints against the practice or provider for personal misconduct

Cultural assessment is complex and involves moving past ethnocentric assumptions. For example, the title of aunt or mother to a child of some cultures may not be restricted to biological or family roles. Assess the patient and family perceptions of space, time, sex roles, kinship ties, and family relationships. Nonverbal communication, gestures, and facial expressions are not credible measures for understanding what is really happening and are misinterpreted often by members of differing cultures. Evaluate for specific biological or genetic conditions that are associated with certain heritages. Collection of data about cultural phenomena takes time and a trust relationship.

Giger and Davidhizar (2004) list six cultural phenomena that are evident in all cultural groups in varying degrees of application. These are communication, space, time, biological variations, environmental control, and social organization. Assessment and intervention are enriched with these kinds of data. Self-care differences among cultural groups are important for rehabilitation nurses to identify before instituting plans for care or engaging in mutual goal setting with patients and families.

Variables based on religious beliefs and practices may become more important when patients encounter chronic, disabling conditions. Ask the patient to describe their religious designation, identify leaders of the group, and how they should be involved in care.. The best rule is to ask what is important for them to have happen and what must never happen based on their religious practices. Incorporate this information into the team record, and validate it with the patient and family. In some instances, religious rules are suspended or altered for those who are ill or receiving medical care. Not only is there wide variation among and within religious groups, but a patient may subscribe to a particular religion, yet not engage in many of the practices. The handling of body fluids or parts and decisions about medical directives predictably have religious importance. Do not assume that a person who refers to spiritual experiences is religious, or vice versa.

Assessing the Therapeutic Relationship. Many patients or families continue to rely on cultural, lay, or folk remedies or CAM therapies during their time in rehabilitation. Essentially, they incorporate CAM therapies into their daily life and as a result formulate their own plan of care, which may be integrated or set apart from the rehabilitation program, especially upon returning to the community. A rehabilitation nurse who has developed a trusting therapeutic relationship with the patient and family is better prepared to assess their plans for CAM or cultural interventions. Assess whether their plans are related to religious beliefs or practices and are compatible with mutual rehabilitation goals. Are there elements in the rehabilitation plans that are misunderstood or not acceptable? Determine whether the plan is safe, reasonable, or feasible; if it is legally and ethically sound; and if there are any apparent detrimental, harmful, or adverse effects. Finally, assess whether the patient and family are informed fully and understand both benefits and consequences of the actions. Their decisions become part of the team record.

Goals

Goals for rehabilitation nurses are to become culturally competent, sensitive, and relevant and to be able to serve as a broker between patient and family cultures and the culture of rehabilitation.

Interventions

Use strategies of the culture broker role to bridge or mediate between the patient culture, the conventional rehabilitation system, and traditional and/or alternative medical systems.
- Clarify information, values, and expectations.
- Broker concepts, such as self-care, among patient and team members.
- Encourage building trust and therapeutic relationships.
- Ensure patient and family fully comprehend information and consent.
- Discuss problems, misconceptions, and disagreements openly.
- Facilitate using conflict resolution and negotiation skills.
- Integrate family and religious and cultural values and beliefs into the person's plan for care as safely as possible.
- Arrange for interventions with sensitivity to variations in perceptions, such as for time, space, lifestyle, dietary needs, and communication.

Use translators cautiously. Age, sex, intraethnic animosities, class issues, and prohibitions about sharing personal information may lead to collecting inaccurate data as a patient's experiencing mistrust or even fear of harm. Consider how many persons are able to speak a language fluently or conversationally but remain unfamiliar with medical terminology or correct descriptions of health problems.

Many therapeutic interventions that are considered CAM practices are performed commonly by rehabilitation nurses. Learn patient expectations of a rehabilitation nurse, especially for self-care and therapeutic relationships, then explain nursing roles. Learn what experiences the patient has had with assistive devices, prostheses, or technology. Examples of interventions known to have benefits include relaxation response, massage, diet and nutrition, and meditative approaches. Rehabilitation nurses may choose to pursue education and training for practicing shiatsu, reflexology, biofeedback, behavioral management, herbal medicine, acupuncture, therapeutic touch, Reiki, healing touch, and other specific healing methodologies. Other chapters in the text may contain information about specific interventions for particular conditions as appropriate.

Outcomes

Outcomes are for cultural competence and sensitivity in rehabilitation practice. The therapeutic relationship is built well when the perceptions and expectations of patient, family, and providers are based on mutual trust.

Evaluation

Rehabilitation nurses may encounter issues with regulations and standards of practice. "Many (CAM) strategies have long been in the purview of nursing practice. Regulatory changes in nurse practices acts and the professional practice acts of other professionals related to (CAM) differ by state and must be carefully monitored by nurses" (Cohen 2003).

Evidence-based practice, such as that guided by information from the CC, international studies, and findings from NCCAM-sponsored research programs, will evaluate methods, techniques, and interventions from alternative and conventional medical systems by their quality, safety, and efficacy. Preventive, as well as restorative and maintenance, benefits from therapeutics, processes, and principles that constitute rehabilitation also hold interest for alternative research. For example, Engstrom and Hauser (2000) found physical rehabilitation not only improved motor scores on the Functional Independence Measure, but also changed perceptions of quality of life for persons with multiple sclerosis. Mitka (1999) found persons who participated in a cardiac rehabilitation program not only improved their overall health, exercise capacity, and energy levels, but also reduced their depression. Other CAM-related issues important to rehabilitation continue to arise, such as findings from the human genome project or therapeutic use of marijuana.

SUMMARY: NURSING AND INTEGRATED CARE

Nurses were among the first professionals to promote alternative and complementary modes of health and healing. A holistic approach is central to nursing, nurses understand care apart from cure, and nurses encourage self-care in the therapeutic process. They recognize that at times healing arises from the person's own participation, whether from biological, psychosocial, spiritual, or other resources. Many techniques identified as alternative or complementary have been embraced by and integrated within professional nursing. Relaxation techniques, stress reduction or smoking cessation programs, lifestyle management, and therapeutic exercise are long-time nursing interventions, whereas Krieger's work (1979)

on therapeutic touch remains an extension of practice for many nurses.

Nurses may use all of these techniques and approaches as interventions in various rehabilitation settings when appropriate for the plan of care. Nurses also are comfortable working with patients from diverse backgrounds and with using proven alternative therapeutics to complement conventional practices. They understand how body, mind, and spirit interrelate so that a person may have mental and spiritual health alongside a terminal body condition.

Prevention is in vogue. The goals of *Healthy People 2010* include helping individuals to maintain optimal functional abilities and promoting healthier, longer lives. However, despite progress in funding toward finding cures for chronic, disabling conditions, efforts that target prevention and early intervention still receive minimal support. Ideally, funds will support conducting research to find ways to prevent or control chronic conditions early and to provide the best care, rather than only seeking cures after the disease or condition occurs. Clearly safety, efficacy, and quality must be rigorously pursued in evidence-based research. Perhaps nurse advocates will direct more attention to improving the physical and social environment, potential for self-healing, and life satisfaction for patients with chronic, disabling, or developmental conditions.

The call is for an integrated health system, rather than conventional, alternative, or complementary medicine and therapeutics (Fontanarosa & Lundberg, 1998; Sobel, 1979). Many treatments, interventions, and therapeutics originating outside conventional medicine have been proven to be safe and to have merit, especially when practiced by a trained practitioner in appropriate situations. Similarly, more open global relationships have resulted in regard for and acceptance of the results of rigorous and controlled research conducted by professionals in other countries. Efforts by WHO and NIDRR to collect and manage international data on health, disability, and function provide additional support for global research.

Case Study

Jill Milner, MSN, RN, CRRN, CHTP

Jane Carter, CRRN, visits Mija Groenwald, a 66-year-old home health care patient with a history of hypertension and type 2 diabetes. Mrs. Groenwald incurred multiple traumas during an automobile accident and has a hip-to-ankle cast. The hospital discharge planner recommended institutional skilled nursing admission, including physical therapy, but the patient refused. Her new diagnoses are a torsion fracture of the left femur (status post open reduction), multiple lacerations and contusions on forearms and face, and back and neck sprain. Ms. Carter's assessment will identify appropriate postsurgical nursing services.

Ms. Carter is greeted by Mr. Groenwald and two adult daughters with three active toddler grandchildren. Mrs. Groenwald's 85-year-old mother, who appears to be of Asian descent, offers comments from her seat in a recliner. The patient, a petite woman of Philippino or Hispanic descent, is wearing a soft neck brace. She is in the bed unable to maneuver with the heavy cast and unable to raise her leg independently or ambulate. The dressed wounds on her face and arms are from windshield glass cuts. Ms. Carter changes the dressings using prescribed wound care; she observes healing without signs of infection.

Continued

Case Study—cont'd

During the cultural assessment Mrs. Groenwald relates that her mother was born in Japan and her father, deceased, was Mexican American. Her husband is "Anglo" (European American descent) and is at work at the family shop. "I know I don't look like a Groenwald," she laughs. "I surprise a lot of people." As Mrs. Groenwald usually cares for her elderly mother, the daughters have taken time off from their part-time employment and are juggling care for three generations of family.

The automobile accident occurred when she lost consciousness during a hypoglycemic event. Before the accident she was taking steroidal medication for persistent back and neck pain and had started insulin to help control her blood glucose level. She no longer takes either medication because her blood glucose level was stabilized during hospitalization. Before the accident she monitored herself only sporadically and disliked having to take insulin. Now she uses a new blood glucose monitoring machine four times daily. "I hate to poke myself, which may seem silly, as acupuncture works for me, so they gave me this kind that doesn't need much blood."

Ms. Carter learns that Mrs. Groenwald occasionally visited an acupuncture clinic and also saw a family friend for chiropractic treatments for her back and neck pain. "Our friend used to just give me a spine adjustment on the living room floor when he visits. Hope he can still help me someway now." She feels that regular acupuncture helped, "For balance, you know," and will resume it when able to travel to the clinic. The family finds routine massage helpful. "I taught my daughters how to rub my neck and back and feet like my mom taught me. I like a regular all-body massage, not that Shiatsu with the pressure points."

Medications include hydrochlorothiazide 25 mg bid, glimepiride (Amaryl) 2 mg daily, calcium as Tums 4 tablets a day, and fentanyl

patch daily. The patch is a new treatment method that she feels works well, but she is nervous about not having an oral medicine should her pain worsen; she asks to take Aleve in that event. She rates her current pain as a 2, "aching" in her cast, and some "stinging" pain from the dressing changes. Ms. Carter asks, "What other methods do you use for pain control or to encourage healing? For example, do you use herbs, supplements, healers, prayer, or any other treatment methods?"

Mrs. Groenwald goes to both her medical internist and a Chinese herbalist, as did her Japanese mother while she was growing up. Mrs. Groenwald displays bags of herbs that the herbalist instructed her to boil twice in a clay pot and then mix into a tea. "This is to cleanse my system and build me up," but Mrs. Groenwald states that these usually result in a bowel cleanse of diarrhea, and she is reluctant to use these while immobile. "I'm not really sure that one works. I think I got dehydrated last time, not stronger. My mother had a bad back too, and when she was in Japan she had little herb balls put on her spine and then burned. They left a scar! I'm not doing that."

The daughters have many questions about their mother's diabetes testing regimen and prescribed 1500-calorie, 2-g sodium diet. Their mother is "almost a vegetarian" taking a varied diet ranging from organically grown salads, to vegetables and tofu stir fried with soy sauce and oriental flavorings, to homemade Mexican dishes. As instructed by their matriarchal grandmother, they want her to eat more red meat "to build up her blood." The hospital dietician suggested dairy products for more calcium, but she tends to experience bloating and diarrhea. A "comfort food" Mrs. Groenwald enjoys is "okyu," soupy rice mixed with egg, a traditional food for a person when ill.

TABLE 6-2 Nursing Diagnoses, Interventions, and Outcomes Applicable to Mrs. Groenwald   **NIC/NOC**

Nursing Diagnosis	Nursing Interventions	Nursing Outcomes
Ineffective health maintenance with deficient knowledge diabetes and hypertension	*Instruct patient and family caregivers in present health management regimen related to diabetes and hypertension, including medication regimen and signs and symptoms of hypoglycemia and hyperglycemia. *Instruct patient and family in 2-g sodium, 1500-calorie diabetic diet incorporating cultural, vegetarian, lactose-free food choices. Obtain nutritionist consultation as indicated. *Monitor blood glucose and blood pressure. Instruct patient and family caregivers in technique, rationale, and acceptable parameters. *Determine, as able through pharmacy and resource consultation, potential side effects and drug interactions of patient herbs, and discuss any areas of potential concern with patient/family and physician.	Patient/family caregivers describe and properly manage medications and symptoms of blood sugar imbalance. Patient/family caregivers describe and demonstrate through a food log basic understanding of prescribed diet related to their customary foods habits. Patient/family caregivers return demonstrate proper techniques and log of monitoring as ordered. Undesirable drug/herb side effects and interactions are prevented. Family confirms health practices and beliefs have been respected.
Impaired skin integrity	*Assess cognitive and physical abilities of patient and family members to perform wound care. *Teach safety/surveillance procedures for wound, skin, and extremity circulation.	Patient/family caregivers verbalize understanding of wound care. Identify parameters for notification of nurse/physician

Case Study—cont'd

Nursing Diagnosis	Nursing Interventions	Patient Outcomes
	*Teach relationship of nutrition, hydration, immobility, and diabetes management to wound healing.	of complications. Specify and demonstrate in daily management actions to promote skin integrity related to diabetes, immobility, and nutritional health.
Risk for infection	*Observe and monitor for signs and symptoms of infection. Obtain cultures, as indicated. *Instruct patient/family caregivers in parameters for notification of nurse/physician, increased risk due to diabetes. *Demonstrate asepsis, and instruct patient/family caregivers in aseptic technique.	Infection is prevented or controlled promptly. Identify parameters for notification of nurse/physician of complications, understanding of patient increased risk. Return demonstrate aseptic technique.
Chronic back and neck pain exacerbated by recent injuries	*Assess pain levels using rating scale and patient descriptors. Assess effectiveness of current pain regimen and integrative therapies. Confer with physician concerning pain control, adjunctive oral agents, including possible use of NSAIDs, nonpharmacological use of heat and cold, and integrative therapies as indicated. *Instruct in positioning to prevent edema and pain in leg and foot, and pain in back and neck. Instruct patient/family caregivers in fentanyl patch use. Monitor side effects, particularly related to mentation and patient safety. *Discuss and implement nonpharmacological options for pain control incorporating familial, cultural, and spiritual beliefs. Teach environmental management and comfort measures for pain prevention and relief, particularly back and neck pain management.	Patient reports pain is controlled. Pain does not compromise patient activities, life enjoyment. Falls and injuries are prevented. Patient/family describes and demonstrates methods for ongoing pain prevention and management post discharge.
Impaired physical mobility; risk for injury	*Clarify with physician current ambulation/activity limitations. Obtain therapy consultation and treatment as indicated. *Maintain and instruct patient/family caregivers in proper positioning of extremities, turning techniques. *Assess safety and effectiveness of current patterns of movement and positioning during care. Instruct in safe, effective methods. *Reinforce activity/exercise within limitations.	Demonstrates safe bed mobility, transfers, and eventual ambulation. Injuries, including skin breakdown, back and neck trauma, falls, and caregiver injury, are prevented. Demonstrates increased endurance and mobility.
Self-care deficit: activities of daily living	*Problem solve methods for patient to maintain maximum possible independence with ADLS during recovery process, beginning with sitting activities. Encourage self-care activities within cultural mores. *Discuss energy management techniques. *Obtain therapist consultation and treatment as indicated.	Patient progresses to preinjury level of self-care or higher.
Risk for caregiver strain	*Determine individual, family, and cultural expectations as to responsibilities for care management of grandmother, patient, and grandchildren. Encourage patient incorporation in sharing of care, such as sitting activities with grandchildren.	Family implements a plan to minimize caregiver strain within cultural and familial norms. Caregivers report disruption of relationships and other role responsibilities has

Continued

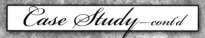

Case Study—cont'd

Nursing Diagnosis	Nursing Interventions	Patient Outcomes
	*Identify areas of caregiver strain and assist patient/family in problem solving concerning available family and community resources and task sharing. Obtain social services consultation as indicated. *Teach energy and stress management techniques for caregivers.	been decreased by resource identification and sharing. Caregivers describe and demonstrate energy and stress management techniques they can use to decrease caregiver strain.

ADLs, Activities of daily living; *NSAIDs*, nonsteroidal antiinflammatory drugs.

Plan of Care

Due to the strong familial involvement, nursing diagnoses in this case are focused on the family unit as the identified patient:

- Ineffective health maintenance related to diabetes and hypertension management: deficient knowledge related to diet, oral agents, blood sugar and hypertension monitoring and management
- Impaired skin integrity related to wounds, contusions and cast
- Risk for infection related to loss of skin integrity and diabetes
- Chronic pain related to fractured left femur, tissue injury, and back and neck sprain.
- Impaired physical mobility
- Self-care deficit: activities of daily living, secondary to injuries
- Risk for caregiver role strain

The interventions and outcomes in the community setting include both patient and family education and involvement:

CRITICAL THINKING

1. What priorities would the nurse identify in this case for teaching and interventions related to patient safety that need to be initiated in this first visit?
2. How does this case demonstrate the importance of the nurse's avoiding assumptions about a patient's health practices based on ethnic background?
3. How could the nurse incorporate the patient's self-help practices into a pain and diet management plan?

REFERENCES

Barnes, P. M., Powell-Griner, E., McFann, K., & Nahin, R. L. (2004). *Complementary and alternative medicine use among adults: United states, 2002* (Advance Data No. 343). Hyattsville, MD: National Center for Health Statistics. Retrieved November 27, 2005, from http://www.cdc.gov/nchs/data/ad/ad343.pdf.

Baron, M. (2004). Clinical weight-loss programs. *Health Care Food & Nutrition Focus, 21*(11), 6-8.

Berman, B. M., Swyers, J. P., & Ezzo, J. (2000). The evidence for acupuncture as a treatment for rheumatologic conditions. *Rheumatic Diseases Clinics of North America, 26*(1), 103-115.

Blumenthal, M., Goldberg, A., & Brinckman, J. (2000). *Herbal medicine: Expanded Commission E monographs.* Newton, MA: Lippincott Williams & Wilkins.

Callahan, E. J., Bertakis, K. D., & Azari, R. (2000). The influence of patient age on primary care resident physician-patient interaction. *Journal of the American Geriatric Society 48*, 30-35.

Chan, K., Qin, L., Lau, M., Woo, J., Au, S., & Choy, W., et al. (2004). A randomized, prospective study of the effects of Tai Chi Chun exercise on bone mineral density in postmenopausal women. *Archives of Physical Medicine and Rehabilitation, 85*(5), 717-722.

Cheuk, D. K. L., & Wong, V. (2005). Acupuncture for epilepsy. *Cochrane Database of Systematic Reviews, 4.*

Choi, J. H., Moon, J., & Song, R. (2005). Effects of Sun-style Tai Chi exercise on physical fitness and fall prevention in fall-prone older adults. *Journal of Advanced Nursing, 51*(2), 150-157.

Clark, P., Tugwell, P., Bennett, K. et al. (2006). Injectable gold for rheumatoid arthritis. *Cochrane Library* [serial on-line], 4. Available at http://www.cochrane.org.

Cohen, M. H. (2003). Complementary and integrative medical therapies, the FDA, and the NIH: Definitions and regulation. *Dermatologic Therapy, 16*(2), 77-84.

Cucherat, M. Haugh, H. C., Gooch, M., & Boissel, J. P. (2000). Evidence of clinical efficacy of homeopathy: A meta-analysis of clinical trials. *European Journal of Clinical Pharmacology, 56*(1), 27-33.

Cuellar, N. G. (2005). Hypnosis for pain management in the older adult. *Pain Management Nursing, 6*(3), 105-111.

Dickersin, K., Straus, S. E., & Bero, L. A. (2007). Evidence based medicine: Increasing, not dictating choice. Available from http://www.cochrane.org.

Dochterman, J. M., Bulechek, G. M., & Iowa Intervention Project. (2004). *Nursing interventions classification (NIC)* (4th ed.). St. Louis, MO: Mosby.

Douglas, R. M., Hemila, H., Chalker, E., D'Souza, R. R. D., & Treacy, B. (2005). Vitamin C for preventing and treating the common cold. *Cochrane Database of Systematic Reviews, 4.*

Eccles, N. K. (2005). A critical review of randomized controlled trials of static magnets for pain relief. *Journal of Alternative and Complementary Medicine, 11*(3), 495-509.

Eisenberg, D. M. (1997). Advising patients who seek alternative medical therapies. *Annals of Internal Medicine, 121*, 61-69.

Eisenberg, D. M., Kessler, R. C., Foster, C., Norlock, F., Calkins, P., & Delbanco, T. (1993). Unconventional medicine in the United States. *New England Journal of Medicine, 328*, 246-252.

Engstrom, J. W., & Hauser, S. L. (2000). Physical rehabilitation improves disability and quality of life perception in patients with multiple sclerosis. *Harrison's online* [Online]. New York: McGraw-Hill. Available from http://www.medscape.com/HOL/articles.

Fadiman, A. (1997). *The spirit catches you and you fall down: A Hmong child, her American doctors, and the collision of two cultures.* New York: Farrar, Straus and Giroux.

Fiscella, K., Franks, P., Clancy, C. M., Doescher, M. P., & Banthin, J. S. (1999). Does skepticism towards medical care predict mortality? *Medical Care, 37*(4), 409-414.

Fontaine, K. L. (2005). *Complementary & alternative therapies for nursing practice* (2nd ed.). Upper Saddle River, NJ: Pearson Prentice Hall.

Fontanarosa, P. B., & Lundberg, G. D. (1998). Alternative medicine meets science. *Journal of the American Medical Association, 280*(18), 1618-1619.

Franks, P., Fiscella, K., Beckett, L., Zwanziger, J., Mooney, C., & Gorthy, S. (2003). Effects of patient and physician practice socioeconomic status on the health care of privately insured managed care patients. *Medical Care, 41*(7), 842-852.

Freeman, L. W. (2004). *Mosby's complementary & alternative medicine: A research-based approach* (2nd ed.). St. Louis, MO: Mosby.

Gelberg, L., Andersen, R. M., & Leake, B. D. (2000). The behavioral model for vulnerable populations: Application to medical use and outcomes for homeless people. *Health Sciences Research, 34*(6), 1273-1314.

Geller, S. E., & Studee, L. (2005). Botanical and dietary supplements for menopausal symptoms: What works, what does not. *Journal of Women's Health, 14*(7), 634-649.

Giger, J. N, and Davidhizar, R E. (2004). *Transcultural nursing* (4th ed.). St. Louis, MO: Elsevier.

Green, S., Buchbinder, R., & Hetrick, S. (2005). Acupuncture for shoulder pain. *Cochrane Database of Systematic Reviews, 4.*

Haddad, L. G., & Hoeman, S. P. (2000). Home healthcare and the Arab-American client. *Home Healthcare Nurse, 18*(3), 189-197.

Hart, J., Kanner, H., Gilboa-Mayo, R., Haroeh-Peer, O., Rozenthul-Sorokin, N., & Eldar, R. (2004). Tai Chi Chuan practice in community-dwelling persons after stroke. *International Journal of Rehabilitation Research, 27*(4), 303-304.

Hemila, H. (2004). Vitamin C supplementation and respiratory infections: A systematic review. *Military Medicine [NLM - MEDLINE], 169*(11), 920.

Hoeman, S. P. (1989). Cultural assessment in rehabilitation nursing practice. *Nursing Clinics of North America, 24,* 277-289.

Hoeman, S. P. (Ed.). (1992). *Proceedings of the interdisciplinary rehabilitation delegation to the People's Republic of China, March, 1992.* Spokane, WA: People-to-People International, Citizen Ambassador Program.

Hoeman, S. P. (1996). Intraethnic diversity. *Home Healthcare Nurse, 14*(7), 32.

Hoeman, S. P. (1997). Alternative health and complementary therapies: Application to advanced practice nursing in rehabilitation. In K. Johnson (Ed.), *Advanced practice nursing in rehabilitation: A core curriculum* (pp. 64-72). Glenview, IL: Rehabilitation Nursing Foundation.

Hoeman, S. P. (1998). Dynamics of rehabilitation nursing. In G. Goldstein & S.R. Beers (Eds.), *Rehabilitation* (pp. 71-87). New York: Plenum Press.

Hoeman, S. P., & Nordin, B. (2003). *Children with complex medical situations and their families in Sweden and the United States.* Research presented at the second International R.N.C Rehabilitation & Intermediate Nursing Forum, Dublin, Ireland.

Hsu, S. (2005). Green tea and the skin. *Journal of the American Academy of Dermatology, 52*(6), 1049-1059.

Hyde, C. A. (2004). Multicultural development in human services agencies: Challenges and solutions. *Social Work, 49*(1), 7.

Izzo, A. A., Di Carlo, G., Borrelli, F., & Ernst, E. (2005). Cardiovascular pharmacotherapy and herbal medicines: The risk of drug interaction. *International Journal of Cardiology, 98*(1), 1-14.

Jonas, W. B., Kaptchuk, T. J., & Linde, K. (2003). Academia and clinic. A critical overview of homeopathy. *Annals of Internal Medicine, 138*(5), 393-399.

Jordan, K. M., Sawyer, S., Coakley, P., Smith, H. E., Cooper, C., & Arden, N. K. (2004). The use of conventional and complementary treatments for knee osteoarthritis in the community. *Rheumatology, 43*(3), 381.

Kelly, M. L., & Fitzsimmons, V. M. (2000). *Understanding cultural diversity: Culture curriculum and community in nursing.* Boston: Jones & Bartlett.

Klein, P. J., & Adams, W. (2004). Cardiopulmonary physiotherapeutic application of Taiji. *Cardiopulmonary Physical Therapy Journal, 15*(4), 5-11.

Klein, P. J., & Adams, W. D. (2004). Comprehensive therapeutic benefits of Taiji: A critical review. *American Journal of Physical Medicine & Rehabilitation, 83*(9), 735-745.

Kleinman, A., Eisenberg, L., & Good, B. (1978). Culture, illness and care: Clinical lessons from anthropologic and cross-cultural research. *Annals of Internal Medicine, 88,* 251-258.

Kohler, S., Funk, P., & Kieser, M. (2004). Influence of a 7-day treatment with ginkgo biloba special extract EGb 761 on bleeding time and coagulation: A randomized, placebo-controlled, double-blind study in healthy volunteers. *Blood Coagulation & Fibrinolysis, 15*(4), 303-309.

Krieger, D. (1979). *The therapeutic touch.* Englewood Cliffs, NJ: Prentice-Hall.

Kroeling, P., Gross, A., Goldsmith, C. H., & Cervical Overview Group. (2005). Electrotherapy for neck disorders. *The Cochrane Library (Oxford),* (4).

Kwapien, C. A., & Kulakowski, K. P. (2005). The complementary modalities of healing touch and reiki for the oncology population. *Oncology Nutrition Connection, 13*(1), 11-13.

Lagnado, L. (2000, March 22). Laetril makes a comeback on the Web. *Wall Street Journal,* Section B, p. 1.

LeMaire, B. (2004). 5 minutes with Elena Avila, on curanderismo folk healing. *NurseWeek (South Central), 9*(1), 7.

Li, F., Harmer, P., Fisher, K. J., & McAuley, E. (2004). Tai Chi: Improving functional balance and predicting subsequent falls in older persons. *Medicine and Science in Sports and Exercise, 36*(12), 2046-2052.

Lin, J. T., & Lane, J. M. (2005). Falls in the elderly population. *Physical Medicine and Rehabilitation Clinics of North America, 16*(1), 109-128.

Linde, K., Kruppel, L. (2005). Large scale observational studies of *Hypericum* extracts in patients with depressive disorders: A systematic review. *Stuttgart, 1/2*(12), 148-158.

Mackenzie, E. R., Taylor, L., Bloom, B. S., Hufford, D. J., & Johnson, J. C. (2003). Ethnic minority use of complementary and alternative medicine (CAM): A national probability survey of CAM utilizers. *Alternative Therapies in Health and Medicine, 9*(4), 50.

Magci, S. K., Yusuf, A., Ozan, K. et al. (2005). *The effect of biofeedback treatment on voiding and urodynamic parameters in children with voiding dysfunction.* Baltimore: Williams & Wilkins.

Manson, J. J., & Rahman, A. (2004). This house believes that we should advise our patients with osteoarthritis of the knee to take glucosamine. *Rheumatology, 43*(1), 100-101.

Margolin, A., Avants, S. K., & Kleber, H. D. (1998). Investigating alternative medicine therapies in randomized controlled trials. *Journal of the American Medical Association, 280*(18), 1628-1629.

McDonald, H. L. (2005). Patients who wore standard magnetic bracelets reported reduced pain from osteoarthritis of the hip or knee compared with patients wearing placebo bracelets. *Evidence-Based Nursing, 8*(3), 89.

Micozzi, M. S. (Ed.). (1996). *Fundamentals of complementary and alternative medicine.* New York: Churchill Livingstone.

Miller, S. C. (2005). Echinacea: A miracle herb against aging and cancer? Evidence *in vivo* in mice. *Evidence-Based Complementary and Alternative Medicine, 2*(3), 309-314.

Mitka, M. (1999). Therapeutic marijuana use supported while thorough proposed study done. *Journal of the American Medical Association 281*(16), 1473-1475.

Modlin, S. J. (2000). Service dogs as interventions: State of the science. *Rehabilitation Nursing, 25*(6), 212-219.

Moorhead, S., Johnson, M., & Maas, M.. (2004). *Nursing outcomes classification (NOC)* (3rd ed.). St. Louis, MO: Mosby.

Murray-Garcia, J. L., Selby, J. V., Schmittdiel, J., Grumbach, K. & Quesenberry, C. P., Jr. (2000). Racial and ethnic differences in a patient survey: Patients' values, ratings, and reports regarding physician primary care performance in a large health maintenance organization. *Medical Care 38*(3), 300-310.

NANDA International. (2007). *Nursing diagnosis: Definitions and Classifications: 2007-2008.* Philadelphia: Author.

National Center for Complementary and Alternative Medicine. (2002). Available from http://www.NCCAM.nih.gov.

National Center for Complementary and Alternative Medicine. (2005). Available from http://www.NCCAM.nih.gov.

National Institute on Disability Rehabilitation Research. (2005). Available from http://www.ed.gov/osers/nidrr.

Neal, L. J., & Guillett, S. E. (2004). *Care of the adult with a chronic illness or disability: A team approach.* St. Louis, MO: Elsevier Mosby.

Parsons, T. (1951). *The social system.* New York: Free Press.

Paul, B. D. (Ed.). (1955). *Health, culture, and community: Case studies of public reactions to health programs.* New York: Russell Sage Foundation.

Piscitelli, S. C., Burstein, A., Chaitt, D., Alfaro, R., & Falloon, J. (2000). Indinavir concentration and St. John's wort. *Lancet, 355,* 541-548.

Richardson, M. A., Allen, C., Ezzo, J., Lao, L., Ramirez, G., & Ramirez, T., et al. (2005). Acupuncture for chemotherapy-induced nausea or vomiting among cancer patients. *Cochrane Database of Systematic Reviews, 4.*

Richeson, N. E. (2003). Effects of animal-assisted therapy on agitated behaviors and social interactions of older adults with dementia: An evidence-based therapeutic recreation intervention. *American Journal of Recreation Therapy, 2*(4), 9-16.

Sampson, W. (2005). Studying herbal remedies. *The New England Journal of Medicine, 353*(4), 337.

Šimánek, V., Kren, V., Ulrichová, J., & Gallo, J. (2005). The efficacy of glucosamine or chondroitin sulfate in the treatment of osteoarthritis: Are these saccharides drugs or nutraceuticals? *Biomedical Papers, 149*(1), 51-56.

Smith, C. E., Holcroft, C., Rebeck, S. L., Thompson, N. C., & Werkowitch, M. (2000). Journal writing as a complementary therapy for reactive depression: A rehabilitation teaching program [Review] [76 refs]. *Rehabilitation Nursing, 25*(5), 170-176.

Sobel, D. S. (Ed.). (1979). *Ways of health: Holistic approaches to ancient and contemporary medicine.* New York: Harcourt Brace Jovanovich.

Starr, P. (1982). *The social transformation of American medicine.* New York: Basic Books.

Suarez-Almazor, M. E., Bennett, K. J., Bombardier, C., Clark, P., Shea, B. J., Tugwell, P., et al. (2005). Injectable gold for rheumatoid arthritis. *Cochrane Database of Systematic Reviews, 4.*

Thompson, J. (2004). Glucosamine modifies effects of knee osteoarthritis. *Community Practitioner, 77*(5), 194.

Tsang, W. W. N., & Hui-Chan, C. W. Y. (2005). Comparison of muscle torque, balance, and confidence in older tai chi and healthy adults. *Medicine & Science in Sports & Exercise, 37*(2), 280-289.

Wellin, E. (1985). Water boiling in a Peruvian town. In B. D. Paul (Ed.). *Health, culture & community: Case studies of public reactions to health programs* (pp. 71-103). New York: Russell Sage Foundation.

Wetzel, M. S., Kaptchuk, T. J., Haramati, A., & Eisenberg, D. M. (2003). Complementary and alternative medical therapies: Implications for medical education. *Annals of Internal Medicine, 138*(3), 191-196.

Williams, K.A., Petronis, J., Smith, D. et al. (2005). Effect of Iyengar yoga therapy for chronic low back pain. *Science Digest,* 1-2(115), 107-117.

Wong, A. M., Lin, Y., Chou, S., Tang, F., & Wong, P. (2001). Coordination exercise and postural stability in elderly people: Effect of Tai Chi Chuan. *Archives of Physical Medicine and Rehabilitation, 82*(5), 608-612.

Woods, D. L., Craven, R. F., & Whitney, J. (2005). The effect of therapeutic touch on behavioral symptoms of persons with dementia. *Alternative Therapies in Health and Medicine, 11*(1), 66-74.

Zborowski, M. (1958). Cultural components in response to pain. In E. G. Jaco (Ed.), *Patients, physicians, and illness.* Glencoe, IL: The Free Press.

Ziporyn, T. (1992). *Nameless diseases.* New Brunswick, NJ: Rutgers University Press.

Zola, I. K. (1991). Bringing our bodies and ourselves back in: Reflections on a past, present, and future "medical sociology." *Journal of Health and Social Behavior, 32*(March), 1-16.

Zwick, D., Rochelle, A., Choksi, A., & Domowicz, J. (2000). Evaluation and treatment of balance in the elderly: A review of the efficacy of the Berg balance test and Tai Chi Quan. *NeuroRehabilitation, 15*(1), 49-56.

7

Pharmacology for Rehabilitation Nursing

Joyce Brewer, PhD, CNM, CFNP

Pharmacotherapeutics is an important adjunct in the management of patients during rehabilitation. The information contained in this chapter is intended to assist rehabilitation nurses in pharmacological management for patients. This is not a complete presentation of the issues of pharmacology in rehabilitation medicine, nor is it intended to replace comprehensive pharmacology texts or drug references. Objectives for this chapter are to define terminology, to explain principles of drug action, to describe pharmacokinetic functions and principles of pharmacodynamics, to identify adverse drug reactions, and to apply this knowledge to decisions in clinical practice. Appropriate prescribing, administering, and monitoring are instrumental in minimizing medication adverse effects and errors.

PHARMACEUTICS

Pharmaceutics evaluates the physical and chemical principles involved in the design, formulation, manufacture, and stability of drug delivery systems and the application of this knowledge to the bioavailability of medications in various routes of administration.

A medication is a chemical that interacts with a living organism to produce a biological response. In general medications have the following characteristics:

1. Medications do not bestow any new function on a tissue or organ in the body—they only modify existing functions. *Example*: Enzyme inhibition with angiotensin-converting enzyme (ACE) inhibitors for blood pressure or congestive heart failure.
2. Medications generally exhibit multiple actions rather than a single effect. Consequently, medications have incidence of side effects in addition to therapeutic effects. Therefore choosing an agent that is more selective for a particular receptor could minimize this. *Example*: First-generation antihistamines, such as diphenhydramine (Benadryl), have more anticholinergic side effects (e.g., dry mouth, blurred vision, confusion, and sedation) than the newer antihistamines, such as loratadine (Claritin), which are more selective.
3. Medication action results from a physiochemical interaction between the drug and an important molecule in the body. This molecule could be a receptor or a component of a membrane structure.

PHARMACOKINETICS

Pharmacokinetics (PK) evaluates the absorption, distribution, metabolism, and elimination of medication. In essence, it is what the body does to the medication. Many variables can affect PK and are discussed throughout this chapter. The processes associated with pharmacokinetics include absorption, bioavailability, distribution, metabolism, elimination, clearance, and half-life. These processes ultimately affect the concentrations available.

Absorption

Medications have 100% absorption when administered intravenously. All other forms of administration depend on the physiochemical properties of the drug, dosage form, and anatomy and physiology of the absorption site. For instance, older individuals have thinner skin with a reduced amount of fat in the subcutaneous layer; ultimately, this affects the absorption of hydrophilic medications, such as nitroglycerin patches. How food affects medication is presented in Chapter 16.

Bioavailability

Bioavailability measures the rate and extent of therapeutically active medication that reaches the systemic circulation. When the bioavailability is rated less than 1 (or 100%), this means that either the dosage form did not release all of the medication or that some of the medication was eliminated or destroyed by stomach acid or other means before it reached the systemic circulation.

Some medications have very low bioavailability, such as alendronate (Fosamax). Administering these drugs correctly is very important. Check references for any drug-food interactions, and determine whether the medications must be taken with food to increase bioavailability. Just as important, some medications must be taken on an empty stomach.

Rehabilitation nurses need to understand the meaning of the term *bioequivalence* when explaining brand-name versus generic medications. A medication is deemed bioequivalent when the area under the concentration-time curve (AUC), maximum of serum or blood concentrations (C_{max}), and the times that C_{max} occur (T_{max}) are neither clinically nor statistically different. When this occurs, the serum concentration versus time curves for the two dosage forms could be superimposed and therefore identical. The United States Food and Drug Administration (FDA) publishes the *Orange Book*, which contains lists of agents that are bioequivalent. This information is crucial when a patient changes from a brand-name medication to a generic form, especially with narrow therapeutic agents. Therapeutic index is the difference between where the concentration of a drug reaches the therapeutic level and the level of concentration where the drug becomes toxic. Many drugs have a wide therapeutic index, but some such as Coumadin, Depakote, or Dilantin have a narrow therapeutic index, so small changes in the dosage level could cause toxic results.

Distribution

When medication is absorbed, the drug molecules are carried throughout the body by the systemic circulation, which carries them to the target site of action (receptor) as well as other tissues and organs. The passage of a drug molecule across a membrane depends on the chemical makeup of the drug. Small molecules permeate cells, organs, and tissues quickly; however, lipophilic medications deposit in fat tissues that release the medication slowly. Medications bound to proteins, such as albumin, may become too large for easy diffusion. The volume of distribution is the amount of drug in the body compared to the concentration measured in plasma, serum, or blood.

Metabolism

Drug metabolism is the process in the body that makes a chemical molecule more polar to hinder its reabsorption and facilitate elimination. The four main processes of drug metabolism are grouped into phase I (oxidation, hydrolysis, and reduction) and Phase II (conjugation). Phase I reactions include the cytochrome P-450 system, which is an enzyme system in the liver that metabolizes drugs. Enzymes involved in the biotransformation are located primarily in the liver; however, other tissues, such as the kidney, lung, small intestine, and skin also contain enzymes. New findings about the multiple interactions within these various enzymes are being reported, and a summary of the known information alone would be extensive (Ament, Bertolino, & Liszewski, 2000). One interaction to highlight is that of grapefruit juice because it inhibits intestinal cytochrome P-450. As a result, it increases levels of drugs metabolized by intestinal CYP 3A4, such as alprazolam (Xanax), cyclosporine (Neoral, Sandimmune), felodipine (Plendil), and nifedipine (Procardia).

Elimination

Elimination is the irreversible removal of drug from the body by all routes. The main organ in this process is the kidney. Most commonly, renal function is expressed by the degree of creatinine clearance. Some drug dosages must therefore be adjusted based on the creatinine clearance. As rehabilitation nurses, it is important to evaluate an individual's renal function to appropriately evaluate dosages of some medications. There are various formulas used to calculate creatinine clearance, but one of the most common is the Cockcroft-Gault. This formula is as follows:

$$\text{Creatinine clearance} = (140 - \text{Age}) \times \text{Weight in kg} \div (72 \times \text{Serum creatinine})$$

For women, multiply by 0.85.

Clearance

The rate at which a drug is eliminated by the body is an important parameter that can be affected by many variables. Physiologically, it is determined by the blood flow to the organ that metabolizes (i.e., liver) or eliminates (i.e., kidney) the medication and the efficiency of the organ in extracting the medication from the body (Craig & Stitzel, 2004). High-clearance medications, such as propranolol, are extensively metabolized by the liver. With low-clearance medications, such as warfarin, elimination is equal to the fraction of unbound, "active," medication in the blood and the intrinsic ability of the organ to clear these medications from the body. These issues become important when introducing drugs that increase or decrease the metabolism of certain substrates or displace binding of highly protein-bound medications. This is especially the case with anticonvulsants, such as phenytoin and valproic acid.

Half-Life

The half-life ($t_{1/2}$) is the amount of time it takes the plasma concentration of a medication to decrease by one half after completing absorption and distribution. This important parameter provides the rehabilitation nurse with insight into when a medication reaches steady state (approximately 3 to 5 half-lives). Many factors affect PK principles and need to be taken into consideration, including age (e.g., pediatric and geriatric changes), gender, body build, drug-drug, drug-disease, and drug-food interactions.

PHARMACODYNAMICS

Pharmacodynamics (PD) is the study of biochemical and physiological effects of medications and their mechanism of action (i.e., what the drug does to the body). Core definitions and concepts aid in understanding these processes.

Core Components

Protein targets for drug binding include enzymes (e.g., cyclooxygenase), carrier molecules (e.g., Na/K pump), ion channels (e.g., voltage gated calcium channels), and receptors (usually proteins designed by nature to confer a response or transduce a signal to a naturally occurring ligand). Some references group all of the aforementioned protein targets as receptors. A specific example is the dopamine receptors.

Medications act selectively on a particular tissue or cell, a process termed *drug specificity.* For example, angiotensin acts selectively on vascular smooth muscle and kidney tubule but has little effect on other smooth muscle. Most drugs do not act with complete specificity, therefore side effects may occur. Medications bind to receptors differently, as described in the following:

1. At equilibrium, binding is related to drug concentration.
2. Higher-affinity or selective drugs need lower concentrations to approach saturation of the receptors and clinically can result in fewer adverse side effects.
3. Competitive antagonism occurs when two or more medications compete for the same receptors, and one may reduce the affinity or selectivity of the other.

After binding to the receptor site, the following different responses can occur:

1. *Agonists* initiate changes in cell function, producing various effects. The potency depends on affinity (tendency to bind to receptors) and efficacy (ability once bound to produce an effect). Full agonists produce maximal effect and have high efficacy; partial agonists produce only submaximal effect and intermediate efficacy.
2. *Antagonists* bind to receptors without initiating changes. Types of antagonisms include the following:
   - Chemical antagonism, such as when a chelating agent binds to a heavy metal
   - Pharmacokinetic antagonism, such as cytochrome P-450 inducers (e.g., carbamazepine, phenobarbital) that increase the metabolism of a substrate such as warfarin
   - Noncompetitive antagonism (i.e., blocking a receptor-effector linkage), such as omeprazole (Prilosec), a proton pump inhibitor
   - Physiological antagonism, wherein two agents balance each other, such as with acetylcholinesterase inhibitors and anticholinergics

Receptor Level Changes

Receptor level changes describe a change in conformational state or a loss of receptors, such as what happens with beta receptors. As beta receptors are exposed to beta-blocking agents, more receptors are activated. This is one reason that it is common to have to increase a beta-blocking agent after a period of time. It also explains the importance of never abruptly stopping an agent such as a beta blocker. If the beta blocker is discontinued, a gradual decrease allows the beta receptors to adjust along with the gradual decrease of the blocking agent. Knowing the basic pharmacodynamic principles assists rehabilitation nurses in understanding how long medications require to reach efficacy and what to expect concerning side effects or toxicity.

UNDERSTANDING PHARMACOLOGICAL CHANGES ACROSS THE LIFE SPAN

Pediatric Considerations

A patient younger than 18 years of age is considered pediatric for the purposes of this text. Physiological changes occur as the child ages. This affects the process of drug absorption, distribution, metabolism, and elimination, as described below.

Effects on Absorption

1. Full-term infants have a stomach pH of 6 to 8 at birth, which decreases to 1 to 3 within 24 hours. The change in pH increases the bioavailability of acid-labile penicillins. Premature infants have an elevated gastric pH level as a result of their immature acid secretion.
2. Gastric emptying is slower in a premature infant as compared to a full-term infant.
3. Intramuscular (IM) injections are rarely used for infants because of the great variability in absorption.
4. An infant's skin has increased permeability secondary to an underdeveloped epidermal barrier (stratum corneum).

Effects on Distribution

1. The proportion of the body that is composed of water is 94% in a fetus, 85% in premature infants, 78% in a full-term infant, and 60% in adults. Water-soluble drugs, such as gentamicin and tobramycin, have an increased volume of distribution in bodies with higher water content.
2. Protein binding is decreased in newborns secondary to their decreased plasma concentration, lowered binding capacity, and decreased affinity.
3. Body fat is substantially lower in neonates than in full-term infants.

Effects on Metabolism. Glucuronidation (phase II) is not developed at birth; therefore avoid use of chloramphenicol because it cannot be metabolized.

Effects on Elimination. The processes of glomerular filtration, tubular secretion, and resorption determine the efficiency of renal excretion. These processes may take several weeks of life to begin to develop and fully develop after 1 year of age.

Geriatric Considerations

Elders are the most rapidly growing segment of the U.S. population. All rehabilitation nurses need to heighten their awareness about medications and the elderly. Many medications are more likely to produce adverse effects and lead to negative outcomes in older persons. A review of the

PK differences in this population helps with understanding the processes.

Effects on Absorption. Changes in absorption are not usually clinically significant. However, older persons have decreased gastric acidity and decreased gastrointestinal tract blood flow. They also have delayed gastric emptying and a reduced lipid content of their skin.

Effects on Distribution. Changes in distribution in the elderly include the following:
1. Decreased total body water, which increases potential dehydration, especially when taking diuretics.
2. Body fat increases from 15% to 30%, and lean body weight decreases in proportion to total body weight. The result is an increase in the volume of distribution and half-life of agents such as diazepam (Valium).
3. There is a decreased serum albumin level, leading to an increase in concentrations of highly protein-bound drugs (e.g., phenytoin).
4. There is a decrease in cardiac output, resulting in reduced hepatic blood flow, which can lead to a slowed rate of metabolism for medications such as warfarin that increase risk for bleeding.

Effects on Metabolism. Metabolism is altered in the elderly by the following:
1. There is a decrease in liver mass.
2. Phase I oxidative process by cytochrome P-450 appears to be decreased.
3. No changes have been noted in the phase II coupling of a parent drug or phase by glucoronidation, sulfation, or acetylation

Effects on Elimination. Elimination of medications is affected by a decrease in the size of the kidney (20%) accompanied by reduced renal blood flow, glomerular filtration rate, and tubular excretory capacity.

ADVERSE DRUG REACTIONS

The Joint Commission (TJC) (2002) defines an adverse drug reaction (ADR) as "any incident in which the use of a medication (drug or biologic) at any dose, a medical device, or a special nutritional product (e.g., dietary supplement, infant formula, medical food) may have resulted in an adverse outcome in a patient." It is important to note that ADRs have been reported as the fourth leading cause of death in the United States, following heart disease, cancer, and stroke (Lazarou, Pomeranz, & Corey, 1998).

Health care providers, including rehabilitation nurses, must advocate for a prospective, ongoing, and concurrent surveillance system that mandates reports of suspected ADRs, as well as screening for high-risk indicators. Patients at high risk for ADRs include, but are not limited to, pediatric

and geriatric aggregates and persons with hepatic or renal failure. High-risk medications extend beyond aminoglycosides, digoxin, heparin, phenytoin, and warfarin. Application of the pharmacology principles discussed in this chapter is an initial step to minimize ADRs in rehabilitation practice.

There are many examples of interactions between medications and nutrients. Refer to Chapter 16 for more information about medications and nutrient interactions.

ORGANIZATION OF THE DRUG TABLES

The following tables give examples of drugs commonly used in rehabilitation and generally follow the chapter organization of the textbook. Table 7-1 covers drugs that affect the central nervous system, including anticonvulsants, antiparkinsonian drugs, and antidepressant agents. Table 7-2 contains drugs used to improve pulmonary function, including bronchodilators, anticholinergics, inhaled antiinflammatory agents, mediator-release inhibitors, and leukotriene modifiers. Additional information is found in Chapter 17. Table 7-3 covers drugs that are used to control urinary incontinence and facilitate bowel elimination. Chapters 18 and 19 provide additional information. Table 7-4 presents drugs that are used to treat autoimmune diseases and pain and/or improve mobility and includes muscle relaxants, disease-modifying drugs, antiinflammatory agents, and analgesic agents. See Chapters 20 and 23 for additional discussion of these drugs. Table 7-5 contains common cardiovascular, anticoagulant/antiplatelet, and cholesterol-lowering agents. The information about cardiovascular medications is presented by classifications because of length considerations. For individual dosage, pregnancy category, metabolism, excretion, and half-life, refer to information specific to that medication. Table 7-6 presents the topical agents used in the care of burn injuries. Table 7-7 covers drugs used in the treatment of diabetes mellitus, including oral sulfonylureas, alpha-glucosidase inhibitors, thiazolidinediones, and insulins. Table 7-8 contains human immunodeficiency virus/acquired immunodeficiency syndrome (HIV/AIDS) drugs, including nucleoside and nucleotide analog reverse transcriptase inhibitors, protease inhibitors, nonnucleoside reverse transcriptase inhibitors, and fusion inhibitors. Chapter 35 provides additional information on these HIV/AIDS medications.

These tables are not comprehensive but include information about medications from different classes common to practice. If you are interested in the specifics of a certain drug, please refer to a drug handbook for details. The individual book chapters contain information about applications of medications and treatments specific to their content. All drug information has been obtained from the following sources: http://www.drugs.com, http://www.pdr.net, and *Lexi-Comp's Drug Information Handbook for Advanced Practice Nursing* (Turkoski, Lance, & Bonfiglio, 2005).

Text continued on page 123

TABLE 7-1 Drugs Acting With in the Central Nervous System

Drug Name	Normal Adult Dose	Therapeutic Use	Major Adverse Effects/Cautions	Comments
Antidepressants *Tricyclic* Included in this group are doxepin (Sinequan), clomipramine (Anafranil), amitriptyline (Elavil), maprotiline (Ludiomil), desipramine (Norpramin), nortriptyline (Pamelor)	Varies with specific medication.	Depression Numerous other uses for this class such as peripheral neuropathy, obsessive-compulsive disorder, enuresis.	**Adverse Effects:** all agents, some more than others, produce anticholinergic side effects such as blurred vision, confusion, delirium (especially in the elderly), irregular heartbeat.	Numerous agents in this class. Look at PK and PD difference plus indication for use when choosing a tricyclic antidepressant. Onset of effect occurs in 2-3 weeks. Metabolism: liver. Excretion: urine. Half-life varies for each specific medication.
Selective Serotonin Reuptake Inhibitors (SSRIs) Included in this class are citalopram (Celexa), escitalopram (Lexapro), fluvoxamine (Luvox), paroxetine (Paxil), fluoxetine (Prozac, Sarafem), sertraline (Zoloft)	Based on individual drug.	First-line therapy in the treatment of mild to moderate depression, obsessive-compulsive disorder, panic disorder.	**Adverse Effects:** sexual dysfunction, dizziness, drowsiness, serotonin syndrome, nausea, vomiting, anorexia, stomach or abdominal cramps, agitation or nervousness, abnormal movements or tremor. Some side effects are dose related.	Takes 2-4 weeks to see full effects. Do not abruptly stop treatment. Do not use with or within 5 weeks of an MAO inhibitor. Close supervision for suicide risk. Lowers seizure threshold.
Others mirtazapine (Remeron)	Start 15 mg PO at bedtime Increase to therapeutic dose up to 45 mg/day.	Major depressive disorder.	**Adverse Effects:** constipation, dizziness, drowsiness, dryness of mouth, increased appetite, and weight gain.	Good for patients needing help with sleep. At lower doses has more antihistaminic properties and causes sedation.
venlafaxine (Effexor)	Start 37.5 mg PO bid × 4 days. Increase to therapeutic dose up to 375 mg/day.	Major depressive disorder.	**Adverse Effects:** headaches, sexual dysfunction, abnormal dreams, anorexia, weight loss, dizziness, increase in blood pressure.	Available in extended release as well; do not open capsules. Dosage adjustments needed for renal or hepatic impairment.
bupropion (Wellbutrin)	Start 100 mg PO bid. After 3 days, increase to therapeutic dose up to 450 mg/day, with no single dose exceeding 150 mg.	Major depressive disorder, nicotine dependence.	**Adverse Effects:** agitation, anxiety, headache, abdominal pain, decrease in appetite, nausea or vomiting, dryness of mouth, insomnia.	Note importance of no single dose greater than 150 mg secondary to decreased seizure threshold. Also available in extended release.
Anticonvulsants *First Generation* phenytoin (Dilantin)	Start 300-400 mg PO divided once daily to tid.	Seizure disorder, status epilepticus.	**Serious Adverse Effects:** VFib, hepatotoxicity, thrombocytopenia, megaloblastic anemia.	Check albumin levels in individual who is poorly nourished secondary to increased likelihood for

TABLE 7-1 Drugs Acting With the Central Nervous System—cont'd

Drug Name	Normal Adult Dose	Therapeutic Use	Major Adverse Effects/Cautions	Comments
	Individualized therapeutic levels 10-20 mcg/ml.		**Common Adverse Effects:** nausea, vomiting, rash, CNS toxicities, gingival hyperplasia.	increased free levels and toxicities. Metabolism: liver; CYP450: 2C9. Excretion: bile, urine. Half-life: 22 hr.
carbamazepine (Tegretol)	Up to 1200 mg/day. Plasma level for seizure prophylaxis: 6-12 mcg/ml.	Partial seizures with simple or complex symptoms, generalized tonic-clonic seizures, mixed, trigeminal neuralgia, bipolar disorder.	**Adverse Effects:** CNS toxicity, blood dyscrasias, hyponatremia, diarrhea, GI irritation, increase in liver function, hypocalcemia.	Numerous drug interactions, autoinduction of metabolism. Take with food to minimize irritation. If using liquid via G-tube, must be spaced out from other medications.
valproic acid (divalproex, Depakote, Depakene)	Up to 60 mg/kg body weight/day (50-100 mg/ml). Therapeutic plasma level: 50-100 mcg/ml.	Simple and complex, absence (petit mal), mixed, and tonic-clonic seizures; bipolar disorder, migraine headache prophylaxis.	**Adverse Effects:** CNS toxicity, blood dyscrasias, GI irritation, worsening liver function, sedation.	Highly protein bound. May use higher levels in patients with bipolar disorder. Assess for drug interactions.
Second Generation topiramate (Topamax)	Start 25 mg PO at bedtime for 1 week. Increase by 25-50 mg/day weekly to a maximum of 400 mg/day. Usual therapeutic dose: 200 mg/day.	Adjunct therapy in adults and children 2 years and older with partial and generalized seizures.	**Serious Adverse Effects:** acute glaucoma and visual abnormalities, nephrolithiasis. **Common Adverse Effects:** fatigue, dizziness, nausea, somnolence, impaired concentration, ataxia, weight loss, aggression.	Topiramate clearance increased by phenytoin and carbamazepine. Topiramate may increase phenytoin levels. Monitoring serum levels not necessary. Use lower doses in individuals with renal impairment.
gabapentin (Neurontin)	Start 300 mg PO day 1, bid day 2, then tid. Up to 3600 mg/day.	Adjunct in treatment of partial seizures with or without secondary generalization in adults and adolescents older than 12 years.	**Common Adverse Effects:** dizziness, fatigue, somnolence, ataxia, tremor.	Titrate slowly to minimize CNS toxicities. Elimination: urine Do not need to monitor serum levels. Little potential for drug interactions. To discontinue, taper over 7-day period.
Antiparkinsonian carbidopa/levodopa (Parcopa, Sinemet, Sinemet CR)	Initially: 50/200 mg controlled release bid. (Should wait 3 days before dosage adjustments.) Up to 1 g/day.	Parkinsonism. Controversial as to when to start. Assess patient; if younger patient, may want to start with a dopamine agonist secondary to motor complications associated with levodopa.	**Serious Adverse Effects:** dyskinesia, bradykinesia, orthostatic hypotension, syncope, arrhythmias, depression, suicidal ideation, hallucinations, psychosis, melanoma, GI bleed. **Common Adverse Effects:** dyskinesia, nausea and vomiting, hallucinations, confusion,	Monitor for food-drug interactions. High-protein meals can interfere with absorption of levodopa across GI endothelium and across blood-brain barrier; timing of meals may be clinically important as the disease progresses. Symptoms unresponsive to levodopa:

Continued

TABLE 7-1 Drugs Acting With the Central Nervous System—cont'd

Drug Name	Normal Adult Dose	Therapeutic Use	Major Adverse Effects/Cautions	Comments
			dizziness, depression, UTI, headache, dry mouth, anxiety, nightmares, insomnia, diarrhea, fatigue, anorexia, dystonia, constipation.	Motor: postural instability, freezing, speech abnormalities. Mental changes: dementia, depression, sensory phenomena, olfactory changes. Autonomic: constipation, sexual dysfunction, urinary problems, sweating.
Anticholinergics benztropine (Cogentin)	Start 0.5-1 mg PO/IM/IV q at bed time; increase 0.5 mg q 5-6 days with a maximum of 6 mg/day.	Parkinsonism, extrapyramidal reactions, dystonic reactions, multiple sclerosis.	**Serious Adverse Effects:** tachycardia, psychosis, anticholinergic. **Common Adverse Effects:** constipation, dry mouth, sedation, urinary retention, blurred vision, tachycardia, dyspnea, nausea, vomiting, flatulence, anorexia, rash, abdominal pain, pruritus, dizziness, headache, edema.	All equally effective. Not recommended in patients older than 60. Metabolism: unknown. Excretion: urine, feces. Half-life: unknown. Method of action: antagonizes acetylcholine and histamine receptors.
trihexyphenidyl (Artane)	Start 1 mg PO × 1 day, then 2 mg daily. Increase by 2 mg q 3-5 days as needed to a maximum of 15 mg/day.	Parkinsonism, extrapyramidal reactions.	**Serious Adverse Effects:** narrow-angle glaucoma, blindness, hyperthermia, tardive dyskinesia, psychosis. **Common Adverse Effects:** anxiety, blurred vision, confusion, constipation, constipation, cycloplegia, dizziness, drowsiness, dry skin, headache, nausea, parotitis, tachycardia, urinary retention, xerostomia.	Metabolism: unknown. Excretion: urine. Half-life: 5.5-10 hr.
selegiline (Eldepryl)	Usual dosage 5 mg PO bid given at breakfast and lunch. Maximum dose 10 mg/day.	Parkinsonism. Useful in early disease for symptomatic management (possibly neuroprotective).	**Adverse Effects:** augments levodopa toxicities, insomnia (give in AM), confusion, agitation, hypomania, diarrhea, sweating, shivering, serotonin syndrome, hyperreflexia, myoclonus, hypertension, incoordination.	Drug interactions: antidepressants, MAO inhibitors and SSRIs, meperidine. Metabolism: liver and GI tract; CYP450: 1A2, 3A4 substrate. Excretion: urine. Half-life: 40 hr.

TABLE 7-1 Drugs Acting With the Central Nervous System—cont'd

Drug Name	Normal Adult Dose	Therapeutic Use	Major Adverse Effects/Cautions	Comments
Other Classes amantadine (Symmetrel)	100 mg daily if taking other meds for parkinsonism treatment. Maximum daily dose: 400 mg.	Parkinsonism, extrapyramidal disorders. As an antiviral is also used in the treatment or prophylaxis of influenza A.	**Serious Adverse Effects:** CHF, arrhythmias, cardiac arrest, psychosis, coma, visual impairment, respiratory failure, pulmonary edema. **Common Adverse Effects:** nausea, dizziness, insomnia, depression, anxiety, irritability, hallucinations, dry mouth, ataxia, constipation, dependent edema, headache.	Not recommended in patients older than 60 years because of cognitive effects; however, there is increasing use in older patients, but dose adjustments are required because of renal impairment. Tolerance may develop. Stop, then restart; sensitivity may be restored. Do not stop abruptly because of possible rebound of symptoms. Modestly effective. Used in early therapy or adjunctive later in treatment. Metabolism: conjugation. Excretion: urine. Half-life: 17 hr (longer in elderly).
Dopamine Agonists		Monotherapy in early disease to delay starting levodopa. When added to carbidopa-levodopa, dopamine agonists may decrease dyskinesia, prolong "on" time, reduce "off" time, and reduce wearing-off complications.	Poorly tolerated by about 30% of patients for following reasons: allergy, palpations/sinus tachycardia, agitation, dizziness/fainting (especially when initiating treatment or increasing doses).	When adding dopamine agonists to carbidopa-levodopa, the dose of carbidopa-levodopa needs to be reduced.
Ergot Derivatives bromocriptine (Parlodel)	Start 1.25-2.5 mg PO at bedtime. Increase q 3-7 days to a maximum of 100 mg/day. Should be taken with food.	Parkinsonism, hyperprolactinemia, acromegaly, neuroleptic malignant syndrome.	**Serious Adverse Effects:** seizures, stroke, syncope, HTN, MI, arrhythmias, hallucinations. **Common Adverse Effects:** nausea, fatigue, diarrhea, abdominal cramps, headache, dizziness, nasal congestion, constipation, anorexia, dyspepsia, ataxia, elevated ALT, AST, elevated alkaline phosphatase.	Metabolism: liver; CYP450: 3A4 substrate. Excretion: bile, urine. Half-life: Up to 15 hr.

Continued

TABLE 7-1 Drugs Acting With the Central Nervous System—cont'd

Drug Name	Normal Adult Dose	Therapeutic Use	Major Adverse Effects/Cautions	Comments
Nonergot Derivatives				
ropinirole (Requip)	Start 0.25 mg PO tid and increase weekly to a maximum of 24 mg/day. Usual dosage 3 mg PO tid. Take with food.	Parkinsonism, restless leg syndrome.	Ropinirole may cause drowsiness, dizziness, or insomnia. Some people have reported falling asleep during activities such as talking or driving. Use with caution when driving, operating machinery, or performing other hazardous activities until patient determines drug's effects.	Metabolism: liver; CYP450: 1A2 substrate. Excretion: urine. Half-life: 6 hr.
pramipexole (Mirapex)	Start 0.125 mg PO tid × 7 days, then 0.25 mg PO tid × 7 days, then increase by 0.25 mg tid every 7 days to a maximum of 4.5 mg/day.	Parkinsonism.	**Common Adverse Effects:** dizziness, light-headedness, or fainting, especially when standing up; drowsiness; hallucinations; nausea; trouble in sleeping; twitching, twisting, or other unusual body movements; unusual tiredness or weakness.	Excretion: urine. Half-life: 8-12 hr.

ALT, Alanine transaminase; *AST*, aspartate transaminase; *CHF*, congestive heart failure; *CNS*, central nervous system; *CYP450*, cytochrome P-450; *GI*, gastrointestinal; *G-tube*, gastrostomy tube; *HTN*, hypertension; *IM*, intramuscular; *IV*, intravenous; *MAO*, monamine oxidase; *MI*, myocardial infarction; *PD*, pharmacodynamics; *PK*, pharmacokinetics; *PO*, by mouth; *bid*, twice a day; *tid*, three times a day; *SSRI*, selective serotonin reuptake inhibitor; *UTI*, urinary tract infection; *VFib*, ventricular fibrillation.

TABLE 7-2 Drugs Used to Improve Pulmonary Function

Drug Name	Normal Adult Dose	Therapeutic Use	Major Adverse Effects/Cautions	Comments
Bronchodilators—Beta Adrenergics				
albuterol (AccuNeb, Proventil, Ventolin, Vospire ER)	90 mcg per spray by metered dose inhaler (MDI). 2.5 mg/3 ml, 5 mg/ml nebulized treatment (NEB). 2.5 mg NEB tid-qid; 2-4 puffs q 4-6 hr. Maximum: 12 puffs per day by MDI or 10 mg/day NEB. 108 mcg/inhalation dry powder inhaler (DPI) 2 puffs q 4-6 hr oral tablets 2, 4 mg; 2-4 mg 3-4 times daily. Oral syrup 2 mg/5 ml. Extended-release tablets 4.8 mg q 12 hr to a maximum of 32 mg daily.	Bronchospasm.	**Serious Adverse Effects:** urticaria, angioedema, angina, arrhythmias, HTN, hypokalemia, seizures. **Common Adverse Effects:** throat irritation, cough, tremor, nausea, headache, nervousness, tachycardia, palpitations.	Metabolism: liver. Excretion: urine, feces. Half-life: 2.5-6 hr.
Levalbuterol (Xopenex)	MDI and nebulizer every 6-8 hr.	Bronchospasm.		
epinephrine (Adrenalin)	0.2-1 mg Sub-Q (preferred) or IM q 4 hr prn.	Severe acute bronchospasm.	**Serious Adverse Effects:** arrhythmias. **Common Adverse Effects:** nervousness, tremor, insomnia, nausea, tachycardia, headache	Metabolism: liver. Excretion: urine. Half-life: 1 minute.
formoterol (Foradil)	12 mcg cap DPI. Usual dosage: 12 mcg INH q 12 hr.	Maintenance of asthma or COPD, exercise-induced bronchospasm.	**Serious Adverse Effects:** exacerbation of asthma, anaphylaxis, angioedema, hypokalemia, arrhythmias. **Common Adverse Effects:** nervousness, tremor, tachycardia, dizziness, insomnia, nausea, dyspepsia, muscle cramps, HTN.	Metabolism: liver; CYP450: 2A6, 2C9/19, 2D6 substrate. Excretion: primarily urine, some feces. Half-life: 10 hr.
metaproterenol (Alupent)	10 mg, 20 mg; 10 mg/5 mL sol; MDI, NEB. Usual dosage: 2-3 puffs INH q 3-4 hr up to 12 puffs/day.	Asthma, COPD.	**Serious Adverse Effects:** MI. **Common Adverse Effects:** nervousness, tremor, headache, tachycardia, nausea, dizziness, insomnia.	Metabolism: liver. Excretion: urine. Half-life: unknown.
terbutaline (Brethine)	Sub-Q: Start 0.25 mg q 20-30 min up to a maximum of 1 mg/4 hr. PO: Start 2.5-5 mg tid to a maximum of 15 mg daily. Inhaled: 2 puffs by MDI q 4-6 hr.	Bronchospasm, tocolysis.	**Serious Adverse Effects:** hypersensitivity reaction, HTN, arrhythmias, pulmonary edema, seizures. **Common Adverse Effects:** headache, tremor, nausea/vomiting, muscle cramps, nervousness, hypokalemia, hyperglycemia.	Metabolism: GI tract when taken PO, liver. Excretion: urine. Half-life 3-4 hr.

Continued

TABLE 7-2 Drugs Used to Improve Pulmonary Function—cont'd

Drug Name	Normal Adult Dose	Therapeutic Use	Major Adverse Effects/Cautions	Comments
salmeterol (Serevent Diskus)	50 mcg INH. Usual dosage: 50 mcg INH q 12 hr. DPI: 1 puff q 12 hr.	Asthma maintenance, COPD maintenance, exercise-induced bronchospasm.	**Serious Adverse Effects:** exacerbation of asthma, anaphylaxis, angioedema, laryngospasm, arrhythmias, HTN. **Common Adverse Effects:** headache, mouth and throat irritation, nasal congestion, rash, palpitations, tachycardia, tremor.	Metabolism: liver. Excretion: feces. Half-life: 5.5 hr. Not for acute management of asthma exacerbations.
pirbuterol (Maxair Autohaler)	0.2 mg/spray. 1-2 puffs q 4-6 hr prn.	Bronchospasm.	**Serious Adverse Effects:** arrhythmias, anorexia, HTN, angina. **Common Adverse Effects:** tremor, nausea/vomiting, diarrhea, nervousness, headache.	Metabolism: liver; CYP450. Excretion: urine. Half-life: 2 hr.
Anticholinergics Used in Respiratory Conditions				
ipratropium (Atrovent, Atrovent HFA)	18 mcg/spray MDI, 500 mcg NEB. HFA-17 mcg/spray MDI 2-4 puffs q 4-6 hr.	Bronchospasm, COPD.	**Serious Adverse Effects:** hypersensitivity reaction (rare), anaphylaxis (rare), angioedema (rare), laryngospasm (rare), paradoxical bronchospasm, (rare), narrow-angle glaucoma. **Common Adverse Effects:** cough, nervousness, nausea, dry mouth, GI upset, dizziness, headache, COPD exacerbation, oral irritation, rash/ urticaria, metallic taste, blurred vision.	Metabolism: hydrolysis. Excretion: predominately feces; some urine. Half-life: 2 hr.
tiotropium inhaled (Spiriva HandiHaler)	18 mcg/cap. DPI 1 puff q 12 hr. HFA-17 mcg/spray MDI.	Bronchospasm, COPD.	**Serious Adverse Effects:** hypersensitivity reaction, angioedema, paradoxical glaucoma, bronchospasm. **Common Adverse Effects:** URI symptoms, dry mouth, pharyngitis, chest pain, UTI, dyspepsia, rhinitis, abdominal pain, edema, constipation, myalgia, vomiting, epistaxis, rash, tachycardia, candidiasis.	Metabolism: minimally in the liver; CYP450: 2D6, 3A4 substrate. Excretion: feces predominately, 14% urine. Half-life: 5-6 days.
Antiinflammatory—Corticosteroids				
beclomethasone (Qvar) (Nasal—Beconase AQ)	40, 80 mcg/spray INH; MDI, DPI. Nebulized 42 mcg/spray.	Asthma maintenance. Allergic and nonallergic rhinitis.	**Serious Adverse Effects:** bronchospasm, osteoporosis, glaucoma, cataract formation, growth suppression in children.	Metabolism: liver, lung; CYP450: 3A4 substrate. Excretion: predominately feces, some urine. Half-life: 2.8 hr. Spacer helps control.

TABLE 7-2 Drugs Used to Improve Pulmonary Function—cont'd

Drug Name	Normal Adult Dose	Therapeutic Use	Major Adverse Effects/Cautions	Comments
			Common Adverse Effects: headache, hoarseness, rhinitis, sinusitis, cough, oral candidiasis.	Candidiasis, also rinse mouth/gargle after use.
budesonide inhaled (Pulmicort Turbuhaler)	200 mcg/spray INH. 1-2 puffs daily bid to a maximum of 4 puffs bid.	Asthma maintenance	As above.	Metabolism: liver; CYP450: 3A4 substrate. Excretion: urine, feces. Half-life: 2-3 hr.
triamcinolone (Azmacort)	100 mcg/spray INH. Usual dosage: 2 puffs tid-qid.	Asthma maintenance.	**Serious Adverse Effects:** angioedema, osteoporosis, osteoporosis, cataracts, growth suppression in children. **Common Adverse Effects:** pharyngitis, cough, sinusitis, fatigue, eczema, pruritus.	Metabolism: liver. Excretion feces, urine. Half-life: 1.5 hr.
flunisolide (AeroBid)	250 mcg/spray INH. 2 puffs INH bid to a maximum of 8 puffs/day.	Asthma maintenance.	**Serious Adverse Effects:** adrenal insufficiency. **Common Adverse Effects:** nausea, diarrhea, vomiting, headache, sore throat, nasal congestion.	Metabolism: liver. Excretion: urine, feces. Half-life: 1.5-2 hr.
Nasal spray (Nasarel)	29 mcg/spray. 2 sprays per nostril bid-tid to a maximum 8 sprays per nostril per day.	Allergic rhinitis, prophylaxis for nasal polyps.		
fluticasone (Flovent HFA)	Start 88 mcg INH bid. Increase to a maximum of 440 mcg INH bid.	Asthma maintenance.	**Serious Adverse Effects:** adrenal suppression, bronchospasm, angioedema, growth suppression in children, osteoporosis. **Common Adverse Effects:** headaches, sore throat, sinusitis, oral candidiasis, cough.	Metabolism: liver. Excretion: feces. Half-life: 7.5-8 hr.
Nasal spray (Flonase)	Nasal spray: 50 mcg/spray. 2 sprays per nostril daily to a maximum of 4 sprays daily.	Allergic rhinitis, prophylaxis for nasal polyps.		
Mediator-Release Inhibitors				
cromolyn sodium (Intal)	800 mcg/spray MDI; 20 mg/ 2 ml NEB. 2 puffs INH qid.	Asthma maintenance, exercise-induced asthma.	Used for prophylaxis not for acute treatment. **Serious Adverse Effects:** bronchospasm, anaphylaxis. **Common Adverse Effects:** sore throat, bad taste in mouth, cough, nausea, headache.	Excretion: feces, urine, bile. Half-life: unknown.
nedocromil (Tilade)	1.75 mg/spray INH. 2 puffs INH qid.	Asthma maintenance.	As above.	Excretion: urine, feces. Half-life: 3.5 hr.
Leukotriene Modifiers				
montelukast (Singulair)	4 mg, 5 mg CH, 10 mg. Usual dosage: 10 mg PO at bedtime.	Asthma maintenance. Allergic rhinitis.	**Serious Adverse Effects:** angioedema, anaphylaxis. **Common Adverse Effects:** headache, stomach pain, cough, fatigue, rash, fever, GI upset, pruritus, elevated liver enzymes.	Metabolism: liver; CYP450: 2C9, 3A4 substrate; 2C8 inhibitor. Excretion: bile, feces, urine. Half-life: 2.5-5.5 hr.

Continued

TABLE 7-2 Drugs Used to Improve Pulmonary Function—cont'd

Drug Name	Normal Adult Dose	Therapeutic Use	Major Adverse Effects/Cautions	Comments
zafirlukast (Accolate)	10, 20 mg tabs. Usual dosage: 20 mg PO bid.	Asthma maintenance.	**Serious Adverse Effects:** hepatic failure, angioedema. **Common Adverse Effects:** headache, nausea, stomach pain, diarrhea, elevated liver enzymes.	Metabolism: liver, CYP450: 2C9 substrate; 2C9, 3A4 inhibitor. Excretion: bile, feces, urine. Half-life: 8-16 hr.
Combination Agents fluticasone/salmeterol inhaled (Advair Diskus)	**Asthma:** 1 dose INH bid Start: 100/50-250/50 mcg INH bid if not on inhaled steroid, 100/50-500/50 mcg INH bid if on other inhaled steroid. **COPD with chronic bronchitis:** 250/50 mcg INH bid.	Asthma maintenance, COPD.	**Serious Adverse Effects:** bronchospasm, paradoxical asthma exacerbation, death, asthma-related (rare) laryngospasm, angioedema, growth suppression (pediatrics), adrenal suppression, cushingoid features, severe ventricular arrhythmia (rare), severe hypokalemia (rare), glaucoma (rare), cataracts (rare), Churg-Strauss syndrome (rare). **Common Adverse Effects:** URI, headache, pharyngitis, cough, sinusitis, nausea/vomiting, dyspepsia, bronchitis, hoarseness, dysphonia, throat irritation, dizziness, palpitations, tremor, taste changes, diarrhea, dermatitis, hypokalemia, oral candidiasis.	Pregnancy category: C. Lactation: safety unknown. Metabolism: see individual drugs. Excretion: see individual drugs. DEA/FDA: Rx.
albuterol/ipratropium inhaled (Combivent)	1-2 puffs INH qid. Maximum: 12 puffs/day.	COPD.	**Serious Adverse Effects:** bronchospasm, paradoxical arrhythmias, angioedema (rare), anaphylaxis (rare), narrow-angle glaucoma. **Common Adverse Effects:** bronchitis, URI, headache, dyspnea, cough, pain, nausea.	Pregnancy category: C. Lactation: safety unknown. Metabolism: see individual drugs. Excretion: see individual drugs.
Smoking Cessation Nicotine Substitutes nicotine transdermal (Nicoderm CQ, Nicotrol)	7 mg, 14 mg, 21 mg/24 hr patch. Begin by using a 21-mg patch daily for 6 weeks, then 14-mg patch daily for 2 weeks, then 7-mg patch daily for 2 weeks. In patients who smoke <10 cigarettes/day, begin with 14-mg dose/24 hr patch.	Smoking cessation.	**Common Adverse Effects:** skin reaction due to irritation from patch, rash, withdrawal symptoms, headache, palpitations, tachycardia, HTN, nausea, flatulence, insomnia.	Important to discontinue use of tobacco products when using this product. Method of Action: binds to nicotine receptors. Pregnancy category: D. Metabolism: liver, kidney, lung. Excretion, urine. Half-life: 3-4 hr.

TABLE 7-2 Drugs Used to Improve Pulmonary Function—cont'd

Drug Name	Normal Adult Dose	Therapeutic Use	Major Adverse Effects/Cautions	Comments
nicotine gum (Nicorette)	2-, 4-mg gum. Begin by chewing 2 mg q 1-2 hr for 6 weeks, then q 2-4 hr for 3 weeks, then q 4-8 hr for 3 weeks. Maximum: 30 pieces/day. Chew gum to activate, then hold in between gum and cheek. Light smokers use 2-mg gum; heavy smokers use 4-mg gum.	As above.	As above.	As above.
nicotine (Commit)	2-, 4-mg lozenge. Begin by using 4 mg PO q 1-2 hr for 6 weeks, then 4 mg PO q 2-4 hr for 3 weeks, then 4 mg PO q 4-8 hr for 3 weeks. Do not chew lozenge; allow to dissolve in mouth.	As above.	As above.	As above.
nicotine inhaler (Nicotrol Inhaler)	4 mg/cartridge. 6-16 cartridges per day during weeks 1-12. Taper over weeks 13-24. Maximum: 16 cartridges per day.	As above.	As above.	As above.
nicotine nasal spray (Nicotrol NS)	0.5 mg/spray. 1-2 sprays each nostril every hour. Maximum: number of sprays— 10 sprays or 5 mg/hr; 80 sprays or 40 mg/day. After 6-8 weeks gradually wean over 4-6 weeks.	As above.	As above.	As above.
Other bupropion (Zyban)	150 mg SR. Begin 150 mg PO daily for 3 days, then 300 mg daily. Discontinue smoking after 5 to 7 days of beginning Zyban.	As above.	**Serious Adverse Effects:** seizures, arrhythmias, tachycardia, Stevens-Johnson syndrome, hallucinations, mania, suicidal ideation, HTN, depression. **Common Adverse Effects:** insomnia, dry mouth, headache, agitation, nausea, constipation, tinnitus, anorexia, abdominal pain, diarrhea, anxiety, rash, palpitations, myalgia, urinary frequency.	Metabolism: liver; CYP450: 2B6 substrate, 2D6 inhibitor. Excretion: urine, feces. Half-life: 21 hr.

bid, Twice a day; *CH*, chewable tablet; *COPD*, chronic obstructive pulmonary disease; *CYP450*, cytochrome P-450; *DEA*, Drug Enforcement Administration; *FDA*, Food and Drug Administration; *GI*, gastrointestinal; *HTN*, Hypertension; *hs*, at bedtime; *IM*, intramuscular; *INH*, inhalation; *MI*, myocardial infarction; *PO*, by mouth; *prn*, as needed; *qid*, four times a day; *Rx*, prescription; *Sub-Q*, subcutaneous; *tid*, three times a day; *URI*, upper respiratory infection; *UTI*, urinary tract infection.

TABLE 7-3 Drugs That Regulate Bladder and Bowel Elimination

Drug Name	Normal Adult Dose	Therapeutic Use	Major Adverse Effects/Cautions	Comments
Bladder Incontinence				
Anticholinergic Agents				
oxybutynin (Ditropan, Ditropan XL, Oxytrol)	Tabs: Begin 2.5 mg PO bid. Increase to effective dose. Maximum 5 mg PO qid. SR: Begin 5-10 mg PO daily. Increase by 5 mg/week to a maximum of 30 mg/day. Transdermal: 1 patch (3.9 mg/day) q 4 days. Apply to abdomen, buttocks, or hip. Rotate sites.	Bladder incontinence.	**Serious Adverse Effects:** heat intolerance. **Common Adverse Effects:** dry mouth, constipation, abnormal vision, diarrhea, abdominal pain, nausea, fatigue, flatulence, headache, rash, decreased sweating, impotence, lactation suppression. Transdermal may also cause local skin irritation.	Metabolism: liver; GI tract; CYP450: 3A4 substrate. Excretion: urine. Half-life: 2-3 hr; extended-release tabs: 13 hr; transdermal patch: 2-5 hr.
tolterodine (Detrol, Detrol LA)	Tabs: 1 mg PO bid. Maximum 4 mg/day. SR: 4 mg PO daily. May decrease to 2 mg PO if effective.	Bladder incontinence.	**Serious Adverse Effects:** anaphylactoid reactions, psychosis, angioedema. **Common Adverse Effects:** dry mouth, headache, constipation, dyspepsia, dry eyes, dizziness, blurred vision, somnolence, urinary retention.	Metabolism: liver; CYP450: 2D6, 3A4 substrates. Excretion: urine, feces. Half-life: 2-3 hr.
Tricyclic antidepressants (TCAs)		Bladder incontinence.	Anticholinergic effects.	TCAs are generally reserved for patients with an additional indication such as depression or neuralgia. Do not use in patients with urinary obstruction. Do not use with MAO inhibitors or within 14 days of MAO use.
nortriptyline (Pamelor)	Usual dosage: 25-100 mg/day (with water or juice).	Bladder incontinence.	As above.	Pregnancy category: D. Metabolism: liver; CYP450: 2D6 substrate. Excretion: urine, feces. Half-life: 18-44 hr.
imipramine (Tofranil, Tofranil-PM)	Usual dosage: 25-100 mg/day (with water or juice).	Bladder incontinence.	As above.	Pregnancy category: D. Metabolism: liver; CYP450: 1A2, 2C19, 2D6, 3A4 substrates. Excretion: urine, bile, feces. Half-life 11-25 hr.
doxepin (Sinequan)	Usual dosage: 25-100 mg/day (with water or juice).	Bladder incontinence.	As above.	Pregnancy Category: C. Metabolism: liver; CYP450: 2C9/19, 2D6 substrates. Excretion: urine. Half-life: 6-8 hr.

TABLE 7-3 Drugs That Regulate Bladder and Bowel Elimination—cont'd

Drug Name	Normal Adult Dose	Therapeutic Use	Major Adverse Effects/Cautions	Comments
Estrogen				
conjugated estrogen (Premarin)	0.5 g vaginal cream 3 times/ week, up to 8 months; repeat course if symptoms recur. OR, estradiol vaginal insert/ring (2 mg per ring). Replace ring after 90 days, if needed; if ineffective, start systemic therapy with conjugated estrogens, 0.3-0.625 mg/day PO. Take immediately after food to decrease nausea. OR, Estraderm patch (0.05 mg/day)—1 patch 2 times per week.	Bladder incontinence.	Few **adverse effects** with cream and vaginal inserts. **Adverse effects** of systemic therapy are headache, vaginal spotting, edema, breast tenderness, possible depression.	Systemic therapy should not be used if there is suspected or confirmed breast or endometrial cancer, or active or past thromboembolism with past oral contraceptive, estrogen, or pregnancy. NOTE: It is necessary to also use Progestin in patients with an intact uterus. Pregnancy category: X. Metabolism: liver; CYP450: 3A4 substrate. Excretion: urine. Half-life 4-18 hr.
Alpha-Adrenergic Agonists				
pseudoephedrine (Sudafed)	Usual dosage: 15-60 tid taken with food, water, or milk.	Stress incontinence.	**Adverse Effects:** anxiety, insomnia, agitation, palpitations, headache, angina, cardiac dysrhythmia, hypertension, tremor. Should not be used in patients with obstructive syndromes and/or hypertension.	Metabolism: liver. Excretion: urine. Half-life: 9-16 hr.
Alpha-Adrenergic Antagonists				
terazosin (Hytrin)	Usual dose: 1 mg at bedtime. Increase by 1 mg q 4 days to a maximum of 5 mg/day.	Overflow (because of enlarged benign prostate).	**Adverse Effects:** postural hypotension, syncope in supine position, heart palpitations, edema, headache, dizziness, vertigo, drowsiness, weakness. **Interactions:** antihypertensives may increase hypotension.	Possible benefit in men with obstructive symptoms of benign prostatic hyperplasia. Monitor sitting and standing blood pressures with first dose and with dose increases. May worsen female stress incontinence.
doxazosin (Cardura, Cardura XL)	1 mg at bedtime, with first dose in supine position. Increase by 1 mg q 7-14 days to 8 mg/day, as needed.	As above.	As above.	As above.
tamsulosin (Flomax)	0.4 mg/day. Increase after 2-4 weeks, if needed, to 0.8 mg/day.	As above.	**Adverse Effects:** as above except fewer incidences of orthostatic hypotension.	As above.

Continued

TABLE 7-3 Drugs That Regulate Bladder and Bowel Elimination—cont'd

Drug Name	Normal Adult Dose	Therapeutic Use	Major Adverse Effects/Cautions	Comments
Antiandrogens finasteride (Proscar) (Propecia)	5 mg PO daily. Can crush, but do NOT handle if pregnant or possibly pregnant. 1 mg PO daily.	As above.	**Common Adverse Effects:** decreased libido, decreased ejaculate volume, impotence, gynecomastia.	Maximum therapeutic effect after 6-12 months. Causes 50% decrease in PSA test. Interactions: Falsely decreased prostate-specific antigen concentration. Pregnancy Category: X. Metabolism: liver; CYP450: 3A4 substrate. Excretion: feces, urine. Half-life: 6 hr.
Phytotherapy _Serenoa repens_ (saw palmetto)	160 mg bid.	As above.	**Common Adverse Effects:** headaches, GI upset, HTN, decreased libido, erectile dysfunction.	Long-term efficacy and safety unknown.
Cholinergics bethanechol (Urecholine)	Start 5-10 mg PO q 1 hr until response up to 50 mg.	Urinary retention and overflow (because of atonic bladder).	**Adverse Effects:** nausea, vomiting, abdominal cramps, diarrhea, bradycardia, bronchoconstriction, hypotension. **Interactions:** decreased effect by anticholinergics.	Avoid use in patients with asthma or heart disease. Short-term use only.
Laxatives **_Bulk Forming_** psyllium (Metamucil)	Powder. Usual dosage 1-2 tsp PO daily-tid dissolved in a full glass of liquid such as water or juice.	Constipation.	**Common Adverse Effects:** bowel or esophageal obstruction, diarrhea, constipation, abdominal cramps.	Important for patient to drink adequate fluids. Excretion: feces.
calcium polycarbophil (Konsyl Fiber Tablets, FiberCon)	Dosage required will vary according to diet, exercise, previous laxative use, and degree of constipation.	Constipation.	As above.	As above.
Emollients docusate sodium (Colace)	Usual dose: 100 mg PO daily divided into one to four doses. Mix liquid with fruit juice or milk.	Constipation.	**Common Adverse Effects:** diarrhea, abdominal cramps, electrolyte disorders.	As above.
docusate potassium	100-300 mg/day until bowel movements are normal.	Preventing constipation.	As above.	As above.
docusate calcium	240 mg/day until bowel movements are normal.	As above.	As above.	As above.

TABLE 7-3 Drugs That Regulate Bladder and Bowel Elimination—cont'd

Drug Name	Normal Adult Dose	Therapeutic Use	Major Adverse Effects/Cautions	Comments
Stimulants bisacodyl (Dulcolax)	Usual dosage: 5-15 mg in a single dose once per day. Up to 30 mg has been used for bowel preparation for special procedures of the lower GI tract.	Constipation.	**Adverse Effects:** chronic use can lead to electrolyte imbalance or abdominal cramping.	Should be used intermittently.
senna (Senokot)	Tablets (187 and 217 mg): 2 tablets (up to 8/day). Tablets (374 mg): 1 tablet at bedtime (up to 4/day). Granules: 1 tsp (up to 4 tsp/day). Suppositories: 1 at bedtime; repeat in 2 hr if necessary. Liquid: 15-30 ml with or after meals or at bedtime. Syrup: 10-15 ml at bedtime (up to 30 ml/day).	Constipation.	As above.	As above.
Hyperosmolar glycerin	Suppositories: Insert 1 suppository high in the rectum and retain 15 minutes; it need not melt to produce laxative action. Rectal liquid: With gentle, steady pressure, insert stem with tip pointing toward navel; squeeze until nearly all the liquid is expelled, then remove; a small amount of liquid will remain in unit.	Constipation.	As above.	As above.
lactulose (Chronulac, Constilac, Kristalose)	15-30 ml (10-20 g lactulose)/ day. Increase to 60 ml/day if necessary.	Constipation.	As above.	Sorbitol is as effective as lactulose yet less expensive.
Saline Products magnesium citrate (Citrate of Magnesia)	1 glassful (approximately 250 ml/day), as needed.	Acute evacuation of the bowel.	**Adverse Effects:** fluid and electrolyte imbalance.	

bid, Twice a day; *CYP450,* cytochrome P-450; *GI,* gastrointestinal; *HTN,* hypertension; *MAO,* monoamine oxidase; *PO,* by mouth; *PSA,* prostate specific antigen; *qid,* four times a day; *SR,* sustained release; *tid,* three times a day.

TABLE 7-4 Drugs Used to Treat Autoimmune Diseases, Pain, and/or Improve Mobility

Drug Name	Normal Adult Dose	Therapeutic Use	Major Adverse Effects/Cautions	Comments
Muscle Relaxants/Antispastics				
baclofen (Kemstro)	Start 5 mg PO tid × 3 days. Increase 15 mg/day every 3 days to a maximum of 80 mg/day in divided doses (tid-qid).	Muscle spasticity; multiple sclerosis.	**Adverse Effects:** seizures, muscle weakness, constipation, dizziness, headaches, drowsiness.	Side effects minimized by titrating slowing and administering lower doses in patients with renal impairment. Do not abruptly stop, rather withdraw slowly.
tizanidine (Zanaflex)	Start 4 mg PO × 1. Increase by 2-4 mg q 6-8 hr until effective dose to a maximum of 36 mg/day (no more than 3 doses or 12 mg/dose).	As above.	**Adverse Effects:** hypotension, sedation, somnolence.	Monitor LFTs at baseline, 1, 3 and 6 months, then periodically.
Disease-Modifying Drugs				
methotrexate (Rheumatrex)	Oral or IM: 7.5-20 mg weekly.	Rheumatoid arthritis, psoriasis, multiple sclerosis.	**Adverse Effects:** myelosuppression, cirrhosis, proteinuria, rash, stomatitis, nausea and vomiting, diarrhea, increased liver enzymes, pulmonary infiltrates.	The DMARD of choice, but not used in pregnant or nursing patients. Give additional folic acid because methotrexate is a folic acid antagonist.
hydroxychloroquine (Plaquenil)	PO. Induction 400-600 mg daily. Maintenance 200-400 mg daily.	Rheumatoid arthritis, SLE, malaria.	**Adverse Effects:** macular damage, rash, diarrhea, abdominal cramps. Increased risk of retinal toxicity if dose exceeds 6 g/kg.	Main benefit is lack of myelosuppression. Used alone does not slow disease progression. Take with food.
sulfasalazine (Azulfidine)	500 mg bid then increase to a maximum of 1 g bid.	Rheumatoid arthritis, ulcerative colitis, Crohn's disease.	**Adverse Effects:** myelosuppression, rash, nausea, vomiting, abdominal discomfort, diarrhea, anorexia.	Can cause urine and skin to turn yellow orange. Periodic monitoring for leukopenia is recommended.
leflunomide (Arava)	100 mg daily for 3 days, then 10-20 mg daily.	Rheumatoid arthritis.	**Adverse Effects:** diarrhea, elevated liver enzymes, alopecia, rash, headaches, risk of infection.	Comparable efficacy to sulfasalazine and methotrexate.
etanercept (Enbrel)	25 mg Sub-Q twice weekly.	Ankylosing spondylitis, psoriasis, psoriatic arthritis, rheumatoid arthritis.	**Adverse Effects:** injection site irritation, upper respiratory infections.	Second-line treatment option FDA approved for monotherapy or in combination with methotrexate. Expensive.
infliximab (Remicade)	3-10 mg/kg IV q 8 weeks or 3-5 mg/kg IV q 4 weeks.	Ankylosing spondylitis, Crohn's disease, ulcerative colitis, rheumatoid arthritis, psoriasis.	Monitor carefully for signs of infection.	Inhibits interleukin-1. FDA approved as second-line therapy.
anakinra (Kineret)	100 mg Sub-Q daily.	Rheumatoid arthritis.	Monitor carefully for signs of infection.	Inhibits interleukin-1. FDA approved as second-line therapy. May be used in combination with other DMARDs except TNF-blocking agents.

NOTE: Take patient variables, administration, comorbid conditions, and cost into account when planning.

TABLE 7-4 Drugs Used to Treat Autoimmune Diseases, Pain, and/or Improve Mobility—cont'd

Drug Name	Normal Adult Dose	Therapeutic Use	Major Adverse Effects/Cautions	Comments
Antiinflammatory **Nonsteroidal Antiinflammatory** **Drugs (NSAIDs)**				Some studies suggest that NSAIDs are associated with hypertension.
Naproxen (Aleve)	440 mg PO daily to a maximum of 660 mg/day.	Osteoarthritis, rheumatoid arthritis, mild-moderate pain, dysmenorrhea, ankylosing spondylitis, acute gouty attacks, inflammation, fever.	**Serious Adverse Effects:** GI bleed, GI ulcers, GI perforation, MI, stroke, thromboembolism, HTN, CHF, nephrotoxicity, hepatotoxicity, anaphylactoid reaction, bronchospasm, Stevens-Johnson syndrome, anemia, prolonged bleeding time. **Common Adverse Effects:** dyspepsia, nausea, abdominal pain, constipation, diarrhea, headache, dizziness, drowsiness, pruritus, skin eruptions, ecchymosis, fluid retention, peripheral edema, tinnitus, dyspnea, elevated liver transaminases.	Metabolism: liver; CYP450: 2C9 substrate. Excretion: urine. Half-life: 12-17 hr.
(Anaprox, Anaprox DS)	550 mg PO bid to a maximum of 1650 mg/day × 6 mo.			
(Naprelan)	750-1000 mg PO daily to a maximum of 1500 mg/day ×6 mo.			
(Naprosyn)	250-500 mg PO bid to a maximum of 1500 mg/day ×6 mo.			
nabumetone (Relafen)	1000-2000 mg PO daily 1-2 doses to a maximum of 2000 mg/day.	As above.	As above.	Metabolism: liver. Excretion: urine, feces. Half-life: 24 hr.
indomethacin (Indocin)	25 mg PO bid-tid. Increase by 25-50 mg every 7 days to a maximum of 200 mg/day.	As above.	As above.	Metabolism: liver; CYP450: 2C9 substrate. Excretion: urine, bile, feces. Half-life: 4.5 hr.
(Indocin SR)	75 mg PO daily to a maximum of 75 mg PO bid.			
ketoprofen (Oruvail)	100-200 mg PO daily to a maximum of 200 mg/day.	As above.	As above.	Metabolism: liver. Excretion: urine. Half-life: 5-6 hr.
COX II Inhibitors				
celecoxib (Celebrex)	100-200 mg PO bid to a maximum of 400 mg/day.	Osteoarthritis, rheumatoid arthritis, acute pain (short-term use only), ankylosing spondylitis, dysmenorrhea.	As above.	Metabolism: liver extensively; CYP450: 2C9 substrate. Excretion: feces, urine. Half-life: 11 hr.
Antiinflammatory Steroids **Corticosteroids:** triamcinolone (Aristocort), hydrocortisone (Cortef), hydrocortisone sodium succinate (Solu-Cortef), dexamethasone (Decadron),	See individual drug.	Inflammatory disorders, adrenal insufficiency, multiple sclerosis, pneumocystis pneumonia, SLE, nephrotic syndrome.	**Serious Adverse Effects:** adrenal insufficiency, steroid psychosis, immunosuppression (long-term use), peptic ulcer, CHF, anaphylaxis, osteoporosis (long-term use), pancreatitis. **Common Adverse Effects:** nausea,	NOTE: Steroids are not a cure of the disease process, but offer only symptomatic relief of swelling, redness, pain, and effusion. Metabolism, excretion, and half-life vary by individual drug.

Continued

TABLE 7-4 Drugs Used to Treat Autoimmune Diseases, Pain, and/or Improve Mobility—cont'd

Drug Name	Normal Adult Dose	Therapeutic Use	Major Adverse Effects/Cautions	Comments
prednisolone (Orapred, Pediapred, Prelone) prednisone (Deltasone, Sterapred), methylprednisolone acetate (Depo-Medrol), methylprednisolone sodium succinate (Solu-Medrol), fludrocortisone (Florinef Acetate), methylprednisolone (Medrol)			vomiting, dyspepsia, appetite change, edema, headache, dizziness, mood swings, insomnia, anxiety, hypokalemia, HTN, hyperglycemia, cushingoid features (long-term use), menstrual irregularities, ecchymosis, acne, skin atrophy (long-term use), impaired wound healing (long-term use).	
Analgesics				
acetaminophen (Tylenol)	320-1000 mg PO q 4-6 hr to a maximum of 4 g/24 hr.	Mild to moderate pain, fever.	**Serious Adverse Effects:** hepatotoxicity, cholestatic jaundice, hepatic necrosis, renal tubular necrosis, acute analgesic, nephropathy, chronic anemia, hemolytic pancytopenia, thrombocytopenia, leukopenia, neutropenia, hypersensitivity reaction, angioedema, anaphylaxis. **Common Adverse Effects:** nausea, urticaria, rash	Metabolism: liver; CYP450: 1A2, 2E1 substrate. Excretion: urine. Half-life: 2-4 hr.
morphine sulfate (Avinza) (Kadian) (MS Contin, Oramorph SR) (Roxanol)	30-120 mg/day to a maximum of 1600 mg/day (in opioid-tolerant patients). 20 mg PO per day. Increase to a maximum of 100 mg/day in opioid-tolerant patients. 15-30 mg PO q 8-12 hr. 10-30 mg PO q 4 hr.	Moderate to severe pain, acute MI.	**Serious Adverse Effects:** respiratory depression, apnea, hypotension, cardiac arrest, shock, bradycardia, paralytic ileus, toxic megacolon, seizures, increased ICP, dependency, withdrawal syndrome. **Common Adverse Effects:** somnolence, constipation, nausea and vomiting, dizziness, hypotension, euphoria, sweating, edema, abdominal pain, pruritus, flushing, dry mouth, asthenia, paresthesias, urinary retention.	Metabolism: liver; GI tract; CYP450: 2D6 substrate. Excretion: urine, bile, feces. Half-life: 2-4 hr. Dosage adjustments are required in patients with renal dysfunction.
hydromorphone (Dilaudid)	PO 2-4 mg q 3-4 hr. IM 0.5-1 mg q 3-4 hr. Rectal 2-4 mg q 3-4 hr.	Moderate to severe pain, cough. More potent than morphine. Can be used in patients with renal dysfunction.	**Serious Adverse Effects:** respiratory depression, apnea, respiratory arrest, hypotension, circulatory depression, shock, cardiac arrest, syncope, bradycardia, arrhythmias, QT prolongation, urinary retention, intestinal	Metabolism: liver. Excretion: urine, bile. Half-life: 2-3 hr.

TABLE 7-4 Drugs Used to Treat Autoimmune Diseases, Pain, and/or Improve Mobility—cont'd

Drug Name	Normal Adult Dose	Therapeutic Use	Major Adverse Effects/Cautions	Comments
			obstruction, paralytic ileus, biliary spasm, hallucinations, delirium, increased ICP, seizure disorder, blood dyscrasias, pancytopenia, agranulocytosis, allergic reactions, withdrawal syndrome, dependency. **Common Adverse Effects:** constipation, nausea and vomiting, asthenia, headache, somnolence, pruritus, dizziness, vasodilation, tachycardia, xerostomia, dysphagia, flatulence, abdominal pain, anorexia, weight loss, sweating, rash, peripheral edema, confusion, insomnia, anxiety, myalgia, urinary retention, euphoria.	
oxymorphone (Numorphan)	IM 1-1.5 mg q 4-6 hr. IV 0.5 mg initially. Rectal 5 mg q 3-4 hr.	Moderate to severe pain, obstetrical analgesia.	As above.	Metabolism: liver. Excretion: urine. Half-life: unknown.
levorphanol (Levo-Dromoran)	PO 2-4 mg q 6-8 hr. IM 2 mg q 6-8 hr. IV 2 mg q 6-8 hr.	Moderate to severe pain. Useful in patients with cancer.	As above.	Metabolism: liver. Excretion: urine. Half-life: 11-16 hr.
codeine sulfate	PO 15-60 mg q 3-4 hr. IM 15-60 mg q 3-4 hr. IV 2 mg q 6-8 hr.	Mild to moderate pain, antitussive. Commonly used with NSAIDs, aspirin, or acetaminophen.	As above.	Metabolism: liver primarily; CYP450: 2D6 substrate. Excretion: urine. Half-life 2-4 hr.
hydrocodone	PO 5-10 mg q 3-4 hr.	Moderate or severe pain. Only available in combination with NSAIDs, aspirin, or ibuprofen.	As above.	Metabolism: liver extensively; CYP450: 2D6, 3A4 substrate. Excretion: renal. Half-life: 3-4 hr.
oxycodone (ETH-Oxydose, OxyFast, OxyIR, Roxicodone) (OxyContin)	PO 5-10 mg q 3-4 hr. Increase to a maximum of 160 mg PO q 12 hr. Controlled release 10-80 mg q 12 hr.	Moderate to severe pain. Most effective when used with NSAIDs, aspirin, or acetaminophen.	As above.	Metabolism: liver; CYP450: 2D6 substrate. Excretion: urine. Half-life: 3.5 hr.
fentanyl (Sublimaze, Duragesic, Actiq)	IM 0.05-0.1 mg q 1-2 hr. Transdermal 25-100 mg/hr q 72 hr. Transmucosal 200-1600 mcg unit PO prn—maximum 4 units/day. IV 50-100 mcg IV q 1-2 hr.	Moderate to severe pain, preoperative analgesia, adjunct to regional anesthesia.	As above.	Metabolism: liver; CYP450: 3A4 substrate. Excretion: urine. Half-life: 3.5-4 hr.
propoxyphene (Darvon) (Darvon-N)	65 mg PO q 4 hr to a maximum of 390 mg/24 hr. 100 mg q 4 hr to a maximum of 600 mg/24 hr.	Mild to moderate pain. Weak analgesia; most effective when used with NSAIDs, aspirin, or acetaminophen.	As above.	Metabolism: liver; CYP450: 2D6 substrate/inhibitor. Excretion: urine. Half-life: 6-12 hr.

Continued

TABLE 7-4 Drugs Used to Treat Autoimmune Diseases, Pain, and/or Improve Mobility—cont'd

Drug Name	Normal Adult Dose	Therapeutic Use	Major Adverse Effects/Cautions	Comments
				Do not use in elderly patients.
tramadol (Ultram)	50-100 mg q 4-6 hr. Maximum dose 400 mg/24 hr.	Moderate to severe pain.	As above.	Metabolism: liver; CYP450: 2D6, 3A4 substrate. Excretion: urine. Half-life: 6.5 hr.

bid, Twice a day; *CHF*, congestive heart failure; *CYP450*, cytochrome P-450; *DMARD*, disease-modifying antirheumatic drug; *FDA*, Food and Drug Administration; *GI*, gastrointestinal; *HTN*, hypertension; *ICP*, intracranial pressure; *IM*, intramuscular; *IV*, intravenous; *LFT*, liver function test; *MI*, myocardial infarction; *PO*, by mouth; *prn*, as needed; *qid*, four times a day; *SLE*, systemic lupus erythematosus; *Sub-Q*, subcutaneous; *tid*, three times a day; *TNF*, tumor necrosis factor.

TABLE 7-5 Common Cardiovascular, Anticoagulant/Antiplatelet, and Cholesterol-Lowering Agents

Drug Name	Normal Adult Dose	Therapeutic Use	Major Adverse Effects/Cautions	Comments
Common Cardiovascular Medications				
Angiotensin-Converting Enzyme (ACE) Inhibitors Includes the following medications: benazepril (Lotensin) captopril (Capoten) enalapril (Vasotec) fosinopril (Monopril) lisinopril (Prinivil, Zestril) moexipril (Univasc) perindopril (Aceon) quinapril (Accupril) ramipril (Altace) trandolapril (Mavik)	Dose depends on specific agent.	CHF, HTN.	**Serious Adverse Effects:** of this entire class include anaphylactic reaction, angioedema, hypotension, Stevens-Johnson syndrome. **Common Adverse Effects:** cough, rash, pruritus, hyperkalemia, renal dysfunction, fetal harm or death, hypotension, dizziness, fatigue, hyperkalemia, nausea/vomiting, elevated BUN and/or creatinine, URI symptoms, musculoskeletal pain.	Pregnancy category: D. Work by decreasing the resistance of the blood vessels by interfering with the body's production of angiotensin. Metabolism, excretion, and half-life depend on specific agent.
Beta Blockers Includes the following medications: acebutolol (Sectral) atenolol (Tenormin) betaxolol (Kerlone) bisoprolol (Zebeta) metoprolol (Lopressor, Toprol XL) nadolol (Corgard) propranolol (Inderal, Inderal LA) timolol (Blocadren)	Dose depends on specific agent.	HTN, ventricular arrhythmias, angina, previous MI, migraine prophylaxis.	Do not stop taking any beta blocker medication abruptly, because this can cause rebound hypertension. **Serious Adverse Effects:** CHF, bradycardia. **Common Adverse Effects:** fatigue, dizziness, headache, constipation, diarrhea, dyspepsia, nausea, dyspnea, insomnia, urinary frequency, blurred vision,	Reduce heart rate and lower cardiac output. Drug of choice for patients with a history of angina or heart attack, but are contraindicated in patients with chronic lung diseases. Pregnancy category, metabolism, excretion, and half-life depend on specific agent.

TABLE 7-5 Common Cardiovascular, Anticoagulant/Antiplatelet, and Cholesterol-Lowering Agents—cont'd

Drug Name	Normal Adult Dose	Therapeutic Use	Major Adverse Effects/Cautions	Comments
			arthralgias, myalgias, edema, chest pain, depression, rash, sexual dysfunction.	
Calcium Channel Blockers Includes the following medications: amlodipine (Norvasc) felodipine (Plendil) isradipine (Dynacirc) nifedipine (Adalat CC, Procardia, Procardia XL) diltiazem (Cardizem, Cardizem LA, Cardizem CD, Cartia XT, Tiazac, Dilacor-XR, Diltia XT) verapamil (Calan, Isoptin, Calan SR, Verelan, Verelan PM)	Dosage depends on specific agent.	HTN, angina, SVT, migraine prophylaxis.	**Serious Adverse Effects:** CHF, arrhythmias, syncope, worsening of angina, pancreatitis, angioedema, leukopenia, thrombocytopenia. **Common Adverse Effects:** edema, headache, fatigue, palpitations, dizziness, nausea, flushing, peripheral edema, hypotension, reflex tachycardia, gingival hyperplasia, rash.	Reduce heart rate and relax blood vessels by interfering with the movement of calcium. Most are pregnancy category C, but check specific drug. Metabolism, excretion, and half-life depend on specific agent.
Diuretics				Decrease water and sodium retention.
Thiazide Includes the following medications: hydrochlorothiazide (Esidrix, HydroDIURIL, Microzide, Oretic) chlorothiazide (Diuril)	Dosage depends on specific agent.	Edema, HTN.	**Serious Adverse Effects:** hypokalemia, electrolyte imbalance, arrhythmias, pancreatitis, anaphylaxis, renal failure, erythema multiforme, exfoliative dermatitis, pancytopenia, agranulocytosis, thrombocytopenia, aplastic anemia. **Common Adverse Effects:** hyponatremia, hypokalemia, metabolic alkalosis, hyperuricemia, hyperglycemia, hypercalcemia, hyperlipidemia, hypomagnesemia, hypotension, dizziness, anorexia, diarrhea, abdominal pain, headache, weakness, muscle cramps, photosensitivity, rash, sexual dysfunction.	Pregnancy category, metabolism, excretion, and half-life depend on specific agent.
Loop Diuretics Includes the following medications: bumetanide (Bumex) furosemide (Lasix)	Dosage depends on specific agent.	Diuresis for heart failure, renal or hepatic failure, edema, hypercalcemia, HTN. Potassium supplements may be needed.	**Serious Adverse Effects:** renal failure, thrombocytopenia. **Common Adverse Effects:** dizziness, headache, orthostatic	Pregnancy category, metabolism, excretion, and half-life depend on specific agent.

Continued

TABLE 7-5 Common Cardiovascular, Anticoagulant/Antiplalelet, and Cholesterol-Lowering Agents—cont'd

Drug Name	Normal Adult Dose	Therapeutic Use	Major Adverse Effects/Cautions	Comments
		Do not use in patients with sulfa allergy.	hypotension, nausea, vomiting, dyspepsia, dry mouth, impotence, rash, hypokalemia, ototoxicity, muscle cramps.	
Potassium-Sparing Diuretics spironolactone (Aldactone)	25-200 mg PO daily to a maximum of 400 mg/day.	Edema, HTN, hyperaldosteronism, hypokalemia, CHF.	**Serious Adverse Effects:** agranulocytosis, anaphylaxis, hepatotoxicity, renal failure. **Common Adverse Effects:** nausea, abdominal pain, diarrhea, headache, confusion, hirsutism, gynecomastia, sexual dysfunction, menstrual irregularities, fever, rash, hyperkalemia, metabolic acidosis.	Pregnancy category: D. Metabolism: liver extensively. Excretion: urine, bile. Half-life: 1-2 hr.
Angiotensin Receptor Blockers (ARBs) Includes the following medications: candesartan (Atacand) eprosartan (Teveten) losartan (Cozaar) olmesartan (Benicar) valsartan (Diovan)	Dosage depends on specific agent.	HTN, CHF.	**Serious Adverse Effects:** angioedema, severe hypotension, hyperkalemia, renal dysfunction or failure, leukopenia, neutropenia, agranulocytosis, fetal/neonatal harm or death (in utero exposure), rhabdomyolysis, hepatitis. **Common Adverse Effects:** dizziness, URI symptoms, back pain, diarrhea, fatigue, dyspepsia.	Blocks the effects of angiotensin. Pregnancy category: D Metabolism, excretion, and half-life depend on specific agent.
Antiplatelet/Anticoagulants Aspirin	325-1300 mg/day.	Antiplatelet.	**Serious Adverse Effects:** anaphylaxis, angioedema, bronchospasm, bleeding, GI ulceration, GI bleed, anemia, iron deficiency, thrombocytopenia, leukopenia, nephrotoxicity, hepatotoxicity, Reye's syndrome. **Common Adverse Effects:** dyspepsia, GI irritation, nausea, abdominal pain, anorexia, rash, urticaria, ecchymosis, bleeding, tinnitus.	Metabolism: GI tract, plasma, liver. Excretion: urine. Half-life: 15 minutes.
warfarin (Coumadin)	Start 2-5 mg PO daily. Adjust dosage every 2-4 days according to INR.	Anticoagulant. Also recommended in atrial fibrillation.	**Serious Adverse Effects:** hemorrhage, skin or tissue necrosis, gangrene, purple	Pregnancy category: X. Metabolism: liver; CYP450: 1A2, 2C8,

TABLE 7-5 Common Cardiovascular, Anticoagulant/Antiplalelet, and Cholesterol-Lowering Agents—cont'd

Drug Name	Normal Adult Dose	Therapeutic Use	Major Adverse Effects/Cautions	Comments
			toes syndrome, hypersensitivity reaction, drug-induced hepatitis, vasculitis. **Common Adverse Effects:** bleeding, easy bruising, abdominal pain, nausea/vomiting, diarrhea, flatulence, fatigue, lethargy, asthenia, headache.	2C18, 2C9, 2C19, 3A4 substrate. Excretion: urine. Half-life: 20-60 hr. Assess carefully for drug interactions. Contraindicated in severe liver or kidney disease, open wound ulcers, or malignant hypertension.
clopidogrel (Plavix)	75 mg PO daily.	Antiplatelet.	**Serious Adverse Effects:** hemorrhage, purpura, thrombocytopenia. **Common Adverse Effects:** nausea, dyspepsia, diarrhea, abdominal pain, hemorrhage, cough, bronchitis, dizziness, headache, fatigue, arthralgias, epistaxis, UTI.	Contraindicated in peptic ulcer disease. Metabolism: liver; CYP450: 2C9 inhibitor. Excretion: urine, feces. Half-life: 8 hr.
ticlopidine (Ticlid)	250 mg bid.	Not used often secondary to blood dyscrasias.	**Common Adverse Effects:** GI complaints, bone marrow suppression, rash, diarrhea, elevated serum cholesterol, neutropenia (2%).	Contraindicated or used with caution in active bleeding disorders, neutropenia, or thrombocytopenia, severe liver disease.
aspirin/dipyridamole (Aggrenox)	25/200 SR: 1 tab daily.	Stroke prevention.	**Common Adverse Effects:** headache, dyspepsia, abdominal pain, nausea and vomiting, diarrhea.	Contraindicated in bleeding disorders, hypersensitivity to agents.
Cholesterol-Lowering Agents				
HMG-CoA Reductase Inhibitors Includes the following medications: atorvastatin (Lipitor) simvastatin (Zocor) lovastatin (Mevacor) fluvastatin (Lescol, Lescol XL) pravastatin (Pravachol) rosuvastatin (Crestor)	Dosage depends on specific agent.	Hypercholesterolemia.	Muscle weakness, elevated liver enzymes. **Serious Adverse Effects:** myopathy, rhabdomyolysis (rare), hepatotoxicity, pancreatitis, hypersensitivity reaction, Stevens-Johnson syndrome. **Common Adverse Effects:** myalgia, headache, rhinitis, diarrhea, arthralgias, rash, allergic reaction, flatulence, constipation, elevated CPK, elevated liver transaminases.	Atorvastatin can be administered as a single dose at any time of day, with or without food. Simvastatin, lovastatin, and fluvastatin should be administered in the evening. Analyze lipid levels within 2-4 weeks. Adjust the dosage accordingly. Adjust dose at intervals of 4 weeks or more. Renal function impairment: initiate therapy with 5 mg/day and monitor closely.

Continued

TABLE 7-5 Common Cardiovascular, Anticoagulant/Antiplalelet, and Cholesterol-Lowering Agents—cont'd

Drug Name	Normal Adult Dose	Therapeutic Use	Major Adverse Effects/Cautions	Comments
				LFTs at baseline, 12 weeks, then periodically. CYP3A4 substrate.
Fibric Acid Derivatives colestipol (Colestid) gemfibrozil (Lopid)	Dosage depends on specific agent.	As above.	**Serious Adverse Effects:** fecal impaction, GI bleed. **Common Adverse Effects:** constipation, abdominal pain, bloating, flatulence, dyspepsia, elevated liver enzymes, myalgia, rash, headache.	Numerous drug interactions. Pregnancy category, metabolism, excretion, and half-life depend on specific agent.
niacin (Niaspan, nicotinic acid, Slo-Niacin)	Usual dosage 1-3 g tid with or after meals. Maximum dose: 8 g/day.	As above.	**Serious Adverse Effects:** arrhythmias, hepatotoxicity. **Common Adverse Effects:** pruritus, rash, flushing, nausea, diarrhea, vomiting, vasodilation.	Give aspirin 325 mg 30 minutes before niacin to decrease side effects.

bid, Twice a day; *BUN,* blood urea nitrogen; *CHF,* congestive heart failure; *CPK,* creatine phosphokinase; *CYP450,* cytochrome P-450; *GI,* gastrointestinal; *HTN,* hypertension; *INR,* International Normalized Ratio; *LFT,* liver function test; *MI,* myocardial infarction; *PO,* by mouth; *SR,* sustained release; *SVT,* supraventricular tachycardia; *tid,* three times a day; *URI,* urinary tract infection; *UTI,* urinary tract infection.

TABLE 7-6 Drugs Used in the Treatment of Burns

Drug Name	Normal Adult Dose	Therapeutic Use	Major Adverse Effects/Cautions	Comments
silver sulfadiazine 1% (Silvadene)	Apply under sterile conditions 1-2 times/day to a thickness of approximately 1/16 inch to the clean and debrided wound.	Prevention and treatment of infection in second- and third-degree burns.	**Serious Adverse Effects:** erythema multiforme, neutropenia, leukopenia. **Common Adverse Effects:** pain, rash, pruritus, skin necrosis, skin discoloration.	Hypersensitivity to drug. Metabolism: body fluids, liver. Excretion: urine.
mafenide (Sulfamylon)	8.5% cream. 50-g powder package. Apply 5% solution (50 g powder in 1000 ml sterile water or saline) q 6-8 hr to keep dressings wet.	As above.	**Serious Adverse Effects:** coagulation disorder, superinfection. **Common Adverse Effects:** skin irritation where applied, burning, excoriation, bleeding, rash, erythema, edema, pruritus.	Metabolism: liver. Excretion: urine. Contraindicated or use with caution in patients with sulfite allergies or with renal failure.

TABLE 7-7 Drugs Used in the Treatment of Diabetes Mellitus

Drug Name	Normal Adult Dose	Therapeutic Use	Major Adverse Effects/Cautions	Comments
Oral Sulfonylureas				Method of action: work by increasing insulin release from the beta cells of the pancreas.
glipizide (Glucotrol, Glucotrol XL)	Usual dosage 10-20 mg once or in divided doses.	Type 2 diabetes.	**Serious Adverse Effects:** hypoglycemia, aplastic anemia, hemolytic anemia, thrombocytopenia. **Common Adverse Effects:** diarrhea, nausea, hypoglycemia, dizziness, flatulence, headache, rash, drowsiness.	Metabolism: liver: CYP450: 2C9 substrate. Excretion: urine, feces. Half-life: 2-5 hr. Contraindicated in patients with sulfa allergy.
glyburide (Micronase, DiaBeta)	Start 2.5-5 mg PO once per day. Increase to a maximum of 20 mg/day. Give with first meal of the day.	As above.	As above.	As above. Half-life: 10 hr.
glyburide micronized (Glynase PresTab)	Start 1.5-3 mg PO once per day. Increase to a maximum of 12 mg/day. Take with first meal of the day.	As above.	As above.	As above.
glimepiride (Amaryl)	Start 1-2 mg PO once per day with first meal of the day. Maximum: 8 mg/day.	As above.	As above.	As above.
Alpha-Glucosidase Inhibitors				Method of action: work by slowing the digestion of carbohydrates.
acarbose (Precose)	Start 25 mg tid to a maximum of 100 mg tid. Take at beginning of each meal.	As above.	**Common Adverse Effects:** diarrhea, flatulence, abdominal pain, elevated liver enzymes, jaundice.	Take with first bite of meal to reduce postprandial blood glucose level.
miglitol (Glyset)	Start 25 mg tid to a maximum of 100 mg tid. Take at beginning of each meal.	As above.	As above.	As above.
Thiazolidinediones (Glitazones)				Method of action: increases insulin sensitivity.
rosiglitazone (Avandia)	Start at 4 mg once per day or 2 mg bid. Increase to a maximum of 8 mg/day in one or two doses.	As above.	**Serious Adverse Effects:** hepatotoxicity, CHF, pleural effusion, pulmonary edema. **Common Adverse Effects:** URI, headache, fluid retention, edema, weight gain, anemia.	Recent research suggests a potential risk for myocardial infarction; additional research is needed to determine the extent and nature of that risk. Monitor liver function Metabolism: liver; CYP450: 2C8, 2C9 substrate. Excretion: urine, feces. Half-life: 3-4 hr. Use with caution in patients with CHF.
pioglitazone (Actos)	Begin 15-30 mg PO once per day. Increase to a maximum of 45 mg/day.	As above.	As above.	Obtain baseline ALT and monitor at 12 weeks, then periodically. Metabolism: liver; CYP450: 2C8, 3A4. Excretion: urine, bile. Half-life: 3-7 hr; 15-24 hr for metabolites.

Continued

TABLE 7-7 Drugs Used in the Treatment of Diabetes Mellitus—cont'd

Drug Name	Normal Adult Dose	Therapeutic Use	Major Adverse Effects/Cautions	Comments
metformin (Glucophage, Glucophage XR, Glumetza, Riomet, Fortamet)	Start 850-1000 mg PO bid. Adjust as needed. Maximum 2550 mg/day. Take with meals. Maximum dose for XR formulation: 2000 mg daily.	As above.	As above.	Obtain baseline creatinine levels, repeat annually. Excretion: urine. Half-life 17-19 hr. Do not use in males with a serum creatinine >1.5 or in females with serum creatinine >1.4.
Insulin				
insulin injection regular—(R) (Humulin R, Novolin R)	Primarily given Sub-Q. Dosage according to laboratory values and individual patient needs. Usual total insulin requirement 0.5-1 units/kg/day; give 30-60 min before a meal or per sliding scale; may be given IM or IV. Most common to use multiple injections daily.	Diabetes mellitus requiring the use of insulin.	**Serious Adverse Effects:** severe hypoglycemia, hypokalemia, hypersensitivity reaction, generalized anaphylaxis (rare). **Common Adverse Effects:** hypoglycemia, injection site reaction, lipoatrophy at injection site, pruritus, rash, weight gain.	Information for Sub-Q injection. Onset approximately 30 minutes. Peak 2-4 hr. Duration 6-8 hr. Pregnancy category: B. Lactation: safety unknown. Metabolism: liver, kidney, fat; CYP450: none. Excretion: urine 30%-80%. Half-life: 1-1.5 hr.
insulin isophane suspension (NPH) (Humulin N, Novolin N)	Primarily given Sub-Q, but may be given IM or IV. Dosage according to individual patient needs. Usual total insulin requirement 0.5-1 units/kg/day. Most common to use multiple injections daily.	Diabetes mellitus requiring the use of insulin.	**Serious Adverse Effects:** Severe hypoglycemia, hypokalemia, hypersensitivity reaction, generalized anaphylaxis (rare). **Common Adverse Effects:** Hypoglycemia, injection site reaction, lipodystrophy at injection site, pruritus, rash, weight gain.	Information for Sub-Q injection. Onset approx 1-2 hr. Peak 4-12 hr. Duration 18-24 hr. Pregnancy category: B. Lactation: probably safe. Metabolism: liver, kidney, fat; CYP450: none. Excretion: urine 30%-80%. Half-life 1-1.5 hr.
insulin isophane suspension (NPH)/insulin regular (R) Humalog Mix (75/25, Humalog Mix 50/50, Humulin 70/30, Humulin 50/50)	Given Sub-Q only. Dosage according to individual patient needs. Usual total insulin requirement 0.5-1 units/kg/day. May use multiple daily injections. Give 30-60 minutes before a meal.	Diabetes mellitus requiring the use of insulin.	Same as above.	Onset approximately 15-30 minutes. Peak 30-90 minutes. Duration up to 24 hr. Pregnancy category: B. Lactation: probably safe. Metabolism: liver, kidney, fat; CYP450: none. Excretion: urine 30%-80%. Half-life: 1-1.5 hr.
insulin glargine (recombinant) (Lantus)	Sub-Q once daily at the same time each day. Dosage according to individual patient needs. Usual total insulin requirement 0.5-1 units/kg/day. May need to use rapid- or short-acting insulin before each meal in type 1 diabetes mellitus. May be used with oral therapy or rapid- or short-acting insulin in type 2 diabetes mellitus; do not mix with other insulins in same syringe.	Diabetes mellitus requiring the use of insulin.	**Serious Adverse Effects:** Severe hypoglycemia, hypokalemia, hypersensitivity reaction, generalized anaphylaxis (rare). **Common Adverse Effects:** hypoglycemia, lipodystrophy at injection site, injection site reaction, pruritus, rash, weight gain, sodium retention, edema.	Onset 1.1 hr. No pronounced peak. Duration 24 hr or longer. Pregnancy category: C. Lactation: probably safe. Metabolism: liver, kidney, fat; CYP450: none. Excretion: urine. Half-life: 1-1.5 hr.

ALT, Alanine transaminase; *bid*, two times a day; *CHF*, congestive heart failure; *CYP450*, cytochrome P-450; *IM*, intramuscular; *IV*, intravenous; *PO*, by mouth; *Sub-Q*, subcutaneous; *tid*, three times a day; *URI*, upper respiratory infection.

TABLE 7-8 Drugs Used to Treat HIV/AIDS

Drug Name	Normal Adult Dose	Therapeutic Use	Major Adverse Effects/Cautions	Comments
Nucleoside and Nucleotide Analog Reverse Transcriptase Inhibitors				
zidovudine (Retrovir) AZT	100 mg, 300 mg; 50 mg/5 ml Usual dosage: 300 mg PO bid.	HIV infection; prophylaxis to prevent maternal-fetal transmission.	**Serious Adverse Effects:** lactic acidosis, hepatotoxicity, neutropenia, myopathy, aplastic anemia, rhabdomyolysis, Stevens-Johnson syndrome. **Common Adverse Effects:** headache, malaise, nausea, fatigue, constipation, anemia, diarrhea.	Metabolism: liver. Excretion: urine. Half-life: 5-3 hr.
lamivudine (Epivir) 3TC	150 mg; 10 mg/ml solution. Usual dosage: 150 mg PO bid.	HIV infection.	Generally well tolerated. **Serious Adverse Effects:** lactic acidosis, hepatotoxicity, severe anemia. **Common Adverse Effects:** headaches, nausea, fatigue, nasal symptoms, cough, diarrhea, vomiting, insomnia, anorexia, depression, elevated liver and pancreas enzymes.	Metabolism: intracellular. Excretion: primarily urine. Half-life: 5-7 hr. Method of action: Inhibits reverse transcription.
zidovudine/lamivudine (Combivir) AZT/3TC	300 mg/150 mg. Usual dosage: 1 tab PO bid.	HIV infection.	As above.	As per individual drugs as listed above.
didanosine (Videx) ddI	125 mg, 200 mg, 250 mg, 400 mg, 25 mg, 50 mg, 100 mg, 200 mg CH; 2, 4 g powder. Usual dosage: 400 mg daily or 200 mg bid on empty stomach; may use 250-mg packets of powder as equivalent or 200 mg chewable tablets.	HIV infection.	**Serious Adverse Effects:** pancreatitis, peripheral neuropathy, hepatotoxicity, optic neuritis. **Common Adverse Effects:** diarrhea, nausea, headache, vomiting, rash, elevation of liver and pancreatic enzymes, anorexia, myalgia.	Metabolism: intracellular. Excretion: urine. Half-life: 1.5 hr (longer in renal disease).
zalcitabine (Hivid) ddC	0.375 mg, 0.75 mg Usual dosage: 0.375-0.75 mg tid.	HIV infection.	**Serious Adverse Effects:** lactic acidosis, hepatotoxicity, pancreatitis, peripheral neuropathy. **Common Adverse Effects:** peripheral neuropathy, liver dysfunction, elevated amylase, anemia, fatigue.	Metabolism: intracellular; minimally in the liver. Excretion: urine, feces. Half-life: 2 hr.
stavudine (Zerit) d4T	15 mg, 20 mg, 30 mg, 40 mg, 1 mg/ml. Usual dosage: 20-40 mg bid for immediate release. Extended release: 75-100 mg daily.	HIV infection.	**Serious Adverse Effects:** lactic acidosis, hepatotoxicity, pancreatitis, peripheral neuropathy, leukopenia.	Metabolism: intracellular. Excretion: urine. Half-life: 1.2-1.6 hr.

Continued

TABLE 7-8 Drugs Used to Treat HIV/AIDS—cont'd

Drug Name	Normal Adult Dose	Therapeutic Use	Major Adverse Effects/Cautions	Comments
			Common Adverse Effects: headache, diarrhea, rash, nausea, vomiting, elevated liver and pancreatic enzymes, fever, chills, anorexia.	
abacavir (Ziagen) ABC	300 mg; 20 mg/ml solution. Usual dosage: 300 mg bid or 600 mg PO daily.	HIV infection.	**Serious Adverse Effects:** hypersensitivity reaction, anaphylaxis, liver or renal failure, severe hypotension, ARDS, respiratory failure, Stevens-Johnson syndrome. **Common Adverse Effects:** nausea, headache, fatigue, vomiting, diarrhea, depression, rash, anxiety.	Metabolism: liver. Excretion: urine, feces. Half-life: 1.5 hr.
zidovudine, lamivudine, abacavir (Trizivir) AZT/3TC/ABC	1 tablet bid.	HIV infection.	See individual components above.	See individual components above.
emtricitabine (Emtriva)	200 mg; 10 mg/ml. 200 mg PO daily or 240 mg solution PO daily.	HIV infection.	**Serious Adverse Effects:** lactic acidosis, hepatomegaly, hepatotoxicity, neutropenia. **Common Adverse Effects:** rash, diarrhea, headaches, nausea, cough, rhinitis, vomiting, insomnia, myalgia.	Metabolism: oxidation, conjugation with glucuronic acid. Excretion: urine, feces. Half-life: 10 hr.
tenofovir (Viread)	300 mg. Usual dosage: 300 mg daily.	HIV infection.	**Serious Adverse Effects:** lactic acidosis, hepatomegaly, hepatotoxicity, nephrotoxicity, renal failure, pancreatitis, dyspnea, allergic reaction. **Common Adverse Effects:** nausea, diarrhea, vomiting, flatulence, rash, depression.	Not recommended as monotherapy. Metabolism: intracellular. Excretion: primarily urine. Half-life: 17 hr.
emtricitabine/tenofovir (Truvada)	200/300 mg. Usual dosage: 1 tablet PO daily.	HIV infection.	See individual components.	See individual components.
abacavir/lamivudine (Epzicom)	600/300 mg. Usual dosage: 1 tablet PO daily.	HIV infection.	See individual components.	See individual components.
Protease Inhibitors saquinavir (Invirase)	200 mg, 500 mg Usual dosage: 1000 mg PO bid with meals.	HIV infection.	**Serious Adverse Effects:** hepatotoxicity, diabetes mellitus, pancreatitis, seizures, Stevens-Johnson syndrome, hemolytic anemia, acute renal failure.	Use only in combination with ritonavir 100 mg PO bid. Usually well tolerated. Ritonavir increases half-life. Metabolism: liver;

TABLE 7-8 Drugs Used to Treat HIV/AIDS—cont'd

Drug Name	Normal Adult Dose	Therapeutic Use	Major Adverse Effects/Cautions	Comments
			Common Adverse Effects: nausea, vomiting, diarrhea, abdominal pain, fatigue, pneumonia, flatulence, pruritus, fever, rash.	CYP450: 3A4 substrate, inhibitor. Excretion: feces, urine. Half-life: 12 hr.
ritonavir (Norvir)	100; 80 mg/ml solution. Start with 300 mg bid and increase by 100 mg bid every 2-3 days to full dose of 600 mg bid. In combination with other protease inhibitors: 100 mg bid.	HIV infection.	**Serious Adverse Effects:** thrombocytopenia, seizures, hepatotoxicity, diabetes, neutropenia. **Common Adverse Effects:** nausea, vomiting, diarrhea, asthenia, rash, myalgia, neuralgia.	Commonly used as 1 or 2 capsules bid with other protease inhibitors. Metabolism: liver; CYP450: 2D6, 3A4 substrate; 2C9,/19, 2D6, 3A4 inhibitors; 1A2, 2C9, 3A4 inducers. Excretion: feces, urine. Half-life: 3-5 hr.
indinavir (Crixivan)	100 mg, 200 mg, 333 mg, 400 mg. Usual dosage 800 mg q 8 hr on an empty stomach.	HIV infection.	**Serious Adverse Effects:** acute renal failure, diabetes mellitus, pancreatitis, anaphylactoid reaction, MI, depression, liver failure. **Common Adverse Effects:** nausea, abdominal pain, kidney stones, GI upset, malaise, taste change, dry mouth.	Important to drink at least 1.5 L/day. Metabolism: liver; CYP450: 3A4 substrate/inhibitor. Excretion: feces, urine. Half-life 1.8 hr.
nelfinavir (Viracept)	250 mg, 625 mg; 50 mg/g powder. Usual dosage 1250 mg bid or 750 mg tid with food.	HIV infection.	**Serious Adverse Effects:** seizures, suicidal ideation, hepatitis, jaundice, hypersensitivity reaction. **Common Adverse Effects:** diarrhea, abdominal pain, nausea, rash, anemia, arthralgia, elevated liver enzymes, myalgias, pruritus.	Metabolism: liver; CYP450: 2C19, 3A substrate; 3A4 inhibitor. Excretion: feces, urine. Half-life: 3.5-5 hr.
fosamprenavir (Lexiva)	700 mg. Usual dosage: 1400 mg bid.	HIV infection.	**Serious Adverse Effects:** neutropenia, Stevens-Johnson syndrome, severe skin reactions, fat redistribution, hemolytic anemia. **Common Adverse Effects:** diarrhea, headache, nausea, vomiting, depression, abdominal pain, rash, urticaria, elevated liver and pancreatic enzymes.	Used commonly in treatment-naïve patients. Metabolism: gut, liver; CYP450: 3A4 substrate/inhibitor/ inducer. Excretion: urine, feces. Half-life 7.5 hr.

Continued

TABLE 7-8 Drugs Used to Treat HIV/AIDS—cont'd

Drug Name	Normal Adult Dose	Therapeutic Use	Major Adverse Effects/Cautions	Comments
lopinavir/ritonavir (Kaletra)	Usual dosage: 400 mg/100 mg PO bid. Alternatively, 800 mg/200 mg PO daily with food.	HIV infection.	**Serious Adverse Effects:** pancreatitis, diabetes mellitus, neutropenia. **Common Adverse Effects:** abnormal stools, fatigue, diarrhea, nausea, vomiting.	Metabolism: see individual drugs. Excretion: see individual drugs.
atazanavir (Reyataz)	100 mg, 150 mg, 200 mg Usual dosage: 400 mg PO daily with food.	HIV infection.	**Serious Adverse Effects:** AV heart block, diabetes mellitus, lactic acidosis. **Common Adverse Effects:** increased bilirubin levels, headache, myalgia, nausea, diarrhea, abdominal pain, rash.	Metabolism: liver; CYP450: 3A4 substrate, 1A2, 2C9, 3A4 inhibitor. Excretion: feces, urine. Half-life: 7 hr.
tipranavir (Aptivus)	250-mg capsules. Usual dosage: 500 mg PO bid with ritonavir 200 mg PO bid.	HIV infection.	**Serious Adverse Effects:** hepatitis, diabetes mellitus. **Common Adverse Effects:** diarrhea, nausea, vomiting, abdominal pain, pyrexia, fatigue, asthenia, bronchitis, headache, depression, insomnia, cough, rash.	Metabolism: liver; CYP450: 3A4 substrate Excretion: feces, minimally in urine. Half-life: 4.8-6 hr.
Nonnucleoside Reverse Transcriptase Inhibitors (NNRTIs)				
nevirapine (Viramune)	200 mg; 50 mg/5 ml suspension. Usual dosage: 200 mg daily × 14 days, then 200 mg bid.	HIV infection.	**Serious Adverse Effects:** hepatotoxicity, Stevens-Johnson syndrome, severe skin reactions, neutropenia, anaphylaxis, angioedema. **Common Adverse Effects:** transient rash, hepatitis, nausea, fatigue, diarrhea.	Metabolism: liver; CYP450: 2B6, 3A4 substrate inducer. Excretion: urine, feces. Half-life: 25-30 hr.
delavirdine (Rescriptor)	100 mg, 200 mg Usual dosage: 400 mg tid.	HIV infection.	**Serious Adverse Effects:** angioedema, leukopenia, thrombocytopenia, pancreatitis, GI bleed. **Common Adverse Effects:** rash, nausea, fatigue, headache, anxiety, URI, diarrhea, elevated liver enzymes.	Multiple drug-drug and drug-food interactions. Metabolism: liver; CYP450: 2D6, 3A4 substrate; 2C9/19, 2D6, 3A4 inhibitor. Excretion: urine, feces. Half-life: 5.8 hr.
efavirenz (Sustiva)	50 mg, 100 mg, 200 mg, 600 mg. Usual dosage: 600 mg daily at bedtime.	HIV infection.	**Serious Adverse Effects:** Stevens-Johnson syndrome, depression, suicide, psychiatric disorders, pancreatitis, seizure activity.	Metabolism: liver; CYP450: 2B6, 3A4 substrate; 3A4 inducer; 2C9/19, 3A4 inhibitor.

TABLE 7-8 Drugs Used to Treat HIV/AIDS—cont'd

Drug Name	Normal Adult Dose	Therapeutic Use	Major Adverse Effects/Cautions	Comments
			Common Adverse Effects: rash, anxiety, insomnia, dizziness, occasional hallucinations, diarrhea, nausea, fever.	
Fusion Inhibitors				The newest class of drugs used to treat HIV act by preventing the virus from fusing to the inside of the cell, thereby preventing it from replicating.
enfuvirtide (Fuzeon)	Sub-Q injection. Usual dosage: 90 mg bid Sub-Q.	HIV infection.	**Serious Adverse Effects:** hypersensitivity reaction, severe injection site reaction, respiratory distress. **Common Adverse Effects:** injection site reactions, diarrhea, nausea, fatigue, weight loss, cough, anorexia, myalgia.	Excretion: unknown. Half-life: 3.5-4 hr.

AIDS, Acquired immunodeficiency syndrome; *ARDS,* acute respiratory distress syndrome; *AV,* atrioventricular; *bid,* twice a day; *CH,* chewable tablet; *CYP450,* cytochrome P-450; *GI,* gastrointestinal; *HIV,* human immunodeficiency virus; *MI,* myocardial infarction; *PO,* by mouth; *Sub-Q,* subcutaneous; *tid,* three times a day; *URI,* upper respiratory infection.

REFERENCES

Ament, P. W., Bertolino, J. G., & Liszewski, J. L. (2000). Clinically significant drug interactions. *American Family Physician, 61,* 1745-1754.

American College of Rheumatology Ad Hoc Committee on Clinical Guidelines. (1996). Guidelines for monitoring drug therapy in rheumatoid arthritis. *Arthritis and Rheumatism 39,* 723-731.

Craig, C. R., & Stitzel, R. E. (2004). *Modern pharmacology with clinical applications* (6th ed.). Philadelphia: Lippincott

Crockgroft, D.W., & Gault, M. H. (1976). Prediction of creatinine clearance from serum creatinine. *Nephron, 16,* 31.

DiPiro, J., Talbert, R., Yee, G., Matzke, G., Wells, B., & Posey, L. (1999). *Pharmacotherapy: A pathophysiologic approach* (4th ed.). Norwalk, CT: Appleton and Lange.

Joint Commission on Accreditation of Healthcare Organizations. (2002). *Sentinel event glossary of terms.* Retrieved from http://www.jointcommission.org/sentinelevents/se_glossary.htm.

Lazarou, J., Pomeranz, B. H., & Corey, P. (1998). Incidence of adverse drug reactions in hospitalized patients: A meta-analysis of prospective patients. *Journal of the American Medical Association, 279,* 1200-1205.

Michalets, E. L. (1998). Update: Clinically significant cytochrome P-450 drug interactions. *Pharmacotherapy, 18*(1), 84-112.

Turkoski, B. B., Lance, B. R., Bonfiglio, M. F. (2005). *Lexi-Comp's drug information handbook for advanced practice nursing* (6th ed.). Hudson, OH: Lexi-Comp.

Administration and Leadership

Aloma R. Gender, MSN, RN, CRRN

ealth care in today's market is focused on the delivery of high-quality, cost-effective, service-oriented, and safe care. Successes in medical rehabilitation are measured by optimal clinical and functional outcomes; high patient, staff, and physician satisfaction ratings; and cost-effective delivery of care. The responsibility to achieve these goals at a unit or work group level rests with the frontline rehabilitation nurse manager or supervisor (Fox, Fox, & Wells, 1999). Nursing leaders have the opportunity to influence the lives of not only their patients and families, but their associates as well.

To cope with the complexity and the changes of today's health care environment, nurse managers must be skilled in both management and leadership techniques (Zenger, Ulrich, & Smallwood, 2000). In executing the manager role, the nurse maintains the work group or unit in a steady state, preserving morale, adhering to budget, and upholding policies and procedures. In a leadership role the nurse manager must be a visionary by anticipating future challenges, taking risks, introducing innovations (Manfredi, 1996), and inspiring staff to motivate themselves toward goal achievement (Studer, 2003). Peters' statement (1987) rings true: "The very essence of leadership is that you have a vision. It's got to be a vision you articulate clearly and forcefully on every occasion. You can't blow an uncertain trumpet" (p. 400).

Success in implementing the leadership role relies on purposeful interaction with others. "The challenge is to be a light, not a judge; to be a model, not a critic" (Covey, 1992, p. 25). The leadership style that a nurse manager chooses ultimately affects the success of the organization (Perra, 2000). Developing leadership skills is foundational to achieving and maintaining high-quality care.

FACTORS ASSOCIATED WITH REHABILITATION NURSING MANAGEMENT AND LEADERSHIP

Expansion of Rehabilitation Nursing Into Other Arenas

Technology and government regulations in the health care market have forced a shift in care delivery from high-cost acute care hospitals to lower-cost ambulatory, community, and home-based settings. This move is evident in rehabilitation environments, where sites for care have shifted from comprehensive inpatient rehabilitation to day hospital, subacute rehabilitation, home health care, and outpatient clinics. With the continued influence of managed care, rehabilitation nurses have expanded into case manager roles with third-party payers. New venues for rehabilitation nurses have been appearing with adult day care services, assisted living, long-term acute care hospitals, and long-term care settings. Chapter 12 discusses community-based rehabilitation in detail.

Future Demand for Rehabilitation Services

The demand for rehabilitation services will increase alongside population growth. On January 1, 2006, the first of approximately 77 million baby boomers (those born between 1946 and 1964) celebrated their sixtieth birthday. Baby boomers make up 42% of all U.S. households and control 50% of all consumer spending (Green, 2005). Baby boomers want to "age in place" by remaining in their homes and staying as active as possible. People 60 years old today can expect to live to 82.3 years (Adler, 2005). Furthermore, the prevalence and impact of more chronic illness will increase as the baby boomers age. One third of all Americans will have a disability at some point in their lives (Williams, 2000). This volume and the demand to stay healthy will create increased demands for rehabilitation services.

Another reason for an increased demand for health care, including rehabilitation services, is the continuous innovation in diagnostic, treatment, and monitoring technologies for all types of problems. In the past, improved technologies have led to the saving of lives that could not be saved before. The field of medical rehabilitation and the practice of rehabilitation nursing have benefited these survivors. As per capita incomes grow, the demand for health services keeps pace. Consumer movements in this country will continue to demand not only the best customer service and quality possible but also the most comprehensive range of services necessary to improve and maintain a functional lifestyle.

National Demographics Related to Nursing as a Profession

Despite an increase of more than 200,000 employed registered nurses (RNs) since 2001, the nursing shortage does not appear to be ending (Buerhaus, Staiger, & Auerbach, 2004). The nursing workforce is projected to peak at 2.3 million in 2012 but shrink to 2.2 million by 2020, at which point it is forecast that 2.8 million RNs will be required (U.S. Department of Health and Human Services, 2002). Approximately one third of the nursing workforce is over 50 years of age. Full-time nursing faculty average 49 years old. The challenge for nursing is to redesign patient care delivery models to support the older workforce, initiate new technology into practice, support the aging nurse with flexibility in scheduling, and create work environments to retain staff (Nevidjon & Erickson, 2001).

FUNCTIONS AND RESPONSIBILITIES OF A REHABILITATION NURSE MANAGER

The American Nurses Association (ANA) (2004) describes the role of the nurse manager as being responsible to a nurse executive and managing one or more defined areas of nursing services. Nurse managers advocate for resources to promote "efficient, effective, safe and compassionate nursing care based on current standards of practice" (p. 7). Furthermore, they promote shared decision making by providing their own and staff's input into executive-level decisions and keep staff informed of executive-level activities. The nurse manager role in rehabilitation has some unique functions beyond those traditionally expected from a frontline nursing manager. In 2003 the Association of Rehabilitation Nurses (ARN) (2003a) revised its role description of the rehabilitation nurse manager. This section expands on those rehabilitation nurse manager functions.

Leadership

At the very heart of the nurse manager role is leadership. Fox et al. (1999) conducted a study to explore which nurse manager activity had the most positive impact on unit productivity levels. They found the leadership role to be most important. Manfredi (1996) states that given the complex nature of the nurse manager's job, leadership skills are essential for survival. Several concepts make up the role of leader.

Vision/Goals. Leadership involves creating a vision or a mental image of a possible and desirable future state for the organization or unit (Manfredi, 1996). A vision tells a story or paints a picture. It bridges the present to the future and is motivating and emotional. A good vision will drive employees' thinking, decisions, and behaviors. It ultimately impacts the bottom line. Nurse managers often carry a vision forward that has been set by the nurse executive, but nurse managers will also have a personal vision for their unit. A vision must be articulated to those being led. In every activity the nurse manager must be clear about the desired end state.

Strategies and Programs for Rehabilitation Nursing Care. Once a vision is set, a strategic plan, with goals and action steps, is mapped out to achieve the vision. Scorecards, often called "dashboards" or "balanced scorecards" can be developed to keep focus and motivation on progress toward goals. Studer (2003) suggests a "Pillar" model to align organizational objectives with individual goals. All leaders are evaluated against one or more of the goals identified. See Figure 8-1 for a rehabilitation example of this model. A leader should produce measurable results and ultimately leave behind a more robust, stronger organization than the one inherited. A leader with vision raises the bar on what an organization expects and helps employees seek ever-loftier goals (Zenger et al., 2000).

As new programs are developed, they must be oriented to supporting positive patient outcomes and satisfaction and should have targeted goals by which the success of the new venture can be evaluated. An example might be the implementation of an interdisciplinary wound team. The team makes weekly skin rounds on all patients with pressure ulcers to monitor wound healing and make suggestions for treatment and equipment needs. The targeted outcome would be a reduction in hospital-acquired pressure ulcers as measured by monthly and yearly reports.

Change. Leadership is about change. Leadership is not required to maintain the status quo. It is required to move an organization forward in a new direction or to a higher level of performance (Zenger et al., 2000). In the past, companies wanted loyal employees. Today's organization calls for flexible employees who can adapt quickly, follow a new direction, and enjoy it again and again (Johnson, 1998). A nurse manager must be a change agent, able to cope with change, explain the rationale for change to the staff, and lead change.

Change theory concepts appear in many theoretical models; classic theories on planned change remain useful when a nurse manager intends to move an organization to a new "desired" state. Lewin (1947) is perhaps one of the easiest theorists to use. Recognition of need to change triggers Lewin's "unfreezing" from the present situation. Before moving to a new level, the driving and restraining forces for the change must be addressed to "unfreeze" the participants and get them motivated to make a change. "Moving" is the implementation phase. When a fit occurs between the change and a new idea or plan, "refreezing" begins. Changes are integrated into lifestyle, relationships, and behaviors, and a sense of closure signifies that the change is completed.

Interpersonal Skills/Emotional Intelligence. Leaders in health care are being charged with the responsibility of becoming more humanistic and with helping to meet staff's emotional needs, as well as helping them to develop better skill sets. When leaders fail, it is often because they lack expertise in the interpersonal side of management. In moving projects forward, the emotional aspect of issues often needs to be analyzed. Anticipating how workers will react to given

Business Literacy	1st Quarter	2nd Quarter	3rd Quarter	4th Quarter	Target
Meet or exceed budgeted % net operating margin. Increase outpatient rehab units of service by 10%.					

Clinical Quality	1st Quarter	2nd Quarter	3rd Quarter	4th Quarter	Target
FIM change will equal or exceed national benchmark. Reduce incidence of patient falls by 50% or more from prior year.					

Service Excellence	1st Quarter	2nd Quarter	3rd Quarter	4th Quarter	Target
Associate satisfaction equal to or greater than 90th percentile. Patient satisfaction equal to or greater than 90th percentile.					

Community Value	1st Quarter	2nd Quarter	3rd Quarter	4th Quarter	Target
Charitable care will be 10% of net patient revenue.					

Figure 8-1 Focus goals. A model to evaluate oraganizational objectives with progress toward individual goals. (Courtesy CHRISTUS St. Michael Rehabilitation Hospital, Texarkana, TX.)

situations and helping them deal with the emotional side of work-related problems are important skills. "Increasingly, successful leaders are recognized as those who lead with the heart" (Kerfoot, 1996, pp. 59-60). Consumers want personalized attentive service. The expectation is for leaders to be more service focused, not only with the external customers, their patients, but with the internal customers as well, especially their staff (Kerfoot, 1996). The most effective leaders have a high degree of emotional intelligence, and its components can be learned as follows:

Self-Awareness. Leaders with emotional intelligence have a deep understanding of their own emotions, strengths, weaknesses, needs, and drives. They are honest with themselves and others.

Self-Regulation. Persons high in emotional intelligence have control over their feelings and impulses. They self-regulate themselves and are able to create an environment of trust and fairness. Politics and infighting are sharply reduced.

Motivation. Emotionally intelligent leaders are driven to achieve for the sake of achievement, not for high salaries or a prestigious company. They have passion for their work, have unflagging energy to do things better, and are restless with the status quo.

Empathy. A leader must be able to sense and understand the viewpoints of every member of the team. An emotionally intelligent nurse manager thoughtfully considers employees' feelings when making decisions. This is important in retaining good talent.

Social Skill. Emotionally intelligent leaders have a wide circle of acquaintances and a knack for finding a common ground with many different types of employees. They work on the assumption that nothing important gets done alone (Goleman, 1998).

Coaching/Mentoring. Another role of a leader is to stimulate growth and development in others (Fox et al., 1999). Everyone should be trained to lead. True leaders help employees perform better than they would have if the leader had not been there. The nurse manager determines what skills are needed in the staff to deliver the explicit results or outcomes for the unit (Zenger et al., 2000). Training content is chosen to target competencies that staff members need for excellence in job performance. Educational and coaching plans are developed to move employees to a desired end point and should be linked with results.

Studer (2003) further suggests re-recruiting top performers, moving middle performers up and low performers either up or out. In order to continue to be successful as an organization, when changes are made that lead to positive outcomes, those not performing must be addressed or the outcomes will decline. The reason for the decline is that the top and middle performers get tired of carrying the weight of the low performers. This usually occurs around 18 months to 2 years into a change if the poor performers are allowed to generate poor quality work and/or behavior.

The workplace has some of the elements of a family in that employees are looking for jobs where they will matter. They come to work where they have a purpose, are able to perform worthwhile work, make a difference, and can be part of decision making (Studer, 2003). They want to work *with* managers, not *for* them. Positive reinforcement, rather than fear and intimidation, is successful. A motivational, rather than autocratic, style produces better results, not only in unit and patient outcomes but also in low staff turnover and high employee morale (Eade, 1996). The supervisor holds the key to high retention (Studer, 2003).

Today's work environment is more unique than at any other time in history. For the first time a nurse leader may have four generations working together on the same unit. Each generation has different expectations and different values. Traditionalists (born between 1900 and 1945) are loyal and want to partner with an organization to get things done. They grew up believing that there was a stigma to changing jobs. Turnover with traditionalists is therefore a good barometer that issues may be serious. They are used to top-down communication and do not expect a lot of praise (Lancaster & Stillman, 2002).

Baby boomers (born between 1946 and 1964) are workers who are optimistic and competitive. They are the "me" generation. They have bonded with traditionalists and generally expect to stay in the same institution for most of their work history because they believe that changing jobs puts them behind in their career. They will leave a job, however, if they can gain ground with their career. Offering growth and mentorships can counteract turnover with this group (Lancaster & Stillman, 2002).

"Generation X" workers (born between 1965 and 1980) grew up in the information age. They learned how to think and communicate in a tidal wave of information (Tulgan, 1999). Having lived in an age where every major American institution was called into question, they have a high degree of skepticism (Lancaster & Stillman, 2002). Generation X workers want meaning in their work and expect to have fun in the workplace. They want constant feedback and short-term rewards. Retirement plans tend not to be of high interest, and they do not feel a strong sense of loyalty to their employers. They want honesty in their relationships with employers and are open to being shown potential career paths in organizations (Cole, 1999).

Persons born between 1981 and 1999 are called the Millennial generation (Lancaster & Stillman, 2002). They compose 26% of the population, whereas generation X workers compose only 16%. This group is steeped in technology. They grew up in an age of great economic optimism. Money is an incentive, and they are more interested in being part of a team (Wellner, 1999). They feel empowered to take action when things go wrong. A key word for this generation is "realistic" (Lancaster & Stillman, 2002). In coaching and developing staff and in providing an environment that will attract and keep rehabilitation nurses, the nurse manager needs to try to meet individual workers' needs and take into consideration what may be motivational factors for specific generations.

Clinical Nursing Practice and Patient Care Delivery

The rehabilitation nurse manager is accountable for excellence in the clinical practice of rehabilitation nursing and the delivery of care on a selected unit or area. Expert clinical nursing practice is achieved only when nurses are willing to take steps toward incorporating current research findings and evidence-based practice into the clinical setting (ARN, 2003).

Rehabilitation Nursing Clinical Roles. The nurse manager supports the rehabilitation nursing staff in performing specific roles and empowers them to become more autonomous. The roles are patient educator, caregiver, counselor, consultant, and patient advocate (ARN, 2003a). All structures, services, systems, and supports must be fully oriented to those the system serves. The patient is at the center of all care. The rehabilitation nurse and the interdisciplinary team support that centerpiece at the point of service. The locus of control for resource use and decision making must be at this point of service.

Institutional and Professional Rehabilitation Nursing Values, Goals, and Objectives. The rehabilitation nurse manager promotes and translates institutional and professional rehabilitation nursing values, goals, and objectives to nursing staff and interdisciplinary team members (ARN, 2003a). To achieve collaborative practice, interdisciplinary team members must also be educated about the body of knowledge that is rehabilitation nursing. The nurse manager can promote this learning and ensure opportunities through new-employee orientation or education programs. Benner (2001) describes how nurses move from novice status to expert roles within the profession as they gain knowledge and experience and invest in their discipline.

Care Delivery System. To establish excellence in clinical practice, the nurse manager, along with the nurse executive, must first define the care delivery system (ARN, 2003a) that will best meet patient needs. Several models have been used successfully in rehabilitation settings.

Team Nursing. Team nursing uses an RN to supervise the clinical care of a large group of patients, usually 15 to 20 patients. The RN performs the professional tasks, and the direct patient care is assigned to nursing assistants or licensed practical/vocational nurses.

Primary Nursing. The primary nurse model often uses an all-RN staff. Each nurse performs total care for a group of patients, usually four to five. In some facilities, a nursing assistant may be available for the unit to assist all of the licensed staff with duties such as passing ice water and making beds.

Modified Primary Nursing. The modified primary nursing model, or modular nursing model, uses a team of licensed and unlicensed nurses to work together in delivering patient care. In this model licensed staff members perform direct patient care as well as licensed procedures, working closely with a nursing assistant. Each team usually cares for 7 to 10 patients, more than with the primary nurse model.

Patient-Focused or Program Model. The patient-focused model of care can be used with any of the above models and incorporates a more transdisciplinary model of care.

Typically, all members of a team report to a single program director, coordinator, or product-line manager. Health care workers may be cross-trained in several disciplines. A nursing assistant may work as a physical or occupational therapy aide or may perform phlebotomies. A housekeeper may be trained to assist with some patient care activities, or respiratory therapists may be cross-trained to perform nursing tasks between treatments. A unit secretary may assist with medical record completion and admission paperwork. Usually, in this model universal duties are established that every member of the team, whether therapist or rehabilitation nurse, is able to perform, such as toileting, transfers, or answering phones and call lights.

The nurse executive, along with the nurse manager, must evaluate unit-specific structures, processes, and the experience level of the staff to determine the best model of care for their unit (Deutschendorf, 2003), which will achieve the highest outcomes and satisfaction for the patient and meet budgeted costs. The model is then implemented and evaluated against targeted results. Chapter 2 contains more information on various types of models and theoretical bases for their use.

Standards of Practice and Competency Guidelines.

The intent of the standards and guidelines of practice for rehabilitation nursing must be established in written policies and procedures. Staff nurses need to be educated in the practices and supervised to ensure competence. Patient assignments are delegated according to the level of education, training, and competency of the personnel and according to state nursing practice acts. The ARN has developed competency tests for rehabilitation nurses that are available online (ARN, 2005).

Standards of Care and Accreditation.

The rehabilitation nurse manager is accountable for staying current on the content and intent of standards of care established by professional organizations such as the ARN and ANA. Also essential are regulations such as those by The Joint Commission (TJC), Commission on Accreditation of Rehabilitation Facilities (CARF), and by government agencies such as the Centers for Medicare and Medicaid Services (CMS) and state departments of health. Nurse managers must be able to determine the regulatory implications for a specific area or unit and to respond by promoting and ensuring compliance (ARN, 2003a).

The Nursing Process.

The nurse manager will encourage use of the nursing process in multiple ways. The nursing process can be used to manage patient care and ensure continuity from admission through discharge and return to family and community (ARN, 2003a). It is useful to facilitate an interdisciplinary approach to care and documentation. The nursing process easily permits interdisciplinary assessments, diagnosis, collaborative patient goal setting, patient and family education, rehabilitation nursing and team interventions, and evaluation of progress toward goals.

Management Information Systems.

Being proficient in the use of the institution's management information systems and understanding related policies and programs are increasingly essential functions of the nurse manager (ANA, 2004). Members of the nursing staff need education and training to become competent in their use of the systems, and they often need assurance and confidence, as well as technical skills.

Nurse managers are often asked to participate in the design and implementation of software programs, such as a documentation or order entry system, tailoring them to meet rehabilitation nursing and/or team needs. They may need to research and write justifications for programs that improve rehabilitation nursing accuracy or efficiency in providing care. Examples might be an automated medication-dispensing system or a program to schedule staffing.

Safe and Caring Environment.

The environment must be maintained as a safe and caring place for patients, conducive to positive health teaching and health maintenance. The work environment should minimize work-related illness and injury (ANA, 2004) for both the patient and the nurse. A safe environment is one in which necessary equipment is ordered and kept in good repair, supplies are appropriate for patient needs and readily available, environmental hazards are avoided, and systems are put in place to provide for accuracy with treatments (see Chapter 10). Some state laws and current research promote the use of algorithms for patient transfers and positioning in order to prevent injuries to caregivers (Nelson & Baptiste, 2004).

A caring environment is created when the nurse manager leads the staff in such a way that nurse satisfaction is positive and excellence in customer service results. Many rehabilitation facilities are adopting customer service models such as the Disney approach (2004).

Aspects of a customer service model may include the following:
- Setting aggressive patient satisfaction goals
- Establishing teams charged with improving key dimensions of patient service
- Defining expected service behaviors for interactions between employees and patients

Patient satisfaction scores and individual comments should be posted weekly for the patient care unit. Key to patient satisfaction is daily nurse manager rounding. Studer (2003) says that when nurse managers make rounds, they should first round for the employee and then the patient. The nurses want a relationship with their manager. This relationship inspires them to provide excellent care and service. Executives should also make routine patient rounds to observe service interventions and to speak with patients and staff. Service reprimands need to occur for violators of service expectations. Poor performers need to be asked to leave. Improved teamwork and interdisciplinary relations will result (Studer, 2003).

Service recovery systems can be developed that include the nurse manager's visiting all newly admitted patients to solicit concerns and complaints and working with staff to resolve problems on the spot. A fix-it fund can be available, consisting of gift certificates, meal tickets, or flowers to correct problems and to acknowledge patient inconvenience.

Another "must have" for patient satisfaction is follow-up phone calls after discharge to check on the patient and answer any questions the patient may have. Studer (2003) contends that this leaves a lasting positive impression with the patient and/or the family about the facility. It is recommended that the nurse manager make the calls for several months and then turn it over to the individual RNs to call on their patients. Responses should be analyzed for trends.

It is important to hire for service aptitude by putting applicants through multiple evaluations designed to assess service orientation (Health Care Advisory Board, 1999). Behavioral-based interviewing, having applicants review a standards agreement, and peer interviewing are all possible components of a hiring process to ensure that the applicant is the right "fit" for the organization (Studer, 2003).

Collaborative Relationships. Because of the broad spectrum of problems and challenges that persons with severe disabilities or chronic illness present, treatment is organized around a team. Responsibility to help patients meet goals is an interdisciplinary effort rather than actions of a single discipline (Halstead et al., 1986). The nurse manager must therefore be able to forge collaborative relationships, be persuasive (Davidhizar & Eshleman, 1999), and facilitate collaborative work among professionals of various disciplines and cooperation with sometimes competing departmental agendas, all to deliver effective quality care (ARN, 2003a).

Treatment team roles and functions are discussed throughout the book. The nurse manager supports the interdisciplinary team model, ensuring that care regimens are coordinated interdependently with all members of the team (ARN, 2003a).

Critical paths or care maps are interdisciplinary tools that outline protocols for care and coordinate the team efforts in a predictable way. The interventions of each team member, as well as the patient outcomes, are integrated into the care map. These tools help strengthen collaboration and teamwork because care delivery relies on mutually set goals and agreed-upon outcomes, timelines, processes, and responsibilities. A patient's health progress can be plotted from admission to discharge, and the variances can be tracked on a care map. Interdisciplinary teaching plans and discharge-planning forms are other useful tools. Interdisciplinary patient-centered goal sheets, established weekly with the patient and signed off by the patient or family member, are another way to coordinate team efforts.

Other role functions of the rehabilitation nurse manager include participating as a member of interdisciplinary committees and participating in planning and in program development (ARN, 2003a). The nurse manager in a rehabilitation setting can expect to meet routinely with directors of medical programs, various therapists, administrators, and

other managers. A collaborative and collegial relationship reflects elements of mutual trust, respect, and support. Input from any and all parties is valued equally, and decisions are made after all perspectives are heard, including those of the patient and family (ARN, 2003a; Velianoff, Neely, & Hall, 1993).

Fiscal Management

Preparation of rehabilitation nurse managers for financial management is frequently on-the-job training. Often the nurse manager's first exposure to fiscal management is preparing a budget or explaining variances. There are excellent texts specifically written to assist the nurse manager in fiscal management. The intent of this section is to provide descriptions of fiscal operations that a rehabilitation nurse manager can expect to perform.

Budget preparation and maintenance is the core of fiscal management for the nurse manager role (ARN, 2003a). A budget is a plan for a designated period, usually 1 year. Budget preparation can be described as short-term fiscal strategic planning. Strategic planning should be completed before budget preparation so that resources are allocated for the identified plans. Budget maintenance is the routine analysis of variances from the fiscal plan that may occur monthly, quarterly, or more often depending on the organization.

Three budget categories are revenue, expense, and capital. An operating budget is a combination of revenue and expense budgets.

Operating Budget

Revenue. The revenue budget projects income for a specific entity or area of responsibility. Although financial report forms vary between settings, typical contents include both current month and fiscal year-to-date information. Sometimes prior year data will also be available. Comparisons of actual income versus predicted income for the current month, and for the fiscal year to date, can be used to identify fiscal trends. "Patient days" are the typical unit of fiscal measurement for inpatient settings. Patient days translate into an average daily census (ADC). Budgets for each year are based on a predicted average daily census (Foley, 2005). Under the prospective payment system for inpatient rehabilitation, established on August 7, 2001 (Department of Health & Human Services Centers for Medicare & Medicaid Services, 2001), patients are classified into a case mix group (CMG). The Functional Independence Measure (FIM) instrument is used to score each patient and determine the CMG (see Figure 11-1 in Chapter 11). Each CMG is allocated a set dollar amount for reimbursement provided the patient is discharged to a community setting (i.e., home or assisted living). The facility is paid per discharge, so the number of patient discharges becomes more important than the number of admissions or the average daily census, although a relationship exits between all three components. Enough admissions are necessary to ensure that a budgeted number of discharges occur. A facility will receive less money for a CMG if the patient leaves too early (discharged before day 5) or is discharged to a noncommunity setting before the patient's Medicare length of stay (LOS). The facility may receive a higher reimbursement if the patient has comorbidities that place the patient into a higher reimbursement tier. Extended patient lengths of stay beyond the Medicare LOS result in additional outlier payments from CMS.

Case mix index (CMI) or severity of disability is a number that helps rehabilitation leadership evaluate the severity of their patients and can be an indication of higher reimbursement. A case mix of 1.0 is considered the average acuity mix for reimbursement. A case mix higher than 1.0 indicates more acute patients, and a case mix less than 1.0 indicates less severity of cases or less intense CMGs.

Accurate documentation within the first 3 days of a patient's stay is critical in order to assign the correct CMG to a patient. The highest burden of care must be recorded by obtaining nursing input on FIM scores over a 24-hour period. Often the patient may be at his or her lowest function and therefore requires the highest burden of care on the evening shift of the first day of admission. A documentation tool to capture this FIM score is critical to appropriate reimbursement and for meeting CMS regulatory compliance for backup documentation to support the FIM scores (Figure 8-2). Ultimately, the scores from each summarized section of this document are used to determine the level of the FIM outcomes using the tool in Figure 11-1.

Length of patient stay becomes important with the new reimbursement system. Revenue per case or CMG divided by the average cost per day will identify a "break-even" LOS for the budget. These break-even points occur when revenues equal expenses. The nurse manager, along with the rehabilitation team, strives to increase revenues and decrease expenses and LOS while maintaining or improving effectiveness and efficiency of patient outcomes. Daily financial reports can assist management and the clinical team, especially case managers, with tracking of CMGs, LOS, CMI, expenses, and revenues.

Expense

Personnel. The expense budget reflects the predictions of annual costs for area-defined expenses. Most costs in the expense budget for inpatient rehabilitation nursing areas are salaries, which include fringe benefits. Salaries frequently exceed 80% to 90% of the total expense budget. This fiscal effect is due to the labor-intensive aspects of rehabilitation and the need for rehabilitation nursing staff with specialized skills and knowledge.

The goal of the staffing function is to provide optimal quality care with the most economic staffing. Staffing in an inpatient setting is a process of determining and providing nursing staff to offer an effective number of nursing hours per patient day (HPPD), that is, the best mix of nursing staff with the correct distribution of personnel over the 24-hour day for 7 days a week. No one correct staffing configuration works for all rehabilitation units or outpatient settings (which may base staffing on the number of visits or units of service performed). A standard system of staffing based on research specific for rehabilitation needs does not exist. Differences in staffing requirements are a result of many variables, including patient populations, physician practices, services available, acuity, and availability of various personnel levels, and these differences make generic staffing approaches unrealistic. Rehabilitation nurse managers should retain input into whatever system is used to promote its appropriateness for their setting (ARN, 1999).

Acuity. Many variables affect staffing, but the primary variable is patient acuity, a measure of each patient's severity of illness and complexity related to the amount of nursing resources needed for care (Finkler & Kovner, 2000). Patient classification systems are used by some facilities to quantify the number or mix of staff needed. A classification system typically divides patients into categories according to the intensity of care each one needs. In turn, the resulting acuity level indicates the mix and number of staff required. A patient classification system must be valid and reliable in order for a manager to make realistic and accountable decisions about staffing. The ARN (2004) is currently conducting research on the development of an acuity tool using FIM scores.

Supplies/Services. The nonsalary budget includes supplies and services or direct expenses not related to employees. They are routine costs to nursing areas such as medical and nonmedical supplies, including rental of equipment. The supplies/services budget accounts may yield opportunities to reduce expenses and improve patient care at the same time through the choice of select products for contracted pricing. The rehabilitation nurse manager must ensure that the products chosen are appropriate for the rehabilitation patient.

Capital Budget. Capital budgets cover such items as equipment, furniture, remodeling, or building project costs. Facility policies direct what is considered a capital budget item. Typically it is an item or project that costs over $1000.00. Capital expense items are intended to be in use for a designated number of years. In planning capital expenditures, the rehabilitation nurse manager takes into account the feasibility of the item in meeting the special needs of rehabilitation patients. Examples include considering bed height conducive to transfer activities or prevention of falls when buying new beds, installing effective safety-lock mechanisms on wheelchair shower chairs for persons who are physically or cognitively impaired, and obtaining dining room tables that have adjustable heights and that are able to accommodate wheelchair leg rests. Nurse managers often can justify a capital equipment purchase if it enhances rehabilitation activities, for example, purchasing hydraulic lifts for safety to help prevent back injuries in staff and families.

Internal Fiscal Monitoring. The effective nurse manager uses internal monitoring to enhance fiscal control. Internal monitoring approaches vary among settings, but their purpose remains constant, to have current knowledge of the financial state of the area of accountability. Internal monitoring could include daily productivity measures (nursing HPPD, number of visits); monthly nursing labor and expense cost reports

**CHRISTUS
ST. MICHAEL**
Rehabilitation Hospital

Patient Label

Interdisciplinary FIM Sheet

					Date								
Room #	Day 1	Day 2	Day 3	D/C	Shift	B	L	D	PT	OT	ST	PSY	LOWEST SCORE
Eating													
Fed self/Opened packages/Cut food/Regular consistency diet					7								
Needed device/Swallow technique/Special food, Fluid consistency/Extra time/Inserted own dentures					6								
Independent with tube feed/IV hydration/Fluids (including set-up)					6								
Supervision/Cues/Needed staff to open packages or cut food					5								
Needed staff to insert dentures					5								
Min-pt fed self 75% or more of effort requiring staff to touch, to assist, or staff checked for food pocketing					4								
Mod-pt fed self 50-74% of effort or staff loaded each bite, patient brought to mouth					3								
Max-pt fed self 25-49% of effort or staff scoops and helps bring to mouth (hand over hand)					2								
Total-pt fed self less than 25% of effort					1								
Staff gave tube feed/IV hydration/Fluids					1								
Activity did not occur this shift					0								

Occupational Therapy D/C Goal Score: ☐

	Shift	N	D	E	PT	OT	ST	PSY	LOWEST SCORE

Grooming - *If patient needs assistance, place check in box for the tasks completed by patient. Cross through boxes for tasks patient doesn't normally perform.*

Day
☐ Washed face   ☐ Washed hands
☐ Cleaned teeth/dentures   ☐ Combed hair
☐ Shaved/applied make-up (optional)

Evening
☐ Washed face   ☐ Washed hands
☐ Cleaned teeth/dentures   ☐ Combed hair
☐ Shaved/applied make-up (optional)

					Shift	N	D	E	PT	OT	ST	PSY	LOWEST SCORE
Independent/Patient obtained all articles needed					7								
Needed device or extra time/Patient obtained all articles needed					6								
Supervision/Needed staff to obtain articles, apply toothpaste, plug in razor, hand items to patient. Staff adjusted water temperature.					5								
Staff inserted, removed dentures					4								
Min-pt did 3 of 4, or 4 of 5 tasks		5 tasks if shaved or applied make-up			4								
Mod-pt did 2 of 4, or 3 of 5 tasks					3								
Max-pt did 1 of 4, or 2 of 5 tasks					2								
Total-pt did 0 of 4, or 1 of 5 tasks					1								
Activity did not occur this shift					0								

Occupational Therapy D/C Goal Score: ☐

Figure 8-2 Interdisciplinary FIM sheet. (Courtesy CHRISTUS St. Michael Rehabilitation Hospital, Texarkana, TX.)

Room #　　Day 1　　Day 2　　Day 3　　D/C		Shift	N	D	E	PT	OT	ST	PSY	LOWEST SCORE

Bathing - *(Actual bathing only - no simulation) Note areas that patient bathed independently and do not count areas not appropriate*
(i.e., Amputated limb). (Washing/Rinsing/Drying)

Place check in box for areas patient bathed.	☐ Chest ☐ Abdomen	☐ Peri Area ☐ Buttocks	☐ Right Arm ☐ Left Arm	☐ Right Thigh ☐ Left Thigh	☐ Right lower leg/foot ☐ Left lower leg/foot

Independently bathed (10/10)	7							
Used device, extra time (10/10) _____ device used	6							
Supervision/Set up/Cues - adjusted water temperature, collects supplies (10/10)	5							
Min-pt did 8 - 9 parts or 75+%	4							
Needed steadying assistance	4							
Mod-pt did 5 - 7 parts or 50 - 74%	3							
Max-pt did 3 - 4 parts or 25 - 49%	2							
Total-pt did 0 - 2 parts or less than 25%	1							
Needed assistance of 2 staff members	1							
Activity did not occur this shift	0							

Occupational Therapy D/C Goal Score: ☐

Dressing / Undressing Upper Body - *(Appropriate public clothing only, not hospital gown.)*

Write in # of steps completed out of # of total steps involved in each step. Then calculate the percentage for total steps completed divided by total steps involved.

Day Dressing
☑ Button shirt = 4 steps　　☑ Pullover = 4 steps
☑ Tuck shirt = 1 step (optional)　　☑ Bra = 3 steps

Evening Undressing
☑ Button shirt = 4 steps　　☑ Pullover = 4 steps
☑ Tuck shirt = 1 step (optional)　　☑ Bra = 3 steps

Dressed/Undressed independently/Obtained own clothing	7							
Needed prosthesis, adaptive device or extra time. Used walker, etc. for steadying.	6							
Staff got clothes from closet	5							
Staff applied prosthesis/Orthosis	5							
Supervision/Set-up/Cues	5							
Min-pt did all but fasteners or needed steadying assistance/Pt did 75+%	4							
Mod-pt did 50-74%	3							
Max-pt did 25-49%	2							
Total-pt did less than 25%	1							
Activity did not occur this shift	0							

Occupational Therapy D/C Goal Score: ☐

Dressing / Undressing Lower Body - *(Appropriate public clothing only, not hospital gown.)*

Write in # of steps completed out of # of total steps involved in each step. Then calculate the percentage for total steps completed divided by total steps involved.

Day Dressing
☑ Underpants = 3 steps　　☑ Elastic waist pants = 3 steps
☑ Button/zip pants = 4 steps　　☑ L-Shoe = 1 step for each
☑ L-Sock = 1 step for each　　☑ R-Shoe = 1 step for each
☑ R-Sock = 1 step for each　　☑ Fastening shoe = 1 step

Evening Undressing
☑ Underpants = 3 steps　　☑ Elastic waist pants = 3 steps
☑ Button/zip pants = 4 steps　　☑ L-Shoe = 1 step for each
☑ L-Sock = 1 step for each　　☑ R-Shoe = 1 step for each
☑ R-Sock = 1 step for each　　☑ Fastening shoe = 1 step

Dressed/Undressed independently/Obtained own items	7							
Needed prosthesis, adaptive device or extra time	6							
Staff applied prosthesis/orthosis/elastic hose	5							
Supervision/Set-up/Cues-Set out clothes or assistance devices	5							
Min-pt did all but fasteners or needed steadying assistance/Pt did 75+%	4							
Mod-pt did 50-74%	3							
Max-pt did 25-49%	2							
Total-pt did less than 25%	1							
Activity did not occur this shift	0							

Occupational Therapy D/C Goal Score: ☐

Figure 8-2, cont'd

**CHRISTUS
ST. MICHAEL**
Rehabilitation Hospital

Patient Label

Room #	Day 1	Day 2	Day 3	D/C	Date Shift	N	D	E	PT	OT	ST	PSY	LOWEST SCORE
Toileting													
(1) Adjusted clothing before using the toilet, (2) hygiene, (3) adjusted clothing after toileting. Score on continent episodes only.													
Patient did all 3 parts independently					7								
Needed device, extra time, grab bars to steady as pulled pants up or down (no helper)					6								
Supervision/Set-up/Cues					5								
Min-pt needed steadying assistance					4								
Needed help with zipper/buttons (3 of 3 with help)					4								
Mod-pt did 2 of 3 parts					3								
Max-pt did 1 of 3 parts					2								
Total-pt did 0 parts - staff did all 3					1								
No continent B/B events this shift					0								
Activity did not occur this shift					0								

Occupational Therapy D/C Goal Score: ☐

Bladder - Level of Assistance *(3 days - Complete/intentional control)*													
Independent (or dialysis/no voids) - No accidents - No meds					7								
Medication for bladder control					6								
Independent with pad, pull-up, diaper					6								
Patient emptied urinal, foley bag, BSC					6								
Supervision/Set-up/Cues for placing or emptying of bladder equipment (i.e. bedpan, urinal, BSC)					5								
Staff emptied urinal/BSC/bedpan					5								
For items below: How much did the patient assist with wet clothes/linens, catheter, diaper/pad, urinal?													
Min-pt did 75+% of clothes/linens clean-up, cath, or tasks					4								
Mod-pt did 50-74% of clothes/linens clean-up, cath, or tasks					3								
Max-pt did 25-49% of clothes/linens clean-up, cath, or tasks					2								
Total-pt did less than 25% of clothes/linen clean-up, cath, or tasks					1								
Staff provides foley catheter care					1								

Nursing D/C Goal Score: ☐

Bladder - Frequency of Accidents *(7 day total) (Wetting of clothes or linen)*													
Look in documentation or ask sending unit nurse for number of accidents last 4 days before Rehab admission _____													
Record the total number of accidents on shift													
No accidents, no meds, no devices used					7								
No accidents, uses devices such as a cath, urinal, BSC, meds, pad					6								

Nursing D/C Goal Score: ☐

Figure 8-2, cont'd

Room # Day 1 Day 2 Day 3 D/C	Shift	N	D	E	PT	OT	ST	PSY	LOWEST SCORE
Bowel - Level of Assistance *(3 days - Complete/intentional control)*									
Independent (No BM) - No accidents (may use prunes, fiber) - No meds	7								
Medication for bowel control - taken by self	6								
Independent with pad, pull-up, diaper	6								
Patient emptied ostomy, bedpan, BSC	6								
Supervision/Set-up/Cues for placing/Emptying equipment (i.e. bedpan, urinal, BSC)	5								
Needed staff to assist to empty BSC, ostomy, bedpan	5								
For items below: How much did the patient assist with soiled clothes/linens, enema/ostomy, digital stimulation, suppository?									
Min-pt did 75+% of clothes/linens clean-up or bowel care	4								
Mod-pt did 50-74% of clothes/linens clean-up or bowel care	3								
Max-pt did 25-49% of clothes/linens clean-up or bowel care	2								
Total-pt did less than 25% of clothes/linens clean-up or bowel care, staff gave enema	1								

Nursing D/C Goal Score: ☐

	Shift	N	D	E	PT	OT	ST	PSY	LOWEST SCORE
Bowel - Frequency of Accidents *(7 day total) (Soiling of clothes or linen)*									
Look in documentation or ask sending unit nurse for number of accidents last 4 days before Rehab admission _____									
Record total number of accidents on shift									
No accidents, no meds, no devices used	7								
No accidents, uses devices (colostomy, bedpan, BSC, diaper, meds)	6								

Nursing D/C Goal Score: ☐

	Shift	N	D	E	PT	OT	ST	PSY	LOWEST SCORE
Bed/Chair/Wheelchair Transfer									
(Include how patient does sit to supine and supine to sit)									
Transferred independently, ambulatory or wheelchair without other device or help	7								
Needed sliding board, walker, rails, chair arms, extra time, or raised own HOB (no helper)	6								
Supervision/Set-up/Cues	5								
Needed help with foot/arm rests or staff locks brakes	5								
Needed steadying or help with 1 limb or min A	4								
Needed boost or help with 2 limbs or mod A	3								
Max assist (needed much lifting)	2								
Total assist/Hoyer lift/2 staff members/Pt did less than 25% of effort	1								
Activity did not occur this shift	0								

Physical Therapy D/C Goal Score: ☐

Figure 8-2, cont'd

**CHRISTUS
ST. MICHAEL**
Rehabilitation Hospital

Patient Label

					Date								
Room #	Day 1	Day 2	Day 3	D/C	**Shift**	N	D	E	PT	OT	ST	PSY	LOWEST SCORE

Toilet Transfer

		N	D	E	PT	OT	ST	PSY	LOWEST SCORE
Transferred independently, ambulatory, or wheelchair without other device or help on and off a standard toilet	7								
Used raised toilet seat, grab bars, sliding board, rails, BSC, or extra time with no help	6								
Supervision/Set-up/Cues/Staff positioned sliding board, locked brakes of wheelchair, lifted foot rests of wheelchair	5								
Needed steadying or help with 1 limb	4								
Needed boost or help with 2 limbs	3								
Max assist (Needed much lifting)	2								
Total assist/Hoyer lift/2 staff members/pt did less than 25% of effort	1								
Activity did not occur this shift	0								

Occupational Therapy D/C Goal Score: ____

Tub / Shower Transfer (   ) Tub   (   ) Shower *(Wet transfer only - no dry simulation)*

		N	D	E	PT	OT	ST	PSY	LOWEST SCORE
Transferred independently, ambulatory, or wheelchair without other device or help	7								
Used grab bars, sliding board, rails, tub/shower bench or extra time (no help)	6								
Supevision/Set-up/Cues/Staff positioned sliding board, locked brakes of wheelchair, lifted foot rests of wheelchair	5								
Needed steadying or help with 1 limb	4								
Needed boost or help with 2 limbs	3								
Max assist (Needed much lifting)	2								
Total assist (or 2 staff members)	1								
Staff rolled patient into shower	1								
Activity did not occur this shift (i.e. bed bath)	0								

Occupational Therapy D/C Goal Score: ____

Walk - *Score this section only for functional mobility (ex: ambulated patient in hallway). Score distance first and then level of assistance.*

		N	D	E	PT	OT	ST	PSY	LOWEST SCORE
Walks minimum 150 ft. independently - without assistance device	7								
Walks minimum 150 ft. with assistance device/extra time	6								
Walks minimum 150 ft. with supervision/Set-up/Cues	5								
Walks minimum 50 ft. with or without device independently (This patient would be a "household ambulator")	5								
Walks minimum 150 ft. with contact guard assistance	4								
Walks minimum 150 ft. with mod assist or helping initiate steps	3								
Walks 50 - 149 ft. with max assist and initiating steps	2								
Total assist to walk/2 staff members - Less than 50 ft.	1								
Activity did not occur this shift	0								

Physical Therapy D/C Goal Score: ____

Figure 8-2, cont'd

Room #	Day 1	Day 2	Day 3	D/C	Shift	N	D	E	PT	OT	ST	PSY	LOWEST SCORE
Wheelchair *(Cannot be a 7)* Score distance first and then level of assistance.													
Propels wheelchair minimum 150 ft. independently					6								
Propels wheelchair minimum 150 ft. with supervision/Set-up/Cues					5								
Operates wheelchair minimum 50 ft. independently (This patient would be at "household mobility")					5								
Propels wheelchair minimum 150 ft. with minimum help around corners, door frames, grades, patient provides 75+%					4								
Propels wheelchair minimum 150 ft. with moderate help to steer, patient provides 50-74% effort					3								
Propels wheelchair 50-149 ft. with maximum help from staff to push and steer, patient provides 25-49% effort					2								
Total assist - Patient provides less than 25% effort (Less than 50 ft). Staff-propelled wheelchair					1								
Activity did not occur this shift					0								

Physical Therapy D/C Goal Score: ☐

Stairs *(One flight is 12-14 stairs)*													
Goes up / down 12-14 steps without handrail or support					7								
Goes up / down 12-14 steps with handrail, support, AFO, assistive device, or extra time, or safety concerns					6								
Goes up / down 4-11 steps independently with or without assistive device					5								
Goes up / down 12-14 steps with supervision, cues, coaxing					5								
Goes up / down 12-14 steps with steadying, touching assisting or needs help with one limb					4								
Goes up / down 12-14 steps performing 50-75% of the activity					3								
Goes up / down 4-11 steps, assist of only 1 person; pt performing 25-49%					2								
Cannot go up 4-6 steps, or needs 2 people, or is carried up the stairs; or refuses to attempt					1								
Activity did not occur this shift					0								

Physical Therapy D/C Goal Score: ☐

						N	D	E	PT	OT	ST	PSY	24 Hour Rating
Comprehension *(In native language)* List mode: Auditory ___ Visual ___ Both ___													
Complex = humor, finances, rationale for medical treatment (hip precautions, pressure relief), religion, current events, discharge planning													
Basic = pain, hunger, thirst, bathroom needs, cold, nutrition, sleep													
Understands complex / abstract conversation / directions. Patient asleep all shift					7								
Understands complex / abstract conversation / directions with extra time, assistance device (glasses, if visual mode or both; hearing aid if auditory mode or both)					6								
Needs cues to understand (Basic tasks)					5								
Understands basic 90% of the time					5								
Needs help to insert / setup hearing aids (Auditory) or apply glasses (Visual) - Needs slowed speech to understand					5								
Understands basic 75-89% - May need words repeated					4								
Understands basic 50-74% - May need parts of sentences repeated					3								
Understands basic 25-49% - Only simple expressions or gestures (waves, hello)					2								
Understands basic less than 25% - Does not respond appropriately					1								
Patient asleep all shifts					N/A								

Occupational Therapy D/C Goal Score: ☐

Figure 8-2, cont'd

CHRISTUS
ST. MICHAEL
Rehabilitation Hospital

Patient Label

					Date								
Room #	Day 1	Day 2	Day 3	D/C	Shift	N	D	E	PT	OT	ST	PSY	24 Hour Rating
Expression *(In native language)* List mode: *Vocal* ___ *Nonvocal* ___ *Both* ___													
Complex = current events, religion, relationships													
Basic = nutrition, fluids, hygiene, sleep, bathroom needs													
Expresses complex / abstract ideas. Patient asleep all shift					*7*								
Expresses complex / abstract ideas with extra time, assistive device (augmentative communication device_____)					*6*								
Needs cues to express basic needs					*5*								
Expresses basic needs or ideas 90% of the time					*5*								
Needs staff member to set up communication device (talk trach valve)					*5*								
Expresses self with assistance from staff member to occlude trach					*4*								
Expresses basic 75-89% of time - Needs to repeat words					*4*								
Expresses basic 50-74% of time - Needs to repeat parts of sentences					*3*								
Expresses basic 25-49% of time - Single words or gestures only					*2*								
Expresses basic less than 25% of time					*1*								
Patient asleep all shifts					*N/A*								

Occupational Therapy D/C Goal Score: ☐

Social Interaction													
Cooperates, getting along and participating in social settings (with staff, family, other patients)													
Interacts appropriately with others - No medications needed. Patient asleep all shift					*7*								
Interacts appropriately with others with medication or extra time (anti-anxiety, antidepressant)					*6*								
Interacts appropriately 90% of time - Needs monitoring or encouragement for participation or interaction					*5*								
Interacts appropriately 75-89% of time - Needs redirection for appropriate language or to initiate interaction					*4*								
Interacts appropriately 50-74% of time - May be physically or verbally inappropriate					*3*								
Interacts appropriately 25-49% of time - Needs frequent redirection					*2*								
Interacts appropriately less than 25% of time - May be withdrawn or combative					*1*								
Patient asleep all shifts					*N/A*								

Occupational Therapy D/C Goal Score: ☐

Figure 8-2, cont'd

Room # Day 1 Day 2 Day 3 D/C	Shift	N	D	E	PT	OT	ST	PSY	24 Hour Rating
Problem Solving									
Safe and timely decisions, sequencing - Recognizes and solves problems									
Complex = balance checkbook, participating in discharge plans, self-administering meds									
Basic = completing daily tasks, dealing with unplanned events or hazards in daily activities									
Solves complex problems (consistently) Patient asleep all shift. Ex: "I would like to use the Home Health service I used before"	7								
Solves complex problems with extra time	6								
Solves complex problems with cues	5								
Solves basic problems 90% of the time. Ex: "I need to go to bed-I'm tired"	5								
Solves basic problems 75-89% of the time	4								
Solves basic problems 50-74% of the time	3								
Solves basic problems 25-49% of the time - needs direction more than half the time to initiate, plan or complete simple activities and may need a restraint for safety	2								
Solves basic problems less than 25% of time - needs direction nearly all the time or does not effectively solve problems and may need a restraint for safety. Bed alarm on at all times.	1								
Patient asleep all shifts	N/A								

Occupational Therapy D/C Goal Score: [ ]

Memory - *(Recognizes familiar faces, recalls routines, executes requests/tasks without repetition)*									
Sample 3 - Step request: "Turn over the paper, hand me the pen and point to your nose."									
Sample 2 - Step request: "Hand me the paper and point to the pen."									
Sample 1 - Step request: "Pick up the pen" "Point to the floor."									
Recognizes, recalls, or executes 3 steps of 3 step request independently. Patient asleep all shift.	7								
Recognizes, recalls, or executes 3 steps of 3 step request with extra time/device (memory book, calendar to remember)	6								
Recognizes, recalls, or executes 3 steps of 3 step request 90% of time (cueing, reminders <10%, loses track of time)	5								
Recognizes, recalls, or executes 75-89% of time 2 steps of 3 step request	4								
Recognizes, recalls, or executes 50-74% of time 2 steps of 2 step request	3								
Recognizes, recalls, or executes 25-49% of time 1 step of 2 step request	2								
Recognizes, recalls, or executes 1 step request less than 25% of time	1								
Patient asleep all shifts	N/A								

Occupational Therapy D/C Goal Score: [ ]

Initials _____	Signature _____	Initials _____	Signature _____
Initials _____	Signature _____	Initials _____	Signature _____
Initials _____	Signature _____	Initials _____	Signature _____
Initials _____	Signature _____	Initials _____	Signature _____

Figure 8-2, cont'd

(including cost of overtime and supplemental staff from outside agencies); and linen, storeroom, or central supply utilization. Involving staff in identifying approaches to cost savings heightens their awareness of financial considerations and builds team "ownership" and accountability. Monitoring the types of tests or procedures ordered is another extremely important way to reduce costs. For example, a follow-up chest x-ray examination that is not critical to a patient's rehabilitation care should be scheduled after discharge. Bringing staff into partnership for fiscal responsibility is a step in team building.

Prioritizing capital equipment purchases may also increase staff awareness of fiscal decision making. Often nursing staff members are unfamiliar with what a wheelchair shower chair, stretcher, or patient lift costs. Knowing the cost of replacing seats for wheelchair shower chairs or slings for patient lifts may encourage staff to take extra care with equipment and heighten the awareness of the benefits of maintenance. Staff meetings should include fiscal information related to monthly salary expenses compared with budget, overtime use, storeroom charges, and other expenses. The rehabilitation nurse manager should share significant variances between actual expenditures and the budgeted amount.

Many external factors have the potential to influence the budget. New regulatory expectations, such as the requirement by the Occupational Safety and Health Administration (OSHA) for the use of "safe needles" nationwide, have a fiscal impact because of the cost of supplies purchased and staff in-service programs. Third-party payment influences the fiscal bottom line because each payer has guidelines for which services, equipment, and supplies will be reimbursed. Financial "caps" to payment mean that a designated number of visits, days, or procedures or a set dollar amount may not be exceeded. External controls, such as federal, state, or accreditation requirements, may affect costs. Fiscal management is an intricate balance of ever-changing factors that enhance or adversely affect the budget bottom line. Vigilance and creativity are necessary if the rehabilitation nurse manager is to manage effectively and efficiently to maintain financial stability.

Performance Improvement

Employees want to do the best job that they are capable of doing. It is incumbent upon managers to create an environment where those closest to the patient are able to adapt work processes and improve quality of care. The nurse manager strives to create a work culture that is committed to performance improvement and learning rather than simply correcting deficiencies or adding another form to meet compliance. Chapter 9 presents a comprehensive overview of the performance improvement/quality process.

The rehabilitation nurse manager has three important functions in the quality process. The manager directs the unit's performance improvement program and continuously seeks to improve the quality of care, institutes practice changes based on evaluation, and supports interdisciplinary performance improvement efforts to improve patient care (ARN, 2003a).

Direction of the Unit's Performance Improvement Program. The nurse manager must direct the unit or area's performance improvement program and continuously seek to improve the quality of care (ARN, 2003a). The status quo must always be challenged. Patient care can be improved only when nurses and team members have both the desire and the authority to find better ways to do their jobs every day.

Priorities for performance improvement are typically set by the organization as a whole. Processes are then measured according to these priorities. Examples in rehabilitation are patient satisfaction surveys and measurements of a patient's functional outcomes on admission, at discharge, and at a predetermined point after discharge. The nurse manager, with the staff's input, may choose to measure other functional areas not identified as organizational priorities. Examples might be measuring a patient's comprehension of teaching about medication regimens or skin care techniques, evaluating alternatives to restraints, or evaluating effectiveness and adequacy of pain control measures.

Implementation of Practice Changes. Once changes that need to be made are identified, the nurse manager implements them into practice (ARN, 2003a). The new practice or system then needs to be evaluated for stability and improvement over time. Evaluation requires examining data using appropriate statistical and analytical tools.

Support of Interdisciplinary Performance Improvement. The interdisciplinary rehabilitation team members must take ownership for their work processes and for improved outcomes. The rehabilitation nurse manager supports interdisciplinary performance improvement efforts (ARN, 2003a) in which processes can be streamlined and made more efficient. Examples are the admission process, the system for patient assessment and goal setting, patient and family education, team conference formats, methods for establishing patient goals, medication administration, and patient scheduling. Communication among team members helps ensure consistency of care and follow-through 24 hours a day, 7 days a week. Performance improvement includes scrutinizing the steps of processes to identify those that can be eliminated to reduce errors or streamlined to improve flow of operations.

The rehabilitation nurse manager encourages nursing and other team members to become partners in improving the processes and outcomes. Staff members can identify concerns, become involved in endeavors to improve performance, assist with evaluating data, and implement changes. The manager who routinely shares data, recognizes teamwork, and celebrates with staff when changes lead to improved practice and outcomes also is building morale and developing staff.

Nursing Staff Development

In collaboration with a clinical nurse specialist or an educator, the rehabilitation nurse manager ensures that licensed and unlicensed staff involved in providing direct care receive education and training (ARN, 2003a). Four steps in defining content of the education program begin with identifying what resources are available to support or provide education. Educational resources may be manpower, such as the manager, nurses with experience or special expertise, clinical educators or faculty, other rehabilitation professionals, vendors of specialty items or adaptive equipment, and experts from community agencies or organizations, such as the Multiple Sclerosis Society. Educational resources include books and journals, equipment or supply instructions, and audiocassettes, videotapes, or computer programs. Financial resources include funds for educational conferences or support for staff to obtain credentials.

The second step is to identify educational priorities related to the unique needs of the patients being served, staff and facility needs, and regulatory or accreditation requirements. The third step, educational needs assessment, can identify goals and objectives for staff development. Responses to a questionnaire or open discussions in staff meetings may yield information about learning needs that are important to staff. Outcome data and observations of clinical practice, as well as new programs or services, may also contribute to staff development needs.

Without the fourth step of creating a supportive environment, education may be futile. The rehabilitation nurse manager serves as a role model to demonstrate continuous education through expectations and actions. By setting an example to enhance the value of ongoing education, the manager and staff are able to share ownership of an increase in knowledge and skills and the value of both. Chapter 5 contains information about all aspects of patient and family education.

Staff Education. The nurse manager as role model, mentor, and coach provides opportunities for nursing staff to acquire clinical rehabilitation nursing skills and expertise (ARN, 2003a). Staff education has three categories: orientation, in-service programs, and continuing education programs. Staff education processes address the learning needs of a variety of staff members, licensed and unlicensed, who work in the nurse manager's area of responsibility. Competency, both knowledge and skill, is an educational responsibility. Competency measurements must assess whether a staff member can apply specific knowledge and skills, not simply identify or list them. The rehabilitation nurse manager plans for staff to achieve competencies necessary for them to carry out their responsibilities in rehabilitation care. Excellent resources are available for teaching nursing assistants about restorative care in subacute, long-term care, and home settings (Hoeman, 1990; Tracey, 1999).

Orientation. Orientation is the process of transitioning a new staff member into a work area. Because rehabilitation nursing is not typically covered as an elective in most nursing programs, many new employees have no prior rehabilitation nursing experience. Without this experience, nurses and other staff members may need education about the unique "culture" of rehabilitation nursing, as well as information to clarify misconceptions they may have developed from lack of exposure to the specialty (Ruiz, 2000). Orientation is critical for transmitting rehabilitation nursing theory and concepts. The nurse manager sets a tone with current staff about the importance of orientation and the value of new employees. Following principles for teaching adult learners, the nurse manager intersperses classroom work with application opportunities. A preceptor, coach, or mentor program is often a good way to help new staff enter the field of rehabilitation nursing. In a preceptor model, the new nurse follows the experienced nurse for several days, learning unit policies and procedures and methods for delivering care. In a coach model, the new RN delivers the care with the coach providing oversight and asking critical questions to ascertain learning and critical thinking. A mentor may be assigned to a new RN to help introduce the nurse into the system and guide the new staff member in his or her new role.

In-Service Programs. In-service programs, a second category, help staff members keep current on new practices, procedures, products, or knowledge. In-service programs can be given in short blocks of time by lecture or discussion, mobile learning carts, computer programs, posters or flyers, or self-learning study packets, to name a few methods. Creativity is essential to ensure that staff members receive and engage in ongoing education with their busy nursing practice schedule.

Continuing Education Programs. Continuing education programs are planned learning experiences for staff development beyond the basic nursing curriculum. Programs may include such diverse areas as advanced assessment parameters for a specific patient population, critical thinking skills, cultural diversity, or identification of acute medical complications in a rehabilitation patient. Ideally, continuing education programs will offer contact hours as continuing education units needed to maintain certification in the nursing specialty.

Typically there are more ideas for educational activities than there is time for staff members to attend or resources to provide them. Although educational activities are planned to meet staff development criteria, in reality they are offered within the context of a busy work area where patient needs are priorities. When educational programs are interrupted continually or not attended, it becomes a quality issue and the manager intervenes. Some facilities plan most of their educational offerings either before or after a shift and pay nurses to attend, in order to not interfere with the shift duties.

Educational activities are evaluated to identify how well attendees learned and the effect of learning on patient outcomes or clinical decision making. Evaluation is important on several levels. Results of evaluations will indicate how well the program was conducted and whether it was cost-effective. Another measure is participants' self-reports of their learning as a result of having attended the program. Over time, education programs are expected to influence changes in participants' behaviors or improve competencies in their professional practices. Only when educational evaluation data demonstrate results can programs be promoted as cost-effective and an appropriate use of resources.

Lifelong Education for Professional Nursing.
It is appropriate for nurse managers to assume professional responsibility for lifelong learning and to promote this among their staff. With the rapid explosion of knowledge and technology in nursing, rehabilitation, and health care, it is impossible to maintain expertise in practice without actively pursuing ongoing learning.

The standards for professional rehabilitation nursing performance include a mandate to acquire and maintain current knowledge and competency in nursing practice (ARN, 2000). Within this standard are criteria that address a nurse's responsibility for participating in ongoing educational activities related to clinical knowledge and professional issues, as well as interdisciplinary team concepts and practice.

Many strategies can be used to pursue lifelong professional learning. Continuing education programs are available in a variety of formats, such as seminars, workshops, conferences offered on site, or Internet courses. Continuing education also is available in independent study modules or through various journals. Regularly reading and critiquing professional materials and books and discussing how to use research findings published in journal articles are popular activities of a staff journal club. Professional associations, health organizations, and government agencies sponsor resources available on the World Wide Web, including health references and continuing education programs.

Learning needs may also be met when nurses participate in formal education programs to seek advanced preparation in the care of individuals with physical disabilities and chronic illnesses and to demonstrate excellence in the rehabilitation nursing specialty through certified rehabilitation registered nurse (CRRN) certification (ARN, 2003a). Certain career goals or positions may lead nurses to complete an academic graduate program of study and seek an advanced practice certification.

Education is an important component of rehabilitation nursing practice because it constitutes a significant portion of what rehabilitation nurses do in providing quality care to individuals with disability and chronic illness. The nurse manager who seeks to maintain a competent staff will encourage staff to participate in educational opportunities; arrange for continuing education programs; inform staff about support for education and tuition; budget funds for educational activities, conferences, and professional literature; and reward and encourage staff members who attend continuing education programs.

Unlicensed Assistive Personnel/Multiskilled Workers.
The preparation and ongoing education of unlicensed assistive personnel and multiskilled workers are areas in which the rehabilitation nurse manager may have significant impact. Although these two groups of workers have differing task assignments in the work area, both are involved in support of patient care.

Unlicensed Assistive Personnel. The ARN position statement (ARN, 2003b) addresses qualifications, scope of care at a basic and secondary level, and settings of care for unlicensed assistive personnel (UAPs). This document identifies UAPs' duties that occur in the rehabilitation area under the direction of an RN. UAPs have either received a nurse's aide certificate or completed at least 4 weeks of on-the-job training. UAPs provide care based on the patient's plan of care and within demonstrated competencies.

Multiskilled Workers. The multiskilled worker is qualified to work in more than one task area. Multiskilled workers may perform technical tasks, such as phlebotomy or electrocardiograms, or may work in different settings, such as inpatient care units, rehabilitation clinics, or outpatient programs, at different times of the day or week.

Student Support.
The nurse manager encourages an environment that supports nursing and allied health students as they learn rehabilitation skills (ARN, 2003a). Nurse managers often interface with student nurses on their rotation for clinical or leadership experiences or when teaching rehabilitation principles to students as part of scheduled lectures.

There are three reasons that nurse managers should encourage students to have experiences in a rehabilitation setting. First and foremost, experiences during basic education are opportunities to expose students to the specialty of rehabilitation nursing. Second, students who become interested in rehabilitation nursing may be recruited as staff. Third, when nursing students understand rehabilitation nursing principles and practices, regardless of their future areas of practice, they will be more likely to incorporate rehabilitation principles and practices into all areas of nursing, helping patients from onset of illness or injury throughout their care. The nurse manager shares student clinical objectives with the nursing staff so they can work together to achieve the objectives and enrich the student experience.

Principles and functions that student nurses need to learn about the unique aspects of rehabilitation nursing include the following:
- Understanding the roles and functions of other disciplines that participate in rehabilitation teams and how those roles interface with rehabilitation care
- Applying the holistic approach to rehabilitation care that includes the patient's family and environment
- Encouraging patient and family involvement as part of the interdisciplinary team in care and lifelong care planning, with a focus on maximizing function, preventing complications, and maintaining optimal health
- Understanding the continuum of physical, psychosocial, and emotional adjustment to disability or chronic illness
- Incorporating knowledge of and adjustments to the patient's home, work, educational, and/or social environments and support systems in the rehabilitation plan
- Encouraging and educating patients and families to learn to do for themselves and apply problem-solving techniques,

rather than expecting the various health care providers to do care that the patient is capable of completing

- Providing education, preventive interventions, and maintenance care as opposed to cure behaviors and even predicting needs beyond the immediate care setting
- Acknowledging the physical and emotional demands on staff inherent to the specialty practice of rehabilitation nursing

Human Resource Management

The rehabilitation nurse manager is on the front line to influence staff job satisfaction so that the objectives of the organization can be accomplished. As a frontline manager, the rehabilitation nurse manager is the individual primarily responsible for acquiring, developing, and retaining staff. A major function of the role is facilitating the work performance of a number of employees with a variety of preparation levels, experiences, and personal preferences. The rehabilitation nurse manager constantly seeks balance in providing a caring, nurturing environment with standardization of conditions so that the work is completed effectively and efficiently.

According to the ARN (2003a), the rehabilitation nurse manager is accountable for the management of personnel functions of the nursing and support staff in the area or unit. The nurse manager is well served by investing time and effort to identify and obtain support through the organization's human resources or personnel department. Broad categories of support from human resources that are helpful include employment, compensation, benefits administration, and employee relations.

Employment. The rehabilitation nurse manager strives to recruit, interview, hire, and retain a skilled mix of qualified, competent, patient-oriented personnel to deliver care and achieve the functional outcomes desired. With sparse exposure to rehabilitation, nurses may be unfamiliar with concepts unique to rehabilitation nursing. Nurses who prefer to concentrate on interpersonal interactions, teaching, counseling, supporting, and coordinating care across a continuum are well suited. Rehabilitation nurses, however, must also be competent in medical/surgical knowledge and skills because persons with significant disability, multiple diagnoses, or extensive complex medical needs are prevalent in many rehabilitation settings. CMS requires that a certain percentage of the inpatient rehabilitation population fall into 13 diagnoses in order to be classified as an inpatient rehabilitation facility (Department of Health & Human Services Centers for Medicare & Medicaid Services, 2004). These diagnoses, such as stroke, spinal cord injury, and brain injury, tend to be more complicated than cardiac or orthopedic diagnoses. Furthermore, as lengths of stay in the acute medical hospitals decline, rehabilitation facilities and units are admitting patients much sooner after their disability or illness.

The rehabilitation nurse manager is best served by giving a clear picture of each position and its performance expectations during the interviewing process. The specific job description,

the orientation process, ongoing development availability and expectations, performance evaluation time frames, hours of work, compensation and benefits, as well as employment and employee expectations should be clearly delineated and agreed on. Behavioral questions during the interview help the nurse manager determine if the candidate will meet the facility standards. An example of a behavioral question might be, "Tell me about a time when you couldn't complete all of your assignments by the end of the shift. What did you do?" Or "In your position, how do you define doing a good job?"

Human resource departments offer support to the manager's employment function by advertising positions, sponsoring career days or job fairs, arranging nursing school visits, and using other recruitment techniques. Human resources may be responsible for orientation to the organization and may screen applicants to provide background and reference checks, conduct a second interview, schedule physicals, extend employment offers, determine compensation, and assist with any relocation information or support.

Compensation. Compensation is typically supported through human resources, and the nurse manager works with human resource personnel to ensure that employees receive appropriate credit for previous experience or education. The nurse manager keeps human resources aware of local market trends, provides updates to job descriptions, and ensures that staff members are clearly aware of performance expectations and how they affect their compensation.

Benefits. Benefits are discussed separately, even though they are part of the overall compensation of an employee. The rehabilitation nurse manager becomes knowledgeable about all aspects of the benefits package available to employees. Employees often have questions regarding benefits, and the manager's ability to provide a rapid and accurate response may deescalate a potentially negative situation for the employee. Employees do not always equate the monetary equivalent of benefits as a substantial part of their compensation. The rehabilitation nurse manager can use actual dollar amounts or percentages to illustrate the worth of benefits as diverse as child care discounts; free parking; life, dental, or optical insurance; meal discounts; credit union membership; and a variety of elective and provided retirement plans. This information may assist in recruitment and retention. Alternatively, the nurse manager may work with human resources by identifying which benefits hold significant value for retaining employees, saving the high cost of turnover.

Employee Relations. Employee relations is a broad category that incorporates many aspects of interaction between the organization and employees. Interactions may be employee recognition programs or activities such as picnics and banquets, assisting employees with problems, or addressing employees who demonstrate negative performance or other behaviors.

Human resource personnel can help the rehabilitation nurse manager ascertain the appropriate assistance for an employee, interpret policies, and apply their provisions or expectations uniformly. Most organizations require managers to review planned disciplinary actions with human resources before meeting with an employee. Human resource personnel assist with grievance mechanisms and serve both employees and managers to achieve fair and equitable resolution to concerns or violation of the organization's rules and policies. The confidential nature of any employee disciplinary action or personal situation must be respected without exception. Even if an employee chooses to share information, the rehabilitation nurse manager must not do so.

The rehabilitation nurse manager can be proactive in creating a positive environment for employee relations, beginning with soliciting ideas from staff and sharing information in a timely manner. Weekly, biweekly, or monthly staff meetings should be held to communicate information and solicit feedback and concerns. Nurse managers often vary their work hours or work different shifts to be in touch with issues that affect all staff members and resolve problems early on. Morale is enhanced and turnover rates reduced when employees and management are involved together in decision-making processes.

Advocacy

Advocacy for persons with disabilities is another role of the rehabilitation nurse manager (ARN, 2003a). Advocacy may take several directions. The rehabilitation nurse may advocate for patients through involvement in professional nursing organizations or interdisciplinary groups. Alternatively, the manager may pursue advocacy by participating in and supporting national disability advocacy groups, such as the National Head Injury Foundation or the Spina Bifida Association of America. Chapter 3 discusses advocacy and ethical matters pertinent to rehabilitation.

The nurse manager may assist those with disabilities or chronic conditions through awareness programs or media promotions. Advocacy may be legislative, by selecting candidates to support, promoting causes with a positive impact for individuals with disabilities or chronic illnesses, and participating in telephone trees or mailings regarding advocacy issues to elected representatives. The nurse manager, through example and organizational support, may introduce staff members to mechanisms of advocacy and encourage them to identify their own niche in supporting individuals with disabilities or chronic illnesses.

Research

The role of the rehabilitation nurse manager in research is to ensure that current rehabilitation research findings and rehabilitation nursing practices are incorporated into clinical practice and the delivery of care (ARN, 2003a). Evidence-based research and consensus statements, such as those produced for poststroke rehabilitation, treatment of pressure ulcers, and urinary incontinence in adults by the Agency for Health Care Policy and Research (now the Agency for Healthcare Research

and Quality; http://www.ahc.gov), should be implemented in the clinical setting. Guidelines published by the Consortium for Spinal Cord Medicine (see Chapter 14) on acute management of autonomic dysreflexia, neurogenic bowel management, and prevention of thromboembolism are other examples. As new research develops and is published, policies and procedures on delivering care must be updated. The nurse manager encourages staff to search for increasingly better methods of delivering care (Stetler et al., 1998).

A research-based professional practice model of care based on one of the nursing theories can also be used, depending on the setting. Chapter 2 provides discussion of theorists and functional models commonly used for practice in rehabilitation nursing.

Not all practice in a health profession is based on science. In some cases researchers have yet to accumulate a sufficient body of knowledge to dictate nursing practice in a given direction. In other cases "a different frame of reference provides the appropriate rationale for action" (Stetler et al., 1998, p. 47), such as ethical decision making.

The nurse manager should also support research activities and studies in the general field of rehabilitation, as well as rehabilitation nursing (ARN, 2003a). This support can be demonstrated by participation in actual studies, financial support to research, or response to surveys regarding practice that adds to the knowledge base.

IMPLICATIONS

The field of medical rehabilitation, while continuing to grow and expand into different settings, is facing a shrinking labor pool of nurses and a decrease in reimbursement for services. This is coupled with a vast movement in which consumers are demanding top-notch service or they will take their business elsewhere. Rehabilitation nurses and rehabilitation nurse leaders can make the difference that will be needed to provide high-quality, customer-focused, cost-efficient care.

Rehabilitation nurse managers must lead by instilling enthusiasm for their organization and its mission in everyone with whom they work. In an ideal world, a nurse manager who demonstrates true leadership skills and abilities will be able to direct the staff toward high employee morale and career development, low turnover rates, and satisfied customers. Those who understand the goals and purpose of the unit are able to work together, are enthusiastic and mutually supportive, and have a sense of achievement and belonging. Furthermore, functional outcomes for their patients will improve and be sustained or increased after discharge. In an ideal world, costs are kept below expenses and are in line with the budget. The nurse manager continually sets ever-higher targets in all of these areas and develops action plans with the staff on ways to reach targeted goals. Rehabilitation nurse leaders are at the forefront, poised to make a difference in the lives of those they serve.

Case Study

The nurse manager on a 30-bed spinal cord injury and orthopedic unit has been receiving complaints about her evening charge nurse, Margi Prescott, for the past 3 months. The concerns brought forward by several nurses were that Margi sat at the desk all evening and rarely left to make patient rounds or to help the nurses with patient care or answering call lights. They also stated that Margi would disappear at times and was noticed making a lot of personal phone calls.

The nurse manager had spoken to Margi about this and recorded it in her files as a verbal counseling. During the past 2 weeks nearly all the evening staff expressed dissatisfaction with Margi Prescott, stating that the behavior was continuing. The nurses commented that they respected Margi's clinical skills and generally liked her but felt that her leadership and role modeling was poor.

The evening nurses were asked whether they would be comfortable meeting with the nurse manager and Margi to discuss these issues openly. The nurses all agreed to the meeting. The nurse manager arranged the meeting the next day and informed Margi of the purpose, which was to discuss charge nurse issues and expectations.

The nurse manager led the meeting. The staff nurses were open in telling Margi what they liked and did not like about her actions. They stated that they respected her clinical skills but needed her to be more available as a resource to new staff or inexperienced nurses who need to improve their competency in rehabilitation skills. An example was given of a new nursing assistant who transferred a patient incorrectly from the wheelchair to the bed. Margi's supervision and help were needed in this situation to ensure that neither the staff member nor the patient encountered harm during the transfer. Margi's presence on the unit would have a positive impact on staff morale and on patient satisfaction if care was supervised so that rehabilitation principles and practices were being followed.

Margi listened constructively to the concerns, understood what they were saying, and agreed to make a change in behavior. The nurse manager reviewed the charge nurse shift routine with Margi, which called for making patient rounds three times a shift, answering call lights, and helping out with patient care, especially during the busy shift times. Margi agreed to follow the guidelines. The expectations were outlined in an action plan for improvement, which Margi signed. A follow-up meeting was scheduled in 2 weeks with the staff and Margi to review progress.

The follow-up meeting was positive on both sides. The staff nurses felt that Margi had made a definite change and that she was now part of their team and a leader with whom they could work positively and continue to respect. Margi thanked the nurse manager for pointing out the issues and for helping her to further develop as a leader and to contribute to the success of the unit and institution.

CRITICAL THINKING

1. As a nurse manager, what steps would you take to ensure that Margi Prescott is continuing to grow in the charge nurse role?
2. What functions of a leader would you discuss with Margi and expect that she carry out on her shift?
3. Discuss the emotional intelligence components that Margi needs to strengthen.

REFERENCES

Adler, J. (2005, November 14). The boomer files: Turning 60. *Newsweek*, 50-58.

American Nurses Association. (2004). *Scope and standards for nurse administrators* (2nd ed.). Washington, DC: Author.

Association of Rehabilitation Nurses. (1999). *Factors to consider in decisions about staffing in rehabilitation settings: Position statement*. Skokie, IL: Author.

Association of Rehabilitation Nurses. (2000). *Standards and scope of rehabilitation nursing practice*. Glenview, IL: Author.

Association of Rehabilitation Nurses. (2003a). *Rehabilitation nurse manager: Role description*. Glenview, IL: Author.

Association of Rehabilitation Nurses. (2003b). *The role of unlicensed assistive personnel in the rehabilitation setting: Position statement*. Glenview, IL: Author.

Association of Rehabilitation Nurses. (2004). President's message: ARN's strategic plan. *ARN Network*, 20(3), 3.

Association of Rehabilitation Nurses. (2005). *ARN competencies assessment tool*. Retrieved November 11, 2005, from http://www.rehabnurse.org/Basiccomp.html.

Benner, P. (2001). *From novice to expert: Excellence and power in nursing practice* (Commemorative 1st ed.). Upper Saddle River, NJ: Prentice Hall.

Buerhaus, P. I., Staiger, D. O., & Auerbach, D. I. (2004, November 17). New signs of a strengthening U.S. nurse labor market? *Health Affairs*. Retrieved October 29, 2005, from http://content.healthaffairs.org/cgi/reprint/hlthaff.w4.526.

Cole, J. (1999, November). The art of wooing Gen Xers. *HR Focus*, 7-12.

Covey, S. R. (1992). *Principle-centered leadership*. New York: Simon & Schuster.

Davidhizar, R., & Eshleman, J. (1999). The friendly art of persuasion. *Health Care Manager*, 18(2), 41-46.

Department of Health & Human Services Centers for Medicare & Medicaid Services. (2001, August 7). *Final Rule in Federal Register*. Retrieved November 11, 2005, from http://www.access.gpo.gov/su_fedreg/a01807c.html.

Department of Health & Human Services Centers for Medicare & Medicaid Services. (2004, June 25). *CMS manual system. Pub. 100-14 Medicare Claims Processing. Transmittal 221*. Retrieved November 11, 2005, from http://www.cms.gov/manuals/pm_trans/r221cp.pdf.

Deutschendorf, A. (2003). From past paradigms to future frontiers. Unique care delivery models to facilitate nursing work and quality outcomes. *Journal of Nursing Administration*, 33(1), 52-59.

Eade, D. M. (1996, November/December). Motivational management: Developing leadership skills. *Clinician Reviews*, 115-125.

Finkler, S. A., & Kovner, C. T. (2000). *Financial management for nurse managers and executives* (2nd ed.). Philadelphia: W. B. Saunders.

Foley, R. (2005). Learn to speak finance. *Nursing Management*, 36(8), 28-33.

Fox, R. T., Fox, D. H., & Wells, P. J. (1999). Performance of first-line management functions on productivity of hospital unit personnel. *Journal of Nursing Administration*, 29(9), 12-18.

Goleman, D. (1998). *Working with emotional intelligence*. New York: Bantam.

Green, K. (2005, September 26). When we're all 64. *The Wall Street Journal*, pp. R1, R4.

Health Care Advisory Board. (1999). *Hardwiring for service excellence*. Washington, DC: The Advisory Board Company.

Hoeman, S. P. (1990). *Rehabilitation/restorative care in the community*. St. Louis, MO: Mosby.

Johnson, S. (1998). *Who moved my cheese?* New York: G. P. Putnam's Sons.

Kerfoot, K. (1996). Today's patient care unit manager. *Nursing Economics*, 14(1), 59-61.

Lancaster, L. C., & Stillman, D. (2002). *When generations collide.* New York: HarperCollins.

Lee, F. (2004). *If Disney ran your hospital: 9½ things you would do differenty.* Bozeman, MT: Second River Healthcare Press.

Lewin, K. (1947). Frontiers in group dynamics: Concept, methods, and reality in social science. *Human Relations, 1,* 5-41.

Manfredi, C. M. (1996). A descriptive study of nurse managers and leadership. *Western Journal of Nursing Research, 18*(3), 314-329.

Nelson, A., & Baptiste, A. (2004, September 30). Evidence-based practices for safe patient handling and movement. *Online Journal of Issues in Nursing, 9*(3). Retrieved February 18, 2006, from www.nursingworld.org/ojin/topic25/tpc25_3.htm.

Nevidjon, B., & Erickson, J. I. (2001). The nursing shortage: Solutions for the short and long term. *ANA Continuing Education.* Retrieved October 27, 2005, from http://nursing world.org/mods/archive/mod270/ceshfull.htm.

Perra, B. M. (2000). Leadership: The key to quality outcomes. *Nursing Administration Quarterly, 24*(2), 56-61.

Peters, T. (1987). Develop an inspiring vision. In *Thriving on chaos* (pp. 399-408). New York: Alfred A. Knopf.

Ruiz, M. (2000). Rehabilitation nursing: Another increasing shortage. Excellence in clinical practice. Indianapolis, IN: Sigma Theta Tau, International.

Stetler, C. B., Brunell, M., Giuliano, K. K., Morsi, D., Prince, L., & Newell-Stokes, V. (1998). Evidence-based practice and the role of nursing leadership. *Journal of Nursing Administration, 28*(7/8), 45-53.

Studer, Q. (2003). *Hardwiring excellence.* Gulf Breeze, FL: Fire Starter Publishing.

Tracey, C. A. (1999). *Restorative nursing: A training manual for nursing assistants.* Glenview, IL: Association of Rehabilitation Nurses.

Tulgan, B. (1999, May). Gen Xers: Will the workplace ever be the same? *Health Management Technology,* 8-9.

U.S. Department of Health and Human Services. (2002, July). *Projected supply, demand, and shortages of registered nurses: 2000-2020.* Retrieved October 29, 2005, from ftp.hrsa.gov/bhpr/nationalcenter/rnproject.pdf.

Velianoff, G. D., Neely, C., & Hall, S. (1993). Developmental levels of interdisciplinary collaborative practice committees. *Journal of Nursing Administration, 23*(7/8), 26-29.

Wellner, A. (1999, February 12). Get ready for generation next. *Training,* 44-48.

Williams, J. (2000, March 20). The new workforce. *Business Week,* 64-70.

Zenger, J., Ulrich, D., & Smallwood, N. (2000, March). The new leadership development. *Training & Development,* 22-27.

9

Quality: Indicators and Management

Pamela M. Duchene, DNSc, RN, CRRN

According to the report by the Institute of Medicine (IOM) (Kohn, Corrigan, & Donaldson, 1999), there are between 44,000 and 98,000 deaths annually in the United States due to medical errors. Such errors occur throughout the continuum of care, including rehabilitation. When breaches in quality occur in succession in any health care setting, the initial response often is defensiveness and fault finding. Blaming and finger pointing are futile in correcting underlying system problems.

In health care, control of quality has often been viewed as the responsibility of a single person, with lapses in quality attributed to the nurse, the physician, the therapist, or patient noncompliance. In such situations the solution is perceived as the need to retrain, write or revise a policy, provide discipline, threaten litigation, and treat the quality failure as a moral issue by naming, blaming, and shaming the clinician involved in the error (Reason, 2000).

The application of this theory is to trace the development of a pressure ulcer to the shift when a nurse or assistant failed to provide pressure relief. In contrast, quality may be viewed as the integrity of a system, where quality control is established through defenses, safeguards, and barriers. The elements may be both human and nonhuman (equipment, technologies, etc.). In this theory the development of a pressure ulcer could be traced back to the shift when the patient was not repositioned, but rather than blaming a nurse or nursing assistant, work environment and system factors would be explored. If the nursing assistant worked a double shift to cover for an absence and was caring for 10 patients as opposed to the usual 7, the defect that led to the pressure ulcer would be considered to be a system problem, with fatigue and workload the causative factors that resulted in the lack of pressure relief. Other causative factors would also be considered, including nutrition, support surfaces, and clinical leadership in providing education and training on the prevention of pressure ulcers.

The above example is offered as an illustration of the complexity of quality. Presented in this chapter is a discussion of quality indicators and management within rehabilitation nursing practice. It includes specific illustrations of how to use quality information.

MEANING OF QUALITY

Quality is a matter of perception. What represents quality to one individual may not to another. For example, a complete head-to-toe nursing assessment is an indicator of quality to many acute care nurses. In rehabilitation, however, the focus of the assessment shifts from physical findings to functional assessment, independence, and therapeutic teaching. Neither perspective is entirely incorrect. Both are perceptions of quality care that are grounded in experience, education, and patient needs. From a consumer perspective, quality care may be more closely linked to how frequently the water pitcher is filled, how quickly the call light is answered, and whether or not the floor is swept clean, rather than the completion of a head-to-toe assessment. In studies comparing and contrasting nursing perceptions of quality care with patient perception of quality care, nurses rate technical aspects of care higher than patients, whereas patients focus on environmental aspects of care as reflective of nursing quality (Durieux, Bissery, Dubois, Gasquet, & Coste, 2004; Idvall, Hamrin, Sjöström, & Unosson, 2002).

Defining quality health care is an arduous task. In 1998 the Vice Presidential Planning Committee for the Forum for Health Care Quality Measurement and Reporting was initiated (Department of Health and Human Services for the Domestic Policy Council, 1998). The agency is now known as the National Quality Forum (NQF) (Lang & Kizer, 2003). The NQF, funded by private and public funds, is a not-for-profit organization. Much of the funding for NQF is from organization membership dues. The charge of the NQF is to develop and implement a national reporting and measurement strategy for health care quality (National Quality Forum, 2005). The NQF provides means for measuring health care quality and is developing standardized measures and mandated data collection and reporting structures. The NQF endorses core measures for standardized health care quality reporting (National Quality Forum, 2002a). The NQF has identified three broad indicators of quality issues: error rates, overtreatment, and undertreatment. The NQF evaluates and recommends specific measures of quality that meet the following requirements:

- The measure is condition specific (e.g., chronic pain) or for a cross-cutting priority area (e.g., inpatient acute care through home health care).
- The acute care hospital is directly able to control or influence the process of care measured and reviewed.
- The measure is not structure or utilization based unless clearly linked to quality.
- The measure is not a proprietary type of measure; it is available for public use.

Error Rates

According to, another source, the NQF, as many as 180,000 deaths are attributable to medical errors, with up to 30% of hospitalized patients and 20% of chronically ill patients receiving contraindicated care. Mortality, morbidity, and health care burdens, complications, and expense are increased through inadequate diagnosis and treatment. The NQF (2002b) identifies 27 serious adverse events that include such items as the following:

- Surgical events:
  - Surgery on the wrong body part
  - Surgery on the wrong patient
- Product or device events resulting in death or disability:
  - From the use of contaminated drugs or devices
  - From misuse of a device or product
- Failure of patient protection
  - Suicide
  - Discharge of an infant to the wrong person
- Care management issue
  - Hemolytic transfusion reaction
  - Medication error resulting in death or disability
  - Hospital-acquired stage III or IV pressure ulcer
- Environmental issues resulting in death, such as
  - Restraint or bed rail use
  - Fall
- Criminal acts resulting in patient injury or death, such as
  - Patient abduction
  - Sexual or physical assault of patient

This list has been commonly renamed the "never list," because it contains events that all hope never happen in any health care organization (Kizer & Stegun, 2002). Although some of the 27 items are specific to acute care hospitalization, there are many that are applicable to rehabilitation. The quality of rehabilitation nursing has been linked with prevention of pressure ulcers, patient falls, and thromboembolic events (Congdon & Magilvy, 2004). Development of pressure ulcers, complications of a fall, or thromboembolic event are visible to referral facilities and community agencies and will have an impact on the reputation of the rehabilitation program if such issues seem to be a trend.

Another example of medical errors is that of medication errors, which occur throughout the health care continuum. In a landmark study Morimoto, Gandhi, Seger, Hsieh, and Bates (2004) found 19% of medication administrations contained an error. The cost of such errors and of adverse drug events is estimated at $2,162 (Senst et al., 2001). When one applies this expense to a large facility, the total costs of medication errors occurring during hospitalization is estimated at $1.7 million. If this rate is applied to all hospitals within the nation, the estimated expense of in-hospital medication errors is over $2 billion annually. One key strategy to prevent medication errors is medication reconciliation. Rehabilitation nurses are in a unique position within the health care continuum in that they are in a key role to review medications the patient will be continuing to take after a frequently long and complex stay.

Overtreatment

The second category of quality concerns identified by the NQF is overtreatment (NQF, 2002a). The NQF estimates that 20% to 30% of health care treatments are not necessary. Overtreatment leads to a risk of complications and expense and negatively affects productivity. Overtreatment with antibiotics, for example, adds expense and may precipitate antibiotic-resistant strains of illness. The prevalence of methicillin-resistant *Staphylococcus aureus* (MRSA) is a result of antibiotic overuse. This has a direct impact on rehabilitation expense, with the admission of some units including a routine screening for MRSA (Manian, Senkel, Zack, & Meyer, 2002). Another example in rehabilitation is the unnecessary duplication of discipline evaluations. In many rehabilitation programs, patients are asked the same questions by each discipline because each has a specially designed form to meet their needs. Such duplicative, repetitive evaluation systems waste the patient's time as well as health care dollars that are better spent with interdisciplinary evaluations. The conversion to electronic medical records offers a means to substantially decrease duplication of documentation, resulting in more cohesive, integrated interdisciplinary records.

Undertreatment

The third category of quality issues identified by the NQF is that of undertreatment. According to the NQF (2002a), only 50% of patients receive the preventive care that has been recommended by providers. Because rehabilitation centers on preventive care, a primary area of concern for rehabilitation providers is the lack of access to rehabilitation services and care (Rao, Boradia, & Ennis, 2005). The implementation of prospective payment systems for rehabilitation juxtaposed with the change in the 75% rule to control access to acute rehabilitation is resulting in a change in admitting criteria, with patients denied acute rehabilitation and referred to long-term care, subacute care, or home health care. The 75% rule is a regulation within the Conditions of Participation through the Centers for Medicare and Medicaid Services (CMS) for distinct part of inpatient rehabilitation programs, which requires 75% of admissions to fall within 14 diagnostic groups. The full impact of these changes has yet to be experienced as of the writing of this text. In the first 12 months under the new 75% rule regulations, the number of admissions for acute rehabilitation declined by 34,000 (American Hospital Association, 2005).

The indicators of error rates, overtreatment, and undertreatment assist in the definition of quality health care. The IOM formed a committee in 1998 (Kohn, Corrigan, & Donaldson, 1999) to identify quality improvement strategies. The committee members identified quality as equated with patient safety and error prevention. In health care, as illustrated in the opening examples, lapses in patient safety and errors are frequently seen as the result of one person's failure to prevent injury or risk. As stated by Deming (2000), quality improvement is possible only through correcting processes. One of Deming's 13 points was, "Drive out fear, so that everyone may work effectively for the company." The statement points to the need for a just culture, rather than fault finding, in an effort to improve performance and quality outcomes. It is critical that health care organizations adopt this strategy, rather than the traditional fallback of fault finding. Rehabilitation, like most areas within health care, is susceptible to the temptation to try to assign blame when events do not go as planned. Errors are most often a result of less visible systems processes. Rehabilitation nurses are often at the sharp end of health care, where the terminal error is visible. As an example, a physician may write an order for a high-risk intravenous medication that is outside of safe parameters. The pharmacist may question the order but proceed to fill it. The nurse who hangs the infusion is in the last (sharp) position to protect the patient from the error (Husch et al., 2005).

UNIVERSAL INDICATORS OF QUALITY

Other than actual errors, what are the indicators of quality? As with the definition of quality, indicators of quality vary substantially from person to person. In a letter to a chief executive nurse, a patient complained that she had suffered a bruise on her upper arm from the use of a thigh-sized cuff. The patient, who was a large individual, believed the standard of a practice was breached because a cuff that should be used on the thigh was used used on her arm. The nurse had commented to the patient that the cuff was a "thigh" cuff, rather than nothing that she needed an appropriately sized cuff. To the patient, the perceived failure of the nurse to obtain a large cuff was a sign of poor quality. In reality, the nurse acted appropriately in selecting a cuff the right size for the patient's arm, but could have avoided the problem by not referring to the cuff as "thigh sized," which the patient found offensive.

Given the public and media demand for quality health care, several agencies have identified key indicators of quality. The Agency for Healthcare Research and Quality (AHRQ) (2005), now known as the Agency for Health Care Research and Quality (AHRQ), published a system for consumers to quickly review the quality of health care systems. Quality health care is "doing the right thing, at the right time, in the right way, for the right person—and having the best possible results" (AHRQ, 2005, p. 3). Quality health care includes reviewing outcome measures, patient satisfaction reports, accreditation reports, and clinical performance measures when making decisions on providers and health care systems. Transparency of health care quality ensures that consumers have information about health care providers and organizations, yet such information may be overwhelming and confusing and still leave the interpretation of quality reports to the discretion of the consumer.

Comparing rehabilitation facilities through the use of outcome management systems is confusing to professionals and is likely to result in confusion of consumers as well. The Commission on Accreditation of Rehabilitation Facilities (CARF) (2005) requires that organizations disclose information on outcomes and accreditation status to consumers. Rehabilitation programs that are not CARF accredited may not be compliant with CARF standards. As a result, consumers may be confused over the quality of rehabilitation programs, assuming that programs do not differ substantively.

COMMON HEALTH CARE INDICATORS OF QUALITY

Indicators of health care quality vary among regulatory groups, professional nursing associations, advocacy groups, and consumer groups. Application of the concepts of health care errors, overtreatment, and undertreatment is effective in assisting professionals and consumers in identifying quality rehabilitation programs. Beyond this general point, however, the amount of information and the number of opinions on health care quality are staggering. In this section regulatory perspectives, professional nursing perspectives, and advocacy group and consumer group perspectives on quality health care indicators will be addressed, with application to rehabilitation nursing.

Regulatory Perspectives

Regulatory agencies, such as the Centers for Medicare and Medicaid Services (CMS) and The Joint Commission (TJC), play a significant role in identifying health care indicators of quality. CMS is active in development of quality standards for programs that participate in Medicare and Medicaid reimbursement. CMS controls quality violations by assessing fines and barring programs that violate quality from participation in Medicare and Medicaid reimbursement. TJC provides and monitors accreditation status based on compliance with regulatory standards. Failure to meet TJC standards results in a potential loss of accreditation status, which may limit insurance payment for services provided.

One method for assessing quality in a systematic manner is through comparison of actual practice with clearly defined standards. A standard is a norm for an agreed-on level of practice. TJC (2005) identifies standards that set maximum achievable performance expectations for areas that affect health care quality. Standards do not explain or prescribe *how* to achieve compliance, but compliance must be clear to those reviewing practice: surveyors, consumers, and clinicians. Standards provide a direction for organizations, but leaders within the organization require vision to use the standards to achieve compliance.

In addition to TJC, other organizations are involved in establishing health care standards. The American Osteopathic Association, through their Healthcare Facilities Accreditation Program, accredits around 160 of the country's 6,000 acute care facilities. As with TJC, HFAP has deeming status through CMS, meaning that the organizations are able to survey for compliance with the Medicare Conditions of Participation; therefore their survey replaces the need for a survey by CMS.

The Center for Medicare and Medicaid Services was initiated as the Health Care Finance Authority in 1977. Through both Medicare and Medicaid, CMS provides health care coverage for 85 million Americans and identifies health care quality standards for 228,200 facilities, including laboratories, nursing homes, hospitals, home health care agencies, ambulatory surgery centers, and hospices. Through state inspection teams, CMS surveys health care suppliers and providers for compliance with federal health, safety, and quality standards of care. As with TJC and HFAP, CMS does not detail how to achieve compliance. Through their website (http://www.cms.hhs.gov/) clinicians and providers can access the Sharing Innovations in Quality site (SIQ) at http://www.cms.hhs.gov/medicaid/survey-cert/siqhome. asp. SIQ is a project providing collaboration between the CMS and state surveyors with professional, consumer, and industry representatives for health care. Creative ideas are collected and freely distributed throughout the country. Through the SIQ program, many suggestions for care improvement are shared. For example, one of the suggested protocols listed is that of prevention and treatment of constipation, authored by the Association of Rehabilitation Nurses.

TJC, HFAP, and CMS publish standards for varied health care environments. CARF publishes standards specific to rehabilitation environments. There are 38,000 CARF-accredited facilities in the world. CARF began standard development for medical rehabilitation programs in 1966. It is a private, nonprofit, nongovernmental standard-setting agency (CARF, 2005). CARF brings third-party payers, consumers, advocacy group representatives, and providers together to determine standards. After standard identification, CARF sends draft standards to payer representatives, consumers, advocacy group representatives, and providers throughout the country for review. CARF standards are recognized on an international level as reflective of rehabilitation quality. CARF promotes outcome-driven, value-based programs for individuals with disabilities and chronic illnesses.

Medicare is the in the process of transitioning quality measures for hospitals to a pay-for-performance system (Duff, 2002; Ebler, 2005). The Hospital Quality Initiative has two overall goals. First, the program is intended to provide consumers with information on care quality so that they are empowered to make informed decisions. Second, CMS (2005) hopes that providers will be encouraged to improve health care quality. The quality measures included in the quality initiative correspond with diseases that tend to cross specialty areas within the acute care hospital. Extensive debate exists over the problems and limitations of pay for performance, with providers and clinicians expressing dissatisfaction with the systems. Concerns include increased costs with data collection and questions regarding whether or not the changes will in fact change the quality of care. One clinician refers to the system as "pain for performance" (Susman, 2005). According to CMS (2005), initial trial of the pay-for-performance system is working to influence improvements in health care systems. At present the quality initiative does not impact rehabilitation programs. However, given that data, including quality data, are already submitted electronically to CMS, it is logical to assume that CMS will expand to the measurement of specific quality measures for inpatient rehabilitation.

Nursing Perspectives

Regulatory agencies mandate compliance with standards and requirements—even when the regulation may not be logical or in accordance with a specific patient need. Although there are many evidence-based reasons for the standards established by TJC and other regulatory agencies, rarely is the best reason for implementing a change that "TJC requires it." Quality standards established by CMS and TJC are not best practices, but minimal expectations. In contrast, nursing perspectives of quality include identification of best practices. Presented in this section is a discussion of the quality of nursing care.

The quality of nursing care has long been linked with caring, as demonstrated through identifying, responding to, and attending to the needs of patients (Carroll, 2005). The focus of nursing care is that of caring and the use of nursing knowledge to provide evidence-based nursing actions and interventions that will result in the optimal patient outcomes (Gunther & Alligood, 2002). Much study has been conducted on the impact of nurse staffing levels, registered nurse (RN) ratios, and patient acuity on patient outcomes and the quality of nursing care (Page, 2004). Studies have primarily been based in acute care settings, so the impact of RN ratios and staffing levels on quality and safety for rehabilitation units is not clear (Aiken, Clarke, Sloane, Sochalski, & Silber, 2002). According to the ARN (2006), nurse staffing should be based on a review of census, admissions, discharges, and intensity of nursing care required, in addition to the environmental architecture and geography, technology, and educational preparation and experiences of the nurses.

Through the California Nursing Outcome Coalition (CalNOC) project, data from 130 California facilities are routinely collected to evaluate nurse-sensitive outcomes measures, including specific nurse-patient ratios, nursing care delivery models, and nursing practice interventions (Seago, 2001). A similar project is underway with the Veterans

Administration. The Veterans Administration's Nursing Outcome Database (VANOD) will soon be a national project inclusive of all Veterans Administration hospitals (Aydin et al., 2004).

The impact of nursing care on patient outcomes is well documented. Nurse-sensitive indicators of quality have been defined by many researchers (Needleman, Buerhaus, Mattke, Stewart, & Zelevinsky, 2002) and are indicators that have a direct impact on patient outcomes. Nurse-sensitive indicators include urinary tract infection, pneumonia, shock, upper gastrointestinal bleeding, length of stay, failure to rescue, sepsis, deep venous thrombosis, falls, restraint use, and pressure ulcers.

The National Database of Nursing Quality Indicators (NDNQI) is a database of the American Nurses Association (ANA). It is the result of the ANA's Safety and Quality Initiative established in 1994 to identify the links between patient outcomes and nursing quality. The Safety and Quality Initiative resulted in the publication of *The Nursing Care Report Card for Acute Care*, which identified 21 measures with possible relationships to patient outcomes. After substantial evaluation and research, the national database indicators were selected. The NDNQI nurse-sensitive indicators are listed in Box 9-1 (Gallagher & Rowell, 2003).

Each of these indicators is applicable to the acute and subacute rehabilitation setting (Brillhart, 2005). Focus on nurse-sensitive indicators presents much potential to lead to significant positive changes in key areas of rehabilitation nursing. The quality of nursing care provided in rehabilitation settings has long been linked with the prevalence of pressure ulcers, urinary tract infections, and falls. The work on identification and measurement of nurse-sensitive indicators provides a framework for benchmarking rehabilitation nursing quality.

BOX 9-1 Nurse-Sensitive Indicators of Patient Outcomes

- Patient falls
- Pressure ulcers
- Physical/sexual assault
- Pain management
- Peripheral IV infiltration
- Staff mix:
  - Registered Nurses (RNs)
  - Licensed Practical/Vocational Nurses (LPNs/LVNs)
  - Unlicensed assistive personnel (UAP)
- Nursing care hours provided per patient day
- RN education/certification
- RN Satisfaction Survey

Permission to print requested from National Database of Nursing Quality Indicators. (2005). *About NDNQI*. Kansas City, KS: University of Kansas Medical Center.
IV, Intravenous.

Consumer Perspectives

Just as regulatory agencies and nurses have perspectives on indicators of quality, consumers of health care have different perspectives. The consumers' perspective of quality care includes care that is accessible, with high accountability for providers of health care. Consumers are demanding that providers act with their needs in mind and that quality information be transparent (Morath, 2003).

Although consumers have immediate access to a broad spectrum of information about health care organizations and quality, many do not review it and even fewer comprehend the information available. Health information literacy is limited for many consumers, with individuals embarrassed about their lack of understanding of information (Speros, 2005). The AHRQ provides extensive information for consumers, including MedlinePlus and Healthfinder (http://www.ahrq.gov/consumer/), yet there are numerous health care information Internet sites that are commercial in nature and do not present evidence-based perspectives. Health care consumers need to have education on identification of credible websites and health care information.

Identification of Quality Indicators Specific to Rehabilitation Nursing Practice

As noted previously in this chapter, quality indicators are identified through regulatory agencies; nursing groups such as NDNQI, CalNOC, and VANOD; and health care consumers. Quality indicators specific to rehabilitation nursing practice have not been identified. Rehabilitation units reporting to NDNQI submit nursing-sensitive outcome measures including skill mix, staffing ratios, patient falls, and pressure ulcers. Figure 9-1 presents possible quality indicators for rehabilitation nursing practice in a scorecard.

MEASUREMENT OF QUALITY INDICATORS

Quality Must Be Measurable

According to the ancient Roman lyric poet and satirist Horace, "There is a measure in everything" (http://www.quotationspage.com/quote/29249.html). Quality measures provide a system for quantification of care aspects against a specific criterion. Clinical performance measures are one form of quality measures. The National Quality Measures Clearinghouse (2005) identifies five key quality measures: access, outcome, process, structure, and patient experience (Box 9-2). Quality indicators must be measurable, and measurements must be valid and reliable to be meaningful. With respect to establishing measurable indicators of rehabilitation nursing quality, suggested measures are listed in Figure 9-1.

Standardized Tools for Quality Measurement

Many different tools are available for measurement of quality that are applicable to rehabilitation. These are described in the following section.

St. Hopeful Hospital

Nursing Scorecard

Indicator	Definition	Benchmark Information	Benchmark	Q2-03	Q3-03	Q4-03	Q1-04	Q2-04	Q3-04	Q4-04	Q1-05	Q2-05	Comments
Pressure Ulcers													
Pressure Ulcers	Quarterly prevalence study of hospital-acquired pressure ulcers	NDNQI benchmark: expressed as ratio for mean of peer hospitals	Ratio <1	1.1	1.2	0.7	0.6	1	0.9	0.5	1.4	0.5	
Medication Safety													
Medication safety	Process audit: review of medication process completed appropriately	Internal benchmark: expressed as number of positive observations divided by total number of observations	100%	N/A	N/A	N/A	N/A	N/A	N/A	100%	100%	100%	Part of CHS Quality Dashboard
Hospital Acquired Infection Prevention													
Hand hygiene	Compliance with hand hygiene policy	Internal benchmark: Expressed as number of positive observations divided by total number of observations	100%	1	N/A	N/A	N/A	53%	N/A	N/A	N/A	78%	
MRSA	Incidence of iatrogenic MRSA	National Nosocomial Infection Surveillance: 0.31 per 1000 patient days	<0.31	N/A	N/A	N/A	N/A	1.00	1.33	0.67	0.00	2.33	
VRE	Incidence of iatrogenic VRE	National Nosocomial Infection Surveillance: 0.15 per 1000 patient days	<.15	N/A	N/A	N/A	N/A	0.00	0.00	0.00	0.00	0.00	
Fall Prevention													
SCI Unit falls	Rate of falls per 1000 patient days	NDNQI benchmark: expressed as ratio for mean of peer hospitals	Ratio ≥1	1	1	1	1	1	1	1	1	0.459	
BI Unit falls	Rate of falls per 1000 patient days	NDNQI benchmark: expressed as ratio for mean of peer hospitals	Ratio ≥1	0.878	0.65	0.878	0.852	0.834	1.236	0.944	0.57	0.776	
Gero-rehab Unit falls	Rate of falls per 1000 patient days	NDNQI benchmark: expressed as ratio for mean of peer hospitals	Ratio ≥1	0.66	0.74	0.9	0.45	1.1	0.8	0.56	0.817	1.647	Added to NDNQI 2005
Ortho rehab Unit falls	Rate of falls per 1000 patient days	NDNQI benchmark: expressed as ratio for mean of peer hospitals	Ratio ≥1	1	1	0.8	1	1	1	0.9	0.667	0.906	Will be added to NDNQI mid-2005

Figure 9-1 Application of concepts: nursing scorecard. Because of the recognition of the impact of nursing care on patient outcomes, routine assessment of nursing quality is essential. Nurse-sensitive indicators of patient outcomes recommended through the National Database for Nursing Quality Indicators (NDNQI) provide information and benchmarking.

BOX 9-2 Types of Quality Measures

Type of Measure	Description	Rehabilitation Example
Access	These quantify ability of patients to receive health care in a timely and appropriate manner.	Ability for patient meeting admission criteria to obtain placement in rehabilitation program.
Outcome	Assessment of the impact of health care services on the outcome experienced by the patient.	Discharge to home independent in dressing, following a cerebrovascular accident.
Structure	Collection of information related to the capacity of the organization to provide quality health care.	Measurement of the nurse-patient ratio for a rehabilitation unit.
Process	Measurement of the components or elements of care provided to the patient.	Audit of the medication administration process.
Patient experience	Assessment of the patient perception of the health care experience.	Collection of patient satisfaction ratings and the likelihood of recommending the facility to friends and family members.

National Quality Measures Clearinghouse. (2005). *Using measures*. Rockville, MD: Author.

Functional Independence Measure. Developed by the Uniform Data System for Medical Rehabilitation (UDSMR) (2005), the Functional Independence Measure (FIM) is used to measure rehabilitation patient outcomes in facilities throughout the world, and it is considered a standard and reliable measure of patient outcomes. Over 800 comprehensive inpatient rehabilitation programs and more than 130 postacute rehabilitation programs in the United States participate in the UDSMR database. The data obtained through FIM allow evaluation of rehabilitation service efficiency and efficacy. In addition, the FIM instrument is a key component of the Inpatient Rehabilitation Facility–Patient Assessment Instrument (IRFPAI), which is used to determine prospective payment rates for all rehabilitation patients with Medicare as the payer. More information on FIM is available in Chapter 11 and online at http://www.udsmr.org.

Minimum Data Set. The Minimum Data Set (MDS) is a component of the Resident Assessment Instrument (RAI). Initiated in 1990 by the Centers for Medicare and Medicaid Services for regulatory purposes, the RAI provides a means for integration of clinical data into regulatory oversight. The MDS is a standardized, regulated assessment database that is used by clinical staff members in long-term care to plan and organize the care that is provided. In 1998 the MDS became the tool through which long-term care facilities receive their Medicare reimbursement determination in the prospective payment system for long-term care. The MDS contains elements that are linked with quality of care (Zimmerman, 2003). Twenty-four indicators cover 12 care aspects: accidents, clinical management, incontinence, cognitive patterns, nutrition, skin care, quality of life, physical functioning, psychotropic drug use, sensory functioning, emotional functioning, and infection control. Through the electronic submission of the MDS, CMS is able to review the quality of care given to the nation's 2 million nursing home residents, living in over 17,000 facilities (Meiller, 2001). The process is explained in

Chapter 11. The MDS can be accessed through the HCFA website (http://www.cms.hhs.gov/medicaid/mds20/).

Health Status Questionnaires. The Medical Outcomes Trust (2001) is a Massachusetts-based not-for-profit organization involved in the development and standardization of outcome measurement instruments for health care. The SF-36 is one of the instruments developed by the Medical Outcomes Trust and is intended for assessment of health status or quality of life. It contains 36 items that are reflective of health status and outcomes from the patient's perspective. The instrument measures limitations in physical activities, usual role activities, body pain, health perceptions, vitality, limitations in social activities, and mental health. It can be administered by telephone, by computer, or in person. The SF-36 can be accessed at http://www.sf-36.org/. The SF-36 has limitations for use in the rehabilitation population unless the physical activity scale is appropriately worded for persons using wheelchairs. The survey has been modified into shorter versions (SF-12, SF-8) and has been translated into 50 languages. All forms of the survey have been extensively studied and validated in many different ethnic groups. The tools are easy to use and are available in either electronic or paper forms.

Disability-Specific Rating Scales and Outcome Scales. Many global and specific rating scales exist for varied aspects of rehabilitation, disability, and functional impairment. For example, for assessment of individuals with traumatic brain injury, the following scales exist:
- Prognostic Score of Ong et al. for Predicting Poor Outcome After Pediatric Head Injury
- Outcome Prediction Score of Combes et al. for Adults With Severe Head Injury
- Risk Factors for Death or Severe Disability in Comatose Patients
- The Rappaport Disability Rating Scale (DRS)
- The Supervision Rating Scale (SRS)

- Differential Outcome Scale (DOS) After Head Injury
- The Rancho Los Amigos Cognitive Scale After Brain Injury (Levels of Cognitive Functioning Scale)
- The Extended Glasgow Outcome Scale

A limitation with some of these and other scales is the amount of testing done for validity and reliability. Rehabilitation nurses should review the literature associated with specific scales to ensure the test is valid and reliable. A comprehensive listing of scales, including links to the scale and scoring information, is available through the Medical Algorithms Project (Svirbely & Iyengar, 2006). The project includes 9600 algorithms, with access provided to 340 algorithms. Registration is free through http://www.medal.org/visitor.

Outcome and Assessment Information Set. The Outcome and Assessment Information Set (OASIS) is a comprehensive assessment system for adult home health care patients. Developed by CMS and implemented in 1999, OASIS includes sociodemographic, environmental, support system, functional status, and health status information for adults receiving home health care. This tool is intended to provide the CMS with quality and outcome information for home health care patients throughout the nation (Kinatukara, Rosati, & Huang, 2005). OASIS can be accessed at http://www.cms.hhs.gov/oasis/.

Compliance and Integrity

Beyond quality and standard attainment are issues with compliance and integrity. A top priority of CMS is the integrity of the Medicare and Medicaid programs. The compliance and integrity efforts of the CMS are directed toward paying the right providers the right amount for reasonable, necessary, covered services. Antifraud efforts are a major focus of the Office of the Inspector General, with $268 million recovered in Medicare fraud through fines, restitutions, penalties, settlements, and 1,096 convictions. In light of such issues, it is imperative that health care organizations work diligently to demonstrate quality initiatives, error prevention strategies, patient safety efforts, and organizational integrity programs.

QUALITY DATA COLLECTION

Data collection processes typically involve patient interviews, surveys, record reviews, and observations. In the Six Sigma process of data collection, the following steps are used (Parker, 2003):

1. *Rationale for data collection is clear to those responsible for obtaining data.* Staff members need to know why data are being collected and what will be done with the data once they are collected. As an illustration, in one organization the nurse manager was concerned about the amount of overtime required by staff members. She asked each nurse to document why overtime was needed. The nurses became upset because they felt the nurse manager was concerned with a misuse of overtime. When the nurse manager noticed the tension among staff members, she asked them why they were upset. She explained that she requested the data because she was actually worried about their need for overtime. She hoped to provide better supports so that nurses would be able to leave work at the scheduled time. Once this was corrected, she was able to complete the study.

2. *Whenever possible, use a noninvolved individual for data collection.* Using individuals who are not members of a particular unit or department may provide more reliable results because they are less apt to be influenced by the need for a particular outcome. As an example, if audits of the medication administration process are completed, the data will be less susceptible to bias if collected by staff members from others departments.

3. *Ensure that stratification of data collected by shift, location, or supplier is considered before data collection.* As an example, one organization targeted a falls prevention program for the night shift, because they believed more patients fell during the night. The data were reviewed and stratified by shift and location, and it was discovered that more falls occurred toward the end of the evening shift. Given this information, the strategies for fall prevention were altered and the focus was modified to the evening shift.

4. *Keep collection processes as simple as possible.* The more cumbersome the process, the less apt individuals are to be able to complete it accurately.

5. *Use columns for data collection, rather than rows to facilitate data transposition.* Using columns should enable easy input from collection form to the data analysis form.

6. *Provide training for those collecting data.* As an example, an organization recently changed to an all-electronic system. During the initial audit of the records, some of those auditing did not understand the new forms and were not able to accurately audit the records. This resulted in poor results. The results were more due to an ineffective audit process rather than the change to an electronic record.

7. *Complete a trial of the data collection tool before full implementation.* Data collection requires time. It is better to collect a few samples and then modify the tool than to collect substantial amounts of data that do not have utility for analysis.

QUALITY CONTROL AND IMPROVEMENT TOOLS

Benchmarking

Benchmarking is a tool used to identify best practices for specific indicators. In rehabilitation the incidence of hospital-acquired pressure ulcers is an indicator that sometimes is used for benchmarking. Rehabilitation nurses within the organization use the information and strive to be better than average and to excel to best-practice level. The NDNQI provides an opportunity for rehabilitation units to benchmark information on nursing hours per patient day, skill mix, patient falls, and pressure ulcers with other units. Benchmarks may be displayed in many styles, including graphs, control charts, and radar diagrams. Presented in Figure 9-2 is a radar diagram of fall rates against a national benchmark. The oraganization's results in July indicate a significant increase in fall rates.

When the nursing quality committee drilled into the increase, the staff nurses on the committee reported that the organization had changed brands of a slipper socks. One of the nurses complained that two of her patients had fallen because of the slipper socks. Nurses from the quality committee took pairs of the new slipper socks home and learned that only 2 hours of consistent use was needed to wear off the tread from the socks. The original change in product had been done based on expense savings, but the product had not been tested before purchase. Based on the nursing feedback and the results of the nursing quality committee trial, the product was removed from stock and the former product was reinstated. As a result, falls within the organization in August returned to the prior rate.

Audits

Audits are a key method of quality of care assessment. Often, the only way to identify trends or issues is through a careful audit of records. In a recent quality issue, a rehabilitation program manager was concerned that four of the recent admissions to rehabilitation from acute care required transfer to intensive care within 24 hours of admission. On audit of the records, it was noted that each of the patients had been evaluated for admission more than 72 hours before transfer. In each case, a call before discharge from acute care services might have alerted the program manager to changes in status that would affect the individual's ability to safely participate in 3 hours or more of daily therapy. The issue was corrected through incorporating such screening calls.

Brainstorming

One technique that has been used for many years in looking at problem resolution to quality issues is brainstorming.

The rules for brainstorming sessions are simple: members of the quality team suggest as many solutions and alternatives as possible without critique. During brainstorming sessions, participants gain momentum by contributing ideas quickly and without debate. All suggestions are written and evaluated at a later time. In this manner, individuals are able just to focus on creative solutions without concern about rejection.

Cause-and-Effect Diagramming

The cause-and-effect, or "fish bone," diagram is a quality control tool (Figure 9-3). It is used for identification of causes of a quality problem and often is used in combination with a brainstorming session. A cause-and-effect diagram method identifies basic categories that can help reduce irrelevant discussion and complaints.

Check Sheets

A fundamental tool for quality control is a check sheet used for data collection (Figure 9-4). The check sheet provides a standardized method of systematically collecting and recording facts. Review of completed check sheets is done to analyze data, determine patterns, and arrive at conclusions.

Flowchart

With many quality control issues, it is difficult to determine why a problem exists. Flowcharts document all steps included in a process from start to finish. Once the flowchart is complete, each step is reviewed for possible problems and opportunities for improvement (Figure 9-5).

Pareto Chart

Asserted in the Pareto principle is that 20% of the problems are responsible for 80% of the effects. Using a Pareto chart enables the user to focus on the primary issues or defects rather than trying to tackle all problems. A Pareto chart is created by listing (in descending order of frequency) all problems occurring in a process (Figure 9-6).

CAUTIONS WITH QUALITY IMPROVEMENT EFFORTS

Retrospective Versus Prospective Quality Reviews

One may complete quality reviews of processes and records either after the event is completed (retrospective) or as events are occurring (prospective). Retrospective reviews typically involve closed records and collected data and are relatively easy to complete. Such reviews require time for document perusal but do not necessitate extensive tracking systems because the individuals completing the review identify the files with appropriate information before the data collection period. In contrast, prospective reviews require tracking of information as it occurs. This can be difficult, particularly in inpatient settings, where there are three shifts of nurses spanning 24 hours of care. Although retrospective reviews are sometimes easier to complete, the information gleaned may be

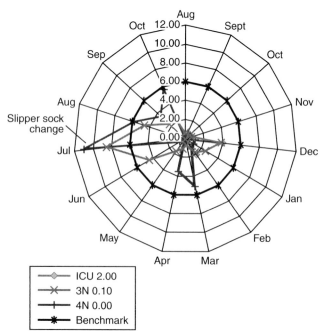

Figure 9-2 Radar diagram of fall rates.

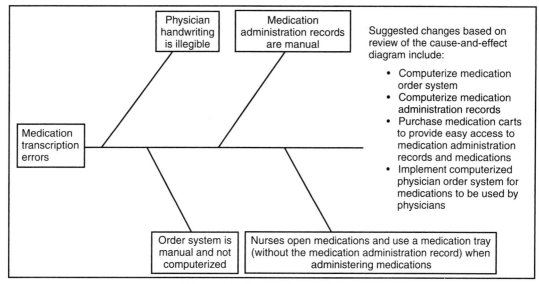

Figure 9-3 Cause-and-effect diagram.

Pain management audit	Pain assessed and documented on admission (1 = yes; 0 = no)	Pain assessed with every assessment of vital signs (No. of times pain/vital signs assessed)	Pain assessed before administration of analgesics (No. of times pain assessed/ analgesics administered)	Pain relief assessed after administration of analgesics (No. of times pain assessed/ analgesics administered)
MR #1234567	1	10/12	3/5	3/5
MR #2345678	1	5/13	3/3	2/3
MR #1345678	1	4/20	4/6	4/6
MR #3452345	1	20/24	4/7	3/7
MR #5899657	1	30/30	2/2	2/2
MR #0986389	0	3/3	1/1	0/1
Summary	5/6 = 83%	72/102 = 70.5%	17/24 = 71%	14/24 = 58%

Figure 9-4 Check sheet example.

less conclusive than those data collected through prospective reviews. Clinicians tend to find information through retrospective reviews that is easily detectable. For example, identifying the incidence of documented complications to anticoagulation therapy through retrospective review would entail reviewing records for evidence of deep venous thrombosis, hematomas, and gastrointestinal bleeding. Such a review would not be difficult to complete. Taking a prospective look at the same issue, however, can result in a more comprehensive picture of the efficacy of anticoagulation therapy. As an example, in a prospective review of anticoagulation therapy, a data collection sheet would be developed through a team

effort to identify as many components and contributing factors to complications with anticoagulation therapy as possible. The data collection sheets would be completed by members of the rehabilitation team and forwarded for analysis to the team leader or facilitator.

Costs

Although it is no longer accepted that higher quality is equated with higher cost, one must not assume that quality does not have a price. Expenses are associated with quality care. As an example, in a spinal injury program at a large freestanding rehabilitation hospital, the nurses place at-risk patients

Issue: Patients complain that breakfast trays are cold and that they do not have time to eat breakfast. Therapists find patients are frequently late for the first therapy session.

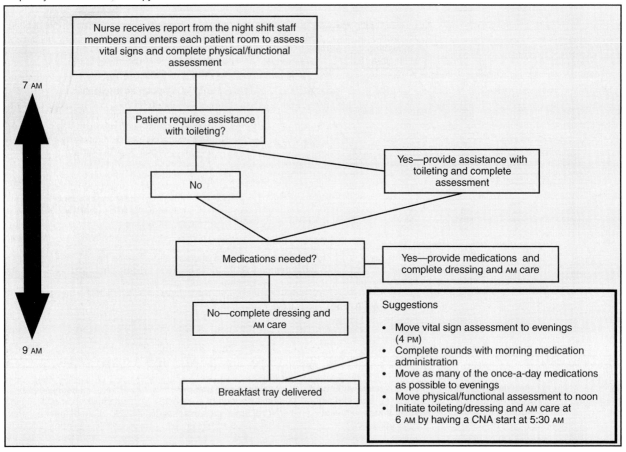

Figure 9-5 Flowchart example.

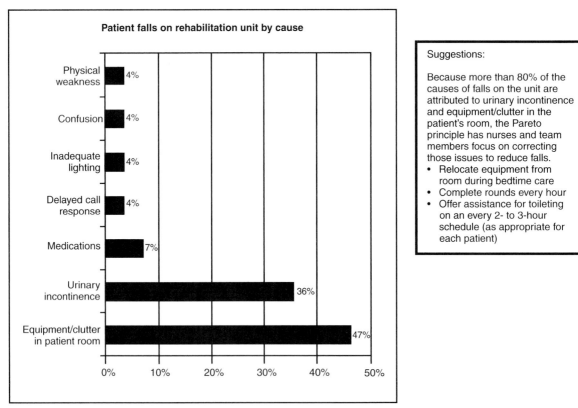

Figure 9-6 Pareto chart example.

in specially designed pressure-relief boots. The boots cost about $150 for each boot, or $300 per pair. The incidence of rehabilitation hospital–acquired heel pressure ulcers is 0%. Although the cost is high, it is thousands of dollars less than the cost of time, care, and treatment associated with a pressure ulcer. It is sometimes necessary to spend a few dollars to save many. This is an example of the importance of research on the cost benefit of treatments and preventive measures (see Chapter 4).

OUTCOME ASSESSMENT

Most aspects of quality control and improvement apply to all health care programs; however, two additional methods— outcome management and functional outcome measurement— are somewhat uncommon but key to the rehabilitation field. Outcome management systems provide a holistic glimpse of the rehabilitation program. Functional outcome studies contribute the "so what?" data for rehabilitation or, in other words, provide substantiation that the rehabilitation expense results in functional gains.

Functional Outcome Studies

Studies on functional outcomes provide information on the essence of rehabilitation results. Although not every individual who enters a rehabilitation program will ambulate and return home, outcome studies give data on the probability of such occurrences. Outcome studies may link the individual's length of stay in a program with the cost and efficacy of the program. Review of such information should weigh the cost of the program against the benefit of the functional gain. At one time in rehabilitation (15 to 20 years ago), the criteria for continued treatment included continued progress, even if this progress was quite slight. However, in this age of health care reform, it is not acceptable to continue creating expense for functional gains that do not enhance the level of independence and lessen the dependence on the health care system.

Related to the legitimate concerns about the cost of rehabilitation and to the proliferation of rehabilitation programs and types of programs, functional outcomes from rehabilitation must be substantiated. In assessing outcomes from a rehabilitation program, one must consider the amount of experience with specific disability types and basic outcome quality indicators. Specifically the outcomes of patients with regard to quality of life, discharge disposition, and self-care independence should be appraised.

Outcome studies are not new to health care or to nursing. Perhaps the first individual to consider health care and nursing outcomes seriously was Florence Nightingale. The outcome measure by which she looked at success was mortality. After she began work with British soldiers, she found a 30% reduction in mortality levels within 6 months (Nutting, Dock, & Dock, 1907) through the incorporation of hand washing and promotion of infection control measures.

Specific outcomes for rehabilitation nursing practice have been documented in the literature. Higgins and Daly (2005) studied failure to thrive in adult patients admitted for long-term rehabilitation and found that the difference in discharge destination was linked with mood, age, nutritional status, cognitive impairment, and physical function. They found that the better the functional outcome, the more likely the patient was to return home. Failure to thrive was linked with depression, low plasma albumin, and inability to return home. Higgins (2005) studied time of entry into cardiac rehabilitation programs. Prompt admission to cardiac rehabilitation was correlated with lower patient anxiety levels. These studies are just two of many linking rehabilitation nursing care with a positive impact on functional outcomes and cost-effectiveness.

SUMMARY

Quality control and improvement have become an integral part of health care and rehabilitation nursing during the past two decades. As administrators and clinicians focus on defining quality and identifying customer satisfaction with services provided, standard-setting agencies such as TJC work toward redefining the quality assessment process. Clinical application of research into practice is critical for improvement in quality and safety (refer to Chapter 4). The time lag between clinical research and patient care may be years; it can be shortened through incorporating review of releevent research with quality improvement projects.

Issues with quality control have shifted to patient safety, as is discussed in Chapter 10, with an emphasis on outcomes and compliance with federally mandated standards. A primary challenge to clinicians is to transcend traditional departmental boundaries and work to refine processes. One current trend is to look at a 24-hour team for quality improvement (Bader, Palmer, Stalcup, & Shaver, 2002). In the 24-hour quality-improvement program the key elements are captured through the mnemonic *FOCUS-PDCA*:

F ind a need for improvement
O rganize knowledgeable staff members into a team
C larify current information about the system
U nderstand causes of problems in the system
S elect methods for improvement and
P lan
D o
C heck
A ct

It is imperative in the current and future climates of financial exigencies that rehabilitation nurses constantly focus on doing more with less expense. Basic concepts of any quality control program include an organizational commitment to quality and patient safety, a focus on patient satisfaction, an empowerment of clinicians and staff members, a loss of department "territoriality" or specific links between quality threats or improvements and patient outcome, and rewards for quality improvement. Rehabilitation nursing has made steps toward identifying positive outcomes of rehabilitation nursing on patients. However, extensive work is needed in identifying and monitoring the outcome of rehabilitation nursing care. Rehabilitation nurses must not lose the focus on function and ability during this era of safety.

Case Study

Toni, a 91-year-old woman from Houston, was visiting her daughter in Boston. On the first Sunday night of her visit, Toni experienced a cerebrovascular accident involving the left hemisphere of her brain and resulting in right-sided hemiplegia and mild dysphagia. The stroke was witnessed by her daughter, who is a nurse. An ambulance was called, and within 32 minutes Toni was seen in the local emergency department. Based on the Cincinnati Stroke Scale, the paramedics identified Toni as having three abnormal ratings within the three items on the scale. This information was provided in the patch given by the paramedics to the hospital emergency department. The diagnosis of stroke was validated in the emergency department through performance of the NIH Stroke Scale, on which Toni scored 15.

An intravenous infusion of normal saline at a rate of 100 ml/hour was initiated. A computerized tomography scan was completed, showing no evidence of intercerebral bleeding. Because Toni was from out of town and had no local primary care provider, the hospitalist was consulted and determined admission to be necessary.

Although she was 91 years of age, Toni had no preexisting health care problems. Her only daily medication was a multivitamin. Before the stroke Toni was functionally independent and lived alone in an elderly housing apartment in Houston. Because the occupancy within the hospital was quite high on the night she was admitted and her electrocardiogram (ECG) showed normal sinus rhythm, Toni was placed on a general medical unit.

Two days after her admission, Toni's granddaughter, a physician from Emory University Hospital in Atlanta, called to express concern about her grandmother's care. She stated that the nurses had been quite attentive; however, she had concerns about the medical care received by her grandmother. She stated that Toni repeatedly rubbed her chest to indicate that she had pain, and she did not understand why she was not on telemetry monitoring. She wanted to know why Toni had not received tissue plasminogen activator (TPA) for her stroke, because her arrival and time seen by the emergency physician was well within the 3-hour limit. In addition, she had concerns with the hospitalist, who had not returned her calls, and with the neurologist, whom she had difficulty understanding and who refused to order testing that was considered standard at Emory. The granddaughter wanted to know if the hospital had a specialty program for

stroke and if her grandmother would receive rehabilitation, which at Emory would have been initiated by this point in her stay. She stated that her grandmother's treatment for stroke seemed reflective of ageism and a lack of quality within the organization.

Following review of the situation, a cardiologist was consulted and Toni was placed on telemetry monitoring. She had a pattern of paroxysmal atrial fibrillation, which had not been identified on the intermittent ECGs. Toni was placed on atenolol to lower her heart rate and Coumadin to reduce the risk of further thromboembolic events.

Returning to the opening case study and Toni's situation, an interdisciplinary team was organized to review care provided within the organization for patients with acute stroke. The American Heart Association's Get With the Guidelines for Stroke was reviewed. In addition, the guidelines from TJC for acute stroke programs were analyzed, and a gap analysis was completed. The CARF standards for stroke rehabilitation programs were reviewed, and a gap analysis was completed. The protocol for the stroke response team was revised. A special code was implemented with mock codes completed to promote education. One year later, the team was able to apply for CARF and TJC accreditation for the organization's stroke program.

CRITICAL THINKING

1. Stroke is the third leading cause of death. It is treated within all acute care settings. There are many initiatives the TJC and AHA programs, to improve the care provided to individuals experiencing stroke. The case study illustates the problems in assuming that stroke is just another illness and that care will be the same in any emergency setting. Discuss ways of introducing research literature (e.g., on the use of tPA) to clinical improvement committees.

2. Few rehabilitation units have access to telemetry monitoring. As an example of quality improvement, discuss pros and cons of telemetry monitoring for acute inpatient rehabilitation.

3. The concept of "designated stroke unit" is an accreditation conundrum. Does the strategy of accreditation program designation, etc. improve the care and outcome of patients? How?

In the preceding case, the questions of quality and system failures are appropriate—for example, in the administration of TPA. Although Toni had a witnessed stroke and an appropriate assessment by the responding paramedics indicating stroke, with the use of the Cincinnati Prehospital Stroke Scale (Nor et al., 2004), the stroke team at the hospital was not activated. Had the stroke team been activated, Toni would have been seen by the neurologist in the emergency department, rather than the following day. In review of the case, the paramedics did not activate the stroke team, because they were both new to the ambulance service and did not know that the hospital had a stroke team. Due to Toni's advanced

age of 91 years, the emergency department staff members did not activate the stroke team arrival at the hospital. Although the landmark study completed by the National Institute of Neurological Disorders and Stroke (NINDS) (2000) study group indicated the risk of adverse reaction to TPA could be increased with advanced age, recent studies have questioned this result (Mouradian et al., 2005), with case reports of successful treatment with TPA for individuals as old as 100 years (Gorman, Tanne, & Lewandowski, 2002). Although the timing of Toni's care was appropriate, the neurological consult was delayed, and she was not considered for TPA administration because of out-of-date guidelines in the hospital's emergency department protocol for acute stroke. Given her excellent premorbid health and low risk factors (aside from advanced age), TPA administration might have made a difference in her overall outcome. Demaershalk and Yip (2005) note in the study from the Mayo Clinic that only 2% of the 616,000 new ischemic stroke patients who might benefit from TPA actually receive the medication. Intervention with TPA is not done more often for a variety of reasons, most frequently due to a failure to seek timely emergency care. The researchers estimate that $600 would be saved for each TPA-treated patient. Therefore, if the percentage of appropriately treated stroke patients increased to just 20%, the annual cost savings in the country would be $74 million. Given such information, the granddaughter was accurate in questioning the quality of the care Toni received on admission to the hospital.

The organization's response to the above incident included a full review of the literature and evidence-based practices. Stroke team activations were reviewed, and the protocols were rewritten. As a result of Toni's incident, practices within the organization were examined, reviewed, and revised.

REFERENCES

Agency for Healthcare Quality and Research. (2005). *Guide to healthcare quality: How to know it when you see it* (AHRQ Publication No. 05-0088). Rockville, MD: Author.

Aiken, L., Clarke, S., Sloane, D., Sochalski, J., & Silber, J. (2002). Hospital nurse staffing and patient mortality, nurse burnout, and job dissatisfaction. *Journal of the American Medical Association, 288*(16), 1987-1993.

American Hospital Association. (2005). AHA comment letter on Medicare Inpatient Rehab Facility PPS for FY 2006 Proposed Rule. Accessed October 15, 2005, from http://www.hospitalconnect.com/aha/key_issues/rehab/content/20050718comment.pdf.

Association of Rehabilitation Nurses. (2006). Factors to consider in decisions about staffing in rehabilitation nursing settings. Accessed July 4, 2006, from http://www.rehabnurse.org/profresources/pstaff.html.

Aydin, C., Bolton, L., Donaldson, N., Brown, D., Buffum, M., Elashoff, J, et al. (2004). Creating and analyzing a statewide nursing quality measurement database. *Journal of Nursing Scholarship, 36*(4), 371-378.

Bader, M., Palmer, S., Stalcup, C., & Shaver, T. (2002). Using a FOCUS-PDCA quality improvement model for applying the severe traumatic brain injury guidelines to practice: Process and outcomes. *The Online Journal for Knowledge Synthesis in Nursing, 9*(4C).

Brillhart, B. (2005). Pressure sore and skin tear prevention and treatment during a 10-month program. *Rehabilitation Nursing, 30*(3), 85-91.

CARF. The Rehabilitation Accreditation Commission. (2005). *2005 Medical rehabilitation standards manual.* Tucson, AZ: Author.

Carroll, V. (2005). Is patient safety synonymous with quality nursing care? Should it be? A brief discourse. *Quality and Management in Health Care, 14*(4), 229-233.

Centers for Medicare & Medicaid Services. (2005). *Hospital quality initiative overview.* Baltimore, MD: Author. Available from http://www.cms.hhs.gov/quality/hospital/overview.pdf.

Chen, C., Iguchi, Y., Grotta, J., Garami, Z., Uchino, K., Shaltoni, H., et al. (2005). Intravenous TPA for very old stroke patients. *European Neurology, 54*(3), 140-144.

Congdon, J., & Magilvy, J. (2004). Hallmarks of quality: Generating knowledge to assist consumers of long-term care. *Community Nursing Research, 37*, 37, 39-49.

Demaershalk, B., & Yip, T. (2005). Economic benefit of increasing utilization of intravenous tissue plasminogen activator for acute ischemic stroke in the United States. *Stroke, 36*(11), 2500-2503.

Deming, W. E. (2000). *Condensation of the 14 points for management.* Washington, DC: W. Edwards Deming Institute. Available from http://www.deming.org/theman/teachings02.html.

Department of Health and Human Services for the Domestic Policy Council. (1998, June 17). *The challenge and potential for assuring quality health care for the 21st century* (Publication No. OM 98-0009). Washington, DC: Author.

Duff, S. (2002). Paying more for results: CMS tries to enlist Premier to tie hospital reimbursement to quality performance. *Modern Healthcare, 32*(37), 9.

Durieux, P., Bissery, A., Dubois, S., Gasquet, I., & Coste, J. (2004). Comparison of health care professionals' self-assessment of standards of care and patients' opinions on the care they received in hospital: Observational study. *Quality and Safety in Health Care, 13*(3), 198-202.

Ebler, J. (2005). The next payment model: Reimbursement based only on quality of care is coming soon. *Modern Healthcare, 35*(22), 22.

Gallagher, R., & Rowell, P. (2003). Claiming the future of nursing through nursing-sensitive quality indicators. *Nursing Administration Quarterly, 27*(4), 273-284.

Gorman, M., Tanne, D., & Lewandowski, C. (2002). Centenarian stroke treated with tissue-type plasminogen activator. *Cerebrovascular Diseases, 13*(4), 285-287.

Gunter, M., & Alligood, M. (2002). A discipline-specific determination of high quality nursing care. *Journal of Advanced Nursing, 38*(4), 353-359.

Harrison, R. (2005). Psychological assessment during cardiac rehabilitation. *Nursing Standard, 19*(27), 33-36.

Higgins, P., & Daly, B. (2005). Adult failure to thrive in the older rehabilitation patient. *Rehabilitation Nursing, 30*(4), 152-159.

Husch, M., Sullivan, C., Rooney, D., Barnard, C., Fotis, M., Clarke, J., et al. (2005). Insights from the sharp end of intravenous medication errors: Implications for infusion pump technology. *Quality and Safety in Health Care, 14*(2), 80-86.

Idvall, E., Hamrin, E., Sjöström, B., & Unosson, M. (2002). Patient and nurse assessment of quality of care in postoperative pain management. *Quality and Safety in Health Care, 11*(4), 327-334.

Joint Commission on Accreditation of Healthcare Organizations. (2005). *Comprehensive accreditation manual for hospitals: The official handbook (CAMH).* Oakbrook Terrace, IL: Author.

Kinatukara, S., Rosati, R., & Huang, L. (2005). Assessment of OASIS reliability and validity using several methodological approaches. *Home Health Care Service Quarterly, 24*(3), 23-38.

Kizer, K., & Stegun, M. (2002). Serious reportable adverse events in healthcare. In *Advances in patient safety: From research to implementation* (Vol. 4, AHRQ Publication No. 050021-4, pp. 339-352). Rockville, MD: Agency for Healthcare Research and Quality. Available from http://www.ahrq.gov/qual/advances/.

Kohn, L., Corrigan, J., & Donaldson, M. (Eds.). (1999). *To err is human: Building a safer health system.* Washington, DC: National Academy Press.

Lang, N., & Kizer, K. (2003). Public policy: National quality forum, an experiment in democracy. *Journal of Professional Nursing, 19*(5), 247-248.

Manian, F., Senkel, D., Zack, J., & Meyer, L. (2002). Routine screening for methicillin-resistant *Staphylococcus aureus* among patients newly admitted to an acute rehabilitation unit. *Infection Control Hospital Epidemiology, 23*(9), 516-519.

Medical Outcomes Trust. (2001). *The Trust home page.* Boston, MA: Medical Outcomes Trust.

Meiller, R. (2001). *Quality indicators keep nursing care on track.* Madison: University of Wisconsin-Madison.

Moncur, M. (2005). *The quotations page,* http://www.quotationspage.com/quote/29249.html.

Morath, J. (2003). Changing the healthcare culture: The consumer as part of the system of care. *Front Health Service Management, 19*(4):17-28.

Morimoto, T., Gandhi, T., Seger, A., Hsieh, T., & Bates, D. (2004). Adverse drug events and medication errors: Detection and classification methods. *Quality and Safety in Health Care, 13*(4), 306-314.

Mouradian, M. S, Senthilselvan, A., Jickling, G., McCombe, J. A., Emery, D. J., Dean, N., et al. (2005). Intravenous rt-PA for acute stroke: Comparing its effectiveness in younger and older patients. *Journal of Neurological and Neurosurgical Psychiatry, 76*(9), 1234-1237.

National Quality Forum. (2002a). *Hospital care national performance measures (group 1).* Washington, DC: National Forum for Healthcare Quality Measurement and Reporting.

National Quality Forum. (2002b). *Serious reportable events in healthcare: A consensus report.* Washington, DC: National Forum for Healthcare Quality Measurement and Reporting.

National Quality Forum. (2005). *NQF: Mission.* Available from http://www.qualityforum.org/mission/home.htm.

National Quality Measures Clearinghouse. (2005). *Using measures.* Rockville, MD: Author.

Needleman, J., Buerhaus, P., Mattke, S., Stewart, M., & Zelevinsky, K. (2002). Nurse staffing levels and the quality of care in hospitals. *New England Journal of Medicine, 346*(22), 1715-1722.

NINDS. (2000). Effect of intravenous recombinant tissue plasminogen activator on ischemic stroke lesion size measured by computed tomography. NINDS; The National Institute of Neurological Disorders and Stroke (NINDS) rt-PA Stroke Study Group. *Stroke, 31*(12), 2912-2919.

Nor, A., McAllister, C., Louw, S. J., Dyker, A. G., Davis, M., Jenkinson, D, et al. (2004). Agreement between ambulance paramedic- and physician-recorded neurological signs with Face Arm Speech Test (FAST) in acute stroke patients. *Stroke, 35*(6), 1355-1359.

Nutting, M., Dock, A., & Dock, L. (1907). *A history of nursing.* New York: G.P. Putnam's Sons.

Page, A. (Ed.). (2004). *Keeping patients safe: Transforming the work environment of nurses.* Washington, DC: Institute of Medicine of The National Academies Press.

Parker, K. (2003). Asking the right questions is the key to data collection. *iSix Sigma.* Available from http://www.isixsigma.com/library/content/c031117a.asp.

Rao, P., Boradia P., & Ennis, J. (2005). Shift happens: Using outcomes to survive conditions under PPS. *Topics in Stroke Rehabilitation, 12*(2), 1-3.

Reason, J. (2000). Human error: *Models and management. BMJ, 320*(7237), 768-770

Seago, J. (2001, July). Nurse staffing, models of care delivery, and interventions. In *Making health care safer: A critical analysis of patient safety practices. Evidence report/technology assessment: Number 43* (AHRQ Publication No. 01-E058). Rockville, MD: Agency for Healthcare Research and Quality. Available from http://www.ahrq.gov/clinic/ptsafety/.

Senst, B., Achusim, L., Genest, R., Cosentino, L., Ford, C., Little, J., et al. (2001). Practical approach to determining costs and frequency of adverse drug events in a health care network. *American Journal of Health System Pharmacists, 58*(12), 1126-1132.

Speros, C. (2005). Healthcare literacy: Concept analysis. *Journal of Advanced Nursing, 50*(6), 633-640.

Susman, J. (2005). P4P—Pain for performance? *Journal of Family Practice, 54*(8), 648.

Svirbely, J., & Iyengar, M. (2006). *The medical algorithm project.* Retrieved July 4, 2006, from http://www.medal.org/visitor/.

Uniform Data System for Medical Rehabilitation. (2005). *Uniform Data System for Medical Rehabilitation.* New York: U. B. Foundation Activities.

Zimmerman, D. (2003). Improving nursing home quality of care through outcomes data: The MDS quality indicators. *International Journal of Geriatric Psychiatry, 18*(13), 250-247

10

Patient Safety for Persons With Disabilities

Audrey Nelson, PhD, RN, FAAN

The goal of rehabilitation is to continually reduce the burden of illness, injury, and disability and to improve health and functional status (Institute of Medicine [IOM], 2001). Medical errors and preventable adverse effects seriously jeopardize attainment of this goal. Errors and adverse events may potentiate illness or injury, delay rehabilitation, impede healing and rehabilitation progress, and compromise patient safety, with resulting deleterious effects on patient functional status and quality of life.

Patient safety emerged as a national health care priority in 1999, when the report *To Err Is Human* was published by the Institute of Medicine (1999). Findings from this report can be summarized by six key points:

1. Medical errors and adverse events are serious problems occurring in even the best facilities and involving the most competent and caring health care professions.
2. Although there is a natural tendency to blame the direct care provider involved with an error or adverse event, these problems are more often the result of poorly designed health care systems and organizational policies that detract from patient safety and "set up" the provider to fail.
3. Lessons to be learned and best practices can be applied to health care from other complex, high-risk industries, such as aviation and nuclear power.
4. The sciences of human factors engineering and cognitive social psychology show great promise in identifying and resolving risks in health care.
5. Recognizing that health care is a high-risk industry, efforts are needed to support a culture change that incorporates a "blame-free" environment where safety is valued at the same level of organizational enthusiasm as productivity. This culture of safety encourages staff to report unintended errors and identify root causes of errors and actively engages staff in redesigning safety hazards.
6. More research is needed to promote patient safety targeting vulnerable patient populations, including the elderly and persons with disabilities.

For decades, nursing participated in health care systems where mistakes were hidden, individuals were blamed for errors, and the role of complex systems in producing errors was largely ignored. Nurses have a responsibility to play an active role in reshaping rehabilitation systems to make them safer for the patient populations served. The intent of this chapter is to provide an overview of the challenges of promoting patient safety in rehabilitation settings and to highlight ways that nurses can make rehabilitation services safer. A conceptual model will be presented to explain why errors or adverse events occur in rehabilitation and what can be done to reduce the incidence and severity of these events. Evidence-based approaches will be identified, including recommendations outlined in three critical patient safety reports: *To Err Is Human* (IOM, 1999), *Crossing the Quality Chasm* (IOM, 2001), and *Keeping Patients Safe: Transforming the Work Environment of Nurses* (IOM, 2004).

Challenges for Promoting Patient Safety in Rehabilitation

As described in previous chapters, rehabilitation has undergone a significant transformation over the past two decades, with cost as a critical driver of change. Rising health care costs have been attributed to the aging population; increased patient demand for new services, technologies, and drugs; and inefficient use of resources; however, medical errors and adverse events have also contributed to costs (IOM, 2001). The rapid rate of change in health care systems has detracted from quality care and patient safety. The growing complexity of science and technology, increase in comorbidities and chronic conditions, a poorly organized delivery system, and limited use of available information technology (e.g., electronic medical records) combine to increase the risk of errors and related adverse events (IOM, 2001). Our current rehabilitation care systems "set up" providers to fail, regardless of their level of dedication or how hard they try (IOM, 2001). The following are a few of the challenges to patient safety in rehabilitation:

- Rehabilitation processes are overly complex, requiring multiple steps and a synchronization of care. Every patient rehabilitation program is individualized, based on impairments, age, physical condition, comorbidities, and personal goals. Rarely are rehabilitation actions flawlessly executed, making rehabilitation progress uneven and disjointed. Our cumbersome rehabilitation processes waste resources, create unaccountable gaps in services, result in loss of patient information, and fail to build on the many strengths of rehabilitation nurses (IOM, 2001). The end result is an increased vulnerability to medical errors and preventable adverse events.

- The direct relationship between rehabilitation nursing actions and patient outcomes is far from precise (Ternov, 2000), making it difficult for nurses to anticipate risk, learn from their errors, or prevent adverse events in vulnerable patients.

- Although rehabilitation professionals pride themselves on great teamwork, the many autonomous disciplines are often not synchronized in rehabilitation care delivery and communication gaps can exist, to the patients' detriment. Shorter lengths of stay for patients and higher levels of staff turnover compound this challenge.

- Rehabilitation nurses care for a vulnerable patient population. Patients in rehabilitation are admitted for diverse problems; many are elderly and have multiple comorbidities. The stress of a new traumatic injury or coping with a disability over time can interfere with the patient's ability to adhere to treatment plans, further increasing risk for adverse events. Impairments in cognition or communication can limit patients' ability to protect themselves by deflecting errors or avoiding adverse events.

- An increase in patient risk occurs when patients are transferred across care settings (e.g., from neurology to rehabilitation to long-term care). These "patient handoffs" create vulnerable transitions for patients, whether it is between shifts, units, or facilities. Patient handoffs create multiple opportunities for errors and adverse events. Information can be lost, important actions fall through the cracks, or care becomes disjointed.

- Like other services, rehabilitation safety goals are often sacrificed in favor of goals related to productivity/efficiency and cost containment. Nurses are expected to care for more patients, who are more acutely ill, in shorter periods of time. These organizational expectations result in higher workload demands, which can contribute to adverse events and errors. Professionals need to view productivity and safety as two sides of a scale and find creative ways to balance the goals without sacrificing either.

- Lengths of acute rehabilitation inpatient stays have been reduced dramatically over the past decade. This shift has resulted in a transfer of risk for adverse events from the hospital setting to the home, where adverse events can go undetected and result in more serious consequences for the patient. Monitoring 30- and 60-day readmissions is one marker for assessing this vulnerability; another is to examine adverse events that occur immediately following acute rehabilitation.

A Conceptual Model for Patient Safety

Accidents are inevitable, and the likelihood of accidents increases in organizations that exhibit complex processes and synchronization of care across many disciplines (Perrow & Langton, 1994), a description that is well suited to rehabilitation. *Patient safety* is defined as freedom from *accidental injury* resulting from either a medical error or preventable adverse event. Although medical errors are very frequent in health care, not every error results in harm to the patient (IOM, 2001). A *medical error* is either failure of a planned action to be completed as intended or use of a wrong plan to achieve an aim (IOM, 2001). Errors can lead to *preventable adverse events*, defined as unintentional errors that result in negative consequences for the patient, including falls, pressure ulcers, or infections.

To prevent patient harm it is important to differentiate between active and latent errors. *Active errors* show up immediately and are committed by direct care providers (Reason, 1994). Examples include giving the wrong medication, failing to assess a change in patient condition, or not intervening to prevent a patient fall. There is a natural tendency to want to blame someone when an error is discovered. However, blaming is not effective in reducing errors or adverse events and focuses attention on the last and probably least remedial link in the accident chain—the provider (Reason, 1994). Known as the "shame and blame" mentality, this common response has resulted in "sweeping errors under the carpet," where others cannot learn from the mistake and the error is likely to be repeated. A poignant description of the cycle of blame and victimization related to errors and adverse events in health care was cited by Dr. Wu (2000):

> Although patients are the first and obvious victims of medical mistakes, doctors are wounded by the same errors; they are the second victims (p. 728). Nurses, pharmacists and other members of the healthcare team are also susceptible to error and vulnerable to its fallout. Given the hospital hierarchy, non-physician providers have little latitude to deal with their mistakes; they often bear silent witness to mistakes and agonize over conflicting loyalties to the patient, institution and team. They too are victims. (p. 729)

Latent errors are delayed consequences of administrative decisions related to the policies, design, and staffing levels. Using the same examples of active errors provided above, we can identify several latent errors that may have contributed to the error (Table 10-1). Examples include the design and construction of the environment and equipment, the structure of the organization, planning and scheduling, training and selection of staff, forecasting, information management, budgeting, and allocating resources. These risks may lie dormant for a long time until activated by more apparent actions in the system, when some unsuspecting rehabilitation care provider makes an error (Bogner, 1994). The number of latent factors embedded in organizational systems can align

TABLE 10-1 Differentiating Between Active and Latent Errors

Error/Adverse Event	Contributing Factors	Active Error	Latent Errors
Medication error (The patient was given the wrong medication.)	• The unit was chronically short staffed with no additional help available. • The nurse manager on the unit is new and her time schedules have consistently left gaps in coverage. • The nurse who made the error was a new graduate, without adequate supervision; she was unfamiliar with the patients on the unit. A new graduate, she was inefficient and was rushing to manage her workload so her colleagues would not think badly of her. • The medication was labeled similarly to another medication, and they were kept side-by-side on the shelf. This was the third error on this unit in which these two medications were confused.	Nurse A gives the patient the wrong medication.	• Staffing levels are inadequate. • Nursing time schedule is inadequate. • Supervision for new graduates is lacking. • There is poor labeling and storage of look-alike medications.
Failure to rescue (The patient's condition deteriorated without being noticed, and he coded at the beginning of a shift.)	• Physical environment is such that this room is at the end of the hall and the bed is not readily visible to nurses unless they enter the room. • The nurse assigned to this patient went home sick, and it was unclear who was to have taken over this patient assignment. • The patient was confused and not able to communicate needs; he was unable to activate the nurse call system.	The nurse assigned to this patient failed to monitor this patient as often as needed or failed to recognize signs that the patient's condition was changing.	• Physical environment detracts from patient observation, and there were no cameras or other monitoring devices available. • There is an inadequate system for handing off patients within the unit (shift to shift).
Fall prevention (The patient falls while trying to get to the bathroom and fractures a hip.)	• The patient had just been transferred from neurology, where she had fallen several times, but this information was not readily available to the evening nurse caring for her. • There was no structured toileting program on the unit to assist patients who needed assistance. • The floor had just been mopped to clean up a spill, making the floor slippery.	Nurse C failed to prevent the high-risk patient from falling.	• Improved system for handing off patients between units is needed. • Fall risk assessment protocol is lacking. • Bed fall alarm systems were requested but not included in the budget for lack of funds. • Toileting protocol is lacking. • Environmental services needs to use signage when floors are wet.

and result in accidents (Reason, 1990, 1997, 2000). Moreover, the link between latent risk factors and an error are more difficult to prove compared to the more obvious link between errors and the actions of direct care providers (Reason, 1994).

Patient safety is viewed as the result of the interaction among complex systems (Perrow, 1984). The conceptual model in Figure 10-1 helps to explain why errors or adverse events occur in rehabilitation and what can be done to reduce their incidence and severity.

Hazard Conditions. Risk factors address the underlying causes of injury and are organized into four categories. Each will be briefly described. *Patient risk factors* can contribute to

errors/adverse events, with some patients more vulnerable to errors/adverse events than others. These risk factors include age, impairments, comorbidities, and others. Patient risk factors are categorized as *nonmodifiable* (e.g., age, gender) or *modifiable* to target which risk factors are most amenable to interventions. *Situational risk factors* include characteristics of the nurse, such as years of experience or familiarity with the patient or the interactions of clinicians given the circumstances of a situation or their interaction with patients. Providers commit unintentional unsafe acts, such as "work arounds," for example, when nurses use broken equipment or devise shortcuts to get the job done. *Organizational risk factors* (latent risk factors/conditions), as described earlier, impede problem solving or delay error detection; they include erroneous

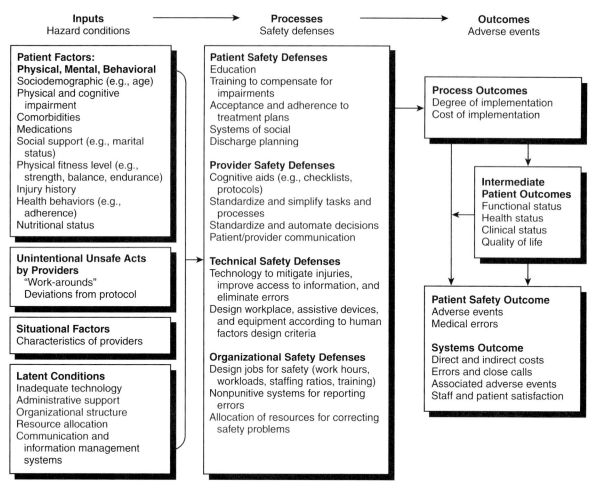

Figure 10-1 **Conceptual framework.** (Modified from Nelson, A., & Powell-Cope, G. [2005]. Nursing care priority area: Patient safety. In J. C. McCloskey & H. K. Grace [Eds.], *Current Issues in Nursing* [pp. 270-282]. St. Louis, MO: Mosby.)

administrative decisions, inadequate staffing or scheduling, excessive workload demands, inadequate training, chaotic implementation of a change in practice or new technology, and outdated equipment, to name a few (Wagenaar, Hudson, & Reason, 1990). These factors may have a delayed impact on how well the system resists errors, prevents adverse events, or mitigates injuries to the patient (Feldman & Roblin, 1997). Latent risk factors suggest that managers and administrators, who have no direct contact with patients, can create unsafe practice environments, setting up direct care providers to make errors.

Safety Defenses. Safety defenses are forces that intervene to prevent an active failure from progressing to a medical error, or they can be planned interventions that target identified risk factors, thus reducing the likelihood of an adverse event. Although it is impossible to design a flawless system, interventions to prevent errors/adverse events involve designs to create or strengthen safety barricades. These interventions can be directed toward the patient, provider, technology, or the organization. Safety defenses can be weak or strong, multidimensional or focused, and involve ability to absorb

the effect of or prevent active failures. Figure 10-1 identifies examples of safety defenses targeting patients, providers, technology, and organization. *Patient safety defenses* are aimed at changing modifiable patient risk factors through psychoeducational efforts ultimately to reduce the occurrence and severity of adverse events. *Provider safety defenses* focus on overcoming human limitations imposed by memory, practice variations, complex processes, fatigue, and provider/patient communication. *Technology safety defenses* focus on overcoming limitations in technology imposed by equipment or lack of proper equipment or proper maintenance. Although technology is often identified as a safety defense (e.g., electronic medical records, fall alarm systems), providers must have knowledge and skills to safely use technology or it could pose additional safety risks. *Organizational safety defenses* are aimed at changing organizational structures and processes that contribute to adverse events. Further research is needed to delineate safety solutions targeting rehabilitation care delivery systems.

Outcomes. To evaluate the effectiveness of safety defenses, outcomes could include three levels: process, intermediate, and long term. *Process evaluation* allows us to determine how and why the safety barrier resulted in the intermediate and ultimate outcomes (Sidani & Braden, 1998). *Intermediate outcomes* represent the more direct impact of interventions on patients, providers, and organizations, compared to ultimate outcomes (*long term*) that are markers of effectiveness, such as quality and cost. In rehabilitation we are ultimately concerned with improving quality of care by decreasing medical errors/adverse events, improving the work environment and retaining a high-quality and productive rehabilitation workforce, and developing high-performing organizations that embrace a positive culture of safety (Refer Chapter 9.).

Proactive Approaches to Promote Patient Safety in Rehabilitation

The first step is to identify high-risk/high-volume rehabilitation processes and create safety defenses. A high-risk process is defined as any health care delivery activity that (1) has a high probability of error, (2) occurs with sufficient frequency, and (3) would result in severe patient injury if an error were made (Ferraco & Spath, 2000). Examples of high-risk processes in rehabilitation nursing include the following:

- Monitoring patients during and immediately following high-risk interventions (e.g., restraints)
- Medication administration (prescribing, preparing, dispensing) and monitoring the effects of medications
- Screening and risk assessment for falls, pressure ulcers, wandering, combative behavior, etc.
- Surveillance and monitoring changes in patient condition
- Transfer of patient care responsibilities between caregivers and facilities (patient handoffs)
- Communication (among nursing staff, between nurses and other health care providers, and between caregivers and patient/significant others)

Efforts to create safer rehabilitation environments can include use of five proactive approaches to redesign high-risk processes (Reason, 1997; Spath, 2000a, p. xxvii).

- *Eliminate errors:* Some errors can be completely eliminated through the use of "forcing functions" that only allow the caregiver to perform the task safely. For example, the size and fitting at the end of a tube will prevent the nurse from inserting it in the wrong outlet for oxygen.
- *Reduce the numbers of errors*: It is not always possible to eliminate errors, so the goal may be to decrease the number of errors by adding backup functions. For example, two people need to match a unit of blood to the right patient before a transfusion. Another strategy might be to have intravenous solutions mixed centrally instead of on the unit, where interruptions and distractions could contribute to errors.
- *Catch errors before harm occurs*: Because not all errors can be prevented, it is wise to develop strategies to detect errors before an injury occurs. For example, protocols that require nurses to monitor vital signs every 15 minutes after certain drugs are administered is a way to detect problems before serious adverse events occur.
- *Contain errors to mitigate error-related adverse outcomes*: You can reduce the severity of error-related injuries

by designing protocols for timely and effective responses once an error has been discovered. For example, if the wrong eye drops are administered, quickly flushing the eyes could prevent serious harm; if a patient falls to the floor, checking for injuries before trying to move the patient may prevent further harm. Another mitigation strategy would be to use hip protectors, minimizing risk of a hip fracture should a patient fall.

- *Review errors and learn from them*: Recognizing that errors are inevitable, creating a work culture that encourages nurses to report and talk about errors can create a learning environment that prevents others from making the same mistake or allows others to design a solution so the error is not repeated (Spath, 2000b).

Recommendations

Rehabilitation is a complex endeavor embedded within complex organizations and processes of care, requiring synchronization and execution among many disciplines. To promote patient safety, all disciplines must work together to redesign the rehabilitation care processes most fraught with human error or those likely to cause injurious adverse events. Rehabilitation nurses have the opportunity to provide leadership in redesigning rehabilitation services and care processes. Rehabilitation nurses should take a leadership role in preventing nurse-sensitive adverse events, such as pressure ulcers, patient falls, infections, elopements, and pain, to name only a few.

Rehabilitation nursing should declare the promotion of patient safety a serious goal, creatively designing solutions with clearly articulated operational plans. We need to support each other, moving away from several outdated approaches, including (1) the "shame and blame" mentality of errors and adverse events, (2) relying heavily on retrospective review of errors, and (3) a feeling of powerlessness to change our rehabilitation processes. Rather, we need to progress toward (1) a positive culture of safety, (2) a prospective evaluation of hazardous conditions, and (3) redesigning nursing care delivery systems to fix underlying system problems to prevent future occurrences. We need proactive approaches for monitoring and analyzing high-risk rehabilitation nursing tasks and processes to identify where additional safeguards are needed to reduce the likelihood of errors or adverse events (Spath, 2000a, p. xxv).

Further research is needed to advance knowledge in five areas: (1) examine the epidemiology and cost of high-risk/high-volume adverse events in rehabilitation; (2) develop models to predict adverse events in specific impairments; (3) develop and validate screening tools, risk assessment tools, and safety outcome measures in rehabilitation; (4) improve technological safety defenses through human factors engineering and other principles of design; and (5) design and test interventions to strengthen safety defenses.

It is time to take action. The Institute of Medicine (IOM) identified six areas to enhance patient safety as a way to begin to make our care delivery systems safer, and these actions apply to rehabilitation settings across the care continuum:

(1) design care processes that more effectively address the needs of chronically ill patients—coordinated seamless care across settings and clinicians and over time; (2) make effective use of information technologies to automate clinical information; (3) enhance the knowledge base and competencies of providers; (4) improve coordination of care across patient conditions, services, and settings over time; (5) promote the effectiveness of health care teams; and (6) incorporate process and outcome measures into daily work (IOM, 2001, pp. 11-12). Although some actions to promote patient safety require resources, many high-risk nursing tasks can be redesigned with little or no cost. Solutions that address workload demands, staffing deficits, and use of technology (e.g., electronic medical records or bar code medication administration) will require substantial fiscal resources. The benefits of work redesign to promote patient safety have obvious advantages for improving patient outcomes and quality of life, but most will also have hidden advantages associated with nurse recruitment/retention, quality of care, patient satisfaction, and cost savings.

A systems approach to improving patient safety is essential to ensuring that mechanisms are repeatable, reliable, and provide minimal variation. This approach ensures that all team members have the necessary information about the patient when and where they need it and the tools to minimize or eliminate the risk for errors. Chapters 9 and 11 contain more information about quality and outcomes.

Case Study

A 74-year-old woman was admitted to the acute care medical unit of a large tertiary care hospital with onset of a left-hemisphere stroke. The patient was not a candidate for immediate thrombolytic therapy and had a slow but uneventful recovery in the hospital with the following resulting conditions:

- Right-sided paresis involving the arm and leg, including slight facial droop
- Some dysphagia associated with the facial paresis
- Atrial fibrillation rate controlled with digoxin
- Coumadin therapy for atrial fibrillation and prophylaxis to prevent further stroke
- Osteoporosis and placed on Fosamax
- Mild hypertension controlled with a diuretic
- Allergy to eggs
- Oriented with some difficulty expressing self and needing reminders

The patient had been active and independent at home before the stroke and was considered a good candidate for rehabilitation to a level of care that would allow independence with living arrangements to be made with her daughter rather than an assisted-living facility. Evaluation during the rehabilitation period would determine if the patient was able to achieve specific goals to live with her daughter. Rehabilitation would include gait training, mobility using a wheelchair (including transfer techniques), speech therapy, and activities of daily living (ADLs) (e.g., dressing, bathing, feeding, and toileting).

The patient was identified at risk for the following safety issues:
- High risk for falls and high risk for injury
- Risk for microaspiration and pneumonia
- General risk for medication error
- Risk of injury associated with anticoagulant therapy
- Risk for handoff problems associated with transfer from acute care to rehabilitation and from one treatment team to another team
- Risk for cardiac surveillance failures associated with atrial fibrillation, hypertension, and recent stroke

The interdisciplinary plan of care includes the following:
- Speech therapy assessment and therapy
- Nutritional consult for swallowing—food consistency
- Physical therapy consult for strength training, gait training, and use of assistive device
- Occupational therapy consult for ADLs (feeding self with assistive device, dressing self, toileting)

- Falls precautions
- Bowel and bladder routine
- Evaluation of the home to accommodate the patient's access, assistive devices, and safety

One Saturday, after a particularly tiring physical therapy session, the transporter is called to return the patient to her room. The therapist is short staffed due to the weekend and has several more patients to be seen. The patient is placed back in bed, so the patient can rest, by a transporter who only works weekends, and the transporter is immediately paged to transport another patient. The nurse is not immediately notified that the patient has returned from therapy, because staffing on the unit is also minimal on a weekend. The patient needs to use the bathroom (on a diuretic) and, because the patient has been doing well in therapy, becomes overconfident in her ability to get up unassisted, even though she has been instructed in fall precautions and the need to call for assistance. She does not want to bother the nurses. She attempts to stand with a walker next to the bed but is weakened after a tiring session with physical therapy and subsequently falls. The factors of Coumadin therapy, osteoporosis, and a fall from a standing position combine to cause a fractured hip on the already affected right side with significant bruising and bleeding into the area.

The patient's injury is identified, and the patient is taken to surgery for repair of the hip fracture and returned to the acute care hospital to a surgical unit. By the time this all takes place, the next shift has come on duty. The nurses on the surgical unit have not received information about the stroke, only the current hip fracture and repair. During the postoperative recovery period the patient is given fluids and left to drink unassisted. The patient needs fluids thickened to reduce aspiration risk, and, because the new team has not been fully involved yet due to the weekend, the patient aspirates, subsequently develops pneumonia, and continues on a downhill course with a prolonged complicated hospitalization. Eventually the patient arrests because of the pneumonia and prolonged bedrest and dies.

The fall with fracture triggers a sentinel event report and root cause analysis (RCA). In reviewing the patient's record and follow-up care in the hospital, the RCA team considers the entire episode of care in the hospital, rehabilitation facility, and return to the hospital. The team identifies all of the failures that contributed to the patient's poor

Case Study—cont'd

outcome and determines the following "system solutions" to improve safety of patients:

1. *Team communication using standardized, structured tools to ensure that patient activities, transports, and changes in condition are communicated and coordinated throughout the day. Standardized methods of communication between staff on the unit and other personnel (e.g., transporters, dietary aides)*

2. *Handoffs using a structured tool at each critical transition (not just shift to shift but from one setting in the hospital to the rehabilitation facility and back), so that all necessary information is included in a written format, as well as verbal interaction for questions*

3. *Formalized falls prevention program, including identification of high-risk patients, use of hip protectors, floor mats, height-adjustable beds, frequent toileting rounds for patients (especially those on diuretics or laxatives), and other interventions from research and toolkits*

4. *Medical record alerts for patients on high-risk medications (e.g., Coumadin) or for special conditions (falls, risk of aspiration) that notify all caregivers of the patient's status*

5. *Automated medical records so that the patient's entire history, physical, and progress notes can be accessed by all team members regardless of setting*

6. *Use of barcoding system for medication administration to eliminate medication errors*

7. *A systemwide rapid response team to intervene early when a patient's condition changes but the patient has not arrested*

8. *Staffing plans that ensure a sufficient level throughout all shifts of the day and days of the week*

CRITICAL THINKING

1. Research shows that hand-offs are areas in which there is a potential gap in knowledge that may result in patient issues. What are the key elements rehabilitation nurses need to consider when obtaining a patient hand-off from an acute care setting?

2. Patient falls are a nurse sensitive indicator of quality outcomes. The incidence of falls (number of falls per 1000 patient days) is typically higher for rehabilitation settings than for acute care settings. What are five key strategies to prevent falls for any patient admitted to an acute rehabilitation unit?

3. What is the single most effective method of preventing the development of hospital-acquired infections? How can rehabilitation nurses encourage patients and family members to comply with this method?

4. A critical result of an INR of 10 is reported to a rehabilitation nurse at 0900. The nurse calls the physician to report the result within 10 minutes of result reporting. The physician is very busy and does not respond with new orders, but tells the nurse that he will "stop by and see the patient." At this point, a failure to communicate exists, because clearly the physician did not comprehend the critical aspect of the situation. What actions must the nurse take to ensure the patient receives the necessary intervention?

REFERENCES

Bogner, M. S. (1994). Introduction. In M. S. Bogner (Ed.), *Human error in medicine* (pp. 1-11). Hillsdale, NJ: Lawrence Erlbaum Associates.

Feldman, S. E., & Roblin, D. W. (1997). Medical accidents in hospital care: Applications of failure analysis to hospital quality appraisal. *Joint Commission Journal on Quality Improvement, 23*(11), 569.

Ferraco, K., & Spath, P. L. (2000). Measuring performance on high risk processes. In P. L. Spath (Ed.), *Error reduction in health care* (pp. 17-95). San Francisco: Jossey-Bass.

Institute of Medicine (IOM). (1999). *To err is human: Building a safer health system.* Washington, DC: National Academy Press.

Institute of Medicine (IOM). (2001). *Crossing the quality chasm.* Washington, DC: National Academy Press.

Institute of Medicine (IOM). (2004). *Keeping patients safe: Transforming the work environment of nurses.* Washington, DC: National Academy Press.

Perrow, C. (1984). *Normal accidents: Living with high risk technologies.* New York: Basic Books.

Perrow, C., & Langton, J. (1994). The limits of safety: The enhancement of a theory of accidents. *Journal of Contingency Management, 2,* 212-220.

Reason, J. T. (1990). *Human error.* New York: Cambridge University Press.

Reason, J. T. (1994). Foreword. In M. S. Bogner (Ed.), *Human error in medicine.* Hillsdale, NJ: Lawrence Erlbaum Associates.

Reason, J. T. (1997). *Managing the risks of organizational accidents.* Brookfield, VT: Ashgate Publishing.

Reason, J. T. (2000). Human error: Models and management. *BMJ, 320,* 768-770.

Sidani, S., & Braden, C. (1998). *Evaluating nursing interventions: A theory-driven approach.* Thousand Oaks, CA: Sage Publications.

Spath, P. L. (Ed.). (2000a). *Error reduction in health care.* San Francisco: Jossey-Bass.

Spath, P. L. (2000b). Reducing errors through work system improvements. In P. L. Spath (Ed.), *Error reduction in health care* (pp. 199-234). San Francisco: Jossey-Bass.

Ternov, S. (2000). The human side of medical mistakes. In P. L. Spath (Ed.), *Error reduction in health care* (pp. 109-110). San Francisco: Jossey-Bass.

Wagenaar, W. A., Hudson, P. T., & Reason, J. T. (1990). Cognitive failures and accidents. *Applied Cognitive Psychology, 4*(4), 273-294.

Wu, A. W. (2000). The doctor who makes mistakes needs help too. *BMJ, 320,* 726-727.

11

Evaluation of Function and Application of Outcome Measures

Margaret Kelly-Hayes, EdD, RN, CRRN, FAAN
Marion A. Phipps, RN, MS, CRRN, FAAN

The goals of rehabilitation are to prevent complications, minimize impairments, and improve function (Duncan et al., 2005; Skinner & Turner-Stokes, 2006). The process by which these goals are met includes comprehensive assessment and diagnosis, identification of expected outcomes, and planned interventions (American Nurses Association [ANA], 2004). Within rehabilitation there is a mandate to standardize the methods of assessment based on a conceptual framework. This chapter identifies a variety of evaluative approaches and methods from a rehabilitation nursing perspective. Comprehensive assessment of patients is essential for appropriate clinical management, and functional evaluation is central to the planning and execution of restorative care. The integration of a person's health condition with functional performance and level of social support allows for the construction of a comprehensive data set that profiles the whole individual. In this era of standardization in rehabilitation, evaluation using reliable and valid measures must be a part of the rehabilitation nursing process. Functional evaluation can be viewed as an extension of the traditional components of nursing assessment. Thus functional evaluation provides a framework for the review of essential components deemed important to independent life. In some cases, functional status may be as reliable in documenting overall health as knowing disease categories.

Functional evaluation is a means to incorporate the results of assessment into patient-centered care plans. This in turn has a direct influence on nursing diagnosis, nursing intervention, and nursing-specific outcome criteria. Nurses assess patients' abilities to meet their personal and rehabilitative goals. Nursing assessment of function, based on validated and objective measures, contributes in a significant way to interdisciplinary evaluation and care planning.

The incorporation of evaluation of functional status into the interdisciplinary process of rehabilitation provides a common denominator for the team effort, an essential component in rehabilitation. Rehabilitation is a collaborative effort, with each member accountable for his or her own profession-specific interventions. Regardless of the health condition of the patient population being served, the rehabilitation team completes an interdisciplinary evaluation following discipline-specific assessments, develops mutually agreed-on goals, and initiates an intervention plan. Evaluation of function is an important component in each of these elements and is the responsibility of the nurse as well as other members of the rehabilitation team.

Several specific assessment measures commonly used by rehabilitation professionals are presented. The types of instruments described in this chapter are general measures of function, including cognition and mood, activities of daily living, and determinants of quality of life. Because the status of the patient does change over time, the type, frequency, and utilization of assessment need to reflect this dynamic. All of the presented instruments are appropriate for inclusion in a patient-centered evaluation.

DISABILITY FRAMEWORK FOR EVALUATION

The focus of rehabilitation is to provide interventions to maximize function and to limit the impact of disability. The spheres of measurement to evaluate these interventions in rehabilitation have evolved from the conceptual framework of disablement. The term *disability* is used to refer to a physical or mental limitation within a social context, the gap between a person's capacity and the demands of the environment.

In a study of the meaning of disability for older adults, the word *disability* was considered multidimensional, inclusive of function and changes in health and social status (Kelley-Moore, Schumacher, Kahana, & Kahana, 2006). Although by definition *disability* assumes interaction between the individual and the environment, it is frequently equated with separate and specific impairments. The relationship between severity of disability and independent living is apparent; however, many times the terms *impairment, disability,* and *handicap* are used interchangeably without consideration of their specific differences. These inconsistencies can pose obstacles to the appropriate use of terminology, correct measures specific to outcomes, and the evaluation of interventions.

The conceptual underpinnings for evaluation of function are based on the seminal works of Nagi and the World Health Organization (WHO). In Nagi's model of disablement (Nagi, 1965; Clifton, 2006), the three major potential consequences of active pathologic condition or disease are impairment or physiologic abnormalities, functional limitations, and disability. Nagi defines *disability* as an inability to perform or a limitation in performing expected social roles. Disability occurs when conditions interfere with the performance of an individual in personally, socially, or culturally expected roles. The WHO (1980) *International Classification of Impairments, Disabilities, and Handicaps* (ICIDH) has been revised to the *International Classification of Functioning, Disability and Health* (ICF) (2001). The new classification system provides health outcomes in terms of body, person, and social function. One of the major changes in the model is the elimination of the term *handicap* because of its negative connotation. In the new system, *impairment* is defined as problems in body function, *activity* as the execution of specific tasks, and *participation* as encompassing life situations. For example, for a person with a stroke, the lower extremity hemiparesis would be the impairment, difficulty walking the activity limitation, and the interference with work the participant restriction. The ICF provides an international framework for disablement that goes beyond disease to focus on how people live with their conditions.

MEASUREMENT OF DISABILITY IN REHABILITATION

Applying disability theory and definitions to rehabilitation has been a difficult task because of the complexities in measurement of functional abilities and limitations. The classic approach devised by Kane and Kane (1981) conceptualized health and disability as a hierarchical structure: the first level is general health or the absence of illness, the second level is basic performance of self-care and mobility activities that are critical for independence, and the third level is the ability to perform and maintain those complex activities and roles associated with a meaningful life. Kane and Kane's conceptualization of disability addresses the wide range of functional performances, from basic self-care to community reintegration. Within this structure, outcome measures guide treatment and interventions at each level.

Evaluation of function provides the information needed to assess and plan interventions and should include all parameters that affect "active life" functioning. This should include the measurement of all domains that constitute independent life routinely assessed as part of the rehabilitation process. Today it is standard practice in rehabilitation to use many assessment instruments to document impairments, basic activities of daily living (ADLs), performance of instrumental activities of daily living (IADLs), and quality-of-life parameters. The combination of these instruments provides the evaluation of critical components that make up independent active life. For rehabilitation nursing, assessment domains include physical, cognitive, affective, social, and quality-of-life measures (Association of Rehabilitation Nurses, 2000).

ASSESSMENT MEASURES: GENERAL CONSIDERATIONS

Information from assessment instruments is most commonly used to describe, evaluate, and/or predict outcome. Descriptive measures document the type and severity of impairments, functional limitations, or disabilities at a given time. Evaluative components measure clinically sensitive changes over time and treatment course. Predictive evaluation is used to establish goals and plan treatments. Ideally an assessment instrument should be practical, be simple to administer, and yield meaningful results.

The guiding principles for selecting a functional assessment instrument include validity, reliability, sensitivity to clinically important changes, and sensibility (Dittmar & Gresham, 2005)

These characteristics are defined as follows:
- *Validity.* Validity is the ability of an instrument to measure what it is intended to measure. An instrument's criterion validity is determined by comparing its results with a standard accepted within the field.
- *Reliability.* Interobserver reliability is the technique in which two individuals administer the same test to the same patient and obtain similar results. Test-retest reliability refers to whether repeated use of a measure yields consistent results in the absence of a change in the patient.
- *Sensitivity.* The sensitivity of an instrument is its ability to detect clinical change.
- *Sensibility.* Sensibility refers to applicability and use.

Each assessment instrument should be able to measure the domain of interest; monitor progress; enhance communication between disciplines, patients, and families; measure effectiveness of treatment; and determine the benefits of rehabilitation interventions. Because assessment instruments are used repeatedly during the course of a person's rehabilitation, the data should be a reliable and valid measure of the condition being treated.

It is important to remember that the method of administration of the assessment instrument can influence the results obtained. Methodological differences in administration of the assessment tool and the type of populations being assessed are two sources for discrepancies in results. Often measures do not clearly differentiate between the presence of a functional impairment that makes an activity impossible to carry out and the actual performance of an activity. Because disability reflects performance within a sociocultural context, one could expect that daily performance would be strongly influenced by social as well as physical factors.

Assessment should determine daily performance, not the capacity to perform an activity. Behavior that is executed in an ideal setting under controlled circumstances may not be an accurate measure of the extent of disability experienced in day-to-day life. Lack of motivation as well as environmental factors can impede the performance of certain activities conducted independently in the rehabilitation setting, but not when a person returns home. These factors need to be considered as part of any evaluation because of their influence on measurement.

Domains and Definition of Functional Assessment

Many assessment instruments are used to document the full range of domains affected by disability. These measures can be generic to rehabilitation in general or disease specific, depending on the intended use of the data. In general, most documentation of disability is determined with generic tools.

The general purposes of functional assessment in rehabilitation are to determine functional status, document the need for interventions and services, devise a treatment plan, and assess and monitor progress. A measure of physical functioning can be derived from many different combinations of items. One of the earliest definitions of functional assessment, defined by Lawton (1972), describes objective measurement in a variety of areas such as physical health, emotional status, and quality of self-maintenance. Dittmar and Gresham (2005) state that functional assessment is a method for describing abilities and limitations to measure an individual's use of a variety of skills included in performing tasks necessary to daily living, leisure activities, vocational pursuits, social interactions, and other required behaviors. Quantitative measurements across multidimensional function areas are apparent in both definitions, demonstrating that assessment is not one dimensional but rather evolves along with the underlying philosophy of rehabilitation.

Self-care and mobility status are two measurements of function that are central to rehabilitation assessment. However, this focus does not adequately describe the actual range of interventions necessary for an independent life. Although functional skills are important parameters in reducing dependence on others, the repertoire of behaviors required to lead a meaningful life is obviously much broader. Therefore rehabilitation programs incorporate measures of physical, cognitive, emotional, perceptual, social, and vocational functioning into the patient evaluation.

SELECTED DISABILITY SCALES

Functional assessment and evaluation instruments are designed to capture domains and constellation of domains involved in an independent life. The framework represents impairments,

disability, and participation. The following section and Table 11-1 describe validated scales that have met standards for measurement in rehabilitation setting. Each has descriptive and evaluative properties in the clinical setting. The utility of these instruments is that they provide a description of overall functioning and can be appropriately used to follow broad measures of a clinical course. These instruments expand across disease categories and physical impairments to address the resultant disability targeted by rehabilitation efforts. Although other assessment measures are available, the instruments presented here were chosen because of the extensive testing and validation in the rehabilitation field.

Measures of Activities of Daily Living and Functional Assessment

ADLs refer to those basic skills that one must possess to care for oneself independently. ADL skills usually include assessment of self-care (eating, dressing, bathing, grooming, etc.), transfers, continence, and in most cases, locomotion (see Chapter 14). These activities are hierarchical, from basic functions such as eating to higher-level functions like stair climbing. Although many functional assessment instruments have been developed for use in rehabilitation hospitals, currently the most widely applied scales are the Functional Independence Measure (FIM) instrument and the Barthel Index.

The FIM (Uniform Data System for Medical Rehabilitation, 2006), included in the Inpatient Rehabilitation Facility Patient Assessment Instrument (IRF-PAI) tool, is designed to document frequency and severity of disability in a uniform and reliable method. It has been extensively tested for reliability, validity, and sensitivity. As seen in Figure 11-1, the FIM is an 18-item assessment that measures self-care, sphincter management, transfers, locomotion, communication, and cognitive (communication and social cognition) skills. Using a seven-level scoring system, a FIM score ranges from a maximum score of 126 points, representing complete independence in all performance areas, to a minimum score of 18, representing dependence in all areas evaluated. The conceptual basis for the scale is that the level of disability should indicate the burden of care or the cost to the individual or society for that person not to be functionally independent (Uniform Data System for Medical Rehabilitation, 2006). One of its unique strengths is the ability to measure communication and social cognition. The measure is used to establish criteria for admission, discharge, and maintenance of rehabilitation gains. Those who practice rehabilitation and who have been trained in its use can administer the instrument. Refer to Chapter 8 (for application in practice).

The Barthel Index is a worldwide-administered ADL outcome measure (Mahoney and Barthel, 1965). It is a weighted scoring system that measures basic activities of ability in mobility, self-care, and continence. With a score ranging from 0 to 100, a score of 100 indicates complete independence in all 10 domains measured, and 0 indicates complete dependence in all 10 domains. To be considered independent, the patient does not require human assistance in any of the measured activities.

TABLE 11-1 Selected Assessment Instruments for Rehabilitation

Type	Name and Source	Description	Strengths/Time
Level-of-consciousness scale	Glasgow Coma Scale (Teasdale, 1974)	3 sections scoring eye opening, motor, and verbal responses to voice commands or pain. Each section scored separately.	Simple, valid, reliable. (2 min)
Mental status screening	Mini-Mental State Examination (MMSE) (Folstein & McHugh, 1975)	7 domains: orientation to time and place, registration of words, attention, calculation, recall, language, and visual construction.	Widely used for screening; sensitive. (<10 min)
Measures of basic activities of daily living (ADLs)	Barthel Index (Mahoney & Barthel, 1965)	10 items: bowels, bladder, feeding, grooming, dressing, transfer, toilet use, mobility, stairs, bathing. Appropriate for screening and monitoring progress.	Well-established validity and reliability. (10 min)
	Functional Independence Measure (FIM) (Granger, 1986)	Measures physical and functional communication. Subscores for motor function and cognition. Domains for self-care, sphincter control, transfers, locomotion, communication, and social cognition.	Widely used in rehabilitation. (<40 min)
Instrumental ADLs	OARS (Duke University, 1978)	Multidimensional assessment with 105 questions in 5 domains: social resources, economics, mental health, physical health, ADLs.	Assesses broad array of activities necessary for independent life. (20 min)
Depression	Center for Epidemiologic Studies Depression (CES-D) (Radloff, 1977)	20-item questionnaire investigating perceived mood and level of functioning within the past week.	Brief, easily administered, useful in elderly. (<10 min)
Health status/quality-of-life measures	Medical Outcomes Study (MOS—SF-36) (Ware, 1992)	Domains: Physical functioning, role limitations due to physical or emotional problems, social functioning, bodily pain, mental health, vitality, and general health perceptions.	Generic health status scale. Brief, can be self-administered. (<30 min)
Skilled nursing facility/ community	MDS (CMS, 2006)	300-item tool that measures physical, psychological, and social functioning for nursing home residents.	Valid and reliable when administered by trained assessors. (60 min)
	OASIS (CMS, 2006)	Provides continuous quality improvement measures for health, function, and support status.	Broad assessment of components for community living. (60 min)

CMS, Centers for Medicare and Medicaid Services; *MDS*, Minimum Data Set; *OASIS*, Outcome and Assessment Information Set; *OARS*, Older American Resources and Services Scale; *PGC*, Philadelphia Geriatric Center Instrumental Role Maintenance Scale.

Measures of Instrumental Activities of Daily Living

Beyond the basic performance of ADLs, the ability to accomplish certain activities that make full participation in independent living possible are the IADL measures. Activities include a variety of tasks, including using a telephone, shopping, preparing meals, and managing money. These skills are often part of rehabilitation retraining but are difficult to evaluate until the individual returns home. IADL scales may be rated either by an interviewer or by the individual, depending on the disability and circumstances. The IADL tool listed here is the Older American Resources and Services Scale (OARS) (Duke University, 1978).

Cognition and Mood Assessment

Cognitive status evaluation is an integral part of the rehabilitation assessment. Assessment of the ability to acquire and retain new information, the underpinning of the rehabilitation process, can be obtained by observation of the patient's interactions, responses to questions, and general knowledge (Kelly-Hayes, Jette, Wolf, D'Agostino, & Odell, 1992). In addition, incorporation of a mental status test as part of the assessment process can serve as a guide in planning outcome goals and identifying those at risk for difficulty in adapting to disability as well as teaching strategies. The Mini-Mental State Examination (MMSE) (Folstein & McHugh, 1975) has been widely used in a variety of populations and is well validated, reliable, and brief. The MMSE is recommended by the 2003 U.S. Preventive Services Task Force for assessment of cognitive function in individuals with suspected impairment (Thibault & Steiner, 2004).

Affect is a powerful determinant of successful rehabilitation. Depressive symptoms can often be exacerbated by loss of physical well-being and independence. In some conditions

DEPARTMENT OF HEALTH AND HUMAN SERVICES
CENTERS FOR MEDICARE & MEDICAID SERVICES

INPATIENT REHABILITATION FACILITY – PATIENT ASSESSMENT INSTRUMENT

Function Modifiers*

Complete the following specific functional items prior to scoring the FIM™ Instrument:

	ADMISSION	DISCHARGE
29. Bladder Level of Assistance (Score using FIM Levels 1 - 7)	☐	☐
30. Bladder Frequency of Accidents (Score as below)	☐	☐

7 - No accidents
6 - No accidents; uses device such as a catheter
5 - One accident in the past 7 days
4 - Two accidents in the past 7 days
3 - Three accidents in the past 7 days
2 - Four accidents in the past 7 days
1 - Five or more accidents in the past 7 days

Enter in Item 39G (Bladder) the lower (more dependent) score from Items 29 and 30 above.

	ADMISSION	DISCHARGE
31. Bowel Level of Assistance (Score using FIM Levels 1 - 7)	☐	☐
32. Bowel Frequency of Accidents (Score as below)	☐	☐

7 - No accidents
6 - No accidents; uses device such as an ostomy
5 - One accident in the past 7 days
4 - Two accidents in the past 7 days
3 - Three accidents in the past 7 days
2 - Four accidents in the past 7 days
1 - Five or more accidents in the past 7 days

Enter in Item 39H (Bowel) the lower (more dependent) score of Items 31 and 32 above.

	ADMISSION	DISCHARGE
33. Tub Transfer	☐	☐
34. Shower Transfer	☐	☐

(Score Items 33 and 34 using FIM Levels 1 - 7; use 0 if activity does not occur) *See training manual for scoring of Item 39K (Tub/Shower Transfer)*

	ADMISSION	DISCHARGE
35. Distance Walked	☐	☐
36. Distance Traveled in Wheelchair	☐	☐

(Code items 35 and 36 using: 3 - 150 feet; 2 - 50 to 149 feet; 1 - Less than 50 feet; 0 – activity does not occur)

	ADMISSION	DISCHARGE
37. Walk	☐	☐
38. Wheelchair	☐	☐

(Score Items 37 and 38 using FIM Levels 1 - 7; 0 if activity does not occur) See training manual for scoring of Item 39L (Walk/Wheelchair)

*The FIM data set, measurement scale and impairment codes incorporated or referenced herein are the property of U B Foundation Activities, Inc. ©1993, 2001 U B Foundation Activities, Inc. The FIM mark is owned by UBFA, Inc.

39. FIM™ Instrument*

	ADMISSION	DISCHARGE	GOAL
SELF-CARE			
A. Eating	☐	☐	☐
B. Grooming	☐	☐	☐
C. Bathing	☐	☐	☐
D. Dressing - Upper	☐	☐	☐
E. Dressing - Lower	☐	☐	☐
F. Toileting	☐	☐	☐
SPHINCTER CONTROL			
G. Bladder	☐	☐	☐
H. Bowel	☐	☐	☐
TRANSFERS			
I. Bed, Chair, WheelChair	☐	☐	☐
J. Toilet	☐	☐	☐
K. Tub, Shower	☐	☐	☐
LOCOMOTION (W - Walk, C - wheelChair, B - Both)			
L. Walk/Wheelchair	☐ ☐	☐ ☐	☐
M. Stairs	☐	☐	☐
COMMUNICATION (A - Auditory, V - Visual, B - Both)			
N. Comprehension	☐ ☐	☐ ☐	☐
O. Expression (V - Vocal, N - Nonvocal, B - Both)	☐ ☐	☐ ☐	☐
SOCIAL COGNITION			
P. Social Interaction	☐	☐	☐
Q. Problem Solving	☐	☐	☐
R. Memory	☐	☐	☐

FIM LEVELS

No Helper
7 Complete Independence (Timely, Safely)
6 Modified Independence (Device)

Helper - Modified Dependence
5 Supervision (Subject = 100%)
4 Minimal Assistance (Subject = 75% or more)
3 Moderate Assistance (Subject = 50% or more)

Helper - Complete Dependence
2 Maximal Assistance (Subject = 25% or more)
1 Total Assistance (Subject less than 25%)

0 Activity does not occur; Use this code only at admission

Form CMS-10036 (01/06) 2

Figure 11-1 Portion of the Inpatient Rehabilitation Facility Patient Assessment Instrument (IRF-PAI) including the Functional Independence Measure (FIM).

such as stroke, depression actually may be a feature of the disease. In a study of 303 survivors of stroke, depression was linked with a more generalized effect on quality of life than basic functional abilities (Kwok et al., 2006). If not recognized and treated, depression can have a profound negative impact on all rehabilitation efforts. The U.S. Preventive Services Task Force (2002) recommends routine screening for depression. Formal screening tools are available (Beck Depression Inventory, the Center for Epidemiological Studies–Depression Scale, the Zung Depression Scale); however, two quick questions will provide the rehabilitation nurse with an indication of depression: (1) During the past 2 weeks, have you felt down, depressed, or hopeless? and (2) During the past 2 weeks, have you felt little pleasure or interest in doing things? (U.S. Preventive Services Task Force, 2002).

Quality-of-Life Measures

Quality-of-life measures capture a wide range of capabilities, symptoms, and psychosocial characteristics that describe function and satisfaction with life. Components of quality of life include social roles and interactions, functional performance, intellectual functioning, perceptions, and subjective health. Indicators can include standards of living and general satisfaction with life. Although there is controversy over the measurement of quality of life, it is a strong indicator of successful rehabilitation (Resnick et al., 2005). Several measures have been developed, but few of these have been as well validated as the Medical Outcome Study (MOS) Short Form Health Surveys. These standardized surveys are available online and in 36-item (SF-36), 12-item (SF-12), and 8-item (SF-8) formats. The SF-36, designed by John Ware, requires 5 to 10 minutes for completion and is intended for self-administration. It is available online for no cost to individuals at http://www.sf-36.org/. The tool is particularly useful because it is available in 29 languages and is considered valid and reliable across socioeconomic levels for individuals age 14 and older (Grandek, Sinclair, Kosinski, & Ware, 2004).

Timing of Assessment for Rehabilitation Patients

As stated earlier, the systematic assessment of disability is the major means of describing, monitoring, and evaluating specific interventions essential at each stage of the recovery process. Equally important is assessing an individual at the appropriate times along the rehabilitation continuum (Box 11-1). Assessment should initially take place at the first clinical contact, usually at the time of admission to an inpatient facility, an outpatient facility, or a rehabilitation program in the community. Often the first examination is a screening for impairments and disability related to the condition under treatment. This assessment can be used to validate the appropriateness of the referral, formulate treatment goals, confirm the management plan, and provide a baseline for monitoring change. The patient's progress should then be assessed at periodic intervals during rehabilitation. Assessment should

---

BOX 11-1 Case Study Flow Chart for Mr. Wood

Initial Assessment Instruments
- Medical comorbidities
- Level-of-consciousness scale
- Mental status screening
- Basic activities of daily living (ADLs)
- Swallowing assessment
- Skin assessment and pressure ulcers
- Risk of deep venous thrombosis (DVT)

Assessment Instruments for Rehabilitation
- Mental status
- ADLs
- Instrumental ADLs (IADLs)
- Depression screen
- Communication impairment
- Psychosocial assessment and family/caregiver support and adjustment
- Risk of complications/recurrence

Assessment Instruments for Postrehabilitation
- Mental status
- ADLs
- IADLs
- Depression screen
- Quality of life
- Health status
- Long-term and community assessment
- Family/caregiver support
- Risk of complications

---

include a baseline and then a subset of the baseline, which are particular targets of intervention. Well-established, reliable measures are essential to achieving valid comparisons among patients with similar problems. After discharge from rehabilitation, assessment is useful to monitor adaptation to the community and for maintenance of functional gains made during rehabilitation.

Use of Functional Assessment Measures for Reimbursement and Regulation

Following an acute hospitalization for disability or chronic illness, patients are faced with a choice of where to receive rehabilitation. An ample quantity of research on pros and cons of different levels and types of services for rehabilitation is accessible within the literature (New, 2006; Silverstein, Findley, & Bode, 2006). The Centers for Medicare and Medicaid Services (CMS) regulates payment for postacute care of Medicare/Medicaid beneficiaries. Given the high number of patients requiring rehabilitation who have insurance through Medicare or Medicaid, the activities and requirements of CMS strongly influence admission criteria and discharge disposition of patients. Scoring on data collection instruments designed through CMS determines the patient's admission eligibility and payment rates. Refer to Chapter 8 for more discussion on regulation and reimbursement. The data collection instruments used for postacute assessment include the Minimum Data Set (MDS) and Resident Assessment Instrument (RAI) for long term care and subacute care, the Outcome and Assessment Information Set (OASIS), and the IRF-PAI. In 2006 CMS proposed a uniform postacute assessment instrument. The Activity Measure for Post Acute Care (AM-PAC) is currently in beta testing at facilities across the country and is under consideration for adoption as the uniform postacute assessment instrument (Coster, Haley, & Jette, 2006). The following discussion covers development and use of the MDS, OASIS, IRF-PAI, and AM-PAC.

Minimum Data Set. For long-term care the MDS is a core source of assessment information for the RAI. It measures physical, medical, psychological, and social functioning of nursing home residents. This 300-item instrument documents ADLs, continence, communication, behavior, and cognition. It is serially administered for all residents in Medicare- and Medicaid-certified facilities and skilled nursing facilities (CMS, 2006). The MDS is electronically submitted to CMS. Validity and interrater reliability have been demonstrated when administered by trained assessors (Lun, Lin, & Kane, 2005).

The MDS is one component of the federally mandated clinical assessment and planning process. Based on the MDS findings, Resident Assessment Protocols (RAPs) are triggered, resulting in care plans for residents. Included within the MDS are 30 quality indicators/measures. Responses to MDS elements identify residents at risk for functional problems or for complications. The quality indicators/measures are publicly reported by CMS and are used to provide direction to health department surveyors during annual compliance surveys.

Outcome and Assessment Information Set. For home health care agencies the OASIS is used to assess status within the community setting (CMS, 2006). The program provides a set of data items necessary for measuring patient outcomes, monitoring care, and other internal agency applications. The OASIS was developed to provide continuous quality improvement in home health care (Schlenker, Powell, & Goodrich, 2005). OASIS data items include sociodemographic information, environmental information, support system, health status, and functional status.

As with the MDS, OASIS is electronically reported to CMS. It, too, is used for planning care and identifying quality variations such as dehydration, depression, pressure ulcers, and hospital readmissions.

Inpatient Rehabilitation Facility Patient Assessment Instrument. The IRF-PAI contains a version of the Functional Independence Measure. It is used to drive the plan for acute rehabilitation and to determine the level of reimbursement. Because most hospital-based rehabilitation programs have "deemed" status through The Joint Commission (TJC) accreditation, IRF-PAI results are not used for department of health surveys. The IRF-PAI results are used to determine compliance of programs with admission criteria established by CMS.

AM-PAC. The activity measure for post acute fare is intended for outcome measurement within the domain of daily living, basic mobility, and applied cognitive. The tool is appropriate for many post acute settings, including long-term care, outpatient therapy, and home health. It is available online and in hard copy form, free of charge from CRE Care (http://222.crecare.come/index.html).

APPLICATIONS OF FUNCTIONAL EVALUATION IN NURSING PRACTICE AND RESEARCH

There are several purposes of functional evaluation in rehabilitation in general (Dittmar & Gresham, 2005) and for rehabilitation nursing specifically. These include systematic identification of functional limitations requiring preventive, maintenance, and restorative actions; documentation of feedback about progression toward goal achievement; allocation of resources; coordination of care and facilitation of placement decisions; provision of objective data with which to analyze costs, benefits, and quality of care; and assistance for accreditation bodies, program evaluation, health care policy evaluation, and third-party payers.

The specialty practice of rehabilitation nursing is founded on the belief that rehabilitation is a process of restoring and maintaining a patient's optimal health—physiological, emotional, vocational, and social. More poetically, Lena Plaisted, a rehabilitation nursing pioneer, stated that "rehabilitation nursing is nursing with an awareness of the patient's tomorrow and the relationship between what does and what does not happen today and the tomorrows that follow" (McCourt, 1993, p. 13). Rehabilitation nurses help individuals and families adapt to life changes that have been caused by illness and disability.

Rehabilitation nursing is, by its nature, a relationship-based practice. To be effective in this work, the nurse must have a connection with the patient, the family, nursing colleagues, and those in other disciplines. This connection is formed through knowing the patient and family, possessing a strong basis in rehabilitation nursing science and knowledge, and having a deep understanding of the contributions made by all members of the care team.

Knowing the patient begins with an initial assessment. The American Nurses Association's *Nursing: Scope and Standards of Practice* (2004) describes criteria using appropriate assessment techniques and instruments that document essential information in a retrievable form. The baseline information provides the nurse with a rich source of data to examine the patient's status at one time and to measure changes that occur. The inclusion of functional, cognitive, and quality-of-life measures within the nursing assessment enhances the description of the patient. From this initial assessment the rehabilitation nurse can identify patient diagnosis and expected outcomes. Functional assessment can be used as a vehicle to identify patient risk factors.

Assessment data provide the nurse with the means to evaluate patient progress toward the attainment of outcomes. Use of functional assessment as part of this evaluation provides the nurse with a universal language to communicate to other nurses and other health care professionals. This is particularly important in this health care era when patients and families move rapidly between settings of care and providers of health care services.

This evaluative approach is a valuable tool in nursing research. Nurse-sensitive measures of acuity and the need for nursing care must include some measure of functional status in populations of patients being served in particular settings of care. Dependence in self-care and toileting requires that

an individual patient have more assistance and more attention to the prevention of iatrogenic complications. Studies have highlighted the critical nature of the relationship between functional status and illness for hospitalized elderly persons (Covinsky et al., 2000).

As Virginia Henderson (Clark, 2006) so eloquently taught nurses, knowing the patient and family provides the nurse with the tools to help them in their journey through illness, recovery, and adaptation or to find a comfortable and peaceful death. Knowing the patient and measuring the impact of nursing interventions are best accomplished through continual assessment of the patient over time. Evaluating the impact of interventions on populations of individuals requires measurement at particular times. Assessment and evaluation of function is vital to planning nursing care of each person as well as in evaluating nursing approaches to populations of patients.

Case Study

Peter Wood, a 79-year-old retired engineer, fell while attempting to go to the bathroom. His wife called 911, and he was admitted to the emergency department of his local hospital. He was found to have a facial paresis and right arm and leg paralysis, and his speech was limited to yes and no answers. Because he was identified as a nonhemorrhagic stroke within the 3-hour onset window, tissue plasminogen activator (TPA) was administered with some improvement in neurological deficits. Mr. Wood's medical history included hypertension, type 2 diabetes, atrial fibrillation, and coronary artery disease.

TABLE 11-2 Nursing Diagnoses, Interventions, and Outcomes Applicable to Mr. Wood   **NIC/NOC**

Nursing Diagnosis	Nursing Intervention	Nursing Outcome

Impaired physical mobility	Energy management
	Environmental management
	Exercise promotion
	Exercise therapy:
	   Joint mobility
	   Balance
	   Positioning
		Mobility

Self-care deficit
  Bathing
  Dressing
  Grooming
  Toileting
	Self-care assistance
	Self-care assistance: instrumental activities of daily living
	Teaching: prescribed activity/exercise
		Self-care: activities of daily living
		Self-care: instrumental activities of
		  daily living

Impaired swallowing	Swallowing therapy Aspiration precautions	Swallowing status
Impaired verbal communication	Active listening Communication enhancement: Speech deficit	Communication: expressive
Risk for falls	Fall prevention Environmental management: safety Exercise therapy: balance/muscle control Urinary elimination: management	Fall prevention behavior
Deficient knowledge	Teaching: disease process Teaching: individual	Knowledge: disease process
Caregiver role strain	Family support	Caregiver home care readiness Caregiver home care education

Case Study—cont'd

On admission to the neurology unit Mr. Wood's nurse completed an admission assessment. The assessment measures administered were the Glasgow Coma Scale, the Barthel Index, the MMSE, the Morse risk to fall scale, and a swallow evaluation. Mr. Wood was found to be dependent in activities of daily living function, to have difficulty swallowing, and to be at risk to fall. Occupational, physical, and speech therapy consultations were requested. By the fifth day of his hospital stay, Mr. Wood was dependent in bathing, dressing, and transferring into a chair. When he attempted to use the urinal, he frequently was wet from being unable to use the urinal independently. He required pureed foods and assistance with being fed. His speech remained limited to yes and no answers. The nursing plan of care (Table 11-3) was developed, identifying nursing diagnoses, interventions, and outcomes (Dochterman and Bulechek, 2004; Moorhead, Johnson, & Maas, 2004). He was screened for rehabilitation and was transferred to a rehabilitation hospital.

On admission to the rehabilitation hospital Mr. Wood's interdisciplinary team utilized the IRF-PAI including the FIM to assess his functional status and to develop an interdisciplinary plan of care. The team, guided by the assessment findings, addressed physical, cognitive, and language deficits. Over his 21-day rehabilitation hospital stay Mr. Wood progressed to being able to ambulate with a short leg brace and a quad cane. He used adaptive equipment to bathe, feed, and dress himself. His wife assisted him in use of the adaptive equipment and in getting up and down stairs. He was able to use the toilet and was continent of bladder and bowel function. His wife assisted him with his clothing when he used the toilet. His language skills continued to improve, he spoke in short sentences, and his comprehension was intact. His swallowing improved, and he could eat a normal diet and swallow pills without difficulty. Thoughtful assessment by the interdisciplinary team (see the critical thinking questions) guided the nurse in preparing for discharge.

After discharge Mr. Wood continued to receive outpatient therapy. His wife drove him to these visits. His goal was to remain in his own home and resume his passion for gardening.

CRITICAL THINKING

While Mr. Wood was in the rehabilitation hospital, the interdisciplinary team prepared his wife for his discharge.

1. How does the information about a patient derived from assessment of function assist in the recognition of discharge needs?
2. How does the nurse utilize patient information obtained from assessment of function to prepare and educate the patient and family for discharge?
3. Describe the method to communicate the rehabilitation plan of care to clinicians who will care for a disabled patient in the community.

REFERENCES

American Nurses Association. (2004). *Nursing: Scope and standards of practice* (2004 ed.). Washington, DC: American Nurses Publishing.

Association of Rehabilitation Nurses. (2000). *Standards and scope of rehabilitation nursing practice.* Glenview, IL: Author.

Center for Long-Term Care. (2002). *Long-term care facility resident assessment instrument (MDS).* Version 2. Baltimore, MD: Centers for Medicare and Medicaid Services.

Centers for Medicare and Medicaid Services. (2006). *Long term care minimum data set (MDS).* Baltimore, MD: Author. Retrieved September 2, 2006, from http://www.cms.hhs.gov/IdentifiableDataFiles/10_LongTermCareMinimumDataSetMDS.asp.

Centers for Medicare and Medicaid Services. (2006). *OASIS: Overview.* Baltimore, MD: Author. Retrieved September 2, 2006, from http://www.cms.hhs.gov/ OASIS/.

Clark, D. (2006). 30th anniversary commentary on Henderson V. (1978) The concept of nursing. *Journal of Advanced Nursing, 3*(1), 113-130.

Clifton, D. (2006). The functional IME: A linkage of expertise across the disability continuum. *Work, 26*(3), 281-285.

Coster, W., Haley, S., & Jette, A., (2006). Measuring patient-reported outcomes after discharge from inpatient rehabilitation settings. *Journal of Rehabilitation Medicine, 38*(4), 237-242.

Covinsky, K., Palmer, R., Counsell, S., Pine, Z., Walter, L, & Chren, M. (2000). Functional status before hospitalization in acutely ill older adults: Validity and clinical importance of retrospective reports. *Journal of the American Geriatrics Society, 48*(2), 164-169.

Dittmar, S., & Gresham, G. E. (2005). *Functional assessment and outcome measures for rehabilitation.* Austin, TX: MD: PRO-ED, Inc.

Dochterman, J. M., & Bulechek, G. M. (2004). *Nursing interventions classification (NIC)* (4th ed.). St. Louis, MO: Mosby.

Duke University Center for the Study of Aging and Human Development. (1978). *Multidimensional functional assessment: The OARS methodology.* Durham, NC: Duke University.

Duncan, P. W., Zorowitz, R., Bates, B., Choi, J. Y., Glasberg, J. J., Graham, G. D., et al. (2005). Management of adult stroke rehabilitation care: A clinical practice guideline. *Stroke, 36*(9):e100-143.

Folstein, M. F., & McHugh, P. (1975). Mini-Mental State: A practical method for grading the cognitive state of patients for the clinician. *Journal of Psychiatric Report, 12,* 189-198.

Grandek, B., Sinclair, S., Kosinski, M., & Ware, J. (2004). Psychometric evaluation of the SF-36 health survey in Medicare managed care. *Health Care Finance Review, 25*(4), 5-25.

Granger, C (1998). Outcome of comprehensive medical rehabilitation: An analysis based upon improvement, disability and handicap model. *International Rehabilitation Medicine, 7*(2), 45-50.

Gresham, G. E., Duncan, P. W., Stason, W. B., Adams, H. P., Adelman, A. M., Alexander, D. N., et al. (1995, May). *Post-stroke rehabilitation* (Clinical Practice Guideline No. 16, AHCPR Publication No. 95-0662). Rockville, MD: U.S. Department of Health and Human Services, Public Health Service, Agency for Health Care Policy and Research.

Kane, R. A., & Kane, R. L. (1981). *Assessing the elderly: A practical guide to measuring.* Lexington, MA: Lexington Books.

Kelly-Hayes, M., Jette, A., Wolf, P. A., D'Agostino, R., & Odell, P. (1992). Functional limitations and disability among elders in the Framingham study. *American Journal of Physical Rehabilitation, 82,* 841-845.

Kelley-Moore, J., Schumacher, J., Kahana, E., & Kahana, B. (2006). When do older adults become "disabled"? Social and health antecedents of perceived disability in a panel study of the oldest old. *Journal of Health Science Behavior, 47*(2), 126-141.

Kwok, T., Lo, R., Wong, E., Wai-Kwong, T., Mok, V., Kai-Sing, W. (2006). Quality of life stroke survivors: A 1-year follow-up study. *Archives of Physical Medicine and Rehabilitation, 87*(9), 1177-1182.

Lawton, M. P. (1972). Assessing the competence of older people. In D. Kent, R. Kastenbaum, & S. Sherwood (Eds.), *Research planning and action for the elderly.* New York: Behavioral Publications.

Lun, T., Lin, W., & Kane, R. (2005). Use of proxy respondents and accuracy of minimum data set assessments of activities of daily living. *The Journals of Gerontology. Series A, Biological Sciences and Medical Sciences, 60*(5), 654-659.

Mahoney, F. I., & Barthel, D. (1965). Functional evaluation: The Barthel Index. *Maryland State Medical Journal, 14,* 56-61.

McCourt, A. (1993). *Rehabilitation nursing: Concepts and practice— A core curriculum* (3rd ed.). Skokie, IL: Rehabilitation Nursing Foundation.

Moorhead, S., Johnson, M., & Maas, M. (Eds.). (2004). *Nursing outcomes classification (NOC)* (3rd ed.). St. Louis, MO: Mosby.

Nagi, S. Z. (1965). Disability concepts revisited. In M. B. Sussman (Ed.), *Sociology and rehabilitation* (pp. 100-113). Washington, DC: American Sociological Association.

New, P. (2006). Non-traumatic spinal cord injury: What is the ideal setting for rehabilitation? *Australian Health Review, 30*(3), 353-361.

Radloff, S. L. (1977). The CES-D scale: A self-report depression scale for research in the general population. *Applied Psychological Measurements, 1,* 385-401.

Resnick, B., Orwig, D., Wehren, L., Hawkes, W., Hebel, R., Zimmerman, S., et al. (2005). Health-related quality of life: Is it a good indicator of function post THR? *Rehabilitation Nursing, 30*(2):46-54, 67.

Schlenker, R. E., Powell, M. C., & Goodrich, G. K. (2005) Initial home health outcomes under prospective payment. *Health Services Research, 40*(1):177-193.

Seacrest, J. A. (2000). Rehabilitation and rehabilitation nursing. In Edwards, P. (Ed.), *The specialty practice of rehabilitation nursing: A core curriculum* (4th ed.). (pp. 2-16). Glenview, IL: Association of Rehabilitation Nurses.

Silverstein, B., Findley, P., & Bode, R. (2006). Usefulness of the nursing home quality measures and quality indicators for assessing skilled nursing facility rehabilitation outcomes. *Archives of Physical Medicine and Rehabilitation, 87*(8), 1021-1025.

Skinner, A., & Turner-Stokes, L. (2006). The use of standardized outcome measures in rehabilitation centres in the UK. *Clinical Rehabilitation, 20*(7), 609-615.

Teasdale, G., & Jennett, B. (1974) Assessment of coma and impaired consciousness: A practical scale. *Lancet, 2*(7872), 81-83.

Thibault, J., & Steiner, R. (2004). Efficient identification of adults with depression and dementia. *American Family Physician, 70*(6), 1101-1112.

Uniform Data System for Medical Rehabilitation. (2006). *Uniform Data System for Medical Rehabilitation.* Buffalo, NY: Author. Retrieved September 3, 2006, from http://www.udsmr.org/fim2_about.php.

U.S. Preventive Services Task Force. (2002). Screening for depression: Recommendations and rationale. *American Family Physician, 66*(4), 647-652.

Ware, J., & Sherburne, C. (1992). The MOS 36 item short-form health survey (SF-36). I. Conceptual framework and item selection. *Medical Care 30*(6), 473-483.

World Health Organization. (1980). *International classification of impairments, disabilities, and handicaps (ICDIDH).* Geneva, Switzerland: Author.

World Health Organization. (2001). *International classification of functioning, disability and related health: ICF.* Geneva, Switzerland. Available from http://www3.who.int/icf/icftemplate.cfm.

12

Community-Based Rehabilitation

Leslie Neal Boylan, PhD, RN, CRRN, FNP-C
Lisa Cyr Buchanan, MS, RN, C, CRRN

Scientific and technological advances, a growing and aging world population, violence, and greater participation in leisure activities have created a milieu in which more individuals of all ages are living with chronic disabling conditions. Changes in eligibility and state funding for nursing home health care and reimbursement for home health care services, shorter lengths of hospital stay, and fewer hospital beds have resulted in many patients leaving hospitals with complex health care needs to receive care in the community setting (Carter & Wade, 2002). However, the political profile of community rehabilitation has increased during recent years as society has become more aware of disability. Evidence suggests that active rehabilitation reduces dependence and the costs of care and increases quality of life. Support for community rehabilitation has grown as politicians and agencies that fund health care have begun to recognize that rehabilitation can contain and reduce health care expenditures (Wade, 2003). It has been demonstrated that the integration of a community-based approach with the continuum of care results in clinically viable outcomes (Kent, 2002).

The rehabilitation focus has shifted in recent years from a biomedical model to a patient-centered model. Autonomy over both decisions and actions has assumed major significance in this shift in perspective. Rehabilitation nurses and other rehabilitation workers provide an environment that fosters autonomy for the individual with a disability (Cardol, De Jong, & Ward, 2002). Nursing, as a profession, has worked toward patient-centered, holistic care that views the patient as a contributing member of the interdisciplinary team. The person with a disability may feel a lack of emotional support, isolated and abandoned with a need for continued support after discharge into the community. Preparation for life in the real world is integral to a satisfying life in the community (Cott, 2004). The community-based rehabilitation nurse plays a key role in assisting patients with successfully reintegrating into the community.

The community in which rehabilitation of the disabled and chronically ill occurs encompasses the environment, availability of housing, transportation, health care providers, geographic location, resources, and access to community buildings. The social system in the community includes the patterns of communication and interactions among the residents, cultural and spiritual patterns, societal attitudes, leadership style of those in power, and how the individual systems within the community interact to carry out the major functions of the community. Residents of a community will experience health problems as individuals or as members of one or more aggregates. Nurses must be adept at assessing all of the subsystems that influence each community system. Consequently, it is important for nurses to understand the concept of community-based rehabilitation and how it is implemented.

THE COMMUNITY-BASED REHABILITATION MODEL

In 1976, the World Health Organization (WHO) (1976) conceptualized community-based rehabilitation (CBR). Most of the people who participate in CBR programs are significantly and severely disabled and must undergo specialized rehabilitation to maintain or acquire employment (Hagen-Foley, Rosenthal, & Thomas, 2005). The genesis of the CBR model and the independent living program (ILP) movement (Table 12-1 and Box 12-1) were based on the recognition that the traditional rehabilitation models were ineffective in meeting the plethora of problems associated with disability. The CBR model is aligned with the national agenda for health care reform in that there is a focus on prevention and taking responsibility for one's own health. Nursing practice models have shifted to integrate the principles of CBR with the health of entire communities.

Originally the CBR model was linked with the medical model of primary health care. However, it has evolved into a

TABLE 12-1 Components of Independent Living Programs and Community-Based Rehabilitation

Independent Living	International Community-Based Rehabilitation
Established during the 1960s in the United States	Established by WHO during 1978 at the Alma-Ata Conference
Focus: Develop independence in self-care	Focus: Prevent disabilities
Goal: Decrease barriers to access	Goal: Reach a large number of persons
Target: Individuals	Target: Entire communities
Control: Individual consumers with disabilities	Control: Create partnerships
Political: Small number of persons making decisions for others ("elite")	Political: Leaders may be privileged in developing countries ("elite")
Self-help and problem solving	Take responsibility for own health
Reduce environmental barriers	Reduce dependency on professionals
Eliminate discrimination	Cultural sensitivity
Peer counseling	Incorporate volunteers, consumer leaders
Consumer advocacy	Cost-effective approaches
Increased power base of consumers	Professionals may have greater power base in developing countries

Modified from Lysack, C., & Kaufert, J. (1994). Comparing the origins and ideologies of the independent living movement and community based rehabilitation. *International Journal of Rehabilitation Research, 17*(3), 231-240.
WHO, World Health Organization.

> **BOX 12-1 Basic Principles of Community-Based Rehabilitation**
>
> - Cultivate positive attitudes and behaviors toward those with disability.
> - Enable persons with disability to live and function independently in the community by eliminating barriers.
> - Empower persons with disability to access appropriate community resources.
> - Promote development of self-help skills and ownership of self-responsibility for health.
> - Provide recipients of health care services and lay workers in the community with knowledge about prevention, healthy behaviors, and rehabilitation.
> - Provide health care services in the community.

Modified from Peat, M. (1991). Community based rehabilitation—development and structure: Part 1. *Clinical Rehabilitation, 5,* 161-166.

comprehensive social model reliant on the resources in the community. The major principle of CBR is to offer primary care services and rehabilitation assistance to people with disabilities by using resources inherent in their communities (Sharma, 2004). The basic tenets of CBR are as follows:

- Utilization of available resources in the community.
- Transfer of knowledge about disabilities and skills in rehabilitation to people with disabilities, families, and communities.
- Community involvement in planning, decision making, and evaluation.
- Utilization and strengthening of referral services at district, [county], and national levels to those agencies able to perform skilled assessments with increasing sophistication, make rehabilitation plans, participate in training, and supervision.

- Utilization of a coordinated, multisectoral approach (Sharma, 2004, p. 326).

Rehabilitation is an integral part of the WHO model of primary care for all nations and is foundational to the goals of the *Healthy People 2000* and *Healthy People 2010* initiatives. The *Healthy People 2000/2010* initiative includes goals and objectives in the categories of health promotion, health protection, and prevention services (U.S. Department of Health and Human Services [USDHHS], 2000). *Rural Health: A Vision for 2010* establishes a plan for providing health care services to all communities through integrating care, promoting safe environments, integrating culturally appropriate care, and creating partnerships between communities (Federal Office of Rural Health Policy and National Rural Health Association [NRHA], 1998). According to *Healthy People 2010,* "individual health is closely linked to community health—the health of the community and environment in which individuals live, work, and play . . . community health is profoundly affected by the collective behaviors, attitudes, and beliefs of everyone who lives in the community" (USDHHS, 2000, p. 3).

The core of CBR is population based with a community focus. One CBR program will be inherently different from the next because its design incorporates the unique attributes, needs, and resources of a particular community. An effective CBR model will incorporate collaboration and planning among the community, the patient with a disability, health care providers, and the family. CBR services are set in noninstitutional arenas where services are sparse or access is limited for persons with disabilities.

Individuals and communities need the appropriate tools, knowledge, technology, and impetus to empower them to take charge of their own health care. Sharing knowledge with communities promotes their health and empowerment and creates partnerships with health professionals. Partnerships can generate the power necessary to implement changes in the delivery of services to communities and in turn enable institutions, communities, all levels of health care providers, and patients to become efficient and effective in their quest for comprehensive health care services. Much of CBR practice is rehabilitation nursing applied to the home, especially encouraging optimal functional independence and self-care as patients' goals (Neal, 1999). Although nurses and other rehabilitation providers often focus on treating the illness and attaining functional gains, adjustment to illness or disability is the primary concern of the patient and family. The trajectory of the disability loses its focus—how will life change for this patient? When providers step back from medical management to rehabilitation, a clearer picture emerges of what patients and communities need for community reintegration. No medical model can prevent disabling conditions, slow the pace of disability, or change the aging population. CBR nursing practice with prevention and education based on the national initiatives may improve outcomes for many rehabilitation patients.

Ideally, patients are involved in discharge planning, controlling their environments, and becoming responsible for their health maintenance plan and lifestyle behaviors. The community health nurse views the community as a whole and fosters collaboration and communication among all providers. Operating within the environment where the patient lives, nurses should work with (not for) patients, regard their priorities, and provide quality care.

CBR NURSING

CBR nurses define a scope of practice, develop a comprehensive knowledge base, and develop an extensive clinical skill base that relies on core knowledge from public health and case management. The core includes, but is not limited to, epidemiology; population-based care, growth, and development; spiritual beliefs; sanitation of the environment; study of communicable diseases; disease prevention; impact of community values; and biological, physical, and behavioral sciences (Williams, 2004).

Rehabilitation community health nurses are registered nurses with specialty training and experience in rehabilitation; they practice a variety of role functions in different community settings, both in their home countries and abroad. For instance, they provide direct care to patients with (increasingly) high acuity within their homes or offer education and consultation with some direct care to patients in clinics, schools, faith communities, and home settings. Roles include staff nurses, educators, administrators, and advanced practice nurses (APNs) in specialty areas of practice, such as incontinence, wound management, and cardiac rehabilitation as well as physical rehabilitation. Box 12-2 contains a list of skills and knowledge expected of the rehabilitation community health nurse, roles that extend beyond providing direct care to individuals. Excellent skills in communication, negotiation,

---

BOX 12-2   Community-Based Rehabilitation Practice Knowledge and Skill Base

- Adult learning principles
- Advocacy
- Case management
- Change theory
- Cognitive/behavioral models
- Communication skills
- Conflict resolution
- Counseling
- Cultural competence
- Detailed knowledge of anatomy and physiology
- Disability management
- Early intervention
- Education
- Environmental influences
- Family systems theories
- Group dynamics
- Health promotion, prevention
- Legislative mandates
- Management of chronic illness
- Negotiation between competing groups
- Normalization
- Research and application to practice
- Service delivery systems
- Sexuality: counseling and interventions
- Spiritual awareness, support
- Systems theory
- Theoretical framework for clinical practice
- Interviewing

---

and interviewing are essential because community health nurses regularly help individuals and groups to think critically and solve problems.

The ability to manage care and other health care professionals while prioritizing and economizing is particularly valuable in the community because nurses coordinate care delivery, as well as professional and ancillary services in the home. Practice in the community enables rehabilitation nurses to expand their knowledge base, to try new and innovative methods for accomplishing goals, and to be flexible because every community is unique and dynamic.

Rehabilitation nurses who visit patients' homes encounter a new environment with each patient. Plans and services that a rehabilitation nurse coordinates from any institution or community setting always take the patient's home environment and resources into account. Data about home and vocational environments are used in planning or implementing care and evaluating a patient's outcomes.

COMMUNITY REINTEGRATION

The term *community reintegration* is poorly defined in the literature. It has been given a barrage of meanings, hence confusing the issue. However, a concise definition is vital for the purpose of research. Dijkers (1999) defines community reintegration as referring to some aspect of the following:

- Being part of the mainstream of family and community life
- Living independently
- Discharging the roles and responsibilities that are considered normal for someone of a specific age, sex, and culture
- Being an active and contributing member of one's social group and of society as a whole

Discharge Planning

Many challenges face providers, patients, and families in planning for the transition from an acute rehabilitation facility to the community. Rehabilitation nurses and skillful discharge planning can be instrumental in successful community reintegration. The term *discharge planning* is used in different ways, but the process is the same; it begins when a patient is admitted to an institution. The process is aided when nurses have in-depth knowledge about the resources available in a community for the patient's reintegration. Providers can develop and maintain a list of community resources (Box 12-3) that is validated and updated regularly. This is one tool for discharge planners who struggle to arrange proper comprehensive services within a short time when a patient is leaving the institution.

The time just before discharge from an acute hospitalization is critical and involves intense discharge planning efforts if community reintegration is to be successful. Older adults are at risk for failure, especially when preadmission factors such as previous functional status are not included in the plan. Thorough discharge planning considers the home and community environment early in the process. For example, any home modifications must be planned so they can be completed quickly or temporary adaptations arranged until permanent work is completed. The team will not have the luxury of postponing a discharge because of incomplete home modifications.

Shortened lengths of stay in some cases may have generated more efficiency within programs. However, some providers believe that patients are denied the crucial time required to adjust to a catastrophic event or life-changing illness. The patient and family are often grieving while attempting to adjust to role changes, provide personal care, coordinate services and finances, and manage the overall impact of the situation on the family unit. The rehabilitation community health nurse coordinates evaluations from many members of the interdisciplinary team to promote a successful community reintegration.

Comprehensive discharge planning can help prevent readmissions to hospitals. Implementing patient and caregiver involvement in the planning process for community reintegration, extensive patient/caregiver teaching, and coordinating and securing community resources and services before discharge from an institution will contribute to successful community reintegration. The rehabilitation nurse has a vital role in identifying individual, family, and community needs; developing a knowledge base about the availability of community resources and services; developing methods for accessing services; and

planning for ongoing evaluations in the community to ensure that the services are adequately meeting changes in needs. These strategies will facilitate successful community reintegration and prevent hospital readmissions or institutionalization.

Discharge planning includes education about preventing complications or further disability and promoting healthy lifestyles and behaviors. Developing partnerships in the community and a thorough assessment of patient and community needs and resources, access to health services, and barriers to community reintegration are essential components and areas where rehabilitation nurses can be instrumental in improving outcomes.

BOX 12-3 Community Resources

Community Resources Available and/or Needed
- Home health care services
- Attendant care
- Transportation
- Support services/groups
- Support from family/friends/clergy
- Disability-related information
- Respite care
- Outpatient rehabilitation services
- Contingency plan if caregiver is ill or unavailable
- School services
- Early intervention services
- Partnerships
- Employee assistance program
- Supported employment
- Volunteer helpers
- Church and church groups
- Local chapters of national organizations
- Rescue squad and fire department
- Planned recreation
- Providers of alternative therapies
- Legal services
- Adult day care
- Specialized care centers
- Assisted living
- Senior centers and programs
- Pharmacy to special order
- Equipment, supplies, and oxygen vendors
- Special camps

Patient/Caregiver Knowledge Base
- Caregiver training for direct care needs
- Emergency services
- Financial resources
- Health care resources
- Equipment care and repair
- Infection control procedures

Home Evaluation

Access to Community Environment

Home Pass Assessment Before Discharge

THEORETICAL FRAMEWORKS OF CBR

Rehabilitation nursing in the community relies on an eclectic combination of theoretical frameworks. Orem (2001) provides frameworks for delivering care to patients to maximize independence and self-care. Roy's work (Roy & Andrews, 1999) is useful to understand how the rehabilitation community health nurse supports the adaptation of the patient to disability, chronic illness, or an otherwise altered lifestyle. Neuman's Systems Model (2002) is used in CBR because it is based on holism and a systems approach as the patient in the community interacts with multiple systems. Neal's research (2000) deals specifically with home health care nurses but can be generalized to other community health nurses.

Nolan and Nolan (1998) suggest that rehabilitation nurses need specific skills (Table 12-2) to practice within the recommended model. They intend that their model will "more closely align professional practice with the needs of chronically ill and disabled persons and their careers." Theorists are discussed further in Chapter 2.

CBR incorporates the concepts of populations at risk and population-based care and comprehensive assessments of communities. Rehabilitation nurses already bring expert clinical performance and extensive experience in providing in-depth education to other health providers, patients, and families, as well as how to function as a core member of a team and to cultivate a spirit of self-help and self-responsibility within groups. Experience improves not only a nurse's expert care to patients, but also the ability to assess and comprehend the intricate workings of a community. Nurses in CBR can identify obstacles to public health and address solutions to complex health issues.

The credibility of rehabilitation nurses in a CBR practice setting extends beyond clinical expertise, as they practice on patients' turfs. Families have multiple health care, social, economic, and psychological needs and seek expertise to articulate solutions and provide support. Exhausted caregivers need respite care. Children living in inner cities and rural areas may have limited access to primary care because of financial or geographical constraints. Violence and abuse are major health care issues in the nation that influence both causation and the process of reintegration. Rehabilitation nurses' clinical knowledge and skills must join with a passion for understanding, caring, and assisting patients in being as healthy as they can be. CBR nursing is practiced within the context of the patient's environment, culture, and geographical location. The rehabilitation community health nurse considers the impact of these variables in planning for CBR services.

The Environment

In this chapter, *environment* refers not only to the physical setting in which the patient lives, works, and functions but also to the dynamics of family and other support systems that might affect the patient's ability to function independently. The patient's financial status, ability to obtain nutrition and medicine, capability of receiving spiritual care, culture, and own psychosocial state are all influential elements of the environment.

It is not uncommon for the nurse to focus on changing the environment while neglecting to view patients in the context of their environment. The focus perhaps should be to assess how the nurse might assist the patient in making adaptations to function more optimally within the current environment. The person who is chronically ill or disabled is significantly affected not only by the home environment but also by every physical environment encountered. Barriers to access abound and are discussed in detail later in this chapter.

Culture

The term *culture* refers not only to ethnicity or ancestry but also to customs observed by a particular individual or within a family. Regardless of whether the rehabilitation community

TABLE 12-2 Indicative Areas of Knowledge and Skills Necessary for Fulfilling a Variety of Potential Nursing Roles in Rehabilitation

Role	Knowledge/Skills
Assessment of physical condition, delivery of skilled care, and prevention of secondary complications	Detailed physiology and related anatomy and pathology of relevant conditions (e.g., stroke, multiple sclerosis); knowledge of normal physiology and a range of therapeutic interventions; knowledge of a range of measurement indexes and their operational bases
Education/counseling	Detailed knowledge of adult learning and counseling theory, group facilitation, processes, etc.; ability to assess readiness, capacity, and motivation to learn; assessment of preferred learning style
Psychosocial interventions	Ability to assess mood state; understanding of a range of theoretical areas, particularly stress theory; ability to assess appropriateness of coping styles and modify accordingly; use of cognitive behavioral models
Family careers	Detailed knowledge of family systems theories; ability to assess family dynamics
Sexuality	Ability to address sexuality on an individual basis; knowledge and skill in counseling and intervention techniques relevant to identified need
Coordinating role, liaison, and facilitating transitions through the health care system	Detailed knowledge of multidisciplinary working; high level of communication skills, diplomacy, assertiveness; knowledge of service delivery systems

From Nolan, M., & Nolan, J. (1998). Rehabilitation: Scope for improvement in current practice. *British Journal of Nursing, 7*(9), 522-526.

health nurse is functioning in his or her own country or in a foreign country, the patient is viewed within the context of the patient's culture and the nurse attempts to avoid introducing bias into his or her care. The patient's home has its own culture, whereas the vocational setting may have a very different culture. The rehabilitation community health nurse is a guest at either site and is therefore expected to respect the cultural values therein.

Culture often presents and predisposes to barriers to health care. Language differences often interrupt smooth communication. Health as a priority and the definition and influence of community related to health behavior may vary significantly among cultures. The acceptance of particular attitudes and behaviors, such as spousal abuse, may be at odds with the nurse's own cultural views and therefore must be approached with sensitivity. Attitudes and behaviors significantly influence adherence to plans of care because patients must accept the need for a change and understand that the change will make them feel better.

The rehabilitation community health nurse performs a cultural assessment that includes customs; verbal and nonverbal means of communication; the patient's perception of the problem; and the diet, medications, and psychosocial status of the patient. The nurse determines who makes decisions for the patient (if not the patient), relevant sick-role behaviors, and the patient's community resources (Portillo, 2002).

Some community health organizations make efficient use of lay community health workers recruited from within the community to assist in identifying health needs and ensuring access to care. The lay workers can be essential in assisting professionals and patients with overcoming barriers to care from language or culture and act to support the development of partnerships and community resources.

Geographical Location

Both urban and rural populations may have limited access to health care. Urban populations, although being close to centers for health care delivery, commonly experience financial and cultural barriers to care. The millions of persons in this country who are uninsured, as well as the millions more who are underinsured, depend on combinations of programs that remain inadequate to meet health care needs (Thompson-Heisterman, 2004).

In rural areas fewer residents translates into fewer opportunities to socialize, lack of transportation for access to health care, and shortages of health care providers. Rehabilitation community health nurses take advantage of social activities and other informal opportunities that arise within the rural community to offer health teaching. Also, the extended family is considered influential in the patient's health care and is approached by the nurse during meaningful interactions.

SPECIAL POPULATIONS

The challenge to the rehabilitation nurse working in the community is to assist persons with physical and/or mental impairments with reestablishing previous roles as desired, developing new roles, and adapting to the impact of the disability (persons never *accept* disabilities, and providers should delete this notion from their vocabularies); to provide support and education for caregivers; and to provide the patient and family with the skills and knowledge necessary for successful community reintegration. Certain populations of patients are at high risk for failure to reintegrate into the community unless they receive intense follow-up support services including education. Populations at risk include elderly patients; infants and young children with physical or developmental disabilities; and individuals with psychiatric disabilities, acquired traumatic brain injury, autism, and physical disabilities. Education, including written materials that can be used after discharge, is related to patients' successful community reintegration.

Mentally Ill Patients

Persons with a combination of cognitive and physical disabilities have needs that challenge attempts at community reintegration. A comprehensive assessment of cognitive and physical abilities is imperative because providers tend to focus on obvious disabilities and neglect more subtle impairments when planning for community reentry. Rehabilitation nurses may consult with interdisciplinary team colleagues often when planning community reentry for persons with multiple disabilities because managing the complexity requires more than the expertise of one professional discipline, and conditions may be rare and unique.

CBR nurses must understand the scope of mental illness in the communities in which they work. Managed care has and will continue to influence community delivery of services for the mentally ill, and insufficient funds and social services may continue to limit resources available to the mentally ill (Thompson-Heisterman, 2004). Agency networking, collaboration among and between agencies, and partnerships with patients and other providers can assist the rehabilitation nurse in improving quality patient care (Coddington, 2001).

Pediatric Patients

One out of seven children in the United States has no health insurance coverage (National Center for Health Statistics [NCHS], 2002). Approximately 200,000 to 800,000 children and teenagers are homeless at any point in time (NCHS, 2002). Injuries are the primary cause of death for children until the age of 21 years, and 20% to 25% of children suffer a problem related to injury (Cowan, 2004). However, technological advances in medicine have enabled more children to survive chronic health problems. Many children with chronic illness or disabilities are cared for at home.

Geriatric Patients

Health care reform is being pushed in part by the demographical trends in our nation. The number of adults over the age of 75 years is growing faster than any other segment of society (Remsburg & Carson, 2002). These trends will have economic, medical, and social consequences. In fact, there are rapidly increasing numbers of persons living in the community who will require some type of rehabilitation services for the rest of their lives. In a milieu of decreasing resources, managed care, and increasing numbers of those requiring community resources, rehabilitation nurses and other allied health professionals must become skilled at ensuring successful community reentry and become politically active to ensure that services to persons with disabilities are continued.

Older adults make up the largest population of patients in the community. Because of their high incidence of functional impairments and effects on their quality of life, the expertise of rehabilitation community health nurses is essential to quality care. One fifth of elderly Americans cannot independently perform at least one basic activity of daily living (NCHS, 2000).

A physician who incorrectly assesses a patient's functional ability may not order home visits or order too few visits to assist the patient to maximal independence within the home. Reimbursement for essential home health care services would then be reduced or eliminated. Rehabilitation nurses can influence changes in this situation because they are skilled at assessing functional ability, can articulate goals and rationales appropriate within reimbursement guidelines, can accurately predict the composition of the interdisciplinary team needed to meet the patient's needs, and are respected by physicians for their specialized knowledge.

Other obstacles for elderly populations are their inability to access transportation, their income status, and the unavailability of services. In addition, older adults tend to have a higher incidence of mental health problems than found in the general population, impairments that can interfere with functional ability. The elderly tend to use many over-the-counter medications. Polypharmacy increases the risk of medication mismanagement and, consequently, adverse effects, some of which can be related to altered functional ability. A medication assessment provides essential information when formulating a comprehensive picture of the patient's status and potential for independence and self-care. The rehabilitation community health nurse assesses a patient's physical environment and ability to navigate the environment, leave the home, and obtain and finance health care and nutrition, as well as the psychosocial status and support systems in the environmental context.

BARRIERS TO COMMUNITY REINTEGRATION

Multiple barriers to receiving health care prevent or affect patients' reintegration (Kim & Fox, 2004), especially when they have chronic or disabling conditions. One barrier to receiving home health care occurs when the patient is unqualified because of ineligibility to receive services. Each person who receives home health care must satisfy requirements, such as being homebound or medically stable. If caring for a patient in the home imposes "an undue administrative or financial burden" on the home health care agency (e.g., because of lack of reimbursement), the agency may refuse to provide care. No legislation, including the Americans With Disabilities Act (ADA), rules that an agency must provide care if doing so overly taxes the agency's resources. Another barrier to care is a patient's need for a service that may not be available within the agency.

Cultural or attitudinal prejudices and socioeconomic status are other potential obstacles to community reintegration. (See Chapter 6 for more information regarding culture.) Transportation, attendant care, employment, housing, caregiver concerns, and reimbursement practices are additional barriers.

Emerging disability groups include people who are sick or living with pain, are not accepted by the medical world as disabled, and may be invisible to society while possessing a high degree of recognition for their own disabilities. These groups appear indistinguishable from others in society because their disabilities are hidden. This contributes to a life of uncertainty, difficulty receiving medical services, a lack of understanding by employers of their need for time off for illness, and difficulty receiving accommodation or disability benefits (Kim & Fox, 2004).

Transportation

Transportation can make the difference between community reintegration and institutionalization for many patients. The ADA of 1990 required that public transportation be accessible. Rehabilitation community health nurses are advocates for accessible, affordable transportation for their patients. Some forms of public transportation still have specific criteria for access, for example, through levying extra or special charges or requirements, such as an attendant to accompany patients during the ride.

Attendant Care

Many adults with disabilities or chronic illnesses live at home and function independently or with minimal assistance. However, there is a population for whom an attendant may make the difference between being able to live at home and going to school or work and becoming institutionalized. Attendants' training, qualifications, and functions vary according to the patient's needs, financial status, preferences, and insurance coverage. A number of persons with disabilities are ineligible for attendant programs or are not covered by certain programs for the extended hours of care they require, leaving responsibilities of caregiving with family members or friends. At a recent conference, family members of patients with chronic diseases discussed their needs for attendant care. They identified the need for flexible nurses and aides, attendants who could provide caregivers respite, and attendants and other caregivers who could develop a relationship with the patient and family that went beyond paying for a professional service. They expected the attendant to be able to communicate with the patient and family, display a positive attitude, and be knowledgeable about community resources (National Association for Home Care, 1999).

"Cluster care" is a program that was first instituted in New York City. This program "enables an elderly person to use an aide for a minimum number of hours because the aide is shared with others who require assistance and who live in the same building or nearby" (Rosengarten, Milburn, & Ryan, 1996, p. 640).

TABLE 12-3 Housing Options for Disabled Persons

Type	Description
Congregate	Segregated community living developed for individuals with mobility impairments
Residential	Support services shared by a group of persons with disabilities living in proximity; services managed by others
Independent living center	Persons with disabilities assisted with housing referral, attendant referral, attendant training, advocacy, equipment repair, and other services; services not managed in a single setting
Institution	Person receives individualized care according to nursing care plan 24 hours per day
Boarding home	Private or state run; person usually required to perform own personal care and must demonstrate ability to be mobile in environment with or without assistive device
Supervised environmental living facility	Supervised apartment program for chronically mentally ill persons; provides comprehensive, supportive, and rehabilitative services to promote community reentry
Integrated housing: private residence or rental	Independent living; may receive support services from the community such as home health care, attendant care
Group home	Supervised living environment; persons with similar disabilities live together
Assisted living	Persons have their own rooms within a building or complex but are offered services such as meals, medication, personal care, and screening services; persons are unable to live alone without some supervision

Employment

Although the ADA prohibits employers from asking questions that might reveal a potential employee's disability, employers are permitted to question prospective employees about their ability to fulfill the requirements of the job. A medical examination can be required only once a job is conditionally offered. In addition, it is not clear per the ADA what does and does not meet the requirement of reasonable accommodation. According to a study of job discrimination among people with disabilities, there is more discrimination regarding access to jobs for people with disabilities than for people with disabilities (Perry, Hendricks, & Broadbent, 2000). Although employment for people with disabilities has risen, "employers are reluctant to hire someone with physical disabilities; too much technology is required; [and] employers won't pay for accommodation . . ." (Mast, 2001).

Housing

Insufficient housing is a barrier for many persons in the community and especially for those with impairments or disabilities. They lack affordable, accessible, or federally funded housing options and encounter housing discrimination. People with disabilities may be treated unfairly in some community-based housing programs. People with disabilities must be able to choose where they wish to live and the services they need.

The individual's ability to make decisions about housing is severely hampered by the government view that everyone with a similar diagnosis has the same needs for services and that affordability and access can be acquired only by mandating that they have their living arrangements set up for them (Table 12-3). Traditionally the medical model of CBR has led to segregation and institutionalization for persons with disabilities (Kim & Fox, 2004). Rehabilitation community health nurses can serve as advocates for patients seeking fair and accessible housing in their communities.

The Rehabilitation Act Amendments of 1992 and 1993 revised the funding process for the Centers for Independent Living programs (CILs) in an attempt to increase access to rehabilitation services for persons with severe disabilities (Kim & Fox, 2004). These centers are based in the community, non-profit, and managed by persons with disabilities. CILs strive to provide patient advocacy, promote community reintegration and participation, be consumer based, provide a range of services above and beyond housing, and serve persons with a variety of disabilities. Factors influencing the choices individuals make regarding community living are listed in Box 12-4.

Effective CILs are proactive, rather than reactive, when identifying and eliminating social, environmental, and economic barriers in the community. Trained, available, and knowledgeable staff work with persons as they reenter their homes and communities, but control and management is by the consumers (Kim & Fox, 2004).

Caregiver Issues

Family members, congregations, and neighbors are increasingly burdened with providing care for persons they care about who reside in community settings. During a time when extended family rarely reside in the same town and family members commonly work full-time while caring for elderly parents and young children, it is not uncommon for disabled and chronically ill persons to be attended by professional caregivers and hired companions.

Often a family caregiver's social/interpersonal, physical, psychological, and financial circumstances are influenced by the caregiving role. Inadequate sleep and fewer opportunities for social interaction, as well as a changed relationship with the person being cared for, compromise the caregiver's quality of life. Unfortunately, issues related to the person for whom care is being provided often are overridden by the multiple concerns and issues confronting the caregiver. Caregivers may

BOX 12-4 Factors Influencing Choices of Community Living Alternatives

- Financial resources
- Type of disability
- Geographical location
- Availability and need for social support systems
- Need for skill acquisition and training
- Availability of attendant care in the community
- Availability and affordability of transportation services
- Ability to manage own finances
- Ability to hire, train, and supervise attendants
- Access to primary care providers and health care facilities

experience emotional problems, changes in their own health, stress-related alterations, and guilt. The health of the caregivers is threatened by their own health problems, fatigue, and inadequate attention to their own needs (Martinson, 2004).

Violence and Abuse

Women, children, individuals with disabilities, and elderly persons are at risk for abuse and violent assaults (Children's Defense Fund, 2001; USDHHS, 2000). Concurrently, individuals may use substance abuse as a means of coping with a disability. Violence and abuse are national issues. "Alcohol and illicit drug use are associated with child and spousal abuse; sexually transmitted diseases, including HIV infection; teen pregnancy; school failure; motor vehicle crashes; escalation of health care costs; low worker productivity; and homelessness" (USDHHS, 2000, p. 20). Public policies, emigration of populations to other neighborhoods, and housing overcrowding can lead to degradation of communities. Substance abuse, unemployment, and psychosocial stress can precipitate violence in the workplace or community.

Rehabilitation nurses must be cognizant of the risk factors for violence and abuse in any community setting and report incidents according to agency policies and Occupational Safety and Health Administration guidelines. Recognition is the first step toward ensuring safe communities and workplace environments.

Reimbursement Practices

Reimbursement for home health care services has changed along with government regulations for patients qualifying for and receiving home health care services. New mandates for methods of measuring and ensuring quality services have resulted in more than 2500 home health care agencies closing since 1997 and the loss of many home health care jobs across the nation.

Nurses working in community settings visit approximately eight patients per day. Patients are discharged from the hospital with an increasingly high level of acuity after short stays, so the community nurse must provide care at levels that used to be the responsibility of the hospital staff and in the same number of visits per day.

Managed care limits the numbers of allowable home health care visits significantly. Services may be further restricted due to perceived need or the particular contract for care. Some insurance companies do not pay for occupational therapy or medical social work services in the home. However, many managed care companies have loosened their restrictions, and this is partially attributable to replacing non–health care professional case managers with nurses. Restrictions have forced home health care professionals to become more efficient with visits. A positive effect is maximizing the care provided per visit. However, care for the elderly, those who require more time to learn, or patients with chronic, disabling conditions can be shortchanged with this increased efficiency.

The Health Plan Employer Data and Information Set (HEDIS) defined outcomes to provide a standard of quality for managed care companies despite community differences. However, health care needs and issues do vary among communities, and managed care organizations must be responsive to the specific demographics and needs of the community.

Managed care, Medicare, and Medicaid typically rely on homebound status (i.e., the patient cannot leave the home without great difficulty or the assistance of another person) as the main criterion for care. Nursing documentation must indicate that there are skilled needs in the home and that the patient cannot easily access other health care options (such as an outpatient clinic) to receive care. The payer readily refuses to reimburse for care without confirming need.

Medicare recognizes "restorative" care as a skill. However, although physical therapy, occupational therapy, and speech therapy are reimbursable services, rehabilitation nursing is subsumed by nursing and is not recognized as a specialty. This incidentally is the case with most nursing specialties offered in home health care. Managed care does provide opportunities to plan for healthy communities. However, there is no guarantee that the community's health will improve. Managed Medicaid does not guarantee care to the poor, nor does managed Medicare.

In 1999 the Centers for Medicare and Medicaid (CMS) mandated the collection of outcome data by home health care organizations regardless of the patient's payer. The collection tool is called the Outcome and Assessment Information Set (OASIS). All nurses and therapists are required to collect OASIS data on every patient they admit to home health care services. These data are then coded and transmitted to the CMS. Agencies receive feedback regarding the aggregated data, and this information is then used for quality improvement.

The OASIS in its longest form is 79 questions. It is administered in some form on admission to service, on discharge, when the patient is due for recertification, and when the patient resumes care after an inpatient stay midservice. Most of the questions are related to functional ability despite the inadequate knowledge of the generalist nurse regarding assessment of functional ability. Other questions include inquiries regarding patient demographics, wound status, and pain management. It typically takes an experienced nurse 1 to $1\frac{1}{2}$ hours to complete the full-length OASIS. The Outcomes Based Quality Improvement (OBQI) program mandated by CMS is based on indicators chosen as foci (by each agency) when reviewing OASIS data.

NURSING INTERVENTIONS

Community-based rehabilitation should take place within the context of the interdisciplinary team (Box 12-5). Ideally the patient and family are at the center of the team. Other core members should include the physician, registered nurse, physical therapist, occupational therapist, speech therapist, social worker, clergy, psychologist, and dietitian when available and appropriate. The team may include these traditional healers as well as providers of alternative complementary services (e.g., acupuncturist). In the community the team may be expanded to include the school nurse, rescue squad, department of human services, and neighbors. The rehabilitation nurse may be the builder and coordinator of the team. However, the reimbursement structure may dictate the team's structure and format.. In underserved areas (rural or city) there may be too few professionals and or there may be an increased cost generated for team meetings. These factors may prevent the team from meeting formally. Team members will need to be creative in collaborating and communicating and in planning, implementing, and evaluating patient care.

The goal of the team is the same whether in the institution or in the community: to work collaboratively in meeting the physical, emotional, social, vocational, cultural, spiritual, and economic needs of patients, caregivers, and family members in the community. The complexity of care provided to patients in the community warrants an expert level of functioning by all team members. Health care professionals must be adept at identifying barriers; facilitating the strengths of the patient, family, and community; procuring services; and empowering patients and their support systems through education and the acquisition of skills. These skills will promote successful community reintegration.

Attendant Care

Funding sources for attendant care may be obtained through a variety of programs. The patient will be required to meet eligibility requirements specific to each program. Some of these programs include Medicare, Medicaid, workers' compensation, private health care insurance, health maintenance organizations (HMOs), Veterans Affairs benefits, preferred provider organizations, and auto liability policies. It is imperative that rehabilitation professionals assist patients and caregivers with identifying individual needs relative to attendant care requirements—specific tasks requiring assistance, number of hours per day—and to obtain the resources required to promote independent community living. The patient and family must learn to work with and replace attendants.

In the wake of managed care changes in the Medicare/Medicaid eligibility for home health care and other services, it is a challenge for case managers and discharge planners to obtain the needed resources for patients and caregivers. Case managers must be proactive and current about regulations and guidelines.

OUTCOMES, EVALUATION, AND RESEARCH

The current focus of health care delivery is on evidenced-based practice, measurement of outcomes in the community and in clinical practice, development of models for specific populations of patients, and program evaluation. Evidence-based practice models of health care delivery require careful scrutiny because they must demonstrate research-based clinical outcomes and improved quality. Legislators, consumers, and payers are demanding efficiency, effectiveness, and accountability from providers. Striving to meet the public health goals of health promotion, health protection, and preventive services of the *Healthy People 2010* initiative goes hand in hand with developing valid and reliable instruments for measuring clinical outcomes in CBR practice settings.

To maximize outcomes of the quality and cost-effectiveness of health care delivery, skills in critical thinking and methods based on evidence are essential. Research that has clinical relevance combined with clinical expertise and patient preference leads to effective and individualized quality care. Rosswurm and Larrabee (1999) developed a model that is useful for CBR evidence-based practice and research. The following steps are from the model:

1. Assess need for change in practice.
2. Link problem, interventions, and outcomes.
3. Synthesize best evidence.
4. Design practice change.
5. Implement and evaluate change in practice.
6. Integrate and maintain change in practice.

Nurses find a rich source of researchable issues and problems in their community practice. The broad range of uncontrolled variables makes research within the community setting challenging and interesting. Research initiatives may come from the agency or the community, or the nurse may identify research questions from clinical practice. Rehabilitation community health nurses, for example, may form research questions centered on improving outcomes for persons with chronic illnesses, impairments, or disabling conditions and altered levels of functional abilities. They may examine the effectiveness of interventions designed to assist patients in managing their own care.

BOX 12-5 Team Building

- Interdisciplinary model used
- Leader chosen based on communication skills, ability to resolve conflict, and clinical expertise
- Unity within group promotes establishing specific goals
- Group process facilitates cohesiveness between members
- Collaboration provides direction in developing comprehensive patient care plans
- Change process implemented when required to enhance team functioning
- Role clarity established

SUMMARY

The rehabilitation community health nurse is a vital player in CBR. Within the community, the rehabilitation nurse offers a perspective that differs from that of nurses who practice within institutional settings and builds on public health nursing principles. The roles of the rehabilitation community health nurse are varied, and the potential for creativity is almost limitless. Whether assisting patients with community reintegration, forming partnerships with patients and community, identifying resources to maximize patients' independence, promoting the nation's primary initiatives, or participating in research, rehabilitation community health nurse roles are likely to expand as more patients receive care in community settings. Multiple issues affect definitions of CBR nursing practice. The knowledge base and skills required of a rehabilitation nurse will vary with the setting, the characteristics and needs of the community, and the types of impairment or disability. A review of the issues and critical needs of patients, families, and communities contributes to development of innovative and appropriate practice models, especially when the need is for comprehensive care plans across the life span.

Case Study

Adam Broward is a 46-year-old man who sustained a T11 spinal cord injury (SCI) as a result of a fall from a tree at his home. Mr. Broward has a long history of alcohol and drug abuse, risk-taking behaviors (reports he has had a combination of 25 motorcycle and motor vehicle accidents in his lifetime), and more recently he has suffered from depression. He feels (and his wife confirms) that his antidepressant medication has not been helpful. He has hepatitis B and C. Mr. Broward was incarcerated for 3 years for smuggling cocaine and was released 2 years ago. He has been free from alcohol and drug use since his release from prison. Adam has a wife (Julie) and two teenage children. Julie Broward works for an agency that requires she be gone overnight from Monday at 8 AM until Wednesday at 2 PM. The teenage children both attend high school and are involved in many activities.

Because he has managed care insurance coverage, Adam Broward was discharged to his home before the modifications were completed. A ramp was built and doorways replaced, but there was no access to his bathroom or the second floor. His family converted the dining room into a bedroom for him. He must wear his thoracic lumbar sacral orthosis (TLSO) brace for another 2 months. Home health care services are provided for 2 to 3 weeks. Adam has had difficulties with the initial transition to the community. The following sections address Adam's specific health care issues. Later, a nursing care plan for a spinal cord injured patient is presented.

Elimination Pattern: Urinary Retention

Adam Broward is on an intermittent catheterization program (ICP) every 6 hours. He learned how to use a clean technique during his acute rehabilitation stay but has required antibiotics for urinary tract infections (UTIs). He is unable to reach his bathroom to empty his own urinal and does not measure intake and output at home. He had catheterization volumes above 500 ml four to five times per week during his acute rehabilitation stay. Julie Broward has not performed the catheterization procedure.

Goals

Patient will:
1. Identify and report signs and symptoms of a UTI
2. Demonstrate knowledge about the purpose, action, and side effects of medications

3. Have catheterization volumes of less than 500 ml
4. Demonstrate knowledge of managing fluid intake to regulate bladder volumes
5. Demonstrate knowledge about preventing UTIs

Interventions

1. Teach regarding prevention of UTIs, medications (purpose, action, side effects), and signs and symptoms of a UTI.
2. Instruct patient to avoid fluids that act as irritants, are diuretics, or cause an increase in the pH of urine.
3. Demonstrate clean, intermittent catheterization technique, and have patient's wife provide return demonstration.
4. Instruct patient to monitor intake, output, and catheterization volumes for the first 2 to 3 weeks.

Bowel Incontinence

Adam Broward was in acute rehabilitation for 2½ weeks. He takes docusate sodium (Colace) 100 mg three times per day and psyllium hydrophilic mucilloid (Metamucil) 1 packet every day at bedtime. He has a morning program (his premorbid pattern) and uses only digital stimulation and a custom-made adaptive device. He has hard stools and difficulty completing his hygiene independently after an occasional accident.

Goals

Patient will:
1. Have a bowel movement every day while on the commode and without accidents
2. Demonstrate knowledge of factors promoting bowel continence: timing of program; nutritional intake; digital stimulation technique, frequency of use, managing with adaptive equipment; exercise; fluid intake; and effects of medications
3. Manage own hygiene

Interventions

1. Teach about techniques to promote bowel continence: digital stimulation; fluid intake and balance intake with catheterization volumes; use of exercise to facilitate evacuation, such as range-of-motion exercises, forward bends, and Valsalva maneuver; and nutritional intake.

Case Study—cont'd

2. *Teach about managing own hygiene: keep TLSO on, use skin inspection mirror, elevate head of bed, have hygiene equipment within reach, use adaptive equipment from the occupational therapist for attaching washcloths, do hygiene independently each time, and ask for help only if absolutely necessary.*

Readiness for Enhanced Family Coping: Potential for Growth

Adam and Julie have had marital problems and no sexual relations for 2 years. Julie has no desires and says she wants to get Adam settled at home and then reevaluate their marriage. They have had marital counseling previously. However, Julie is not ready for Adam to come home, and their children have mixed feelings about his parenting, which they describe as his "barking" orders at them. Julie says she is comfortable telling him when his communication style is inappropriate. The family dynamics and the disability are overwhelming. Julie Broward states, "I really wanted everything to be done before he came home. It would have made make things a lot easier."

Goals

Adam and the family will:
1. *Express feelings and emotions freely*
2. *Demonstrate knowledge about psychosocial adjustment to a spinal cord injury*
3. *Demonstrate an understanding of resources available in the community and methods by which to access them*
4. *Seek professional assistance when required*

Interventions

1. *Evaluate impact of disability on family roles, and facilitate patient/family description of changes in roles for each family member.*
2. *Teach patient and family about the grieving process, psychosocial adjustment after an SCI, methods to use for communicating appropriately with family members and others, constructive outlets for feelings of frustration and anger.*
3. *Encourage social and community activities.*
4. *Encourage Adam to foster relationship with Mike Collier, a 39-year-old man who lives in the same community and who visited the Adam twice during his rehabilitation admission.*
5. *Assist patient and family with identifying available support systems and counseling options.*

Ineffective Role Performance: Change in Physical Capacity to Resume Role

Adam Broward (except while incarcerated) was employed for less than a year as a painter at a local paper mill. His employer has agreed to pay his salary for 6 months; he has no short- or long-term disability insurance. Adam built a home and maintained the building and grounds. He is considering selling his home and building one that is accessible. He wants to return to work.

Goals

Adam will:
1. *Identify specific changes in roles that have been affected by the disability*
2. *Demonstrate the ability to perform family role behaviors*
3. *Return to work and perform work role behaviors*

Interventions

1. *Provide family support.*
2. *Initiate referral for vocational rehabilitation.*
3. *Encourage participation in social and community activities.*
4. *Initiate referral to advocacy group for peer support and counseling.*
5. *Evaluate employment and job retraining opportunities in current employment situation.*

Ineffective Sexuality Pattern

Julie and Adam had no sexual relations for 2 years before the SCI and had a history of marital discord. Adam promised his sister before she died that he would stay with his wife for the children. Julie states that she is not interested in having a sexual relationship and plans to wait until the family has adjusted to Adam's return home and then work on their marriage. Both are amenable to seeking counseling again. Adam says one issue is managing changes in body image; Julie has concerns about renewing intimacy with the discord in their relationship. She wants to renew marriage vows if they decide to continue their relationship. Adam received extensive teaching and counseling regarding sexuality while in rehabilitation.

Goals

Adam and Julie will:
1. *Express positive psychosocial adjustment to the life change caused by the disability*
2. *Identify issues causing marital discord*

Interventions

1. *Facilitate patient/wife participation in a support group.*
2. *Arrange for marital counseling.*
3. *Provide sexual counseling.*
4. *Teach regarding sexual functioning and sexuality after an SCI.*

CRITICAL THINKING QUESTIONS

1. What should be the priorities for nursing care from most important to least important?
2. Identify and describe safety issues that exist for this patient.
3. Who are the most appropriate members of the interdisciplinary team to care for this patient, and what will they do?
4. Recalling growth and development milestones and behaviors, how should the nurse integrate the patient's children into the plan of care?

Continued

Case Study—cont'd

Nursing Care Plan for a Patient With a Lower Motor Neuron Spinal Cord Injury

Nursing Diagnosis	Plan/Interventions	Expected Outcomes
Decreased cardiac output r/t immobility	Perform ROM of lower extremities at least every 8 hr.	No deep venous thrombosis or pulmonary emboli.
Impaired skin integrity r/t immobility and poor tissue perfusion	Inspect all areas of skin (particularly over bony prominences) every day, instruct patient to perform seat pushups every 15 minutes, teach patient about adequate nutritional intake, maintain hygiene of skin, teach patient/family about risk of pressure ulcers.	Skin will remain intact, no pressure ulcers.
Constipation	Auscultate bowel sounds at each visit, note nausea and vomiting, begin bowel program that includes suppositories every other day and stool softeners; teach patient and wife about adequate food and food intake, including bulk and fiber, encourage exercise (ROM) to facilitate evacuation.	Established bowel program, bowel movement every day or every other day.
Urinary retention r/t injury and limited fluid intake	Teach patient/family intermittent catheterization (to be done every 6 hr), teach patient/family to maintain intake and output records, encourage fluid intake (2-4 L/day), teach patient/family about signs/symptoms of UTI.	No urinary retention, able to perform self-catheterization.
Impaired physical mobility r/t spinal cord injury	Assess motor and sensory function at each visit, teach family and patient to perform passive ROM on lower extremities, teach use of splints and orthoses to prevent contractures.	No complications of immobility.
Imbalanced nutrition: less than body requirements r/t increased metabolic demand	Encourage high-protein, high-carbohydrate, high-calorie diet with high bulk; weigh patient at each visit (weekly).	Weight loss <10 lb.
Risk for injury r/t sensory deficit	Assess environment for potential safety hazards, teach patient/family to anticipate possible threats to safety within the home and community settings.	No injuries.
Interrupted family processes r/t change in the functional ability of a family member	Assess dynamics of family and roles and responsibilities of family members, encourage open communication and discussion of long-term planning, encourage understanding of each family member's feelings by other family members, assist in design of plan to meet the patient's needs, include patient and family in team approach to meeting the needs of the family.	Family makes maximum use of individual and collective strengths to adapt to altered lifestyle.
Risk for ineffective individual family coping r/t loss of control	Assess for inability to accept diagnosis/prognosis, provide support and acceptance of patient's feelings, assist with problem solving, encourage use of support systems to solve problems, offer accurate information and answer questions honestly, teach positive coping behaviors and behavioral techniques to reduce stress.	Patient expresses ability to cope.
Disturbed body image r/t paralysis	Encourage patient to discuss feelings about altered body image, allow patient to grieve losses, foster social interaction with others, encourage family members to support patient, refer for counseling as appropriate.	Patient verbalizes feelings about self and adaptation to altered body image.

r/t, Related to; *ROM*, range-of-motion exercises; *UTI*, urinary tract infection.

REFERENCES

Cardol, M., De Jong, B. A., & Ward, C. D. (2002). On autonomy and participation in rehabilitation. *Disability and Rehabilitation, 24*(18), 970-974.

Carter, N. D., & Wade, D. T. (2002). Delayed discharge from Oxford city hospitals: Who and why? *Clinical Rehabilitation, 16,* 315-320.

Children's Defense Fund (2001). *The state of America's children yearbook.* Washington, DC: Author.

Coddington, D. G. (2001). Impact of political, societal, and local influences on mental health center service providers. *Administrative Policy Mental Health, 29*(1), 81.

Cott, C. A. (2004). Patient-centered rehabilitation: Patient perspectives. *Disability and Rehabilitation, 26*(24), 1411-1422.

Cowan, M. K. (2004). Child and adolescent health. In M. Stanhope & J. Lancaster (Eds.), *Community and public health nursing* (pp. 616-651). St. Louis, MO: Mosby.

Dijkers, M. (1999). Community integration: Conceptual issues and measurement approaches in rehabilitation research. *Journal of Rehabilitation Outcomes Measurement, 3*(1), 39-49.

Federal Office of Rural Health Policy and National Rural Health Association. (1998, January). *Rural health: A vision for 2010.* Rockville, MD, and Kansas City, MO: Authors.

Hagen-Foley, D. L., Rosenthal, D. A., & Thomas, D. F. (2005). Informed consumer choice in community rehabilitation programs. *Rehabilitation Counseling Bulletin, 48*(2), 110-117.

Kent, A. (2002). The evolution of home and community-based rehabilitation. *Inside Case management, 8*(10), 6-7.

Kim, K., & Fox, M. H. (2004). Knocking on the door: The integration of emerging disability groups into independent living. *Journal of Vocational Rehabilitation, 20,* 91-98.

Mast, M. (2001). Employment and physical disability. *Journal of Vocational Rehabilitation, 16,* 1.

National Association for Home Care. (1999). Caregiving: Into the minds and hearts of family caregivers. *Caring, 18*(7), 34.

National Center for Health Statistics. (2000). http://www.cdc.gov/nchs/.org.

National Center for Health Statistics. (2002). *FASTSTATS* [Online]. Retrieved October 31, 2005, from www.cdc.gov/nchs.

Neal, L. J. (1999). Research supporting the congruence between rehabilitation principles and home health nursing practice. *Rehabilitation Nursing, 24*(3), 115-121.

Neal, L. J. (2000). The "R" word and the new millennium. *Home Healthcare Nurse, 18*(1), 35-37.

Neuman, B. (2002). The Neuman Systems Model. In B. Neuman & J. Fawcett (Eds.). *The Neuman Systems Model* (4th ed., pp. 1-34). Upper Saddle River, NJ: Prentice-Hall.

Nolan, M., & Nolan, J. (1998). Rehabilitation: Scope for improvement in current practice. *British Journal of Nursing, 7*(9), 522-526.

Orem, D. E. (2001). *Nursing: Concepts of practice* (6th ed.). St. Louis, MO: Mosby.

Peat, M. (1991). Community based rehabilitation—development and structure: Part 1. *Clinical Rehabilitation, 5,* 161-166.

Perry, E. L., Hendricks, W., & Broadbent, E. (2000). An exploration of access and treatment discrimination and job satisfaction among college graduates with and without physical disabilities, *Human Relations, 53*(7), 923-955.

Portillo, C. J. (2002). Cultural competence in home care. In I. M. Martinson, A. G. Widmer, & C. J. Portillo, *Home health nursing care* (2nd ed., pp. 197-205). Philadelphia: Saunders.

Remsburg, R. E., & Carson, B. (2002). Rehabilitation. In I. M. Lubkin & P. D. Larson (Eds.), *Chronic illness: Impact and interventions* (5th ed., pp. 555-583). Sudbury, MA: Jones and Bartlett.

Rosengarten, L., Milburn, F., & Ryan, M. C. (1996). Helping home care aides work with newly dependent elderly in a cluster care setting. *Home Healthcare Nurse, 14*(8), 638-646.

Rosswurm, M. A., & Larrabee, J. H. (1999). A model for change to evidence-based practice. *Image, 31*(4), 317-322.

Roy, C., & Andrews, H. A. (1999). *The Roy adaptation method* (2nd ed.). Upper Saddle River, NJ: Prentice-Hall.

Sharma, M. (2004). Viable methods for evaluation of community-based rehabilitation programs. *Disability and Rehabilitation, 26*(6), 326-334.

Thompson-Heisterman, A. (2004). Mental health issues. In M. Stanhope & J. Lancaster (Eds.), *Community and public health nursing* (pp. 826-847), St. Louis, MO: Mosby.

U.S. Department of Health and Human Services. (1991). *Healthy children 2000: National health promotion and disease prevention objectives related to mothers, infants, children, adolescents, and youth* (DHHS Publication No. HRSA-M-CH 91-2). Washington, DC: U.S. Government Printing Office.

U.S. Department of Health and Human Services. (2000). *Healthy people 2010: Conference edition* [Online]. Available from http://web.health.gov/ healthy-people/document.

Wade, D. T. (2003). Community rehabilitation, or rehabilitation in the community? *Disability and Rehabilitation, 25*(15), 875-881.

Williams, C. A. (2004). Community-oriented population-focused practice: The foundation of specialization in public health nursing. In M. Stanhope & J. Lancaster (Eds.), *Community and Public Health Nursing* (pp. 2-21), St. Louis, MO: Mosby.

13

Case Management

Patricia L. McCollom, MS, RN, CRRN, CDMS, CCM, CLC

Case management has emerged as a key strategy and innovative approach to improving patient care within a rapidly changing health care delivery system. Providing a framework for planning, implementing, and evaluating care, case management is an effective tool for dealing with the increasing complexity, fragmentation and constraints of the delivery of health services.

Case management is not a profession in itself, but rather a functional area of practice within rehabilitation nursing, with various and complex transdisciplinary relationships. Case management processes benefit patients, families, communities, providers, and payers by assisting individuals with chronic or complex illness, injury, or disability to utilize appropriate resources and to reach their potential for independence and for gaining satisfaction with quality of life.

The processes of case management contribute to a new focus within health care: consumer involvement, with goals of prevention and health. Shifting from a medical model of diagnosis/treatment/cure, case management offers a method of forging partnerships within the community and among providers to improve quality of service and access to care. This new focus has evolved due to a restructuring of the U.S. health care system brought about by the need for economic accountability and by the need for measurements of the results of care and treatment.

ORIGINS OF CASE MANAGEMENT

Case management began in the early 1900s with professionals interested in coordinating community services. Legislation for the disabled began to impact the public sector, resulting in the insurance industry's assuming a more proactive role in addressing rising health care costs. Case management became the term of choice as the concept of "cost control" was implemented.

The Vocational Rehabilitation Act of 1943, which funded professional training and research for persons with disabilities, served to establish vocational case management. This area of case management was strengthened by the Workers' Compensation Rehabilitation Law of 1960, the Rehabilitation Act of 1973, and subsequent amendments.

The insurance industry was a leader in development, implementation, and application of case management principles. In 1945 Liberty Mutual Insurance began hiring nurses to coordinate care and assist injured workers in returning to work. In 1970 the Insurance Company of North America began the first private sector rehabilitation company, International Rehabilitation Associates. Nurses and vocational rehabilitation counselors were hired to coordinate care and to create long-term plans to address the needs of persons with disabilities. Crawford and Company, then the largest insurance adjusting company, followed into this field. By the mid-1970s, thousands of smaller companies had been spawned from these pioneers.

As the insurance industry contributed to the growth and development of case management outside the traditional boundaries of health care delivery systems, within facilities the effects of cost control and external influences on care delivery became apparent. Nurse case management, as a professional practice model within hospitals, was introduced in the 1980s to allow a mechanism to avoid duplication of services, to evaluate care, and to contain costs while improving the effectiveness of care (Cohen & Cesta, 2005). Models of hospital-based case management promote outcome-based care and integration of clinical and community services, which support quality and consistency of care across the continuum of service delivery.

The U.S. government has developed case management programs within Children's Medical Services, Title V of the Social Security Act, and the Older Americans Act of 1973. Further, the Department of Veterans Affairs and TRICARE, health insurance for military dependents and retirees, employ case management as the method of choice to maximize services and achieve quality care.

DEFINITIONS

The definition of case management varies depending upon the arena of practice. The Case Management Society of America (CMSA), a nonprofit, multidisciplinary society of case management professionals, promotes professional development of health care case management practitioners in various settings. In 2002 the CMSA board of directors approved and published the following definition:

> Case management is a collaborative process of assessment, planning, facilitation and advocacy for options and services that meet an individual's health needs through communication and available resources to promote quality cost-effective outcomes (CMSA, 2002, p. 5).

This definition is considered by CMSA as the foundation for their Standards of Practice. The group sees the case manager as the advocate and link among patient, providers, and payer.

The American Nurses Credentialing Center (ANCC) defines case management as

> A dynamic and systematic collaborative approach to providing and coordinating health care services to a defined population. It is a participative process to identify and facilitate options and services for meeting individuals' health needs, while decreasing fragmentation and duplication of care and enhancing quality, cost-effective clinical outcomes. The framework for nursing case management includes five essential functions: assessment, planning, implementation, evaluation, and interaction (ANCC, 2004, p. 10).

Practitioners within health care delivery systems have developed alternative definitions, usually associated with the model of case management used. Cesta and Tahan (2003) suggested that nursing case management is

- A nursing care delivery system
- A role and process focusing on procuring, negotiating, and coordinating care, services, and resources throughout an episode of illness
- A system of health care delivery designed to facilitate achievement of outcomes and decrease fragmentation within health care
- A process of care delivery

When compared, the various definitions are similar and contain the same essential functions of the case management process: assessment, planning, implementation, coordination, monitoring, and evaluating.

MODELS OF CASE MANAGEMENT

As health care has continued to evolve, the need for case management has grown in a wide variety of practice settings. Case managers from numerous disciplines work in private practice, corporations, insurance companies, managed care organizations, health maintenance organizations (HMOs), clinics, and physician practice groups. Case managers work in hospitals, long-term care facilities, specialty care facilities, home health care, and public/community settings. Those involved with facility-based case management may be involved with critical pathways for care, analysis of variances, and outcomes management. Data gathering and analysis, then, becomes the means for decision making and improvement of care.

Case managers serve diverse populations who are in need of medical, vocational, psychosocial, and other coordinated care.

The practice in all settings and models involves consumer/family involvement, availability of resources and services, and development of a mutually agreed-upon plan to achieve goals promoting health, well-being, and satisfaction with health care services (Box 13-1).

ESSENTIAL FUNCTIONS OF CASE MANAGEMENT PRACTICE

Patient Identification

Case managers must identify individuals or groups appropriate for intervention. Specification of criteria signaling need for case management services is based upon the relationship between diagnosis, complications, potential cost, and geographical availability of needed resources.

Assessment

Data gathering from all available resources is necessary to identify the individual's needs, potential resources, and anticipated goals. Meeting with the individual, the family, and care providers and reviewing medical records provide understanding of the patient's status, patient/family knowledge of the treatment plan, and anticipated outcomes. Box 13-2 represents a listing of categories necessary for case management assessment.

Planning

Development of a case management plan is evidence based and patient centered. Case management plans identify long- and short-term needs and methods for meeting the patient's needs. The plan is mutually agreed upon with the patient, family, and treatment team and considers available resources to achieve goals. Stating expected outcomes, the plan may involve a care pathway or other management tool as a guide toward quality care.

Implementation

This process involves setting the case management plan into action. Appropriate authorizations and approvals must be carried out, in collaboration and communication with the providers. As an advocate for the patient, the case manager is placed in the position of managing financial aspects of accessing care, avoiding duplication of services, using community resources, and/or obtaining approval for contract exceptions within a group health contract. Documentation of all activities and communications is essential to promote

---

BOX 13-1 Outcomes of Case Management Plan

- Mutually agreed-upon plan with patient/family
- Goal identification
- Defined resources and alternatives
- Health promotion emphasized

plan implementation and to protect patient progress along the plan of care.

Coordination

The case manager acts as a pivotal point for communication, monitoring of actual services, and follow-up for implementation of the case management plan. Research and assessment of

---

BOX 13-2 Case Management Assessment Categories

Health Status
- History
- Review of systems
- Current status
- Medications (include pharmacist)
- Nutritional status
- Eating habits
- Height
- Weight

Functional Skills
- Self-care
- Cognition
- Communication
- Behavior
- Mobility
- Elimination
- Safety
- Community involvement

Psychosocial Status
- Family/friends
- Patient/family values
- Community support
- Mood/affect
- Coping mechanisms
- Stressors
- Substance use/abuse
- Sleep patterns
- Vocational experience
- Avocational interest

Environment
- Architectural barriers
- Geographical barriers
- Health hazards
- Need for modification
- Transportation

Financial Status
- Income
- Assets
- Monthly costs
- Insurance
- Guardian/conservator
- Power of attorney
- Living will

---

various financial and community resources available to assist in meeting patient needs is critical to maintaining coordination of care. Identification of community resources is an ongoing activity, due to the dynamic nature of public and private agencies, in a time of economic volatility. Case managers must also define methods of linking patients and resources within case management plans. This involves the development of relationships and networking with community agencies and services and communication with the patient/family.

This component of case management distinguishes the practice from other health care practices and requires extensive documentation and direct involvement in service delivery.

Monitoring

The case manager's role includes ongoing assessment of the patient's ability to adhere to the plan of care and reviewing achievement of benchmarks along the plan. Such close observance allows awareness of developing problems and opportunities for plan revision as needed and for documentation of variances.

Evaluation

Case management practice demands a measurement of the patient's response to care and services, as well as the quality of care and services. This evaluation process is interrelated to continuous monitoring and demands the autonomous ability to proactively make decisions regarding alterations to the case management plan. The result of evaluation is clear documentation of outcomes achieved, cost efficiency, and patient/system benefits.

STANDARDS OF PRACTICE

Standards of professional practice are designed by a profession (1) to define the parameters of the practice, (2) to provide a basis for evaluation of practice, (3) to stimulate the development of the practice, and (4) to encourage research to validate the practice. Standards provide a baseline for knowledge, skill, and behavior.

Case management is a transdisciplinary specialty practice, yet it is estimated that over 70% of professionals identified as case managers are professional nurses (CCMC, 2005). This represents an interesting phenomenon because nurses are accountable for practice as described by the American Nurses Association (2004). Nurses who are case managers are accountable for nursing practice standards *and* case management practice standards, defined by CMSA. CMSA Standards of Practice (2002) clearly outline practice and performance standards expected from case managers. Therefore nurses who are case managers must be knowledgeable about both sets of standards.

For rehabilitation practice the Association of Rehabilitation Nurses has published *Standards and Scope of Rehabilitation Nursing Practice* (2000). A nurse practicing in rehabilitation case management has three layers of standards for which there are definitions and direction for accountability. These publications all define process and declare professional responsibility for acting in the patient's best interest, assuming responsibility for care delivery, and practicing with accountability and advocacy. The essential elements of case management practice presented here are consistent with current published standards of practice in nursing, case management, and rehabilitation nursing.

CASE MANAGEMENT PROCESS

The case management process is a series of activities applied to the management of patient care. The case management process emphasizes a systematic approach to patient care delivery and management of health care resources (Cesta & Tahan, 2003).

As a result of application of the essential functions of case management, within the parameters of the Standards of Practice, four major processes of case management are identified:

1. Care coordination
2. Quality management
3. Outcomes management
4. Cost management

Care Coordination

In all practice settings it is the case manager who is the coordinator of the work of the care team. This coordinator role results in both clinical and financial accountability.

From a clinical perspective the case manager coordinates and collaborates to meet patient needs and achieve goals outlined in the plan of care. Coordination activities include provision of day-to-day care, discharge planning, patient/family education, and movement through the health system into appropriate follow-up services within the community, promoting community reintegration.

The coordinated clinical activities represent a foundation for financial coordination. Coordination of necessary care results in cost efficiency, elimination of duplication, and decreased fragmentation of services. Ongoing coordination of care and services also supports early intervention to avoid problems and complications. The case manager is in the position to act to change the plan of care, to avoid delays in treatment or discharge, and to access appropriate services. An advantage of case management services is highlighted in the following example.

Example of Case Management Services. Case managers involved in a capitated elder care program that spanned the health care continuum from inpatient facility to outpatient community-based program implemented a new protocol for health status evaluation. Eager to improve the quality of patient health and prevent inpatient stays, case managers enrolled their patients in the new program. Subsequently, funding for the project was lost in a budget reforecast. With the administrative staff the case managers worked to continue the project by developing a clinic approach to the health status evaluation of patients and by reaching out to collaborate on the project with local church parish nurses who provided patient monitoring. By assuming accountability for the well-being of their patients, these case managers devised a creative, collaborative solution to a problem arising from budgetary constraints.

Quality Management

The term *quality* has evolved over time to a broader meaning. Quality now includes aspects of availability and accessibility of care, improvement in the health of an individual, the level of community reentry, and the patient/family's perceived satisfaction with services. Case management affects quality in health care through the process of care coordination. The case manager is in a unique position to carry out these processes over the course of care, therefore promoting necessary and timely care, treatment, and services.

In case management, quality measurement is both a concurrent and retrospective process (Huber, 2006). Concurrently, case managers continually evaluate care and response, intervening when the plan of care requires adjustment. This critical monitoring function promotes consistency and positive, durable outcomes. Retrospectively, the case manager is able to identify problem areas, process limits, and feasible options for improved care/services. The important synthesis and surveillance elements of case management services relate directly to cost-effective outcomes. This is illustrated in the next section.

Example of Cost-Effective Outcomes. A managed care plan determines that a patient with severe osteoporosis should not be approved for nontraditional pain management treatment but is willing to continue reimbursement for narcotic administration and the surgical implantation of a morphine pump. The patient feels little benefit from the narcotic and requests assistance. A case manager discusses options for pain management under consideration by the individual and gathers data to objectively evaluate options, which are provided to the managed care plan. The outcome is approval for the nontraditional treatment, which controls the patient's pain.

Cost Management

Managed costs are clearly an outcome of case management. Case managers purchase, negotiate, and coordinate care and services, resulting in effective use of resources. Within the processes of case management, there is the opportunity for creativity and development of nontraditional options to meet patient needs. Such flexibility is necessary for achieving cost-effectiveness.

In general, positive cost management results from care coordination by eliminating duplication of services and decreasing fragmentation. The outcome of case management, simply stated, is use of available funding and resources in the patient's best interest. This goal is explained in the next section.

Example of Cost Management. Nurses working in a rural rehabilitation facility note that patients receiving benefits from a specific plan are not receiving durable medical equipment from local providers, but instead from an approved mail-order provider. The nurses' options are to accept the plan's restrictive approval or to gather data demonstrating the effect this decision is having on their patients. The nurses gather data on repair costs, parts availability, and service. They include data about services in rural communities and the impact of downtime on patients when equipment has to be sent in for servicing. Their concern for the patients' well-being results in a change by the payer, to local provider approval.

Outcomes Management

Outcomes are defined as the end results obtained from the efforts directed toward accomplishing a goal (Huber, 2006). Outcomes management focuses on the results of the delivery of health care to individuals and groups, based on specific measurements.

Outcomes management combines care coordination, quality, and cost management processes into a systematic research effort to improve clinical practice and care provision and reduce costs. Emphasizing quality, outcomes management programs recognize the importance of accurate data collection and analysis and move case management into the arena of research-based practice. Research efforts have created a national database for outcomes in health care. The Agency for Healthcare Research and Quality offers a website (http://www.ahrq.gov/clinic/outfact/htm) that provides current outcomes research and discusses the impact of certain practices on patients, their quality of life, and economic issues.

Outcomes measurement is the foundation for outcomes management. Measurement of outcomes serves to assist professionals in achieving goals, internally, externally, or with specific individuals or groups. Key data elements in all sectors include trends, history, clinical decisions, and identification of patterns.

Categories of measurement of patient outcomes are physiological, psychosocial, functional, behavioral, knowledge, home functioning, family strain, safety, symptom control, quality of life, goal attainment, patient satisfaction, utilization of service, and nursing diagnosis resolution (Cohen & Cesta, 2005). These categories may be easily applied by case management practitioners to clarify and specify the results of intervention for individuals and groups.

CASE MANAGEMENT AND REHABILITATION NURSING

The concept of case management practice is readily adapted to rehabilitation nursing. A coordinated effort among all care providers and across disciplines correlates with the long-accepted model of the rehabilitation team. There are two additional members of the team: (1) the payer source, approving or denying services, and (2) the community, providing alternate resources.

Case management enhances patient and family involvement, because long- and short-term needs must be identified for both to attain the objective of appropriate use of available resources. With the increased communication inherent in case

management, the patient and family have greater knowledge about care, services, and options. Energies may then be directed to urgent health issues and to rehabilitation efforts.

ISSUES IN CASE MANAGEMENT

The system of health care delivery in the United States is in dire need of ongoing reform. Change has been occurring at a rapid pace, and challenges stand before us to meet the needs of a new practice environment. The challenges for case management are those that exist for nursing as well. However, because case management practice is carried out in various settings by a variety of professionals with differing expectations, the future of case management will depend on the ability of this transdisciplinary group to come to a consensus about definition, goals, purposes, and outcomes. Agreement about the fundamentals of case management practice creates a foundation for moving forward with progress toward resolving other practice issues and answering legal and ethical dilemmas.

Certification

Certification is a nationally recognized method for documenting an individual's abilities to serve the needs of his or her patients, based on a predetermined set of criteria outlining required education and experience. Typically, certification is voluntary. Professional disciplines see certification as a major method for ensuring individual practitioner's competence. As a result, jobs may require certification as a condition of employment.

Certified Case Manager. The certification process to obtain the designation "Certified Case Manager" (CCM) is administered by the Commission for Case Manager Certification. As of January 2006 over 24,000 practitioners have been certified through this process, which includes passing an examination. The examination is researched based and reflects the transdisciplinary practice of case management.

The American Nurses Credentialing Center (ANCC) published a certification for nurse case managers. Focused on facility-based practice, the application criteria require a minimum of a bachelor's degree in nursing (ANCC, 2004).

Accreditation

Accreditation is the process of critical review of a program, service, facility, or health system as compared to national standards that have been approved by peers within the field.

Two accreditation processes exist for case management facilities or agencies. The Commission on Accreditation of Rehabilitation Facilities (CARF) developed standards for medical rehabilitation case management that were implemented July 1, 1999. CARF believes that case management is an integral part of rehabilitation care. Coordination, communication, and advocacy are primary themes within the CARF standards.

The American Accreditation HealthCare Commission/Utilization Review Accreditation Commission (URAC) developed standards as an accreditation process in 1998, designed to promote innovation and best practice in the case management industry. Convening multiple professional groups to develop standards, the goal was to create a case management accreditation system for health care organizations that promotes a level of structure and processes to further improve patient care quality.

To date, URAC has accredited hundreds of organizations that provide all types of case management services, in both health and workers' compensation settings—helping to ensure that their case management offerings are of the highest quality. The URAC standards cover several critical operational categories for any qualified case management program, including the following:

- Staff structure
- Staff management and development
- Information management
- Quality improvement
- Oversight of delegated functions
- Organizational ethics
- Complaints

Implications for Practice

The nature of the role of case management in any practice setting is complex and difficult. Case managers in varying settings have responsibility to approve care or deny services within a contract, to coordinate community resources and justify expenditures, to implement clinical pathways and design research methodologies, and to meet patient needs and affect outcomes. Case managers are accountable to professional groups, to one another, and to those entrusted to their care. This integrated role in health care creates multiple legal and ethical considerations for case management practice.

Legal issues within case management practice have emerged and are seen as potentially increasing litigation. The concepts of liability and accountability for outcomes of care appear to be the basis for potential litigation involving case managers. Negligent referral and abandonment are other areas for potential litigation. Case management programs with clear documentation of action and consistency with standards and practice guidelines will be better able to respond to legal action.

Ethical issues face case management practitioners on a daily basis. When the element of cost control/containment enters the practice dialogue, there is an inherent ethical dilemma with the case manager's advocate role. As a case manager, does one have the moral right to deny care, speed discharge, or inform a payer about the patient's substance abuse? When case management is practiced by professionals, the guiding principles must be advocacy, acting in the patient's best interest, and proper use of existing resources. (Refer to Chapter 3 for a discussion on ethics.)

SUMMARY

Case management has emerged as a key strategy and innovative approach to improving patient care within a health care delivery system that must respond to economic limits and multiple external influences. Future demands for case management are unlimited, as definitions of practice are refined and new roles for case managers are developed.

Case management practice is evident in multiple practice settings; however, case managers are bonded by consistency in essential elements of practice and process (Figure 13-1). Increased awareness of case management outcomes will prompt tremendous growth in the specialty, particularly in the areas of long-term care, aging, and chronic disease.

Through review of the case management diagram (Figure 13-2), the process of case management may be viewed as a method for organization of care, a tool for evaluation of services, and a framework for resource allocation. An application of these concepts can be used to analyze the following case study.

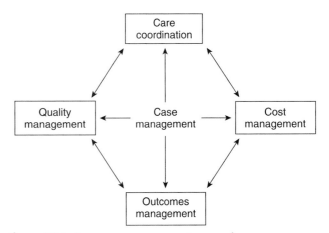

Figure 13-1 Case management as an integrated process.

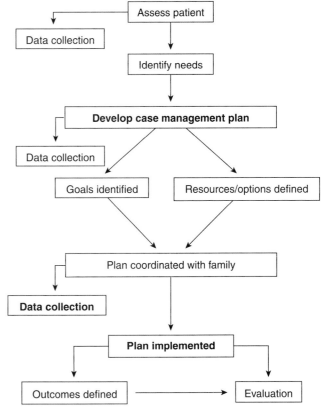

Figure 13-2 Process of case management.

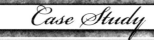

Case Study

Josh Sullivan, 17 years old, was injured in a motor vehicle accident 11 days before initial assessment. His diagnosis was status post severe closed brain injury, with continued coma. His parents were most supportive, and the mother remained at his bedside continuously. Acute rehabilitation had been initiated.

Initial Assessment

Josh (patient) was observed and his family interviewed for assessment purposes on July 31, 2005.

Date of injury: July 20, 2005.

Medical diagnosis: Status post severe head injury; emergency and intensive care treatment completed at Comprehensive Medical Center, Chicago, Illinois. Coma is noted in medical records as 10 days. Acute rehabilitation was initiated and is in process at a free-standing rehabilitation center.

Current Status

Age: 17.

Sex: Male.

Marital Status: Single.

Living relatives: Father, mother, brother, paternal grandparents.

Role in family: Oldest child.

Occupation: Student.

Recreational interest: School sports; participated in football, music.

Housing: Josh Sullivan requires total care for his health, wellness, and safety. He is maintained at QC Rehabilitation Center, participating in a full rehabilitation program.

Josh responds inconsistently to verbal, visual, and environmental stimuli. He participates in a full rehabilitation program daily. He is wheelchair dependent for mobility with full assistance required for transfer. Hypertonicity has developed in bilateral lower extremities. Physical therapy promotes sitting tolerance, balance, range of motion, and increased endurance. Daily psychological therapy focuses on verbal and visual stimulation; visual perception cannot be assessed at this time. Speech therapy focuses on consistent use of a voice output communication aid.

Josh experiences generalized seizures one to two times daily; continuous drooling was noted, right side of mouth. Skin breakdown at the coccyx and right hip was noted. He is dependent in mobility, dressing, and personal hygiene. He is independent in oral intake with prompting and adaptive equipment. A gastrostomy for feeding was placed July 30, 2005.

Health History

Josh had the usual childhood diseases; fractured his left wrist June 2000; is allergic to house dust, molds; and completed desensitization October 1999.

Current Medications

As noted on chart.

Education

One semester tenth grade.

Work History

Not applicable.

Family Status

Josh's parents have been actively involved in all facets of their son's care. His mother has resigned from work as a legal secretary to participate in care. Both parents have participated in brain injury education programs provided by the facility; they are attending the Head Injury Association support group weekly. Josh's father is employed as a regional supervisor for sales of farm equipment (annual salary, $48,000); health and accident coverage is Blue Cross/Blue Shield of Illinois. Josh has $2,000 in a savings account. Because of his personal savings, he has been declared ineligible for Supplemental Security Income (SSI) Medicare funding.

Medical Records Reviewed

Comprehensive Medical Center
1. Records of emergency care
2. Consultation reports
3. Operative reports
4. Discharge report to QC Rehabilitation Center

Additional Information

A meeting was held July 31, 2005, with the following in attendance: J. Jerry, MD; K. Olson, speech therapist; T. Davis, PhD, psychologist; M. Goode, MSW, social worker; T. Strong, PT. The following needs were discussed: (1) further evaluation of uncontrolled seizures, (2) assistance to family for home modifications, and (3) clarification of insurance benefits.

CRITICAL THINKING

1. Josh Sullivan has experienced a significant closed head injury, resulting in a persistent vegetative state. The family has chosen to modify their home and provide care for their son at home. Discuss the case manager's role in accessing resources and assisting the family in providing quality care.
2. Discuss three goals for rehabilitation care for Josh.
3. Identify the case manager's role in each of the following areas: relationship with the family, interaction with the payer, and identification of community resources.
4. List three nursing diagnoses that will affect implementation of the case management plan.

REFERENCES

American Nurses Association. (1999). *Modular certification examination catalog.* Washington, DC: American Nurses Credentialing Center.

American Nurses Association. (2004). *Nursing: Scope and standards of practice.* Washington, DC: American Nursing Publishing.

American Nurses Credentialing Center (ANCC). (2004). *ANCC certification: Specialty nursing, nursing administration (basic, advanced), clinical nurse specialist (community health, home health)* (p. 10). Washington, DC: ANCC.

Case Management Society of America. (2002). *Standards of practice for case managers.* Little Rock, AR: Author.

Cesta, T., & Tahan, H. (2003). *The case manager's survival guide: Winning strategies for clinic practice* (2nd ed.). St. Louis, MO: Mosby.

Cohen, E., & Cesta, T. (2005). *Nursing case management from essentials to advanced practice applications* (4th ed.). St. Louis, MO: Elsevier.

Commission for Care Manager Certification (CCMC). (2005). Results of the Role and Function Study, Research and Examination Committee. Unpublished data. Schaumberg, IL: CCMC.

Huber, D. (Ed.). (2005). *Disease management: A guide for case managers.* St. Louis, MO: Elsevier.

Huber, D. (Ed.). (2006). *Leadership and nursing case management* (3rd ed.) (pp. 827, 870). St. Louis, MO: Saunders.

14

Functional Mobility With Activities of Daily Living

Shirley P. Hoeman, PhD, MPH, RN, CS
Karen Liszner, BSN, MHA, CRRN
Joan Alverzo, PhD, MSN, CRRN

This chapter addresses the complex topic of movement and mobility from two perspectives relevant to rehabilitation nurses. In the first view it relates function with activities of daily living (ADLs) and instrumental activities of daily living (IADLs). The theory-based interventions can be used wherever rehabilitation nursing practice spans the continuum of care. The illustrations of movement and ADLs can be used in all care settings and to instruct students or family members. Another view is on movement theories and practice frameworks and focuses on the neurological foundations of motor function with attention to upper and lower motor neuron syndromes. The case study discusses spinal cord injury in detail.

Rehabilitation nurses working with patients and their families in facilities and in community settings need to understand the theoretical basis of movement, as well as the structure and function of muscles, joints, bones, and nerves. A complete and integrated assessment of the musculoskeletal and nervous systems enables the nurse to formulate diagnoses and set realistic goals with patients that complement the interventions of other members of the rehabilitation team. Educating a patient and family about reasons for and methods of optimizing mobility increases the probability of follow-through, maintenance of optimal independence, effective coping and adjustment, and prevention of further disability or complications. Research is needed for examining instances of greater comorbidity, disabilities associated with certain diseases, particular combinations of diseases that may lead to even more complex situations, and interactions among disease processes and their effect on functional outcomes.

MOBILITY AND FUNCTION

Medical prescriptions for rest versus mobility have vacillated since antiquity; conventional medicine prescribed extensive bed rest for healing as recently as the 1940s. Then Olson's classic article (1967) exposed the "hazards of immobility" and raised awareness of how any or all systems of the body, mind, and spirit break down as consequences of immobility, disuse, or even poor positioning, all preventable. Patients are at high risk for problems due to the very nature of their chronic and disabling conditions or multiple traumas, from specific impairments or complications, and even from use of the very assistive device or adaptive equipment that affords them mobility or function. Immobility and functional limitations represent tremendous challenges. They portend depression, disorientation, irritability, lack of energy or interest, incontinence, feelings of imbalance, increased pain or aching, and general malaise. Inappropriate medication regimens, disrupted sleep, lack of sensory or cognitive stimulation, poor nutrition and low fluid balance, social isolation, and feelings of powerlessness may contribute as much toward functional loss and further reduced mobility as does a specific disease or impairment.

Most adults take their ability to move for granted until it becomes painful, restrained, or impaired. Movement is critical to a person's capacity for interaction with the environment; problems resulting from immobility are noticeable quickly even in healthy persons. In the United States more than 54 million persons have some activity limitations due to chronic health problems; that is, more than 12% of persons 65 years or older, a prevalence rate predicted to increase by 50% owing to the disproportionate numbers of very old persons in the population. Chronic conditions contribute to limitations especially for older persons (Centers for Disease Control and Prevention [CDC], 2006). Nearly 3.5 million people need assistance in ADLs, and 6 million, or 1 in 25 persons from age 5, need assistance with IADLs and other means of living independently (National Institute of Disability and

Rehabilitation Research [NIDRR], 2006). The greatest intervention is assistive technology devices (ATDs); 7.4 million people rely on ATDs for help with mobility impairments alone (CDC, 2006). Overall 9.4 million adults age 18 years and older receive assistance with some ADLs and IADLs. Nearly half are younger than 65 years, and 4 of 5 (79%) live in the community (Spector, 2000); another 2.5 million lack funds for assistive technology (LaPlante, Hendershot, & Moss, 1996).

UNIVERSAL DESIGN

Healthy People 2010 goals are to reduce disparities in access to health services (U.S. Department of Health and Human Services, 2000). The National Institute on Disability and Rehabilitation Research (NIDRR) has given high priority to research projects dealing with an approach to improving access, called universal design. It is a vision of ways to prepare, by design, the total environment, equipment, devices, goods and products, and spaces to be as usable to the greatest possible extent by people of any age, ability, or situation and without need for adaptation or specialized design. Broad principles of universal design are equitable, flexible, and intuitive use; perceptible information; tolerance for error; and size and space for approach and use. Other considerations can be incorporated into the practice and process of designs for special populations (Connell & Wolf, 1997).

Although legislation has opened public places to those who can ambulate on a level surface for a short distance, they still may be denied access to the upstairs of their home or the yard. Children may attend school but have difficulty participating in field trips or social activities outside their own controlled environment. Too often health professionals' offices, equipment, or examination rooms are not accessible. Environmental assistive devices contribute in many situations; however, each device must be evaluated critically, considering the patient's lifestyle and environment against cost, maintenance, or storage space.

Examples of improvements include ramps, elevators, permanent and portable lifts, altered or expanded doorways, robotic and electronic controls, and wheelchair-tread devices, and all sorts of modified home spaces, such as modified cooking areas, worktable heights, bathroom accessories, and grooming areas make daily life easier. Modified equipment and outdoor spaces allow persons to participate in recreational and leisure pursuits.

Technology Aids

Advances in technology are a hallmark of universal design. Ergonomic designs are used in the home, school, and workplace. Computers may be outfitted with ergonomic devices, including mouse pads, large and Braille keyboards, padded or shaped frames, special on/off switches, specialty chairs or lumbar wedges, and height adjustment devices. Computer software for augmentative communication, screen readers, remote controls, and voice recognition and instant message systems on the World Wide Web are options.

Improved interactive voice response systems enable patients to receive recorded messages and then contact health providers and others for help or information (Piette, 2000). Computerized systems report a patient's condition, medical and clinical records, images of results, and other data, as well as allow nurses to communicate with colleagues while in the patient's home. A telephone touch-tone keypad or voice recognition technology may change the quality of care and mode of delivery for patients, especially those at home in remote or difficult areas. Internet sites provide extensive information about assistive devices and technology (e.g., http://www.wapd.org/assistive and http://www.abledata.com).

SELF-CARE

Conceptual Bases

Several theories from nursing, along with social science (Chapter 2) and education constructs (Chapter 5), suggest how motivations, beliefs, perceptions, and needs influence a person's self-care participation and practices. Factors such as ethnicity, social support, environment, finances and access to services, and physical, psychological, and spiritual well-being represent some of the barriers and assets that motivate people about self-care.

Responsibility and Self-Care

The organizing framework for this book builds on self-care activities necessary for participation in everyday life. The intent is to understand individual potential and improve patients' self-care, as expressed through performing ADLs and IADLs. Rehabilitation nurses help patients develop their strengths, optimize function, and accept responsibility as part of their participation in the rehabilitation team process.

Performing self-care is a personal matter beginning with rituals, habits, timing, and ways learned in childhood from families and cultures. Ideally, patients will choose to perform self-care to the limits of their ability. Nurses advocate for patients' maximum autonomy, independence, and participation by setting appropriate goals that promote life quality and satisfaction. A goal may be modified so patients can direct others to perform care according to their preferences; indeed, some cultural norms dictate that others perform care for the person. Conversely, assertiveness training enables others to accomplish their objectives effectively. Although ability to learn (memory) and personal motivation (executive function) both have direct effects on performance, multiple factors influence functional mobility outcomes as shown in Table 14-1.

Heavy reliance on goals established only by standardized plans, or by third-party payer targets, may detract from those mutually set by patients and providers. Shortened lengths of stay in rehabilitation facilities and minimal services in other levels of care challenge rehabilitation teams to find ways to ensure that patients and families are prepared to continue to perform self-care skills when patients return to home and the community and to reduce undue reliance on caregivers or learned helplessness.

TABLE 14-1 Factors Influencing Functional Mobility

Factor	Influence on Functional Mobility
Descending motor systems of peripheral nervous system (PNS)	These control muscle tone, reflexes, movement, coordination, balance, motor development, and system status.
Musculoskeletal system	This system is the source for muscle strength, range of motion, joint stability, body alignment and postural control, and positioning; all moderated with endurance or fatigue and affected by nutrition, sleep, stress, and general health status.
Central nervous system: the senses	Visual-auditory-olfactory-tactile sensations are related to coordination, pain and proprioception, and spatial orientations and supply visual support for balance, sensory intake, stimulation, and expression.
Cognition perception	Selective attention, declarative memory including orientation; concept formation for comprehension, judgment, and planning; and executive attention networks for vigilance, detection, and working memory. Perceptual deficits affect hand-eye coordination and figure-ground or depth perception and manifest as agnosia, apraxia, or neglect with distortion of body image.
Psychosocial and emotional situation	Coping behaviors and style, concerns or fears, and motivation affect self-care attitude and responsibility.
Environment and technology	Architectural barriers, unsafe communities or home conditions, or lack of assistive devices and/or poorly prescribed adapted equipment deter self-care.
Social, cultural, and economic factors	Beliefs, including stigma and cultural practices, inability to access services, and insufficient resources may foster distrust.
Other	Overall health status, comorbidity or specific problems, age and developmental stage are factors.

Exercise as Self-Care

Both aerobic exercise and strength training may forestall, even reverse, age-related changes in muscle function, as well as increase endurance and improve overall health status. Weight-bearing exercise improves muscle strength, postural stability and control, alertness, and ability to pay attention. It helps reduce falls associated with reduced bone density, muscle mass, range of motion (ROM), strength, and balance and increased frailty of older persons. Weight-training exercises may increase strength and performance for those with postpolio syndrome, progressive neuromuscular disease, and myasthenia gravis. Persons with osteoarthritis, cystic fibrosis, and multiple sclerosis experienced increased endurance and aerobic exercise capacity. Monitored aerobic exercise has improved fitness and prevented secondary disabilities for persons with mixed physical disabilities. Gait training may help older persons who live independently at home with balance problems, especially weight bearing, and improve dynamic postural stability.

Regular exercise performed appropriate to the patient's situation and functional goals is beneficial. Before a patient is medically stable the intent is to prevent contractures or atrophy; avoid pain or joint damage; and maintain muscle tone, strength, and function. Impaired sensation and cognition present special challenges. The therapeutic level, type, and independence in exercise also are regulated to conserve energy and avoid fatigue. Safety, essential for any mobility or therapeutic exercise program, includes proper body mechanics (Box 14-1).

Specific Conditions and Self-Care

Specific conditions and impairments predictably affect self-care as evidenced in ADL and IADL capabilities. Some movements are outright contraindicated for certain conditions, such as following amputation or total hip replacement surgeries.

BOX 14-1 Principles of Body Mechanics

- Maintain good posture with back straight, knees slightly bent, and weight over center of body.
- Maintain a wide base of support using both sides of the body equally.
- Bend from the hips and knees, and do not use the back muscles to perform work.
- Move in close to the object or person; hold them close in to the body; do not reach in front or above the head.
- Push or pull instead of lifting, making smooth, fluid movements.
- Do not twist the body, pivot, or shift the feet to turn.
- Get help if necessary, and use aids such as lifting sheets, mechanical lifts, trolleys, or carts.
- Use transfer or gait belts, seat belts, transfer boards, and other safety devices.
- Evaluate the environment for any potential tripping, slipping, or other hazards before moving or lifting.
- Report any injury or problems, and seek evaluation and treatment early.

Self-care ADLs consist of multiple components and specific skills to complete a task; some steps may be readily achievable, whereas others are difficult or not possible. Patients with conditions that vacillate, such as fibromyalgia, are trauma based, such as repetitive motion problems, or are progressive or sequela, such as postpolio syndrome, may exhibit varied performance. Or a patient may be physically able to perform an activity but unable to produce the necessary purposeful, organized movement such as with certain types of dyspraxia or apraxia as presented in Table 14-2.

TABLE 14-2 Dyspraxias and Apraxias

Types	Description	Location
Ideomotor apraxia	Impairment in selecting, sequencing, and spatial orientation of movements involved in gestures (spatial and temporal production errors)	Left parietal cortex (angular gyrus) or supramarginal gyrus
Posterior form	Difficulty performing in response to command and imitation; cannot discriminate well between poorly performed and well-performed acts	Left parietal cortex (angular gyrus or supramarginal gyrus) lesion
Anterior form	Performs poorly to command and imitation but comprehends and discriminates pantomime	Lesions anterior to the supramarginal gyrus, which disconnects visual kinesthetic motor engrams from premotor and motor areas
Conduction apraxia	Greater impairment in performance when imitating movements than when pantomiming to command; comprehends pantomime and gesture but cannot perform the movements	Location unknown at this time
Disassociation apraxia	Inability to gesture normally to command and required verbal mediation; has good performance with imitation and actual tools and objects	Callosal abnormalities but not all locations known
Ideational apraxia	Inability to carry out an ideational plan or series of acts in the proper sequence	Location unclear at this time
Conceptual apraxia	Cannot recall type of action associated with specific tools, utensils, or objects (content and tool selection errors; may be unable to recall which tool is associated with a specific object or may have impaired mechanical knowledge)	Bilateral frontal and parietal dysfunction

From McCance, K. L., & Huether, S. E. (2006). *Pathophysiology: The biologic basis for disease in adults and children* (5th ed.). St. Louis, MO: Mosby.

Sequelae to Congenital Conditions

Certain mobility problems occur later in life as sequelae to congenital conditions. Children with a tethered cord are at risk for loss of motor strength with mixtures of spasticity and flaccidity, asymmetrical involvement of the lower extremity, paraplegia, scoliosis or kyphosis, and other complex problems affecting mobility. The involvement of hips, knees, feet, and spine intensifies with development and aging, making energy conservation important. Interventions include bracing and orthotics, supplemented by crutches or special canes, and adaptive devices.

MOVEMENT THEORIES

In the context of each patient's unique situation and environment, concepts and principles from movement theories are useful to promote recovery and enhance compensation for altered or impaired functional abilities. According to classic movement theories, motor development is a maturation process of the central nervous system (CNS). Pioneers in the field identified specific developmental sequences and incorporated certain behaviors of early motor development into various treatment programs. Because of their belief that motor development ended with neural maturation, it became a marker for completed developmental processes, or *milestones*. In contrast, a life span concept views the processes of age-related changes in motor behaviors, such as learning, maturation, and aging, as lifelong phenomena. Behavioral change then results from interactions among intrinsic and extrinsic factors, such as physical growth and neural maturation, and supportive versus risk environments.

In the hierarchy of reflex models, the primitive reflexes are the baseline unit for motor control. The higher cortical and subcortical brain centers regulate and control the lower centers in a hierarchical fashion. Motor development matures in a ranked order from primitive reflex control regulated by the spinal cord to control in the brainstem and midbrain, such as high-level righting and equilibrium actions. In this scheme, a child does not walk until sequentially higher levels of the CNS mature sufficiently to allow independent balance and locomotion; equilibrium represents a still higher level of maturation. Damage to a higher control center relegates motor control to a lower, more primitive reflex level. As the higher levels deteriorate with aging, they default to primitive reflex controls.

Sensorimotor Models

Sensorimotor approaches to movement theory rely on assumptions from the reflex and hierarchical models. Five program models are noteworthy for their use in rehabilitation: Rood (1956), the Brunnstrom (1970) movement therapy approach, the proprioceptive neuromuscular facilitation approach (PNF) (Voss, Ionta, & Myers, 1985), the Feldenkrais method (Jackson-Wyatt, 1997), and the neurodevelopmental treatment model (NDT) or Bobath program (1991). The PNF program, a neurophysiological approach, features moving the extremities in patterned spiral and diagonal movements and a rapid stretch technique.

The Feldenkrais method, a neuropsychomotor approach, is based on the patient's perceptions and lifestyle and includes strategies for sensory, emotional, cognitive, and movement components. Sr. Kenny used similar principles in her treatment for poliomyelitis. The notion is that personal habits of movement occur unconsciously. When lost or altered, they can be reconstituted through sensory and motor systems learning and adapting. All the models propose that their treatments influence muscle tone and that sensory stimulation can be used to evoke a motor response and to develop motor skills.

The Bobaths recognized the brain's ability for neuroplasticity, that is, a capacity to reorganize and learn, even to adapt, by developing new synaptic pathways. By setting goals that promote a patient's abilities for recovering movement, encouraging participation, enhancing their quality of life, and use of the involved extremity, they hoped to capitalize on brain plasticity. A large body of funded research has been built around the brain's neuroplasticity. Bobath principles are incorporated into many ADL interventions in this chapter.

Active participation to promote the potential for recovery is a focus during a consistent 24-hour monitored Bobath program. Patients practice devoting attention to improved movement, use of the involved extremity, and retaining learned motor skills, rather than to compensate for deficits. The notion is to focus on the sensation of movement in the involved extremity, not the movement itself. When brain damage occurs and sensation is altered or impaired, sensation is shunted to developing abnormal patterns of posture and movement that are incompatible with performing normal activities. Patients attempt to halt or break the abnormal patterns by regaining control over motor output, rather than by modifying sensory input. Initially nurses provide stimuli to enable patients to learn basic postural and movement patterns that elicit the righting and equilibrium responses while inhibiting abnormal patterns. Eventually these patterns can be elaborated on so the patient can perform functional skills. Every skilled activity is conducted within the context of patterns for postural control, righting, equilibrium, and other protective reactions. Sensory input from the corrected motor patterns is essential for the person to develop improvement in motor control.

Dynamic Systems Models

The hierarchical approaches have proven inefficient to manage the complexities of the CNS. The dynamic systems model (distributed control model) identifies movement as a product of complex interactions of multiple systems and proposes that change in any system affects all subsystems. The person is active, as well as reactive, in a continually changing environment, but the physiological body also is a mechanistic mass subject to the forces of gravity and inertia. All parts interact to support the patient's abilities to act and participate, and the results are motor control and movement. The CNS is one part of the multiple interwoven systems and subsystems that share in the control process, and connections are highly sensitive; movement is one outcome. As a nonlinear concept, the systems are complex, dynamic, adaptive to the environment, and emerging.

A task-oriented approach that promotes solving problems fits with the dynamic systems model. The argument for constraint-induced movement therapy as an intervention for motor recovery is that nonuse of an extremity after stroke becomes a learned behavior. Finding movement difficult or simply forgetting to do so, the patient neglects to use the involved extremity. Nonuse is further supported or reinforced by teaching compensatory movements to a patient before evidence of any spontaneous recovery. Constraint-induced therapy causes the patient to use the involved extremity while the unaffected extremity is immobilized; ideally the cortical areas reorganize more rapidly. The practice of shaping, or using the involved extremity to achieve small successful gains in motor function that improve performance of ADLs, may help reverse learned nonuse.

Dynamic pattern theory (DPT) is another nonlinear example familiar to rehabilitation nurses. As the name implies, DPT focuses on movement patterns and how or why changes in the pattern occur and then how to make them retrievable or available again. Interactions among the CNS and other (e.g., peripheral) nervous systems lead to patterns. Some patterns may be instinctive, and others may be learned, but they vary in stability and with the environment or situation. That is to say, patients can find more than one way to perform activities depending on their physical and cognitive abilities and the environment. Thus a rehabilitation nurse assists a patient with medication to manage pain that prohibited transfer from a wheelchair and then installs support bars and elevates the toilet seat to facilitate transfer to the commode, resulting in improved independent function. Complex systems models explain changes in balance across the life span and underlie certain interventions for imbalance and postural control.

Behavioral Approaches

Behavioral approaches include *kinesic* and *somatic* interventions to assist patients with stress reduction or pain management, such as biofeedback, therapeutic massage, progressive relaxation, or therapeutic touch. Biofeedback is a method of autonomic nervous system control through self-regulation. Patients receive continuous data feedback about their biological function (heart rate, body temperature, or muscle activity) via auditory or visual signals, such as those emitted from electromyelograms (EMGs). As patients perceive the workings of their internal biological systems, they attempt to control them by incorporating themselves into the system as part of a "feedback loop." Their efforts are complementary with exercise programs.

Some approaches are argued to be paradigm shifts in conceptual frameworks for movement science and therapy. The Pilates method, based on synergistic principles, incorporates holism, including breathing, centering, and concentrating, among others. Many complementary techniques employ technology, such as electrical stimulation. These are topics for rehabilitation nurses to examine in research and to carefully evaluate for utilization in practice.

NORMAL MOVEMENT

The basics of involuntary, voluntary, and normal movement are precursors to understanding movement dysfunction. Rehabilitation nurses, as well as physical and occupational therapists, collaborate using these principles and when educating patients and families about ways to improve outcomes, independence, and continued well-being.

The nursing assessment of a deficit or undesirable state of altered mobility (i.e., immobility) identifies a diagnosis and interventions to improve mobility. Normal neurological and musculoskeletal system mechanisms enable purposeful movement and prevent the consequences of immobility, such as pressure ulcers, pneumonia, contractures, and other negative outcomes. Although rehabilitation nursing practice has an extraordinary investment in mobility, few studies pursue it as a theoretical concept. For the most part, nurses have regarded mobility in the physical sense, which is, focusing on ability or impairment and the level of assistance a patient needs.

Movement represents a key component in a person's ability to interact with the environment and adapt. It is dynamic in that its capacities change with development, health status, and other multiple dimensions. In a holistic view, movement has physical, cognitive, social, spatial, political, temporal, or environmental parameters (Chan & Heck, 2000). In this view, functional abilities, as expressed through performing ADLs and IADLs, are measures that incorporate the environment, mental competence, and some social interaction in addition to physical actions.

Motor Development

Human motor development proceeds from birth in an orderly and purposeful fashion. Cephalocaudal development means from the head to the feet and from the center to the periphery of the body. The infant learns to support the head before developing the trunk strength necessary to sit, and development of the legs follows, enabling the infant to crawl and stand. Gross motor movements develop central and earlier, as with the extremities, where gross motor movements emerge before the more peripheral hands can perform fine motor skills. As the nervous system matures, genetically based movement patterns become more elaborate, and primitive reflexes disappear, being replaced by higher-level responses. Thus an infant's Moro and tonic neck reflexes are expected to disappear before righting and equilibrium responses emerge.

In normal development, skills are acquired at certain specified stages and become less random and coarse; they develop into sequences that are more purposeful and synchronized, forming the basis for stability and posture. Posture and movement are intertwined for learning motor skills and producing goal-directed activities. Once learned and perfected through practice, motor skills become nearly automatic and unless the pathways are disrupted, require little conscious thought to execute correctly.

Musculoskeletal Structures

The musculoskeletal system is a dynamic body system, accounting for more than 50% of the body's weight. The bony skeletal structure protects vital organs of the body and provides a frame for the skin and muscles with their underlying contents. Muscle movement depends on neurological direction and stimulation and cognitive goals. In a physical sense, movement consists of an involuntary action, a reflex process, or a conscious and deliberate choice to have muscles act on bones, joints, and ligament and tendon structures.

Bones manufacture red blood cells, store salts and minerals, and bear the weight of the body. Calcium metabolized with vitamin D is essential to bone health and repair; the parathyroid hormone acts to regulate the process. Loss of bony structure and osteoporosis occur with non–weight-bearing status, inadequate nutrients to mineralize the bone, chronic conditions or disuse, or trauma that may induce heterotopic ossification. Bones are constructed and joined in configurations that allow certain types of movements in concert with muscle actions.

Cartilage is a firm gel composed of strong but flexible fibers that contain no blood vessels, lymph tissue, or nerves, rendering it insensitive to pain. It does not self-repair after injury and so depends on nutrients supplying the synovial membrane during movement at the joint. The amount of fiber increases with aging (e.g., the elastic hyaline cartilage [articular] found at the ends of bones becomes more fibrous). Fibrous cartilage composes the intervertebral disks.

Joints are categorized by the amount of movement and the type of connective tissue they contain. They enable flexibility and movement, and movement maintains joints and instigates the flow of synovial fluid that nourishes the hyaline cartilage. It is important for ROM exercises, as well as for positioning and alignment. Situations that restrict or immobilize joints, such as casting, severe guarding due to pain, paralysis, non–weight-bearing status, altered or reduced muscle control, or abuse and trauma, are detrimental to function and lead to deterioration of the joint structures, notably cartilage.

Tendons are strong, fibrous tissue bands without elasticity that attach muscles to bones at their origin and insertion. Fibrous tendons sheathe each muscle in complex joints, such as the wrist and ankle. As tough, flexible bands of fibrous tissue, ligaments connect the ends of bones to provide stability and limit movement that may injure joints, such as the knees.

Ligaments have some elasticity, enabling them to connect bones and cartilage, bridge visceral organs, and secure joints, such as limiting movement in certain directions to prevent injury; some are part of joint synovial membranes. Synovial fluid, plasma from blood vessels, lubricates and adds stability at the insertion sites. The longitudinal collagen fibers that make up tendons and ligaments often are overlooked until they evoke pain or immobility. Recovery from damage or disuse of tendons and ligaments is a lengthy process. With contractures, tendons and ligaments are involved with immobility of muscles, joints, and surrounding tissues.

The fibrous connective tissue that encapsulates muscles, nerves, and blood vessels is the fascia; it has surface and deep layers. Bursa are connective tissue sacs filled with synovial fluid that serve as buffers between muscles, tendons, and bones, or bones and skin. They are found most often at the hips, knees, elbows, and shoulders. Injury, infection, or prolonged pressure may cause bursa to become inflamed and painful, limiting movement; bursitis may become chronic with repeated trauma.

Skeletal muscles are of interest in this chapter, especially their abilities to contract and extend. A skeletal muscle is formed from a multitude of thin cell fibers with unique cell properties. The fibers extend the length of the muscle and have several nuclei, a plasma membrane or sarcolemma, and cytoplasm. Several distinct networks of tubules and sacs are involved; some allow calcium ion storage and actions, and others assist intramuscle electrical impulses. Myofibrils are bundles of many minute fibers (myofilaments) found only in the skeletal muscle. They are interspersed with a fluid, the sarcoplasm. The sarcomere portion of a myofibril is the skeletal muscle unit capable of contraction. They appear as darker bands or stripes (striated) interspersed and alternated with paler-colored muscle bands, Z lines and I bands, for example. The process of muscle innervation is discussed later in the chapter.

Neurological System Classifications

The nervous system is composed of the brain, spinal cord, and nerves. In a familiar classification, the CNS contains the nerve cells encompassed within the physical brain and spinal cord, and the peripheral nervous system (PNS) contains the nerve cells and their branches that extend into the other parts of the nervous system. The main parts of the CNS and their components can be thought of as having functional steps; at the highest step is the cortical brain followed by the subcortical brain, with the spinal cord at the lowest level. The PNS includes the twelve cranial nerves (see Chapter 23) that start in the brain and the 31 pairs of spinal nerves (with their branches and ganglia) that form in the spinal cord. Spinal nerves have a dorsal and ventral root and are named according to the level of the vertebra where they exit the spinal column (e.g., cervical, lumbar). They are mixed, in that they have both motor and sensory neurons. The anterior spinal nerves join in various combinations to create plexuses. From these networks, nerve fibers extend to innervate a specific area of the body. The four pairs of key plexuses are cervical, brachial, lumbar, and sacral. Injury at a specific nerve level influences functional outcomes as shown in Table 14-12. (The thoracic nerves differ, because they reach through the intercostal spaces and innervate the thorax.)

Because both the CNS and PNS systems contain one-direction nerve pathways that carry data into or away from the centers, a second classification of the nervous system uses the end points or effectors as the organizing criterion. Sensory or afferent information is gathered via peripheral nerves and conducted to sensory centers in all levels of the spinal cord,

the reticular activating system in the brain, the cerebellum, thalamus, and parts of the cerebral cortex. Motor or efferent information is transmitted from higher neurons through the synapses and conducts action back to the appropriate effector (e.g., contraction of a specific skeletal muscle). Skeletal muscles have levels of control throughout the CNS; the lowest are located in the spinal cord, then the reticular system of the medulla, pons, and midbrain, and the basal ganglia, with higher levels in the cerebellum and the motor cortex. The higher the level, the more voluntary and complex are the movements.

The autonomic nervous system (ANS) operates parallel to the motor nerve pathways; however, it controls autonomic effectors, such as cardiac and smooth muscles and glands. Although a person can affect the actions of the ANS, most of its actions occur in seemingly involuntary ways. Afferent pathways of the ANS are involved in sensing body regulatory functions and movements, such as control of smooth muscle contractions and chemical secretions essential for glands. Efferent pathways of the ANS are subdivided into the parasympathetic and sympathetic divisions. Parasympathetic pathways, concerned with maintaining resting equilibrium, leave centers at the brain or lower sections of the spinal cord. The sympathetic pathways leave from the midsection of the spinal cord and handle immediate threats to the person, the "fight or flight" response.

Neurological Structures

Neurons. The many billions of neurons that populate the CNS are also the most basic units. In its simplest form, a neuron consists of a soma (cell body) with a nucleus, cytoplasm, mitochondria for cell energy, and a Golgi apparatus that stores and processes proteins for the neuron. Proteins that are used to transmit nerve impulses between neurons are neurotransmitters. Examples of neurotransmitters are acetylcholine; amines such as dopamine, epinephrine, norepinephrine, serotonin, and histamine; amino acids such as gamma-aminobutyric acid (GABA); and neuropeptides. Neurotransmitters are essential for nervous system functions and are discussed in Chapter 21. Figure 14-1 illustrates synapse actions that occur at the neuromuscular junction.

Each neuron cell body has stringlike extensions, that is, an axon that extends to the peripheral nerve and one or more dendrites that send fingerlike extensions into the spinal cord area, as well as the rest of the CNS (see Figure 21-4). Many tiny presynaptic terminals, or knobs, are situated on the dendrites, some on the soma, of motor neurons. They are essential in the complex chemistry of neurotransmission. Neurons also are classified by configuration. Sensory unipolar neurons have one extension, less common bipolar neurons have one axon and a branched dendrite, and the numerous multipolar neurons with one axon and several dendrites are found in the brain and spinal cord.

Neurons service specific routes in the nervous system. Sensory (afferent) neurons send nerve impulses toward the brain or spinal cord, whereas motor (efferent) neurons send nerve impulses away from the brain or spinal cord and toward

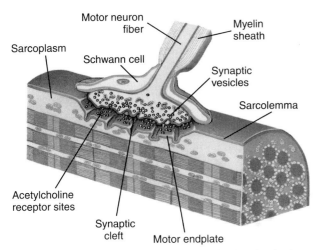

Figure 14-1 Neuromuscular junction (NMJ). The sketch shows a side view of the NMJ. Note how the distal end of the motor neuron fiber forms a synapse, or "chemical junction," with the adjacent muscle fiber. Neurotransmitter molecules (specifically acetylcholine) are released from the neuron's synaptic vesicles and diffuse across the synaptic cleft. There they stimulate receptors in the motor end plate region of the sarcolemma. (From Thibodeau, G. A., & Patton, K. T. [2007]. *Anatomy and physiology* [6th ed.]. St. Louis, MO: Mosby.)

muscles or glands. Although most nerves contain both sensory and motor nerve fibers, they are classified by whichever type is more prominent.

The interneurons are inside the brain and spinal cord. Their role is to conduct sensory neuron signals to motor neurons within an area called a synapse, where the chemical actions of neurotransmitters occur; both excitatory and inhibitory actions are involved. These are one-direction transmissions, which heightens their ability to send numerous and specific information to the target. (Electrical synapses do not occur in the nervous system.) The simplest example of neuron function is the reflex arc during which signals are sent to and from the brain or spinal cord in response to a stimulus.

Neurons generally do not regenerate or replace themselves. Owing to the interconnectedness of the neuron networks, damage to one part of a nerve fiber (e.g., severing axons) may result in a full nerve pathway becoming inoperative. Major research efforts are directed toward ways to restore damaged neurons and other parts of the nervous system.

Glia. Glia (neuroglia) and neurons are the primary nerve cells in the nervous system. Until recently glia were thought to be secondary, mere supportive actors, in the nervous system despite their great numbers, in the billions. Glia cells are able to divide and thus replace themselves, an area of neurobiological research. A brief comment on the five most prominent glia and their contributions follows. The star-shaped astrocytes, found only in the nervous system, are active in neuron nutrition and have roles in the blood-brain barrier, as well as in neuron circuitry. Microglia operate as phagocytes of the nervous system.

Ependymal cells create linings for fluid-filled cavities in the brain and spinal cord.

Oligodendrocytes gather or clump around nerve cell bodies and between nerve fibers, binding them together. These are important for their role in producing part of the myelin sheath, the fatty covering around nerve fibers. With multiple sclerosis, the myelin is lost or damaged throughout the white matter of the CNS and replaced with a hardened plaque formation that disrupts nerve conduction. Layers of Schwann cells also form a myelin sheath as they wrap themselves around and around a peripheral nerve fiber in layers or serve to bundle nerve fibers together. Bundled myelinated fibers constitute the white matter of the nervous system; neuron cell bodies and unmyelinated fibers form the gray matter and are called ganglia in the peripheral nerves. Peripheral nerves are gathered together with their blood supply and supported with layers of connective tissue.

Spinal Column and Spinal Cord

The 24 vertebral bones (plus the sacrum and coccyx) that surround the spinal cord form a segmented vertical column. The vertebral disks, set between the adjacent joints of the vertebral bones of the spinal cord, are composed of fibrous tissues and cartilage that encloses an elastic puttylike center. Disks are bound in place by ligaments and stabilize the vertebrae while allowing flexible movements in many directions.

From a lateral view, the curved vertebral bones have a central opening or foramen surrounding the spinal cord. The spinal cavity contains the spinal cord, the meninges, tissues, blood vessels, and cerebrospinal fluid. The spinal cord is composed of both a gray and a white matter that extend in separate columns for the length of the cord. Because of the appearance of the gray matter in cross section, it is referred to as the anterior, posterior, and lateral horns. The columns of white matter contain bundled nerve fibers or spinal tracts, which are named for their origin and destination.

The spinal cord serves as a conduit sending and modifying information into the brain via ascending (sensory) tracts and away via descending (motor) tracts. Key motor tracts of the spinal cord are the lateral corticospinal (crossed pyramidal) and anterior corticospinal (direct pyramidal) tracts (upper motor neurons), responsible for voluntary movement and small muscle group contractions; and the reticulospinal, rubrospinal, and the vestibulospinal tracts that control body coordination, posture, and balance during movement. The larger anterior groove (anterior median fissure) of the spinal cord guides fibers of the anterior nerve root that leave the spinal cord with motor information, and a less prominent posterior median sulcus hosts posterior nerve roots bringing in sensory information. Both nerve roots have cell bodies and intersect with the many interneurons found in the spinal cord gray matter core.

The gray matter of the spinal cord also is the reflex center for all of the spinal reflexes. Posterior and anterior nerve fibers mingle to form individual spinal nerves that emerge from both sides of the spinal cord. The lowest spinal nerves fan out below the sacral area resembling a horse's tail (i.e., cauda equine). The spinal reflex arcs may consist of a basic synapse between two neurons or may involve an interneuron and are described in this chapter with muscle innervations.

The Brainstem

For motor movement purposes, the parts of the brainstem are considered collectively as they sit atop the spinal cord in base order, the medulla oblongata, the pons, and the midbrain. Controls of reflex centers for respiratory, vasomotor, and cardiac functions are notable in the medulla, major sensory tracts (spinothalamic) pass through the brainstem structures, and vital cranial nerve reflexes are centered in the midbrain portion. Of interest here for muscle movement are the corticospinal and reticulospinal (motor) tracts and the vestibulospinal tract useful for posture and balance, all found in the white matter columns. The medulla is where fibers from the precentral cortex are formed into pyramid-shaped structures; these cross over before descending in lateral columns of the spinal cord, part of the pyramidal system (upper motor neuron).

The midbrain (mesencephalon) contains several structures concerned with eye movement and righting, balance, and posture as motor movements. It also houses the red nucleus, which serves as an alternate pathway for sending sensory information to the cerebellum and motor information to the cervical spinal cord. There are differences in how the structures in these areas have been classified. Some schemata place part of the basal ganglia, the substantia nigra where dopamine is synthesized, in the midbrain. Other schemata place the cerebellum and the pons (metencephalon) and the medulla oblongata (myelencephalon) in an area termed the hindbrain.

The Cerebellum

The cerebellum sits under and behind much of the cerebrum, separated by a transverse fissure. Grooves (sulci) and foliage-like elevations (folia or gyri) cover the surface. The cerebellum is composed of a left and a right hemisphere joined at the center by a beltlike area called the vermis. Each hemisphere has a designated lateral and an intermediate zone or region. The lateral zone works with the cerebral cortex for coordinating and planning motor movements. The intermediate zone controls specific muscle actions in the distal portions of the extremities (via managing their contractions). The foliage-like white matter in the center of the cerebellum is surrounded by the gray matter of the cortex. Short nerve tracts in the cerebellum communicate impulses from neuron cell bodies in the cerebellar cortex to nuclei internal to the cerebellum. Longer fiber nerve tracts pass through the three pair of peduncles to transfer impulses back and forth with the cerebellum. Each hemisphere contains a pair of dentate nuclei that communicate via tracts with the thalamus and motor cerebral cortex. Despite being smaller than the cerebrum, the cerebellum has more neuron power than any other part of the brain and thus is capable of managing more information than all the rest of the nervous system; it exerts great influence on motor functions.

The cerebellum is a primary accessory to the cerebrum in the processes for planning and conducting important skeletal muscle coordination actions and in maintaining balance. The cerebellum receives motor impulse information from the cerebral premotor cortex and compares it with sensory receptor data arriving from the body via the dorsal and ventral spinocerebellar tracts. For example, the cerebrum instigates a movement, and the cerebellum controls the muscle functions to make it smooth and coordinated, including confirmation with sensory information and ideation, or the "thinking about an action." It dispenses motor information to other parts of the brain via several complex pathways. One pathway from the cerebellum travels through the thalamus and through the basal ganglia and the red nucleus as part of specific muscle contractions. A breakdown of cerebellum functions due to disease or injury leads to symptoms that reflect the loss of coordination, such as ataxia, or tremors, or a compromised gait and issues with balance, but not paralysis.

Diencephalon

The diencephalon is a part of the brain that lies between the midbrain and the cerebrum. It contains the thalamus, hypothalamus, and pineal gland and houses the optic chiasma. Although many important functions are associated with the diencephalon, they are not directly concerned with motor movement.

Basal Ganglia (Nuclei)

The basal ganglia are located in various areas of the brain around the thalamus and have a large presence in the interior cerebral hemispheres. They border the internal capsule of the brain, which is the major trail for most of the motor and sensory nerves that communicate between the spinal cord and the cerebral cortex (i.e., the cortico-spinal-cerebellar system) but exist apart from the pathways, thus the extrapyramidal system.

A number of neurotransmitters function as inhibitors, creating negative cybernetic (feedback) loops between the cerebral cortex and the basal ganglia and thus providing stability to the system. Loss of smooth, coordinated, accurately moving muscle activity results from damage to the cerebellum or basal ganglia and in turn creates imbalance in the extrapyramidal system, threatening righting and equilibrium responses. Delay in carrying out movement or slow initiation signals cerebellum problems because that is where movement parameters are specified and preprogrammed movements are initiated.

Disturbances in these areas of the nervous system result in posture and movement dysfunctions evidenced in the gait, balance, posture, and other disjointed, choppy motions. Gait may be staggering or wide stepped, with marked muscular rigidity and bradykinesia, and coarse tremor accompanied by other involuntary movements, such as chorea, athetosis, and facial grimacing. Tremors may be barely noticeable or so severe as to be disabling; the frequency, location, and action may vary. Postural or resting tremor is a classic movement with Parkinson's disease that may arise with abnormality in the basal ganglia of the brain.

More complex than this discussion allows, these interconnections are essential to control, learned patterns including tasks like writing, and sequences of movements. Thus damage or disruptions in the functions of the basal ganglia are associated with Huntington disease, stroke, and Parkinson's disease.

Cerebrum and Cerebral Motor Cortex

The cerebrum is the largest part of the brain; it is the upper part anatomically and divided into a left and right hemisphere; the basal ganglia lie interior. The layers of the cerebral cortex composed of gray matter containing millions of neurons and synapses form the surface of the cerebrum. This distinctive surface appears as convoluted layers (gyrus) with both shallow (sulci) and deep grooves (fissures) between loops. Like the fissures, the lobes of the cerebrum serve as divisions and landmarks; the lobes are frontal, parietal, temporal, and occipital, also the insula. The cerebral hemispheres are divided as to their control of functions, in addition to location of functions by lobe; and due to nerve crossovers, the right cerebral hemisphere controls motor functions on the left side of the body and vice versa.

Cerebral Tracts

The white matter of the cerebrum is formed by three tracts (basal ganglia constitute the gray matter). Most information is sent within the same hemisphere via association tracts, whereas the fibers that travel between an area in one hemisphere to a place in the other hemisphere are collectively termed the corpus callosum. The corpus callosum is surrounded by structures that constitute the limbic system. The ascending (sensory) spinothalamic tract and descending (motor) corticospinal tract have extensions into the cerebrum forming projection tracts. Thus the functions of the parts of the cerebral cortex are related directly to their communication. The postcentral gyrus is the location for much of the sensory interpretive activity and the termination of the sensory pathways to the brain. The location of specific functions within the cerebral cortex is important for research in neuroplasticity of the brain. Sensory integrative functions, such as the role of the reticular activating system in consciousness, functions for language, speech, and declarative memory are discussed in Chapter 24, and memory is discussed also in Chapter 25.

Complex motor (efferent) pathways are located in the cerebral cortex. Those in the precentral gyrus of the frontal lobe manage specific muscles and another pathway just anterior in the premotor area cause group of muscles to work together; these are of interest in this chapter. For the corticospinal tract, the precentral cortex produces more than half of the corticospinal fibers; the others come from the neuron cell bodies in the sensorimotor area, postcentral cortex. Simply, voluntary motor impulses from the cortex travel through the anterior corticospinal tract or cross at the medulla level and descend through the lateral corticospinal tract to the anterior horn cells and to the skeletal muscles. The fibers meet in the medulla, where three fourths of them cross to descend the opposite side of the spinal cord. The remaining fourth do not cross. One pair of these uncrossed fibers is housed in the white matter of the spinal cord forming the anterior corticospinal tract. Most of the fibers of the corticospinal tracts synapse with interneurons that stimulate the anterior horn neurons that mediate voluntary controlled movement. Injury to these tracts leads to paralysis and paresis, such as following a cerebrovascular accident (CVA).

The cerebral cortex distributes impulses from motor areas via neurons in the spinal cord to skeletal muscles using a number of somatic motor pathways (e.g., the pyramidal pathway). Figure 14-2 illustrates two motor pathways. Damage to these anterior horn motor neurons results in flaccid skeletal muscles that are unable to contract, such as occurs with poliomyelitis.

The precentral gyrus areas of the cerebral cortical regions execute voluntary movement, but the supplementary motor area controls programming of complex sequences into rapid, discrete movements. New motor programs are assembled in the premotor area. The posterior parietal areas direct attention to objects of interest in visual space and form strategies for eye and arm movement and their coordination in space. Cognitive functions related to movement occur in the prefrontal cortex with accessory functions from the basal nuclei (ganglia). With disease or injury the motor cortex cannot stimulate a voluntary motor movement, thus paresis or paralysis results. Muscle spasms also result from the lack of inhibition of the brainstem and spinal cord tone-setting mechanisms. The surplus tone in the muscles of the involved extremities plays out as muscle spasticity.

Altered movement may result from neurological insult to the nervous system. The site and extent of motor impairment correlate with the damage to or acquired lesions of the motor regions of the nervous system. For example, circumscribed cortical lesions, ranging from stroke to gunshot to penetrating wounds, result in dysfunctional motor planning in the related areas of function. The results are problems with planning, sequencing steps, smooth coordination, and timing of movements, as well as potential unpredictable movement based on sensory data. Accompanying deficits in sensory, cognitive, and perceptual processing also alter motor control.

Musculoskeletal Innervation for Movement

In movement the focus is on skeletal or striated muscle, less on visceral and cardiac muscles. Muscles provide heat through contraction, produce motion and strength, help to regulate body temperature, and maintain posture. Strength is greater in larger muscles and in those with wider bulk. Muscle fibers are bundled together and wrapped in connective tissue to form a muscle. Usually fewer fiber branches produce finer muscle movements.

Skeletal muscles are managed through the voluntary motor pathways of the somatic nervous system, a subdivision of the peripheral nervous system. The exception is the sympathetic "fight or flight" response that elicits physiological changes, such as increased oxygen for greater breathing capacity and

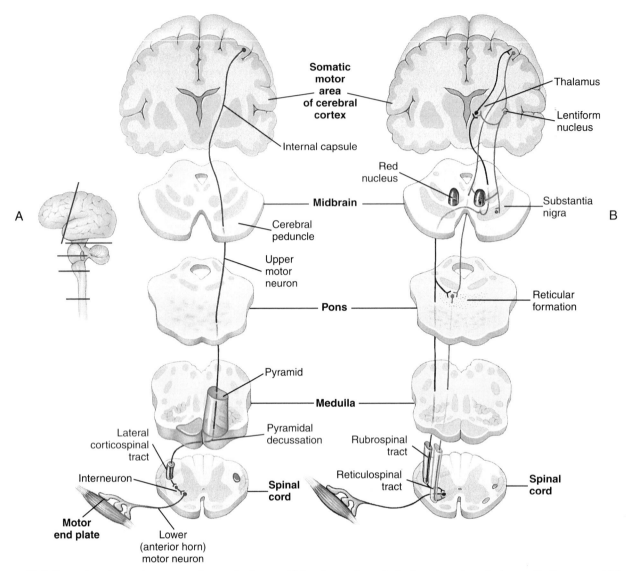

Figure 14-2 Examples of somatic motor pathways. **A,** A pyramidal pathway, through the lateral corticospinal tract. **B,** Extrapyramidal pathways, through the rubrospinal and reticulospinal tracts. (From Thibodeau, G. A., & Patton, K. T. [2007]. *Anatomy and physiology* [6th ed.]. St. Louis, MO: Mosby.)

blood flow and more available glucose that prepares muscles to run or fight at maximum level.

Cranial and spinal nerves form the peripheral nervous system. Skeletal muscles may be controlled from the spinal cord, the brainstem, the basal ganglia, the cerebellum, and the cerebral cortex. When a stimulus to a muscle (effector) causes a nerve impulse to follow a reflex arc, it elicits a reflex response. Reflex arcs located in the brain yield cranial nerve reflexes; those in the spinal cord produce spinal reflexes. Reflex arcs involving somatic motor neurons (anterior horn or lower motor neurons) yield skeletal muscle contractions. Simple somatic reflex arcs occur as a stimulated (afferent or sensory) proprioceptor nerve fiber enters the dorsal root of the spinal cord, synapses via an interneuron with a single motor neuron in the anterior gray horn, and then by way of the ventral nerve root sends a response back to the specific

(effector) skeletal muscle. Examples of reflex arcs are shown in Figure 14-3.

A multitude of variations exist, because the sensory and motor information may enter and leave the CNS on the same side, or enter the CNS on one side and exit on the other. Not all signals complete the arc, and some signals may originate in the brain and not from muscles.

The somatic motor neurons involved are single neurons that extend small branches into the muscle, and their impulses enable the muscles to contract, extend, flex, and demonstrate irritability and elasticity. Muscles respond to stimuli by shortening and thickening, stretching, and returning to the original shape. The strength of muscle contraction is influenced by the number and length of available fibers, the degree of fatigue, the effectiveness of the neuron transmission, the metabolic situation, and the stretch (or load) placed on the muscle.

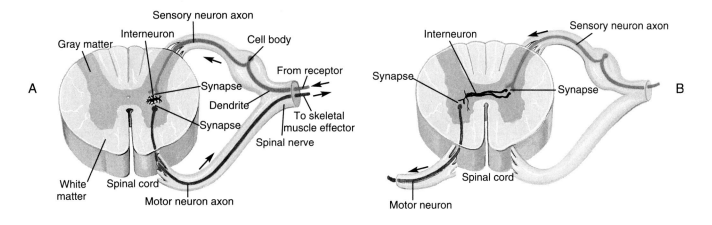

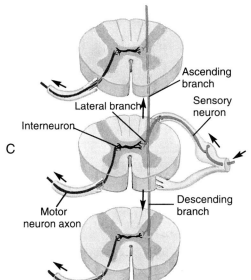

Figure 14-3 Examples of reflex arcs. **A,** Three-neuron ipsilateral reflex arc. Sensory information enters on the same side of the central nervous system (CNS) as the motor information leaves the CNS. **B,** Three-neuron contralateral reflex arc. Sensory information enters on the opposite side of the CNS from the side that motor information exits the CNS. **C,** Intersegmental contralateral reflex arc. Divergent branches of a sensory neuron bring information to several segments of the CNS at the same time. Motor information leaves each segment on the opposite side of the CNS. (From Thibodeau, G. A., & Patton, K. T. [2007]. *Anatomy and physiology* [6th ed.]. St. Louis, MO: Mosby.)

Two sensory proprioceptors (stretch receptors) are the Golgi tendon receptors and muscle spindles. They communicate information about the length of a muscle and its contraction strength to the spinal cord. They do not communicate sensations, such as pain. Motor neurons send the response back to the muscle, where the contraction is adjusted. When the stretch is greater than the muscle capacity, the response is relaxation, thus the stretch reflex.

Golgi tendon organs are located where muscles join tendons. Actually encapsulated dendrites of receptor sensory nerve fibers mingled with collagen fibers from the tendon, they are activated to relax muscles in response to contraction of the muscle. Golgi tendon organs identify muscle tension by transmitting to the spinal cord and by traveling fiber pathways to the cerebellum and cerebral cortex. An inhibitory interneuron

blocks the anterior motor neuron and thus prevents excessive tension on the specific muscle.

Muscle spindles are composed of specialized muscle fibers (intrafusal fibers) that lie alongside basic muscle fibers (extrafusal fibers) and are joined on both ends by connective tissues, as illustrated in Figure 14-4. With stretch on a muscle, the sensory neurons send impulses to the spinal cord and higher center (e.g., the cerebellum or motor areas of the cerebral cortex) to regulate changes in the muscle length. Gamma motor neurons located in the anterior gray horn of the spinal cord elicit muscle contraction of the striated ends of muscle spindle fibers while alpha motor neurons elicit contraction of regular muscle fibers. The centers of the intrafusal fibers do not contract, but the ends do. Once a muscle at rest is lengthened, the middle of the spindle is stretched to a point that it activates the muscle spindles to

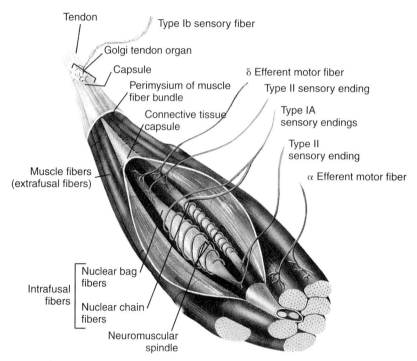

Figure 14-4 Proprioceptors. Muscle length and strength of muscle contraction is dependent on the functions of stretch receptors (Golgi tendon receptors and muscle spindles) and stimulation of sensory and motor nerve fibers. (From Thibodeau, G. A., & Patton, K. T. [2007]. *Anatomy and physiology* [6th ed.]. St. Louis, MO: Mosby.)

shorten the related muscles. This action is a stretch reflex important to posture and body positioning.

The sensory ends of the muscle spindles respond to a rapid stretch of a muscle by signaling the spinal cord, resulting in a response manifested as a swift reflex contraction in the muscle. A less powerful reflex may be sustained to keep the muscle contraction stable, beneficial for control of potentially jerking or oscillating movements and maintaining body position. The knee jerk and Achilles tendon reflexes are examples of diagnostic stretch reflexes.

Muscle Contraction

Muscle contraction and relaxation is described in Box 14-2. Muscle fibers can produce isotonic, isometric, or isokinetic motions, among others. Isotonic contraction shortens the muscle as the fibers contract but without increasing internal tension, leading to movement. Isometric contraction against stable resistance maintains the length of the muscle but increases the tension or force generated by the muscle; thus no body movement occurs. The underlying principle is building strength by lifting or moving and holding weight against the force of gravity while in various positions. Less common, isokinetic muscle movement occurs when muscle contracts maximally throughout its entire ROM and requires special equipment, such as that used in sports training and rehabilitation programs. (Isotonic and isometric contractions are shown in Figure 14-5).

Every muscle movement involves a primary muscle mover, the agonist that is responsible for eliciting a particular movement; synergist muscles assist agonists in their actions. Antagonist muscles work to oppose agonist muscles, just as the name implies. These coordinated functions are due to collaborative performance of the upper portion of the cerebellum and the motor control areas of the cerebrum. When the biceps brachii muscle contracts (agonist) to flex the forearm, the triceps brachii muscle relaxes (antagonist). The coracoid and brachialis muscles function as synergists because they contract to allow elbow flexion. Synergist muscles can be retrained in some instances to perform the function of agonists, such as when optimizing function with paralysis after stroke or spinal cord injury (SCI) or for patients using upper extremity prostheses.

Motor control and movement depend on muscle development and function as evidenced in strength, gross and fine motor coordination, fluidity of planned movements, balance, and cognition. Muscle strength is an important factor in movement often related to factors such as postural control, functional capacity, endurance, bone mass, and overall health status, including falls and mental outlook. Standard muscle strength tests may yield unreliable results for patients who experience pain or immobility at various positions or midway through ROM. The same may occur for those who are fatigued, experience early morning stiffness, take particular medications, or have cognitive or sensory alterations.

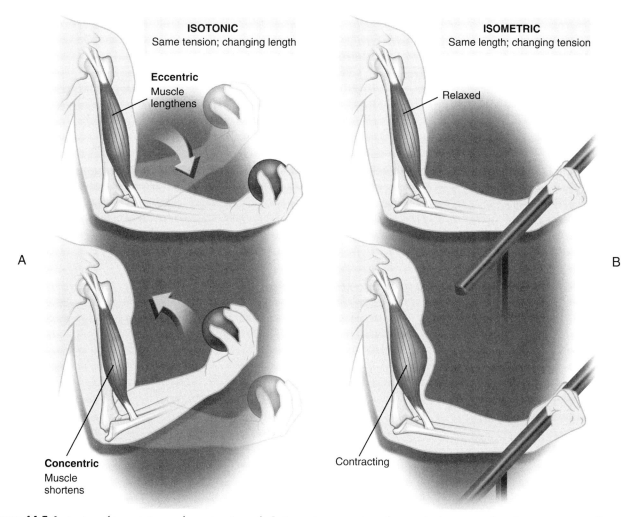

Figure 14-5 Isotonic and isometric muscle contractions. **A,** In isotonic contractions the muscle shortens and produces movement. Concentric contractions occur when the muscle shortens during the movement. Eccentric contractions occur when the contracting muscle lengthens. **B,** In isometric contraction the muscle pulls forcefully against a load but does not shorten. (From Thibodeau, G. A., & Patton, K. T. [2007]. *Anatomy and physiology* [6th ed.]. St. Louis, MO: Mosby.)

A resting muscle has a set level of minimal partial contraction, its tone. Muscle tone can be determined in part by the amount of resistance that occurs when performing passive ROM for a patient who is cooperative and relaxed. With prolonged immobility, muscle fibers shorten and stiffen, predisposing them to reduced ROM, in some instances contributing to contractures. Hypotonia, reduced or lost tone, occurs with damage to lower motor neurons or to the fibers that stimulate muscle spindles. When tone becomes flaccid, as with unconsciousness or coma, muscles correspondingly lose their bouncing stretch capacity, and the resulting stiffness resists extension. This may account for some of the hypertonic stretch response associated with spasticity.

ALTERED MOVEMENT

Upper Motor Neuron Syndrome Deficits

Clinically, upper motor neuron syndrome (UMN) is caused by congenital and acquired diseases, damage, or lesions of the cortical, internal capsule, subcortical, brainstem, and spinal cord areas. The pyramidal motor system is disrupted, resulting in deficits with performance (negative symptoms) that include paresis, weakness and fatigue, and reduced fine motor skills, especially manually; poor tone and loss of strength occur.

The positive symptoms reflect altered motor movements, exaggerated reflex responses (especially hypertonic stretch reflexes), increased muscle tone, and conditions that result from their dysfunction, such as spasticity or chorea. Nurses must anticipate potential responses, such as a mass reflex causing a patient to fall or come out of a chair. Alterations in mobility are described in Table 14-3. Although a pattern of spontaneous recovery of voluntary motor control is possible after stroke, factors such as the degree or amount, particular functions, length of time, and lag time for returns are unpredictable and individual.

At any given time some cells in a muscle are contracted while others are relaxed, resulting in muscle tone required to maintain normal posture. Motor control influences the power of muscle contractions through the number of motor units involved and the frequency of nerve stimulation. Injury or

TABLE 14-3 Definitions of Alterations in Mobility

Movement	Definition	Comments
Akinesia Also a root word for kinesia terms (e.g., hyperkinetic or bradykinesia)	Loss of voluntary muscle movement that may be associated with motor or psychic factors	Kinesiology is the study of movement that is important for an understanding of gait and exercise along with other facets of mobility
Altered Muscle Tone		
Hypotone (flaccidity)	Lack of muscle tone that may result in atrophy and disuse Characterized by soft, weak, and floppy qualities; muscles lack coordination	Indicator of little or no tone, often after lower motor neuron damage or lesions Performance of ADLs, strength, and postural alignment may be compromised
Hypertone (spasticity)	A spasm is an involuntary, transient muscle contraction with sudden onset; often associated with a specific type of spasm may be used to describe a quality of gait, hemiplegia, or paraplegia Muscles that are hypertonic and have increased resistance to stretch demonstrate spasticity Prime locations are flexors of the arms and extensors of the legs; other muscles can be affected Deep tendon reflexes are increased while superficial reflexes are decreased; there may be weakness	Spastic is an old word for certain disability conditions; also was used to describe the neurogenic (spastic) bladder in some situations Spasms vary in intensity and duration Movements are difficult and uncoordinated Pain, weakness, and inability to move properly may impair sleep, medical procedures, and ADLs; may even cause urinary retention Risk is high for damage to skin and development of contractures With conditions such as multiple sclerosis, inhibited function is exacerbated by pain, fatigue, and stiffness (Gelber & Jozefczyk, 2000)
Clonus (also clonic spasm)	Clonus implies involuntary skeletal muscle actions that rapidly alternate between relaxing and contracting	Clonic reflex action occurs as a result of an uninhibited reflex arc that results in stretching skeletal muscles when upper motor neuron lesions are present

TABLE 14-3 Definitions of Alterations in Mobility—cont'd

Movement	Definition	Comments
Rigidity	Increased tension in both agonist and antagonist muscles produces stiff, hard, inflexible muscles that resist movement	Extrapyramidal system lesions such as with Parkinson's disease eventually affect postural reflexes, as evidenced in poor initiation of movement and cogwheel rigidity Affects mobility and function Other examples are with upper brainstem lesions that cause the extremities to stiffen and extend or with resistance to passive range of motion after brain damage and coma
Altered Muscle Movements		
Chorea	Involuntary movements, usually of the proximal limbs, that are rapid, jerky, and forceful; not purposeful and are irregular and arrhythmic	Chorea is also a suffix for specific conditions such as Huntington or Sydenham chorea; associated with excess concentration of or supersensitivity to dopamine within the basal ganglion and may appear with use of dopamine medications Persons may attempt to mask movements by including them in movements for planned actions
Athetoses	Involuntary movements of the distal extremities characterized by slow, writhing activity Patient cannot maintain one position, and movement is essentially continuous	Typically noted with certain cerebral palsy movements or with lesions in the basal ganglia or tabes dorsalis; also seen with dopaminergic medication
Ballism	Violent, uncoordinated jerking or flinging of the proximal extremities	Associated with injury to the subthalamus nucleus of the basal ganglion and extrapyramidal disorders; may occur as hemiballismus
Tremor	Involuntary and repetitive movements described as quivering, quick movements that are rhythmic and nonpurposeful; movements may be fine or coarse Opposing muscle groups, usually the distal limb such as the hand, respond to alternating muscle contraction and relaxation	Resting tremor, often associated with Parkinson's disease; may disappear during planned movements Intentional tremors occur with diseasesof the cerebellum or red nucleus of the brainstem, such as multiple sclerosis, trauma, vascular conditions, are toxin-related, or due to tumors Cause of tremor may be senile, toxic metallic related, or psychogenic (Gillespie, 1991); tremor may be caused by Parkinson's disease, hepatic encephalopathy, metabolic disorders, essential (familial) tremor, cerebellar disease, red nucleus injury, or myoclonus
Dyspraxias and Apraxias (see Table 14-2) **Altered Muscle Reflexes**		
Reflex	Involuntary, unconscious, and immediate reaction or response to stimuli Reflexes are simple or complex and very specific; some are related to stages of development	Neuromuscular reflex responses have specific parameters; inappropriate responses may be part of diagnostic criteria
Hyporeflexia	Reduced quality and response of reflexes	Occurs when there is dysfunction in the muscle spindle system as seen in lower motor neuron disease
Hyperreflexia	Exaggerated quality and response of reflexes	Occurs when higher brain center no longer inhibits lower centers, as with autonomic hyperreflexia associated with spinal cord injury

Data from Anderson, K. N., Anderson, L. E., & Glanze, W. D. (1998). *Mosby's medical, nursing, and allied health dictionary* (5th ed.). St. Louis, MO: Mosby.
ADLs, Activities of daily living.

disease affecting the upper motor neuron pathway produces continued muscle contractions with spastic tone and exaggerated reflexes. The greater-than-normal muscle tone produces spasticity and dysfunctional posture and positioning. Abnormal high muscle tone is characterized as *hypertonic* when stimuli are uninhibited and create a state of imbalance and muscles resist passive movement; overextension and hyperflexion may be evident. Spasticity is associated with brain injury, SCI, multiple sclerosis, cerebral palsy, or stroke.

Spasticity is a concern when it inhibits movement or leads to complications, especially contractures. Spasms may make sitting in a wheelchair not only intolerable but also unsafe, whereas others may experience pain. Dexterity and rest may be compromised when upper body and extremity spasticity occurs, making ADLs or even personal hygiene difficult. The "clasped knife" phenomenon occurs in a spastic extremity when the muscle is stretched. The initial muscle contraction is followed by a sudden relaxation and tension release. Spasticity may enable function such as with muscle weakness or partial paralysis of the lower extremities (paraparesis). For example,

some patients are able to harness momentum from the increased tone in their antigravity muscles and have sufficient power to make a standing transfer (assisted for safety) from the wheelchair to the toilet.

Those with cerebral palsy find their posture, movement, or position may stimulate muscle tone leading to spasticity. Consider how spastic movements can thwart learning for a child sitting in a wheelchair and attempting to attend to classroom instructions. Scissoring steps, due to spasms from the hip and lower extremities, may impair ambulation for some. However, as a child with cerebral palsy develops and grows, it becomes difficult to control muscle tone and provide stretch to appropriate muscles to prevent fixed contractures. Continued flaccid tone leads to muscle atrophy and corresponding loss of muscle mass and reduced strength. This situation can arise from prolonged immobility or result from neurological or muscular disorders.

Figure 14-6 distinguishes disturbances that occur with alterations in upper motor neuron versus lower motor neuron functions.

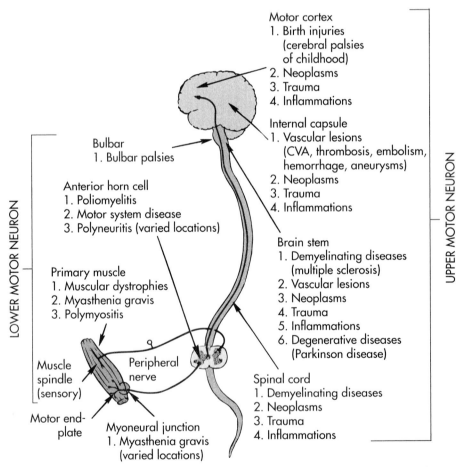

Figure 14-6 Disturbances in motor function. Disturbances in motor function are classified pathologically along upper and lower motor neuron structures. It should be noted that the same pathological condition occurs at more than one site in an upper motor neuron, *above right*. A few pathological conditions involve both upper and lower motor neuron structures, as in amyotrophic lateral sclerosis. Other lesion sites include myoneural junction and primary muscle, making it possible to classify conditions as neuromuscular and muscular, respectively. (From Huether, S., & McCance, K. [2004]. *Understanding pathophysiology* [3rd ed.]. St. Louis, MO: Mosby.)

Lower Motor Neuron Syndrome Deficits

Lower motor neuron syndrome (LMN) reflects damage, disease, or lesions of the anterior horn cell, bulbar myelencephalon and related cranial nerves, peripheral nerves, and muscle spindles or the myoneural junction. When both large and small neuron systems are affected and because the lower motor neuron is the final pathway actually terminating in a skeletal muscle, loss of function through disease or trauma results in flaccid paralysis or loss of both reflex and voluntary movements. Paresis often accompanies amyotrophic lateral sclerosis (ALS), and the motor dysfunction may present as breathing or swallowing deficits.

Recovery Patterns in the Nervous System

Recovery of cortical lesion damage follows a developmental sequence in that it returns from reflex to voluntary control, from mass to discrete movement, from tone before voluntary movements, and from proximal to distal control. Nonpurposeful extensor and flexor synergy patterns of the extremities may occur as a precursor to voluntary motor return, appearing as mass contractions of muscles in upper and lower extremities. Recovery of motor functions may cease at any point or level; recovery speed may indicate the level of function attainable. Cells in the brain that have been destroyed by the insult often do not regenerate, and the specific functions are diminished or altered. Diseases of the cerebellum and basal ganglia are often degenerative. To date, neural recovery is not expected, and the focus is on medication therapy and compensatory function through rehabilitation.

ASSESSMENT

The overall goal of assessment of functional mobility is to determine the patient's level of independence and the optimal environment, aids, or equipment necessary for the patient to safely achieve access and perform personal management. The question is, how much assistance, at what level, for how much time, and at what cost does the patient need for optimal independent function? Integrated neurological and musculoskeletal evaluations are essential to evaluation of movement and mobility and are conducted with levels of ADL and IADL performance in mind. One of the standardized assessment tools is necessary to evaluate levels of function and outcomes. Research-based schemata, such as data from the Functional Independence Measure (FIM) (Granger, 1997) (see Chapter 11) and the classifications of the Omaha System (Martin & Scheet, 1992) (see Chapter 2) are useful for guiding practice, certifying documentation, and managing information. Assessment tools, such as the Barthel Index (Mahoney & Barthel, 1965) and the Katz rating scales (Katz & Akpom, 1976), the Klein-Bell Scale (Klein & Bell, 1982) for self-care, or the Assessment of Motor and Process Skills (AMPS) (Fisher, 1999) and Older American Resources and Services Scale (OARS) (Duke University Center for the Study of Aging and Human Development, 1978) have stood, with modifications, over time. Chapter 31 contains information about the WeeFIM and other pediatric functional assessments. Studies are examining psychometric properties of new scales, such as those designed for persons with specific conditions.

Subjective Assessment

Subjective assessment begins with the history of the specific problem and a review of past function, including performance of ADLs and IADLs in the household and community. Identify assistive devices and adapted equipment, the reason for having them, and how they are used. Elicit patients' perceptions of their function and lifestyle goals for vocation, education, or leisure.

Describe limitations in access or ability, and identify problems related to health status, impairments, or conditions. Inquire about comorbid conditions affecting mobility or self-care, such as pain; sensory, communication, or cognitive impairments; energy or endurance level; sleep hygiene; household or environmental stressors; and safety concerns, such as poor balance. Evaluate psychosocial, emotional, and cultural factors affecting mobility or performance of ADLs. A shortened home and community assessment for patients returning home is detailed in Box 14-3.

A medical history includes surgeries; details of cardiovascular, pulmonary, rheumatological, neurological, or musculoskeletal conditions; and a family history. Describe the type, location, and severity of impairment or injury, along with any comorbid conditions and the potential for infection or other untoward effects. The review of systems focuses on skin, gastrointestinal (GI), respiration, circulation, regulatory control, elimination, eating and nutrition, sexuality, and integrated neuromuscular systems, as well as cognitive and emotional status. Review medications with attention to allergies and adverse effects, multiple medication use, and signs of misuse of medications or substances.

Objective Assessment

The following guidelines are for assessment of musculoskeletal and neurological functions related to movement. However, movement and self-care abilities are complex and involve multiple functions, such as cognition, swallowing, or communication as presented in specific chapters. Recovery occurs in varying degrees and at different rates but in predictable patterns. Baseline assessment data should be documented and patients reassessed at regular intervals or when change occurs. Specialized evaluations, such as a person's ability to return to work or to drive a car, involve expertise from the interdisciplinary team.

Physical Examination. Observe respiratory status, skin color and turgor, and posture and alignment. Note stooped shoulders, involuntary movements, unusual gait or gestures, signs of weakness or pain during activities, and overall appearance. Inspect body for shape, symmetry, length of extremities, abnormalities, redness, and edema (positional). Palpate for turgor, tone, and response of tenderness, pain, or tightness.

Assess joints for ROM, stability, tightness, impingement, pain or grating on movement, edema, heat or redness, and nodules or unusual protrusions. During ROM exercises rehabilitation nurses have opportunities to assess the quality of

---

BOX 14-3 Home and Community Assessment: Access Considerations

- Barrier-free access to community buildings and health providers. Marked handicapped parking, close to entrance, space to maneuver or manage packages
- Access to private or public transportation: distance from home, cost, assistance required, ability to operate own vehicle safely
- Storage of vehicle, access to home and street, vehicle adaptations for driver or passenger
- Access to home: width of doors; ability to turn key, open and close doors; need for ramps, handrails; and location, height, and style of mailbox
- Lighting in entrances, hallways, rooms, and work areas; accessible switches; access to control lights inside and outside home; steps, porch, front door lighted and protected from the weather; nonslip doormat
- Home maintenance and safety program with community support as needed for setting width, height of incline of ramps and walks and snow removal
- House number clearly visible and readable for quick identification during an emergency
- Locks secure with deadbolts and ability to operate; secure mailbox, peephole in door to view visitors
- Smoke detectors: type, location, access; space heaters: type, location of wiring; outlet covers for children
- Location of knobs on stove, safety around stove, cleanliness of stove; ability to use good judgment when cooking and transporting food from kitchen to table
- Ability to dispose of infectious materials safely and pest-free method of trash storage/disposal
- Use of oxygen: precautions and appropriate signs in home
- Ventilation in all rooms; heat and air conditioning, as needed
- Height of sink and toilet, shower/tub, and location of faucets
- Space for maneuvering wheelchair or assistive device
- Threshold for shower; water temperature regulator
- Ability to use facilities safely; nonslip floor, bath seat, location of grab bars, and secure anchors to solid wall
- Height of bed, firm mattress, elevated head, if needed
- Access to closet, ability to reach rods, storage area
- Arrangement of furniture and ability to transfer in and out of bed safely; adequate space around bed space to maneuver and store needed items

---

muscle movements. Appendix 14A is a guide for assessment of a patient's movement based on normal degrees of joint motion conducted before initiating a program of ROM exercises.

Assess muscle strength using a manual muscle test (MMT) to score. Evaluate for relative strength against resistance, when grasping and squeezing, for equality on both sides of the body and in proximal and distal positions, and for ability to flex and relax. Grip the patient's hand as in a handshake, both using right hands; repeat with left hands. Handgrips reveal strength and function. Observe for intact pincer grasp, uneven hand strength, contractions, spasticity, or flaccidity, and note pain. For example, poor triceps muscle strength impairs movement that involves pushing or pulling over the head. The person raises the arm straight overhead, bends at the elbow, and moves the hand behind the head. With the nurse's hand on the forearm, the patient pushes against the resistance. Spasticity, reduced ROM, or weakness may render the push against resistance nonfunctional for activities without modifications.

Assess muscle tone by palpating the muscle and examining neurological responses for spasticity or rigidity. Assess motor stretch reflexes by testing deep tendon reflexes (DTRs), such as by striking tendons over muscle groups and observing for overresponse or underresponse of muscle contractions and involuntary muscle movements. Specific assessments related to selected motor stretch reflexes are listed in Table 14-4. Evaluate reflexes for symmetry, hyporeflex-hyperreflex activity,

TABLE 14-4 Motor Stretch Reflexes

Reflex	Assesses
Biceps reflex	C5-C6 functions
Patellar reflex (knee jerk)	L2-L4 functions
Achilles reflex (ankle)	S1-S2 functions
Triceps reflex	C6-C8 functions
Brachioradial reflex	C5-C6 functions
Abdominal reflex	Lower thoracic cord reflex centers; associated with multiple sclerosis
Plantar reflex	Upper motor neuron damage; Babinski's sign normal during first year of life

abnormal or inappropriate response to stimulus (such as appearance or persistence of primitive reflexes such as reflex grasp or tonic neck), or contraction to adjoining muscles.

Assess cranial nerves for function, with special attention to motor control related to vision and eye control, vestibular operations, speech, and swallowing.

Assess sensory status beginning with sensation on the trunk and extremities. Use side-to-side symmetrical testing beginning distally on the body. Assess superficial and deep pain, pressure, touch, and temperature. Document the findings on a dermatome map or similar figure. (See Figures 14-18 and 21-1.)

BOX 14-4 Potential Problems in Function or Movement

Assess further when a patient is observed improvising or compensating movement by the following:
- Holding onto a handrail to pull the body while going up stairs
- Holding onto a bed side rail or bedcovers to pull to sitting in bed
- Leaning to one side and using both hands on the handrail while going down the stairs or a ramp
- Holding onto furniture or doorways and watching the feet while walking in the house
- Lifting a leg (or arm) by using the other leg (or arm) as support or by lifting with the pants leg (or sleeve)
- Tilting the head to reach the back or side of the hair while grooming
- Pushing up, rocking forward and back, and/or leaning the body over for momentum ("nose over toes") when rising to stand from a chair
- Leaning over from the waist without bending the knees and then using one hand on the thigh, as if it were a prop, to assist in getting upright
- Turning to reach for an object and then using the other arm or an object to support the reaching arm at the elbow or wrist
- Positioning a chair before sitting down by using the front or back of the knees and then using the back of the knees to guide sitting down; using the torso and hips to lean against a table or chair
- Reaching and leaning with the body rather than with an arm
- Walking with a lean to one side, a limp, a waddle, or other variation of gait
- Scanning ineffectively while eating or grooming
- Rolling or scooting the body, sliding forward in a seat, or other maneuvers to move off a bed or out of a chair

---

Sensory and motor qualities and cerebellar function are involved in the ability to actually plan and then carry out movement, as well as the sequence of movements, as with apraxia (see Table 14-2). Therefore include hands-on observation of a person's specific perceptual, motor, or sensory problems when the patient is unable to perform self-care in ADLs.

Assess proprioception and sense of position in space (kinesthesia perception) for upper and lower extremities. Ask the patient to close both eyes while holding his or her thumb between your thumb and forefinger. As you move the thumb up and down, ask the patient to identify the positions. If a position is identified incorrectly, repeat this process with other joints, such as the wrist, elbow, and shoulder. For the lower extremity, begin with the big toe and progress to the ankle, knee, and hip. Next, strike a tuning fork and place it on the most distal bony prominence of the extremities. Patients then report where and when they can feel the vibrations. In addition, assess the patient's ability to identify familiar objects through touch, such as closing the eyes and then recognizing a coin held in the hand as a quarter.

Assess balance and coordination while sitting and during activities. Ask the person to rapidly touch the thumb to each finger or to rotate the hands from supine to prone. Or ask the patient to touch his or her nose and then your finger; move your finger and repeat in several positions. Observe for control of balance at the abdomen and trunk and strength, which are necessary for dressing and household skills, such as cooking. While the patient moves forward in the seat of a chair, observe from behind; cross both arms to fold across the chest with elbows aimed to the front. Observe for compensatory balancing when pushing the upper body side-to-side and front-to-back while seated. The person seated in a chair or at the side of the bed may slump or sway to one side. Assess the ability of a patient to rotate the neck and trunk by looking behind over each shoulder while keeping the hips straight in place. Upper extremity activities can be modified, such as using over-the-head dressing techniques, when trunk rotation is limited.

Assess balance and coordination during mobility activities, such as when moving in and out of the bed, during transfers, and during ambulation. Use the Romberg test for persons able to stand with their eyes closed and feet together. However, use precautions against falls because loss of balance is possible and is a positive sign of cerebellar problems. Observe for swaying, leaning, reeling, or if standing, taking a step backward to maintain balance.

Assess gait pattern, arm swing, balance and steadiness, gait during turns, and whether the patient moves to the intended destination. Observe for involuntary movements or gait patterns associated with specific conditions such as the following:

- **Hemiplegia:** A stiff gait with toes on the affected side scraping the floor due to reduced flexion of the knee and swing from hip. The affected arm does not swing with the unaffected footstep; the shoulder may slouch.
- **Parkinson's disease:** A festinating gait with initial hesitation, followed by small, shuffling steps. Patient may appear to march in place because of difficulty in initiating walking and then be unable to halt once in motion. The body and head appear to lean forward with the arms extended back, not swinging with gait.
- **Multiple sclerosis/cerebral palsy:** A scissor gait may appear; slow steps may be due to bilateral spasticity in the legs.
- **Other:** Persons with lower motor problems may appear to be stepping up stairs although walking on a flat surface. Those with progressive neuromuscular disease may develop a waddling gait.

Assess patient's safety and performance of ADLs and IADLs. Evaluate the level and amount of physical, mental and cognitive, and emotional assistance needed, as well as types of assistive devices. Observe for actions that indicate a patient is using accessory muscles or compensatory movements to aid function. Many of these movements may be effective and purposeful; others are unsafe or detrimental and indicate problems in individual situations. Table 14-5 describes actions that may represent problems or lead to further disabilities.

TABLE 14.5 Nursing Diagnoses, Interventions, and Outcomes Applicable to Functional Mobility

NIC/NOC

Nursing Diagnosis	Nursing Interventions	Nursing Outcomes
Risk for disuse syndrome	Therapeutic exercises Environment management	Risk detection and control
Impaired bed mobility	Body mechanics promotion Prevention of complications	Body mechanics performance
Impaired physical mobility	Positioning specific to situation Active/passive range of motion Teaching prescribed activities Biofeedback Exercise promotion	Body positioning, self-initiated Joint movement and skeletal function Ambulation Immobility consequences, psychocognitive Immobility consequences, physiological
Fatigue	Energy management	Energy conservation
Activity intolerance	Self-care assistance (IADLs)	Activity tolerance Endurance
Risk for falls	Environmental management: safety Exercise therapy: balance	Fall prevention behavior Balance
Impaired wheelchair mobility	Wheelchair positioning and safety Exercise therapy: strength training and muscle control	Transfer performance Coordinated movement Ambulation: wheelchair
Self-care deficit	Self-care assistance for specific tasks Assistive devices and adapted equipment specific to needs Teaching prescribed activities for specific tasks Assistance with health access Self-responsibility facilitation Mutual goal setting	Self-care ADLs Self-care IADLs Bathing Dressing/grooming Eating Toileting Hygiene Oral hygiene Health maintenance Self-direction of care

Data from Moorhead, S., Johnson, M., & Maas, M. (2004). *Nursing outcomes classification (NOC)* (3rd ed.). St. Louis, MO: Mosby; Dochterman, J., & Bulechek, G. M. (2004). *Nursing interventions classification (NIC)* (4th ed.). St. Louis, MO: Mosby; and NANDA International. (2005). *Nursing diagnoses: Definitions and classification, 2005-2006* (6th ed.). Philadelphia: Author.
IADLs, Instrumental activities of daily living; *ADLs*, activities of daily living.

Box 14-5 contains information for the nursing diagnoses, outcomes, and interventions related to functional mobility and focuses on performance of ADLs and IADLs.

Overall Rehabilitation Goals

Patient goals specific to rehabilitation include optimal independence in ADL and IADL activities, prevention of complications and further disability, maximal function and mobility, safety, life satisfaction and effective coping, access to community, and quality social interactions.

NURSING INTERVENTIONS

Therapeutic interventions for mobility and self-care are core principles of rehabilitation nursing practice. Due to the amount of information, interventions in the chapter are separated into those for exercise and mobility, positioning, movement, assistive devices, wheelchairs, and self-care topics. Related content on eating and swallowing, bowel and bladder elimination, and cognition is presented in specific chapters.

Interventions for Maintaining Mobility

The importance of mobility to prevent disuse syndrome and other complications, and for optimal performance of ADLs and IADLs, is established. Detailed interventions for achieving functional outcomes follow.

Therapeutic Exercise. Regular exercise is an essential intervention for persons with or without impaired physical mobility. Assess the person's overall condition, and implement appropriate exercises to prevent contractures or atrophy and maintain muscle tone, strength, and function even if he or she is not able to begin active physical or occupational therapy.

Safety is a consideration for any mobility or therapeutic exercise program. Joint damage is possible with passive or active ROM, especially if sensation to the extremity has been impaired; spasticity and flexion contractures may be aggravated with UMN damage. Exercises use isotonic contractions, producing movement of joint and muscle, or isometric contractions, shortening muscle fibers without apparent movement of the limb or joint. Specific concerns include autonomic dysreflexia (AD) with SCI, altered respiratory and regulatory functions, poor postural response or hypotension, dizziness or fainting, skin damage, impaired cognition, headache and visual disturbance, increased pain, and falls.

When teaching the exercise program to the patient, family, or other caregivers, encourage active participation, demonstrate the exercise program, lead the patient and family through practice, observe the patient and family redemonstrate the exercises, and delegate responsibility for the exercise program to the patient and family as an ADL.

Range-of-Motion Exercises. ROM exercise is a precise set of actions to move the joints through their range, as possible for an individual. ROM can be passive (performed for the person), active (by the person independently), or active with assistance. ROM exercises are isotonic and used to prevent muscle contractures or atrophy; to maintain muscle tone, strength, and function; and to forestall many problems that occur with reduced mobility. Measure the angle of flexion of a joint because damage to the joints, pain, and other problems may result from improperly administered ROM exercises.

Appendix 14A provides visual and written instructions for passive, active, and functional ROM. Rehabilitation nurses have primary responsibility for ensuring that ROM exercises are performed properly, safely, and at regular intervals, as well as for educating others to perform them. Encourage patients to perform as many ROM exercises as independently as possible; ADLs, especially for personal hygiene, can integrate ROM exercises into daily living. Strategize with the team for best ways to perform ROM exercises for those who have chronic disabling conditions, specific impairments, or complications such as contractures, spasticity, pain, or paralysis.

Providers demonstrate learning by performing a "return demonstration" of the exercises, ideally performing the exercises upon one another. In addition to establishing correct movements, they have experience with the exercise movements and of being passive recipients. In the community, family members, volunteers, and other caregivers may learn to perform ROM under supervision.

Patients who perform active ROM may find it easier to learn exercises that are demonstrated first, supplemented with diagrams, and then demonstrate their accuracy and effectiveness. Persons with similar disabilities may be grouped during the day for "range" exercises, or a patient and family member may exercise together. A cable or online facility television station or other media presentations of exercises may stimulate participation.

ROM exercise modifications for persons with specific impairments, such as hemiplegia or paraplegia, incorporate methods that aid movement of extremities using the unaffected extremities. For example, a patient laces the fingers of the unaffected hand through those of the affected hand for support to exercise. Raising one arm above the shoulder supports and raises the other, and flexing and extending the unaffected arm at the elbow assist reciprocal action in the other. To move the legs through their ROM, combine the efforts of the unaffected arm and leg, depending on strength and balance. With paraplegia a person may exercise the legs and feet while sitting in bed, because the bed assists in maintaining balance and supports the legs and feet.

Isometric Exercises. Isometric exercises contract muscle fibers without movement of limbs or joints and thus require voluntary participation. After teaching a patient to perform an activity, monitor and evaluate the results. Energy expenditure, pain, postural stability and balance, cognition, and safety are considerations for any exercise plan. Sometimes referred to as *muscle-setting exercises*, the most common isometric exercises are abdominal-setting, quadriceps-setting, and gluteal-setting exercises. For abdominal-setting exercises, place one hand on the abdomen while the patient tenses the abdominal muscle. The muscle is contracted and held for 10 seconds and then released. Remind patients, especially those who have had myocardial infarctions or brain injuries, to maintain a normal respiratory pattern during the exercise. For quadriceps-setting exercises the person contracts the long muscles in the thighs; for gluteal-setting exercises the buttocks are pinched together. Other muscle groups such as the perineal, biceps, and triceps may be contracted isometrically.

Another type of isometric exercise contracts a muscle group against an object, for example, pushing or plantar flexing the feet against a footboard for 10 seconds or less to prevent circulatory stasis. This isometric exercise is resistive because the footboard provides resistance to the activity of the muscles of the legs and feet.

Alternative and Complementary Measures. An increasing number and variety of alternative interventions are proving effective as exercises or as complementary interventions, such as yoga, tai chi, and various stretching regimens. Biofeedback and/or electrical stimulation, such as with transcutaneous electrical stimulation (TENS), may maintain or increase muscle strength and tone; biofeedback complements isometric exercise.

Prevention Through Fitness. Preventive exercises are important for all, and patient education examples are readily available, including exercises specific to preventing low back pain, osteoporosis, or maintaining overall fitness. Exercise equipment; repetitive motion machines; a wide range of styles and sizes of balls, weights, and balance and posture aids; computer-assisted gait programs; and more are available to support therapeutic exercise to improve or maintain movement.

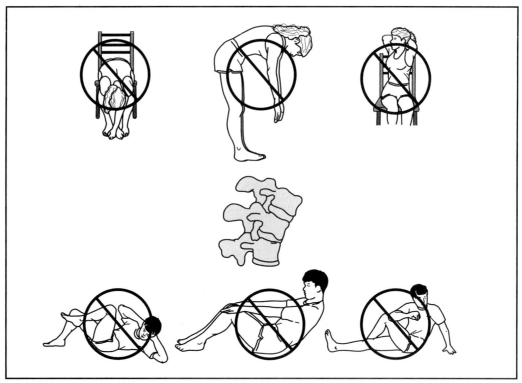

Figure 14-7 Spinal flexion exercises to be avoided by people with osteoporosis. (From Robinson, D., Kidd, P., & Rogers, K. M. [2000]. *Primary care across the lifespan.* St. Louis, MO: Mosby).

Objects common to the home or community are usable, including large, flat elastic bands designed for stretching to exercise the legs and feet, or wooden dowels, a cane, or shortened broom handles to maintain posture and stretch during exercises from the chair. Canned goods as weights, soft pliable balls to squeeze in the hand, and large balls for balance or tossing against a wall or to another person are strategies. Straight-back, steady chairs are good supports and balance while exercising, and mats and cushions help with yoga and floor exercises.

Exercises Specific to Conditions. Therapeutic exercises can be tailored to assist patients with specific conditions and to prevent additional problems. Patients must be able to perform them safely and know when they are contraindicated, such as with osteoporosis (Figure 14-7). Success with exercise begins in everyday activities. For instance, personal hygiene and ADLs are opportunities for performing therapeutic and preventive exercises in a safe environment. Kegel exercises help with certain incontinence problems, relaxation and breathing exercises aid in respiration, and oral-facial movements as detailed in Box 14-5 benefit conditions such as Parkinson's disease. Posture, balance, and strength training with improvement in muscle tone may benefit patients following a stroke, with Guillain-Barré syndrome, after brain injury, or with multiple sclerosis. Those using a wheelchair who have upper body mobility can perform stretching and flexibility exercises

---

BOX 14-5 Oral-Facial Exercises

Repeat each exercise three to five times:
- Slowly open and close the mouth, pressing the lips to close tightly and open widely.
- Pretend to give a kiss, exaggerating puckered lips.
- Smile broadly, let relax, and repeat, pushing up the facial cheeks.
- Open the mouth wide, and with the lips form an "o" shape, keeping the mouth wide; then close lips tightly and repeat.
- Open the mouth and stick the tongue out straight as far as possible; hold it in place without touching the mouth or lips; then pull it back and push out rapidly.
- Stick out the tongue and try to touch the nose, then the chin; next lick all around the lips, touching every corner of the mouth.
- Rapidly repeat sounds for MA-MA, KA-KA, LA-LA, then rest; try combining the sounds, as with KALA-KALA, MALA-MALA.
- Wrinkle nose, raise the eyebrows and wrinkle the forehead, and then relax and repeat.
- Open and close the mouth quickly.
- Mimic exaggerated chewing motions with the mouth opening and closing with each chew.

---

for the head and neck and upper extremities. Patients with postpolio syndrome, Lyme disease, or other fatigue-related conditions need to modify exercises to control for pain and endurance levels; conversely, proper exercise programs may yield gains in strength, tolerance, and respiratory function.

Body Mechanics. Rehabilitation nurses both practice and teach families and other caregivers the principles of proper body mechanics (see Box 14-1), not only for lifting and carrying but for every movement in practice. In a time-sensitive health scene, nurses must take time to perform care effectively and safely for themselves, as well as for patients; rushing a patient is not a standard of care. It takes time to explain; allow the patient to do as much as possible; assess readiness, capability, and understanding of the particular action; conserve energy; avoid pain or contraindicated movement; and ensure safety.

Therapeutic Positioning

Therapeutic positioning is essential for preventing complications when a person has restricted mobility. Positioning involves not only mechanical placement of the body but also changes or repositions, mobility in place, and positions specific to the condition or needs. Prevention of complications begins with a plan for regular position change based on the patient's independence or self-initiated movement, overall physical and mental status, comfort, fatigue, loss of sensation, symptoms such as edema, specific disease or condition factors, and devices or equipment, such as casts, prostheses, or bracing.

General guidelines for positioning also are subject to regulatory guidelines or facility and agency policies. Patients who experience discomfort after 30 to 60 minutes of lying prone need to be repositioned, whereas those able to shift their weight every 20 to 30 minutes and move independently may change total position every 2 to 4 hours. Loss of sensation, paralysis, coma, and edema are indications for position changes every 2 hours or more frequently when the patient is unable to communicate discomfort or pain. Edematous, paralyzed tissue is more sensitive to pressure than normal tissue. Chapter 15 provides detailed information about maintaining skin integrity.

Time of day and comfort or pressure-relief devices may influence repositioning. For instance, when a patient's overall condition permits, positioning every 4 hours during the night may promote a more restful sleep. Post the schedule for all caregivers.

Basic Positions. Classic positions are supine (back-lying), lateral (side-lying), prone (abdomen-lying), semiprone, and thirty-degree lateral (Figure 14-8). Attention to details may influence mobility outcomes, such as specific positions following total hip or knee replacement or below-knee amputation. Specialty beds and devices are discussed in Chapter 15. Aids used in positioning are listed in Table 14-6.

Supine Position. Assist the patient to lie on the back (Figure 14-8, *A*), with a small, flat pillow to support the head, neck, and upper shoulders. The arms lie along the sides with elbows extended and palms down. Vary the upper extremity position by abducting the shoulder slightly using a small pillow, then elevating the forearm and hand. Other upper extremity positions are full abduction of the shoulder with the elbow and wrist extended, or full abduction of the shoulder with a 90-degree elbow flexion and the arm and hand positioned upward or down.

Extend the hips, and support with a trochanter roll. Avoid pressure on the back of the legs, which may damage blood vessels, resulting in phlebitis. Extend or slightly flex the knees, but too great a degree of knee flexion risks flexion contracture and impaired posture and gait. Place the feet perpendicular with the leg. Footboards are not effective against footdrop or contractures; however, maintain some support for the desired flexion, such as adjustable footboards, firmly folded blankets, resting leg splints with footplates, or high-top sneakers. Note precautions in the Positioning Aids section.

Lateral Position. Assist the patient to lie on one side (Figure 14-8, *B*) with a firm pillow to support the head and neck. Position the lower arm at the side with the uppermost arm supported by a pillow to prevent pressure on the chest. Flex the upper leg at the hip and knee, and position on a pillow in front of the lower leg to minimize pressure on the lower leg. Place another pillow behind the back to maintain this side-lying position. After a stroke, the side-lying positioning incorporates the Bobath NDT approach with a patient's lying on the affected side as tolerated. From this position the patient begins to establish weight bearing and lengthens the trunk, which later helps to counteract altered posture while sitting and standing. Positioning the person on the affected side may stimulate improved muscle tone through weight bearing in preparation for the bilateral weight bearing necessary to move up in bed, move on and off the bedpan, and stand.

Generally, in this position the bottom shoulder lies slightly ahead of the rest of the body, with the hip, knee, and shoulder in some degree of flexion. When positioning the individual who has had a stroke in the side-lying position on the affected side, place the head in a neutral position, with the lower shoulder brought forward with the arm extended and the palm facing up and the hips and knees flexed. The shoulder is placed away from the spastic pattern associated with hemiplegic posture. A towel or small pillow under the trunk at waist level helps elongate the affected side.

Prone Position. Before placing a patient in a prone position, assess for any possible contraindications, such as increasing intracranial pressure or cardiopulmonary distress. Assist the person with lying on the abdomen (Figure 14-8, *C*). Turn the head to one side to facilitate breathing and drainage of oral secretions. Place a small pillow under the head for comfort and another between the chest and the umbilicus to relieve pressure on the chest or breasts. Extend the hips and knees and support them on pillows. The feet and toes are supported by another pillow or are positioned between the edge of the mattress and the bed frame to prevent pressure areas. In the prone position a patient may feel most comfortable with arms flexed over the head or extended along the body in a neutral position. The patient is in the semiprone position when resting on the side with the uppermost arm and leg placed farther forward.

Thirty-Degree Lateral Position. Place the patient supine with the pelvis tilted at a 30-degree angle to the

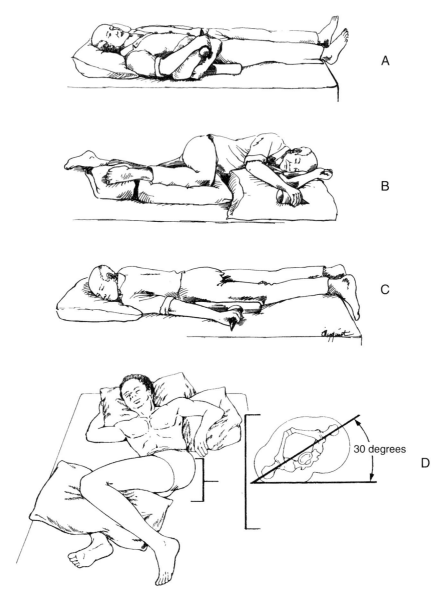

Figure 14-8 Four basic positions. **A,** Supine position with trochanter roll to prevent external rotation of the hips. **B,** Lateral position with hand cone to prevent flexion contraction of the hand. **C,** Prone position with trochanter roll and hand cone. **D,** Thirty-degree lateral position at which pressure points are avoided. (**D** from Bryant, R. A. [2000]. *Acute and chronic wounds: Nursing management* [2nd ed]. St. Louis, MO: Mosby.)

bed (Figure 14-8, *D*). All extremities are flexed at either the elbow or knee and supported on pillows. This position alleviates pressure on points, but a repositioning schedule is important because one hip supports weight. Attention to the patient's lower back and overall proper alignment and support are essential; carefully assess the effects on those with shoulder problems.

Sitting Position. With so much attention placed on mobility, the act of sitting and features of seating are often undervalued. Not only is the ability to sit with balance and trunk control preliminary to transfers, it offers an upright view of the world. All patients should sit with their feet placed flat on the floor and the hips well back in the seat, with weight distributed evenly over the hips. Weight shifts are useful techniques for those with sufficient upper body strength and

function and who are able to perform them safely from a chair or wheelchair, or who have assistance for wheelchair back tilting.

Positioning Aids. Details of a wheelchair and any inserts affect position. Measure the depth, width, and height of the chair for sitting position and to deter the person from leaning to one side or the other. If the chair seat is too wide or too deep to allow the hip and knees to be placed at right angles, use pillows cautiously because they may cause the thighs to roll inward or form lumps, among other problems. Proper seat cushions and back supports improve comfort and alignment. A proper seat is firm and wide and does not slump or sag into a slinglike shape, unless specifically prescribed. Although foam or rubber devices are common, never use doughnut-shaped cushions because they may impair circulation and skin integrity.

TABLE 14-6 Positioning Aids

(Bed support surfaces and specialty beds are discussed in Chapter 15.)

Positioning Aid	Description of Use	Comments on Use
Pillows	Use to position, stabilize, support, or bridge beneath a pressure area; maintain proper alignment. Substitute rolled or folded towels, bath blankets, or foam squares covered with washable material.	Check contents for allergy-eliciting materials. Do not bunch or pack into hard lumps; no foam or rubber seat doughnuts. Pillows must fully support the extremity or body part.
Trochanter rolls	Prevent outward rotation of the hip when lying down. Place the roll just at the hips, from the top of the iliac crest to approximately 6 inches above the knee; form a roll along the outer aspect of the thigh.	Commercial trochanter rolls may be replaced with a flannel sheet or bath blanket folded into thirds lengthwise and rolled under toward the patient. (Figure 14-8, *A* and *C*, shows proper placement.)
Foot supports	Not effective and no longer used; they may initiate spasticity. Patients should wear shoes for protection.	A footboard may keep the bedcovers off the feet; also use specialty boots and sheepskin covers.
Hand rolls	Maintain position and prevent contractures.	Use hard cones, not soft rolled materials.
Splints or orthoses Upper limb and lower limb differ; the most common lower limb orthoses are ankle-foot (short-leg braces). Knee-ankle-foot orthoses (long-leg braces) have joints at the knee. Pediatric orthoses range from a standing frame, parapodium and swivel walker, and reverse walker, to spinal orthoses for scoliosis. Special shoes often are necessary when patients have orthoses.	Two types (includes functional): 1. Static is rigid and provides support without movement. 2. Dynamic allows some movement and may be used to stretch a contracture. The purpose is to improve current and long-term function. Orthoses may be highly specific, as for rheumatoid arthritis, spinal cord injury, burns, scoliosis, carpal tunnel syndrome, and other nerve and joint inflammations. Slings are not used for shoulder subluxation after stroke and when the patient is sitting or lying down.	Orthoses should be as basic as possible, comfortable, and easy to maintain; ideally they will be cosmetic. Patient may wear an orthosis intermittently until it is tolerated but will be more likely to use it if it adds function. Some splints may cover large and sensate areas of the body such as the forearm and hand and thus decrease sensory input; others may work on larger joints using the effects of gravity and weight. A resting splint maintains the wrist, thumb, and fingers in extension. At times, orthoses are used in conjunction with casting.
Casts Casts are composed of various materials, including plaster, plastic, and fiberglass. May cover small or large portions of the body. Casts may be highly specific.	Casts are used in rehabilitation in a variety of situations: after multiple trauma, especially with fractures; to prevent pain and cardiopulmonary complications that may accompany postural problems with scoliosis; and in burn care to prevent contractures with scarring. Casts may help prevent contractures such as with rheumatoid arthritis or with flaccid muscles.	Therapists may use serial casting after x-ray examination of the area; the cast is used to provide additional extension. A new cast is applied each week, but it is removed daily for personal hygiene and observation. Rehabilitation nurses are responsible for maintaining skin integrity, circulation, and other standards of care.
Abductor wedge or pillow	Abductor wedge or pillow is designed specifically for use after total hip replacement surgery; it maintains the legs in abduction to keep the prosthesis positioned until the muscles, soft tissues, and incisions heal. A knee immobilizer may be added to control flexion of the knee to the hip on the prosthesis side. Patient must not exceed an angle of 90 degrees of flexion between the knee and hip, a concern with seating or toileting as recovery progresses.	Patients may wear antiembolism stockings after the surgery; muscle tone and strength, skin integrity, and prevention of thromboses are priorities. Positioning and turning schedules take into account the person's age, comorbid conditions, risk factors such as osteoporosis or obesity, or conditions such as diabetes or rheumatoid arthritis. Schedules for positioning take into account the daily schedule, socialization opportunities, and patient preferences to allow the person as much control as possible while otherwise being immobilized. Early ambulation is monitored closely.

Custom seating systems may be needed to distribute pressure evenly. Consult a professional who has been trained in fitting wheelchairs or an assistive technology specialist before placing an order for a permanent chair. Vendors also may provide information about modifications for their products.

When the chair seat height does not allow the person to place both feet flat on the floor, add a small footstool, or use footrests in a wheelchair. Shoes offer a great deal of protection even when seated. When sitting up in bed or in a chair, instruct patients to avoid positions that encourage spastic patterns to develop, to avoid bending the residual limb at the knee after amputation, and to maintain proper hip angles after hip surgery. Place the affected shoulder forward using a pillow for support, if needed, and avoid a slouching posture. The affected arm rests on a table at a comfortable height or in the wheelchair on an armrest of proper height and support.

Patients With Lower Limb Amputations. Patients who have lower limb amputations may turn prone for care or lie prone for short times. Positioning cautions are listed in Box 14-6. Strengthening activities for the upper body include lifting and turning in bed using an overhead trapeze. During the inpatient time, a patient sitting in a wheelchair or chair extends the residual limb straight and uses a leg rest or residual limb board to support it. Once fitted for their prosthesis, patients will have prescribed positioning.

Activities for Movement

Movement in the Bed. Activities for a person who is in bed consist of turning from side to side; bridging and changing positions to relieve pressure points; moving up and down or to the side of the bed; and, if possible, sitting up in the bed. Patients with total dependence need assistance to move. Those who can move with some assistance or use adaptive equipment can participate provided they are capable of following instructions. Useful devices are an overhead trapeze, bed side rails, ropes or cords tied to foot rails, or other firm and secure places to grasp and pull.

BOX 14-6 Positioning Cautions for Patients With a Lower Extremity Amputation

Patients who have experienced a lower extremity amputation **should NOT:**
- Place a pillow under the hip or knee when in bed
- Lie in bed with knees bent or cross the legs
- Place a pillow under the back when lying supine in bed
- Put a pillow between the thighs
- Elevate the lower end of the bed under the knees
- Allow the residual limb to roll in or turn in toward the other leg
- Let the legs fall outwards while lying supine
- Rest the residual limb over the edge of the bed or a chair
- Sit with the residual limb bent
- Stand with the residual limb resting on the bar of a walker or grip of a crutch

---

Proper body mechanics are essential to move a person who is dependent in, out, or around the bed. Raise the bed to a working height, approximately hip level, by locking the bed casters or bracing it against a wall and elevating it securely on blocks. This coincides with the center of gravity and allows the caregiver to stand with knees slightly flexed and legs positioned in a wide base of support so the large leg and gluteal, not back, muscles are used. Transfer weight from one leg to the other in the direction of the move.

In moving the patient who is dependent toward the top or bottom of the bed, two caregivers are safer and more energy efficient. The method of moving depends on the patient's weight and breadth. For an average weight range, two persons are efficient. Using the hands as levers, with elbows bent, one caregiver slides the arms under the person's upper back; one arm is under the shoulders, the other under the waist. The other caregiver supports the patient's lower back, positioning one arm at the waist, the other below the patient's hips. Both caregivers stand at the same side of the bed and mentally "divide" responsibility for moving a portion of the patient's height and weight. Using their arms as levers, each caregiver stands with knees slightly flexed and one foot forward. At a given count both caregivers transfer their weight to move the patient in one smooth, continuous motion toward the top of the bed, taking care to avoid friction or shearing of the skin.

A person with some upper body strength and lower limb mobility can assist with moving to the head of the bed. The patient grasps the side rails, pulls up with the arms, and pushes the soles of both feet down into the mattress, which thrusts the body upward in bed. The headboard or a trapeze suspended on an over-bed frame is useful for a patient to pull up on, for bedpan positioning, or during bed making, but continued dependence on side rails or a trapeze is discouraged unless options are exhausted.

A single caregiver can move a patient to the side of the bed using the principles of "thirds," and moving a section at a time. Using proper body mechanics, begin moving the patient's head and shoulders, then the waist and hips, and finally the legs and feet.

The patient with hemiplegia or paresis following a stroke is instructed in sequential steps to move to the side of the bed with assistance using the Bobath NDT approach:
1. Clasp the hands, and stretch them forward.
2. Bend the knees.
3. Turn the head, and look in the direction of the turn.
4. Swing the extended arms to the side of the turn.
5. Let the knees follow to complete the turn (Borgman & Passarella, 1991).

Turning. When turning a patient to the side, stand on the bed side toward which they are to be turned. Position the person's arms on the abdomen and cross the far leg over the near leg at the ankle (unless contraindicated, as with total hip replacement). Standing with knees slightly bent and one leg forward, place one hand beneath the patient's far shoulder, and position the other hand beneath the hips on the far side.

Using a smooth, complete motion, transfer weight from the forward leg to the back leg, thereby moving the patient to a side-lying position.

A patient who has hemiplegia or paresis bridges the hips, lifting them off the bed as to get on a bedpan. Ask or help the patient to bend the knees and to place the unaffected foot over the affected one to stabilize it. Place one hand on top of the patient's affected knee to move it down toward the feet and the other hand under the affected hip to direct the lifting movement of the hips (Borgman & Passarella, 1991). Pressure exerted over the knee causes the hip to rise automatically. Bridging is also used with lower body dressing techniques discussed later in this chapter (Figure 14-9).

Encouraging Patient Participation. Encourage participation and provide instruction whenever a patient is able to assist in activities in bed. Teach the patient to turn to the side of the bed by pulling up on the side rail using either upper extremity. Without side rails, the patient carefully positions the immobilized arm when turning onto the affected side; ideally place it on the abdomen so that it is not "left behind" during the turn. Position the affected leg over the other ankle; ensure the leg is in alignment. If one or both legs are mobile, the patient facilitates the turn using the sole (not heel) of the foot to push in the direction of the turn.

Activities Out of the Bed. Patients who are completely dependent or require some assistance are moved out of bed to a chair or wheelchair for a change in position and surroundings and to minimize the effects of immobility. Assess readiness to sit in a chair; monitor vital signs, balance, alertness, and level of comfort before the person moves from a high Fowler's position or dangling; supervise carefully. In the home evaluate the environment. Assess circulation to the lower extremities with the legs dangling; apply compression or antiembolism stockings or elastic bandages, if needed. Place the legs and feet fully

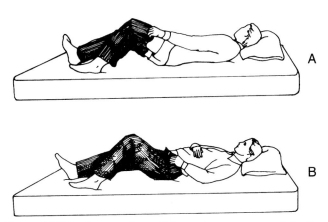

Figure 14-9 Bridging to dress. If the patient cannot stand, he lies down on the bed. **A,** Patient flexes his unaffected knee, keeping his foot flat on the bed. **B,** As the patient pushes down on the bed, his hips elevate. Patient uses his unaffected hand and arm to pull up his pants and fasten them. (From Hoeman, S.P. [1990] *Rehabilitation: Restorative care in the community.* St. Louis, MO: Mosby.)

supported on an elevated wheelchair footrest or on a stool to reduce edema and venous stasis.

Transfers

Patients able to perform transfers can move from the bed to other locations and outdoors. Important transfers are to a chair or wheelchair, the commode or toilet, the bathtub or shower, and perhaps a vehicle and then back to the bed.

Transferring a Person Who Is Dependent for Mobility. Transferring a patient who is dependent from bed to a chair requires mechanical devices or trained personnel using lift transfers or pivot transfers, as described in the following section. Once a person is seated, monitor body alignment and sitting posture and time weight shifts.

Mechanical Devices. A common mechanical device is the pneumatic lift. A person is positioned on a one- or two-piece sling connected by chains to a crossbar on the lift. Pumping the hydraulic mechanism lifts a person in a seated position off the bed. Because the lift is stable and adjustable, the person can be wheeled while suspended in the lift sling from the bed to a chair or commode. As the hydraulic pressure is released slowly, the patient descends into the seat. Depending on a patient's size and impairment, one, two, or three caregivers may be required for a safe transfer to a chair. The lift slings may be removed or left in place beneath the patient until returning to bed. Turn the hooks on the slings away from the patient to prevent injury, and line the sling for hygiene.

Lift Transfer. Two caregivers can transfer patients of average weight from the bed to a chair. Elevate the bed slightly higher than the chair. One caregiver stands at the head of the bed and reaches both arms under the patient's arms and across, using opposite hands to grasp the patient's wrists. The other supports the legs and feet. Using proper body mechanics, on a predetermined count they lift the patient out of bed and glide him or her into the chair. With a heavier person, four caregivers use a sturdy lift sheet, one at each of the person's shoulders and one at each of the knees. At the predetermined count, they use the lift sheet to slide the patient above the bed surface and into the seat.

Pivot Transfer (Assisted). When weight bearing is allowed, patients who are dependent can be pivot transferred from bed to a chair. The patient is helped to sit on the side of the bed and places both arms around the caregiver's neck and shoulder. The caregiver passes both arms under the patient's arms to support the lower back; then with one foot forward flexes the knees and thighs while rocking back and forth with the patient to gain momentum. When both are ready, the caregiver shifts weight, lifting the patient off the bed and turning toward the chair. By shifting weight from the back leg to the forward leg and bending at the hip and knee, the caregiver lowers the patient into the chair.

Positioning in a Chair. The nurse evaluates the patient's seated posture; ideally a straight, slightly relaxed back; hips and knees flexed at 90 degrees; and feet flat on the floor.

Use a footstool if the chair is too high, and examine alignment or any pressure on the legs. When a chair is too wide, pillows at either side prevent leaning; when a chair is too deep, a back pillow prevents "slumping" or "slinging." A low chair leads the patient to flex the hips and knees too acutely, predisposing contractures; try a foam pad or pillow in the chair seat. Teach patients to reposition each hour while in a chair; and when able, to shift weight every 15 minutes by leaning forward, to the right, or to the left. Those with sufficient upper body strength can push up with the arms to raise themselves up off the buttocks several times.

Assisting Transfers. Patients who are independent for short periods or who require minimal assistance may find a pivot transfer useful. Figure 14-10 illustrates the steps in pivot transfer from a wheelchair to the toilet as performed by a person wearing a lower extremity prosthesis. Patients with partial dependence may improve using techniques described in the following section for a patient with paraplegia or hemiplegia using a transfer board. The nurse encourages

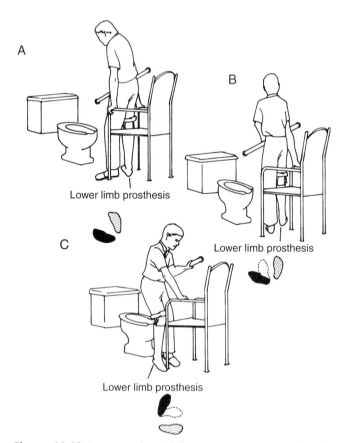

A, Lower limb prosthesis

B, Lower limb prosthesis

C, Lower limb prosthesis

Figure 14-10 Pivot transfer with lower extremity amputation. **A,** Patient is shown wearing a lower limb prosthesis on the affected leg. First, lock any braces or casters; lock the knee of the prosthesis, if applicable. **B,** Patient will pivot with weight on the residual limb (the unaffected leg). **C,** Residual limb provides main support and balance for the transfer. Be sure to assist the patient as necessary for safety. (From Hoeman, S. P. [1990]. *Rehabilitation: Restorative care in the community.* St. Louis, MO: Mosby.)

patient participation, teaches sequential steps for each technique, is available for assistance, and ensures a safe environment and technique, such as using transfer belts or other safety devices.

Patient With Paraplegia. A patient who has paraplegia or limited mobility below the waist, such as with bilateral lower extremity amputation, can use the following transfer. Place the chair perpendicular to the middle of the bed. Lock bed casters and commode or wheelchair wheels, and remove footrests. The patient rises to sit and using upper extremity strength turns the trunk and legs in line with the chair. With the patient's back positioned close to the chair seat, the patient reaches backward with both arms to grasp the armrests, and then moves the hips and legs from the bed backward into the seat of the chair. As the chair is moved away from the bed, the patient lowers the legs carefully. When proficient, a patient may use a push-up and side-to-side transfer.

Patient With Hemiplegia. The person with hemiplegia has less muscle strength and/or sensation on one side of the body, but usually can learn an independent standing transfer (Figure 14-11).

When incorporating the Bobath NDT approach, place the chair at an angle to the bed on the patient's affected side. Lock the chair, and remove the armrest closest to the bed. Assist the patient to the side of the bed, and position the feet flat on the floor with the heels under or slightly behind the knees. The patient clasps the hands and extends the arms, leaning forward until the head and trunk are in position over the feet. The caregiver leans over the patient's back to assist in moving the hips. Rocking to shift weight to the back foot, the caregiver pivots while turning the patient's hips toward the chair, affected side first. The caregiver shifts his or her weight forward, and the patient is lowered gently to the chair (Borgman & Passarella, 1991).

Transfer Board. A transfer board may be used to facilitate movement between many sites (e.g., a chair and the tub or a chair and a toilet) for the patient who has limited function of the lower extremities. A patient may wear a transfer belt for a caregiver to grasp when offering assistance. Generally, a physical therapist initiates upper extremity strengthening and training; the nurse encourages and reinforces, monitors the procedures, and finds ways for the patient to integrate the transfer into daily activities.

Several styles of transfer boards are available; some promote a "lift and bounce" across the board, but the principle is the same. Often referred to as *sliding*, a patient does not slide literally on the transfer board because this would impair skin integrity. Set the bed and wheelchair or chair at the same height, place the wheelchair beside the bed at a 45-degree angle and lock brakes, and if possible, remove armrests. Ideally the bed and chair are the same height. Place the transfer board bridging the chair and the bed; a patient needs a clear path to avoid brushing against the wheel during transfer.

With assistance the patient leans to position a portion of the transfer board under the buttocks and then sits and regains balance. Using the upper extremities, the patient performs

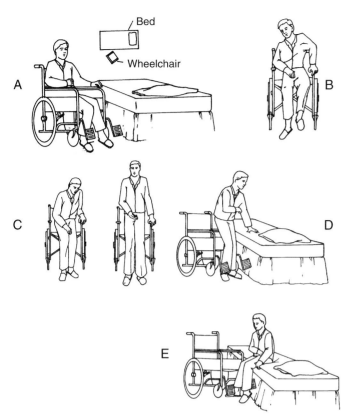

Figure 14-11 Independent standing transfer. **A,** Lock brakes and lift footrests. Angle the wheelchair close to the bed, facing the head of the bed, preferably on the patient's unaffected side. Instruct the patient to place both feet flat on the floor. **B,** Unaffected foot should be placed directly beneath the wheelchair seat (slightly behind the affected foot). **C,** As the patient leans forward on the unaffected foot and pushes on the armrest, he will rise to a standing position. **D,** Patient should continue to use the armrest and keep feet slightly apart for balance and safety. If the patient is tall, an adjustable-height armrest may be needed for the patient to stand erect. **E,** Patient uses his unaffected arm to balance and support himself on the edge of the bed. The patient should be instructed to take short side steps to turn toward the unaffected side. When the patient's back is perpendicular to the side of the bed, he can sit. (From Hoeman, S. P. [1990]. *Rehabilitation: Restorative care in the community.* St. Louis, MO: Mosby.)

a series of "little push-ups" across the board. Those with a great deal of upper body strength may pull themselves toward the far armrest of the chair, but skin friction and shearing must be prevented. Either way, the hips and lower extremities are moved over the transfer board and into the chair. The patient tilts the other way and removes the board.

Ambulation and Gait Training

Goal setting and attainment for functional independence in ambulation is a team effort in which the patient is an active participant. A physical therapist works with the patient to propose a safe ambulation plan that is reinforced in all team areas and in the community. A plan may include isometric and therapeutic exercises designed to prepare the muscles used in walking, provide practice in maintaining sitting and

standing balance, gain ability for passive standing, and select adaptive equipment and assistive devices used with specific gait-training techniques.

Preambulation Activities. Preambulation activities begin early on and are conducted in the bed, including isometric exercises to strengthen upper extremity muscles and muscles of the lower extremities and trunk, including the gluteal and abdominal muscles for standing and walking. Other therapeutic exercises preparatory to walking are modified sit-ups in the supine position and modified push-ups in the prone position. Gaining sitting balance is important. The patient sits at the side of the bed with both feet resting firmly on the floor or supported by a footstool and raises the arms left, right, forward, and upward. Those who are able to maintain balance can begin an ambulation program. When the goal is to walk using crutches, the patient sits in a locked wheelchair or very sturdy armchair and uses both upper extremities to support body weight during push-ups.

Ideally a patient progresses to standing balance. To practice coming to a standing position safely, the patient slides to the edge of the bed or chair, keeping the feet back and under the body, then pushes down with the legs and arms while leaning the trunk forward to come to a standing position. Some need assistance or may compensate by using assistive devices. Initially patients stand near a stable support until they can maintain an erect position and trunk balance while moving the extremities. Fall prevention is important, especially for elderly persons, who may experience imbalance with arm movements, changes in gait patterns, or increased body sway. Activities that increase vestibular stimulation, such as passive rocking in a chair, may improve balance. Passive standing activities precede transfer and standing; they prepare the cardiovascular system to adjust to the change in circulatory demands from recumbent to erect positions.

Assistive Devices for Mobility

Assistive Devices. Everyday assistive devices, such as remote controls, electric appliances, automatic garage door openers, sensor lights, telephone headsets, or computers are familiar. Assistive devices or adapted equipment are used to improve function and access by eliminating barriers in the environment or by creating new environments. Changes in structure, ergonomic and task modification, safety measures, combined therapy approaches, and adjustments in ambiance are examples. Assistive devices can reduce or ameliorate the impact of functional impairments, add support and stability to correct balance, provide strength, improve flexibility and motor control, and increase sensory abilities. Devices can aid in healing, help in performing mobility activities, protect from damage or further injury, or enable return to activity.

Devices and equipment require careful selection. Rehabilitation nurse case managers work with the patient and team to determine appropriate prescriptions within the economic, social, cultural, environmental, and physical parameters. Considerations include not only the initial cost but also maintenance, service, and repair costs; availability of replacement parts; reliability; and durability. Patients may demonstrate a need for a device, but it must fit in the home or workplace, and they must be able to learn to operate it and be safe and comfortable while using it. Equipment must be acceptable and fit the person's lifestyle. If others are to assist with the device, they must be able to maneuver and manage it; portable equipment must fit into vehicles and not be too heavy or unwieldy. The environment is important when equipment requires access to electrical outlets; special supplies and battery chargers tips should not be worn, and all parts must be connected securely. The particular assistive device or piece of equipment selected for a patient depends on the physical limitations, disease or medical status, self-esteem and body image, lifestyle, and financial situation.

Assistive Devices for Standing.

Many assistive devices support passive standing, such as a tilt table or standing frame used in physical therapy. In moving from a supine position, safety straps secure the person to the table as both feet rest on a foot support. After checking baseline blood pressure and pulse, the tilt table is elevated slowly to a 15- to 20-degree angle. The degree of tilt increases in 5- to 10-degree increments until the patient can tolerate a standing position for 10 to 30 minutes. Blood pressure; pulse; dependent edema of the lower extremities; skin mottling; and sensations of faintness, dizziness, or headache are monitored. After prolonged bed rest or with poor cardiovascular response, a patient may wear elastic wraps or stockings or an abdominal binder. Benefits of tilt table activities include relief of pressure on gluteal areas, maintenance of postural reflexes, enhanced bladder and bowel function, unimpeded chest expansion, and psychological motivation to participate in an ambulation program.

A standing frame or table is used for passive standing activities that help a patient adjust to transfer from sitting to immediate upright standing without the incremental increases to erect position of the tilt table. Standing frames have anterior stabilizers, either padded supports at the knees and abdomen or actual tabletop surfaces. Posterior stabilizers include heel cups, knee stabilizers, and pelvic or gluteal supports. With a standing frame the patient can enjoy the physiological and psychological rewards of an erect position, while improving standing balance and leaving upper extremities free for activity. Children may use standing tables in school to practice being upright, to provide visualization and stimulation in learning or performing activities, and to promote inclusion with peers. Specially sized pediatric standing frames are available. When a patient develops functional ability to ambulate, the physical therapist prescribes assistive devices or equipment for the specific disability and initiates patient and family education. In the community, rehabilitation nurses monitor and reinforce the care plan.

Assistive Devices for Ambulation.

Those with full use of and strength in their upper extremities but limited lower extremity function due to amputation, fracture, paraparesis, or paraplegia may use crutches. Broad-based canes or three- or four-footed canes are used for weakness or paralysis of one side of the body. A walker is prescribed when generalized weakness occurs in upper and lower extremities, such as in older persons with arthritis, hip fracture, or neuromuscular diseases. The physical therapist measures a patient's height, weight, and specific needs for each device and piece of equipment; crutches, canes, and walkers are not shared. Rehabilitation nurses monitor the patient's posture, body alignment, endurance, awareness, safety, and technique. Schedule time to evaluate walking in areas typical of daily living; many facilities have realistic virtual lifestyle units.

Patient and family education includes the following:
- Caring for equipment or devices
- Coming to a standing position
- Walking properly (gait training)
- Maneuvering stairs or curbs
- Returning to a sitting position
- Managing after a fall, such as by coming to a sitting or erect position

Crutches. A patient is measured for crutches before attempting crutch walking. Measure crutch length by marking the floor 2 inches out from and 6 inches ahead of the tip of the shoe; the patient holds the crutch handgrip and flexes the elbow at 30 degrees. Measure the distance from 2 inches below the patient's axilla to the mark on the floor. The handgrip, never the axilla, supports body weight.

Gait Patterns With Crutches. Gait patterns depend on individual abilities. Standard patterns are a four-point alternate, a two-point, or a swing gait with the crutch. Regularly examine crutches, canes, and walkers to ensure the tips are not worn and all parts are connected securely.

The four-point alternative gait complements limited muscle strength or questionable balance; a person with a very stable and safe gait pattern may use the four-point gait to ambulate slowly. Begin from a standard crutch stance, elbows slightly flexed and crutch tips placed on the floor 6 inches out from the side of the shoe and 6 inches away from the shoe toes. The crutch axillary bar rests 2 inches below the axilla and is pressed against the chest for lateral stability. The four-point gait pattern is left crutch, right leg, and right crutch, left leg. Repeat until the destination is reached.

The two-point gait resembles a walking gait pattern. Although more rapid than a four-point gait, the two-point gait requires better balance because only two points of contact occur with the floor at any given time. Begin from a standard crutch stance to shift weight to advance the right leg and left crutch simultaneously. Follow through with the left leg and right crutch, and continue the pattern to destination.

Swing gaits are used for persons who have strength and balance, but are unable to bear weight on a lower extremity, such as after hip or leg fracture or amputation. Swing gaits vary from a slow but stable swing-to or step-to gait to a rapid but more complex swing-through gait. In the step-to swing gait, begin from a standard crutch stance, placing no weight on the affected extremity. Lift both crutches to move them forward 4 to 6 inches as one unit; whenever the patient bears weight on the unaffected extremity, weight is shifted onto the crutches. The patient steps up to the crutches and repeats the step-to gait process. In the step-through or swing-through gait, begin from a standard crutch stance. Again move both crutches 4 to 6 inches ahead as a single unit as the patient supports weight on the unaffected extremity. This time, when the patient shifts weight onto the crutches, the unaffected leg is swung through to set down in advance of the other leg, landing ahead of the crutches. Repeat the process to destination.

Canes. Canes are available in many styles with features for specific needs and lifestyles. A straight cane makes a single point of contact with the floor, whereas four- or three-footed canes provide broader bases of support but are bulkier to handle. Canes can be unsafe when selected incorrectly, fitted improperly, or maintained poorly. Environmental hazards (especially wet, slippery, or uneven pavement) may lead to falls.

A person's cane length is equal to the distance between the greater trochanter and the floor. To be measured properly, a patient stands with elbows slightly flexed when the cane tip is set on the floor about 6 inches to the side of the foot.

To walk, the patient stands with weight on both feet and on the hand holding the cane. The cane is held on the unaffected side; patients and caregivers tend to attempt using a cane on the affected side. Advance the cane 4 to 6 inches, move the affected leg up to the cane, and support weight on the affected leg and the cane. Continue by moving the unaffected leg past the cane; repeat the process to destination.

Walkers. Walkers vary in structure and purpose; they are measured as described above for canes. Persons able to maintain balance and arm strength to lift the walker can use a lightweight, adjustable, pickup walker. Reciprocal walkers are suitable for a patient with reduced upper body strength and poor balance who might fall backward when lifting a regular walker. They have adjustable heights and can be hinged so one side moves ahead of the other. Rolling walkers, with or without a seat, may be unstable for some but have appeal because they help conserve energy. Check the environment for potential hazards.

With the pickup walker, the patient advances the walker, steps forward in equal-sized steps using each leg in turn, ensures balance, and repeats by advancing the walker. Alternatively, advance the pickup walker and set it down; step with the right foot, advance the walker, and set it down; and step with the left foot and continue the gait pattern. The patient must attend closely to coordinate movements with placing weight on the walker or the feet, and remember to set the walker down in turn and not to step while the walker is off the floor. A pickup walker is pictured in Figure 20-14.

Weight bearing and upright positioning help enhance body image and self-esteem for children and adolescents. These actions may reduce contractures and help with skin integrity and bowel and bladder function; weight bearing also may reduce obesity, improve balance, and aid muscle and bone strength. The parapodium and its modification, the swivel walker, help with access to socialization and education; however, many rely on a prescribed wheelchair for daily mobility. Children, ages 18 months through 8 years of age, some up *to* 14 years, may benefit from use of a four-wheel reverse walker

that has supports on three sides, including from behind. It has multiple selections for handles, seats, back and forearm supports, and can be used indoors or outdoors. The reverse walker promotes overall gross motor movements, bilateral weight bearing and weight shifting, and aids lower body strength, posture, and balance.

Orthotics and Bracing. These assistive devices are involved with ambulation. A person with hemiplegia may use a short leg orthosis for walking and support of the affected lower extremity. Less frequently, the lower limb orthosis may be attached to the shoe and extend to just below the knee, where it can prevent the ankle from pronating by raising the toes during walking and striking the heel back to the floor. Corrective shoes, inserts, and other devices are routine prescriptions with orthotics. Long leg braces, or knee-ankle-foot orthoses (KAFOs), are hinged at the knee to allow bending. KAFOs provide stability at the knee, ankle, and foot and may combine with crutches or a walker and other devices for functional ambulation, such as with paraplegia; however, the energy expenditure is great.

Although some controversy persists, electrical stimulation and other innovations promote functional ambulation. Research using new technologies as ambulatory aids has dealt with limited groups. New directions in research and technological advances continue to change professional and public views concerning possibilities in movement and function.

Prosthetic Devices. Amputation and prostheses are discussed in detail in Chapter 20. For mobility purposes a prosthetic device after lower limb amputation is more stable and acceptable than a walker or crutches. Techniques for fitting and use of prostheses change with new data and products, but some basic principles apply. Early fitting after surgery may enable ambulation soon thereafter; however, permanent prosthetic devices are not fitted until shrinkage subsides in the residual limb. A prosthetist-orthotist constructs highly individualized prostheses based on prescriptions from the physiatrist. Basically the lower limb prosthesis for a person with an above-the-knee amputation consists of a socket, joints at the hip and knee, a suspension system, and a foot and ankle. Specialized cushioned feet and unique knee joints, as for athletic activities, computer-assisted design, and computer-assisted manufacture (CAD-CAM) represent only a few of the innovations in prosthetics. Because of the diversity of the components available, the prescription and construction are complicated. The prosthesis should be functional and easy to care for while appearing as natural as possible. Prosthetic design takes the following into account:

- Length and condition of the residual limb
- Size of the patient's foot
- Patient's general status
- Patient's age, weight, agility, and endurance
- Patient's lifestyle, social goals, and vocation
- Cosmesis, including shape and skin tone
- Financial status and payment coverage
- Individual motivation and family support

Once fitted with the prosthesis a patient continues gait training using a four-point or swing gait; many maneuver independently while wearing the prosthesis. Patients are taught to avoid the habit of a pelvic tilt while standing and during ambulation. Patient education includes daily inspection of the surgical site and residual limb for redness, abrasions, or irritation. Instruction stresses hygiene, gentle care, edema prevention, positioning to prevent contractures, and care of prosthetic stockings and limb. Patients are cautioned to consult a prosthetist for mechanical alterations or adjustments and for regular maintenance.

Wheelchairs and Mobility

When used 9 hours a day, the average life span of a wheelchair in the United States is about 2 years; children outgrow their wheelchairs much more rapidly. In developed countries the multiple varieties and prescriptions available from manufacturers are refined in style, technology, function, and features. Architectural barriers, village or countryside terrain, social construction of disability, and cost are factors that restrict wheelchairs for persons in many countries; they are a scarce commodity with little regard to fit or condition. As a result persons have restricted access, impaired socialization, and reduced independence and opportunity for self-support. In developing countries a few cottage industries repair or construct wheelchairs, and although significantly less sophisticated, the chairs provide transportation and are available. Although some patients reject a wheelchair, the benefits of access, energy conservation, upright seated posture, and diverse activity usually outweigh issues of self-esteem or a psychological need to ambulate. Competitive sports have entered the mainstream, and wheelchair sports, dancing, and travel promote physical, emotional, and social rehabilitation, as discussed in Chapter 28.

Wheelchair Prescriptions. Wheelchairs are as diverse as the persons who use them. A prescription lists specific recommendations for wheelchair height and width based on the patient's physical dimensions and requirements for seated posture. The back and seat of a wheelchair can be modified to accommodate antipressure devices and additional positioning supports. High backs, reclining backs, and others provide head and neck support or options to an erect seated position. In early transfers from the bed to a wheelchair, a patient may perform a simple sliding transfer into a wheelchair fitted with a back that flattens out completely. Elevating the wheelchair back helps the person into a seated position.

Folding wheelchairs, many with detachable armrests and foot or leg rests to facilitate transfers, are transported easily. Patients with upper body strength learn to load their own wheelchairs into a car. Cars can be fitted with hand controls, and those who pass a driver's examination can operate their own vehicles. Vans equipped with hydraulic lifts and fold-down ramps allow patients to elevate into the vehicle while sitting in the wheelchair. The weight of the chair and the size and type of tires are considerations when traveling within or outside the home. Generally, heavier chairs with durable tires are better suited to the outdoors; those with lightweight frames, high-quality bearings, and tubular tires are designed for sports and racing.

As a rule, modifications in wheelchair design increase costs and maintenance complexity. Manual hand controls, as well as electronic touch and breath control, can propel a wheelchair. Companies are developing energy-efficient components to improve manual propulsion, ergonomic designs, and technological boosters for a variety of needs. Electric wheelchairs with microprocessors and computer technology, and robotics are on the horizon.

Wheelchair Prescription Criteria. Traditionally, rehabilitation nurses evaluated patients and prepared wheelchair prescriptions. Today wheelchair design is a team activity with patient and family and perhaps a case manager, vendor, and others. Criteria for prescription of wheelchairs as the primary mode of mobility include the following:
- Energy expenditure and conservation
- Function, access benefits, and safety
- Cost, maintenance fees, and durability
- Physiological and specific disease factors
- Cosmetic and psychosocial factors
- Growth and development
- Patient lifestyle and occupational and educational goals

Patient Education. Patient education includes learning to
- Transfer to and from the wheelchair
- Change position and shift weight while seated in the wheelchair and check for signs of pressure
- Perform basic wheelchair maintenance
- Propel or operate the wheelchair safely and reliably

Wheelchair Accessibility. Accessibility is an issue. Because the Americans With Disabilities Act (ADA) and universal design are not implemented throughout the community, it is essential to know the environment where the wheelchair will be used. Measure doorways and room dimensions, exits, entrances, and areas for ramp placement; building access, levels of living area, and transportation to and from living areas. Also consider the feasibility of transfer from the wheelchair into a traditional motor vehicle, requirements of specialized or modified vans, and amount and kind of assistance and emergency services available.

INTERVENTIONS FOR SELF-CARE IN ACTIVITIES OF DAILY LIVING

Patients improve their self-esteem when they achieve maximum independence in personal care. A person may need to break tasks into sequential units and complete as many as possible and may require assistance with others. Repetition, practice, and demonstrations help with learning. Limit distractions in the environment, choose a best time for work on activities, and encourage concentration. Findings from the assessment relate directly to the level, style, and type of self-care activity. Patients can be challenged to meet their potential, but the nurse relies on assessment to recognize when impairments interfere and plans modifications or assistance. Safety and energy conservation are ongoing concerns.

The components of self-care discussed in detail in this chapter include performing personal care, dressing, bathing, toileting, and eating. Additional components for self-care status include the person's ability to manage finances, recognize safety issues in the home, adhere to therapeutic medication and exercise regimens, and arrange for obtaining health maintenance, household goods, and personal transportation. Self-care activities may be subject to cultural and ethnic beliefs and practices about washing or bathing and personal care that may vary among individuals or families. Ask patients or families about special rules, customs, or rituals they may use in self-care activities. As a rule, never remove amulets, pins, necklaces, bracelets, or hair ornaments without permission. Do not cut hair or nails without permission; do not dispose of hair, nail trimmings, or other body parts or remnants, except as directed by agency policies in concert with the person or family member.

Personal Care

Personal care activities consist of personal hygiene, grooming, oral hygiene, and menstrual management. In the home setting the patient, family, and nurse may devise and improvise ways to accomplish self-care. Assistive devices for personal care are available commercially or can be constructed in the home; innovations are endless. Suction cups to hold an object, such as a nail clipper, cosmetic jar, or drinking cup in place, built-up handles for those with arthritis or a weak grasp, or pump-style tubes for hair gel or toothpaste are examples. Mirrors, toilet paper holders, shoehorns, various reachers with long and curved handles, and the versatile universal cuff are useful to grip and maneuver many items.

Hair Care. Washing the hair is difficult for those who cannot lean over, raise hands above the head, maneuver the hands, or balance the torso. Patients who can sit on a shower seat wash their hair during a shower. Others may need assistance to lie supine with a shower tray or pan to collect rinse water.

Left-sided hemiparesis or hemiplegia may cause neglect when combing hair at the back of the head, and patients need cues and reminders. Alternatively, a patient with right hemiplegia and agnosia might misconstrue a comb to be a toothbrush and put it in the mouth. Demonstrating use of the comb enables this person to use it properly. Built-up handles or a universal cuff help those with difficulty in gripping or moving smoothly. Loops strapped to items such as brushes enable a patient, even with C5 or C6 SCI, to slide a hand through the space and use the brush.

Nail Care. Nail care is difficult for a person who cannot manage implements or reach the feet, who experiences pain, or who has problems bending or balancing. With aging, nails tend to become thickened or brittle, and calluses and ingrown toenails may develop, placing persons with diabetes or peripheral

vascular problems at risk for complications. Hand and nail care are challenging when a patient has a fixed grasp or closed position, reduced ROM, or pain in the hand. With loss of sensation the person may not be aware of early signs of infection; ingrown nails; or dry, cracked tissues around or in the nail beds. A magnifying glass that can be stabilized or worn about the neck may help those with impaired vision to inspect the nails.

Oral Hygiene. One of the most neglected areas of personal care for patients who cannot brush their teeth adequately is oral hygiene. Older persons have bone loss and thinner oral mucosa that is less resistant to disease. Absent teeth or ill-fitted dentures contribute to difficulty with eating and poor nutrition that is amplified with deficits, such as dysphagia or pocketing of food. Chronic illness, lowered resistance, and medication regimens may lead to poor dental health. Children and young adults who manifest oral defensiveness, excessive drooling, or other responses may need sedation even during routine dental work. The difficulties in finding appropriate dental services and resources for patients with badly damaged teeth or gum disease is compounded when they have impaired mobility or make involuntary movements. Rehabilitation nurses can advocate with dentists about patients' specific needs and ways to make them comfortable and find modifications for care.

Grooming. Grooming activities enhance self-esteem and improve hygiene. Shaving may be unwise for men and women taking anticoagulant medications or who have restricted movement or paresis. Depilatory creams or electrolysis may be solutions when an electric razor is not an option. Deodorant is applied in the supine position when one extremity is flaccid or spastic. Raise the affected extremity over the head using the other extremity to apply deodorant. A patient who can sit at the table can move the flaccid arm forward and, reaching underneath in the space created, apply deodorant.

Cosmetics contribute to body image for some women but may be difficult to open. Use a suction cup to stabilize the base of a jar on a table. Using the unaffected hand, the woman grasps the tube near the screw top and uses the thumb and index finger to twist the cap or flip the top. Alternatively, hold the tube between the knees and use the sides of both hands to twist the top. This technique works with most tubes. Patients with neglect may ignore one side of the face and need feedback for correct application of cosmetics.

Women's Issues

Women with disabilities and chronic conditions remain disadvantaged in access to preventive health services and the quality of health maintenance (Theirry, 2000; NSW Cervical Screening Program, 2006). Menstrual management is one of the most difficult tasks for women with lack of sensation, impaired strength or dexterity, or mobility problems, such as spasticity. It involves multiple steps to position herself to manipulate clothing and underwear, remove and dispose of the soiled tampon or pad, cleanse the perineum area, get up or transfer from the toilet, and rearrange clothing.

Assess the ability to lean forward and maintain postural control to manage the task. With sufficient balance, hand dexterity, and maneuverability to slide her pants forward, she may sit on a raised toilet seat or front edge of the wheelchair seat and insert a tampon. To use sanitary pads, she must bridge the hips upward while leaning against the back of the wheelchair; this will enable her to slide a pad backward. A woman able to transfer from a wheelchair to the toilet may use a long-handled mirror, a grasper similar to an assistive toilet paper holder, and a knee spreader if abduction is difficult. If strength is sufficient but balance is poor, she can lean to one side holding onto a bar or locked wheelchair. The mirror is important when sensation is impaired. Others find managing clothing too cumbersome and choose to change lying down and bridging while in the bed.

A woman having problems with coordination, such as with cerebral palsy, may use a grab bar or find kneeling helps to support a stable position and manage clothing. Even when access is good, these adaptations are difficult to accomplish in public places where privacy, cleanliness, support bars, and paper supplies may be lacking.

Recommended adaptations for managing menstruation include adapted positions and use of mirrors, self-sticking sanitary pads, prepared or packaged wipes, and loose underwear. Replacing the crotch flap in underwear or fashioning a flap that covers the crotch from front to back at the waistband and securing it with Velcro may work. Sew loops in several places on the sides of the underwear to pull up and down.

Dressing

Modifications or designs in clothing, assistive or adapted devices, and dressing techniques enable patients with restricted ROM to achieve optimal independence in dressing. Wearing personal clothing signifies wellness and improves body image; those who are employed need to have a professional appearance. Those who use a wheelchair can evaluate clothing for a nonrestrictive style while sitting and for practical use during transfers. Ideally, adaptive clothing is made from fabrics that are durable and easy care and cut to lay smoothly while seated by fitting over appliances and draping free of wheels.

Persons in casts or traction, with urinary collection devices, or with reduced muscle strength can wear extra-large shirts that pull overhead, skirts or pants with wide tops (10 to 12 inches larger than hip size), longer skirts, and skirts or pants with drawstring or elastic waists. Modify clothing using large buttons or hooks, elastic waists, front closures, zipper pulls, stretch fabrics, loops or extension tabs, and Velcro closures. Hand wash support and prosthetic stockings every other day to eliminate perspiration that leads to skin breakdown and odors. Hang to dry to prolong life of the stocking. Avoid elastic, knee-high stockings and tight tube socks that impede circulation.

Clothing must fit with the person's condition, any sensory impairment, and the weather and environment and must not lead to complications. For example, skin breakdown may occur if the heavy center back seam of jeans cuts or shears the skin during positioning or transfer. Protective clothing, such as headgear and footwear are essential; many have prescriptive footwear. Patients wear shoes with solid toes whenever out of bed; with sensory deficits they do not feel heat, bumping against a chair leg, or pressure on unprotected feet. Shoes with Velcro closures or elastic inserts have replaced most laced shoes, but a one-handed shoe tie is possible. Assistive devices include a long-handled shoehorn and a sock pull. Wear a boot on the unaffected foot to balance a single leg cast or antiembolism stocking. Balance, dexterity, and ROM are key factors in a patient's ability to pull on socks or to put on a front-button shirt as shown in Figure 14-12.

Women experience difficulty with bras when using one hand or with restricted ROM. A regular back-fastened bra may be a better choice than front-fastened or over-the-head sports bras. Figure 14-13 illustrates the steps in bra dressing. If hooks are a problem, cover them with Velcro; however, Velcro may be difficult to manage with one hand, and hooks can irritate the skin. A snap clothespin holding the bra to the top of pants or underwear can mimic a stable handhold while the unaffected hand closes the hooks or the Velcro. If the patient can

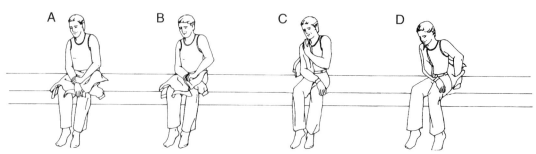

Figure 14-12 Dressing in a shirt (button style). Check your patient's ability to balance before beginning. The patient who has one side of the body affected should sit to don a button-style shirt. **A,** Patient lays the shirt inside-up with the collar at his knees. **B** and **C,** Patient uses his unaffected hand to lift the affected hand into the armhole and pull the sleeve over his affected shoulder. **D,** Patient uses a tossing movement to place the shirt and other sleeve behind him. He can reach behind himself with his unaffected hand and insert it into the shirt sleeve to finish dressing. (From Hoeman, S. P. [1990]. *Rehabilitation: Restorative care in the community.* St. Louis, MO: Mosby.)

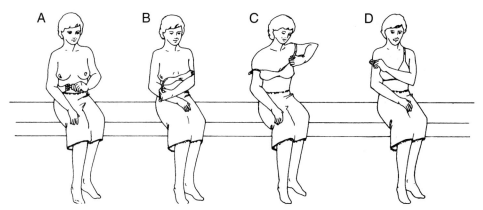

Figure 14-13 Dressing in a back-closure bra. Patient must be able to sit and balance safely. **A,** Patient puts the bra on backwards around her waist. Be sure the cups are positioned correctly. If the patient cannot fasten the hooks, Velcro may work instead. Use a safety strap, if needed. **B,** Patient turns the bra to the front. She uses her unaffected hand to insert the affected arm into the strap. **C,** She inserts her unaffected arm into the other strap and positions the bra. **D,** Patient uses her unaffected hand to position the strap on the affected side and to adjust bra. (From Hoeman, S. P. [1990]. *Rehabilitation: Restorative care in the community.* St. Louis, MO: Mosby.)

maneuver overhead, a sports bra or Lycra stretch bra stitched closed can be pulled down into position. Persons with multiple sclerosis, amputations, hemiplegia, or spinal cord injuries may be able to manage, whereas someone with arthritis may choose to step into a bra and pull it up if stretch is sufficient. Information in Box 14-7 lists goals and suggests dressing aids and other ADL techniques for specific conditions.

Use educational principles adjusted to specific deficits and impairments when a patient is learning dressing techniques. Assess a patient's cognitive, emotional, and physical status with attention to mobility before beginning. If necessary, establish a means of communication, such as with eye blinks, head nods, finger movements, or communication devices. After 30 to 40 minutes of attempts, offer assistance to maintain an atmosphere of encouragement without frustration. Plan to provide cues, repetition, and reinforcement for activities, and keep environmental distraction minimal. Figures 14-9 and 14-14, pp. 227 and 237, illustrate two ways for dressing in pants depending on the person's abilities.

Bathing and Toileting

Independent toileting is a major goal. Despite difficulties, encourage and assist patients who are able to use the bathroom. Modesty, privacy, and dignity are important in any toileting or bathing situation. Safety is important because bathrooms are prime locations for accidents, especially when persons who are wet, soapy, and loosely dressed are moving on or off the hard surface of the toilet or in and out of the shower or tub. Patients may rely on bars to lower into sitting or pull up on bars to rise from a tub or toilet seat.

Structural adaptations such as the following improve safety:

- Countertop space for grooming items
- No electrical razors or hairdryers near water
- Electrical outlets away from the sink

- Insulated or covered hot water pipes under the sink
- Nonslip surfaces on floor, tub, and shower
- Properly installed safety bars (Figure 14-15)
- Controlled hot water temperature
- No clutter, no loose towels, clothing, or rugs
- Open sink without vanity top, for knee space when seated

Access is difficult in bathrooms where space to turn around or complete a transfer is cramped or inaccessible by wheelchair. Narrow bathroom doors can be removed, enlarged, or converted into sliders for access. Lowering the sink, countertop, and mirror and opening space under the counter allows a person to sit in a wheelchair while grooming. A walk-in or roll-in shower stall, with or without a shower seat or table, is an option when a tub is unmanageable and the bathroom can be reconfigured. Wheelchair toileting options include a commode with under-the-seat bucket.

Benches and tub seats are available in a variety of sizes, heights, styles, colors, and adjustable features. A larger seat is preferable for assisting a patient with moving and bathing. Bath mats, hand-held shower hoses, bath mitts and soap bags with nonallergenic products, suction cups or wall-mounted dispensers, universal cuffs with extended holders on Velcro for holding toilet paper or razors, long-handled mirrors and back brushes, and premoistened wipes are only a few of the items available.

Patients able to transfer can use the pivot method (see Figure 14-10) or an independent standing transfer (see Figure 14-11) when moving from the wheelchair to the toilet. Some patients may use a transfer board to move from one seat to another, to transfer to toilet seats that are the height of the wheelchair, and to transfer to the tub (Figures 14-16 and 14-17). Assess the patient's alertness, balance, and motivation. For safety, use a transfer belt and lock the wheels.

BOX 14-7 Goals and Activities of Daily Living Techniques for Specific Conditions

The following goals and techniques are general samples of recommendations for specific conditions and can be adapted for individual patients' situations and preferences.

A. The goal for persons who have limited range of motion (ROM) and decreased strength, such as with arthritis, is to compensate for reduced movement, conserve energy, and reduce pain.

  1. Dressing
      a. Use large buttons and a button hook; or replace buttons, snaps, and hooks with Velcro or big zippers with a loop on the pull tab.
      b. Select loose-fitting, open-front clothing made from slightly stretchable fabric.
      c. Use adapted shoe fasteners, such as Velcro tabs or elastic laces, to avoid bending over to tie shoes.
      d. Use stocking aids to ease on socks; use dressing sticks or reachers to push stockings off the heel and to move clothing up or down the feet and legs.
      e. Use reachers to pick items off the floor or from hangers before and after dressing.

  2. Eating and food preparation
      a. Use utensils with built-up handles and reachers.
      b. Try universal cuffs, straws with clips, or suction cup bases to stabilize items.
      c. Use jar openers, nonsafety caps, and the like to ease opening food packages.
      d. Try precut foods; transfer foods into easy-open, lightweight storage or juice/milk containers.

  3. Grooming and toileting
      a. Use lighter-weight personal care items with enlarged grips, elongated lever handles, stabilized bases, and oversized buttons.
      b. Use electric toothbrushes and razors.
      c. Install flexible handheld shower heads, wall-mounted hair dryer, toilet paper holder aids, raised toilet seat with side support bars, and shower/tub safety bars; and telephone with oversized key pad and emergency call in toilet area.
      d. Add totes for carrying items, such as on bars of walkers.

B. The goal for persons who have neurological disorders and use a wheelchair is to compensate for decreased mobility/ambulation so the person has better access and is able to maneuver and carry items.

  1. Dressing
      a. When dressing from the wheelchair, begin with stockings, then undergarments, any orthotics, pants, shoes, bra, shirt, or dress. Refer to Figures 14-12 through 14-14 for techniques. Some patients need to modify the techniques, such as with imbalance and safety concerns, functional or strength deficits, involuntary movements, or cognitive impairments.
      b. To put on pants and underwear in a wheelchair, lock the wheelchair. Slide to the front of the seat, and then lean against the seat back.
          1. Pull one leg into a flexed position, and put foot into and then through pant leg, pull rest of that pant leg up past knee; repeat with other leg.
          2. Work pants up as high as possible in this forward-seated position while gathering excess pant material in front.
          3. "Push-up" to raise the buttocks and thighs from the seat, including the pant tops, and in the same motion, repositioning buttocks toward the back of the wheelchair seat.
          4. Hold pant waist, and slide or "butt-walk" down into pant tops; repeat a lift/slide motion until pants are positioned properly.
          5. To remove pants, unfasten while sitting in the forward part of the wheelchair seat, hook the waistband with the thumbs, and perform another "push-up" while backing out of the pant top; repeat as necessary.

C. The goal for persons who have hemiplegia or hemiparesis is to individualize the plan of care to enhance optimal function. Assessment includes cognitive and perceptual data. Focus on increasing muscle strength and ROM, improving balance, coordination, and perceptual abilities that lead to better motor control. Techniques maximize use of the involved side, while eliminating inefficient or ineffective movements that cause upset and frustrations. Avoid adverse and unsafe situations, such as pain or fatigue, and incorrect positions or movements that may lead to secondary problems.

  1. Dressing is illustrated in Figures 14-12 through 14-14.
      a. In general, begin with the involved extremity during dressing; speak to the person, and assist from the involved side.
      b. When balance is a concern, encourage the person to dress while balanced against a wall or door frame or while seated in a sturdy armchair or a locked wheelchair; organize clothing within easy reach, or use reachers.
      c. With visual agnosia or apraxia, encourage the person to touch and feel clothing to assist with recognition. For example, trace the line of buttons on a shirt, begin matching buttons from shirt bottom, use labels to find the back and right side, position shirt with buttons face down on bed, touch buttons as pushed through buttonholes, or play name games for items of clothing and matching with body parts.
      d. With unilateral neglect, stimulate awareness and reinforce use of the involved side. For example, teach scanning, use frequent cues, assist from that side, and use the same dressing sequence and triggers to build the person's attention toward the involved side.
      e. With figure-ground visual difficulties, teach the person to proceed slowly and carefully, offer cues to "missing" items. Reduce clutter, and make clear distinctions between the general environment and the objects of interest, such as by laying out clothing on a highly contrasting coverlet. Organize drawers by separating types of clothing, and practice finding them.

  2. Eating and food preparation
      a. Prevent accidents and spills by using precut foods, avoid open-flame gas stoves, and use weighted utensils, tableware, or suction cups on bases.
      b. Set environment to enhance therapeutic techniques, such as scanning; use carts for transporting items.

BOX 14-7 Goals and Activities of Daily Living Techniques for Specific Conditions—cont'd

3. Grooming and toileting
   a. Avoid falls due to imbalance or perceptual problems by using nonskid mats or shower/bath seats; removing rugs and replacing doorsills; and installing ramps, grab bars, and good lighting.
   b. Use assistive items that aid vision and maximize one-handed management, such as bath mitts, liquid soap or soap-on-a-rope, suction base brush for dentures and manicure instruments, toilet paper holders, wall-mounted hair dryer, electric razor, magnified mirror, and the like.

D. The goal for persons who experience incoordination due to movement disorders is to perform fine and gross motor movements and tasks as safely and independently as possible. Most dressing techniques, modifications for eating and grooming, and bathing aids used for the person with hemiplegia are appropriate here.
   1. Sequence and pace tasks, and simplify work; conserve energy.
   2. Support involved upper extremity on a solid surface to stabilize during use; add weight if tolerated.
   3. Ensure safety during ambulation, coach proper gait, and slide objects rather than lifting.
   4. Avoid fatigue, frustration, and fear, and set environment to reduce anxiety.

E. The goal for persons with low vision is to maximize functional independence in a safe manner.
   1. Keep items for daily use and personal care and medications in a set location, and return them to that place. Place food types on plate in clockwise order; add textured labels and markers on foods or microwave that can be identified by touch.
   2. Minimize glare, maximize contrast, and use direct lighting; use scanning, if appropriate.
   3. Eliminate safety hazards (e.g., rugs), and keep furniture in place.
   4. Use magnification devices, technology for "talking" speaker phones, clocks, scales, kitchen devices, and personal safety or responder systems.
   5. Use organizers for medications; specialized products are available for persons who are insulin dependent.
   6. Obtain services for the blind for aid with managing medications, finances, home cleaning and food preparation, transportation, personal safety, and library delivery of books on tape, among other services.

F. The person who has cognitive deficits may exhibit problems with memory, inattention, poor judgment, limited problem solving or lack of insight, poor mental flexibility, or difficulty with abstract thinking. The goal is to function safely and with dignity.
   1. Approach the person with a program that is used by the entire family and caregiver network;. the program is centered on being consistent.
   2. Use consistent cues, such as verbal cues, vocalizing step-by-step actions as a means of self-cuing, memory aids placed in clear view or taped on a mirror or door, and cues the person identifies as meaningful.
   3. Control the amount, type, and duration of stimuli; avoid situations that place the person at risk due to judgment or cognitive limitations.
   4. Reinforce behaviors, such as scanning, responding to cues, and the like.
   5. Incorporate family lifestyle, patient preferences, and cultural aspects into plan.

G. The goal for persons who have an amputation of a limb varies according to the person's general abilities and characteristics and the type, level, cause, and stage of the amputation.
   1. Persons with upper extremity amputations may use some of the same one-handed techniques as those with hemiplegia.
   2. Those with lower extremity amputations may perform dressing using techniques, such as bridging (as shown in Figure 14-9) or bed rolling. Many persons will dress while seated to avoid any difficulty with balance.
   3. Older persons or those with diabetes who have difficulty donning or doffing prostheses and managing shoes and socks may be helped with dressing aids, such as long-handled shoe horns and sock aids.
   4. Box 14-7 lists positioning ***to be avoided*** following lower extremity amputation.

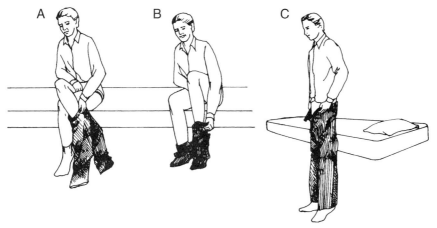

Figure 14-14 Dressing in pants. Check patient's ability to sit or stand and balance safely. **A,** While sitting, the patient uses his unaffected hand to lift his affected leg across his unaffected knee. He pulls his pants leg completely over his affected foot and ankle. If he cannot lift or cross his legs, assist him to elevate his affected leg on a box or stool so that he does not lean over. **B,** Patient inserts his unaffected leg fully through the other pants leg. He uses his unaffected hand to pull the pants up on both legs as high as he is able. **C,** If the patient can safely stand, he holds onto the pants and the waist with his unaffected hand. He pulls the pants on and adjusts the waist and zipper. The patient never bends over to pull his pants. (From Hoeman, S. P. [1990]. *Rehabilitation: Restorative care in the community.* St. Louis, MO: Mosby.)

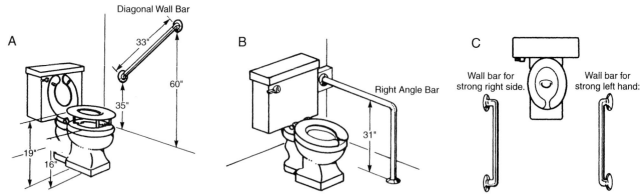

Figure 14-15 Safety grab bar installation. **A,** Diagonal wall bar next to commode. If commode seat is too low, making it difficult for the patient to get up, it may have to be raised by using a raised toilet seat. Be sure the raised seat is secure. **B,** Right-angle wall bar. **C,** Wall bars should be securely fastened to avoid a fall and should be at a 45-degree angle. Bar should be 2 to 4 inches away from the wall on the patient's strong side and must be attached firmly to the studs in the wall. Bathrooms and patients' abilities and needs vary. Refer to http://www. adaptiveaccess.com or similar sites for specific instructions for installing shower and tub grab bars. (From Hoeman, S. P. [1990]. *Rehabilitation: Restorative care in the community.* St. Louis, MO: Mosby.)

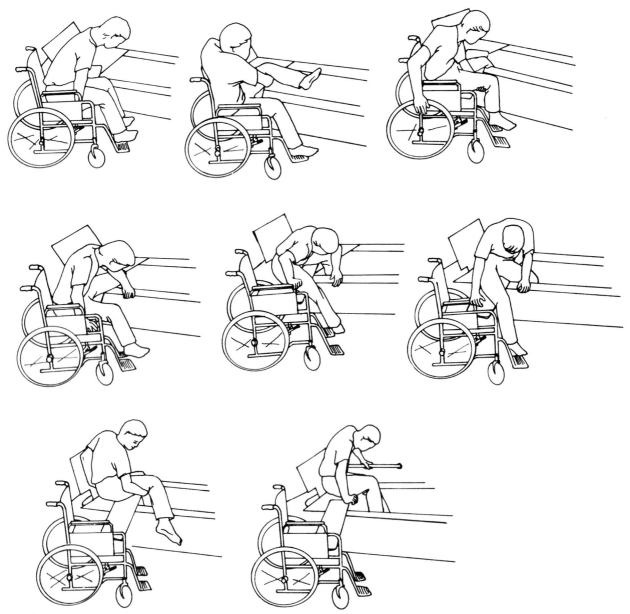

Figure 14-16 Tub transfer. Transfer board may be used to move a patient from a wheelchair onto a bathtub seat. Because the patient's safety is a priority, assistance with the transfer belt may be needed. (From Hoeman, S. P. [1990]. *Rehabilitation: Restorative care in the community.* St. Louis, MO: Mosby.)

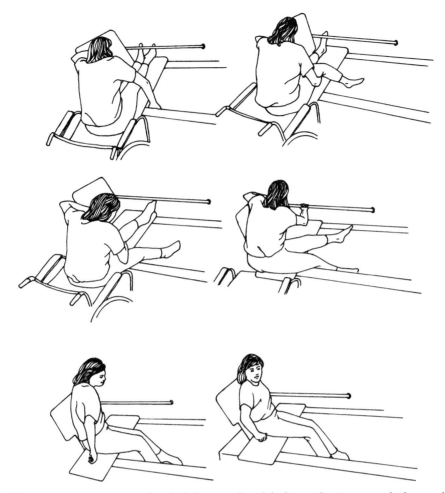

Figure 14-17 Tub transfer variation. Some patients place both feet into the tub before performing a transfer from a wheelchair to a tub. (From Hoeman, S. P. [1990]. *Rehabilitation: Restorative care in the community*. St. Louis, MO: Mosby.)

Demographics of Spinal Cord Injury

According to data from the National Spinal Cord Injury Statistical Center (2005), fewer SCIs are occurring due to trauma; the average age of those sustaining an SCI is 37.5 years, an increase of almost 10 years since the 1970s. Males remain four times as likely to suffer a SCI, and more than half of those incurring a SCI are unmarried. Motor vehicle accidents continue as the leading cause of SCI, but injuries due to falls have increased. The racial distribution for SCI has also changed over the past 30 years, with fewer injuries among whites and increased injuries among minority groups. A persistent seasonal pattern shows the greatest frequency of SCI to be during the summer in the northern United States. Cervical injuries constitute approximately 52% of all injuries. As with Jake's situation, persons with injuries between C1 and C5 have improved survival rates because of better emergency response and medical support immediately following the initial injury. Consequently, more survivors are dependent on mechanical ventilation. Other injuries that frequently accompany traumatic SCI are broken bones (29.3%), loss of consciousness (28.2%), and pneumothorax (17.8%). Box 14-8 summarizes the epidemiology for traumatic SCI in the United States.

Since 1973 the National SCI Database has been tracking causes of death for persons with a SCI. Over the past 30 years renal failure was the most common cause of death; others were pneumonia, pulmonary emboli, and septicemia. Although the life span of persons who have sustained a SCI has increased, the first year post injury represents the greatest risk of mortality. Table 14-7 summarizes life expectancy statistics 1 year post injury.

Types of Spinal Cord Injury

Traumatic spinal cord injury occurs when there is direct or indirect trauma to the vertebral column either from the primary trauma or from sequela to the injury. The primary injury can directly compress, crush, or transect the spinal cord with varying degrees of damage. Depending on the nature and the level of injury, the spinal cord can be damaged in different ways as demonstrated in Box 14-9.

Secondary trauma can be caused by ischemia of the cord, inflammation, cell destruction, and/or apoptosis (programmed cell death). Ischemia occurs when there is reduced circulation from the trauma or from vasospasm when norepinephrine, serotonin, or histamine is released (Kwon, Tetzlaff, Grauer,

---

BOX 14-8 Epidemiology for Traumatic Spinal Cord Injury in the United States

Incidence
11,000 cases per year

Etiology
MVA	47.5%
Falls	22.9%
Violence	13.8%
Sports	8.9%
Other	6.8%

Ethnic Groups
White	62.9%
African American	22%
Hispanic	12.6%
Other	2.5%

Prevalence
250,000

Demographic Profile
Mean age	37.6 years
Gender	79.6% male
Marital status	51.8% never married
Occupational status	60.5% competitive labor
Level of education	60.2% high school

Neurological Level/Extent of Lesion
Incomplete tetraplegia	34.5%
Complete paraplegia	23.1%
Complete tetraplegia	18.4%
Incomplete paraplegia	17.5%

Data from National Spinal Cord Injury Statistical Center. (2005). *Spinal cord injury: Facts and figures at a glance.* Birmingham: University of Alabama.

TABLE 14-7 Life Expectancy for Persons Who Survive at Least 1 Year Post Injury

Age at Injury	No SCI	Motor Functional at Any Level	Paraplegia	Low Tetraplegia (C5-C8)	High Tetraplegia (C1-C4)	Ventilator Dependent at Any Level
14 yr	58.2	53.2	45.9	41.4	37.8	23.1
40 yr	39.3	34.7	28.3	24.4	21.5	10.9
60 yr	22.0	18.1	13.3	10.6	8.7	3.0

Data from National Spinal Cord Injury Statistical Center. (2005). *Spinal cord injury: Facts and figures at a glance.* Birmingham: University of Alabama.
SCI, Spinal cord injury.

Beiner, & Vaccaro, 2004). Inflammation is a result of a release of neutrophils and microphages in response to the trauma (Keane, Davis, & Dietrich, 2006). When cell destruction occurs in the area of injury, a derangement of potassium and sodium, along with a shift of calcium, destroys cell membranes and can cause demyelization (Sekhon & Fehlings, 2001). Apoptosis is a response that contributes to further damage of the spinal cord (Lu, Ashwell, & Waite, 2000).

Nontraumatic spinal cord injury can arise from a number of causes. Tumors or cancer damages the spinal cord when it is directly involved in the pathologic process, when there is pressure on the spinal cord. An infarction or other circulatory pathologic condition can alter the blood supply to the spinal cord. In addition, the spinal cord can be damaged as a result of an infection, arthritis, stenosis, congenital anomalies, Guillain-Barré syndome, multiple sclerosis, or amyotrophic lateral sclerosis. The type and extent of damage to the spinal cord with each of these conditions varies from complete paralysis to paresis and/or weakness.

BOX 14-9 Common Mechanisms of Traumatic Injury

The following may be accompanied by rotation, lateral flexion, or both.

- **Flexion**—neck flexed violently forward; compression force anterior and distraction force posterior (rapid deceleration—MVA and falls)
- **Hyperextension**—head thrown violently backward (fall when face or chin is struck, MVA hit from behind—whiplash)
- **Flexion-rotation**—twisting of head on axis; disrupts ligaments, vessels, tissue, bone
- **Compression (axial loading/vertical compression)**—force on vertebral body to cause "burst" fracture with fragments that may impinge upon cord (falls onto buttocks, diving accidents)
- **Penetration**—direct piercing of cord (foreign body—gunshot/knife wound)

MVA, Motor vehicle accident.

Nursing Assessment Upon Admission to Rehabilitation

With SCI a methodical and thorough assessment is essential because each patient presentation varies substantially. The international standard method of assessing an SCI is the American Spinal Injury Association (ASIA) (2002) Impairment Scale (Figure 14-18). A standardized flow sheet is used to score sensory and motor levels of functioning or neurological level of injury (NLI). The rehabilitation nurse uses the tool to determine the completeness of the injury and the classification of the impairment. The goal is to determine the degree and level of the injury that is the most caudal level where both sensory and motor functioning is preserved bilaterally. An injury of the cervical region that results in the paralysis of all four extremities at T1 or above is termed tetraplegia. Paraplegia is an injury of the thoracic, lumbar, or sacral regions of the cord that results in paralysis of the lower extremities, usually at T2 or below.

Beginning with the sensory examination, 28 dermatomes on each side of the body are tested for pinprick and light touch and scored on a 3-point scale:

0 = inability to distinguish sharp from dull
1 = distinguishes sharp from dull but not the same as the face
2 = normal

The face is used as a control point because sensation on the face is preserved in all spinal cord injuries. Deep anal sensation is tested by digital rectal examination while exerting firm pressure on the rectal wall. The patient reports awareness of sensation as "yes" or "no." The sensory level is the dermatome with reported bilateral normal sensation.

The motor examination tests strength on both sides of the body, including five upper regions and five lower regions, as well as the voluntary contraction of the rectal sphincter. Strength is rated on a scale of 1 to 5 and is reported as, for example, 2/5 or 2 out of 5. The motor level is the most caudal muscle group that is graded as 3/5 or greater, with the requirement that the segment immediately above is graded as 5/5. The NLI is the most caudal level where both motor and sensory are intact.

In a complete injury both sensory and motor function are absent in the lowest sacral segments, or no sacral sparing. With an incomplete injury either sensory or motor functioning is partly preserved below the NLI. This includes sacral sparing, that is, the presence of sensation at the anal mucocutaneous junction in response to a pinprick and light touch, along with voluntary anal contraction or deep anal sensation. These responses indicate that the spinal tracts are not completely interrupted and retain a connection between the brain and the regions below the level of the injury for sensation or motor innervations or both. A complete injury may have a region where the dermatomes and myotomes caudal to the NLI are preserved. But unless there is sacral sparing, the injury is still classified as complete with a zone of partial preservation (ZPP).

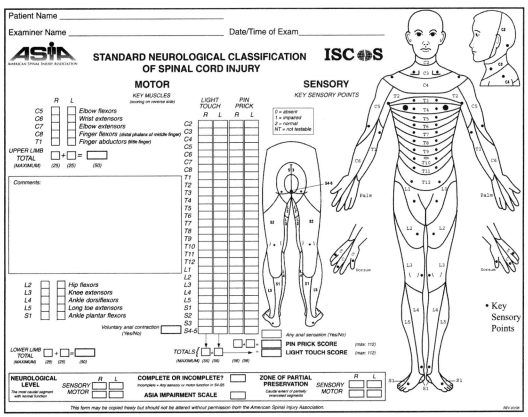

Figure 14-18 Standard neurological classification of spinal cord injury. (Courtesy American Spinal Injury Association.)

An Expanded Case Study

Spinal Cord Injury

One of the most challenging and long-term patient situations in rehabilitation occurs with a patient who has experienced a spinal cord injury. Persons with SCI are at risk for multiple complications depending on the type and level of SCI; impairments in functional mobility always are involved. Complications ranging from pressure ulcers, spasticity, or heterotrophic ossification can cause pain and further restrict activity. The ability to perform ADLs also declines with aging so that those who live longer need more attendant-care services (Liem, McColl, King, & Smith, 2004). The following case study is an example of the critical and complex plan of care required for a person who has experienced an SCI.

Jake, a 29-year-old police officer, was a restrained passenger in a car versus tree collision. Emergency care, including neck collar and backboard placement, was administered at the scene, and Jake was transferred immediately to a nearby medical center. It was questionable whether Jake lost consciousness because he has no recall of the events surrounding the collision; he does recall being transported to the emergency department. The trauma survey revealed a C5 burst fracture with retropulsion of bone into the spinal canal. Jake was started on a steroid protocol and placed in cervical traction. He then presented with decreased oxygen saturation and a cough requiring intubation.

A computed tomography (CT) scan of the chest revealed aspiration pneumonia and a small right anterior and medial pneumothorax. The following day Jake underwent a C5 vertebrectomy with fusion of C3 through C7 anterior and posterior with a plate allied to C4 to C6. He received a chest tube for treatment of the right pneumothorax, and insertion of a Greenfield filter to prevent pulmonary embolus.

Jake's postoperative course was complicated by increased pulmonary secretions and temperature spikes treated with intravenous antibiotics. He subsequently developed a Clostridium difficile colitis, successfully treated with Flagyl. Jake had been extubated postoperatively but needed a tracheostomy when increased pulmonary secretions returned and oxygen saturation decreased. A videofluoroscopic swallowing study showed no evidence of aspiration or penetration, and he began an all-liquid diet. Jake was incontinent of bladder and bowel functions. He had an indwelling urinary catheter but had not begun a specific bowel program. Jake was transferred to an acute rehabilitation facility 28 days after his initial injury. The chest tube had been removed, but he retained the tracheostomy tube with a speaking valve. Before he left the hospital, a Stage II pressure ulcer measuring 4 by 5 cm was documented on his sacral area.

ZPP is used only in patients with ASIA impairment level A SCI. For example, the NLI may be C5, but the zone of partial preservation may be at the level of T1.

A patient who has an incomplete injury with some spinal cord tracts preserved may develop one of a number of clinical syndromes in SCI with a specific pattern of injury, as described in Table 14-8.

The comprehensive nursing assessment of a patient with spinal cord injury not only determines the level and classification of the SCI, but also the phase of recovery the patient is experiencing. The standard of care for all patients is to assess conditions associated with the injury or preexisting conditions. The nurse assesses the patient's function in detail, especially regarding mobility, skin, elimination, and autonomic regulation and comfort, including adjustment and pain. Findings from the assessment guide the interventions and comprehensive plan of care that will assist the patient toward maximal levels of health and functioning.

Jake's ASIA Classification

The motor strength in Jake's upper extremities was assessed at 3+/5 in the right biceps and 1/5 in left biceps. All 10 key muscles groups of the bilateral upper and lower extremities were 0/5. There was no voluntary anal contraction. Sensation to pinprick was intact in the C2-C4 dermatomes bilaterally and was absent in C5 through S4-S5 bilaterally. Light touch sensation was intact in the C2-C4 dermatomes bilaterally, was present but impaired in right C5, and was absent in left C5 and bilateral C6 through

S4-S5 dermatomes; there was no anal sensation detected to light touch or pinprick, nor was there deep anal sensation. Based upon the motor examination of the 10 key muscle groups, including anal contraction, the NLI was determined to be C4. Based upon the sensory examination, the sensory level was determined to be the same at C4. It was determined that there was absent motor and sensory function below NLI, including sacral segments S4-S5 (there was no sacral sparing); therefore Jake's injury was classified as complete with an ASIA impairment scale of A. No zone of partial preservation was determined.

Jake's General Assessment

Jake was awake, alert, and oriented to time, place, and person when he was admitted to the SCI rehabilitation unit. He displayed no deficits in communication or with long- or short-term memory. Jake's pupils were equal, round, and reactive to light, and cranial nerves II through XII were intact. The integument was warm, moist, and of normal coloration upon inspection. A stage II pressure ulcer noted at the sacrum measured 4 by 5 cm, the area was beefy red, with no drainage or tunneling. No other skin areas showed redness or breakdown. Jake scored as high risk for pressure ulcer on the Braden Scale (see Chapter 15). His skin was at risk due to his limited sensory perception, decreases in sensation, activity, and mobility, and a potential for damage from friction and shear; tone was decreased in the bilateral upper and lower extremities. A trace of bilateral pedal edema was noted, but without lower extremity redness, warmth, or tenderness. Jake exhibited intermittent

TABLE 14-8 Spinal Cord Syndromes (ASIA 2002)

Syndrome	Type of Injury	Resulting Impairment
Central cord syndrome	Hyperextension of the neck causing a lesion, usually in the cervical region	Greater weakness in the upper extremities than lower extremities; sacral sparing; bowel and bladder dysfunctions common
Brown-Séquard syndrome	Injury to one side of the spinal cord (hemisection), often the result of a penetration injury	Loss of ipsilateral proprioception, motor function, deep touch sensation and contralateral light touch, pain, temperature, and sensitivity
Anterior cord syndrome	Acute compression of the anterior portion of the spinal cord (either a flexion injury or from retropulsed bone fragments)	Loss of motor function and sensitivity to pain and temperature, though preserving sensation for position, vibration, and touch
Posterior cord syndrome	Absence of all doral column function; least common of spinal cord injury syndromes (omitted from recent versions of ASIA)	Varying degrees of motor preservation with preservation of pain, temperature, and touch; prognosis for ambulation is poor
Conus medullaris syndrome	Injury of the sacral and lumbar nerve roots	Produces a reflexive bowel, bladder, and lower extremities; sacral segments may show preserved bulbocavernous and micturition reflexes
Cauda equina syndrome	Injury to the lumbosacral nerve roots	Produces a reflexive bowel, bladder, and lower limbs; sensation may be spared in the perineum or lower extremities with complete paralysis; extent of recovery varies depending on the number of nerve roots damaged

Data from American Spinal Injury Association. (2002). *International standards for neurological and functional classification of spinal cord injury.* Atlanta, GA: Author.
SCI, Spinal cord injury; *ASIA*, American Spinal Injury Association.
*Separation of conus and cauda equina lesions is difficult because clinical features overlap.

spasticity in the lower extremities, but he denied increased pain or difficulty sleeping.

Inspection showed no redness on the external meatus of the penis, no drainage or bleeding, and no excoriation, macerations, or lesions to the genital area. Jake had a No. 16 Foley catheter due to incontinence; it was draining clear yellow urine. His bladder was not distended, but he was unable to feel bladder fullness or sense any urge to void (neurogenic bladder). Before the injury, Jake had daily bowel movements after breakfast, without aid of stool softeners or laxatives. At the time of the examination he was incontinent of stool (involuntary) and unaware of the need to defecate. Jake reported that his bowel movements were very loose and watery that morning, and a subsequent rectal examination found hardened stool in the anal vault. Bowel sounds were present, and the abdomen was distended moderately and was nontender to palpation; Jake denied having abdominal pain, nausea, or vomiting. At this assessment Jake's medications included narcotics for pain management, iron sulfate, and an oral stimulant (Bisacodyl).

Jake's respiratory rate was 18 breaths per minute with a cuffed Shiley tracheostomy tube in place; the site was clean with no drainage. Oxygen saturation was 94% on room air with no central or peripheral cyanosis. Upon auscultation the lungs exhibited diminished breath sounds bilaterally along with adventitious breath sounds. The breaths were shallow but symmetrical; a weak but functional cough was noted. Jake reported dizziness and light-headedness when brought to an

upright sitting position; his blood pressure decreased, and his pulse rate increased. During the night he felt "hot and sweaty."

Jake was married and had a 1-year-old daughter; his wife was a homemaker. They lived in a single-family home. He has no history of drug or alcohol abuse. Jake said he is very anxious regarding his current prognosis, loss of control, and decreased independence. He denied depression but shared that he is extremely concerned about the ongoing stability of his marriage, as well as for being able to support his family financially.

Nursing Care Plan

The goals for patients can change substantially based on their potential for function, on the particular phase of recovery, and on their individual resilience and resources. Tables 14-9 and 14-10 outline changes in patient goals for functional areas during three phases of recovery as a framework for the nursing plan of care. Jake's goals are presented in the first section because he had an upper motor neuron level injury.

Nursing diagnoses, interventions, and anticipated outcomes for Jake's altered mobility are listed in Table 14-11; Table 14-5, on p. 220, contains additional nursing diagnoses, outcomes, and interventions relevant to functional mobility for Jake.

Alterations in Function and Mobility

Based on Jake's assessment, the rehabilitation team can make general predictions about his expected levels of functioning, as well as the type of equipment and amount of attendant care

TABLE 14-9 Goals for Stages of Recovery Following a Spinal Cord Injury

Spinal Shock	Acute Rehabilitation	Long Term
Upper Motor Neuron Injuries		
Goals for Spasticity		
Utilize good body alignment and posture in all positioning and movement	Identify triggers for spasticity and develop strategies to reduce their occurrence	Establish plan to reduce spasticity triggers and manage symptoms after discharge
Goals for Skin Integrity		
Reduce the risk of skin breakdown by evaluating risk, using alternate mattresses and surfaces, and establishing turning and positioning schedules	Establish weight-shifting strategies and schedule while in W/C and turning schedule while in bed with good positioning	Establish weight-shifting and turning schedule and methods to maximize the patient's ability to perform or direct the activity
Goals for Respiratory Function		
Promote full lung expansion and good pulmonary toileting	Artificial airway—wean patient if possible Continue to promote full lung expansion and good pulmonary toileting	Establish home strategies to maximize lung expansion and support pulmonary toileting
Goals for Thermoregulation		
Monitor body temperature to determine any variations and modify the environment to achieve a normal body temperature	Continue environmental modifications to regulate body temperature and facilitate the participation of the patient and/or family in recognizing temperature variations	Educate the patient/family to monitor body temperature and changes in ambient temperature and to initiate strategies to modify
Goals for Autonomic Dysreflexia (AD)		
None	Identify signs and symptoms of AD and initiate protocol or physicians' orders at the first sign of AD to reverse the condition	Establish a plan for early recognition of recognizing the signs and symptoms and a plan for the patient and/or family to initiate interventions quickly to reverse the condition
Goals for Orthostatic Hypotension		
Minimize drop in BP by changing position gradually and through use of abdominal binder and/or elastic wraps	Monitor for any changes in BP with position changes and continue strategies to mitigate the condition	None
Goals for Urinary Elimination		
Establish urine containment system	Implement bladder program to ensure regular and complete bladder emptying	Establish bladder program directed and/or performed by the patient that is feasible at home
Goals for Bowel Elimination		
Establish and maintain a "clean" bowel	Implement daily bowel program including nutritional support, medications, and interventions for a complete daily bowel evacuation	Establish bowel program that will be effective in the home environment and is directed and/or performed by the patient
Goals for Adaptation		
Establish a trusting relationship to facilitate regular and ongoing communication	Identify patient willingness to direct and/or participate in self-care activities and implement consistently	Utilize support systems and networks in the community to enhance community reintegration and adaptation
Goals for Comfort Related to Neurogenic Pain		
Utilize good posture and body alignment to reduce the risk of neurogenic pain	Identify factors that increase or decrease neurogenic pain and incorporate them into the plan for pain management	Establish pain management strategies for long-term management of neurogenic pain

he will need to support his maximal independence. Predictions and expectations must be individualized for the unique needs and characteristics of each patient. For instance, predicting functional deficits when an SCI is incomplete is especially difficult, because motor recovery can vary regardless of injury level. Muscle recovery is dependent on the level of motor strength a patient demonstrates within the first few months post injury. Although many variables are involved, motor recovery has not occurred below the level of injury when the SCI is complete, such as with Jake's injury (Fisher et al., 2005). Table 14-12 summarizes the motor and sensory effects of each injury level and the associated functional potential.

Problems and Interventions

The following alterations in health patterns and resulting problems are discussed in terms of Jake's situation with SCI. The accompanying interventions apply to nursing management of these problems and complications that commonly occur for patients with SCI.

Spasticity. Spasticity is a common and potentially disabling phenomenon that occurs when inhibitory and excitatory impulses become imbalanced. The movement usually manifests during the acute rehabilitation phase after spinal shock is resolved (see Table 14-3 for definition of spasticity). Spasticity appears in 65% to 78% of patients who have SCI and is the most frequent cause of rehospitalization after the initial phase of rehabilitation (Paker et al., 2006). It occurs most frequently with upper motor neuron lesions and tends to be more severe with cervical injuries (Skold, Levi, & Seiger, 1999). Spasticity is increased by certain postures and movements and may increase when the patient experiences pain or has pressure ulcers, urinary tract infections, abdominal pathologic processes, hemorrhoids, or fecal impaction. Emotional and physical stress increases the incidence of spasticity. Some drugs used to treat comorbid conditions, such as antidepressants, also have been reported to increase spasticity (Stolp-Smith & Wainberg, 1999). Complications of spasticity include contractures, pain, skin breakdown, sleep disturbance, and impaired function. Clinical rating scales are available to assess the severity of spasticity, but a single assessment without patient self-rating may be unreliable (Lechner, Frotzler, & Eser, 2006).

An individualized management plan for Jake identifies potential sources of spasticity for assessment with the intention of decreasing spasticity over the long term. Interdisciplinary management of spasticity begins with establishing correct posture, position, and alignment to be used wherever Jake encounters a surface, such as a bed or wheelchair footrest, and whenever he changes position or makes a transfer

TABLE 14-10 Goals for Stages of Lower Motor Neuron Injuries: Recovery Following a Spinal Cord Injury

Spinal Shock	Acute Rehabilitation	Long Term
Goals for Skin Integrity Initiate turning and positioning to ensure relief on pressure areas at least every 2 hours in bed and every hour in W/C	Establish strategies for patient to initiate and perform weight shifts and repositioning on an established schedule	Develop a plan for weight shifting and positioning on all surfaces in accordance with normal daily routines and activities in the home
Goals for Urinary Elimination Establish urine containment system	Establish routines for urine containment and initiate strategies for the patient to perform skills with nursing supervision	Educate patient to manage urine containment, to identify symptoms of urinary tract infections, and to seek medical care
Goals for Bowel Elimination Establish and maintain a "clean" bowel	Implement daily bowel program with the patient actively participating and directing care	Establish a bowel program to minimize incontinence and schedule bowel evacuations in accordance with lifestyle
Goals for Comfort Related to Neurogenic Pain Utilize good posture and body alignment to reduce the risk of neurogenic pain	Identify factors that increase or decrease neurogenic pain and develop a pain management plan	Establish a pain management program for long-term management of neurogenic pain
Goals for Adaptation Establish a trusting relationship to facilitate regular and ongoing communication	Identify patient willingness to direct and/or participate in self-care activities and implement consistently	Utilize support systems and networks in the community to enhance community reintegration adaptation

W/C, Wheelchair; *BP*, blood pressure.

(Albert & Yelnik, 2003). Standing activities and use of the tilt table or the standing frame provide a prolonged muscle stretch and may decrease spasticity. Stretching and ROM exercises, performed at least twice a day, diminish excessive tone (Kirshblum, 1999). Modalities such as cold and topical anesthetics may reduce reflex excitability, lessen clonus, improve ROM, and facilitate increased motor function (Jozefczyk, 2002; Price, Lehmann, Boswell-Bessette, Burleigh, & deLateur, 1993).

Casting, splinting, and orthotic management of muscles and joints at risk for contracture may reduce tone (Hinderer & Dixon, 2001; Kirshblum, 1999). Electrical stimulation (ES) has shown marked short-term improvement (Aydin, Tomruk, Keles, Demir, & Okun, 2005) but has not demonstrated long-term benefits in spasticity management (Albert & Yelnik, 2003; Jozefczyk, 2002). Surgical interventions may be considered as a final resort to control spasticity, most taking place at the muscle or tendon; selective surgical procedures may only

TABLE 14-11 Nursing Diagnoses, Interventions, and Outcomes Applicable to Altered Mobility **NIC/NOC**

Nursing Diagnosis	Nursing Interventions	Nursing Outcomes
Risk for impaired skin integrity	Skin surveillance Skin care: topical treatments Pressure ulcer prevention	Tissue integrity: skin and mucous membranes
Impaired skin integrity—sacrum	Pressure ulcer care Wound care Nutrition management	Wound healing: primary intention
Reflex urinary incontinence Impaired urinary elimination	Urinary catheterization: intermittent	Urinary elimination
Constipation	Constipation/impaction management Bowel management	Bowel elimination
Bowel incontinence	Bowel training Bowel incontinence care	Bowel elimination Bowel continence
Ineffective breathing pattern	Respiratory monitoring Airway management Airway suctioning Chest physiotherapy	Respiratory status: patent airway
Ineffective tissue perfusion secondary to orthostatic hypotension	Vital signs monitoring Hemodynamic regulation Pressure management Embolus precautions	Tissue perfusion: peripheral Tissue perfusion: abdominal organs
Risk-prone health behaviors	Mutual goal setting Coping enhancement Role enhancement	Adaptation to physical disability

Data from Moorhead, S., Johnson, M., & Maas, M. (2004). *Nursing outcomes classification (NOC)* (3rd ed.). St. Louis, MO: Mosby; Dochterman, J., & Bulechek, G. M. (2004). *Nursing interventions classification (NIC)* (4th ed.). St. Louis, MO: Mosby; and NANDA International. (2005). *Nursing diagnoses: Definitions and classification, 2005-2006* (6th ed.). Philadelphia: Author.

TABLE 14-12 Spinal Cord Injury Levels, Effects, and Functional Potential

Injury Level	Motor/Sensory Effects	Functional Potential
Upper Motor Neuron Injuries		
C1 through C3	No voluntary movement or sensation below the level of the injury. Minimal muscular function allowing limited head and neck movement Paralysis of diaphragm and intercostal muscles Sensory losses of occipital region of head, ears, and some areas of face	Ventilator dependent Completely dependent for care Limited mobility potential with voice-, chin-, or breath-controlled wheelchair
C4	As above and neck accessory muscle function intact with some potential for partial function of diaphragm Limited shoulder movement	May be able to breathe without ventilator for intervals May have limited self-feeding ability with adaptive sling

TABLE 14-12 Spinal Cord Injury Levels, Effects, and Functional Potential—cont'd

Injury Level	Motor/Sensory Effects	Functional Potential
C5	Deltoid and biceps function present, adding shoulder strength, elbow flexion, and control of head and neck Unopposed trapezius and levator scapulae action with ability to raise shoulders Full sensation to head, neck, upper back, and chest and lateral parts of upper arms Phrenic nerve intact to diaphragm	Independent breathing but limited tidal volume of 300 ml Improved hand-to-mouth coordination permitting self-feeding, oral care, dressing of upper body, with assistive aids Dependent in other areas of care Assistance needed to transfer Electric wheelchair for mobility
C6	Action of brachioradialis added, permitting wrist dorsiflexion with some grasp and wrist extension Unopposed action of biceps and deltoids abducts and flexes arms Sensation over lateral aspects of entire arm, thumb, and index finger	Independent in eating and grooming with adaptive equipment—assists with dressing, transfers, and elimination Independent manual wheelchair Driving with hand controls
C7	Diaphragm and accessories compensate and support normal breathing Elbow flexion and extension present; wrist flexion and some finger control Sensation to middle finger and part of ring finger	Potential for independent living Can achieve independence in eating, bathing, dressing, transfer, wheelchair mobility, and elimination care
C8	Addition of adductor and internal rotator muscles eliminate abnormal arm and shoulder positions Full sensation to hand; finger flexion	Moderate to full control of shoulders, arm, wrist, and fingers Able to live independently
T1 through T5	No voluntary movement or sensation below the level of the injury Full control of upper extremities Some intercostal and thoracic muscle function Sensation intact to arms and midchest/midback	Pulmonary function within acceptable norms; tidal volume 500-700 ml Independent in self-care; balance improves with each segment of abdominal muscles Independent with manual wheelchair Potential for full-time employment
T6 through T10	Increasing control over abdominal and trunk muscles Sensation steadily increasing to level of umbilicus and midback	Balance improves with each segment of abdominal muscles No interference with respiratory function Full independence in care; manual wheelchair Employment reasonable expectation, can participate in sports activities

Lower Motor Neuron Injuries

Injury Level	Motor/Sensory Effects	Functional Potential
T11 through L5	Progressively adds function of hip flexors, knee extension, knee flexion, and ankle dorsiflexion Slight foot movement added at L4 Sensation intact to lower abdomen, hips, anterior surface of legs, selected sections on posterior of legs No sensation present in groin, genitals, anus, or portions of buttocks	Independent in self-care Ambulation with long leg braces possible but will tire easily
S1 Through S5	Progressive return of full control to legs, ankles, and feet Progressive control of bowel, bladder, and sexual function; sensory function to groin, anus, and posterior aspects of legs and feet	Independent in self-care Independent ambulation; short braces may be used for support

reduce pain related to spasticity (Bucheil & Hsu, 2001). Overall, interventions proceed from least to most invasive weighing the risk-benefit ratio (Hinderer & Dixon, 2001).

Acute episodes of spasticity require pain management, and a plan should be in place to manage pain in advance of activities known to trigger increased spasticity for a patient. Several medications are used to treat spasticity, but none is universally beneficial because drug actions may target spasticity only as related to the bladder, bowel, or movement. Patients are carefully monitored for side effects because most medications have some sedation properties. Peripheral nerve or motor point nerve blocks may be useful adjuncts to medications for managing spasticity.

Skin Integrity. Pressure ulcers are a major complication. Following SCI, the losses of mobility, sensation, and autonomic function create a tremendous risk for skin breakdown. A prime cause is the slow flow of blood that delays oxygen and nutrients reaching an area of skin where there has been pressure; it also intensifies the ulceration process. Regular assessment of Jake's skin integrity included monitoring risk factors and recognizing any change in his overall health status. The challenge was to institute specific interventions and teach Jake and his family to conduct systematic skin inspections to prevent pressure ulcers from developing; knowledge and vigilance are critical to preserving skin integrity. See Chapter 15 for detailed discussion of pressure areas, intrinsic and extrinsic factors influencing skin integrity, the incidence and prevalence in persons with SCI, pressure ulcer risk assessment tools, guidelines, and preventive management strategies.

Respiratory Function. The respiratory system function depends on four muscle groups innervated by spinal nerves: accessory muscles innervated at C2-C8 expand the chest and rib cage, muscles of the diaphragm innervated at C3-C5 are used for inspiration, intercostal muscles innervated at T1-T8 facilitate coughing, and abdominal muscles innervated at T6-T12 are used in expiration and coughing. The level of the SCI and completeness of the injury determine the respiratory capacity. Patients with injuries above C4 because of paralysis of respiratory muscles, or who experience severe respiratory compromise, may require mechanical ventilation. Injuries like Jake's, located between C4 and T6, usually require aggressive pulmonary management, but eventually the person may be weaned from mechanical ventilation. Injuries between T6 and T12 result in some degree of paralysis and may not require an intensive daily respiratory program.

Many respiratory complications are associated with SCI, including atelectasis, pneumonia, and respiratory failure. Higher injury level, more complete injury, and older age increase the likelihood of complications (Chen, Apple, Hudson & Bode, 1999; Linn et al., 2001). Patients are immobile overall and cannot produce an effective cough because innervation of the respiratory musculature (T12 and above) is lost. Jake's interventions began as soon as possible post injury beginning with a baseline assessment of breath sounds, which

would be assessed for changes before and after any interventions. His pulmonary secretion management included medication and respiratory treatments and adequate hydration. He required mechanical ventilation and measures to increase lung inflation and compliance, such as a deep breathing regimen designed for his level of SCI injury. Once his spine was stabilized, he received chest physiotherapy, with postural drainage and percussion. Many patients learn assistive coughing, such as "quad cough"; however, this technique is contraindicated for patients with newly inserted inferior vena cava filters, such as in Jake's case. A different suctioning technique, preferred by patients with SCI (Garstang, Kirshblum, & Wood, 2000; Liszner & Feinberg, 2006); this one uses a mechanical insufflator/exsufflator device. This device delivers deep positive pressure to the airway followed by high negative pressure, which produces a high expiratory rate that simulates a cough. Incentive spirometry in conjunction with exercises to increase innervated inspiratory musculature strength can improve pulmonary functioning (Liaw, Lin, Cheng, Wong, & Tang, 2000). Refer to Chapter 17 for more pulmonary discussion.

Autonomic Regulation. Jake's autonomic regulation was altered because of interrupted communication between receptor organs and brain centers. Immediately following his SCI during the phase of spinal shock, the sympathetic nervous system, with its preganglionic and postganglionic fibers (innervated by cell bodies located between T1 and L2), shut down. He may have had direct damage to this region because autonomic dysfunction continued after the resolution of spinal shock. The initial presentation during spinal shock could have included altered thermoregulation, orthostasis, cardiac arrhythmia, autonomic dysreflexia, and thrombophlebitic disorders.

The typical elements of spinal shock include hypotension, bradycardia, and hypothermia (Ditunno, Little, Tessler, & Burns, 2004). Hypotension results from the initial loss of sympathetic tone, a decrease in vascular resistance, and dilation of venous vessels. Hypovolemia caused by hemorrhage or inadequate hydration may be a contributing factor, and treatment often includes fluid replacement and vasopressors (Campagnolo & Heary, 2002). Careful nursing monitoring of overhydration is important to prevent pulmonary edema. Once spinal shock has resolved, a subset of patients with injuries at T6 or above may develop autonomic dysreflexia.

Bradycardia. Bradycardia occurs most often with lesions above the T5 level owing to insufficient supraspinal control of the sympathetic nervous system, as well as unrestricted vagal tone. Activities that may contribute to bradycardia are those that stimulate the vagus nerve, including tracheal suctioning, defecation, positional turning, or bringing the patient to a prone position. Although bradycardia usually improves with resolution of spinal shock, during this period Jake was carefully monitored when performing these activities. For the most part, bradycardia does not require intervention unless it is severe or the patient becomes symptomatic; then a cardiac pacemaker is an option (Gilgoff, Ward, & Hohn, 1991).

Thermoregulation. Thermoregulation (i.e., adjustments in core body temperature) is regulated by the hypothalamus. It triggers shivering to generate heat and vasoconstriction to minimize heat loss, or sweating and vasodilatation to facilitate heat loss (see Chapter 35). Its ability to regulate the periphery is reduced following SCI, and patients with lesions above T5 may become poikilothermic, that is, they adapt to the temperature of their environment. For example, a hot room or sun exposure may cause a patient to have a high core temperature that is mistaken as a fever and/or an infection. Problems with thermoregulation usually occur during the period of spinal shock, although they can persist, such as with autonomic dysreflexia precipitating increased sweating with heat loss and a drop in body temperature. The patient's ability to correct the drop in body temperature with shivering is impaired. The change in body temperature indicates a need for nursing assessment to distinguish between a thermoregulation problem and a medical condition, such as an infection.

Nursing interventions for Jake are to maintain a proper ambient temperature and ensure he is well hydrated. Strategies include using proper clothing, bedding, or blankets; ventilation; and independent heating or cooling sources to allow quick adjustment of ambient temperatures. Jake and his family need education to recognize signs and learn how to prevent hyperthermia or hypothermia.

Orthostatic Hypotension. Jake experienced orthostatic hypotension during the acute SCI phase, most often when he was moved upright from a lying position, a common situation with complete SCI above T6. His symptoms included dizziness and light-headedness, but no syncope, nausea, facial pallor, and/or numbness. Normally when a person moves to an upright position, the carotid and aortic baroceptors perceive the fall in blood pressure and trigger the sympathetic nervous system to call for vasoconstriction and tachycardia to increase blood flow to the heart and brain. Because Jake's efferent pathways were disrupted, the diminished sympathetic response led to orthostasis from the pooling of venous blood in the lower extremities and the splanchnic vessels in the abdomen. This phenomenon lessens over time, possibly due to increased sensitivity of baroreceptors and catecholamine receptors, improved autoregulation of cerebrovascular circulation, and development of spasticity (Claydon, Steeves, & Krassioukov, 2006; Teasell, Arnold, Krassioukov, & Delaney, 2000).

Nursing management was to prevent orthostatic hypotension and implement strategies to reduce or eliminate it when it occurs. Jake was adequately hydrated, and his blood pressure and pulse were monitored before any movement while he was supine and again when he was moved upright. Any movement to an upright position, whether to sit or stand, was performed gradually. Because orthostatic hypotension has been a problem for Jake, interventions to mitigate venous pooling may include elastic wrap or compression stockings to the lower extremities and abdominal binders donned before his sitting upright. Should orthostatic hypotension occur, the immediate nursing intervention is to tilt Jake back to a lower level until symptoms resolve. In the case of syncope, he may need to be placed in a supine position with the legs elevated.

Autonomic Dysreflexia. AD is a potentially life-threatening event that can occur in a subset of SCI patients after the resolution of spinal shock; it is marked by a sudden and dangerous increase in blood pressure. Estimates vary, but 48% to 98% of persons with SCI experience this phenomenon (Campagnolo & Merli, 2002; Schmitt, Midha, McKenzie, & Narla, 2001). Timely action is essential, because the longer the hypertension continues, the greater the risks. Bradycardia may be a response to the arterial pressure rise or vagal stimulation but does not affect the blood pressure appreciably. (See Chapter 18, Appendix 18-A for an extensive discussion of AD.)

Management of an episode of AD requires immediate recognition of symptoms and a rapid assessment to eliminate the source of the noxious stimuli (Teasell et al., 2000; Consortium for Spinal Cord Medicine, 2001). Monitor the patient's blood pressure at 5-minute intervals, at a minimum. Interventions to avoid noxious stimuli include ensuring the bowel program is effective and the patient does not have a distended bladder, that clothing and bedding are smooth and not constricting, and that patients receive appropriate skin and wound care and podiatric care. Any time Jake needs an invasive procedure, particularly one involving the genitourinary or gastrointestinal system, nursing management includes monitoring and possibly medication management before the procedure. Education for Jake, his family, and caregivers regarding the risks, symptoms, and prevention of AD was crucial.

Thromboembolic Disorders. Thromboembolic disorders, deep venous thrombosis (DVT) and pulmonary embolism (PE), are recognized as potential complications following SCI. Incidence rates fluctuate greatly, but fewer reported cases may be due to more effective prophylaxis and diagnostic procedures (Green, Sullivan, Simpson, Soltysik, & Yarnold, 2005). DVT usually develops within the first 2 weeks post injury, with the incidence decreasing after 8 weeks. PE has been reported in 5% of patients during the acute SCI phase and is a leading cause of death in the first year post injury (McKinley, Jackson, Cardenas, & DeVivo, 1999). (See Chapter 33 for risk factors.)

The Consortium for Spinal Cord Medicine (1999) recommends a method of mechanical prophylaxis for at least 2 weeks post injury (pneumonic compression devices or compression hose), as well as anticoagulant prophylaxis for at least 8 to 12 weeks. Jake received a vena cava filter because he had contraindications to anticoagulation therapy. As soon as he was medically stable, Jake began early mobilization and exercise. A nursing physical assessment was conducted twice daily to detect signs and symptoms of unilateral lower extremity edema, pain/tenderness, or low-grade fever of unknown origin. However, clinical signs of a DVT in a SCI patient may be unreliable because of sensory loss and dependent edema. The gold standard for diagnosing a DVT is via contrast venography, but it is typically not performed because of its invasiveness. Although limited, the common diagnostic technique is a duplex ultrasound.

Nursing management includes monitoring for symptoms of pulmonary embolus, including difficulty breathing, a heavy feeling in the chest or pain, apprehension, cough, and/or fever. Patients are monitored for signs of bleeding secondary to anticoagulation therapy, including hematuria, epistaxis, hematomas, and/or decrease in hemoglobin or hematocrit levels. Also monitor the intake and balance of fluid to avoid dehydration. The selected compression modality and the underlying skin need to be inspected for any evidence of compromise. Interventions specific to circumventing venous obstruction or venous hypertension are proper positioning and wearing nonrestrictive garments. DVT is discussed in detail in Chapter 33.

Urinary Elimination. With SCI, normal bladder function is often disrupted. Jake needed an effective bladder management program to normalize his body functions, promote his quality of life, and prepare him to go home. The bladder management plan was individualized for the level and extent of his SCI and considering his risk for complications, such as infection, bladder stones, and renal failure. Risk of bladder complications increases with aging (Drake, Cortina-Borja, Savic, Charlifue, & Gardner, 2005). Bladder programs are dynamic; changing needs and medical conditions throughout Jake's life span will necessitate lifelong modifications and adjustments. (See Chapter 18 for details and management of a neurogenic bladder.)

Nursing management (for an upper motor neuron bladder) included regular, complete bladder emptying using scheduled self-intermittent catheterizations during the hospital stay and continued at home, which eliminated the need for an indwelling catheter. Patients like Jake, who have upper extremity function and an injury at C5 or below, can effectively use self-catheterization equipment and techniques. Medications assist in regulating bladder emptying, particularly for patients who have detrusor sphincter dyssynergia. A number of patients may need an indwelling catheter, which must be managed to avoid associated risks of infection and stone formation. In some cases surgical procedures, including the placement of a neuroprosthesis and/or a posterior sacral rhizotomy, may enhance the patient's ability to manage a neurogenic bladder (Creasey et al., 2001). Repeated diagnostic tests such as laboratory work, cystoscopies, and urodynamics and urological surgeries are part of lifelong urological management.

Unlike Jake, patients who have a flaccid bladder and sphincter and are unable to store urine (a lower motor neuron bladder) still can set a self-care goal to perform and manage their bladder program. The central objective is urine containment. Although an indwelling catheter may be necessary, other less-invasive options should be pursued. A man may find an external catheter and drainage system to be a good option;

however, an indwelling catheter is often the only option for women. Adult briefs are not an optimal strategy; their use is associated with a high risk for skin breakdown.

Bowel Elimination. Altered bowel function is the most frequent gastrointestinal problem following an SCI. Jake needed an effective bowel program to have a sense of control over his bodily functions and reduce the fear and potential embarrassment of incontinence and to avoid medical complications (Coggrave, 2004). Achieving an effective program is more challenging for patients with a lower motor neuron bowel compared to those with an upper motor neuron bowel (Yim, Yoon, Lee, Rah, & Moon, 2001) (see Chapter 19). Risk for autonomic dysreflexia increases the importance of an effective bowel program with regular, planned bowel evacuations.

Because of competing priorities, bowel function was not initially addressed during Jake's acute hospitalization, but it should have been, given the alterations in his GI tract innervation and diminished motility during spinal shock. Jake was at high risk for constipation and fecal impaction. A "clean" bowel is essential before initiating a bowel program because increased bowel motility and frequent or loose stools interfere and add to the challenge.

Patients, like Jake, who have an upper motor neuron injury are likely to have a reflex (upper motor neuron or neurogenic) bowel once spinal shock has resolved. Although conscious control of bowel emptying is not possible, triggers such as the gastrocolic reflex, distending the rectal cavity, and inserting a suppository or other artificial stimulant promote reflex emptying. The associated hyperreflexia that often accompanies upper motor neuron injuries can challenge bowel continence, but the parasympathetic innervation of the sphincter that creates tone tends to reduce the risk of fecal incontinence. The goal of an upper motor neuron bowel program is to establish a pattern of regular, reflexive bowel emptying and continence. For Jake, a bowel program was conducted at a regular time each day.

Patients with a lower motor neuron injury have an autonomous neurogenic bowel with a loss of motor tone and a flaccid rectal sphincter. This, in combination with reduced peristalsis, increases the risk of constipation and stool impaction. The flaccid rectal sphincter makes bowel incontinence a major concern, which may be worsened by the consistency and volume of the stool. Nursing management includes hydration, dietary modifications, and medications to support motility that will move the bolus of food through the patient's GI tract efficiently to produce a firm stool. Instituting strategies and a schedule for bowel evacuations mitigates the risk of incontinence.

Neurogenic Pain. While not a problem for Jake, neurogenic pain is common with SCI; however, the causative factors are understood poorly. Neurogenic pain includes pain related to injury of nerve roots, the spinal cord, or the cauda equina (Bryce & Ragnarsson, 2000) and is associated with incomplete injuries (Norrbrink Budh et al., 2003) and younger patients (Putzke, Richards, Hicken, & DeVivo, 2002). The high frequency of shoulder pain among persons with tetraplegia is thought to be due to sensation at the level of the injury combined with impaired movement and posture (Dyson-Hudson & Kirshblum, 2004).

Neurogenic pain generally presents within the first 6 months following the injury. Prolonged sitting, muscle spasms, and fatigue contribute (Widerstrom-Noga & Turk, 2004), and patients who express a negative mood or a limited sense of control in their lives tend to have more pain issues. Cold weather and sudden movements may produce neurogenic pain. For some, it can be overwhelming, interfering with their ability to perform the simplest of tasks. The degree to which the pain interferes with ADLs can be predictive of its effect on quality of life.

The nursing management of neurogenic pain focuses on interventions to prevent pain, as well as those to treat the pain directly. Posture and positioning with proper body alignment in the wheelchair, bed, or any other surface to decrease the risk of muscle spasms is an important first step. Patients need frequent periods of adequate rest between activities and reduced fatigue. The nurse and patient must collaborate to develop an optimal schedule for administering medications to manage pain and spasticity. This incorporates early interventions for predictable patterns of pain that are related to activities.

Heterotrophic Ossification.
Heterotrophic ossification (HO) can have a significant impact on mobility, performance of functional activities, and comfort and quality of life. HO is the overgrowth of bone in the soft tissue surrounding a joint; it develops distal to the level of injury. Between 13% and 37% of persons with SCI develop HO, usually within the first 6 months post injury (van Kuijk, Geurts, & van Kuppevelt, 2002). An early symptom is a red and swollen joint with decreased ROM, possibly accompanied by pain, low-grade fever, malaise, and increased spasticity. In extreme cases the joint may progress to ankylosis.

Nursing interventions are pain management, appropriate positioning to prevent skin compromise arising from increased bone pressure or changes in posture secondary to the extra bone, and alternative strategies to promote self-care. After the acute inflammatory phase, gentle active-assisted and passive ROM with stretching can be initiated. Pharmacological management can reduce inflammation, as well as reduce bone growth. Patients with severely limited ROM that impedes functional activity may be candidates for surgical intervention.

Osteoporosis.
Osteoporosis, bone reabsorption that exceeds formation, is active in the first year post SCI but slows in following years. Decreases in bone density are correlated with completeness of the SCI (Garland, Atkins, Rah, & Stewart, 2001) and raise the risk for lower extremity fractures. Loss of weight-bearing activity and immobility are major contributing factors. A 26% loss of upper extremity bone mass occurs with tetraplegia, 25% loss in the proximal femur, 40% loss in the distal femur, and a somewhat higher loss in the proximal and distal tibia. No difference was found between patients with paraplegia or tetraplegia regarding lower extremity bone loss (Kiratli, Smith, Nauenberg, Kallfelz, & Perkash, 2000).

Interventions to minimize Jake's bone loss included weight-bearing activities, functional electric stimulation (FES), and pharmacological agents. FES has shown some preventive benefits but has not been found to reverse bone loss once it has occurred (Belanger, Stein, Wheeler, Gordon, & Leduc, 2000). Weight-bearing activities, namely standing and ambulation, have not shown a consistent increase in bone density, although performing them early on may be beneficial (Needham-Shropshire et al., 1997). Pharmacological agents have demonstrated some benefit and are a subject of ongoing research. From an interdisciplinary perspective, mobility and exercise interventions that support a patient's functional abilities help to prevent bone loss and preserve muscle tone.

Emotional and Social Adjustment.
A patient's sense of loss can be profound and may be related to changes in physical abilities, functional abilities, social relationships, financial resources, and/or personal identity. The journey of each patient is unique. A patient's internal resilience and past history of coping help predict the ability to adjust; this is a devastating injury. Nurses are with patients and their families a full 24 hours a day over 7 days a week and are able to observe how a patient's mood state and personal strategies for coping vary with what is being asked of them, and their realization of the extent of their injury. Adjustment to a SCI continues long after a patient's stay in a rehabilitation unit and has a profound impact on the quality of life (Jang, Wang, & Wang, 2005).

To maximize Jake's ability for self-care, an interdisciplinary evaluation made the distinction between activities that he could perform, and at what level of independence, and activities that he could direct a caregiver to perform. Jake had an opportunity to make decisions about participation. Jake, his family, and the nurse set mutual goals and interventions that were important to his overall recovery, which enhanced his sense of self-control and improved his quality of life. This therapeutic relationship required all of them to cultivate trust, listen without judgment, educate one another, and encourage active participation in personal and social activities. Jake's ability to adapt and adjust were part of the nursing assessment at every stage of recovery.

Depression.
Depression, common after a SCI, is challenging to treat. A combination of modalities may include medications, treatment groups, and individual psychotherapy, as well as alternative interventions (Kemp, Kahan, Krause, Adkins, & Nava, 2004). Nursing assessment for signs and symptoms of depression and any evidence of suicidal ideation is ongoing through all phases of recovery. It is difficult to distinguish between normal grieving associated with loss and clinical depression; careful, supportive listening is both necessary and therapeutic. The incidence of self-medication using alcohol or illegal drugs is quite high, particularly for those whose preinjury behavior included these activities (Osteraker & Levi, 2005). Visitors may supply drugs or alcohol to patients while in the rehabilitation hospital, a situation that must be observed for, discussed with the team, and reported according to policies of the institution.

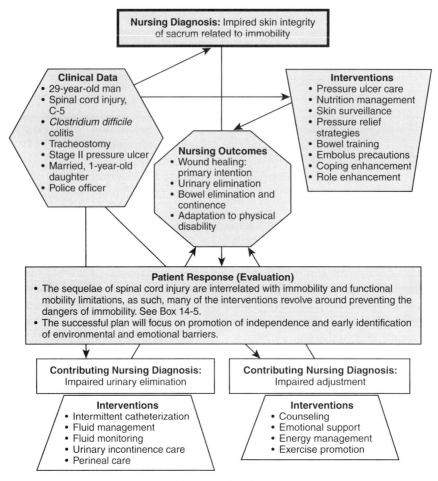

Concept Map. Jake's primary problem is that of the immobility related to the spinal cord injury. Interventions are needed to promote healing of the pressure ulcer while promoting urinary and bowel management. The rehabilitation nurse will focus on coordinating interventions to achieve the outcomes of wound healing, promotion of tissue integrity, tissue perfusion, and self-care.

CRITICAL THINKING

1. What are the key components of a bowel program for Jake to ensure daily, effective bowel evacuations?
2. What level of care and/or assistance and what type of wheelchair will be needed for Jake upon discharge (based on his ASIA classification) to maximize his mobility and function?
3. Based upon the admission assessment for the case study, what specific respiratory interventions would be initiated?
4. What strategies should be put in place to prevent an episode of autonomic dysreflexia?

REFERENCES

Albert, T., & Yelnik, A. (2003). Physiotherapy for spasticity. *Neurosurgery, 49,* 239-246.

American Spinal Injury Association (ASIA). (2002). *International standards for neurological and functional classification of spinal cord injury.* Atlanta, GA: Author.

Aydin, G., Tomruk, S., Keles, I., Demir, S., & Orkun, S. (2005). Transcutaneous electrical stimulation versus baclofen in spasticity: Clinical and electrophysical comparison. *American Journal of Physical Medicine and Rehabilitation, 84*(8), 584-592.

Belanger, M., Stein, R., Wheeler, G., Gordon, T., & Leduc, B. (2000). Electrical stimulation: Can it increase muscle strength and reverse osteoporosis in spinal cord injured individuals. *Archives of Physical Medicine and Rehabilitation, 81,* 1090-1098.

Bobath, B. (1991). *Adult hemiplegia: Evaluation and treatment* (3rd ed.). London: Heinemann.

Bohannon, R. (1993). Tilt table standing for reducing spasticity after spinal cord injury. *Archives of Physical Medicine and Rehabilitation, 74,* 1121-1122.

Borgman, M. F., & Passarella, P. M. (1991). Nursing care of the stroke patient using Bobath principles: An approach to altered movement. *Nursing Clinics of North America, 20,* 1019-1035.

Brunnstrom, S. (1970). *Movement therapy in hemiplegia.* New York: Harper & Row.

Bryce, T. N., & Ragnarsson, K. T. (2000). Pain after spinal cord injury. *Physical Medicine and Rehabilitation Clinics of North America, 11*(1), 157-168

Buchiel, K., & Hsu, F. (2001). Pain and spasticity after spinal cord injury: Mechanisms and treatment. *Spine, 248,* s146-s160.

Campagnolo, D., & Heary, R. (2002). Acute medical and surgical management of spinal cord injury. In S. Kirshblum, D. Campagnolo, & J. A. DeLisa (Eds.). *Spinal Cord Medicine.* Philadelphia: Lippincott Williams & Wilkins.

Campagnolo, D. I., & Merli, G. J. (2002). Autonomic and cardiovascular complications of spinal cord injury. In S. Kirshblum, D. Campagnolo, & J. A. DeLisa (Eds.). *Spinal Cord Medicine.* Philadelphia: Lippincott Williams & Wilkins.

Centers for Disease Control and Prevention. (2000). *Disability and health.* Atlanta: Division of Birth Defects, Child Development, and Disability and Health. Available from http://www.cdc.gov/nceh/cddh.

Centers for Disease Control and Prevention, National Center for Health Statistics. (2006). *National health interview survey* (Table 58, Family Questionnaire). Hyattsville, MD: Author.

Chan, A., & Heck, C. S. (2000). Mobility in multiple sclerosis: More than just a physical problem. *International Journal of MS Care [serial online], 3,* 35-40. Available from http://mscare.com.

Chen, D., Apple, D., Hudson, L., & Bode, R. (1999). Medical complications during acute rehabilitation following spinal cord injury—current experience of the Model Systems. *Archives of Physical Medicine and Rehabilitation*, 80, 1397-1401.

Claydon, V., Steeves, J., & Krassioukov, A. (2006). Orthostatic hypotension following spinal cord injury: Understanding clinical pathophysiology. *Spinal Cord*, 44, 341-351.

Coggrave, M. (2004). Effective bowel management for patients after spinal cord injury. *Nursing Times*, 100(20), 48-51.

Connell, B. R., & Wolf, S. L. (1997). Environmental and behavioral circumstances associated with falls at home among healthy elderly individuals: Atlanta FICSIT Group. *Archives of Physical Medicine and Rehabilitation*, 78(2), 179-186.

Consortium for Spinal Cord Medicine. (1999). *Prevention of thromboembolism in spinal cord injury*. Washington, DC: Paralyzed Veterans of America.

Consortium for Spinal Cord Medicine. (2001). Acute management of autonomic dysreflexia. Washington, D.C.: Paralyzed Paralyzed Veterans of America. Available from http://www.NCSCIMS.org/home/systemsofcare/RehabilitationMedicine/tabid/146/default.aspx.

Creasey G. H., Grill, J. H., Korsten, M., U, H. S., Betz, R., Anderson, R., & Walter, J. (2001). An implantable neuroprosthesis for restoring bladder and bowel control to patients with spinal cord injuries: A multicenter trial. *Archives of Physical Medicine and Rehabilitation*, 82(11), 1512-1519.

Ditunno, J., Little, J., Tessler, R., & Burns, A. (2004). Spinal shock revisited: A four phase model. *Spinal Cord*, 42, 383-395.

Dochterman, J., & Bulechek, G. M. (2004). *Nursing interventions classification (NIC)* (4th ed.). St. Louis, MO: Mosby.

Drake, M. J., Cortina-Borja, M., Savic, G., Charlifue, S. W., & Gardner, B. P. (2005). Prospective evaluation of urological effects of aging in chronic spinal cord injury by method of bladder management. *Neurourological Dynamics*, 24(2), 111-116.

Dyson-Hudson, T. A., & Kirshblum, S. (2004). Shoulder pain in chronic spinal cord injury: Part 1. Epidemiology, etiology, and pathomechanics. *Journal of Spinal Cord Medicine*, 27(1), 4-17.

Fisher, A. G. (1999). *Assessment of Motor and Process Skills (AMPS)*. Fort Collins, CO: Three Star Press.

Fisher, C., Noonan, V., Smith, D., Wing, P., Dvorak, M., & Kwon, B. (2005). Motor recovery, functional status, and health-related quality of life in patients with complete spinal cord injuries. *Spine*, 30(19), 2200-2207.

Garland, D., Atkins, R., Rah, A., & Stewart, C. (2001). Bone loss with aging and the impact of SCI. *Topics in Spinal Cord Rehabilitation*, 61(3), 47-60.

Garstang, S., Kirshblum, S., & Wood, K. (2000). Patient preference for in-exsufflation for secretion management in spinal cord injury. *Journal of Spinal Cord Medicine*, 23, 80-85.

Gerber, D. A., & Jozefczyk, P. B. (2000). The management of spasticity in multiple sclerosis. *International Journal of MS Care [serial online]*, 1(1), 5-11. Available at http://www.mscare.com.

Gerhart, K., Bergstrom, E., & Charlifue, S. (1993). Long-term spinal cord injury: Functional changes over time. *Archives of Physical Medicine and Rehabilitation*, 74, 1030-1034.

Gilgoff, I., Ward, S., & Hohn, P. (1991). Cardiac pacemaker in high spinal cord injury. *Archives of Physical Medicine and Rehabilitation*, 72, 601-603.

Gillespie, M. M. (1991). Tremor. *Journal of Neuroscience Nursing*, 23(3), 170-174.

Granger, C. V., Hamilton, B. B., & Sherwin, F. S. (1997). *Guide for the use of the uniform data set for medical rehabilitation (version 5.1)*. Buffalo, NY: Uniform Data System of Medical Rehabilitation Project Office.

Green, D., Sullivan, S., Simpson, J., Soltysik, R., & Yarnold, P. (2005). Evolving risk for thromboembolism in spinal cord injury (SPIRATE Study). *American Journal of Physical Medicine and Rehabilitation*, 84, 420-422.

Hinderer, S., & Dixon, K. (2001). Physiologic and clinical monitoring of spastic hypertonia. *Physical Medicine and Rehabilitation Clinics of North America*, 12(4), 733-746.

Hoeman, S. P. (1997). Primary care for children with spina bifida. *Nurse Practitioner*, 22, 60-72.

Hogan, D. P., Rogers, M. L., & Msall, M. E. (2000). Functional limitations and key indicators of well-being in children with disability. *Archives of Pediatric and Adolescent Medicine*, 15, 1042-1048.

Jackson-Wyatt, D. (1007). Feldenkrals method and rehabilitation. In Davis, C. M. (Ed.), *Complementary therapies in rehabilitation* (pp. 189-197). Thorofare, NJ: Slack.

Jang, Y., Wang, Y. H., & Wang, J. D. (2005). Return to work after spinal cord injury in Taiwan: The contribution of functional independence. *Archives of Physical Medicine and Rehabilitation*, 86(4), 681-686.

Jozefczyk, P. (2002). The management of focal spasticity. *Clinical Neuropharmacology*, 25, 158-173.

Katz, S., & Akpom, A. (1976). A measure of primary sociobiological functions. *International Journal of Health Sciences*, 6, 493-506.

Keane, R., Davis, A., & Dietrich, W. (2006). Inflammatory and apoptotic signaling after spinal cord injury. *Journal of Neurotrauma*, 23(3-4), 335-344.

Kemp, B. J., Kahan, J. S., Krause, J. S., Adkins, R. H., & Nava, G. (2004). Treatment of major depression in individuals with spinal cord injury. *Journal of Spinal Cord Medicine*, 27(1), 22-28.

Kemp, B., & Thompson, L. (2002). Aging and spinal core injury: Medical, functional and psychosocial changes. *SCI Nursing*, 19(2), 51-60.

Kiratli, B., Smith, A., Nauenberg, T., Kallfelz, C., & Perkash, I. (2000). Bone mineral and geometric changes through the femur with immobilization due to spinal cord injury. *Journal of Rehabilitation, Research, and Development*, 37(2), 225-233.

Kirshblum, S. (1999). Treatment alternatives for spinal cord injury related spasticity. *Journal of Spinal Cord Medicine*, 22(3), 199-217.

Klein, R. M., & Bell, B. (1982). Self care skills: Behavioral measurement with Klein-Bell ADL scale. *Archives of Physical Medicine and Rehabilitation*, 63(7), 335.

Knight, M. M. (2000). Cognitive ability and functional status. *Journal of Advanced Nursing*, 31(6), 1459-1468.

Kwon, B., Tetzlaff, W., Grauer, J., Beiner, J, & Vaccaro, A. (2004). Pathophysiology and pharmacologic treatment of acute spinal cord injury. *Spine*, 4(4), 451-464.

LaPlante, M., Hendershot, G., & Moss, A. (1996). Assistive technology devices and home accessibility features: Prevalence, payment need, and trends. In *Advance data from vital and health statistics* (No. 217). Hyattsville, MD: National Center for Health Statistics.

Lechner, H., Frotzler, A., & Eser, P. (2006). Relationship between self-and clinically rated spasticity in spinal cord injury. *Archives of Physical Medicine and Rehabilitation*, 87(1), 15-19.

Liaw, M., Lin, M., Cheng, P., Wong, M., & Tang, F. (2000). Resistive inspiratory muscle training in subjects with acute complete cervical cord injury. *Archives of Physical Medicine and Rehabilitation*, 81, 752-756.

Liem, N., McColl, M., King, W., & Smith, K. (2004). Aging with spinal cord injury: Factors associated with the need for more help with activities of daily living. *Archives of Physical Medicine and Rehabilitation*, 85, 1567-1577.

Linn, W., Spungen, A., Gong, H., Adkins, R., Bauman, W., & Waters, R. (2001). Forced vital capacity in two large outpatient populations with chronic spinal cord injury. *Spinal Cord*, 39, 263-268.

Liszner, K., & Feinberg, M. (2006). Cough assist strategy for pulmonary toileting: Ventilator-dependent spinal cord patients. *Rehabilitation Nursing*, 31(5), 218-221.

Lu, J., Ashwell, K., & Waite, P. (2000). Advances in secondary spinal cord injury: Role of apoptosis. *Spine*, 25(14), 1859-1866.

Mahoney, F. I., & Barthel, D. (1965). Functional evaluation: The Barthel Index *Maryland State Medical Journal*, 14, 56-61.

Martin, K. S. (2005). *Th Omaha System: A key to practice, documentation, and information management*. St. Louis, MO: Saunders.

McKinley, W., Jackson, A., Cardenas, D., & DeVivo, M. (1999). Long term medical complications after traumatic spinal cord injury: A regional model systems analysis. *Archives of Physical Medicine and Rehabilitation*, 80(11), 1402-1410.

Moorhead, S., Johnson, M., & Maas, M. (Eds.). (2004). *Nursing outcomes classification (NOC)* (3rd ed.). St. Louis, MO: Mosby.

National Institute of Disability and Rehabilitation Research. (2000). Available at http://www.ed.gov/ossers.nidu.

National Spinal Cord Injury Statistical Center. (2005). *Spinal cord injury: Facts and figures at a glance*. Birmingham: University of Alabama.

Needham-Shropshire, B., Broton, J., Klose, K., Lebwohl, N., Guest, R., & Jacobs, P. (1997). Evaluation of a training program for person with SCI paraplegia using the Parastep 1 ambulation system: Part 3. Lack of effect on bone mineral density. *Archives of Physical Medicine and Rehabilitation*, 78, 799-803.

Norrbrink Budh, C., Lund, I., Ertzgaard, P., Holtz, A., Hulting, C., Levi, R., et al. (2003). Pain in a Swedish spinal cord injury population. *Clinical Rehabilitation*, 17(6), 685-690.

NSW Cervical Screening Program (2006). Preventative women's health care for women with disabilities: Guidelines for general practitioners—Background and literature review. Alexandria, New South Wales, Australia: Author. Available at http://www.csp.NSW.gov.au.

O'Connor, K., & Salcido, R. (2002). Pressure ulcers in spinal cord injury. In Kirshblum, S., Campagnolo, D., & DeLisa, J. (Eds.), *Spinal cord medicine*. New York: Lippincott Williams & Wilkins.

Olson, E. V. (1967). The hazards of immobility. *American Journal of Nursing*, 67, 779-797.

Osteraker, A. L., & Levi, R. (2005). Indicators of psychological distress in postacute spinal cord injured individuals. *Spinal Cord*, 43(4), 223-229.

Parker, N., Soy, D., Kesiktas, N., Nueparkdak, A., Erbil, M., Ersoy, S., & Ylmaz, H. (2006). Reasons for hospitalization in patients with spinal cord injury: 5 year's experience. *International Journal of Rehabilitation Research*, 29(1), 71-79.

Pendleton, H. M., & Schultz-Krohn, W. (2006). *Pedretti's occupational therapy practice skills for physical dysfunction*. St. Louis, MO: Mosby.

Piette, J. D. (2000). Interactive voice response systems in the diagnosis and management of chronic disease. *American Journal of Managed Care* 6(7), 817-827.

Price, R., Lehmann, J., Boswell-Bessette, S., Burleigh, A., & deLateur, B. (1993). Influence of cryotherapy on spasticity at the human ankle. *Archives of Physical Medicine and Rehabilitation*, 74, 300-304.

Prysak, G., Andresen, E., & Meyers, A. (2000). Prevalence of secondary conditions in veterans with spinal cord injury and their interference with life activities. *Topics in Spinal Cord Rehabilitation*, 6(1), 34-42.

Putzke, J. D., Richards, J. S., Hicken, B. J., & DeVivo, M. J. (2002). Interference due to pain following spinal cord injury: Important predictors and impact on quality of life. *Pain*, 100(3), 231-242.

Rood, M. (1956). Neurophysiological mechanisms utilized in the treatment of neuromuscular dysfunction. *American Journal of Occupational Therapy*, 10(4).

Schmitt, J., Midha, M., McKenzie, N., & Narla, S. (2001). Autonomic dysreflexia. In I. Eltorai & J. Schmitt (Eds.), *Emergencies in chronic spinal cord injury patients* (3rd ed.). Jackson Heights, NY: Eastern Paralyzed Veterans Association.

Sekhon, L., & Fehlings, M. (2001). Epidemiology, demographics, and pathophysiology of acute spinal cord injury. *Spine*, 26(24 Suppl), S2-12.

Skold, C., Levi, R., & Seiger, A. (1999). Spasticity after traumatic spinal cord injury: Nature, severity, and location. *Archives of Physical Medicine and Rehabilitation*, 80, 1548-1557.

Spector, W. (2000). *Characteristics of long term care users* (Publication No. 00-0049). Washington, DC: Agency for Healthcare Research and Quality.

Stolp-Smith, K., & Wainberg, M. (1999). Antidepressant exacerbation of spasticity. *Archives of Physical Medicine and Rehabilitation*, 80, 339-342.

Teasell, R. W., Arnold, J. M., Krassioukov, A., & Delaney, G. (2000). Cardiovascular consequences of loss of supraspinal control of the sympathetic nervous system after spinal cord injury. *Archives of Physical Medicine and Rehabilitation*, 81(4), 506-516.

Thibodeau, G. A., & Patton, K. T. (2007). *Anatomy and physiology* (6th ed.). St. Louis, MO: Mosby.

Thierry, J.M. (2000). Promoting the health and wellness of women with disabilites. *Journal of Women's Health*, 7(5), 505-507.

Thompson, L., Waters, R., & Kemp, B. (2001). Functional changes in long-standing spinal cord injury: The need for multi-disciplinary intervention. *Journal of Spinal Cord Medicine*, 24(1), S6.

Thompson, L., & Yakura, J. (2001). Aging related functional changes in persons with spinal cord injury. *Topics in Spinal Cord Rehabilitation*, 6(3), 69-82.

U.S. Department of Health and Human Services. (2000). *Healthy People 2010*. Retrieved April 27, 2006, from http://web.health.gov/healthypeople.

van Kuijk, A., Geurts, A., van Kuppevelt, H. (2002). Neurogenic heterotrophic ossification in spinal card injury. *Spinal Cord*, 40, 313-326.

Voss, D. E., Ionta, M. K., & Myers, B. J. (1985). *Proprioceptive neuromuscular facilitation* (3rd ed.). Philadelphia: Harper & Row.

Widerstrom-Noga, E. G., & Turk, D. C. (2004). Exacerbation of chronic pain following spinal cord injury. *Journal of Neurotrauma*, 21(10), 1384-1395.

Yim, S. Y., Yoon, S. H., Lee, I. Y., Rah, E. W., & Moon, H. W. (2001). A comparison of bowel care patterns in patients with spinal cord injury: Upper motor neuron bowel vs lower motor neuron bowel. *Spinal Cord*, 39(4), 204-207.

APPENDIX 14A: RANGE OF MOTION: PASSIVE, ACTIVE, AND FUNCTIONAL

I. Terms: range of motion (ROM; amount of movement present in a joint)
   A. Types of ROM
      1. Flexion: bending of joint
      2. Extension: straightening of joint
      3. Adduction: motion away from midline
      4. Adduction: motion toward midline
      5. Circumduction: circular movement
      6. Internal/external rotation
      7. Pronation/supination of elbow
      8. Plantar flexion: downward motion of foot at ankle joint
      9. Dorsiflexion: upward motion of foot at ankle joint

   B. Passive ROM: nurse moves the extremity so that full motion occurs at the joint
   C. Active ROM: patient uses muscles to do the moving
   D. Functional activities of ROM: many activities of daily living produce full ROM (e.g., rolling over in bed, sitting up, getting dressed); ROM can be done in conjunction with bed bathing, bed positioning, and mobilization activities
   E. Progressive resistive exercises: muscles begin to work against gravity, enhancing the strength of the muscle

II. General nursing interventions
   A. Explain all activities to patient and ensure safety
   B. Reinforce all teaching to patient and family
   C. Move patient's arms and legs gently during ROM, and move within patient's tolerance and flexibility
   D. Support the extremity above and below the joint being treated
   E. Give passive ROM when patient is in the supine position
   F. Perform each exercise 5 to 10 times during each treatment
   G. Assess the motion of the involved side against the ROM of the uninvolved side
   H. Perform ROM on all extremities if patient is immobilized
   I. Nurse should use proper body mechanics

III. Specific ROM exercises: upper extremity
   A. Shoulder flexion/extension
      1. Support the arm at the wrist and elbow; shoulder is in extended position

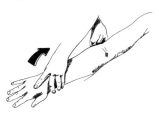

      2. Lift the arm straight over patient's head; flexion occurs as the arm is lifted up and back

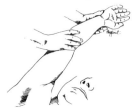

      3. Rest the arm flat on the bed above the head
      4. Bend patient's elbow if there is not enough room for the entire motion
   B. Shoulder abduction/adduction
      1. Support the arm at the wrist and elbow, with patient's palm facing his or her body
      2. Slide the arm sideways away from the body, which produces shoulder abduction; sliding the arm toward the body produces shoulder adduction

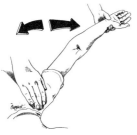

3. Allow the arm to roll or turn over when it reaches about a 90-degree angle with the shoulder
4. Bend the patient's elbow if there is not enough room for the entire movement

C. Shoulder external/internal rotation
1. Support patient's hand and shoulder
2. Bring the arm away from the patient's side, forming a 90-degree angle with the body
3. Keep the elbow bent 90 degrees and the arm supported on the bed
4. Press down on the shoulder toward the bed
5. Move the patient's hand backward until the back of the hand touches the bed; as the forearm is brought up and back, external rotation occurs at the shoulder joint

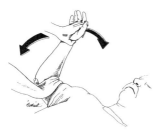

6. Move the patient's hand forward until the palm touches the bed; as the forearm is brought down, internal rotation occurs at the shoulder joint

D. Elbow flexion/extension
1. Support the elbow and wrist
2. Bend the patient's arm to touch the hand to the shoulder, producing elbow flexion

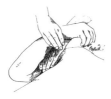

3. Straighten the arm toward the bed, producing elbow extension

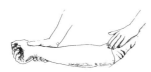

E. Forearm: pronate/supinate
1. Support the upper arm and wrist

2. Turn the palm of the patient's hand toward the feet; rolling the forearm downward places it in pronation

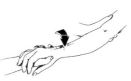

3. Turn palm of patient's hand upward from the feet; this places the forearm in supination

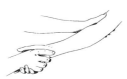

F. Wrist
1. Support the patient's wrist and hand, and hold patient's fingers in the other hand; bend wrist forward and make a fist, producing wrist flexion

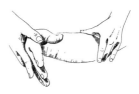

2. Bend wrist backward and extend fingers, producing wrist extension

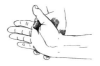

3. Move the wrist laterally, producing radial and ulnar deviation

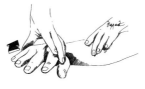

G. Fingers
1. Support patient's hand by holding the palm of the hand
2. Bend all fingers at once into a closed fist, producing flexion

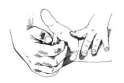

3. Straighten all fingers at once (described as an open fist), producing extension

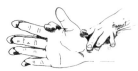

4. Each finger is separated (abducted) and brought back together (adducted)

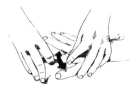

H. Thumb
   1. Support the patient's hand by holding the fingers straight with one hand
   2. Thumb flexed toward and extended away from the fourth digit

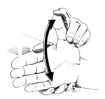

3. Pull the thumb away from the palm; thumb is abducted and adducted in relation to the other fingers

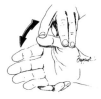

4. Stretch the web space between the thumb and index finger

I. Thumb opposition
   1. Support the hand as in thumb abduction
   2. Move the thumb toward the little finger in opposition to the base of each of the other four digits

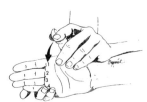

3. Move the thumb through a semicircle design

IV. Specific ROM exercises: lower extremity
   A. Hip flexion/extension
      1. Support under the patient's knee and heel
      2. Raise the knee toward the chest, producing flexion

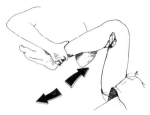

3. Bend the hip as much as possible; allow the knee to bend slightly or within patient's tolerance
4. Sliding the leg forward produces extension
   B. Hip flexion/strength
      1. Support under patient's knees and heel
      2. Lift patient's leg straight and as high as possible
      3. Hold for count of 5
      4. Lower the leg gently
   C. Hip abduction/adduction
      1. Support patient's knee and heel, keeping the leg in "toes up" position
      2. Move the leg away from the midline of the body, abducting the hip

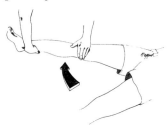

3. Move the leg toward the midline of the body and cross over the other leg, adducting the hip

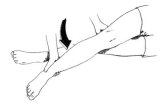

D. Hip internal/external rotation
   1. Support under patient's knee and heel
   2. Bend the hip up to 90 degrees, and bend the knee up to 90 degrees
   3. Turn the lower leg toward you, keeping the hip and knee in place
   4. Turn the lower leg away from you, keeping the hip and knee in place
   5. Do not force this motion
E. Hip internal/external rotation
   1. Support patient's leg by placing hand on top of patient's knee and ankle
   2. Roll the leg inward

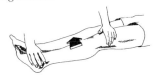

3. Roll the leg outward

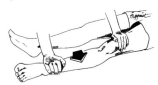

F. Knee flexion/extension
　1. Support the leg as necessary at the heel and behind the knee
　2. Flex the hip high 90 degrees
　3. Bend the knee in a position of flexion

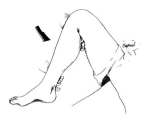

　4. Movement of lower leg upward produces knee extension; hip is also in extension

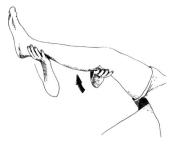

G. Heel cord stretching
　1. Support patient's calf with one hand and press downward on patient's leg with the other hand
　2. Pull down on the heel
　3. Press your forearm against the patient's foot, pushing it toward the leg

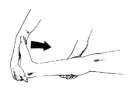

　4. Hold for count of 5 and relax

H. Toe flexion/extension
　1. Support patient's foot
　2. Bend all toes downward, producing flexion
　3. Push all toes backward, producing extension
I. Ankle
　1. Support patient's leg with one hand, and hold the foot with the other hand
　2. Pressure with the palm of the hand against the ball of the foot produces ankle dorsiflexion

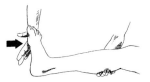

　3. Pressure against the top of the foot produces ankle plantar flexion

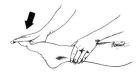

　4. Turning the foot inward produces ankle inversion

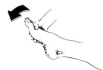

　5. Turning the foot outward produces ankle eversion

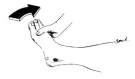

15

Skin Integrity

Maureen Preston, MSN, APRN, BC, CRRN, CWOCN
Cherisse Tebben, MSN, CWOCN, CFNP
Kelly M. M. Johnson, RN, MSN, CRRN, CNNA

Nurses in rehabilitation settings frequently encounter clinical challenges related to maintaining skin integrity. For this reason it is imperative that the rehabilitation nurse have a sound understanding of the physiological basis of skin management. Furthermore, evidence-based nursing practice enables nurses to select appropriate and effective interventions that will prevent alterations in skin integrity. This chapter addresses management of skin integrity utilizing the nursing process: assessment, diagnosis, intervention, and evaluation of outcomes.

SCOPE OF THE PROBLEM

Incidence and Prevalence

Despite the increased awareness of the incidence and prevalence of pressure ulcers and chronic wounds in health care, improvement in assessment of risk, extensive research on prevention and management, and ongoing development of prevention and treatment options, pressure ulcers remain one of the most common and costly complications in health care. The development of pressure ulcers and chronic wounds in rehabilitation patients is multifactorial. Aging, chronic illness, such as cardiovascular disease and diabetes mellitus, and wear and tear of skin in individuals with neurological compromise all contribute to acute pressure ulcers and chronic nonhealing wounds. Approximately 2 million people in the United States are affected by pressure ulcers, most of them elderly (Beitz & Goldberg, 2005). With the burgeoning growth of the older adult population, increased knowledge and understanding of the chronic wound experience is vital for caregivers, nurses, and other health care professionals.

The incidence of pressure ulcers varies greatly by clinical setting. Incidence rates of 0.4% to 38% for hospitals and 2.2% to 23.9% for long-term care settings have been reported (Lyder & Torpy, 2003). Wound care interventions are frequently provided in the home health care setting. Wounds account for 31% to 36% of patients in home health care, with approximately half of these patients having more than one wound

(Buckley, Adelson, & Hess, 2005). Varying pressure ulcer prevalence rates have been reported from surveys in health care institutions in different countries, ranging from 10.1% to 23.1%. Because there is a lack of standardized methods for determining incidence and prevalence rates, these studies are not always comparable. Among the confounding factors are the severity of illness of the patients surveyed, how pressure ulcers have been defined, and the methods used in data collection (Gunningberg & Ehrenberg, 2004).

Special Populations at Risk

There are several definitive risk factors for development of pressure ulcers. These risk factors are higher in select groups, and incident rates are not distributed evenly across populations. For example, persons with hip fractures are at greater risk than those admitted to hospitals for elective orthopedic procedures. However, in some studies, hospital nurses were found not to recognize the high risk and did not document preventive measures or begin treatment until after the pressure ulcers formed in patients with hip fractures.

Patients with disabilities are at higher risk for pressure ulcer formation. The reported prevalence of pressure ulcers in persons with disabilities varies widely in the rehabilitation literature. This variation is due to unclear ulcer staging, the use of multiple formulas to calculate prevalence, differing case mixes, dissimilar data sources, and other issues. Databases indicate that between 1990 and 2000, pressure ulcer prevalence for stages I to IV in postrehabilitation patients was 12% to 27% and ranged from 15.2% to 30% among spinal cord injury (SCI) patients (Brillhart, 2005).

The literature is replete with studies describing variables associated with incidence and prevalence of pressure ulcers in patients with SCI. Individuals with SCI have reduced mobility, activity, and sensory perception, which may impact skin integrity. Pressure ulcers occur more frequently in patients with more extensive paralysis and completeness of SCI, longer duration of SCI, and less functional independence. Aspects of physical and psychosocial well-being associated with the occurrence of pressure ulcers include lack of responsibility for skin care, poor nutrition, use of tobacco, alcohol and drug abuse, low self-esteem, and feelings of dissatisfaction with life and one's activities (Consortium for Spinal Cord Medicine, 2000). Pressure ulcers have been implicated as one of the most common complications of individuals with SCI living in the community, with a 33% prevalence rate (Brandeis, Berlwitz, Hossain, & Morris, 1995). Prevention of recurrence of pressure ulcers remains a challenge because 35.2% of initial pressure ulcers recur in the SCI population, and 42.2% recur in those who also smoke (Eastwood, Hagglund, Ragnarsson, Gordon, & Marino, 1999).

In addition to pressure ulcers, many Americans, primarily the elderly, are affected by venous, arterial, and neuropathic extremity ulcers. It is reported that as many as 2 million people in the United States have venous ulcers. In addition, between 1 and 2 million diabetic patients have neuropathic foot ulcers (Bietz & Goldberg, 2005). In total, venous, arterial, and neuropathic ulcers may affect as many as 5 million older Americans. Diabetes is projected to increase to total 366 million people by 2030, with the largest demographic change in people over 65 years of age (Wild et al., 2004). Given the projected increase in the number of individuals with diabetes, health care providers need to understand the chronic wound experience (Dellefield, 2004).

Economic and Psychosocial Impact of Alterations in Skin Integrity

Pressure ulcers are a costly phenomenon in regard to human suffering, financial expense, and human resource utilization across health care settings. In the United States close to $1.6 billion are spent annually on care of pressure ulcers (Moody, Gonzales, & Cureton, 2004). Pressure ulcers are especially costly for hospitals, resulting in increased length of stay and related costs, and impose significant effects on patients who must endure the suffering associated with a pressure ulcer. The estimated cost per hospital stay associated with each pressure ulcer ranges from $200 to $3000 for stage I, II, and III ulcers and up to $70,000 for a complex, full-thickness stage IV ulcer (Arnold, 2003). Increased lengths of stay in the hospital may cause patients, especially the elderly, to lose their independence, delay rehabilitation, and weaken normal social networks of support, making independence at discharge more difficult (Young, Evans, & Davis, 2003). The National Pressure Ulcer Advisory Panel (NPUAP) recommends that the following elements be considered when calculating pressure ulcer costs: physician fees, care-related devices, equipment, supplies, laboratory fees, drugs, and room and board associated with lengths of stay, nursing care, and nutritional interventions (Brillhart, 2005).

In addition to direct wound care costs and possible hospital admission, patients may also sustain psychosocial and emotional difficulties, especially when they are placed on bed rest because of their pressure ulcer. Patients on bed rest experience multiple hardships including missed work time and reduced leisure time. Increased need for personal care attendants to assist with activities of daily living, meal preparation, household errands, housekeeping, and other activities are a potential impact of bed rest that has far-reaching financial implications. Patients on bed rest may also experience compromised social interaction, decreased quality of life, and depression with the potential need for initiation of antidepressant or antianxiety medication. The potential onset of secondary complications related to the relative immobility of confinement to bed includes deconditioning and pneumonia. Other factors to be considered by individuals on prolonged bed rest include negative effect on functional status, relationships, and vocational and avocational activities (Brillhart, 2005). Pressure ulcers are a significant source of morbidity that seriously affects quality of life in persons with disabilities.

In home health care settings rehabilitation nurses may encounter the full range of chronic wounds, such as pressure ulcers, venous and arterial ulcers, neuropathic ulcers, nonhealing surgical wounds, and skin tears. Management of chronic wounds in the home health care setting is costly, and costs may be further increased by ineffective wound care practices, such as inaccurate or inconsistent wound assessments and failure to use appropriate wound care products or bed support surfaces. These factors may lead to prolonged healing times, lower healing rates, increased number of home health care visits, and more frequent hospitalizations secondary to complications (Buckley et al., 2005).

Ethnic Considerations

Patients often have a diversity of skin tones, which can pose a challenge to clinicians assessing patients for signs of blanchable and nonblanchable erythema (Bethell, 2005). Nonblanchable erythema of intact skin must be recognized as a warning sign that tissue death will quickly result unless pressure is completely removed from the area. In patients with darkly pigmented skin, erythema is often difficult to visually detect, but the effected skin is generally darker and warmer than the surrounding tissue. Edema or induration may also be indicators of stage I ulcers. In patients with more lightly pigmented skin, a stage I pressure ulcer may appear as a dark purple or red area that does not blanche under fingertip pressure (Folkedahl, 2002).

Edema and induration may also be indicators of stage I pressure ulcers in patients with lightly or darkly pigmented skin. It has been noted that photographs give better skin definition in patients with darkly pigmented skin, because the flash from the camera helps to visualize the area (Bethel, 2005). Because the usual signs of redness that characterize blanching and nonblanching erythema are difficult to detect in patients with darkly pigmented skin, it is important that an assessment be made by trained practitioners . Although it may be useful to ask the patient or caregiver to describe what they perceive as alterations in the skin, it is important to remember that caregivers who are not of the same ethnic background as the patient may be less sensitive to slight changes in the skin (Bethel, 2005).

ANATOMY AND PHYSIOLOGY

Understanding the anatomy and physiology of the skin, phases of the wound healing process, types and classifications of wounds, and wound repair is essential for recognizing factors that may complicate or delay wound healing. Each of these considerations plays a key role in the assessment and management of various wound types.

The skin is made up of two major layers, the epidermis and the dermis. Each layer is composed of different types of tissue and has different functions. A cross section of the skin is represented in Figure 15-1.

The outermost layer of the skin is the epidermis. Its primary functions are to maintain skin integrity and to act as a physical barrier. When the epidermis is intact, it prevents microorganisms from penetrating the skin. The epidermis has five sublayers: the outermost stratum corneum, the stratum lucidum, the stratum granulosum, the stratum spinosum, and the innermost stratum germinativum, or basal cell layer. The epidermis is vascular and relatively uniform in thickness throughout the body. Complete epidural renewal occurs every 2 months (Wysocki, 2007).

The dermis provides strength, support, blood, nutrients, and oxygen to the skin. This layer contains blood vessels, hair follicles, lymphatic vessels, sebaceous glands, and sweat glands. The tough, fibrous connective tissue of the dermis supports the epidermis. Tough, elastic, and flexible, this layer contains fibroblasts that synthesize and secrete collagen and elastin. Collagen is a protein that gives skin its tone and tensile strength, and elastin provides elastic recoil (Wysocki, 2007).

Subcutaneous tissue is composed of adipose and connective tissue, as well as major blood vessels, nerves, and lymphatic vessels. The thickness of the epidermis, dermis, and subcutaneous tissue varies from person to person and from one part of the body to another (Wysocki, 2007).

The skin is the largest organ of the body and has six functions. It provides **protection** against the outside environment. Nerve endings in the skin provide **sensation** and allow a person to feel pain, pressure, heat, and cold. Skin regulates body temperature, or **thermoregulation,** through vasoconstriction, vasodilation, and sweating. Waste products, such as electrolytes and water, are excreted through the skin, thereby aiding thermoregulation. Vitamin D is synthesized in skin exposed to sunlight, which activates metabolism

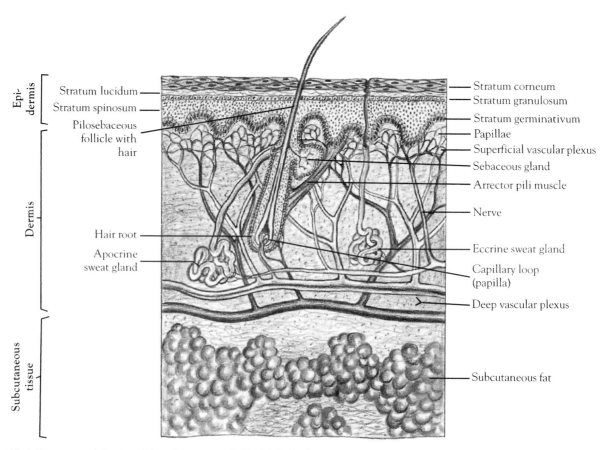

Figure 15-1 Structures of the skin. (From Thompson, J. M., McFarland, G. K., Hirsch, J. E., & Tucker, S. M. [1997]. *Mosby's clinical nursing* [4th ed.]. St. Louis, MO: Mosby.)

of calcium and phosphate. Finally, skin functions as a mode of identification and communication (Wysocki, 2007).

FACTORS INFLUENCING SKIN INTEGRITY

To better understand causal factors contributing to skin breakdown in the neurologically impaired patient, it is helpful to differentiate between extrinsic and intrinsic factors (Figure 15-2).

Extrinsic Factors

Four primary extrinsic factors contributing to alteration in skin integrity have been identified: pressure, shear, friction, and moisture. Of these, pressure is the most important causal factor. Pressure is a mechanical force that leads to the formation of pressure ulcers. The duration of pressure on tissue is an important factor considered along with intensity of pressure in determination of the amount of tissue damage (Pieper, 2007). *External pressure* applied to the skin for prolonged or unrelieved periods and in amounts in excess of capillary closing pressure will produce ischemia in underlying tissue. The blood vessels dilate in response to anoxia, leakage of fluid from the blood vessels causes interstitial edema, and forward flow of blood is impeded. The cells continue to produce metabolic byproducts that accumulate because they cannot be transported out as a result of vessel compromise.

The old adage "where there is no pressure, there is no pressure ulcer" remains true today (Priebe, Martin, Wuermser, Castillo, & McFarlin, 2003). Muscle is most sensitive to pressure-induced ischemia due to its high metabolic activity and ease of blood vessel compression. The time between the onset of pressure and the occurrence of tissue damage may be as

little as 1 hour of constant pressure. Tissues can tolerate much higher cyclic pressures than constant pressures. If pressure is relieved intermittently every 3 to 5 minutes, higher pressures can be tolerated (Kosiak, 1959). Pressure needs to be relieved frequently over time and reduced over the surface-skin interface. This translates to the clinical practice of weight shifting every few minutes to extend safe sitting times and the use of 2-hour minimum turning times in bed, or frequent small position changes in bed to provide pressure relief (Panel for Prediction and Prevention of Pressure Ulcers in Adults [PPPPUA], 1992).

Even when initial signs of pressure damage are recognized early and relief measures are initiated, deep muscle and fat necrosis may have already occurred (Priebe et al., 2003). Neurologically impaired patients who have microcirculation abnormalities resulting in decreased resting blood flow are at increased risk for pressure ulcer development.

Shear contributes to pressure areas and other skin injuries. Shear injury occurs when the skin remains stationary and the underlying tissue shifts (PPPPUA, 1992). Shearing forces (Figure 15-3) are produced when adjacent surfaces slide over one another (Bryant & Clark, 2007). Shearing forces cause blood vessels to become angulated, disrupting the arteries of the skin from the blood supply of the muscle. The typical shear injury presents as a wound with a large amount of undermining. Common causes of shearing are spasticity, poor sitting posture, poor bed positioning, and sliding rather than lifting the patient. When the head of the bed is elevated between 30 and 90 degrees, the patient may slide down, producing shearing forces. The sacrum, with the attached muscle and fascia, slides down while the skin stays in place; this causes shearing (Bryant & Clark, 2007). Shearing is frequently responsible for the triangular shaped ulcers overlying the sacrum and coccyx.

Friction is a mechanical force that occurs when the skin moves against a support surface, such as when extremities are brushed across a mattress. These movements can be inadvertent, as in spasticity, or due to carelessness. In its mildest form, friction produces skin tears: abrasions limited to the epidermal and dermal layers (Bryant & Clark, 2007). Friction decreases

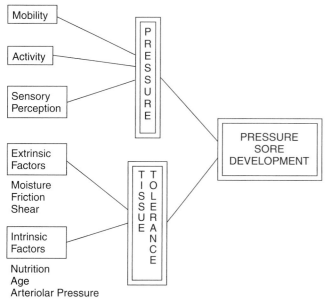

Figure 15-2 Braden and Bergstrom's conceptual schema of pressure sore risk factors. (From Braden, B., & Bergstrom, M. [1989]. A conceptual schema for the study of the etiology of pressure sores. *Rehabilitation Nursing, 14*[5], 258.)

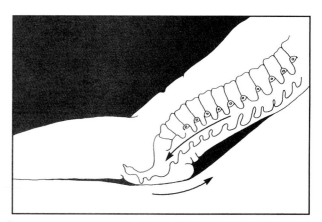

Figure 15-3 Shearing force. (From Bryant, R. A. [Ed.]. [2000]. *Acute and chronic wounds* [2nd ed]. St. Louis, MO: Mosby.)

the amount of external pressure required to produce a pressure ulcer, and when pressure combines with shear, friction contributes to extensive injury (PPPPUA, 1992). Skin breakdown related to friction often occurs over elbows and heels in patients on bed rest, because patients may use their elbows and heels to aid in movement. Elbows and heels are also subject to friction when a patient is agitated or experiencing spasticity or seizure activity (Arnold, 2003).

Skin tears occur when forces of minor friction or shearing cause the epidermis to separate from the dermis at the dermal-epidermal junction. These most commonly occur on the extremities of older adults (Payne & Martin, 1993a, 1993b). Skin tears can result from such varied activities as grasping an extremity, dressing, bathing, performing a transfer, and scraping against objects such as a table or chair (Bryant & Clark, 2007). Epidemiological studies suggest that at least 1.5 million skin tears occur each year in adults who are institutionalized (Thomas, Goode, LaMaster, Tennyson, & Parnell, 1999).

Evidence supports the premise that *moisture* alone can make the skin more susceptible to injury (PPPPUA, 1992). Moisture causes weakening of the connective tissue of the skin, making it five times as likely to become ulcerated as dry skin (Maklebust & Sieggreen, 1996). When exposed to prolonged moisture from sweating, urinary and fecal incontinence, and wound drainage, the skin can become macerated and develop a rash or become infected, predisposing it to pressure ulcer formation. Incontinence is a major risk factor and the most reliable predictor for pressure ulcer formation, especially fecal incontinence (Allman, Goode, Burst, Bartolucci, & Thomas, 1999) or urinary incontinence occurring with both friction and neurological disorders (Haalboom, den Boer, & Buskens, 1999). Conversely, skin that becomes excessively dry due to dehydration, lack of environmental humidity, or extended periods of cold is also susceptible to damage (Priebe et al., 2003).

Radiation can damage the epidermis, presenting with dry skin due to destruction of sweat and sebaceous glands. Radiation reduces fibroblasts and destroys the cell nucleus, which can result in wide, shallow, irregularly bordered wounds. Radiation-induced ulcers appear after being latent for 7 months to 8 years (Goldberg & McGinn-Byer, 2000). Irradiated skin requires continual assessment for changes and care to protect against mechanical and chemical assault.

Intrinsic Factors

Factors that occur throughout the body, intrinsic factors, may also contribute to alterations in skin integrity. These factors include neurological impairments, chronic diseases, poor nutritional status, vascular insufficiencies, immunosuppression, the aging process, and smoking. Paralysis and loss of protective sensation results in a decreased awareness of the effects of tissue ischemia. In fully sensate patients, early detection of an uncomfortable sensation results in a shift of body weight. In patients with decreased or absent sensation, this does not occur unless the patient has been taught to reposition body weight at frequent intervals or a care provider assists with frequent weight shifts or repositioning (Priebe et al., 2003).

Chronic diseases such as anemia, coronary artery disease, peripheral vascular disease, diabetes mellitus, and cancer adversely affect wound healing. Such diseases must be monitored and managed in order to heal wounds. Many wounds associated with chronic disease heal slowly, if at all. Fevers caused by acute or chronic disease increase metabolic demands and result in increased risk for pressure ulcer development (Priebe et al., 2003).

Malnutrition and vitamin or mineral abnormalities lead to increased risk of pressure ulcer development and decreased ability of the body to heal. Vitamins C, A, and E; zinc; protein; and individual amino acids all have been identified as necessary for prevention of pressure ulcers and for adequate wound healing (Thomas, 1997). Malnutrition has been reported in 52% to 85% of institutionalized elderly persons (Zulkowski, 1999). Hypoproteinemia leads to interstitial edema, which impairs the cellular transport of oxygen and nutrients. Vitamin C deficiencies can lead to capillary fragility and an impaired immune system (Ayello, Thomas, & Litchford, 1999; Stotts, 2000). Low serum albumin levels have been highly associated with pressure ulcer development (Bates-Jensen, 1998).

Two prospective studies show evidence that poor diet, especially inadequate intake of calories, protein, and iron, is a causative factor in pressure ulcer development (Bergstrom & Braden, 1992; PPPPUA, 1992). However, obese persons have many nutritional deficits and may have malnutrition despite their adequate calorie intake (Gallagher, 1997). Those with long-term tetraplegia are often in a hypometabolic state and frequently restrict their intake to control their weight, but they also have a significant increase in resting energy expenditure when a pressure ulcer is present (Lui, Spungen, Fink, Losada, & Bauman, 1996). Table 15-1 displays the role of select nutrients in wound healing. Figure 15-4 contains the Agency for Health Care Policy and Research (AHCPR), now known as the Agency for Healthcare Research and Quality (AHRQ), algorithm of recommendations for nutritional assessment and support for a patient who has an existing pressure ulcer.

Vascular insufficiencies affect the lower extremities, causing arterial, diabetic, venous, and pressure ulcers. These ulcers, caused by decreased blood supply, must be properly identified, and appropriate treatment must be initiated.

Immunosuppression, caused by disease or medication, may result in delayed wound healing. Many classifications of medications can affect the skin: corticosteroids interfere with epidermal proliferation, and others medications, such as specific antibiotics, have photosensitizing effects. A thorough review of the medication profile of every patient is essential to assess for possible medication effects on the skin.

Integumentary changes associated with aging result in thinner skin and associated increased risk of skin breakdown. Aging skin is less resilient against trauma and shear, and wounds in the elderly heal more slowly than those in younger patients (Bryant & Clark, 2007; Priebe et al., 2003).

Smoking is a risk factor for alteration in skin integrity. Studies examining the role of smoking in development of

TABLE 15-1 Role of Selected Nutrients in Wound Healing

Nutrient	Function
Protein	Cell multiplication, antibody production, wound remodeling; promotes angiogenesis and collagen synthesis
Carbohydrates	Provide energy to leukocytes and fibroblasts; cofactor for synthesis of fatty acids and some amino acids
Vitamin A	Promotes epithelialization and collagen synthesis; factor in inflammatory response
Vitamin B complex	Promotes protein synthesis; enhances antibody formation to promote immunity; cofactor in enzyme systems and cellular development; amino acid metabolism
Vitamin C	Hydroxylation of amino acids; immune reaction; promotes collagen synthesis for scar formation, capillary formation, and capillary permeability
Vitamin D	Absorption and metabolism of calcium from small intestine necessary for collagen maturation
Vitamin E	Antiinflammatory action; role in wound healing poorly understood
Vitamin K	Protein synthesis; prothrombin synthesis; synthesis of blood clotting factors VII, IX, X
Amino acids	Protein synthesis
Albumin	Maintenance of capillary colloid osmotic pressure
Essential fatty acids	Provide energy to leukocytes and fibroblasts; building blocks for prostaglandins; provide cellular membrane integrity
Copper	Component of enzyme systems in collagen maturation strength; hemoglobin synthesis
Iron	Hydroxylation of amino acids for collagen synthesis; supports oxygen transport via red blood cell formation
Magnesium	Activates enzymes for protein synthesis
Zinc	Role in vitamin A transport and plasma vitamin A concentration; promotes collagen and noncollagen protein activity in granulation tissue; stabilizes cellular membranes; cofactor in enzyme systems

From Andrychuk, M. A. (1998). Pressure ulcers: Causes, risk factors, assessment and intervention. *Orthopaedic Nursing, 17*(4), 65-82.

pressure ulcers for individuals with SCI found a correlation; the more a person smoked, the greater the incidence of pressure ulcers (Niazi, Salzberg, Byrne, & Viehbeck, 1997).

ASSESSMENT

Pressure Ulcer Risk Assessment

The purpose of a risk assessment tool is to identify patients at risk for pressure ulcer development, to target specific risk factors, and to define early intervention strategies for prevention (PPPUA, 1992). Although current risk assessment scales offer standardized measures of risk, their predictive value in rehabilitation populations, such as those with neurological deficits, requires continued investigation. In adults the Norton and Braden scales are two of the most common tools clinicians utilize to analyze a patient's risk for pressure ulcer development. The Norton scale has been tested extensively and consists of five parameters: physical condition, mental state, activity, mobility, and incontinence. Each parameter is rated on a scale from 1 to 4. The sum of the rating for all five parameters (range 5 to 20) is utilized to assess risk. Lower scores indicate higher risk. The "onset of risk" begins with a score of 12 or less.

The Braden scale is composed of six subscales that conceptually reflect degrees of sensory perception, skin moisture, physical activity, nutritional intake, friction, shear, and ability to change and control body position. All subscales are rated from 1 to 4, except for the friction and shear subscale, which is rated from 1 to 3. Each rating is accompanied by a brief description of criteria for assigning the rating. Potential scores range from 6 to 23. Initial studies found that a score equal to 16 or lower on the Braden scale provided the most accurate prediction of patients at risk for pressure ulcer development.

Recent studies indicate that a score of 18 or less may be more appropriate for patients who are older, physiologically unstable, or have less access to individualized care. The cumulative evidence suggests that a patient in any setting with a score of 18 or below should be considered at risk for pressure ulcer development (Bielan, 2005).

In the population of patients with SCI, values for sensory perception, activity, mobility, and friction/shear are all affected. Thus a person with tetraplegia can achieve a maximum possible score of 15, putting the person at high risk for pressure ulcer development without consideration of any other factors. Risk assessment scales specific to SCI have been proposed but have limited testing for validity or reliability (Priebe et al., 2003).

Epidemiological data indicate that infants and children who are significantly premature, are critically ill, have neurological impairments, have nutritional deficits, have poor tissue perfusion or oxygenation, or are exposed to prolonged pressure from hospital apparatus or tubes are at increased risk of pressure ulcer development. Pediatric skin assessment tools are currently being developed and tested for validity and reliability, including the Braden Q scale for children and Neonatal Skin Risk Assessment Scale for neonates. Until the validity and reliability of these scales can be further verified, their use should be combined with individualized and subjective risk assessment and combined with appropriate prevention strategies (Gray, 2004).

The frequency of risk assessment will vary according to the physical status of the patient and the care setting. Risk assessment scales cannot stand alone in predicting pressure ulcers in patients; thus a routine skin assessment for early signs of pressure injury is an essential adjunct to risk assessment.

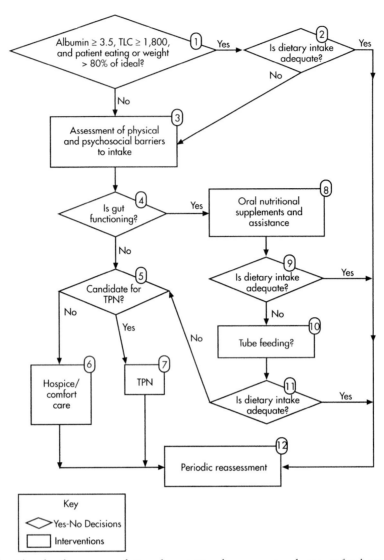

Figure 15-4 The AHCPR algorithm details recommendations for nutritional assessment and support for the patient who has an existing pressure ulcer. *TLC*, Total lymphocyte count; *TPN*, total parenteral nutrition. (From Bergstrom, N., Bennett, M. A., Carlson, C. E., et al. [1994]. *Treatment of pressure ulcers* [Clinical Practice Guideline No. 15, AHCPR Publication No. 95-0652]. Rockville, MD: U.S. Department of Health and Human Services, Agency for Health Care Policy and Research.)

Regardless of the care setting, frequency of skin assessment may need to be increased if the patient's status deteriorates.

Assessment of the Individual With a Pressure Ulcer

Individuals who present with a pressure ulcer should have a comprehensive assessment that includes the following: complete history; physical examination and laboratory tests; psychosocial status, cognitive status, and cultural beliefs; self-care abilities and utilization of personal care attendants; financial resources; mechanism of pressure ulcer development; posture, positioning, and equipment evaluation; and transfer techniques, frequency and type of weight shifts, and methods for short- and long-distance mobility.

Adequate nutritional support is critical for patients with pressure ulcers. A baseline nutritional assessment includes height and weight, calculation of body mass index (BMI), clinical indicators of malnutrition, laboratory studies, determination of current nutrient intake, and determination of nutrient needs (Evans, 2005). The prealbumin level is considered a sensitive indicator of nutritional status, particularly in the hospitalized patient. Prealbumin has a 2-day half-life and is more reflective of nutritional status than albumin, which can be affected by hydration status and has a 21-day half-life. Additional laboratory tests that can be used to complement the prealbumin and albumin levels include a complete blood count (CBC), C-reactive protein (CRP), erythrocyte sedimentation rate (ESR), and total lymphocyte count (TLC) (Evans, 2005).

Common Sites of Pressure Ulcers

Pressure ulcers most frequently occur over bony prominences including the sacrum, ischium, trochanter, and calcaneus (Figure 15-5). In acute care hospitals the most common sites for patients to develop pressure ulcers are the sacrum and heels (Blaszcyk, Majewski, & Sato, 1998; Tourtual, Riesenberg, Korutz, Semo, Asef, & Gill, 1997), but pressure ulcers can occur in any location where soft tissue in compressed. The most common cause of pressure ulcer formation is positional pressure (47.4%), followed by pressure from cervical collars (23.7%) and tracheostomy/endotracheal tubes (10.5%) (Watts et al., 1998). Pressure ulcer formation in patients with SCI is greatest on the ischium (28%), sacrum (21%), and trochanter (20%) (Priebe et al., 2003). In the immediate acute trauma period for SCI, the most common areas of pressure ulcer formation are on the sacrum (57%) and on the heels (22%) (Carlson, King, Kirk, Temple, & Heinemann, 1992). The sacrum is the most common site for severe pressure ulcers in patients with SCI, due in part to time spent on the spine board or the operating room table (Main, 1996).

In the pediatric population the most common skin breakdown locations are in the sitting area (35%), foot (20%), and upper extremities (18%). The sitting area includes the buttocks, sacrum/coccyx, scrotum, and hip. The most common types of skin breakdown beyond pressure ulcers are excoriation/ diaper dermatitis (42%), skin tear (17%), and intravenous (IV) extravasations (15%) (Gray, 2004).

Wound Assessment

Comprehensive evaluation of a pressure ulcer includes assessment of the wound stage, size and depth, and additional characteristics such as drainage and presence of eschar. The condition of the surrounding tissue is an element of wound assessment. Presently there is no universal classification system for pressure ulcers.

Classification of Wounds by Staging. Pressure ulcers are classified by a standardized measurement system termed staging. Staging systems identify wounds by the layers of tissue involved. Staging does not describe all elements of a wound and is only a representation of the wound depth. In 2007, the National Pressure Ulcer Advisory Panel (NPUAP) published definitions of pressure ulcers and the stages of pressure ulcers (Figure 15-5). The staging definitions include the original four stages, adding two stages relative to deep tissue injury and unstageable pressure ulcers (NPUAP, 2007). Pressure ulcer stages and definitions are given in the following section (NPUAP, 2007).

Stage I pressure ulcers present as intact skin, with nonblanchable redness or erythema, a localized area usually over a bony prominence. Stage II pressure ulcers represent partial-thickness loss presenting as a shallow, open ulcer with a red-pink wound bed, without slough. A stage II ulcer may also present as an intact or open/ruptured serum-filled blister. Stage III pressure ulcers represent full-thickness tissue loss. Stage III ulcers may have undermining and tunneling. The depth

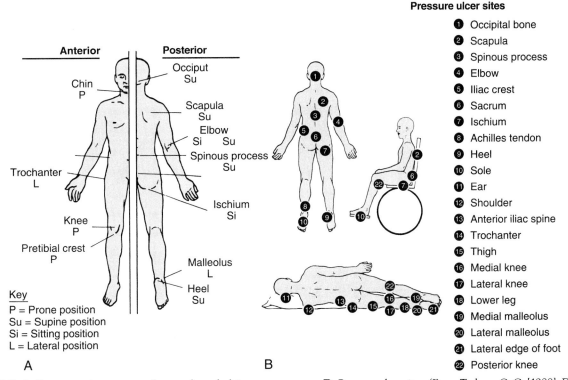

Figure 15-5 A, Bony prominences most frequently underlying pressure sores. **B,** Pressure ulcer sites. (From Trelease C. C. [1988]. Developing standards for wound care, *Ostomy/Wound Management 26*[50], 1998.) Used with permission of *Ostomy/Wound Management.*

Staging of Pressure Ulcers

Suspected deep tissue: Purple or maroon localized area of discolored intact skin or blood-filled blister; surrounding tissue may be painful, firm, mushy, boggy, or warmer or cooler compared to adjacent tissue.

Stage I—characterized by an observable alteration of intact skin, which may include the following:
- Skin temperature (warmth or coolness)
- Tissue consistency (firm or boggy feel)
- Sensation (pain, itching)

The ulcer area is defined by persistent redness in lightly pigmented skin; in darker skin a persistent red, blue, or purple tone is visible.

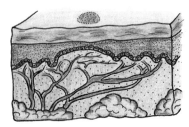 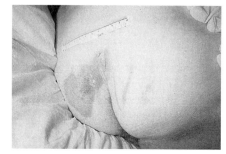

Stage II—characterized by partial-thickness skin loss involving epidermis and/or dermis. Superficial ulcer appears as an abrasion, blister, or shallow crater.

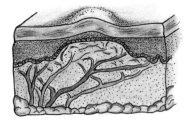 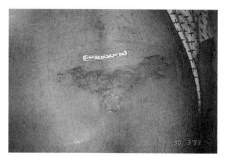

Stage III—characterized by full-thickness skin loss involving damage to subcutaneous tissue down to, but not through, fascia. The ulcer appears to be a deep crater and may include undermining of adjacent tissue.

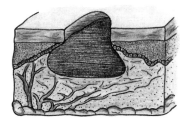 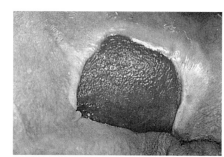

Stage IV—characterized by full-thickness skin loss with extensive destruction including tissue necrosis; damage to muscle, bone, tendons, joint capsule; and undermining and sinus tracts.

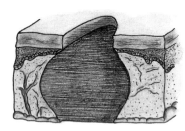 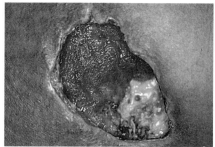

Unstageable ulcer: Full-thickness tissue loss in which the base of the ulcer is covered by slough (yellow, tan, gray, green, or brown) or eschar (tan, brown, or black) in the wound bed. Until enough slough or eschar is removed to expose wound base, the true depth and therefore stage cannot be determined.

Figure 15-6 Assessment of pressure ulcers is not possible if eschar is present. Once the eschar has sloughed or the wound is debrided, an accurate assessment may be completed. (Data from National Pressure Ulcer Advisory Panel. [2007]. Pressure ulcer prevalence, cost and risk assessment: Consensus development conference statement, *Decubitus* 2[2], 24, 1989.

of a stage III pressure ulcer varies by anatomical location. The bridge of the nose, ear, occiput, and malleolus do not have subcutaneous tissue, and stage III ulcers can be shallow. In contrast, areas of significant adiposity can develop extremely deep stage III pressure ulcers. Bone or tendon is not visible or directly palpable. Stage IV pressure ulcers represent full-thickness skin loss with exposed tendon or muscle. Slough or eschar may be present on some parts of the wound bed. Often these wounds have undermining and tunneling. The depth of a stage IV pressure ulcer also varies by anatomical location. Stage IV ulcers can extend into muscle and supporting structures (e.g., fascia, tendon, or joint capsule), making osteomyelitis possible. Exposed bone or tendon is visible and directly palpable.

Suspected deep tissue injury is defined as a purple or maroon localized area of discolored intact skin or blood-filled blister due to damage of underlying soft tissue from pressure or shear. The area may be preceded by tissue that is painful, firm, mushy, boggy, warmer, or cooler compared to adjacent tissue. Deep tissue injury may be difficult to detect in individuals with dark skin tones. Evolution may include a thin blister over a dark wound bed. The wound may further evolve and become covered by a thin eschar. Evolution may be rapid, exposing additional layers of tissue even with optimal treatment.

An unstageable pressure ulcer is defined as full-thickness tissue loss in which the base of the ulcer is covered by slough (yellow, tan, gray, green, or brown) or eschar (tan, brown, or black) in the wound bed. Until enough slough or eschar is removed to expose the base of the wound, the true depth, and therefore stage, cannot be determined.

Wound Size. Wound size is used to measure a patient's progress toward healing and provides information about the efficacy of the wound treatment being performed. A number of techniques have been developed to measure wound size. The three-dimensional linear technique is the most common. This technique measures wound length, width, and depth. A long-handled cotton-tipped applicator and disposable ruler are the tools for measuring the wound length, width, and depth of the cavity. Undermining and tracking in the wound bed are also measured. Undermining is defined as an extension of the wound under the skin surface that is parallel to the skin surface. Tracking is defined as a tract heading away from the wound in any direction. Undermining and tracts are best documented as components of the face of a clock (e.g., 30-mm tract at 2 o'clock or undermining from 3 o'clock to 6 o'clock) (Priebe et al., 2003).

Another common approach to wound measurement is by tracing the wound diameter. The consistency with which these measurements are taken affects the reliability of the measurements. Wounds can be difficult to trace depending on their location, because a patient's position can alter the shape of the wound opening (Cooper, 2000).

Photographic wound images may provide powerful support to linear measurements. Photography should be considered as a part of the pressure ulcer assessment. If photographs are used, then consistent methodology in obtaining the photograph is essential. For example, because background can improve the clarity of the image, extraneous clutter around the area to be photographed should be removed. To provide an optimal photograph, a background drape of medium blue or white should be used; avoid colors such as black or gray. Another technique, which supports comparative measures and assessments, is to include a disposable tape measure in centimeters marked with the patient's identification number and body part (Buckley et al., 2005). Documenting the distance from which the photograph was taken is extremely important, because different distances can distort the true size of the pressure ulcer (Lyder & Torpy, 2003). Ultrasonic scanners can capture and reproduce images of soft tissue at high resolution via laptop computers; the images are then stored or e-mailed to other clinicians for interpretation (Salcido, 2000).

Wound characteristics that are more difficult to photograph, such as undermining and tunneling, can be captured with the use of cotton-tipped applicators, one placed within and the other parallel to it outside the wound. This photography technique also allows the viewer to appreciate the depth and angle of tunnels and tracts. Edema presents another clinical finding that is difficult to photograph. A distant image of an edematous extremity may help clarify the extent and location of edema, which can be masked in close-up images of the wound. Photographs of the opposite extremity may also benefit as a comparison to help assess the severity of the edema (Buckley et al., 2005).

Wound Base. The type of tissue in the wound base can range from viable tissue to nonviable tissue. Viable tissue includes granulation, epithelialization, subcutaneous tissue, and muscle and must be distinguished from nonviable tissue (Nix, 2007a). Slough is a form of nonviable tissue and is identified by soft yellow, brown, or gray material that is characterized by its stringy adherent quality. A necrotic ulcer may appear hard and dry in the form of eschar or soft with nonviable tissue in the wound base. Both sloughing and necrotic tissue require debridement. The amount of slough and necrotic tissue should be documented as an estimated percentage of coverage in the wound base. Underlying support structures, such as bone, tendon, or joint capsule, may be visible or palpable in the wound (Priebe et al., 2003).

Wound Exudate. The type and amount of wound exudate, including color, provides information about the phase of wound healing, as well as the presence or absence of infection. Terms used to describe exudate include creamy, tan, yellow, green, purulent, sanguineous, serous, and serosanguineous (Arnold, 2003). Increased exudate is frequently an indicator of bacterial colonization and is a major determinant in choice of dressing material utilized. Copiously draining wounds are those producing more than 50 ml per day (Priebe et al., 2003).

Wound Edges. Assessment and documentation of the condition of the wound edges can provide information regarding the condition of a wound. Ideally, advancing epithelium would be seen at the wound edge, migrating across a healthy bed of granulation tissue. If the wound margins or edges of a wound are rolled, this suggests that the wound is chronic in nature (Priebe et al., 2003).

Periwound Skin. Periwound skin assessment is an additional component of wound assessment. The condition of the skin surrounding a wound can assist in determination of the state of wound healing. Inflammation may present as erythematous, edematous, or warm skin surrounding a wound and may indicate the presence of infection. Maceration of the periwound skin may indicate excess drainage of the wound and indicate a need for a more absorbent dressing material (Arnold, 2003).

Wound Healing Assessment Tools

Several tools have been developed and validated to assess the healing of pressure ulcers. The two most widely used tools are the Pressure Sore Status Tool (PSST) and the Pressure Ulcer Scale for Healing (PUSH). The PSST is a data collection form designed to describe the status of a pressure ulcer over time. Thirteen items are scored on a Likert scale. The indicators that are measured include wound size, depth, edges, undermining, necrotic tissue, exudate type, exudate amount, skin color surrounding the wound, peripheral tissue edema, peripheral tissue induration, granulation tissue, and epithelialization. The sum of the 13 items provides a numerical indicator of the assessment of the wound. One of the advantages of the PSST is that it can be used to assess any chronic wound. Several disadvantages are that the PSST requires more time to complete than other tools, requires training to obtain reliable measurements, and has not been tested in the population of patients with disabilities (Mullins, Thomason, & Legro, 2005).

The PUSH tool is a data collection form developed by a task force of the NPUAP (2005). The PUSH tool was designed to assess the progression of an ulcer over time. The tool has three subscores: length by width, exudate amount, and tissue type. The total score consists of the sum of the three subscores. The score is displayed by two graphing formats. The graph of the patient's accumulated PUSH score reflects the trajectory of change of the wound over time (NPUAP, 2005). The advantages of the PUSH tool are that it takes less than 1 minute to complete, provides a graphic format to review healing over time, and has been tested for validity and reliability in multiple samples. Several disadvantages are that the PUSH does not include elements of undermining or tunneling and does not specifically measure necrotic eschar, slough, granulation, or epithelial tissue (Mullins et al., 2005).

Documentation

Consistent documentation of wounds is essential to monitor progress in wound healing or deterioration of the wound over time. Elements to be documented include etiology and type of ulcer; anatomical location of the ulcer; ulcer measurement in millimeters or centimeters; stage of the ulcer; description

of the wound edges; measurement of undermining, tunneling, or sinus tracts; and a description of the wound bed, including notation of the presence or absence of necrotic or granulation tissue, exudates, and odor, and description of the periwound skin.

FACTORS INFLUENCING WOUND HEALING

Phases of Wound Healing

When alteration in skin integrity occurs and a wound develops, the healing process begins. There are three phases of wound healing: inflammatory, proliferative, and maturation.

The first phase of wound healing is the **inflammatory phase**, characterized by edema, erythema, hyperemia, and in sensate patients, pain. The inflammatory phase typically lasts 4 to 6 days. The second phase of wound healing is the **proliferative phase**. Granulation tissue is generated during the proliferative phase. Granulation tissue appears as beefy red, shiny, and granular. In this phase, collagen is produced, which gives tissue its tensile strength. The wound bed fills with granulation tissue, causing the wound margins to contract, which results in a decrease in the size of the wound surface. This phase lasts from 4 to 24 days. The last phase of wound healing is the **maturation phase.** The maturation phase results in epithelialization of the wound, thereby sealing the skin from the external environment. This phase results in scar formation, remodeling, and increasing tensile strength. This process continues until the scar has regained about 80% of the skin's original strength, which can last from 21 days to 2 years. Scar tissue will always be at risk for breakdown, because its tensile strength is less than that of uninjured skin (Black & Black, 2007).

Increased bacterial load is a common complication that causes wounds to stagnate during the healing process. Bacterial load may lead to local or systemic infection. Signs of wound infection include fever, leukocytosis, erythema, hyperemia, edema, induration, odor, and increased drainage. When treating chronic wounds that do not progress, infection may be the primary culprit (Montroy & Eltorai, 2003).

Wound Repair

There are three types of wound repair: primary, secondary, and tertiary intention. Acute wounds, such as surgical incisions, are closed by primary intention, with the skin edges touching one another, which results in less risk of infection, and healing usually occurs with minimal scarring in 4 to 14 days. Chronic wounds, such as pressure ulcers, heal by secondary intention with the wound edges not approximating or touching. These wounds result in greater tissue loss, higher rate of infection, and longer healing time. Healing by tertiary intention occurs when there is delayed primary closure. Significant infection is a common reason for closure by tertiary intention. Closure or approximation of the wound is delayed to allow edema or infection to resolve (Doughty & Sparks-Defriese, 2007).

WOUNDS COMMONLY MANAGED BY REHABILITATION NURSES

Nurses in rehabilitation settings most often encounter three categories of wounds: pressure ulcers, neuropathic ulcers, and arterial and venous ulcers. Pressure ulcers can occur over any bony prominence or anywhere on the body where there is unrelieved pressure. Lower extremity ulcers may be caused by pressure or by other chronic disease, including diabetes mellitus, or arterial or venous insufficiency.

Lower Extremity Ulcers

Neuropathic Ulcers. Patients with diabetic peripheral neuropathy experience varying degrees of symptoms from sensory, motor, or autonomic origins, or a combination. Loss of sensation is most problematic because it predisposes the foot to trauma and skin breakdown. Musculoskeletal abnormalities may be present that result in muscular atrophies of the foot, thinning under the metatarsal heads, bony deformity and other changes that may lead to undue stress on the foot and leading to pressure, shear, friction, and potential for development of ulcers (Driver, Landowski & Madsen, 2007).

Arterial and Venous Ulcers. Some patients have both arterial and venous ulcers, and treatment for one type of ulcer may exacerbate the symptoms or alter the healing of the other type. Insufficient arterial perfusion to an extremity causes arterial ulcers (Doughty & Holbrook, 2007). Less common than venous ulcers, they are more difficult to manage with the complexity of disease processes and complications. The lack of perfusion to the lower extremity creates great difficulty for wound healing. Peripheral vascular disease is the associated disease entity with arterial insufficiency. It involves the arteries, veins, and lymphatics.

Venous insufficiency leads to venous ulcers that result from disorders of the deep venous system. Most commonly the origin is damage to incompetent valves from thrombosis in the deep or superficial veins (Doughty & Holbrook, 2007). Damage occurs to the veins or calf muscle pump, resulting in high venous pressure in the deep veins (venous hypertension). Precursors include clinical conditions that trigger a sequence of events promoting edema and perhaps dermal ulceration (Doughty & Holbrook, 2007). When a disease process alters the flow of blood forward, dysfunction ensues, resulting in increased hydrostatic pressure and venous hypotension, leading to dermal ulceration.

NURSING DIAGNOSIS

As with any area of nursing practice, nursing diagnoses are useful to the rehabilitation nurse in describing clinical assessments about health-related conditions, projecting outcomes, and planning interventions. Examples of nursing diagnoses applicable to maintaining skin integrity in patients requiring rehabilitation nursing services are listed in Table 15-2. The primary diagnoses are impaired skin integrity and risk for impaired skin integrity. The associated or contributing diagnoses might include deficient knowledge: skin management and nutritional management; impaired physical mobility; impaired bed mobility; impaired transfer ability; impaired wheelchair mobility; and self-care deficit (Dochterman & Bulechek, 2004).

REHABILITATION NURSING INTERVENTIONS

Nursing interventions to promote, maintain, and manage skin integrity target three primary aspects of care: prevention strategies, treatment considerations, and patient education.

Prevention

Nursing intervention for skin management is targeted primarily at prevention. As mentioned previously, the risk for alteration in skin integrity is an integral component of health assessment and will guide the prevention efforts of the rehabilitation nurse. Identified risk factors should be incorporated into the plan of care. The AHRQ recommends four target goals: (1) identify at-risk individuals who need prevention and the specific factors placing them at risk; (2) maintain and improve tissue tolerance to pressure in order to prevent injury; (3) protect against the adverse effects of pressure, friction, and shear; and (4) reduce the incidence of pressure ulcers through educational programs (PPPPUA, 1992).

Additional recommendations for prevention and treatment of pressure, mechanical loading and support surfaces, and educational programs for the prevention of pressure ulcers are outlined in Boxes 15-1, 15-2, and 15-3 (American Hospital Association, 1997).

Support Surfaces. Bed support surfaces are an important element of available preventative strategies. A support surface is "a device that redistributes pressure" and may also reduce shear friction and moisture (Nix, 2007b, p. 535). Support surfaces can be described as pressure-relieving or pressure-reducing devices. Pressure-relieving and reducing devices are surfaces that create a skin-resting surface interface pressure to near capillary closing pressure and therefore less likely to interrupt or occlude capillary blood flow. Pressure relieving surfaces are products that present skin-resting surface interface pressures consistently below 32 mm Hg. Pressure-reducing surfaces are those that lower the skin-resting surface interface pressure to a pressure above 32 mm Hg but lower than a standard hospital mattress (Nix, 2007b).

Support surfaces can also be categorized as to whether the support surface is dynamic or static. Dynamic systems are electrically powered to alternate inflation and deflation of the support surface channels/baffles and thus reduce pressure from body surfaces. Static devices reduce pressure by spreading the body weight over a larger area.

In addition, support surfaces can be categorized as overlays, replacement mattresses, and specialty beds. Overlay mattresses are products that lie on top of the standard mattress. Mattress replacements are used in place of the standard hospital mattress and are placed on the hospital bed frame. Both overlay mattresses and mattress replacements help with pressure

TABLE 15-2 Nursing Diagnoses, Interventions, and Outcomes Applicable to Skin Management

NIC/NOC

Nursing Diagnosis	Nursing Interventions	Nursing Outcomes
Risk for impaired skin integrity	Pressure management Skin surveillance Positioning Pressure ulcer prevention Risk identification Nutritional management/therapy Self-care assistance Foot care intervention Health education	Risk reduction Risk control Tissue integrity Tissue perfusion Immobility consequences Nutritional status Risk reduction/control
Impaired skin integrity	Health education Pressure ulcer assessment/care Skin surveillance Infection control/protection Support surfaces to protect the skin or aid in healing Skin care: Topical treatment Pressure management/positioning Initiate consultation of a certified wound, ostomy, continence nurse as needed	Tissue integrity Wound healing Tissue perfusion Nutritional status Self-care Fluid balance Immobility consequences Treatment behavior
Deficient knowledge: skin management	Health education Learning facilitation Learning readiness enhancement Teaching: pressure ulcer prevention, development, treatment, pressure points Teaching: prescribed diet and nutrition management	Knowledge: skin care and treatment regimen Knowledge: prevention of pressure ulcers
Imbalanced nutrition: less than body requirements	Fluid/electrolyte management Nutritional counseling Nutritional management Nutrition therapy Nutritional monitoring Teaching: prescribed diet Encourage intake of protein and supplements as needed Consult dietician as needed	Nutritional status: nutrient intake
Impaired physical mobility/impaired bed mobility	Exercise promotion Exercise therapy Positioning Self-care assistance Fall prevention Bed rest care Pain management Skin surveillance	Body positioning: self-initiated Immobility consequences Neurological status

Data from Moorhead, S., Johnson, M., & Maas, M. (Eds.). (2004). *Nursing outcomes classification (NOC)* (3rd ed.). St. Louis, MO: Mosby; Dochterman, J. M., & Bulechek, G. M. (2004). *Nursing interventions classification (NIC)* (4th ed.). St. Louis, MO: Mosby; and NANDA International. (2005). *Nursing diagnoses: Definitions and classification, 2005-2006* (6th ed.). Philadelphia: Author.

BOX 15-1 Recommendations for Skin Care and Early Treatment of Pressure Ulcers

- Inspect the skin of all at-risk individuals at least once a day, but ideally with every patient turn for erythema or areas of breakdown; pay particular attention to bony prominences.
- Document results of skin inspection.
- Cleanse the skin at the time of soiling and at routine intervals; individualize the frequency of skin cleansing according to need and/or patient preference.
- Avoid hot water, and use a mild cleansing agent that minimizes irritation and dryness of the skin.
- During cleansing, take care to minimize the force and friction applied to the skin.
- Minimize environmental factors leading to skin drying, such as low humidity (less than 40%) and exposure to cold; treat dry skin with moisturizers.
- Avoid massage over bony prominences.
- Minimize skin exposure to moisture due to incontinence, perspiration, or wound drainage.
- Minimize skin injury due to friction and shear forces through proper positioning, transferring, and turning techniques; friction injuries may be reduced by the use of lubricants, protective films, protective dressings, and protective padding.
- When apparently well-nourished patients develop an inadequate dietary intake of protein or calories, first attempt to discover the factors compromising intake and offer support, including nutritional supplements, as needed; for nutritionally compromised individuals, implement a plan of nutritional support and/or supplementation.

Data from American Hospital Association. (1997, November). Here are highlights of pressure ulcer guideline. *Healthcare Benchmarks*, 162-163.

BOX 15-2 Recommendations for Management of Mechanical Loading and Support Surfaces

- Reposition any individual in bed who is assessed to be at risk for developing pressure ulcers at least every 2 hours if consistent with overall patient goals; teach patients using wheelchairs to shift their weight every 15 minutes.
- For individuals in bed, use positioning devices such as pillows or foam wedges to keep bony prominences from direct contact with one another.
- Maintain the head of the bed at the lowest degree of elevation consistent with medical conditions and other restrictions; limit the amount of time the head of the bed is elevated.
- Use lifting devices such as a trapeze or bed linen to move (rather than drag) individuals in bed who cannot assist during transfers and position changes.
- Place any individual at risk for developing pressure ulcers on a pressure-reducing device, such as a foam, static air, alternating air, gel, or water mattress, when he or she is lying in bed.
- For chair-bound individuals, use a pressure-reducing device; do not use doughnut-shaped devices.

Data from American Hospital Association. (1997, November). Here are highlights of pressure ulcer guideline. *Healthcare Benchmarks*, 162-163.

BOX 15-3 Recommendations for Educational Programs for the Prevention of Pressure Ulcers

- Be structured, organized, comprehensive, and directed at all levels of health care providers, patients, and family caregivers.
- Include information on cause of and risk factors for pressure ulcers, risk assessment tools and their application, skin assessment, selection and/or use of support surfaces, development and implementation of an individualized program of skin care, demonstration of positioning to decrease risk of tissue breakdown, and instruction on accurate documentation of pertinent information.
- Identify persons responsible for pressure ulcer prevention, describe each person's role, and be appropriate to the audience in terms of level of information presented and expected participation.

Data from American Hospital Association. (1997, November). Here are highlights of pressure ulcer guideline. *Healthcare Benchmarks*, 162-163.

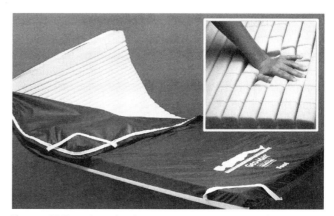

Figure 15-7 Bed overlay. (Courtesy Span-America Medical Systems, Greenville, SC.)

reduction but do not provide complete pressure relief. Full-framed products are called specialty beds and replace the entire bed unit, including the mattress and its frame.

Overlays and mattress replacements are the most common types of support systems and are made of foam, air, alternating air, and gel materials (Figure 15-7). All mattress overlays raise the level of the bed surface, which may create safety issues, such as the patient rolling over the side rails or becoming wedged between the side rails and the overlay. The patient's ability to independently transfer with the increased height of the bed may be problematic. Caregivers must be cautious about utilizing good body mechanics because positioning, turning, and transfers may be difficult with the raised bed height. Because moisture against the patient's skin may occur, air-filled, low air-loss, and alternating air-filled overlays may be the best choice for certain patients. Replacement mattresses are covered with a comfortable bacteriostatic cover that can be cleaned.

Full-framed specialty beds require some form of electric pump and are at the high end of the specialty bed spectrum. The three basic types of beds in this group are high air loss, low air loss, and kinetic therapy. High air-loss beds are also called fluid-air beds and use high air flow through silicon beads to provide pressure relief to most body surfaces. Pressure relief is not absolute on high air-loss beds because studies have continued to report heel pressure on these surfaces (PPPPUA, 1992). These surfaces generally can provide pressure relief on patients who cannot be turned, have stage III or IV pressure ulcers on one or more turning surfaces, or for protection of the surgical site the first several weeks after myocutaneous flap surgery. Disadvantages in utilizing this type of support surface include patient dehydration, wound drying, heat generation for the patient and the ambient environment, and disorientation. High air-loss beds are not recommended for patients with spinal instability or pulmonary disease (Nix, 2007b).

Low air-loss beds consist of a hospital bed frame that holds a series of interconnected air-filled pillows surrounding the bed. The amount of pressure in the pillows can be controlled to provide maximum pressure reduction for the patient. Low air-loss beds are superior to air overlays because they offer significant inflation, which protects the patient from "bottom-out" against the bed frame (Priebe et al., 2003).

Kinetic therapy is provided by some specialty beds. These beds are designed to counteract the effects of immobility by continuous passive motion or oscillation therapy. Some beds are a combination of oscillation therapy and low air loss. Oscillation therapy is believed to provide mobilization of respiratory secretions and decrease the incidence of atelectasis and pneumonia.

The heels are known to be particularly vulnerable to pressure, even on pressure-reducing support surfaces (Blaszczyk et al., 1998). To protect heels when the patient is in the supine position, pillows should be used to support the entire length of the legs, ending at the ankles and suspending the heels above the mattress. The heels must be checked frequently to ensure that, as the pillows compress, they remain free of pressure. If use of the pillows is not effective in protecting the heels, a number of commercially available pressure-reducing devices are available. Sheepskin and foam boots can help protect the heels from shearing and friction or bumping the feet during transfers. Multi Podus boots that completely elevate the foot from the support surface are most effective when pressure relief is needed.

The bariatric population requires appropriate equipment as well as adequate personnel to meet their patient care needs. Bariatric patients are at increased risk for skin breakdown and present a challenge to clinicians and facilities in terms of providing care such as turning and transferring that is crucial to optimal patient outcomes. Access to equipment that can accommodate a patient's weight and size is an important consideration for patient care (Wright & Bauer, 2005).

Wheelchair Cushions. Wheelchair cushions are considered a primary intervention (Figure 15-8). Wheelchair

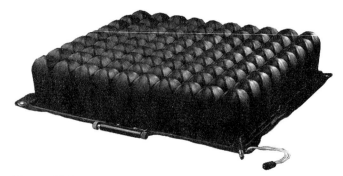

Figure 15-8 Wheelchair cushion. (Courtesy The ROHO Group, Inc., Belleville, IL.)

cushions are critical for protecting the skin over bony prominences, especially for patients who have motor sensory deficits and use a wheelchair for mobility. Physical therapists are trained to evaluate a patient's needs and recommend an appropriate wheelchair cushion.

The purpose of a cushion is to distribute pressure loads over the entire sitting surface and keep excess pressure off bony prominences. Pressure, shear, heat, moisture, and postural control can all contribute to the development of a pressure ulcer and must be considered in selection of a cushion or seating system (Rapple, 1998). Patients with cognitive ability and upper strength are taught to shift their weight every 15 minutes when sitting in a wheelchair. When selecting a wheelchair cushion, consideration should be given to the patient's body weight and habitus, ease of transfer from the cushion, continence status, reimbursement by the patient's insurer, and durability of the cushion.

Treatment

Management of skin integrity focuses primarily on pressure reduction, prevention of shear and friction, and moisture control. These factors were discussed previously with prevention strategies. Intrinsic factors, also mentioned previously, must be managed. This section will focus on wound management once a pressure ulcer develops. The AHCPR algorithm for treatment of pressure ulcers (Figure 15-9) illustrates a conceptual overview (PPPUA, 1994).

Local Wound Care. Local wound care involves cleansing and debriding the wound, treating infection, and selecting an appropriate dressing.

Wound Cleansing. The AHRQ recommends using normal saline solution with enough irrigation pressure to enhance wound cleansing without causing trauma to the wound bed (PPPPUA, 1994). Trauma inflicted by the cleansing process must be justified by the effectiveness of the procedure. Extremely necrotic wounds require more mechanical force. However, as the wound becomes cleaner, the mechanical force and cleanser strength can be decreased proportionally.

Antiseptic cleansers such as povidone-iodine, acetic acid, Dakin's solution, and hydrogen peroxide should not be used

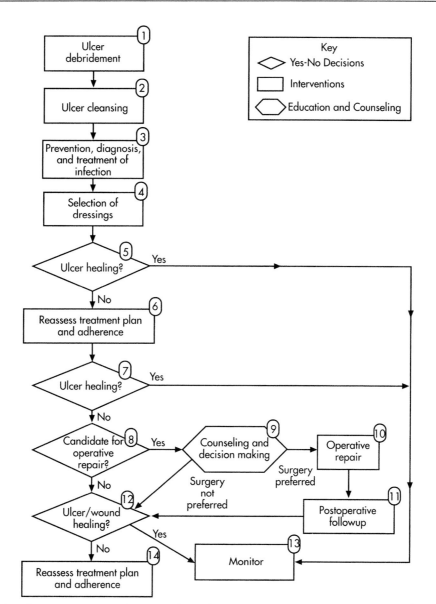

Figure 15-9 The AHRQ algorithm for treatment of pressure ulcers. (From Bergstrom, N., Bennett, M. A., Carlson, C. E., et al. [1994]. *Treatment of pressure ulcers.* [Clinical Practice Guideline No. 15, AHCPR Publication No. 95-0652]. Rockville, MD: U.S. Department of Health and Human Services, Agency for Health Care Policy and Research.)

for routine wound cleansing because of their harmful effects on healing tissue (Rolstad, Ovington, & Harris, 2000). Povidone-iodine damages granulation tissue and may cause iodine toxicity (Eaglstein, 1986). Acetic acid is effective against *Pseudomonas aeruginosa* but also damages proliferating tissue. Dakin's solution is irritating to granulation tissue as well as surrounding tissue. Although hydrogen peroxide provides mechanical cleansing, it is harmful to new tissue, and the air bubbles formed can cause air emboli if introduced into sinus tracts.

Debridement. Necrotic tissue prolongs the inflammatory process and promotes bacterial growth, and therefore necrotic tissue must be debrided. Debridement can be accomplished with selective methods, which remove only nonviable tissue, or by nonselective methods. Selective methods include surgical or sharp, autolytic, and enzymatic debridement.

Nonselective methods include wet-to-dry dressings, pressurized irrigation, and whirlpool. Surgical or sharp debridement uses a scalpel, scissors, and forceps.

Autolytic debridement is facilitated by covering the wound with a moisture-retentive dressing such as a hydrocolloid or transparent film. Usually within 72 to 96 hours of occlusion the necrotic tissue begins to liquefy as the polymorphonuclear leukocytes, macrophages, and bacteria in the wound fluid provide endogenous enzymes to continue autodigestion. Enzymatic debridement involves topical application of an exogenous enzyme that digests necrotic tissue. Santyl and Accuzyme are examples of topical enzymatic debriding agents that break up the collagen fibers that hold the necrotic tissue within the wound base. Eschar is removed or cross-hatched to improve the penetration of debriding agents.

Nonselective methods such as wet-to-dry dressings remove necrotic tissue when removed but also remove fragile epithelial cells and newly formed granulation tissue and increase patient discomfort. Pressurized irrigation and whirlpool are also nonselective and are used to remove necrotic tissue but are discontinued once the wounds are clean and granulation tissue is present (Baharestani, 1999).

Management of Excess Exudate. Wound exudate must be absorbed to prevent maceration of surrounding tissue and dilution of the wound-healing nutrients and wound-healing factors at the wound surface. To prevent periwound maceration, moisture barriers should be used, including ointments, sealants, or solid wafers.

Management of Dead Space. It is important to obliterate the dead space formed by tissue destruction beneath the wound, such as sinus tracts. Dead spaces provide a medium for bacterial growth and can contribute to abscess formation and inhibit the healing process. If the wound is contracting, sinus tracts may prematurely close over a fluid-filled defect, which promotes abscess formation.

Figure 15-9 displays the AHRQ algorithm for treatment of pressure ulcers (PPPPUA, 1994).

Management of Infection. A wound will not heal until infection is eradicated (Stotts, 2007). The goal of treatment is "reduction in bioburden without damaging healthy tissue" (Stotts, 2007, p. 170). Wound infection is managed at four levels. The first level is cleansing the wound. The purpose is to reduce surface contamination and metabolic by-products, not treating the infection. The second level is intervention debridement. Autolysis or chemical or surgical debridement can facilitate wound healing and manage infection through removal of dead tissue and foreign materials. Topical therapy includes antiseptics, topical antibiotics, topical elemental antimicrobials, and other treatments such as negative-pressure wound therapy, electrical stimulation, and hyperbaric oxygen. Each of these third-level treatments play a role in treatment of infected wounds. Systemic treatment of infected wounds may be required when there is a systemic response to infection. Therapeutic level of antibiotics that the organisms are sensitive to is requisite for effective treatment. The goal is to treat with an antibiotic that has an adequate but narrow spectrum of coverage (Stotts, 2007). Culturing of wounds is controversial. In general, wounds are cultured when there are signs of infection: fever, edema, induration of the surrounding wound bed, and erythema. Drainage may be minimal, or it may be copious and foul smelling. All chronic wounds are considered contaminated with the presence of multiple organisms. Cultures (swabs) of the surface of the wound will uncover multiple organisms, but these represent contaminants within the wound bed rather than a pathogenic agent producing a clinically relevant wound infection. When an organism is cultured from the tissue of a wound in a nonimmunocompromised patient, a colony forming unit (CFU) count of more than 10 CFU/ml indicates an invasive wound infection. This culture must be obtained with a wound biopsy specimen (Fowler, 1998). Figure 15-10 reflects the AHRQ recommendations for management of bacterial colonization and infection (PPPPUA, 1994).

Wound Dressings. A primary goal of dressing selection for a wound is to select a product that will promote a moist wound environment. A variety of wound dressings are available to enhance the natural physiological wound environment, but the nurse making a dressing selection must also select a dressing that promotes infection control, pain relief or reduction, ease of use, and patient safety (Rolstad & Ovington, 2007). The type of dressing is selected based on the clinical assessment of wound characteristics matched with the qualities of particular dressings. The depth of the wound and the amount of exudate will help to determine the type and frequency of dressing changes. The ultimate goal is to keep the wound environment moist to allow for wound contraction, granulation, and epithelialization. If a wound fails to progress in healing, it is important to review the factors that may impair wound healing, including wound infection, or other systemic factors. Alternate dressings should be considered if a wound fails to progress in healing after 2 weeks or the wound rapidly worsens. Dressings are classified by the materials utilized for wound protection, absorption, and drainage (Table 15-3).

A variety of tapes and taping methods can be used to prevent removal of epidermis with tape removal. Skin sealant may be applied to the skin before the tape is applied to provide protection from epidermal stripping.

Surgical Management. An ulcer that deteriorates no longer responds to nonsurgical intervention or is a chronic wound and should be considered for surgical repair. Surgical intervention is generally considered after more conservative methods of treatment have been tried and failed. Surgical repair may be considered early in a severe wound as early surgical closure decreases loss of fluid and nutrients, improves the patient's general health status, and lead to earlier mobilization and reentry into society. Unfortunately, rates of recurrence of pressure ulcers and surgical failures are high (Goodman, Cohen, Armenta, Thornby, & Netscher, 1999; Yamamoto, Tsutsumida, & Sugihara, 1996), and therefore patients must have optimum nutrition before surgical intervention. In addition, smokers are at increased risk for perioperative and postoperative complications, because smoking promotes a hypercoagulable state, increases myocardial effort, decreases oxygen delivery, and causes coronary vasoconstriction. Surgeons have long recognized that the healing of surgical wounds may be impaired in smokers, and thus patients should be educated to quit smoking in order to maximize postoperative healing.

Alternative Treatments

Growth Factors. Growth factors have gained popularity in treatment of chronic ulcers, although findings from randomized, controlled clinical trials are variable. Wound bed preparation is critical to the success of growth factor therapy. Wound bed preparation incorporates the principles of viable tissue, treatment of infection or inflammation, moisture balance,

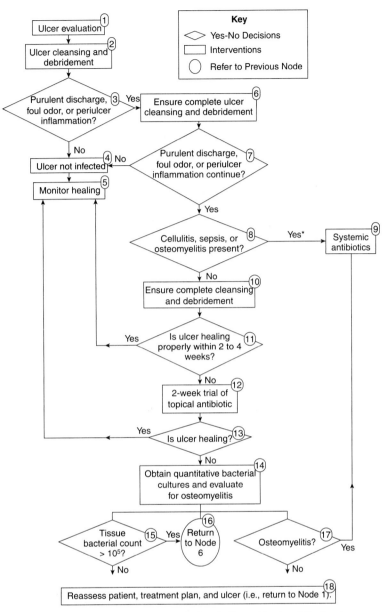

Figure 15-10 Managing bacterial colonization and infection. (From Bergstrom, N., Bennett, M. A., Carlson, C. E., et al. [1994]. *Treatment of pressure ulcers.* [Clinical Practice Guideline No. 15, AHCPR Publication No. 95-0652]. Rockville, MD: U.S. Department of Health and Human Services, Agency for Health Care Policy and Research.)

and a healthy wound edge. Outcomes are variable, and cost-effectiveness has not been widely established (Schultz, 2007). Regranex is the most widely used and studied growth factor approved for this use.

Anabolic Steroids. Systemic use of anabolic steroids is gaining acceptance in wound management. Growth hormone has been shown to increase lean body mass and protein stores and improve the healing rate of wounds. Use of these anabolic steroids has not presented serious side effects (Demling & DeSanti, 1999).

Electrical Stimulation. Electrical stimulation is gaining acceptance as a modality in wound management. The theory

behind this treatment is that when an electrical current is applied, energy transfers to the wound and facilitates healing, because it enhances the body's own bioelectrical system to attract the cells of repair, change the cell membrane permeability, enhance cellular secretion through the cell membranes, and orient cell structures. Electrical stimulation has shown positive effects on increasing blood flow, reducing edema, debriding the wound, controlling infection, improving wound oxygenation, and improving scar formation (Sussman & Byl, 1998).

Negative Pressure Wound Therapy (Vacuum-Assisted Closure). Continuous negative pressure is a modality used to

TABLE 15-3 Classifications and Use of Dressings

Dressing Classification	Description and Potential Uses	Indication of Treatment by Stage
Alginate dressing	Highly absorptive dressing. Manufactured from seaweed, biodegradable	II-IV
Gauze dressing	See-through fabric of open weave, usually made of cotton or synthetics, that is absorptive and permeable to water, water vapor, and oxygen. May be impregnated with petroleum, antiseptics, hydrogels, or other agents	II-IV
Hydrocolloid dressing	A type of dressing containing gel-forming agents and gelatin. In many products these are combined with elastomers and adhesives and applied to a carrier—usually polyurethane foam or film—to form an absorbent, self-adhesive, waterproof wafer	II
Hydrogel dressing	Water-based, nonadherent gel. May contain pectin and sodium carboxymethylcellulose in a clear, viscous vehicle. The dressing has the ability to absorb exudates but does not add moisture to dry necrotic tissue or slough	II-IV
Transparent film dressing	Clear, adherent, nonabsorptive, polymer-based dressing that is permeable to oxygen and water vapor but not to water	I-II
Foam dressing	Spongelike polymer dressing that may be impregnated or coated with other materials and has some absorptive properties	II-IV

remove excess edema in skin surrounding a wound and decrease the bacterial load in a contaminated wound. The removal of excess fluid in a wound bed helps promote moist wound healing and evacuates wound fluid. Negative pressure further assists the body by encouraging angiogenesis. These new blood vessels will carry oxygen and nutrients to the wound bed (Priebe et al., 2003). Vacuum-assisted closure (VAC) is often utilized as an adjunctive therapy to surgical intervention and has been used to increase granulation tissue before surgery.

Hyperbaric Treatment. Hyperbaric oxygen therapy (HBOT) is a mode of therapy in which the patient receives 100% oxygen at pressures greater than normal atmospheric pressure. The principal benefit of HBOT is its ability to increase oxygen tension in the bloodstream and local tissues. This treatment also promotes collagen synthesis and angiogenesis, which are important components of wound healing.

HBOT has been advocated in the literature as adjunctive treatment for a variety of conditions including diabetic foot ulcers, venous ulcers, pressure ulcers, and skin flaps. Currently there is strong evidence that HBOT reduces major amputations in patients with diabetic foot ulcers, but there is insufficient evidence that HBOT is effective in the treatment of venous ulcers and pressure ulcers.

Important considerations in the use of HBOT include the time involved with HBOT. Daily treatments average 90 minutes, and 20 to 40 treatments may be needed. Therefore the time and direct costs of daily travel to and from the treatment center must be considered (Gray & Ratliff, 2006).

Pulsed Lavage. Wound cleansing is an essential component of wound management and is used to facilitate the healing process. Pulsed lavage irrigation removes the surface bacteria and necrotic tissue from the wound, thus cleansing the wound and enhancing granulation. Pulsed lavage irrigation works by delivering an irrigant (usually normal saline)

under direct pressure that is produced by an electrically powered device. Pulsed lavage irrigation refers to the intermittent or interrupted delivery of irrigant to the wound. The number of pulses per second or frequency produced by this method varies among manufacturers. This method of treatment takes approximately 15 to 30 minutes to complete. Other terms for this treatment include *lavage, jet lavage,* and *mechanical lavage.*

Concerns have been raised regarding potential hazards associated with using "high-pressure" pulsed lavage in wound cleansing. Several studies have investigated the potential risks, including the development of bacteremia following lavage of contaminated wounds, trauma to the wound bed, and dissemination of particulate matter or bacteria to the surrounding tissue. Although the studies concluded that these concerns were invalid, there remains caution that high-pressure irrigation may impede tissue defenses against infection and should not be used indiscriminately (Morgan & Hoelscher, 2000).

Education

Staff education for the rehabilitation team is a critical component for maintaining skin integrity. Awareness and educational programs have been shown to reduce the incidence and severity of pressure ulcers. Therefore preventive efforts must be focused on education. In addition, the literature points toward broad, team-based programs where each team member has specific, identified responsibilities.

A comprehensive educational program includes prevention as a key means of improving outcomes. The AHRQ clinical practice guidelines on the treatment of pressure ulcers recommend the development and implementation of educational programs that are focused on three areas: prevention and treatment, assessing tissue damage, and monitoring outcomes (PPPUA, 1994).

Educational programs for patients, caregivers, and health care providers should reflect a continuum of care, beginning with a structured, comprehensive, and organized approach to prevention and should culminate in effective treatment protocols. Information should be presented at an appropriate level for the target audience to maximize retention and ensure carryover into practice. Patients should be encouraged to actively participate in and comply with decisions regarding pressure ulcer prevention and treatment (PPPUA, 1992, 1994).

Assessing tissue damage by accurate staging of pressure ulcers is prerequisite to development and implementation of appropriate and effective treatment protocols and ongoing monitoring of wound healing. Other essential components of an effective educational program include risk assessment, uniform terminology, consistent documentation, individualized wound treatment, and the use of appropriate dressings and support surfaces. Educational programs should be updated frequently to ensure that current information reflects research-based practices.

Evaluation of outcomes serves as the basis for changing practice and improving patient care. Improvement in outcomes depends on knowledgeable nurses and other health care providers who deliver care according to a specific, individualized, and documented plan of care.

NURSING OUTCOMES

An outcome may be defined as the result of an intervention. Outcomes are well-established quality control tools and are objective measurements used to benchmark change as a result of an intervention. Assessing patient outcomes provides clinicians with a means for assessing the effectiveness of an intervention or interventions and providing data to direct changes in treatment modalities and plans (Moorhead, Johnson, & Maas, 2004). Rehabilitation nurses are accountable for a multitude of patient outcomes. Expected outcomes related to skin integrity are listed in Table 15-2.

SUMMARY

Pressure ulcer prediction, prevention, and treatment are national concerns, as evidenced by the attention received from such groups as the NPUAP and the PPPPUA. The costs in morbidity, mortality, and dollars are high. Nurses play a pivotal role in maintaining skin integrity and in predicting, preventing, and treating pressure ulcers. Evidence-based practice is becoming a norm for professional nursing. As information about risk factors is disseminated and incorporated into practice, nurses can influence prevention and outcomes (Gerrish, Clayton, Nolan, Parker, & Morgan, 1999).

Case Study

Mr. Smith was sent to a regional model spinal cord injury health care center for evaluation in an interdisciplinary skin clinic. Upon evaluation by the interdisciplinary team, led by a nurse practitioner, Mr. Smith was found to have a stage IV ischial pressure ulcer.

Mr. Smith is a professional businessman in his mid-50s. He sustained a complete T4 spinal cord injury as a 16-year-old in a rollover motor vehicle accident. Mr. Smith has been extremely healthy all of his life and has experienced no complications from his spinal cord injury until the past 6 months. Mr. Smith has an extensive business travel schedule. He reports that weight shifts have become more difficult to perform due to progressive shoulder pain; however, he does perform them routinely. Mr. Smith performs self skin checks on a daily basis. He noted a discolored area over his right ischium approximately 6 months before the clinic visit. The area of discoloration initially presented as a red, warm area with a hard knot underneath the skin surface. The area progressed and became an open ulcer with serous drainage. Mr. Smith attempted to remain off the area as much as possible and has been covering the ulcer with a dry gauze. Mr. Smith continues to travel so he does not lose his job and the health benefits that are provided by his company. Mr. Smith is very thin and is a one pack-per-day smoker.

When evaluated at the outpatient interdisciplinary skin clinic at a regional model spinal cord injury center, his vital signs were within normal limits, and he was afebrile. His wound was measured and found to be 30 mm × 27 mm × 22 mm deep. A copious amount of serous drainage was present on the gauze dressing, but there was no

odor to the drainage. The wound base had 30% yellow adherent slough, which was removed by sharp debridement by the nurse practitioner. After sharp debridement the wound base was a pale pink. Although there was a thin layer of tissue covering the right ischium, the bony prominence could easily be palpated. The periulcer skin was a dusky gray color, indicative of a yeast infection. The presence of yeast suggested that the exudate was not being properly managed and was spilling onto the skin surrounding the wound.

Samples were drawn for laboratory examination, including a CBC, ESR, TLC, and a prealbumin level to assess Mr. Smith's general medical and nutritional status. His height and weight showed him to be underweight at 6 feet and 135 pounds. His BMI is 18. A medical history and medication profile was obtained, and the patient was found to be in good health with no comorbid conditions. Mr. Smith did report a significant amount of shoulder pain bilaterally, which he was controlling with antiinflammatory medications.

Mr. Smith's social history showed he is married, with good support from his wife and children. He is independent in all of his activities of daily living (ADLs). He is college educated, drinks socially, and smokes approximately one pack of cigarettes per day. He has no specific cultural beliefs or practices that would affect his health care. He is financially secure but is the main source of income for his family and is concerned about taking time off from work.

Physical therapy evaluated the manual wheelchair and wheelchair cushion, and all was found to be in good repair. Mr. Smith reported

Continued

that because of his shoulder pain he had several "bad transfers" in the past 6 months and believes that trauma may have been the initial cause of his pressure ulcer formation. He is currently turning from side-to-side at night and sleeps on a regular mattress. He has a padded toilet seat for his bowel program, which takes only 15 minutes to complete.

Mr. Smith was evaluated by the plastic surgeon and was informed that he had a stage IV pressure ulcer of the right ischium requiring a myocutaneous flap surgery to close the wound. Although he was in agreement with this plan, he needed time to complete some projects at work. His laboratory results were reviewed and were within normal limits.

Because the wound drainage was excessive, a calcium alginate dressing was ordered, with the goal of absorbing drainage. An antifungal ointment was prescribed for the periwound yeast. Mr. Smith was given written information regarding increasing his protein and calories in preparation for surgery. It was also recommended that he begin taking a multivitamin daily.

Mr. Smith was informed that it was imperative that he quit smoking. The relationship between smoking and poor wound healing was discussed. Mr. Smith was provided with a prescription for nicotine patches.

Physical therapy discussed shoulder conservation measures and informed Mr. Smith that a power wheelchair may be a good option in order to protect his shoulders from continued overuse. Transfer techniques were reviewed, and Mr. Smith was encouraged to continue turning from side-to-side at night and to position himself at a 30-degree angle in an effort to protect his trochanters from pressure.

Mr. Smith will continue to be followed by the interdisciplinary team until he is scheduled for surgery.

There are numerous diagnoses applicable to Mr. Smith from the case study. The applicable nursing diagnoses include impaired skin integrity related to stage IV pressure ulcer; chronic pain related to shoulder pain; impaired transfer ability related to chronic shoulder pain; potential self-care deficit related to bed rest; potential alteration in skin integrity of other body surface areas related to bed rest; and knowledge deficient related to shoulder conservation strategies, improper transfer technique, and inadequate pressure ulcer prevention and management.

The expected outcomes for Mr. Smith include wound healing by surgical closure. A major focus of patient education will be related to prevention of pressure ulcers and maintenance of skin integrity.

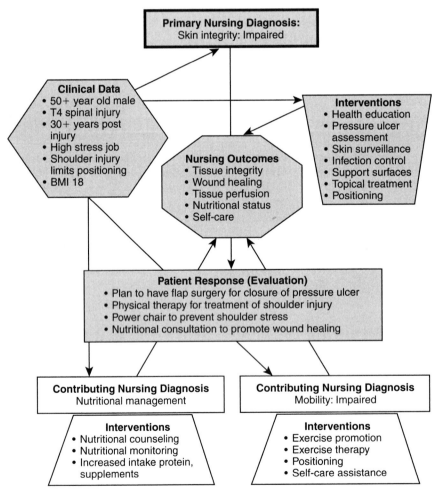

Concept Map. Mr. Smith's primary problem is that of the impaired skin integrity. Interventions are needed to address the contributing issues of nutrition and impaired mobility. The following concept map illustrates the interrelationships between the nursing diagnoses of impaired skin integrity, nutritional management, and impaired mobility. The rehabilitation nurse will focus on coordinating interventions to achieve the outcomes of wound healing, promotion of tissue integrity, tissue perfusion, and self-care.

CRITICAL THINKING

Several critical thinking questions based on the case study follow. The principles of this case analysis would apply to many patients at risk for impaired skin integrity.

1. What risk factors can you identify that placed Mr. Smith at increased risk for impaired skin integrity?
2. What findings during Mr. Smith's assessment were significant in directing nursing interventions?
3. Based on the nursing diagnoses assigned to Mr. Smith in the case study, what interventions and outcomes would you implement for at least one of the diagnoses?

REFERENCES

Allman, R. M., Goode, P. S., Burst, N., Bartolucci, A. A., & Thomas, D. R. (1999). Pressure ulcers, hospital complications, and disease severity: Impact on hospital costs and length of stay. *Advances in Wound Care, 12*, 22-30.

American Hospital Association. (1997, November). Here are highlights of pressure ulcer guideline. *Healthcare Benchmarks*, 162-163.

Arnold, M. C. (2003). Pressure ulcer prevention and management. The current evidence for care. *AACN Clinical Issues, 14*(4), 411-428.

Ayello, E. A., Thomas, D. R., & Litchford, M. A. (1999). Nutritional aspects of wound healing. *Home Healthcare Nurse, 17*(11), 719-729.

Baharestani, M. (1999). Pressure ulcers in an age of managed care: A nursing perspective. *Ostomy/Wound Management, 45*(5), 18-26, 28-32, 34.

Bates-Jensen, B. (1998). *Wound care: A collaborative manual for physical therapists and nurses.* Gaithersburg, MD: Aspen.

Beitz, J., & Goldberg, E. (2005). The lived experience of having a chronic wound: A phenomenologic study. *Dermatology Nursing, 17*(4), 272-275.

Bergstrom, N., & Braden, B. (1992). A prospective study of pressure sore risk among the institutionalized elderly. *Journal of the American Geriatric Society, 40*(8), 747-758.

Bethel, E. (2005). Wound care for patients with darkly pigmented skin. *Nursing Standard, 20*(4), 41-49.

Black, J. M., & Black, S. B. (2007). The role of surgery in wound healing. In Bryant, R. A., & Nix, D. P. (Eds.). *Acute and chronic wounds: Current management concepts* (3rd ed., pp. 461-470). St. Louis, MO: Mosby.

Blaszczyk, J., Majewski, M., & Sato, F. (1998). Make a difference: Standardize your heel care practice. *Ostomy/Wound Management 44*(5), 32-40.

Braden, B., & Bergstrom, M. (1989). A conceptual schema for the study of the etiology of pressure sores. *Rehabilitation nursing, 14*(5), 258.

Brandeis, G. H., Berlowitz, D. R., Hossain, M., & Morris, J. N. (1995). Pressure ulcers: The minimum data set and the resident assessment protocol. *Advances in Wound Care, 8*(6), 18-25.

Brillhart, B. (2005). Pressure sore and skin tear prevention and treatment during a 10-month program. *Rehabilitation Nursing, 30*(3), 85-91.

Bryant, R. A. (2000). Skin pathology and types of damage. In R. Bryant (Ed.), *Acute and chronic wounds: Nursing management* (2nd ed.). St. Louis, MO: Mosby.

Bryant, R. A., Clark, R. A. F. (2007). Skin pathology and types of damage. In Bryant, R. A., & Nix, D. P. (Eds.), *Acute and chronic wounds: Current management concepts* (3rd ed., pp. 100-129). St. Louis, MO: Mosby.

Buckley, K. M., Adelson, L. K., & Hess, C. T. (2005, May/June). Get the picture! Developing a wound photography competency for home care nurses. *Journal of Wound, Ostomy and Continence Nursing, 32*, 171-175.

Carlson, C. E., King, R. B., Kirk, P. M., Temple, R., & Heinemann, A. (1992). Incidence and correlates of pressure ulcer development after spinal cord injury. *Rehabilitation Nursing Research, 1*, 34-40.

Consortium for Spinal Cord Medicine. (2000, August). *Pressure ulcer prevention and treatment following spinal cord injury: A clinical practice guideline for healthcare professionals.* Washington, DC: Paralyzed Veterans of America.

Cooper, D. M. (2000). Assessment, measurement and evaluation: Their pivotal roles in wound healing. In R. Bryant (Ed.), *Acute and chronic wounds: Nursing management* (2nd ed.). St. Louis, MO: Mosby.

Dellefield, M. E. (2004). Prevalence rate of pressure ulcers in California nursing homes: Using the OSCAR database to develop a risk adjustment model. *Journal of gerontological nursing, 30*(11), 13-21.

Demling, R., & DeSanti, L. (1999). Involuntary weight loss and the non-healing wound: The role of anabolic agents. *Advances in Wound Care, 12*(1 Suppl.), 1-14.

Dochterman, J. M. & Bulechek, G. M. (2004). *Nursing interventions classification (NIC)* (4th ed.). St. Louis, MO: Mosby.

Doughty, D. B., & Holbrook, R. (2007). Lower extremity ulcers of vascular etiology. In Bryant, R. A., & Nix, D. P. (Eds.), *Acute and chronic wounds: Current management concepts* (3rd ed., pp. 258-306). St. Louis, MO: Mosby.

Doughty, D. B., & Sparks-Defriese, B. (2007). Wound healing physiology. In Bryant, R. A., & Nix, D. P. (Eds.), *Acute and chronic wounds: Current management concepts* (3rd ed., pp. 56-81). St. Louis, MO: Mosby.

Driver, V. R., Landowski, M. A., & Madsen, J. L. (2007). Neuropathic wounds: The diabetic wound. In Bryant, R. A., & Nix, D. P. (Eds.), *Acute and chronic wounds: Current management concepts* (3rd ed., pp. 397-336). St. Louis, MO: Mosby.

Eaglstein, W. H. (1986). Wound healing and aging. *Dermatology Clinics, 4*, 481-484.

Eastwood, K. A., Hagglund, K. J., Ragnarsson, K. J., Gordon, W. A., & Marino, R. J. (1999). Medical rehabilitation length of stay and outcomes for persons with traumatic spinal cord injury: 1990-1997. *Archives of Physical Medicine and Rehabilitation, 80*(11), 1457-1463.

Evans, E. (2005). Nutritional assessment in chronic wound care. *Journal of Wound, Ostomy and Continence Nursing, 32*(5), 317-320.

Folkedahl, F. R. (2002, May). *Prevention of pressure ulcers.* University of Iowa Gerontological Nursing Interventions Research Center, Research Dissemination Core. Retrieved November 1, 2005, from http://www.guideline.gov/summary.aspx.

Fowler, E. (1998). Wound infection: A nurse's perspective. *Ostomy/Wound Management, 44*(8), 44-52.

Gallagher, S. (1997). Morbid obesity: A chronic disease with an impact on wounds and related problems. *Ostomy/Wound Management, 43*(5), 18-27.

Gerrish, K., Clayton, J., Nolan, M., Parker, K., & Morgan, L. (1999). Promoting evidence-based practice: Managing change in the assessment of pressure damage risk. *Journal of Nursing Management, 7*(6), 355-362.

Goldberg, M. T., & McGinn-Byer, P. (2000). Oncology-related skin changes. In R. Bryant (Ed.), *Acute and chronic wounds: Nursing management* (2nd ed.). St. Louis, MO: Mosby.

Goodman, C. M., Cohen, V., Armenta, A., Thornby, J., & Netscher, D. T. (1999). Evaluation of results and treatment variables for pressure ulcers in 48 veteran spinal cord injured patients. *Annals of Plastic Surgery, 42*(6), 665-672.

Gray, M. (2004). Which pressure ulcer risk scales are valid and reliable in a pediatric population? *Journal of Wound, Ostomy and Continence Nursing, 31*(4), 157-160.

Gray, M, & Ratliff, C. R. (2006). Is hyperbaric oxygen therapy effective for the management of chronic wounds? *Journal of Wound Ostomy Continence Nursing, 33*(1), 21-25.

Gunningberg, L., & Ehrenberg, A. (2004). Accuracy and quality in the nursing documentation of pressure ulcers. *Journal of Wound, Ostomy, Continence Nursing, 31*(6), 328-334.

Haalboom, J. R., den Boer, J., & Buskens, E. (1999). Risk-assessment tools in the prevention of pressure ulcers. *Ostomy/Wound Management, 45*(2), 20-26, 28, 30-34.

Kosiak, M. (1959). Etiology and pathology of ischemic ulcers. *Archives of Physical Medicine and Rehabilitation, 40*, 62-69.

Lui, M., Spungen, A., Fink, L., Losada, M., & Bauman, W. (1996). Increased energy needs in patients with quadriplegia and pressure sores. *Advances in Wound Care, 9*(3), 41-45.

Lyder, C. H., & Torpy, J. M. (2003). Pressure ulcer prevention and management. *JAMA, 289*(2), 223-226.

Main, P. W. (1996). A review of seven support surfaces with emphasis on their protection of the spinally injured. *Journal of Accident and Emergency Medicine, 13*, 34-37.

Maklebust, J., & Sieggreen, M. (1996). *Pressure ulcers: Guidelines for prevention, and nursing management* (2nd ed.). Springhouse, PA: Springhouse.

Montroy, R. E., & Eltorai, I. (2003). The surgical management of pressure ulcers. In V. W. Lin (Ed. in Chief), *Spinal cord medicine: Principles and practice* (pp. 591-612). New York: Demos Publishing.

Moody, P., Gonzales, I., & Cureton, V. Y. (2004). The effect of body position and mattress type on interface pressure in quadriplegic adults: A pilot study. *Dermatology Nursing, 16*(6), 507-512.

Moorhead, S., Johnson, M., & Maas, M. (2004). *Nursing outcomes classification (NOC,* (3rd ed.). St. Louis, MO: Mosby.

Morgan, D., & Hoelscher, J. (2000). Pulsed lavage: Promoting comfort and healing in home care. *Ostomy Wound Management, 46*(4), 44-49.

Mullins, M., Thomason, S. S., & Legro, M. (2005). Monitoring pressure ulcer healing in persons with disabilities. *Rehabilitation Nursing, 30*(3), 92-99.

National Pressure Ulcer Advisory Panel. (2005). *The PUSH tool.* Retrieved November 1, 2005, from http://www.npuap.org.

National Pressure Ulcer Advisory Council. (2007). Pressure ulcer stages. Retrieved March 19, 2007, from http://www.NPUAP.org/documents.

Niazi, Z. B. M., Salzberg, C. A., Byrne, D. W., & Viehbeck, M. (1997). Recurrence of initial pressure ulcer in persons with spinal cord injuries. *Advances in Wound Care, 10*(3), 38-42.

Nix, D. P. (2007a). Patient assessment and evaluation of healing. In Bryant, R. A., & Nix, D. P. (Eds.), *Acute and chronic wounds: Current management concepts* (3rd ed., pp. 100-129). St. Louis, MO: Mosby.

Nix. D. P. (2007b). Support surfaces. In Bryant, R. A., & Nix, D. P. (Eds.), *Acute and chronic wounds: Current management concepts* (3rd ed., pp. 235-248). St. Louis, MO: Mosby.

Panel for Prediction and Prevention of Pressure Ulcers in Adults. (1992). *Pressure ulcers in adults: Prediction and prevention* (Clinical Practice Guideline No. 3, AHCPR Publication No. 92-0047). Rockville, MD: Agency for Health Care Policy and Research, Public Health Service, U.S. Department of Health and Human Services.

Payne, R. L., & Martin, M. L. (1993a). Defining and classifying skin tears: Need for common language. *Ostomy/Wound Management, 39*(5), 16.

Payne, R. L., & Martin, M. L. (1993b). The epidemiology and management of skin tears in older adults. *Ostomy/Wound Management, 26*, 26-37.

Pieper, B. (2007). Mechanical forces: Pressure, shear and friction. In R. A. Bryant (Ed.), *Acute and chronic wounds: Nursing management* (2nd ed.). St. Louis, MO: Mosby.

Priebe, M. M., Martin, M., Wuermser, L. A., Castillo, T., & McFarlin, J. (2003). The medical management of pressure ulcers. In V. W. Lin (Ed. in Chief), *Spinal cord medicine: Principles and practice* (pp. 567-589). New York: Demos Publishing.

Rapple, L. M. (1998). Management of pressure by therapeutic positioning. In C. Sussman & B. M. Bates-Jensen (Eds.), *Wound care: A collaborative practice manual for physical therapists and nurses.* Gaithersburg, MD: Aspen.

Rolstad, B. S., & Ovington, L. G. (2007). Principles of wound management. In R. A. Bryant, & D. P. Nix (Eds.), *Acute and chronic wounds: Nursing management* (2nd ed., pp. 391-426). St. Louis, MO: Mosby.

Rolsted, B., Ovington, L. G., & Hanis, A. (2000). Principles of wound management. In Bryant, R. A. (Ed.), *Acute and chronic wounds: Nursing management* (2nd ed.). St. Louis, MO: Mosby.

Salcido, R. (2000). The future of wound measurements. *Advances in Wound Care, 13*(2), 54-55.

Schultz, G. (2007). Molecular regulation of wound healing. In Bryant, R. A., & Nix, D. P. (Eds.), *Acute and chronic wounds: Current management concepts* (3rd ed., pp. 82-99). St. Louis, MO: Mosby.

Stotts, N. A. (2000). Nutritional assessment and support. In R. Bryant (Ed.), *Acute and chronic wounds: Nursing management* (2nd ed.). St. Louis, MO: Mosby.

Stotts, N. A. (2007). Wound infection: Diagnosis and management. In Bryant, R. A., & Nix, D. P. (Eds.), *Acute and chronic wounds: Current management concepts* (3rd ed., pp. 161-175). St. Louis, MO: Mosby.

Sussman, C., & Byl, N. (1998). Electrical stimulation for wound healing. In C. Sussman & B. M. Bates-Jensen (Eds.), *Wound care: A collaborative practice manual for physical therapists and nurses.* Gaithersburg, MD: Aspen.

Thomas, D. (1997). Specific nutritional factors in wound healing. *Advances in Wound Care, 10*(4), 40-43.

Thomas, D. R., Goode, P. S., La Master, K., Tennyson, T., & Parnell, L. K. S. (1999). A comparison of an opaque foam dressing versus a transparent film dressing in the management of skin tears in institutionalized subjects. *Ostomy/Wound Management, 45*(6), 22-24, 27-28.

Thompson, J. M., McFarland, G. K., Hirsch, J. E. & Tucker, S. (1997). *Mosby's clinical nursing* (4th ed.). St. Louis, MO: Mosby.

Tourtual, D. M., Riesenberg, L. A., Korutz, C. J., Semo, A. H., Asef, A., & Gill, R. D. F. (1997). Predictors of hospital acquired heel pressure ulcers. *Ostomy/Wound Management, 43*(9), 24-34.

Watts, D., Abrahams, E., MacMillan, C., Sanat, J., Silver, R., VanGorder, S., et al. (1998, July/August). Insult after injury: Pressure ulcers in trauma patients. *Orthopedic Nursing,* 84-91.

Wild, S. Roglic, G. Green, A., Sicree R., & King, H. (2004). Global prevalence of diabetes: Estimates for the year 2000 and projection for 2030. *Diabetes Care, 27*, 1047-1053.

Wright, K., & Bauer, C. (2005). Meeting bariatric patient care needs. *Journal of Wound, Ostomy, Continence Nursing, 32*(6), 402-406.

Wysocki, A. B. (2007). Anatomy and physiology of skin and soft tissue. In R. A. Bryant & D. P. Nix (Eds.), *Acute and chronic wounds: Nursing management* (2nd ed., pp. 39-55). St. Louis, MO: Mosby.

Yamamoto, Y., Tsutsumida, A., Murazumi, M., & Sugihara, T. (1996). Long-term outcomes of pressure sores treated with flap coverage. *Plastic and Reconstructive Surgery, 100*(5), 1212-1217.

Young, Z. F., Evans, A., & Davis, J. (2003). Nosocomial pressure ulcer prevention: A successful project. *Journal of Nursing Administration, 33*(7/8), 380-383.

Zulkowski, K. (1999). A conceptual model of pressure prevalence: MDS + items and nutrition. *Ostomy/Wound Management, 45*(2), 36-44.

16

Nourishment and Swallowing

Nancy H. Glenn-Molali, MSN, RN, CRRN

Swallowing is something we do nearly 1000 times a day. If we are healthy and all swallowing mechanisms are functioning properly, we are generally unaware of a large number of our swallows. It is typically only when we are eating or drinking, pleasurable activities, that we focus on our swallows. An adult independently obtains and ingests proper nutrients to maintain health and function. Eating meals occurs during family or social gatherings, celebrations, or events for many cultural groups and has become associated with feelings of sharing, belonging, and friendship. When a person can no longer secure or ingest nutrients in an efficient manner, a biological, social, or psychological crisis may occur. Patients who are no longer able to swallow in a normal manner are said to have dysphagia. Dysphagia may cause patients to aspirate food or fluids resulting in aspiration pneumonia, or they may have frequent choking resulting in frustration, disappointment, and fear, which may lead to reduced nutritional intake, dehydration, and malnutrition. This chapter includes information on nourishment, anatomy and physiology of swallowing, statistics on dysphagia, factors associated with altered deglutition, diagnostic tests, and nursing process with outcome criteria for persons with impairments of eating or swallowing.

NOURISHMENT

The primary purpose of eating and swallowing is to provide the body with necessary nutrients and hydration. All persons need a balanced diet from the major food groups, as recommended by the U.S. Department of Agriculture (USDA) and the U.S. Department of Health and Human Services (USHHS), and adequate hydration (at least eight 8-oz glasses of water a day), unless contraindicated due to a physiological condition.

In 2005 the food guide pyramid was replaced by MyPyramid (Figure 16-1). MyPyramid is part of an overall food guidance system that emphasizes the need for an individualized plan to improve diet and exercise. It incorporates recommendations from the 2005 Dietary Guidelines released by the USDA and USHHS. MyPyramid focuses on the importance of making smart choices in all food groups each day.

The new plan, found at http://mypyramid.gov/, uses interactive technology to let individuals enter their age, gender, and physical activity level to obtain personalized recommendations. A child-friendly version for children 6 to 11 years of age is available at http://mypyramid.gov/kids/index.html.

"We are what we eat" is an old but true saying. Research findings support the contribution of adequate and appropriate nutrition to improved outcomes in healing, strength, tissue regeneration, and cognitive awareness. Metabolic responses to chronic illnesses, such as pulmonary diseases, and to stresses after trauma are increasingly important areas of concern for rehabilitation nurses. Severe deficiencies in several B vitamins affect brain function and behavior, including abnormal electroencephalograms, impaired memory, anxiety, confusion, irritability, and depression. Pyridoxine (vitamin B_6) deficiencies cause abnormal brain electrical activity (Harris, 1996). Cognitive impairment may be caused by a disease, but it can also be caused by dehydration, potassium imbalance, iron-deficiency anemia, and deficiency of water-soluble vitamins. Zinc deficiency is associated with impaired immune function, anorexia, poor wound healing, and development of pressure ulcers (Shuman, 1996).

Nutrition, Medication, and Herbs

Nutritional status and the medications taken by a patient can have direct effects on each other. Medications include prescriptions, over-the-counter medicines, vitamins, minerals, herbs, and dietary supplements. Tables 16-1 and 16-2 give examples of some medications that affect nutritional status and some foods that affect medications. Medications can affect nutritional status by increasing or decreasing appetite, decreasing the senses of smell and taste, affecting absorption of nutrients, or altering metabolism and excretion of nutrients. Food can affect medications by altering absorption, metabolism, and excretion. Any person who takes medication is at risk for a drug-nutrient interaction. Persons at highest risk include those who take multiple medications; consume alcohol; have poor nutrition; take a vitamin, mineral, or herbal supplement; or take medications at mealtimes.

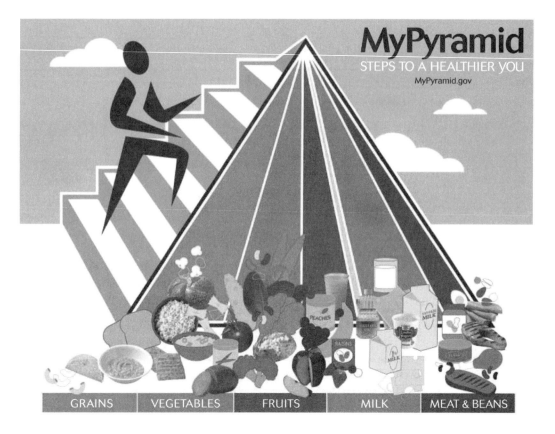

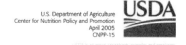

Figure 16-1 MyPyramid.

TABLE 16-1 Examples of Medications Affecting Nutritional Status

Medication	Effect on Nutritional Status
Phenobarbital, phenytoin, primidone	Interfere with intestinal absorption of calcium
Phenytoin	Metabolism requires folic acid and is accelerated by supplementation, which may cause subtherapeutic levels of the medication
Levodopa	Binds with pyridoxine and is excreted; supplemental pyridoxine may decrease effectiveness
Corticosteroids	Deplete body of ascorbic acid
Cholestyramine	Increases excretion of fat-soluble vitamins A, D, E, and K; folic acid; vitamin B_{12}; calcium; and iron
Long-term antacid or potassium	Neutralizes gastric acidity and decreases absorption of folic acid, vitamin B_{12}, chloride use and iron
Furosemide	Increases excretion of sodium, potassium, and calcium

Data from Lutz, C. A., & Przytulski, K. R. (1997). *Nutrition and diet therapy* (2nd ed.). Philadelphia: F. A. Davis; and Burns, R. D., & Carr-Davis, E. M. (1996). Nutritional care in diseases of the nervous system. In L. K. Mahan & S. Escott-Stump (Eds.), *Krause's food, nutrition and diet therapy* (9th ed., pp. 863-889). Philadelphia: W. B. Saunders.

TABLE 16-2 Examples of Foods Affecting Medications

Food	Effect on Medication
Amino acids in protein	Inhibit absorption of levodopa and theophylline; delay action of phenytoin
High-fiber meal	Decreases absorption of digoxin
Milk, alcohol, and hot beverages	Cause premature erosion of enteric coatings
Pectin in jelly and apples	Decreases absorption of acetaminophen
Carbohydrates	Increase absorption of levodopa, phenytoin, and theophylline
Tyramine-containing foods	Cause hypertension crisis when combined with MAO inhibitors
Vitamin K (in food or supplement)	Reverses effects of warfarin

Data from Lutz, C. A., & Przytulski, K. R. (1997). *Nutrition and diet therapy* (2nd ed.). Philadelphia: F. A. Davis; and Burns, R. D., & Carr-Davis, E. M. (1996). Nutritional care in diseases of the nervous system. In L. K. Mahan & S. Escott-Stump (Eds.), *Krause's food, nutrition and diet therapy* (9th ed., pp. 863-889). Philadelphia: W. B. Saunders.
MAO, Monoamine oxidase.

When completing a nutritional assessment, it is important to obtain information regarding intake of vitamins, herbs, and nutritional supplements. Some vitamins, when taken in excess of body requirements, can have negative effects. Excess vitamin A has been associated with liver injury, elevated intracranial pressure, and birth defects after maternal consumption during pregnancy. Vitamin B_6 in excess may lead to ataxia or sensory neuropathy. Excess niacin may produce liver damage, gastrointestinal distress, myopathy, cytopenia, and maculopathy of the eyes (Harris, 1996).

Many persons use herbs to treat various ailments and do not consider them medications. It is important to question patients on the use of herbs because some can cause serious illness. Some herbal preparations used for weight reduction, for example, germander, stephania, magnolia, or ma huang, have caused problems including stroke, hypertension, and severe kidney disease. All patients, at home, in a hospital, nursing home, or residential center, should have a nutritional assessment on admission, then every 6 months, and as their condition changes, such as with weight gain, loss, and disease progression. This is particularly helpful in improving outcomes for patients with infections, impaired skin integrity, loss of muscle tissue, healing bones or wounds (D'Eramo, Sedlak, Doheny, & Jenkins, 1994), and potential malnutrition due to poor absorption or compromised immunity.

Psychological and Sociocultural Factors

Nutritional status is influenced by the physical ability to consume food and by psychological and sociocultural factors. In the United States there are many ethnic groups; each has various food preferences, and each attaches different emotional significance to food. It is important to identify these characteristics and to realize that cultural patterns may affect the patient's nutritional choices. In addition, food is commonly associated with social events and therefore has significant psychological meaning. Traditional foods for holidays are one example. As one ages or becomes ill, the lack of interaction at meals or of other meaningful social interactions can reduce nutritional intake significantly. It is difficult to change lifelong eating habits, and these can hinder the rehabilitation. However, motivated patients can overcome these habits.

When dietary plans and menus are offered to patients from differing cultural groups, the nutritional composition of ethnic or religious food selections may be calculated so these foods are included in the plan. For example, Asian diets have rice as a staple and few dairy products. Pork and chicken are used more than beef. Mediterranean diets are high in olive oil, fruits, vegetables, cheeses, milk, legumes, and wine. Vegetarian diets vary from consuming no animal products to consuming fowl, fish, and dairy products but no red meat.

Malnutrition

Many patients will be at risk for malnutrition. Risk factors for malnutrition include any of the following: cognitive impairment, social isolation, being homebound, frailty, depression, advanced age, low income, exhaustive medical illness, chronic disability, functional disability, poor dentition, polypharmacy, regular alcohol intake, dysphagia, or inadequate food intake. Older patients are at risk for dehydration because the sense of thirst diminishes with age and there is a decrease in water conservation by the kidneys. Many older patients also take diuretics and laxatives, which deplete fluid volume. Some patients with incontinence limit fluid intake to decrease the risk of an accident.

Patients may also have inadequate nutritional intake due to a knowledge deficit. They may be unaware of what foods and nutrients compose an adequate diet, what adaptive equipment is available, or what community resources are available. Some community resources include the Women, Infants, and Children (WIC) program, food stamps, community food programs, food banks, cooperatives, church- or religion-sponsored meal programs, social services, Meals on Wheels, and adult day care programs. Some services also provide shopping and meal preparation for elderly persons.

Diseases and Injuries

Swallowing impairments are common with many neurological diseases and can cause nutritional deficits. Other diseases and injuries, such as Alzheimer's disease, rheumatoid arthritis, and burns, can put a patient at risk for a nutritional deficit.

Barrett-Connor, Edelstein, Corey-Bloom, and Wiederholt, (1996) found weight loss in the elderly may be an early warning sign of Alzheimer's disease. As the disease progresses, patients may have an insatiable appetite with weight gain, possibly because they forget they have eaten, or, more commonly, they refuse food or forget to eat. These patients need frequent offerings of finger foods. In the late stage the patient may be unable to chew, and a diet with modified consistencies or a feeding tube may be needed.

Patients with rheumatic diseases may have anorexia because of medications, fatigue, and pain; decreased dietary intake; and taste alterations due to xerostomia. If metabolic bone disease is present, calcium and vitamin D supplements are indicated (Touger-Decker, 1996).

Patients with metabolic stress, such as sepsis, multiple trauma, burns, or surgery, require additional calories. The requirements for patients with burns can increase as much as 100% or more, and protein requirements may triple, depending on the size and depth of the injury. This is due to stress, fluid and protein loss through the wound exudates, fever, infection, immobility, and hypercatabolism. Vitamin and mineral requirements may increase to two times the recommended daily allowance, particularly vitamins C and A because they promote wound healing (Moy, 1996; Winkler & Manchester, 1996).

Patients who have acute brain injury are generally well nourished before injury. However, because of the hypermetabolic and hypercatabolic state after injury, nutritional support is needed to prevent rapid loss of lean body mass and immunosuppression. Patients with severe brain injury can require up to twice the normal number of calories, with increased protein demands. Patients also benefit from B vitamins, vitamin C, and zinc (Stanley, 1998; Walleck & Mooney, 1994).

Elderly Patients

Traditionally the term *elderly* refers to persons 65 years and older. There are several factors to consider when working with the elderly: glucose tolerance decreases with age, leading to an increase in plasma glucose; thus the glucose tolerance curve developed for young adults is now recognized as inappropriate for elderly persons. The basal metabolic rate decreases by 20% between the ages of 30 and 90 years because of a decrease in lean body mass, kidney function can decrease by 50% between the ages of 30 and 80 years, acid-base response to metabolic challenges is slowed, lean body mass is replaced with fat and connective tissue, body protein in healthy elderly persons is 30% to 40% less than that of young adults, and bone density is diminished.

Excess Weight

A patient's nutritional status affects nearly all aspects of life, and it is important to consider the effect that extra weight has on a person's life. Excess weight can lead to physical and psychological problems and is the result of diet, physical activity, genetic factors, and health conditions. Eating may be a means to relieve anxiety, stress, depression, loneliness, and to pass the time. Excess weight stresses many of the body's systems in both adults and children. It increases a person's risk for heart disease, high cholesterol levels, stroke, joint disease, hypertension, type 2 diabetes, gallbladder disease, sleep disorders, some cancers, and menstrual irregularities (Barlow & Dietz, 1998; Centers for Disease Control and Prevention [CDC], 2004). It can decrease mobility and level of functioning in all activities of daily living.

The results from two National Health and Nutrition Examination Surveys indicate that among adults aged 20 to 74 years, the prevalence of obesity increased from 15% in the 1976 to 1980 survey to 32.9% in the 2003 to 2004 survey. A person is considered obese if body mass index (BMI) is greater than or equal to 30. The percentage of children ages 6 to 11 years considered overweight was increased from 6.5% to 18.8%. A child is considered overweight if BMI-for-age is at or above the 95th percentile of the CDC Growth Chart. For those aged 12 to 19 years, the prevalence rose from 5% to 17.4% (CDC, 2007).

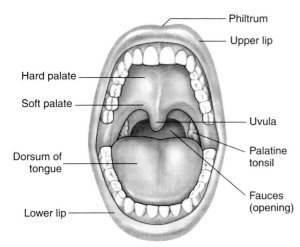

Figure 16-2 The oral cavity. (From Thibodeau, G. A., & Patton, K. I. [2007]. *Anatomy and physiology* [6th ed.]. St. Louis, MO: Mosby.)

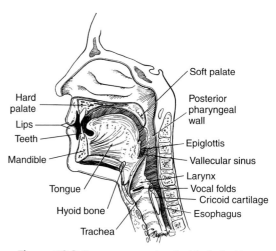

Figure 16-3 Structures associated with deglutition.

Healthy People 2000, the previous prevention agenda for the nation, identified being overweight as "the most significant preventable threat to health." It identified physical activity and fitness and nutrition as the top two priority areas (USDHHS, 1990). *Healthy People 2010*, the new prevention agenda for the nation, lists as its number one goal "to increase the quality and years of healthy life. . . ." A major component is helping people achieve and maintain a healthy weight (USDHHS, 2000).

MECHANICS OF EATING

The ability to eat and swallow food and liquids is dependent on position and function of the oropharyngeal cavity, esophagus, cranial nerves, brain, muscles, and limbs. The mechanics of eating and swallowing comprise the anatomical structures, physiological processes of eating and swallowing, and phases of swallowing discussed in the following material.

Anatomical Structures

Swallowing is a complex neuromuscular process that requires communication between the central and peripheral nervous systems and coordinated actions between the oral cavity, pharynx, esophagus, larynx, muscles, cranial nerves, and brain. Ingestion of food begins in the oral cavity, composed of the lips, cheeks, tongue, teeth, gums, mandible, hard and soft palate, uvula, anterior and posterior faucial arches, palatine tonsils, and salivary glands (Figure 16-2).

The oral cavity is lined with different types of sensory cells that have a role in swallowing. The mechanoreceptive cells cover the largest area and are concentrated most heavily at the tip of the tongue and along the midline of the palate. When the sensory cells on the palate are stimulated with pressure, peristaltic movements of the tongue are produced. The oral cavity is also innervated by thermoreceptive and chemoreceptive cells. The spatial distribution of the

thermoreceptive cells is highest along areas of the palate and tongue that come in contact with each other during swallowing. Chemoreceptive cells are distributed most densely along the tongue (Plant, 1998).

Pharynx

The oral cavity communicates with the pharynx via the oropharyngeal isthmus. The pharynx is a 12- to 14-cm musculomembranous tube extending from the soft palate to the cricoid cartilage, where it connects to the esophagus. It is formed by 26 pairs of striated muscles and is densely innervated with motor fibers. Three striated constrictor muscles, the superior, medial, and inferior, propel food along the pharynx during swallowing. Fibers of the inferior constrictor muscle attach to the sides of the thyroid cartilage, forming the pyriform sinuses and ending at the cricopharyngeal muscle (Logemann, 1983), the most inferior structure of the pharynx (Figure 16-3). At rest, tonic contractions of the cricopharyngeal muscle prevent air from entering the esophagus during respiration and food from refluxing into the esophagus and up to the pharynx. The cricopharyngeal muscle relaxes to allow a bolus of food to enter the esophagus. The pharynx is divided into the nasopharynx above the soft palate, the oropharynx, posterior to the mouth, and the hypopharynx, which extends below the esophagus (Groher, 1997) (Figure 16-4).

Esophagus and Larynx

The esophagus is a hollow, muscular tube approximately 23 to 25 cm long, with a sphincter at each end. The muscles of the upper third of the esophagus are striated; the muscles of the middle third are a mix of both striated and smooth. The lower third, including the lower esophageal sphincter, is smooth muscle. The bolus of food enters the esophagus from the pharynx and is transported to the stomach by the muscular peristaltic action of the esophagus.

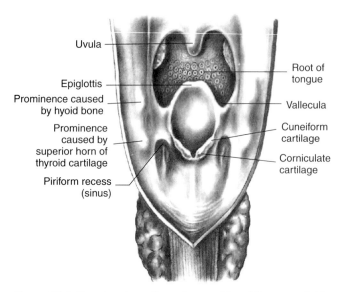

Uvula
Epiglottis
Prominence caused by hyoid bone
Prominence caused by superior horn of thyroid cartilage
Piriform recess (sinus)
Root of tongue
Vallecula
Cuneiform cartilage
Corniculate cartilage

Figure 16-4 Posterior view of hypopharynx. (From Thompson, J. M., McFarland, G. K., Hirsh, J. E., & Tucker, S. M. [2002]. *Mosby's Clinical Nursing* [5th ed.]. St. Louis, MO: Mosby.)

TABLE 16-3 Cranial Nerves Used for Deglutition

Cranial Nerve	Function
Trigeminal (V)	
Motor	Mandibular muscles
Sensory	Maxillary, mandibular
Facial (VII)	
Motor	Submandibular and sublingual salivary glands; facial expression
Sensory	Taste: anterior two thirds of tongue
Glossopharyngeal (IX)	
Motor	Stylopharyngeus muscle
Sensory	Taste: posterior third of tongue; sensation of soft palate and uvula
Vagus (X)	
Sensory	Membrane of larynx and pharynx
Spinal Accessory (XI)	
Motor	Sternocleidomastoid muscle
Hypoglossal (XII)	
Motor	Intrinsic tongue

The upper esophageal sphincter (UES) separates the hypopharynx from the esophagus. It is a high-pressure region, 3 to 4 cm long, which prevents air from entering the stomach during swallowing and limits reflux of gastric contents. There are two muscles running from the cricoid cartilage to the pharynx, the pars obliqua and pars fundiformis. The pars obliqua runs in an oblique direction superiorly and posteriorly from the lateral cricoid and blends with the inferior constrictor fibers. The pars fundiformis runs in a horizontal direction around the posterior pharynx and reinserts on the opposite side of the cricoid. The triangular gap between the pars obliqua and the pars fundiformis is Killian's triangle. The pars fundiformis is referred to as the *cricopharyngeus muscle*. There are five levels of UES activity: relaxation, opening, distention, collapse, and contraction. The forces propelling the food bolus through the UES are generated by the movement of the tongue in the pharynx. The sphincter opening and closing occur during the time of maximum laryngeal elevation (Wisdom & Blitzer, 1998).

The larynx begins at the base of the tongue with the epiglottis. It is anterior to the hypopharynx at the upper end of the trachea. The spaces formed between the base of the tongue and the sides of the epiglottis are the valleculae, where food may collect either before or after the swallow reflex is triggered. The larynx has many cells that respond to liquid stimulation (Plant, 1998). Other structures of the larynx include the aryepiglottic folds and the true and false vocal cords. During deglutition the larynx is elevated, the epiglottis is displaced downward, and the aryepiglottic folds and true and false vocal cords are adducted to protect the trachea (Groher, 1997; Logemann, 1998).

The brain interprets, integrates, and coordinates sensory, motor, and reflex information and activity. Six cranial nerves (V, VII, IX, X, XI, and XII) and the first three cervical nerves are involved in eating and swallowing (Table 16-3).

Stimulation studies show regions in the pons and medulla that evoke a swallowing reflex when stimulated. The motor nuclei for many of the muscles involved in swallowing are located in the brainstem. The cerebral cortex assists in the initiation of the oral and pharyngeal phases of swallowing (Plant, 1998).

Secondary Structures

Secondary structures involved in eating are the eyes, nose, arms, hands, and legs, which are necessary for a person to remain functionally independent, able to locate, secure, and prepare food and deliver it to the oral cavity. Visualizing food may stimulate appetite, and movements such as the arm bringing food to the mouth, presenting food on a utensil, taste, and food texture are important in alerting the body to prepare for swallowing and in triggering the swallow itself (Poertner & Coleman, 1998).

PHYSIOLOGICAL BASIS

The physiological process of eating and swallowing requires four stages: selecting and securing food, preparing food, experiencing the anticipatory stage when food is brought to and placed in the mouth, and swallowing.

A caregiver may select and secure food for a patient without serious physiological consequences. However, social and psychological consequences may result when a person becomes unable to prepare food and self-feed.

The final stage of eating is the act of swallowing; it begins once food enters the oral cavity. Swallowing is a complex function accomplished when activities within the oral cavity, pharynx, larynx, and esophagus are coordinated with interruption of respirations. Afferent, efferent, and central nervous system actions—some volitional and some reflexive—govern the entire swallowing process, which lasts 5 to 10 seconds (Logemann, 1998). Swallowing is divided into four phases: the oral preparatory phase, when food is manipulated, chewed, mixed with saliva, and formed into a bolus; the oral phase, where the bolus is centrally located on the tongue and pushed posteriorly toward the oropharynx; the pharyngeal phase, when the bolus is moved by the swallowing reflex through the pharynx; and the esophageal phase, as peristalsis moves the bolus to the stomach.

Oral Preparatory Phase

The oral preparatory phase is a voluntary phase during which the airway remains open and nasal breathing continues. Food is placed in the mouth, and the labial seal holds it in the oral cavity while it is manipulated. The type and amount of manipulation vary with the consistency of the food. Mastication uses rotary and lateral movements of the tongue and mandible to control and manipulate food while the upper and lower teeth crush food.

Mixed with saliva to form a bolus, the food is collected medially on the tongue before the swallow. Soft food may be held on the tongue or between the tongue and hard palate. Liquids are pooled and cupped between the tongue and anterior hard palate until the oral stage begins. Peripheral nerves give feedback about the position of the bolus to prevent injury to the tongue.

Oral Phase

The oral phase, also voluntary, begins as the tongue moves the bolus posterior toward the oropharynx. The bolus sits in a groove created along the center of the tongue until the tongue squeezes the bolus posteriorly against the hard palate toward the oropharynx (Figure 16-5, A). Within a second the bolus passes the anterior faucial arches, completing the oral phase. Cranial nerves V, VII, and XII control this phase.

Pharyngeal Phase

The most complex part of swallowing is the pharyngeal phase. The person must maintain airway integrity while the bolus moves along the pharynx to the esophagus. Respirations are inhibited during this phase (Wisdom & Blitzer, 1998). Although this phase is reflexive, it must be initiated voluntarily; once initiated, it cannot be stopped. The swallowing reflex in most individuals is activated when the food bolus comes into contact with the anterior faucial arches. However, sensory receptors that can elicit the swallowing reflex are present in the tongue, epiglottis, and larynx (Logemann, 1983).

Once the swallowing reflex has been initiated, the following events occur: the tongue moves up and back to force the bolus into the upper pharynx, the soft palate elevates to assist in closure of the pharyngeal port to prevent entry of food into the nasal cavity, the pharyngeal constrictors initiate pharyngeal peristalsis to carry the bolus past the pharynx, the lateral walls of the pharynx are drawn up, the larynx is elevated and pulled forward to assist in closure of the larynx, and the epiglottis angles down to help protect the airway (Figure 16-5, B). The epiglottis checks the descent of the bolus, and the cricopharyngeal sphincter relaxes to permit the bolus to enter the esophagus (Groher, 1997). Impulses travel to the swallowing center in the brainstem via the glossopharyngeal nerve. Cranial nerves V, VII, X, and XII carry the motor impulses that produce the swallowing reflex. The pharyngeal phase lasts approximately 1 second.

Laryngeal Actions. The larynx is protected in part by the downward movement of the epiglottis at an angle of approximately 135 degrees. This moves the laryngeal opening up and forward under the base of the tongue and epiglottis. Laryngeal movement with contraction of the intrinsic laryngeal muscles temporarily decreases the circumference of the laryngeal vestibule. The true and false vocal cords also adduct, and the aryepiglottic folds close to provide airway protection. The larynx may close at any stage during swallowing but is closed when the bolus leaves the pharynx. This causes any food entering the larynx to be squeezed out. The downward movement of the epiglottis helps protect the laryngeal opening from bolus residue. The negative pharyngeal pressure associated with reinflation of the airway propels any residue up and traps it in the valleculae (Groher, 1997).

Esophageal Phase

Swallowing is completed with the esophageal phase (Figure 16-5, C), which lasts 8 to 20 seconds. As the bolus enters the esophagus at the cricopharyngeal junction, peristaltic waves respond to the swallow reflex by propelling the bolus down the esophagus. The bolus passes through the gastroesophageal juncture into the stomach. The cricopharyngeus exerts a pharyngeal pressure of 15 to 23 mm Hg and must be overcome by the hypopharynx to induce the opening of the UES (Wisdom & Blitzer, 1998).

Maintaining and Protecting Airway Integrity

Both food and air share the pathway of the pharynx. Consequently, to avoid aspiration while eating, respirations (airflow) must cease for approximately a half second during movement of the bolus through the pharyngeal phase. Food is not permitted into the larynx and trachea. Respiration and swallowing are coordinated functions. The following events protect the airway during swallowing: the tongue moves posteriorly to push the bolus into the pharynx; the soft palate elevates to help block the nasopharyngeal opening; and the larynx is elevated and pulled forward, causing the epiglottis to tilt down and help protect the airway. The vocal cords adduct to close off the trachea (Plant, 1998; Groher, 1997). The vocal folds normally close before initiation of the pharyngeal swallow and at the same time as elevation of the larynx. Closure of

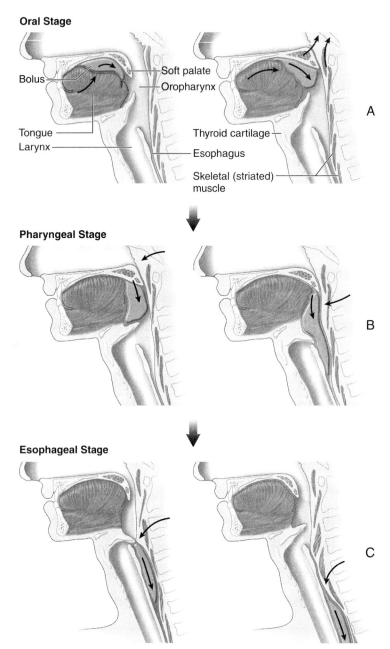

Oral Stage

Bolus
Tongue
Larynx

Soft palate
Oropharynx
Thyroid cartilage
Esophagus
Skeletal (striated) muscle

A

Pharyngeal Stage

B

Esophageal Stage

C

Figure 16-5 Deglutition. **A,** Oral stage. A bolus of food is voluntarily formed on the tongue, pushed against the palate and into the oropharynx. The soft palate helps to prevent food from entering the nasopharynx. **B,** Pharyngeal stage. Once the bolus is in the oropharynx, involuntary reflexes push the bolus down toward the esophagus. The upward movement of the larynx and downward movement of the bolus close the epiglottis, preventing food from entering the respiratory tract. **C,** Esophageal stage. Involuntary reflexes of skeletal and smooth muscle move the bolus through the esophagus. (From Thibodeau, G. A., & Patton, K. I. [2007]. *Anatomy and physiology* [6th ed.]. St. Louis, MO: Mosby.)

the airway starts at the vocal folds and progresses in a superior direction (Groher, 1997).

The gag reflex, a protective mechanism preventing unwanted material from entering the pharynx, larynx, or trachea, does not occur during the normal act of swallowing. Sensory mechanisms that trigger the gag reflex differ from those involved in swallowing. Motor control of the gag reflex is opposite the motor coordination activated in swallowing, because it forces food up and out of the pharynx. Absence of a gag reflex is not a sign of dysphagia. Approximately one third of persons without dysphagia do not have a gag reflex or have a diminished one. A gag reflex does not protect against aspiration. Patients with dysphagia can have a normal gag reflex (Leder, 1996; Perry & Love, 2001).

SWALLOWING CHANGES ACROSS THE LIFE SPAN

Swallowing is a complex neuromuscular process, and many factors can impair its efficiency. Age, neuromuscular impairments, and certain structural deficiencies that may alter swallowing must be understood.

Infants

The fetus begins swallowing in the womb between 10 and 14 weeks' gestation, with most fetuses able to swallow by 15 weeks' gestation. After 18 weeks' gestation the healthy fetus is able to open and close the jaw and perform anterior tongue movements and sucking. There is consistent swallowing between 22 and 24 weeks' gestation (Miller, Sonies, & Macedonia, 2003).

In infants, swallowing continues to develop as sensory inputs from the mouth and pharynx during feeding stimulate development of the regions in the brain that are responsible for feeding movements, which then generate more refined movements (Groher, 1997). Oral feeding is the most complex sensorimotor process the infant undertakes (Rodgers & Arvedson, 2005) An infant must coordinate sucking, swallowing, and breathing. Respirations in the sucking pattern follow in a sequence of inhalation, swallow, and exhalation. In some term infants, preterm infants, and neurologically compromised infants, feeding apnea may lead to hypoxia or bradycardia.

For term infants the sucking reflex, present at birth and throughout the first 7 months, begins the swallow. Anatomy and swallowing patterns of infants differ from those of adults. An infant's oral cavity is smaller, causing the tongue to fill a greater part of the mouth and to rest more interiorly. The larynx is suspended higher in the pharynx; the jaw, tongue, cheeks, and lips move as a single unit. The tongue elevates during sucking and thrusts the liquid to the posterior oral cavity. These actions are coordinated with the pharyngeal swallow. The anterior to posterior sucking movements of the tongue make the intake of soft solids difficult before the third to fourth month (Derkay & Schechter, 1998; Groher, 1997).

As the infant grows, the lower jaw extends downward and forward, and sucking pads are reabsorbed, increasing the intraoral space. The infant learns new voluntary suck patterns and suppresses the reflexive suckle patterns. The rooting reflex, initiated by touching the corner of the mouth, causes the infant to turn its head toward the touch; the rooting reflex disappears between 3 and 6 months. Tongue protrusion and transverse reflexes occur when the tongue or lips are touched. The tongue protrusion reflex disappears between 4 and 6 months. The tongue transverse reflex disappears between 6 and 9 months (Arvedson & Brodsky, 2002). There is an increased closing action of the lips, and tongue motion becomes a raising and lowering of the body of the tongue. This up-and-down motion helps to pull soft food and liquid into the oral cavity. Most infants complete this transition by 9 months of age (Darrow & Harley, 1998).

Children

Development of functional feeding skills is indicative of the achievements in sensorimotor integration of swallowing and respiration, hand and eye coordination, normal muscle tone and posture control, and psychosocial maturation (Arvedson & Brodsky, 2002). To become an independent feeder, gross and fine motor skills must be developed to bring food to the mouth, first with fingers and later utensils. Children develop patterns and behaviors associated with eating as part of the maturation process. A child with impaired swallowing needs to experience eating and food-related events appropriate for culture and age, such as finger foods for toddlers. The same child can be expected to develop food preferences and may use eating as a manipulative tool if too much attention is focused on eating.

Clinicians working with infants and children are aware of the influence that early abnormal feeding performance has on patterns of feeding in the neurologically impaired child. Children who require long-term tube feedings often experience oral feeding difficulties when the tube feedings are no longer necessary. Examples of difficulties include refusal to take any food in the oral cavity or accepting only a small variety of tastes and textures (Mason, Harris, & Blissett, 2005). Pinelli and Symington (2004) concluded, after an extensive literature review, that nonnutritive sucking has a positive effect on the transition from tube feeding to bottle feeding and on bottle-feeding performance. Abnormalities in feeding, respiration, and posture affect the development of the muscles and skeleton in the mouth, pharynx, and larynx, causing further abnormalities and difficulties in feeding and swallowing (Bosma, 1997).

The child with poor head and trunk control, altered or dependent sitting balance, and impaired swallowing, as occurs with cerebral palsy, requires special attention to posture, head position, lip and mouth control, eating and swallowing techniques, and feeding environment. This child may retain oral and swallowing reflexes that are expected to disappear, making risk of aspiration extremely high (Helfrich-Miller, Rector, & Straka, 1986). It is imperative for long-term feeding skills that infants transition to as normal a feeding process as possible. Once an infant is 6 months of age, it is increasingly difficult to establish bottle feeding for the first time (Mizuno & Ueda, 2001).

Adults

Normal healthy adults can experience primary presbyphagia, the age-related changes that occur in swallowing (Robbins et al., 2005) Individuals over the age of 60 have decreased two-point discrimination in the anterior two thirds of the tongue compared with individuals less than 40 years of age. There is a decrease in motor function and strength of the tongue in individuals over 60 years of age (Robbins, Levine, Wood, Roecker, & Luschei, 1994). Because the tongue creates the major propulsive force in moving the bolus through the oropharynx and into the esophagus, the changes can cause a decrease in speed and strength of swallows. Other changes may include loss of dentition, decreased sensation in the oral cavity, reduced pharyngeal peristalsis, with some of the bolus remaining in the pharynx, decreased size of the opening of the cricopharyngeal sphincter, decreased esophageal peristalsis, and increased esophageal transit time (Rademaker, Pauloski, Colangelo, & Logemann, 1998; Yoshikawa et al., 2005). There can also be subtle changes in the coordination of swallowing and respirations (Leslie, Drinnan, Ford, & Wilson, 2005).

DYSPHAGIA STATISTICS

Dysphagia means a difficulty in swallowing or an inability to swallow and is derived from the Greek words *dys* (bad) and *phagein* (to eat). The nature of dysphagia makes it difficult to accurately identify all persons who are affected. Specific statistics on the nature and prevalence of dysphagia are rare, and the statistics that are available for the United States generally pertain to persons older than 60 years.

It is estimated that approximately 15 million Americans have dysphagia (Hansell & Heinemann, 1996), and about 338,393 to 624,757 persons are affected by dysphagia each year as a result of a neurological disorder. The largest group with neurological disorders that has dysphagia is composed of individuals who have had a stroke. Videofluoroscopic studies indicate that 64% to 90% of conscious individuals in the acute phase of a stroke have some degree of dysphagia (Mann, Hankey, & Cameron, 1999). Approximately 213,000 persons with Parkinson's disease are diagnosed with dysphagia each year, and approximately 240,781 persons are affected by dysphagia each year as a result of other neurological diseases (Agency for Health Care Policy and Research [AHCPR], 1999). Studies of residents in nursing homes report the prevalence of dysphagia to be between 53% and 74% (O'Laughlin & Shanley, 1998).

Morris (2005) surveyed 171 patients over the age of 75 from one general practitioner in England and found that 11% reported swallowing problems. There is little information about the prevalence of dysphagia in the community.

These statistics do not address persons younger than 60 years, including the pediatric population; thus it is difficult to truly appreciate the magnitude of the numbers of persons who are affected each year in hospitals, nursing homes, and the community.

Aspiration is the passage of food or liquid through the vocal folds. Individuals who aspirate are at increased risk for pneumonia. Dysphagia is the major pathophysiological mechanism leading to aspiration pneumonia in the elderly. Pneumonia is the third highest cause of death during the first month after stroke, though not all cases can be attributed to aspiration of food or liquids (Ekberg, Hamdy, & Woisard, 2002). Thus the early detection, treatment, and management of dysphagia are critical.

NEUROMUSCULAR DISEASES

Neuromuscular diseases often affect multiple body systems and functions, including swallowing. The complex innervations of

the eating and swallowing process allow multiple variations of impairment to occur, involving minute steps during any one or more phases (Willig, Paulus, Lacau Saint Guily, Beon, & Naavarro, 1994). Major neuromuscular impairments that can affect swallowing are summarized in Table 16-4, along with the phase of deglutition affected and the impairment that results.

Impairments in the oral preparatory phase commonly result from poor sensation and perception about quantity and location of food in the mouth. Impaired motor control of the muscles and tongue during mastication may leave food improperly chewed or pocketed to the side of the mouth.

Impaired pharyngeal motility results in a poorly coordinated swallowing reflex. Food becomes lodged within the valleculae or pyriform sinuses and drains into the trachea, causing aspiration. Aspiration occurs most commonly during the oral phase when the swallowing reflex is delayed and the bolus is allowed to invade the larynx. The most experienced bedside observers do not identify 40% of the patients who aspirate (Logemann, 1983). Patients who have had a cerebrovascular accident may exhibit lingual hemiparesis, which interferes with tongue control and preparation for swallowing.

Patients with the same neurological disease will exhibit different symptoms, and the onset of dysphagia will occur at different stages of the disease. Patients must always be treated as individuals, and the interventions based on specific symptoms.

Specific Neurological Impairments

The most common neurological impairment associated with dysphagia is stroke. It occurs in 67% of brainstem strokes, 28% of left hemispheric strokes, and 21% of right hemispheric strokes. It is more common in bilateral lesions than in unilateral lesions and more common with large vessel injury than small vessel injury. Patients with damage to the left hemisphere are more likely to have impairments in the oral phase, whereas damage to the right hemisphere causes deficits in the pharyngeal phase (AHCPR, 1999).

Patients with amyotrophic lateral sclerosis (ALS) often have difficulty with oral transit and initiating a swallow, thus mealtimes are prolonged. They may also have palatal and pharyngeal weakness and isolated choking with liquids. Interventions include a modified diet and the use of calorie-dense foods with increased taste, temperature, and texture sensation to combat weight loss and food boredom. Patients should also have regular swallowing evaluations to monitor disease progression.

Patients with Parkinson's disease may have difficulty during the oral, pharyngeal, and esophageal phases of swallowing. Severity of the disease does not correspond to severity of dysphagia. Interventions may include feeding and dietary modifications, coordinating medications with mealtimes to maximize their positive effects, and offering small, frequent meals with increased sensory input. Small, frequent meals offer psychological benefits, allowing patients to feel they do not need to finish a large meal in a short time, thus allowing

TABLE 16-4 Neuromuscular Diseases Associated With Poor Deglutition and the Resulting Impairment

Phase of Deglutition/Disease	Impairment
Oral Preparatory	
Cerebral palsy	Poor suck reflex, inappropriate reflexive behaviors
Parkinson's disease; myasthenia gravis; ALS; left, right, bilateral, and brainstem cerebrovascular accidents; multiple sclerosis (when cranial nerve XII is involved)	Poor mastication, foods inadequately chewed
ALS; left, right, bilateral, and brainstem cerebrovascular accidents; Huntington's chorea; myasthenia gravis; Parkinson's disease; head trauma	Poor tongue control and mobility
Oral	
Bilateral and brainstem cerebrovascular accident	Delay in swallow reflex
Huntington's chorea, head trauma, cerebral palsy, Parkinson's disease, multiple sclerosis (when cranial nerve IX is involved)	Choking or coughing
Left, right cerebrovascular accident	Lingual hemiparesis
Pharyngeal	
Parkinson's disease; ALS; multiple sclerosis; left, right, bilateral, and brainstem cerebrovascular accident; poliomyelitis	Impaired pharyngeal motility and peristalsis
Cerebrovascular accident, myasthenia gravis	Residue in valleculae and pyriform sinuses
Myotonic dystrophy, head trauma, ALS, Huntington's chorea	Aspiration

ALS, Amyotrophic lateral sclerosis.

them to enjoy the meal, and it reassures patients that they will not go hungry if they do not finish a meal (Groher, 1997; Wisdom & Blitzer, 1998).

Patients with multiple sclerosis may deny difficulty with swallowing. This can be due to cognitive deficits or because they are not aware of the swallowing difficulty. In the early stages patients may have occasional choking, especially when fatigued. In later stages the swallowing difficulties are in the oral cavity and pharynx, with delayed swallowing reflex and reduced pharyngeal peristalsis. Some patients also report abnormal taste. Interventions include feeding modifications, decreased distractions at mealtime, and increased awareness of sensory cues (Wisdom & Blitzer, 1998).

Patients with myasthenia gravis may have slow, weak tongue movements, fatigue during deglutition, and bolus residue in the oropharynx. Chewing and swallowing abilities may deteriorate during meals. Interventions include coordinating medications with meals and limiting physical activity, including talking, before eating to maintain strength (Groher, 1997).

Neuromuscular impairments typically involve more than one stage of swallowing (Glenn, Araya, Jones, & Liljefors, 1993). Robbins, Logemann, and Kirshner (1986) found all participants of their study who had Parkinson's disease "exhibited abnormal oropharyngeal movement patterns and timing during the volitional oral and pharyngeal phases of swallowing." Patients with chronic, progressive diseases such as cerebral palsy, Parkinson's disease, multiple sclerosis, and amyotrophic lateral sclerosis often have progressive difficulty with swallowing (Acello, 2003).

ANATOMICAL IMPAIRMENTS

Cleft lips and cleft palates, anatomical impairments found in children, require surgical correction. A cleft in the lip may be a small notch or may extend to the floor of the nose. Cleft palates occur alone or in conjunction with cleft lips. Until surgical repair is completed, nasal regurgitation complicates the tasks of sucking and swallowing liquids and nutritional intake is compromised during a stage of rapid growth and development.

Pharyngoesophageal diverticulum, or Zenker's diverticulum, in the cervical esophagus is an abnormal muscular pouch that forms either above the cricopharyngeal muscle through Killian's triangle or below the cricopharyngeal muscle. The cause has not been established. The symptoms include regurgitation of undigested food, foul breath, fullness in the neck, weight loss, and nighttime cough with aspiration. Surgery is usually required to correct this dysfunction (Groher, 1997).

Radical head and neck surgery often contributes to impaired swallowing. Severity of the impairment varies with location and cause of surgery. Other less common causes of dysphagia include prolonged mechanical ventilation (Tolep, Getch, & Criner, 1996); tracheostomy tubes, which can reduce elevation and anterior movement of the larynx; improperly fitting hard cervical collars, which can restrict laryngeal elevation (Houghton & Curley, 1996); neck overextension in patients with halo fixators; excessive neck flexion with Philadelphia collars; and inadequate head support in high-back wheelchairs. Additional causes are cervical spine surgery with an anterior approach (Baron, 2003; O'Brien, Zarro, Gelb, Bhargara, & Ludwig, 2005), cervical osteophytosis (McGarrah & Teller, 1997), and acquired immunodeficiency syndrome (AIDS) (Martinez & Nord, 1995).

FEEDING TUBES

Any patient with dysphagia who is unable to meet his or her nutritional needs orally should be evaluated for nasogastric feedings as soon as possible. A goal for all patients is to avoid the prolonged use of feeding tubes. However, in the early stages of treatment one may be necessary to provide the nutrients needed to maintain or achieve metabolic balance.

For early tube feeding the nasogastric method is commonly used. Huggins, Tuomi, and Young (1999) found that both fine-bore (8 French × 85 cm) and wide-bore (16 French × 122 cm) nasogastric tubes slowed swallowing in healthy persons; however, the small-bore nasogastric tubes slowed swallowing less. The smaller tubes are also less irritating with less nasopharyngeal erosion and less compromise of the gastroesophageal sphincter. A nasogastric tube in a patient with dysphagia can cause increased difficulty with swallowing of saliva, regurgitation of gastric contents, and suppression of the cough reflex. A surgically placed feeding tube is the method of choice for most enteral feeding programs lasting more than 4 weeks, including patients who receive nutritional care at home. The most commonly used tubes are gastrostomy, jejunostomy, esophagostomy, and percutaneous endoscopic gastrostomy (PEG). PEGs can be performed with local anesthesia and result in fewer complications than surgical procedures (Sands, 1999). Children may have a gastrostomy button. Patients and families are taught to recognize and report signs of complications such as postoperative edema, bleeding, tube dislodgment, peritonitis, aspiration, skin irritations, and diarrhea. The most serious complication associated with any method of tube feeding is aspiration. The potential for aspiration is lessened when the patient is sitting up in a chair or in bed with the head elevated at least 45 degrees while being fed and for the hour that follows.

Patients receiving any type of tube feeding should be monitored daily for edema, dehydration, fluid intake and output, and stool output and consistency (including caloric composition and density). A weight should be taken at the same time, in the same amount of clothing (as little as possible), at least 3 times a week. Levels of serum electrolytes, blood urea nitrogen (BUN), creatinine, and blood count should be checked 2 to 3 times a week, and a chemistry profile should be done weekly (Bradford, 1996; Sands, 1999).

Not all medications can be crushed and given via the tube, and some may not be available in a liquid form; thus substitutions may be needed. Some drug forms that should not be crushed are extended release (drugs ending in SR—sustained release, SA—sustained action, XL—extended release, or those having -bid, -dur, -ten, -slow or contin in the name), enteric coated, encapsulated beads, wax matrix, and sublingual. Crushing drugs in these forms causes changes that can greatly affect the

rate of absorption and increase the risk for adverse reactions (Cornish, 2005; Glenn-Molali, 2005). Other forms that should not be crushed include capsules containing a liquid, capsule within a capsule, capsules that are sealed, and compressed tablets (McCann, 2004). Communication between the nurse, physician, and pharmacist is imperative to ensure that proper forms of medication are available and to avoid medication errors. Patient and family teaching regarding medication administration is critical for individuals going home on tube feedings and for whom swallowing pills is difficult.

When a patient is able to take adequate oral nutrition, the tube is removed. Accurate calorie and nutritional data are indicators as to whether a person can maintain adequate oral intake and must be carefully assessed before the tube is removed. Premature removal and subsequent reinsertion of a feeding tube may add to discomfort and be viewed as regression or lead to depression for the patient or family.

NURSING ASSESSMENT

The nursing assessment involves both collection and interpretation of data. It is central to understanding a patient's nourishment patterns and eating process and identifying specific deficits. A complete assessment includes a history of difficulties in eating, a measurable review of food and fluid intake, evaluation of laboratory data, interpretation of findings from diagnostic studies, and a physical assessment.

Nursing History

The purpose of the nursing history is to establish the present eating patterns and the patterns before illness/injury, describe any present difficulties, determine areas of evaluation for physical assessment, and evaluate the patient's need for education. The history should focus on four broad areas: ability of the patient to obtain and prepare food, adequacy of diet and nutritional habits and preferences, ability of the patient to bring food to the mouth, and ability to chew and swallow.

The assessment questions are divided into the four areas listed above. Different questions may be more important depending on where the care is being provided: community, clinic, rehabilitation, acute care, or long-term care setting.

Obtaining and Preparing Food. Caregivers who obtain and prepare food should be present, if possible, when taking the history to offer information regarding nutritional adequacy of the diet, how food is prepared, personal or ethnic rules about food or eating, when foods are served, and similar data that might affect a patient's intake. When a patient shops for and prepares food, ask questions related to transportation to the store and frequency of trips, storage and preparation facilities, difficulties preparing food, accessibility and safety of cooking areas, presence of a fire extinguisher and place for sharp knives, if meals are prepared from a standing or sitting position, adaptive devices used, difficulty with mobility, and strength and dexterity in the arms and hands to manipulate, open, and prepare foods.

Data from Harris, D. R. (1996). *Diet and nutrition sourcebook*. Detroit, MI: Omnigraphics; and Groher, M. (1997). *Dysphagia: Diagnosis and management* (3rd ed.). Boston: Butterworth-Heinemann.

Adequacy of the Diet, Nutritional Habits, and Preferences. Questions related to diet, nutritional habits, and preferences should elicit information regarding the following: special dietary recommendations by physicians and how closely the diet is followed; recent weight changes and possible reasons; meals eaten alone; type of meals prepared in the home and meals purchased or brought in by someone; number of meals and snacks per day; amount and type of fluids consumed, including alcohol; medications (both prescription and over the counter), including vitamins, herbs, and supplements (medications that can affect swallowing are described in Box 16-1); medications taken with meals; cultural or religious preferences; food allergies or food intolerances; and amount of money available for food per week.

Economics and access to affordable fresh foods are important for the types of food available to the patient. Convenience or prepared foods are easier but more expensive and many contain unwanted fat and salt. Fresh foods have more nutrient value but are more difficult to prepare and store, and they may be more expensive out of season. The social aspect of eating may also affect nutritional status; persons who eat alone are at greater risk for poor nutrition.

Ability of the Patient to Bring Food to the Mouth. This area covers the patient's ability to eat independently, adaptive feeding equipment used, ability to open individual food containers/packages, shortness of breath while eating, and sitting position for eating and the time just after eating.

Ability of the Patient to Chew and Swallow Food. The next phase of the history elicits information about the patient's ability to swallow effectively. If the patient answers yes for any of the following symptoms, ask how long the symptom has been present. Factors to be considered include history of aspiration pneumonia or chest infections, pain with swallowing, difficulty chewing, food sticking in the throat, solids being washed down with liquids, difficulty swallowing solid or soft foods, difficulty swallowing liquids, foods needing to be cut into very small pieces, foods or liquids regurgitating nasally, choking/coughing when eating or drinking, modification of foods/fluids, position used when eating or drinking, special techniques/movements used to help with swallowing, and duration of meal times.

Psychosocial Factors. By the end of the history the nurse should be able to assess the following through conversations with the patient: the degree to which loneliness, depression, or swallowing difficulties are contributing to a poor nutritional intake; amount of fear the person has regarding eating; degree to which lifelong eating habits are contributing to a poor nutritional intake; and degree of willingness and motivation the patient has to work in a rehabilitation program.

Physical Assessment

The physical assessment begins with examination of the head and neck and includes assessment of the following: head control in a seated position; facial symmetry; the lips for color, symmetry, and moisture (malignant lesions of the oral cavity may occur on the lips and under the tongue); drooling, indicating poor control of oral fluids; ability to close lips tightly and open mouth; internal symmetry; mucosa of the oral cavity and tongue (with dehydration they appear dry); lacerations, indicating biting while chewing; and teeth for number and condition. If there are dentures, inspect for proper fit, ask the patient to remove them (or remove if patient is unable), and inspect underlying gums.

Test cranial nerve XII (hypoglossal) by inspecting the tongue for irregular movement or asymmetry, both while the tongue is in the mouth and when protruded. Ask the patient to move the tongue side to side and in and out rapidly.

Cranial nerves IX (glossopharyngeal) and X (vagus) are tested by asking the patient to say "ah." The uvula and soft palate should rise. Deviation of the uvula is found with paralysis. When the uvula is touched with a tongue depressor, a gag reflex occurs, indicating intact motor function of the vagus nerve. Although the gag reflex is closely associated with the swallowing reflex, it does not need to be present for the normal swallow to occur. Presence of a gag reflex does not rule out dysphagia. Evaluate the voice for hoarseness or nasal quality. Inspect the pharynx for color, edema, and ulcerations including the anterior and posterior faucial arches and palatine tonsils.

Test cranial nerve V (trigeminal) for strength and symmetry by asking the patient to clench the teeth, chew, and move the lower jaw side to side against the resistance of the examiner's hand. The examiner palpates the temporomandibular area to determine muscle strength during contraction. The sensory component of the nerve is tested by asking the patient to identify sharp and dull sensations on the sides of the face, forehead, and cheeks. The two sides should be compared to each other.

Test cranial nerve VII (facial) throughout the examination by observing for tics and unusual movements or asymmetry of the face. Test motor function by observing the patient's ability to clench the teeth, smile, raise the eyebrows, wrinkle the forehead, purse the lips, whistle, and blow. Dentures should be in place if worn. The sensory component of this cranial nerve is used to identify sweet and salty tastes. Sugar or salt may be placed on the anterior two thirds of the tongue.

Test cranial nerve XI (spinal accessory) by asking the patient to raise the shoulders against resistance of the examiner's hands and to turn the head against resistance. Inability to raise the shoulders indicates damage on the ipsilateral side, and inability to turn the head is indicative of damage on the contralateral side from the head turn (Voss, 1994).

If indicated, test the patient for the presence of primitive reflex behaviors usually seen only in infants and which, when present in later life, indicate a disturbance of the upper motor neuron system (e.g., after a brain injury). These reflexes include the rooting reflex and the tonic neck reflex, sometimes called the fencing position.

Throughout the examination, evaluate the patient's voice. Oral and palatal dysfunctions are highlighted by dysarthria or hypernasality. Ask the patient to cough. If it is not forceful, ask the patient to cough forcefully. Ask the patient to swallow water; observe for a tight seal with the lips, water leakage, difficulty initiating the swallow, and compensatory techniques used. Observe the patient for a moist, wet voice and frequent clearing of the throat after swallowing the water. Check the patient's temperature 30 minutes after eating; an elevation can be indicative of aspiration.

The remainder of the physical examination should focus on the patient's ability to eat independently. The following areas should be assessed: mobility, muscle strength, and control of utensils from the plate to mouth, adequacy of grip and strength holding utensils, presence of tremor or involuntary movements that interfere with coordination, ability to cut food and use both hands, muscle strength and head control to remain sitting upright for meals, and visual acuity. Is vision limited (e.g., hemianopsia)?

The nursing history and physical assessment should provide data to describe the patient's disability and to form the basis for the nursing diagnoses.

Diagnostic Tests

The most commonly used diagnostic tests for identifying dysphagia include the bedside swallow examination (BSE), modified barium swallow with videofluoroscopy, and videoendoscopy.

The **BSE** should be done on all patients considered at risk for dysphagia. It may be done with or without liquids or food. The purpose is to identify patients at risk for aspiration due to an ineffective pharyngeal swallow. The BSE may be an informal examination or a structured assessment. Informal examinations may consist of a few questions and assessing the pharyngeal swallow in the following manner. The clinician's index finger is placed at the base of the tongue in the submandibular

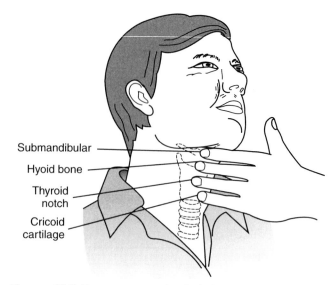

Figure 16-6 Finger position for bedside swallow examination. (From Elkin, M. K., Perry, A. G., Potter, P. A. [2007]. *Nursing interventions & clinical skills* [4th ed.]. St. Louis, MO, Mosby.)

region, the middle finger at the hyoid bone, the ring finger at the thyroid notch, and the little finger at the cricoid cartilage. As the patient swallows, the clinician should feel the tongue and laryngeal structures moving up and forward simultaneously as the swallow occurs (Figure 16-6).

A structured BSE consists of a detailed history regarding the medical condition, surgeries, and medications that may cause dysphagia; a physical examination of the patient's face, mouth, and throat (see Physical Assessment); assessing cognition; and observing the patient swallow without food and with different amounts and consistencies of food and fluid (AHCPR, 1999; Payten, 2005).

Videofluoroscopic swallow study (VFSS) or modified barium swallow, allows viewing of the oral cavity, laryngopharynx, and cervical esophagus. The patient swallows small amounts of a liquid, puree, and/or solid mixed with barium. As the bolus is manipulated in the oral cavity and swallowed, the study is recorded on videotape. Videotaping allows for repeated viewing and slow-motion analysis. Head position, compensatory techniques, and a patient's tolerance for swallowing foods and liquids of different consistencies can be evaluated and all phases of swallowing assessed (Marik, 2003).

Video endoscopic swallow study (VEES)/fiberoptic endoscopic swallow study (FEES) uses a fiberoptic nasopharyngoscope to visually examine a patient's nasopharynx. Swallows are observed as are any secretions that may pool. The sensations of the upper aerodigestive tract may also be assessed. The patient is then given fluids and foods of different consistencies to swallow. Dye may be added to the food to increase its visibility and the study recorded for patient teaching and biofeedback. The equipment is portable, and no radiation is used. The test can also be conducted throughout a meal to identify fatigue factors (Bastian, 1998; Marik, 2003).

Fiberoptic endoscopic evaluation of swallowing with sensory testing (FEESST) combines endoscopic evaluation of swallowing with a technique that determines laryngopharyngeal sensory discrimination thresholds. An air-pulse stimulus is delivered through the endoscope to mucosa innervated by the superior laryngeal nerve. The stimulus elicits a brainstem-mediated airway protection reflex (Aviv et al., 2000).

Manometry is used to study the strength, timing, and sequencing of pressure events in the esophagus during deglutition. A catheter with pressure transducers is positioned within the esophagus; the transducers measure pressures as the patient swallows. Usually the transducers are positioned to measure pressures in the UES, the esophagus, and the lower esophageal sphincter. Manometry is used to identify disruptions in the peristaltic waves through the pharynx and esophagus and to diagnose impairments of the upper or lower esophagus. Manofluorography combines monometry with videofluoroscopy (Bastian, 1998).

NURSING DIAGNOSIS

The priority nursing diagnoses that may be used for eating and swallowing deficits from the nutrition support and respiratory management classes are listed in Table 16-5, along with the suggested Nursing Interventions Classification (NIC) interventions and Nursing Outcomes Classification (NOC) outcomes.

Other nursing diagnoses that may be applicable to the patient with eating and swallowing impairments are the following: Impaired verbal communication, Feeding self-care deficit, Bathing/hygiene self-care deficit, Health-seeking behaviors (specify), Ineffective therapeutic regimen management (specify area), Risk for ineffective therapeutic regimen management (specify area), Effective therapeutic regimen management, Ineffective family therapeutic regimen management, Ineffective health maintenance (specify area), Noncompliance (specify area), and Deficient knowledge in proper nutrition, adaptive equipment, or availability of community resources.

Goals

Goals established by the nurse and patient relate to the nursing diagnoses and are based on information obtained from the patient during the nursing assessment, family members, and home assessment data. The nurse may help decrease the episodes of aspiration and choking for patients by reinforcing compensatory swallowing techniques to make the swallowing process safer. For someone with an impaired swallowing process, liquids are often difficult to swallow. As a result the patient may have a great deal of fear when taking liquids and be fluid-volume deficient. It is important to maximize the safety of swallowing, to provide encouragement, and to increase liquid intake either through alternate forms or by offering fluids more often.

Inadequate caloric intake, particularly of solid foods, necessitates alternate and more frequent feedings. If poor intake is a result of depression, the underlying problem must be addressed. A complete diet history that includes food preferences and the significance of food may be completed to find foods the patient might eat.

The goals for the patient having difficulty with eating and swallowing or for the family may include all or some of the following: maintains adequate nutrition, maintains adequate body weight, demonstrates and uses compensatory postures, demonstrates and uses compensatory swallowing techniques, demonstrates ability to swallow modified foods and fluids, verbalizes understanding of the importance of modifications in consistency of foods and fluids, shows no evidence of aspiration, improves or maintains fluid volume, demonstrates improved ability to feed self, demonstrates ability to use adaptive equipment, demonstrates improved ability to participate in oral hygiene, verbalizes understanding of measures to prevent and alleviate choking, verbalizes understanding of proper nutrition,

TABLE 16-5 Nursing Diagnoses, Interventions, and Outcomes Applicable to Dysphagia `NIC/NOC`

Nursing Diagnosis	Nursing Interventions	Nursing Outcomes
Ineffective airway clearance Risk for aspiration	Aspiration precautions Swallow therapy Aspiration precautions	Aspiration prevention Aspiration prevention Swallowing status
Imbalanced nutrition: less than body requirements	Nutritional therapy	Nutritional status Nutritional status, food and fluid intake Nutritional status, nutrient intake
Impaired swallowing	Aspiration precautions Swallowing therapy	Aspiration prevention Swallowing status Swallowing status: oral phase Swallowing status: pharyngeal phase Swallowing status: esophageal phase

Data from Moorhead, S., Johnson, M., & Maas, M. (Eds.). (2004). *Nursing outcomes classification (NOC)* (3rd ed.). St. Louis, MO: Mosby; Dochterman, J. M., & Bulechek, G. M. (2004). *Nursing interventions classification (NIC)* (4th ed.). St. Louis, MO: Mosby; and NANDA International. (2005). *Nursing diagnoses: Definitions and classification, 2005-2006* (6th ed.). Philadelphia: Author.

verbalizes understanding of importance of following prescribed dietary restrictions, and verbalizes understanding of available community resources to assist in providing adequate nutrition.

NURSING INTERVENTIONS

Once an assessment is completed, nursing diagnoses are formulated, and goals are established, specific nursing interventions must be individualized for the patient. The priority NIC interventions that may be used for eating and swallowing deficits from the nutritional class are listed in Table 16-5 with the nursing diagnosis and NOC outcomes. Other NIC interventions (Dochterman & Bulechek, 2004) that may be applicable to a patient with dysphagia include diet staging, nutritional management monitoring, intravenous therapy, oral health maintenance, teaching: prescribed diet, and health education.

Interventions

All patients need proper body posture and alignment during mealtimes with any necessary modifications for their situation. Proper body alignment helps stimulate the central nervous system. Box 16-2 lists general mealtime recommendations for a patient who is dysphagic and taking a diet with modified food consistencies.

The following suggestions should be altered as necessary for each patient:

- For poor head control when the head falls forward, hold the head up by placing the palm of your hand on the patient's forehead for support.
- Initially use teaspoon-sized bites of soft food that are easy to swallow (custards, purees); observe laryngeal elevation before offering the next bite.
- Place a half teaspoonful on the middle to back part of the tongue; however, if the patient has tongue or facial paralysis or has had a partial laryngectomy, the correct placement is on the unaffected intact side, not midline, to provide maximum sensory stimulation.
- Place the spoon firmly on the tongue to stimulate removal of food from the spoon.
- If swallowing does not occur, remove the spoon and instruct the patient to move the food toward the rear of the mouth.
- Check that the lips are sealed, or the swallowing reflex will not begin; manually seal the lips together, or use a jaw control maneuver to pull the jaws together.
- Medications may need to be given in custard, jelly, or blended flavored gelatin instead of applesauce because it tends to fall apart during swallowing.
- If fatigue is a factor, offer nutritious snacks or small, frequent meals.

Additional interventions for all patients with dysphagia include monitoring weight, hydration, and caloric intake (Box 16-3). Adequate fiber should be offered to prevent constipation.

Dietary Modifications

It is often suggested that thick liquids and pureed foods be offered to the patient with dysphagia; however, these are not always the safest options. Diet modifications must be specific to the physiology of the swallowing disorder.

Patients who have difficulty managing liquids eat a modified diet using liquids of a specified consistency. The texture

---

BOX 16-2 Recommendations for Patients on a Diet With Modified Consistencies

- Place patient in an upright sitting position with head in midline and arms supported on table; use positioning aids if needed; the upright position is the most efficient for eating and drinking for most patients and allows a more adequate swallow to be performed.
- For many patients the head-down/chin-tuck position (so the neck is flexed and the chin is approximately three fourths of the way down toward chest) will provide better airway protection and decrease the risk of aspiration.
- Keep the patient upright for 30 minutes after the meal to decrease esophageal reflux.
- Throughout the meal observe the patient for signs and symptoms of aspiration and change in respiration rate, color, voice quality, and coughing (Groher 1997; Miller & Chang, 1999).
- Room is well lighted with minimal distractions and quiet; conversations are kept to a minimum, although brief conversation allows assessment of the patient's voice quality.
- Encourage the patient to participate in feeding as much as possible.
- Sit down when assisting the patient to eat; this communicates time and willingness to help.
- Allow at least 30 to 45 minutes for feeding a patient with dysphagia.
- Let the patient see and smell the food.

BOX 16-3 Additional Interventions for Patients With Dysphagia

- Weight is a key indicator of the degree of difficulty the patient may have with eating and should be monitored. In the hospital and home, patients should be weighed at least weekly in the same amount of clothing.
- Dehydration, a major concern particularly for those unable to tolerate thin liquids, can lead to electrolyte imbalance and confusion. Liquids of modified consistency should be offered throughout the day and intravenous fluids used if necessary.
- Intake and output (I&O) and calorie counts assist in monitoring nutritional intake. Records should be filled out correctly because this information is often used to determine whether a patient is able to have a feeding tube removed. Most facilities have specific forms for this purpose.

or consistency of the foods eaten may also need to be modified. Most institutions have dysphagia diets that categorize liquids by consistency and foods by texture or consistency. In 2003 the American Dietetic Association (ADA) published the *National Dysphagia Diet* (NDD) to promote standard terminology of dietary texture modifications for liquids and food (Boxes 16-4 and 16-5).

Hot and cold liquids may be thickened by adding a commercial thickening agent or a household food product, such as instant potato flakes and instant baby rice cereal. For commercial thickening agents, refer to the product information for obtaining the proper consistency. Some thickening agents will hold the thickness or consistency as mixed, others will continue to thicken the liquid over time. The persons using the thickening agent (nurses, nursing assistants, dietitians, dietary aides, etc.) must be familiar with the product characteristics and be notified when an institution changes products. There are also many prethickened liquids available and in use by health care settings.

Modifications in food consistency are divided into four levels (see Box 16-5). As a patient progresses to a new level, the foods from the previous level may still be consumed. Most diets of modified consistencies are low in fiber. To prevent constipation, bran may be added to many dishes and prune juice thickened to the necessary consistency.

Choking (a protective maneuver for the airway) is frightening for a patient but unfortunately may be expected to occur at times in persons with swallowing difficulties. If coughing and choking can be minimized, fear and anxiety associated with feeding will be decreased. If food becomes lodged in the larynx, compromising breathing, and the patient is unable to cough forcefully or speak, the Heimlich maneuver should be used.

Compensatory Postures and Swallowing Techniques

Interventions are individualized for each patient. Tables 16-6 and 16-7 list compensatory postures and swallowing techniques and their benefits and the physiological disorders for which they are used. Box 16-6 describes how to do the swallowing techniques.

Sensory Stimulation

Sensory stimulation heightens sensitivity of sensory receptors involved in facilitation, initiation, efficiency, and safety of swallowing. Techniques include placement of food in specific locations within the oral cavity and modification in bolus volume, consistency, temperature, and taste. Because swallowing impairments usually occur in conjunction with impairments of the oral cavity, pharynx, larynx, and esophagus, the sensory stimulation techniques should be tested during radiographic evaluation. Patients with partial or complete sensory loss within the oral cavity or with impaired facial and lingual muscle strength may not be able to safely manage and control the bolus. The bolus may spread throughout the oral cavity and spill out of the lips or fall prematurely over the back of the tongue into the pharynx. The patient with lingual hemiparesis may need the bolus placed on the unaffected side of the tongue. The patient with difficulties propelling the bolus to the back of the oral cavity may require placement of the bolus on the back of the tongue (Martin-Harris & Cherney, 1996).

Modifying the consistency of a bolus can affect the onset and duration of swallowing events. The consistency of the bolus affects the transit time through the oral cavity and pharynx. Thick liquids move more slowly than thin liquids; thus thick liquids are recommended for patients with delayed pharyngeal swallow. Thick liquids may also be suggested for patients with incomplete laryngeal elevation and closure because a thick liquid is less likely to penetrate the unprotected larynx. Thin liquids may be recommended for patients with cricopharyngeal dysfunction or decreased pharyngeal clearance (Martin-Harris & Cherney, 1996).

Modifying the bolus size to a small volume may assist the patient prone to aspiration due to a pharyngeal swallow delay because a small bolus will not enter the pharynx as quickly as a large bolus. A larger bolus may be needed by other patients to initiate oral bolus transit. In addition, larger bolus volumes increase the extent and duration of laryngeal elevation, laryngeal closure, and pharyngoesophageal segment opening (Martin-Harris & Cherney, 1996).

For patients with decreased oral sensation or poor initiation of oral transport, cold stimulus facilitates more rapid

TABLE 16-6 Compensatory Postures: Postural Changes Affect How Gravity Moves Food Through the Pharynx

Position	Benefit	Physiological Disorder
Head-down/chin-tuck position: lowering head so neck is flexed and chin is approximately three fourths of way down toward chest	Widens valleculae; epiglottis covers more of airway, resulting in increased protection and decreased risk of aspiration; decreases pressures at cricopharyngeal muscle	Delayed reflex and reduced laryngeal closure
Head back: gently and slowly tossing head back	Moves food more rapidly through the oral cavity	Reduced tongue movement
Head turned toward affected or less functional side	Increases vocal fold adduction; closes pharynx on side to which head is turned, causing bolus to travel down opposite side of pharynx; reduces resting tone of cricopharyngeal muscle	Unilateral pharyngeal dysfunction, reduced laryngeal closures or unilateral laryngeal dysfunction, cricopharyngeal problems
Head tilted to more functional side	Gravity directs food down more functional side of pharynx	Unilateral damage to tongue and pharynx
Head turned and chin down	Affects direction of bolus and increases airway protection	Reduced laryngeal closure
Head back and turned	Moves bolus quickly through oral cavity; sets direction of bolus	Decreased tongue function, decreased laryngeal closure, unilateral pharyngeal weakness
Lying on one side with head supported	Removes effects of gravity	Reduced peristalsis, reduced laryngeal elevation

Modified from Logemann, J. A. (1991). Approaches to management of disordered swallowing. *Bailliere's clinical gastroenterology, 5,* 269-280; and Miller, R. M., & Chang, M. W. (1999). Advances in the management of dysphagia caused by stroke. *Physical Medicine and Rehabilitation Clinics of North America, 10*(4), 925-941.

TABLE 16-7 Swallowing Techniques

Technique	Benefit	Physiological Disorder
Supraglottic swallow	Increases voluntary airway protection, voluntary closure of glottis before and during swallow, ensures pulmonary air volume for throat clearing	Delayed pharyngeal swallow, impaired vocal cord closure
Mendelson maneuver	Allows voluntary increase in laryngeal elevation time and opening of cricopharyngeal sphincter, prolongs airway closure	Decreased laryngeal elevation or opening of cricopharyngeal sphincter
Effortful swallow	Improves weakness of tongue base	Reduced posterior movements of tongue

Modified from Logemann, J. A. (1991). Approaches to management of disordered swallowing. *Bailliere's Clinical Gastroenterology, 5,* 269-280; and Miller, R. M., & Chang, M. W. (1999). Advances in the management of dysphagia caused by stroke. *Physical Medicine and Rehabilitation Clinics of North America, 10*(4), 925-941.

posterior tongue movements and pharyngeal swallow. Other patients swallow efficiently with a warm bolus. Logemann and Pauloski (1995) demonstrated that patients with pharyngeal swallow delay showed a significant improvement in oral onset of swallow using a sour bolus.

Adaptive Equipment

For the patient who has a self-feeding deficit, the nurse can work closely with occupational and physical therapists in muscle strengthening, coordination, and use of adaptive equipment.

The nurse's role is to assess intake and implement and reinforce the compensatory techniques and use of adaptive equipment. Examples of adaptive equipment include scoop dishes, plate guards, and silverware modified for easy grasp and effective cutting and eating (Figure 16-7). Nonskid pads or a damp cloth may be used under dishes to prevent slipping.

Use of a straw requires complex functioning of the oral musculature and is often not recommended for patients with dysphagia. A patient drinking from a cup must tilt the head back when the cup becomes less than half full. This position increases the risk of aspiration. Specially designed cups are available, or a cutaway cup can be made by cutting a semicircular portion out of a paper cup. This allows the patient to tilt the cup further without tilting the head (Figure 16-8).

BOX 16-6 How to Implement Swallowing Techniques

Supraglottic Swallow (May Be Done With or Without Food in the Oral Cavity)
- If using food, place food in mouth.
- Have patient inhale and hold breath.
- Ask patient to swallow while holding breath (cover tracheostomy tube if applicable).
- Have patient cough or clear throat after swallowing without inhaling again.
- Repeat 10 times, 3 to 4 times per day.

Mendelson Maneuver (May Be Done With or Without Food in the Oral Cavity)
- Ask patient to place hand on larynx.
- Have patient swallow and feel larynx left at its highest position.
- If using food, ask patient to place food in mouth.
- Have patient swallow and again hold larynx in highest position during the swallow; patient then releases hold.
- Repeat 3 to 5 times, 3 to 4 times per day.

From Logemann, J. A. (1991). Approaches to management of disordered swallowing. *Bailliere's clinical gastroenterology, 5,* 269-280.

Oral Hygiene

It is important to remind or assist the patient with maintaining good oral hygiene. Dentures and partial plates should be worn to help support oral structures, give contour to the mouth, and promote normal movements (Miller & Chang, 1999). The oral cavity should be cleaned before and after each meal. The teeth, gums, palate and tongue should all

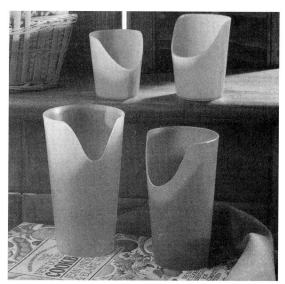

Figure 16-8 Tumbler with a special cutout for the nose allows the patient to drink without tipping the head back. (Courtesy Sammons Preston, a Bissell Healthcare Company, Bolingbrook, IL.)

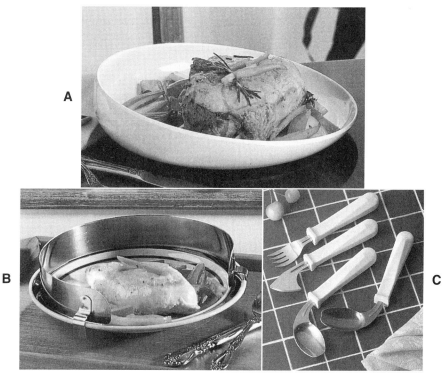

Figure 16-7 A, Scoop dish. **B,** Food guard. **C,** Easy-hold utensils. Knife blade will cut in both slicing and rocking motions. (Courtesy Sammons Preston, a Bissell Healthcare Company, Bolingbrook, IL.)

be brushed. Cleaning the oral cavity helps reduce bacteria in the mouth, that if aspirated, can increase the risk for pneumonia. One study on patients in a nursing home demonstrated that good oral care reduced the incidence of pneumonia (Yoneyama, Yoshida, Ohrui 2002). Another study of patients in a nursing home, found that intensive oral care improved cough reflex sensitivity (Watando et al., 2004). Care providers cleaned the patient's teeth for 5 minutes after each meal for 30 days. Cleaning included brushing palatal and mandibular mucosa and the dorsum of the tongue. Artificial saliva and humidified air may be beneficial to some patients because mouth breathing can cause drying of oral structures and promote bacterial growth. Chapter 30 discusses oral health needs for patients with intellectual/developmental disabilities.

Patient and Family Education

In addition to understanding the exact nature of the eating deficit, the patient and family need to be involved in establishing goals and planning care. Without patient and family cooperation, the rehabilitation process will be less effective. The role of the rehabilitation nurse includes promoting good communication with the family. Throughout the system, between care plan meetings, and elsewhere the nurse is an advocate for the family, explains new treatment approaches, and reports progress. The patient and family should demonstrate knowledge of dietary modifications, the hazards of offering "unsafe" food even when requested by the patient, use of adaptive equipment if needed, the process for feeding, and performance of emergency measures in the event of choking.

When the patient has excessive caloric intake, it is necessary to work with the family and patient. For this patient food commonly is substituted for other activities or used as a reward. Family members may bring food to the patient because it brings pleasure. The nurse can work with the patient and family to develop other positive forms of reinforcement and long-term goals for rehabilitation and to help the patient to see the consequences of overeating.

Rehabilitation Team Interventions

Eating and swallowing deficits are complex, multifaceted disorders that require the nurse to collaborate with other rehabilitation team professionals. All patients presenting with neuromuscular or neurological disorders should be evaluated for a swallowing impairment as early in the assessment process as possible and referred to the necessary team members (Hoeman & Glenn-Molali, 1999). Many facilities now have dysphagia teams or programs that are usually led by a speech-language pathologist, nurse, or occupational therapist (Glenn et al., 1993). The members of the team and their roles vary by institution, but the key members are the physician, nurse, speech-language pathologist, occupational therapist, dietitian, and physical therapist.

The physician is responsible for coordination of the patient's medical management and orders the initial referral to the dysphagia team. The physician also writes orders for dietary modifications.

As noted earlier, physical therapy helps improve muscle tone, strength, and coordination. Treatment is directed at improving muscle tone for the primary eating muscles, as well as secondary muscles of the arms, legs, head, and neck.

The occupational therapist performs self-feeding evaluations, recommends and teaches the use of adaptive equipment and exercises to improve hand control and coordination, and offers assistance in food preparation techniques. The therapist also may recommend meaningful activities for the patient to engage in during the day as a substitute for eating.

The speech-language pathologist may perform a bedside swallow evaluation and determine the need for diagnostic tests. On the basis of results of the screening or testing, the speech pathologist may design a program of exercises for the oropharyngeal musculature and identify what compensatory swallowing techniques and postures are to be used. Speech-language pathologists also work with patients on speech deficits.

The dietitian helps develop a menu plan that meets the nutritional, socioeconomic, and cultural requirements of the patient and teaches the proper diet to the patient and family. The dietitian also monitors nutritional status.

The nurse conducts a complete history and physical assessment and in-depth self-feeding and swallowing assessments. The nurse also monitors the patient's weight, caloric and fluid intake, and laboratory studies for hydration and nutritional status. A primary nursing responsibility is working with the patient and family to reinforce feeding and swallowing skills and to communicate progress to other team members. Demonstrated abilities on the unit or in a feeding group may differ from abilities in a private session with a therapist.

NURSING OUTCOMES

The priority NOC outcomes that may be used for eating and swallowing deficits from the nutritional-metabolic pattern are listed in Table 16-5 with the nursing diagnosis and NIC interventions.

Other nursing outcomes (Moorhead, Johnson, & Maas, 2004) that may be applicable for the patient experiencing difficulty with eating and swallowing include the following: nutritional status: energy; nutritional status: nutrient intake; respiratory status: airway patency; respiratory status: gas exchange; oral hygiene; self-care: hygiene; self-care: eating; knowledge: treatment regimen; knowledge: treatment procedures; and knowledge: diet.

For the patient with a progressive neuromuscular disorder, maintaining the maximum level of independence in eating and attaining adequate nutritional intake are realistic goals.

SUMMARY

Physiologically eating and swallowing are essential to a person's survival. Psychologically food and the ability to eat are important to feelings of self-worth. Socially many activities revolve around food. When one can no longer eat without difficulty, fear is commonly an overriding emotion. It includes not only fear for one's survival and ability to function but also fear of or actual loss of significant social interactions.

The nurse is crucial in identifying patients who may be at risk for or who have an eating or swallowing deficit. The nurse is the primary advocate in assisting these patients and their families in receiving the necessary interventions in all types of settings. The nurse has the knowledge and ability to draw in other rehabilitation team members as needed. The nurse is also the core team member to teach the patient and family about this aspect of rehabilitation that can result in many positive rewards and outcomes for the patient, family, and nurse.

Case Study

Elena Marinatos, a 76-year-old married woman originally from Greece, lives with her husband in a two-story home in a predominately Greek neighborhood. Their three grown children live in the same city. Mrs. Marinatos has just been transferred to the stroke unit of a rehabilitation facility. She is 4 days post left cerebrovascular accident. Upon entering the room, Mrs. Marinatos begins speaking to you. Her speech is slurred and difficult to understand. She is pointing to the lunch tray of her roommate. You greet her and begin the initial assessment. Mrs. Marinatos is drooling out of the right side of her mouth. Halfway through the assessment, Mr. Marinatos arrives, announcing that their daughter has sent fresh baklava, Elena's favorite dessert, to celebrate her leaving the hospital and coming to rehabilitation. Mr. Marinatos kisses his wife and gives her a piece of baklava as he says, "This is where you will get well." Mrs. Marinatos immediately takes the dessert and begins to eat before you can say anything. Bits of baklava are falling out of her mouth. Her husband says that it is good to see her eat real food again.

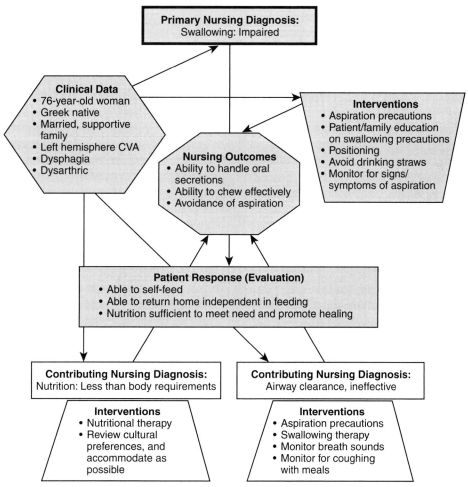

Concept Map. Mrs. Marinatos has a primary problem of impaired swallowing that will overshadow her successful rehabilitation program, if not addressed quickly. Interventions are needed to address the contributing issues of cultural preferences, diet, and family education. The concept map illustrates the interrelationships between the nursing diagnoses of impaired swallowing, less than required nutrition, and airway clearance. To promote independence for Mrs. Marinatos, the rehabilitation nurse will focus on coordinating interventions to achieve sufficient nutrition in a culturally sensitive manner while minimizing the risk of aspiration.

CRITICAL THINKING

1. What questions would be important to ask Mrs. Marinatos and her husband?
2. Which areas of the nursing physical assessment are top priority?
3. Which diagnostic tests are anticipated?
4. What would be important areas for patient/family education?

REFERENCES

Acello, B. (2003). Handling an unwelcome comeback: Postpolio syndrome. *Nursing, 33*(11), 32-35.

Agency for Health Care Policy and Research. (1999, July). *Diagnosis and treatment of swallowing disorders (dysphagia) in acute-care stroke patients* (Evidence Report/ Technology Assessment No. 8. prepared by ECRI Evidence-Based Practice Center under contract No. 290-97-0020, AHCPR Publication No. 99-E024). Rockville, MD: Agency for Healthcare Quality and Research.

Arvedson, J., & Brodsky, L. (2002). *American Dietetic Association: Pediatric swallowing and feeding: Assessment and management* (2nd ed.). Albany, NY: Singular Thomson Learning.

Aviv, J. E. (2000). Prospective, randomized outcome study of endoscopy vs modified barium swallow in patients with dysphagia. *Laryngoscope, 110*(4), 563-574.

Aviv, J. E., Kaplan, S.T., Thomson, J. E., Spitzer, J., Diamond, B., & Close, L.G. (2000). The safety of flexible endoscopic evaluation of swallowing with sensory testing (FEESST): An analysis of 500 consecutive evaluations. *Dysphagia, 15*, 39-44.

Barlow, S., & Dietz, W. (1998). Obesity evaluations and treatment: Expert committee recommendations. *Pediatrics, 102*(3), e29.

Baron, E. M., Solimann, A. M., Gaughan, J. P., Simpson, L., & Young, W. F. (2003). Dysphagia, hoarseness and unilateral true vocal fold motor impairment following anterior cervical diskectomy and fusion. *Annals of Otology, Rhinology and Laryngology, 112*(11), 921-926.

Barrett-Conner, E., Edelstein, S. I., Corey-Bloom, J., & Wiederholt, W. C. (1996). Weight loss precedes dementia in community dwelling older adults. *Journal of the American Geriatric Society, 44*, 1147-1152.

Bastian, R. (1998). Contemporary diagnosis of the dysphagic. *Otolaryngologic Clinics of North America, 31*(3), 489-506.

Bosma, J. F. (1997). Development and impairments of feeding in infancy and childhood. In M. Groher (Ed.), *Dysphagia diagnosis and management* (pp. 289-312). Boston: Butterworth-Heinemann.

Bradford, S. (1996). Methods of nutritional support. In L. K. Mahan, & S. Escott-Stump (Eds.), *Krause's food, nutrition and diet therapy* (9th ed., pp. 425-448). Philadelphia: W. B. Saunders.

Burns, R. D., & Carr-Davis, E. M. (1996). Nutritional care in diseases of the nervous system. In L. K. Mahan & S. Escott-Stump (Eds.), *Krause's food, nutrition and diet therapy* (9th ed., pp. 863-889). Philadelphia: W. B. Saunders.

Centers for Disease Control and Prevention, National Center for Health Statistics. (2004). *National health and nutrition examination survey.* Available from http://www.cdc.gov/nchs/data.

Centers for Disease Control and Prevention. (2007). Overweight and obesity. Available from http://www.CDC.gov/nccdphp/dnpa/obesity/trend/maps/index.htm.

Cornish, P. (2005). Avoid the crush: Hazards of medication administration in patients with dysphagia or a feeding tube. *Canadian Medical Association Journal, 172*(7), 871-872.

Darrow, D. H., & Harley, C. M. (1998). Evaluation of swallowing disorders in children. *Otolaryngologic Clinics of North America, 31*(3), 405-418.

D'Eramo, A. L., Sedlak, D., Doheny, M. O., & Jenkins, M. (1994). Nutritional aspects of the orthopaedic trauma patient. *Orthopedic Nursing, 13*, 13-20.

Derkay, C. S., & Schechter, G. L. (1998). Anatomy and physiology in pediatric swallowing disorders. *Otolaryngologic Clinics of North America, 31*(3), 397-404.

Dochterman, J. M., & Bulechek, G. M. (2004). *Nursing interventions classification (NIC)* (4th ed.). St. Louis, MO: Mosby.

Ekberg, O., Hamdy, S., & Woisard, V. (2002). Social and psychological burden of dysphagia: Its impact on diagnosis and treatment. *Dysphagia, 17*, 139-146.

Glenn, N., Araya, T., Jones, K., & Liljefors, J. (1993). A therapeutic feeding team in the rehabilitation setting. *Holistic Nursing Practice, 7*, 78-81.

Glenn-Molali, N. (2005). Personal communication with pharmacists. Havre de Grace, MD:

Groher, M. (1997). *Dysphagia: Diagnosis and management* (3rd ed.). Boston: Butterworth-Heinemann.

Hansell, D., & Heinemann, D. (1996). Improving nursing practice with staff education: The challenges of dysphagia. *Gastroenterology Nursing 6*, 201-206.

Harris, D. R. (1996). *Diet and nutrition sourcebook.* Detroit, MI: Omnigraphics.

Helfrich-Miller, K. R., Rector, K. L., & Straka, J. A. (1986). Dysphagia: Its treatment in the profoundly retarded patient with cerebral palsy. *Archives of Physical Medicine and Rehabilitation, 67*(8), 520-525.

Hoeman, S. P., & Glenn-Molali, N. (1999). Community approaches for evidence-based practice in dysphagia. *Nutrition in Clinical Practice, 14*(5), S31-S34.

Houghton, D. J., & Curley, J. W. (1996). Dysphagia caused by a hard cervical collar. *British Journal of Neurosurgery, 10*(5), 501-502.

Huggins, P. S., Tuomi, S. K., & Young, C. (1999). Effects of nasogastric tubes on the young, normal swallowing mechanism. *Dysphagia, 14*, 157-161.

Leder, S. (1996, March/April). Gag reflex and dysphagia. *Head and Neck*, 138-141.

Leslie, P., Drinnan, M. J., Ford, G. A. & Wilson, J. A. (2005). Swallow respiratory patterns and aging: Presbyphagia or dysphagia. *Journals of Gerontology Series A Biological Sciences and Medical Sciences, 60*(3), 391-395.

Logemann, J. A. (1983). *Evaluation and treatment of swallowing disorders.* San Diego, CA: College Hill Press.

Logemann, J. A. (1998). *Evaluation and treatment of swallowing disorders* (2nd ed.). Austin, TX: PRO-ED.

Logemann, J. A., & Pauloski, B. R. (1995). Effects of a sour bolus on oropharyngeal swallowing measures in patients with neurogenic dysphagia. *Journal of Speech & Hearing Disorders, 38*(3), 556-564.

Lutz, C. A., & Przytulski, K. R. (1997). *Nutrition and diet therapy* (2nd ed.). Philadelphia: F. A. Davis.

Mann, G., Hankey, G. J., & Cameron, D. (1999). Swallowing function after stroke: Prognosis and prognostic factors at 6 months. *Stroke, 30*(4), 744-748.

Marik, P. E., & Kaplan, D. (2003). Aspiration and dysphagia in the elderly. *Chest, 124*(1), 328-336.

Martinez, E. J., & Nord, H. J. (1995). Significance of solitary and multiple esophageal ulcers in patients with AIDS. *Southern Medical Journal, 88*(6), 626-629.

Martin-Harris, B., & Cherney, L. R. (1996). Treating swallowing disorders following stroke. In L. R. Cherney & A. S. Halper (Eds.), *Topics in stroke rehabilitation* (3rd ed., pp. 27-40). Frederick, MD: Aspen.

Mason, S., Harris, G., & Blissett, J. (2005). Tube feeding in infancy: Implications for the development of normal eating and drinking skills. *Dysphagia, 20*, 46-61.

McCann, J. (2004). *Nursing 2004 drug handbook* (24th ed.). Philadelphia: Lippincott Williams and Wilkins.

McGarrah, P. D., & Teller, D. (1997). Posttraumatic cervical osteophytosis causing progressive dysphagia. *Southern Medical Journal, 90*(8), 858-860.

Miller, J. L., Sonies, B. C., & Macedonia, C. (2003). Emergence oropharyngeal laryngeal and swallowing activity in developing fetal upper aerodigestive tract: An ultrasound evaluation. *Early Human Development, 71*, 61-87.

Miller, R. M., & Chang, M. W. (1999). Advances in the management of dysphagia caused by stroke. *Physical Medicine and Rehabilitation Clinics of North America, 10*(4), 925-941.

Mizuno, K., & Ueda, A. (2001). Development of sucking behavior in infants who have not been fed for 2 months after birth. *Pediatrics International, 43*, 251-255.

Moorhead, S., Johnson, M., & Maas, M. (Eds.). (2004). *Nursing outcomes classification (NOC)* (3rd ed.). St. Louis, MO: Mosby.

Morris, H. (2005). Dysphagia in a general practice population. *Gerontological Care and Practice, 17*(8), 20-23.

Moy, A. (1996). Restorative rehabilitation with burn injuries. In S. Hoeman (Ed.), *Rehabilitation nursing: Process and application* (p. 650). St. Louis, MO: Mosby.

National dysphagia diet: Standardization for optimal care. (2003). Chicago, IL: J American Dietetic Association.

O'Brien, J., Zarro, C., Gelb, D., Bhargava, A., & Ludwig, S. (2005). Dysphagia, aspiration and dysphonia related to cervical surgery. *Current Opinions in Orthopaedics, 16*(3), 184-188.

O'Laughlin, G., & Shanley, C. (1998). Swallowing problems in the nursing home: A novel training response. *Dysphagia, 13*, 172-183.

Payten, C. (2005). Referral, diagnosis and management of dysphagia. *Pulse, 64*.

Perry, L., & Love, C. P. (2001). Screening for dysphagia and aspiration in acute stroke: A systematic review. *Dysphagia, 16*(1), 7-18.

Pinelli, J., & Symington, A. (2004). Non-nutritive sucking for promoting physiologic stability and nutrition in preterm infants. *Cochrane Database Systemic Review, 2.*

Plant, R. (1998). Anatomy and physiology of swallowing in adults and geriatrics. *Otolaryngologic Clinics of North America, 31*(3), 477-489.

Poertner, L., & Coleman, R. (1998). Swallowing therapy in adults. *Otolaryngologic Clinics of North America, 31*(3), 561-579.

Rademaker, A. W., Pauloski, B. R., Colangelo, L. A., & Logemann, J. A. (1998). Age and volume effects on liquid swallowing function in normal women. *Journal of Speech, Language, & Hearing Research, 41*(2), 275-285.

Robbins J., Gangnon, R., Theis, S., Kays, S., Hewitt, A., & Hind, J. (2005). The effects of lingual exercises on swallowing in older adults. *Journal of the American Geriatrics Society, 53*(9), 1483-1487.

Robbins, J., Levine, R., Wood, J., Roecker, E., & Luschei, E. (1994, December). Geriatrics. Swallowing physiology related to normal aging. *Rehabilitation R&D Progress Reports,* 30-31, 108-109.

Robbins, J. A., Logemann, J. A., & Kirshner, H. S. (1986). Swallowing and speech production in Parkinson's disease. *Annals of Neurology, 19,* 283-287.

Rodgers, B., & Arvedson, J. (2005). Assessment of infant oral sensorimotor and swallowing function. *Mental Retardation and Developmental Disabilities Research Reviews, 22,* 74-82.

Sands, J. K. (1999). Management of persons with problems of the intestines. In W. J. Phipps, J. K. Sands, & J. F. Marek, *Medical-surgical nursing* (6th ed., pp. 1313-1372). St. Louis, MO: Mosby.

Shuman, J. M. (1996). Nutrition in aging. In L. K. Mahan & S. Escott-Stump (Eds.), *Krause's food, nutrition and diet therapy* (9th ed., pp. 287-308). Philadelphia: W. B. Saunders.

Stanley, K. (1998). Assessing the nutritional needs of the geriatric patient with diabetes. *Diabetes Educator, 24*(1), 29-36.

Tolep, K., Getch, C. L., & Criner, G. J. (1996). Swallowing dysfunction in patients receiving prolonged mechanical ventilation. *Chest, 109*(1), 167-172.

Touger-Decker, R. (1996). Nutritional care in rheumatic diseases. In L. K. Mahan & S. Escott-Stump (Eds.), *Krause's food, nutrition and diet therapy* (9th ed., pp. 889-898). Philadelphia: W. B. Saunders.

U.S. Department of Health and Human Services. (1990). *Healthy People 2000.* Retrieved 2006 from http://web.health.gov/healthypeople.

U.S. Department of Health and Human Services. (2000a). *Healthy People 2010.* Retrieved 2006 from http://web.health.gov/healthypeople.

Voss, H. (1994). The neurologic assessment. In E. Barker (Ed.), *Neuroscience nursing* (pp. 49-92). St. Louis, MO: Mosby.

Walleck, C., & Mooney, K. (1994). Neurotrauma: Head injury. In E. Barker (Ed.), *Neuroscience nursing* (pp. 324-351). St. Louis, MO: Mosby.

Watando, A., Ebihara, S., Ebihara, T., Okazaki, T., Takahashi, H., Asada, M., et al. (2004). Daily oral care and cough reflex sensitivity in elderly nursing home patients. *Chest, 26,* 1066-1070.

Willig, T. N., Paulus, J., Lacau Saint Guily, J., Beon, C., & Naavarro, J. (1994). Swallowing problems in neuromuscular disorders. *Archives of Physical Medicine and Rehabilitation, 75,* 1175-1181.

Winkler, M. F., & Manchester, S. (1996). Nutritional care in metabolic stress: Sepsis, trauma, burns, and surgery. In L. K. Mahan & S. Escott-Stump (Eds.), *Krause's food, nutrition and diet therapy* (9th ed., pp. 663-680). Philadelphia: W. B. Saunders.

Wisdom, G., & Blitzer, A. (1998). Surgical therapy for swallowing disorders. *Otolaryngologic Clinics of North America, 31*(3), 537-538.

Yoneyama, T., Yoshida, M., Ohrui, T., Mukaiyama, H., Okamoto, H., Hoshiba, K., et al. (2002). Oral care reduces pneumonia in older patients in nursing homes. *Journal of the American Geriatric Society, 50,* 430-433.

Yoshikawa, M., Yoshida, M., Nagasaki, T., Tanimoto, K., Tsuga, K., Akagawa, Y., et al. (2005). Aspects of swallowing in healthy dentate elderly persons older than 80 years. *Journals of Gerontology Series A Biological Sciences and Medical Sciences, 60*(4), 506-509.

17

Respiration and Pulmonary Rehabilitation

Cynthia Gronkiewicz, RN, MS, APRN, AE-C
Lenore Coover, RN, MSN, AE-C

Rehabilitation nurses work with patients who have multiple, complex respiratory conditions.

Respiratory disability has a considerable physical, psychosocial, and financial impact on the patient, family, and society because the nature of impaired breathing is multidimensional. The comprehensive definition of pulmonary rehabilitation is as follows:

> ... an art of medical practice wherein an individually tailored, multidisciplinary program is formulated which through accurate diagnosis, therapy, emotional support, and education stabilizes or reverses both the physio- and psychopathology of pulmonary diseases and attempts to return the patient to the highest possible functional capacity allowed by his pulmonary handicap and overall life situation (American Thoracic Society [ATS], 1981).

There are a variety of respiratory disorders deemed suitable for pulmonary rehabilitation: chronic obstructive pulmonary disease (COPD), chronic asthma, cystic fibrosis (CF), bronchiectasis, interstitial lung disease, restrictive lung disease, postpolio syndrome, muscular dystrophy, Guillain-Barré syndrome, ventilatory dependency, and those patients with preoperative and postoperative lung volume reduction and lung transplantation surgery. Patients with these disorders share the common characteristic of functional limitations despite optimal medical management. Patients who exhibit significant dyspnea, limited tolerance for the activities required for daily life, and a poor quality of life are candidates for pulmonary rehabilitation (Make, 2006).

CONCEPTS FOR PULMONARY REHABILITATION

Pulmonary rehabilitation includes the following patient goals: reduction of symptoms, decreased disability, increased participation in physical and social activities, and an overall improvement in the quality of life of individuals with chronic respiratory disease. All pulmonary rehabilitation programs contain four components: medical evaluation and management, assessment and goal setting, application of therapeutic modalities, and evaluation of outcomes (ATS, 1999). Successful programs can be conducted in hospitals, rehabilitation centers, outpatient settings, or at home.

A key element in the American Thoracic Society (ATS) definition of pulmonary rehabilitation is that of the multidisciplinary program. This is best achieved through a team approach with health care professionals providing services in their area of expertise. Personnel require knowledge and experience in exercise training, psychosocial evaluation and counseling, respiratory medications and oxygen therapy, breathing exercises and retraining, education on the particular lung disease, nutritional issues, energy conservation techniques, smoking cessation strategies, and establishment of an individual, long-term program (Make, 2004).

Extensive research has confirmed the benefits of pulmonary rehabilitation: increased exercise tolerance, reduced dyspnea and fatigue, health promotion behaviors, improved quality of life, and reduced hospitalizations. Outcome measures should be used to guide the development and ongoing evaluation of an individualized, comprehensive program. The need for collaboration and communication is key to excellent outcomes for all.

RESPIRATORY PHYSIOLOGY

Structure and Function

Airways are either conducting airways or respiratory units. Conducting airways extend from the nose through the terminal bronchioles and function as conduits, distributing but not exchanging gases throughout the lungs (Figure 17-1). Respiratory units extend from the respiratory bronchioles to the alveoli

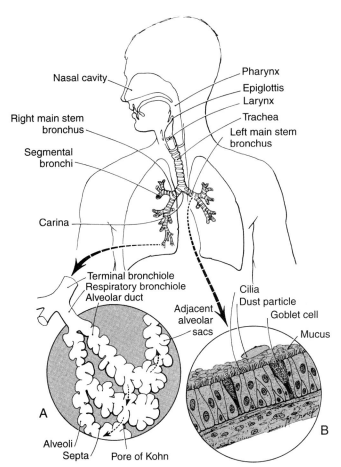

Figure 17-1 Structures of the respiratory tract. **A,** Pulmonary functional unit. **B,** Ciliated mucous membrane. (From Price, S., & Wilson, L. [2003]. *Pathophysiology: Clinical concepts of disease* [6th ed.]. St. Louis, MO: Mosby.)

and are the areas for oxygen and carbon dioxide exchange. The circumference of individual airways decreases with each branching, whereas the surface area increases. In larger airways, inspired air moves by bulk flow, but the velocity of airflow decreases as the aggregate circumference of the airways increases. The velocity of airflow is very slow in the smaller airways, and in the alveoli air moves by diffusion of gases.

Conducting Airway. The mucosa of the nasopharyngeal region is well vascularized, enabling inspired air to be heated to body temperature and humidified by the time it reaches the trachea. Because the airway is lined with ciliated columnar epithelium and mucus-secreting cells and glands, any large airborne particle gets trapped in the mucous layer before it reaches the trachea. The entire tracheobronchial region is lined with ciliated epithelial cells, mucus-secreting cells, and mucous glands (see Figure 17-1). Smaller airborne particles are trapped in the mucous layer in this region, and only the tiniest particles reach terminal respiratory units. The mucus and cilia lining the conducting airways protect the respiratory system and serve as a major defense mechanism, the mucociliary escalator.

The normal volume of secretions is approximately 100 ml/day (Copstead & Banasik, 2005). Closure of the epiglottis, located at the entrance to the larynx, protects the airway from aspiration during swallowing and allows intrathoracic pressure to develop during coughing or the Valsalva maneuver. Sensory fibers in the larynx and tracheobronchial tree are sensitive to chemical and mechanical irritants that stimulate a cough. The cough reflex can be depressed by neurological dysfunction including unconsciousness or anesthesia. It may become less sensitive with age, increasing the risk of infection in the upper respiratory tract.

Gas Exchange Units. The terminal respiratory unit, or acinus, consists of respiratory bronchioles, alveolar ducts, and alveoli. As alveoli begin to appear as outgrowths of the airways in the smaller bronchioles, increasing in number with each generation, they provide a surface area for gas exchange about the size of a tennis court.

Ventilation

Ventilation is the movement of air into and out of the lungs and can be likened to a "pump" for the lungs. The process of ventilation involves the central nervous system, peripheral nervous system, rib cage, and respiratory muscles. When respiratory centers in the brain send messages via the central and peripheral pathways to the respiratory muscles, they contract and generate the pressure differences required for airflow.

Alveolar ventilation is the amount of air that actually reaches the alveoli and participates in gas exchange. Alveolar ventilation is less than the volume of inspired air because the conducting airways, including the trachea and large bronchi, are anatomical dead space not directly communicating with alveoli. Alveolar ventilation is unevenly distributed, with a greater fraction of ventilation flowing to the bases of the lungs in the upright body position.

Mechanics of Breathing

Strength of both inspiratory and expiratory muscles of respiration functions in the same manner as other skeletal muscles. Strength declines with aging, in malnutrition, and with a sedentary lifestyle; in women with less muscle mass than men, there is less muscle strength. The diaphragm is the primary muscle of *inspiration* (Figure 17-2). Innervated by the phrenic nerve arising from C3, C4, and C5, its dome shape is attached peripherally to the lower rib cage. When the diaphragm contracts, it pulls downward on the lungs, decreasing intrapleural, intrathoracic, and airway pressures, creating the pressure gradient for inspiratory airflow. Diaphragm contraction pushes downward on the abdominal cavity, increasing abdominal pressure. Normal *expiration* is passive with elastic recoil of the lungs. Expiratory muscles are recruited to maintain high levels of ventilation during exercise and forced expiratory maneuvers, such as a cough. The accessory muscles of respiration (sternocleidomastoid, trapezius, abdominal) can be overused to the point of exhaustion in patients with COPD. However, in neuromuscular disease and spinal cord injuries, patients are taught to use these muscles to increase vital capacity and assist with phonation (Frownfelter & Dean, 2006).

Lung Compliance. *Compliance* refers to the elasticity of the lungs. Static compliance is the change in pressure necessary to inflate the lungs to a given volume. Normally, lung pressure-volume characteristics are influenced by surfactant that reduces the surface tension of alveoli, increasing their compliance and stabilizing them. Without the stabilizing effect, the smaller alveoli tend to collapse at low lung volumes during expiration. For example, with pulmonary fibrosis the stiff lungs have decreased compliance and resist inflation; therefore alveolar ventilation is harder (Copstead & Banasik, 2005). *Airway resistance* determines the pressure required to generate a given airflow. Resistance to flow is inversely related to the diameter of the airways. Inflammation or obstruction of the airways and increased tone of airway smooth muscle can decrease airway diameter. Increased airway resistance increases the work of breathing, as with COPD, CF, and asthma.

Control of Breathing

Breathing can be modified by involuntary and voluntary control. Involuntary control occurs through activity of respiratory centers in the brainstem, peripheral chemoreceptors, central chemoreceptors, and respiratory motor neurons. Voluntary control arises from the cerebral cortex. The basic spontaneous rhythm of breathing is established in the *respiratory centers.* Chemoreceptors, proprioceptors, and the vagus nerve send afferent input to the respiratory centers, where the sensory information is coordinated and neural output is initiated via the spinal motor neurons and efferent nerves.

Central chemoreceptors are aggregates of cells in bilateral areas of the medulla that are distinct from respiratory center neurons. They are sensitive to elevations in carbon dioxide (CO_2) and the hydrogen ion concentration (H^+) in the surrounding extracellular fluid and respond by increasing the minute ventilation (V_E). *Peripheral chemoreceptors*, located at the bifurcation of the common carotid arteries and along the aortic arch, respond to a decrease in partial pressure of arterial oxygen (PaO_2) of less than 60 mm Hg by stimulating the respiratory centers to increase ventilation. They also respond to decreases in pH and increases in CO_2 by signaling the respiratory center for increased breathing. Voluntary control of respiration is regulated by the *cerebral cortex.* Breathing patterns are modified by conscious control during talking, laughing, crying, and swallowing. This control depends on the patient's degree of wakefulness. The voluntary conducting pathways in the spinal cord are distinct from those involved in involuntary regulation. Fibers from involuntary pathways can be injured even though the voluntary pathways remain intact, and vice versa.

Gas Transport

Oxygen Transport. Most oxygen is transported to the peripheral tissues bound to hemoglobin (Hb); minimal oxygenation is in the form of dissolved O_2 (Copstead & Banasik, 2005).

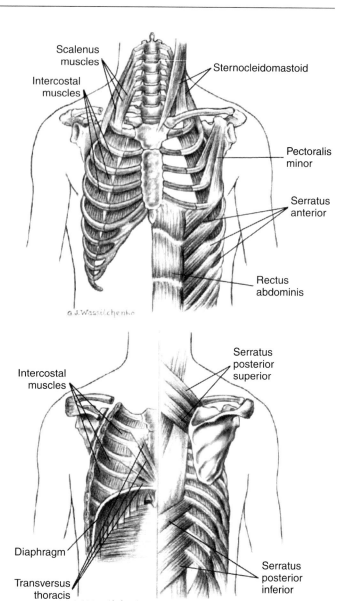

Figure 17-2 Inspiratory muscles of the chest aid in inspiration and expiration. (From Wilson, S. F., & Thompson, J. F. [1990]. *Respiratory disorders.* St. Louis, MO: Mosby.).

The difference in alveolar and pulmonary capillary PO_2 establishes the gradient for the diffusion of O_2 across the alveolar-capillary membrane. The arterial PO_2 in turn drives the binding of oxygen with hemoglobin. Delivery of O_2 to the tissues requires adequate cardiac output and tissue perfusion. As arterialized blood perfuses the tissues, O_2 is unloaded because of the lower PO_2 at the tissue level.

Carbon Dioxide Transport. Carbon dioxide transport deals with the amount of CO_2 produced as an end product of metabolism and depends on metabolic activity and dietary intake. CO_2 is transported from the peripheral tissues as carbonic acid (an insignificant amount), dissolved in plasma (5% to 10% of total), as carbamino compounds (20% to 30% of total), or as bicarbonate (60% to 70% of total). Elimination of

CO_2 via the lungs depends on an adequate level of alveolar ventilation (V_A).

Gas Exchange

Pulmonary Circulation. The pulmonary vascular bed is a low-resistance system. Normal distribution of pulmonary blood flow is influenced passively by posture and exercise. When a person is at rest, perfusion of the pulmonary capillary bed is greatest in the dependent portions of the lungs; when a person is upright, perfusion is greatest at lung bases; and when a person is in the side-lying position, perfusion is greatest in the inferior portion of the dependent lung. This uneven distribution of pulmonary blood flow is caused by hydrostatic pressure differences within the pulmonary vascular system. Due to gravity, hydrostatic pressures are greater in the dependent regions, distending the vessels and increasing the rate of flow. Mild exercise increases both cardiac output and pulmonary blood flow, leveling hydrostatic pressures and blood flow distribution in the pulmonary vascular bed (Copstead & Banasik, 2005).

Diffusion. Oxygen diffuses down its concentration gradient from the alveolar gases, across the alveolar-capillary membranes, through the plasma, across the red blood cell membrane, and within the red blood cell to combine with Hb. The rate of diffusion is directly proportional to the alveolar-capillary gradient of PO_2 (the difference in gas partial pressures between the two sides of the alveoli) and the cross-sectional area of the alveolar-capillary membrane. In addition, the rate of diffusion is inversely proportional to the length of the diffusion path. Theoretically the diffusion capacity can be reduced by destruction of alveolar-capillary surface area, as occurs in COPD, or by a lengthening of the diffusion path, as occurs in interstitial fibrosis. However, multiple factors must be present to impair gas exchange on the basis of a true diffusion defect.

Ventilation-Perfusion Relationships. Efficient gas exchange depends on ventilation of the alveoli, perfusion of the pulmonary capillary bed, and matching ventilation and perfusion. Uniform distribution of ventilation and perfusion throughout the lungs is ideal for gas exchange, but even distribution of ventilation and perfusion is not a normal situation. When an individual is positioned upright, a greater portion of ventilation and perfusion is distributed to the base of the lungs, but the difference is greater for perfusion. Consequently the ventilation-perfusion ratio increases from the base to the apex of the lungs, with an average ratio of 0.8, an alveolar PO_2 of 104 mm Hg, and an arterial PO_2 of 100 mm Hg.

FACTORS ASSOCIATED WITH ALTERED PHYSIOLOGICAL FUNCTIONING

Major changes in physiological functioning are categorized as alterations in gas exchange or alterations in ventilation.

Many chronic lung diseases are characterized by a combination of these alterations, especially in severe or advanced stages. Clinically, patients with chronic lung disease experience a slow, progressive worsening of their condition with episodic acute exacerbations secondary to upper and lower respiratory tract infections (RTIs). When impairment of lung function is mild, clinical evidence of altered functioning may be apparent only during acute exacerbations; when severe, the clinical evidence is readily visible on a daily basis, even without exacerbations.

There are many anatomical and physiological differences in children that may predispose them to respiratory compromise. These special considerations are summarized in Box 17-1.

Aging may also accentuate pulmonary problems, resulting in decreased compliance as tissues stiffen, changes tidal volumes and vital capacity, and the aggravation of underlying lung disease. Increased calcification of rib articulations may interfere with chest expansion: the chest wall stiffens, and accessory muscles are recruited for resting breathing (Bickley, 2004).

Biological variation in the prevalence, morbidity, and mortality of COPD reveals that the incidences of chronic bronchitis and emphysema are higher in men; however, they cause increased mortality in middle-age women when associated with increased smoking exposure. International variability may be explained by differences in smoking habits, types of cigarettes, and methods of diagnosis and death reports. However, genetic susceptibility and other environmental influences on respiratory health are implicated. Indoor and outdoor air quality aggravates chronic respiratory conditions. Poor indoor ventilation combined with strong odors, secondhand smoke and fuel burning, except nuclear, produce carbon monoxide and nitric oxide, which converts to nitrogen dioxide and irritates the airways. When small hydrocarbons from burning fossil fuels and strong sunlight combine into ozone and other photochemical products, this photochemical smog remains until winds disperse it. Changes in weather, especially humidity and rapid temperature drops, are difficult for patients with COPD to tolerate and may exacerbate asthma.

Subjective Assessment

Subjective manifestations of disease may prompt individuals to seek medical attention. Constitutional symptoms such as fever, weight loss, fatigue, and sleep disturbance may be present, justifying a review of body systems. A detailed subjective assessment of the three most common respiratory-related complaints—dyspnea, cough, and activity intolerance—and a history of symptoms and smoking behavior are essential to planning care.

Dyspnea. Dyspnea, the sensation of difficulty with breathing associated with increased effort to breathe, manifests in many ways. Patients use different terms to describe dyspnea—shortness of breath, difficulty breathing, suffocating, and chest tightness. Dyspnea, the primary symptom for many

---

BOX 17-1 Pediatric Anatomy and Physiology of the Respiratory System: Special Considerations in Children

There are many anatomical and physiological differences in children that predispose them to respiratory compromise. In a child with a respiratory disease process or condition, the differences only increase the risk of respiratory compromise.
1. Central nervous system control of breathing is immature in infants.
2. Airways in infants and children are much smaller compared with those of an adult.
3. In children, distal airways develop more slowly than proximal airways, providing increased resistance to airflow.
4. Supportive airway cartilage is not fully developed until school age, making it more prone to collapse.
5. The pediatric larynx is anterior and cephalad.
6. Neonates and infants are obligate nose breathers, so any obstruction of the nasal passages can become a critical threat.
7. The tongue is larger in proportion to the mouth, increasing the likelihood of airway obstruction.
8. There are decreased numbers of alveoli available for gas exchange, which contributes to a decreased respiratory reserve.
9. The chest wall is compliant due to cartilaginous ribs. Furthermore, the chest wall retracts during respiratory distress, reducing the young child's ability to maintain functional residual capacity.
10. The intercostal muscles are not fully developed until school age and may lack power, tone, and coordination, especially during times of respiratory distress.
11. The diaphragm is the primary muscle of respiration; therefore anything that interferes with diaphragmatic movement can compromise ventilation.
12. Oxygen consumption is higher in infants and children (6 to 8 ml/kg/min) compared with that of an adult (3 to 4 ml/kg/min). Therefore, when apnea or inadequate ventilation develops in a child, hypoxia can occur more rapidly.
13. Children suffer an increased number of respiratory infections compared with the adult population.
14. Respiratory compromise accounts for the majority of pediatric arrests, *not* cardiac compromise.

---

patients with cardiopulmonary diseases including COPD, pulmonary fibrosis, asthma, pulmonary hypertension, and congestive heart disease, may occur with obesity, pregnancy, and neuromuscular diseases. Intensity may not correlate with the extent of impairment; some patients with severe lung disease report minimal dyspnea, whereas others with mild lung disease report intense dyspnea. Clinical assessment describes frequency, intensity, history of symptom onset (acute or chronic), precipitating events, duration, associated symptoms, relieving factors, and identifiable patterns.

The Borg CR10 Scale for rating of perceived exertion rates the intensity of dyspnea at rest or during physical activity (Borg, 1998). Patients point to the number on the scale that best describes the intensity of their breathlessness. However, the validity of the scale appears limited. Some patients appear in acute distress while rating their dyspnea as minimal, whereas others use the full range, reporting maximal dyspnea when they appear to be extremely dyspneic. Consequently, the intensity of dyspnea is not comparable across respondents. Patients tend to use the scale consistently when rating changes in their dyspnea over time. To assess the general intensity of dyspnea, rehabilitation nurses might use one of the scales designed for large population studies of lung disease, such as the breathlessness scale from the Recommended Respiratory Disease Questionnaire (Ferris, 1978) (Box 17-2).

Chronic dyspnea contributes to functional disability when activities that produce symptoms or decrease energy are eliminated despite their importance to life satisfaction. Lifestyles and interests may change accordingly at great cost to personal, physical, social, and emotional well-being.

BOX 17-2 Breathlessness Scales From the ATS-DLD Questionnaire

1. Are you troubled by shortness of breath when hurrying on the level or walking up a slight hill?
2. (If yes) Do you have to walk slower than others your age on the level because of breathlessness?
3. (If yes) Do you ever have to stop for breath when walking at your own pace on the level?
4. (If yes) Do you ever have to stop for breath after walking about 100 yards (or after a few minutes) on the level?
5. (If yes) Are you too breathless to leave the house or breathless on dressing or undressing?

Modified from Ferris, B. G. (1978). Recommended respiratory disease questionnaires for use with adults and children in epidemiological research (part 2). *American Review of Respiratory Disease, 118,* 7-53.

Cough. Coughing occurs to clear the airways of secretions and to protect them from aspiration and/or inhalation of noxious substances. A cough can be acute or chronic, associated with other symptoms (e.g., pain, wheezing, dyspnea, syncope), productive or dry, or effective or ineffective (unable to clear secretions). It is abnormal if it is persistent, irritating, painful, or productive. Thus all data about how the cough developed are pertinent. For example, the cough may follow a recent illness or RTI, be exacerbated by seasonal or environmental conditions, or occur only at a certain time of day. Chronic cough tends to worsen when a patient is lying down or arising after lying down for an extended period. A cough during or shortly after eating may indicate aspiration of food or fluid into the tracheobronchial tree. Characteristics of the cough—quality, frequency, and alleviating factors—or a change in usual characteristics of a chronic cough require evaluation. The presence of a cough alone is nonspecific but along with other signs and symptoms may suggest a particular diagnosis or may indicate the disease is not under good control.

Sputum production, quantity, and character should be assessed. Normally, individuals do not produce noticeable amounts of sputum, but persons with chronic bronchitis expectorate small to moderate amounts of mucoid material each day, often in the morning. The volume is greatly increased with bronchiectasis and CF. Clinicians should suspect lower RTI with a change to thick yellow or green sputum. Individuals with COPD, bronchiectasis, CF, and spinal cord injury at the mid-cervical level are predisposed to RTIs. In CF, thick, green, and purulent sputum suggests *Pseudomonas aeruginosa* infection; foul odors in sputum signal anaerobic bacterial infections such as those caused by the *Pseudomonas*.

Hemoptysis generally originates from a problem in the airways, parenchyma, or pulmonary vasculature. Severity varies from blood-streaked sputum, as sometimes seen in chronic bronchitis, to frank bleeding, which may accompany pulmonary infarction. Commonly occurring without a diagnosis, the symptom is worrisome and requires investigation. A small amount of blood streaking in the sputum is not uncommon and is usually self-limiting with CF, especially in older patients, and does not require intervention.

Activity Intolerance. Typically, patients with respiratory disease complain of shortness of breath and easy fatigue with exercise that may relate to the severity of disease. Activity produces an abnormal heart rate, and the time needed to return to the preactivity rate is prolonged. Muscle pain or weakness in peripheral muscles may occur while an individual is engaging in physical activity, but severe dyspnea prevents patients from continuing activity. Exercise is frequently a trigger for asthma but can be controlled by instructing the patient to premedicate 10 to 15 minutes before the activity.

History of Symptoms and Smoking Behavior. A chronology of health data focusing on presenting respiratory symptoms helps the health care provider to establish nursing diagnoses and develop a plan of care. Data collection should include information about past or concurrent medical problems, treatment regimens, compliance behaviors, incidence of respiratory infections, smoking habits, age smoking began, type and amount of tobacco used (cigarettes, cigar, pipe, snuff, chewing tobacco), current smoking habits, successful and unsuccessful attempts to quit and reasons for continuing to smoke or for quitting

The team should ascertain the patient's readiness to participate in a pulmonary rehabilitation program. Information about the psychosocial environment is essential assessment data for developing an appropriate plan of care.

Objective Assessment

A complete physical examination is indicated because respiratory dysfunction often results from other system impairments (Bickley, 2004). The following section details clinical evaluation specific to the respiratory system. When examining the chest, envision the underlying anatomy of the lungs and thorax and compare for bilateral symmetry.

Inspection. Inspection begins during the interview in a well-lighted room. Observe the patient's general appearance, skin color, presence and degree of respiratory distress, character and rate of respirations, quality of voice, pattern of speech, interruptions by coughing or breathlessness, flaring nostrils, use of pursed-lip breathing (PLB), and assumed posture. For the inspiratory to expiratory ratio of breathing (I:E), the inspiratory phase is longer than the expiratory phase over most lung fields. With obstruction, as in COPD, the expiratory phase is prolonged and the I:E ratio may exceed 1:6. With the patient supine and chest exposed, look for asymmetrical movement and expansion of the rib cage with breathing, use of accessory muscles of respiration, splinting secondary to pain, obstructed airflow, or paralysis of the respiratory muscles. Paradoxical motion of the abdomen during quiet breathing may indicate abnormal or absent diaphragm use, as seen with high cervical lesions of the spinal cord.

The patient sits for inspection of chest shape and configuration. The anteroposterior diameter increases slightly with aging but significantly with COPD. The thoracic spine and rib cage are evaluated for deformities or abnormalities that interfere with chest expansion, causing decreased compliance and reduced lung volume. Common deformities contributing to a restrictive defect include kyphosis, scoliosis, and kyphoscoliosis. Ankylosing spondylitis causes a forward angling of the spine and an immobile spinal column that limits expansion of the chest. Trauma can cause a flail chest that appears as a paradoxical movement of a portion of the chest wall.

Cyanosis is best detected in daylight at the nail beds and buccal mucosa. Cyanosis reflects severe hypoxemia of arterial blood to a sufficient degree to desaturate hemoglobin. For this reason, cyanosis is not identified with anemia until hypoxemia is severe, whereas patients with polycythemia may appear cyanotic with less hypoxemia present. The most common cause for cyanosis is generalized hypoxemia (central cyanosis), but cyanosis also may occur secondary to peripheral vasoconstriction.

Palpation. Palpation is used to evaluate the underlying structure and function of the chest, detect areas of tenderness or crepitation, and assess respiratory excursion. Tenderness noted on palpation often is musculoskeletal, but the intercostal spaces are palpated for tumor, swelling, or crepitation that needs evaluation.

A variety of chest conditions alter transmission of sounds. Decreased transmission can be secondary to weakness of the voice; obstruction of the airway; or the collection of air, fluid, or tissue in the pleural space. Increased air retained in the lung, as in emphysema, decreases tactile fremitus, whereas consolidated lung tissue, as with pneumonia or tumor mass, causes increased fremitus if the airway remains patent.

Percussion. Healthy, air-filled lungs produce a more resonant sound with percussion than do fluid-filled lungs or solid tissue. With increased density of lung tissue, resonance fades to dullness as when percussing over solid organs, areas of consolidation, or fluid-filled spaces. Hyperresonance accompanies an increased accumulation of air, such as with hyperinflation or pneumothorax.

Diaphragm location and excursion are evaluated by percussing the lower posterior lung fields until the sound changes. The distances between levels of dullness at deep inspiration and deep expiration are compared to evaluate movement of the diaphragm. Normal excursion ranges from 4 to 6 cm. A low-lying diaphragm with limited excursion often accompanies hyperinflation. Diaphragm paralysis, atelectasis, or pleural effusion may accompany an elevated diaphragm and impaired movement.

Auscultation. Auscultation of the chest is used to evaluate the quality and intensity of breath sounds in all lung fields and adventitious lung sounds that may indicate a respiratory disorder. When possible, the chest is bare and the patient seated, but if the patient is weak or debilitated, have him or her turn from side to side to complete the examination. The clinician should caution patients from rapid breathing that may cause dizziness. Breath sounds are decreased or absent when the rate of airflow is decreased, as seen in persons with increased airway resistance and excessive secretions. Shallow breathing from weakness, obesity, or neuromuscular disorders produces diminished breath sounds, as does excess subcutaneous fat or pleural effusion.

Crackles (rales) are commonly heard with pulmonary edema, atelectasis, pneumonia, and interstitial lung disease. *Wheezes* (rhonchi) are caused by airflow through obstructed airways caused by bronchospasm, secretions, compression, mucosal swelling, and/or a foreign body. When pleural surfaces become inflamed or roughened, a *pleural friction rub*, a grating sound or vibration associated with breathing, can be heard over the site of discomfort. Many conditions are associated with a pleural friction rub, including pleurisy, tuberculosis, pulmonary infarction, pneumonia, and primary and metastatic carcinoma. *Stridor*, a high-pitched sound on inspiration, is caused by an obstruction high in the respiratory tree and is characterized by a prolonged inspiratory phase with an I:E ratio of 3:1 or greater. In infants and children, stridor indicates a serious problem in the trachea or larynx that warrants immediate attention (Bickley, 2004).

Diagnostic Studies

Accurate medical diagnosis of a pulmonary problem includes pulmonary function tests, arterial blood gas studies, radiological studies, and laboratory data. Nurses play a major role in patient and family education throughout the assessment and ongoing evaluation and collaborate with the rehabilitation team to establish a complete profile of information for informed decision making.

Pulmonary Function Testing. Pulmonary function testing that is conducted in a specialized laboratory by trained technicians provides an objective, noninvasive means of documenting pulmonary impairment. Lung volumes determined by body plethysmography or helium dilution establish the extent of hyperinflation with large lung volumes or restrictive lung disease with small lung volumes. *Spirometry* establishes the extent of airflow obstruction and may be tested in outpatient settings to monitor effectiveness of treatment. All spirometers are calibrated regularly to meet ATS standards. The nurse coaches patients to use proper technique to attain the best flow-volume measurements; at least three acceptable efforts are recorded at each testing. The personal effort that meets ATS criteria with the highest sum of forced vital capacity (VC) and forced expiratory volume in 1 second (FEV_1) recorded is the patient's reading for that day. The most useful parameters are VC, FEV_1, functional residual capacity (FRC), residual volume (RV), and total lung capacity (TLC). In the home a peak flowmeter can be useful to determine effectiveness of medications and to indicate early bronchoconstriction and worsening of asthma symptoms.

Arterial Blood Gases. Arterial blood gas values are used to evaluate oxygenation, ventilation, and acid-base balance. Arterial blood gas values are routinely evaluated for PO_2 (80 to 100 mm Hg), PCO_2 (35 to 45 mm Hg), bicarbonate (22 to 26 mEq/L), and pH (7.35 to 7.45). Many persons with pulmonary disease have a complex, mixed picture of abnormalities that can be better understood through periodic monitoring of arterial blood gas values. Blood gas measurements are objective data that determine the need for supplemental O_2.

Pulse Oximetry. Pulse oximetry is used for the continuous, noninvasive monitoring of oxygen saturation. It gives no information about ventilation or carbon dioxide level. When blood perfusion is adequate, saturation levels greater than 70% closely correlate with the saturation measured by an arterial blood gas value. Hence pulse oximetry becomes a very useful tool in monitoring respiratory patients in the rehabilitation setting. Because many of these individuals desaturate during meals, with exercise, or during sleep, continuous monitoring enables the nurse to monitor and titrate supplemental oxygen during these activities. A sensor is applied to the skin over areas with strong arterial pulsatile blood flow: finger, toe, bridge of nose, ear, or forehead. The accuracy of the pulse oximeter can be affected by clinical situations that compromise the arterial signal: hypotension, vasoconstriction, vasoactive drugs, hypothermia, movement of the sensor, or poor skin adherence (Chulay & Burns, 2006).

There are many ways to ensure the accuracy of pulse oximetry, including applying the sensor to a dry finger on the nondominant hand, ensuring adequate pulse wave, rotating application sites and changing sensor per manufacturer's directions, assessing the skin for heat or pressure damage, and comparing the pulse oximeter readings with arterial blood gas values when values do not match the clinical situation (Chulay & Burns, 2006).

Six-Minute Walk Test. The six-minute walk is a simple and practical test to monitor a patient's response to therapeutic interventions and pulmonary rehabilitation. It is a self-paced test at submaximal functional capacity to measure the maximal distance walked by a subject in 6 minutes across an indoor corridor (ATS, 2002). Any desaturation with exercise is noted, and subsequent improvement with titration of supplemental oxygen can be objectively monitored via pulse oximetry, dyspnea scale, heart rate, and the 6-minute walk distance response (Johnson & Weisman, 2006).

Radiographical Examination. A chest x-ray examination is a baseline evaluation and helps rule out other causes for symptoms, such as heart failure with cardiac enlargement, foreign body, or lung lesions from cancers. Computed axial tomography (CAT) scans are used to depict areas of emphysematous tissue and to evaluate patients for surgical therapies.

Laboratory Data. Laboratory data include standard measurements of blood count, serum electrolytes, urea, creatinine, blood glucose, sweat chloride, and immunoglobulin profile. Results assist in ruling out anemias and other abnormalities that may mimic a chronic respiratory disorder.

INEFFECTIVE AIRWAY CLEARANCE

Ineffective airway clearance is defined as the "inability to effectively clear secretions or obstructions from [the] respiratory tract" (Gordon, 2002). Normal, small amounts of secretions cleared by the mucociliary system differ from the excessive secretions produced by patients with a respiratory condition, such as chronic bronchitis, CF, bronchiectasis, or lower respiratory tract infection (LRTI). Problems arise when the volume of secretions is too large to be cleared by deep breathing and coughing because respiratory muscles are too weak to be effective and/or when secretions are too thick to mobilize. Carlson-Catalano et al. (1998) found the following defining characteristics of ineffective breathing, listed in order of importance: difficulty with sputum, abnormal breath sounds, chest congestion, fatigue, cough, and anxiety.

To generate an effective cough, patients must have sufficient muscle strength on inspiration to take a deep breath before the cough and on expiration to generate the sudden rise in intrathoracic pressure during the cough. Respiratory muscle strength is influenced by nutritional status and lean body muscle mass. Some patients with obstructive pulmonary disorders experience daily problems with ineffective airway clearance, whereas others have episodes during exacerbation. Individuals with a significant amount of chronic bronchitis or CF produce excessive secretions, evidenced by a productive cough every morning on arising. Unless they mobilize secretions and clear their airways daily, these patients are at risk for stagnated secretions and bacterial growth. Patients with neuromuscular disease, COPD, and CF who contract a viral or bacterial respiratory infection have further reductions in muscle strength and are at risk for ineffective airway clearance (Seemungal, Donaldson, Bhowmik, Jeffries, & Wedzicha, 2000). Viral infections cause increased secretions and promote a secondary bacterial infection of the lungs, further increasing the work of breathing. Consequently, in patients with severe respiratory muscle weakness the increased work of breathing and reduction in respiratory muscle strength may be sufficient to trigger ventilatory failure.

Episodic problems with airway clearance occur with respiratory muscle weakness secondary to neuromuscular disease and in midcervical or higher level injury of the spinal cord. The respiratory muscles are too weak to produce effective coughing and deep breathing during a respiratory tract infection, and the pathogen can cause further impairment of respiratory muscle strength. Immobility, with shallow breathing and pooled stagnant secretions, compounds problems.

Subjective Assessment

Patients with ineffective airway clearance typically complain of an inability to cough up secretions and chest congestion. They also complain of dyspnea, fatigue, and anxiety.

Objective Assessment

Typically, adventitious breath sounds include low- or high-pitched wheezes and coarse crackles that occur on inspiration or on both inspiration and expiration. Low-pitched wheezes indicate secretions in the airway that generally clear with coughing. A persistent cough and hypoxemia may signal ineffective airway clearance, and sputum suggests pulmonary disease. Sputum characteristics are documented as to amount, color, odor, and consistency and described as being tenacious, viscous, frothy, mucoid, mucopurulent, blood tinged, or having a foul odor.

Goals

The primary nursing goals for the individual with ineffective airway clearance are to establish and maintain a patent airway and adequate ventilation (see Table 17-1). Patient goals include maintaining a patent airway, mastering techniques that can assist in producing an effective cough, mobilizing secretions through a variety of airway clearance modalities, maintaining adequate hydration and humidification, correcting nutritional deficiencies, and appropriately administering pharmacological agents for bronchodilation and secretion clearance.

Interventions for Patients With Actual or Potential Airway Clearance Problems

Nursing interventions to achieve goals augment the patient's natural defense mechanisms. Specific interventions are appropriate pharmacotherapy, hydration, nebulization, inhaled medications, cough techniques, deep breathing exercises,

TABLE 17-1 Nursing Diagnoses, Interventions, and Outcomes Applicable to Ineffective Airway Clearance, Impaired Gas Exchange, and Ineffective Breathing Pattern **NIC/NOC**

Nursing Diagnosis	Nursing Interventions	Nursing Outcomes
Ineffective airway clearance	Cough enhancement Airway management Airway insertion and stabilization Artificial airway management Airway suctioning Asthma management Respiratory monitoring Oxygen therapy Medication administration: Inhalation Smoking cessation assistance	Respiratory status: Airway patency Ventilation Gas exchange
Impaired gas exchange	Positioning Airway management Airway suctioning Oxygen therapy Asthma management Chest physiotherapy Energy management Nutrition management Smoking cessation assistance Ventilation assistance Respiratory monitoring Anxiety reduction	Respiratory status: ventilation Respiratory status: gas exchange Vital signs status
Ineffective breathing pattern	Ventilation assistance Mechanical ventilation Airway suctioning Anxiety reduction Exercise promotion Energy management Asthma management Airway management Respiratory monitoring Smoking cessation assistance Medication management	Respiratory status: ventilation Anxiety self-control Physical fitness Energy conservation Asthma self-management Respiratory status Vital signs Medication response

Data from Moorhead, S., Johnson, M., & Maas, M. (Eds.). (2004). *Nursing outcomes classification (NOC)* (3rd ed.). St. Louis, MO: Mosby; Dochterman, J. M., & Bulechek, G. M. (2004). *Nursing interventions classification (NIC)* (4th ed.). St. Louis, MO: Mosby.; and NANDA International. (2005). *Nursing diagnoses: Definitions and classification, 2005-2006* (6th ed.). Philadelphia: Author.

incentive spirometry, chest percussion, chest vibration, high-frequency wall oscillation, postural drainage, and secretion mobilization modalities. Table 17-1 lists interventions and outcomes based on the nursing diagnosis of ineffective airway clearance.

Although ineffective airway clearance problems can be managed without invasive measures, some disease processes require progressive airway maintenance and ventilatory support. In severe cases, endotracheal intubation via tracheostomy may be indicated.

Pharmacotherapy. The goals of pharmacotherapy in patients with airway clearance problems are to reduce the work of breathing by decreasing airflow obstruction and airway

inflammation, to relieve symptoms of cough and dyspnea, to provide early treatment of acute exacerbations, and to prevent progressive decrease in lung function. The medications most commonly used are bronchodilators, corticosteroids, antibiotics, and vaccinations.

Bronchodilators include beta$_2$-agonists, anticholinergics, and methylxanthines. Beta$_2$-agonists are the preferred agent for treatment of bronchospasm in patients with asthma, COPD, and bronchiectasis. Another group of bronchodilators, the anticholinergics, block contraction of airway smooth muscle and decrease mucous hypersecretion but have a slower onset of action and longer duration than the beta$_2$-agonists. These two bronchodilators are often more effective when used in combination and are available as a combination agent

(National Asthma Education and Prevention Program [NAEPP], 2002; Pauwels, Buist, Calverley, Jenkins, & Hurd, 2001). See Chapter 7 for delivery methods, dosing, and adverse effects.

Methylxanthines are used to provide bronchodilation and increase mucociliary clearance in patients with obstructive lung disease. There is some evidence they improve diaphragm function and can enhance pulmonary vasodilation to improve right ventricular function. Although still a part of the disease treatment guidelines, their popularity has waned because of their narrow therapeutic range and numerous drug interactions. They are available as oral solutions or tablets for stable management of COPD and asthma. The most common side effects are nausea, tremors, arrhythmias, and seizures; hence close monitoring of drug levels is imperative (NAEPP, 2002; Pauwels et al., 2001).

Corticosteroids suppress the inflammatory process in the airways and lungs to decrease mucous hypersecretion and to improve airflow and gas exchange. The inhaled corticosteroids (ICS) are the primary controller medication for asthma and are now indicated for moderate to severe COPD (Global Initiative for Chronic Obstructive Pulmonary Disease [GOLD], 2005; NAEPP, 2002). They are also used in children with bronchopulmonary dysplasia. See Chapter 7 for further information.

As previously mentioned, the bronchodilators and ICS come in a variety of delivery devices. It is critical that the nurse and patient have a thorough understanding of the appropriate technique for a prescribed medication to achieve maximal therapeutic effect with minimal side effects. See Figure 17-3 for metered-dose inhaler (MDI) technique.

Bacteria can contribute to airway damage and accelerate airway obstruction when an acute respiratory illness is superimposed on an underlying chronic respiratory disorder. For this reason, the 2005 Global Initiative for Chronic Obstructive

Pulmonary Disease (GOLD) guideline update recommends the early use of antibiotics for an acute exacerbation of COPD when increased dyspnea, increased sputum volume, and increased purulence are present (GOLD, 2005). However, the National Asthma Education and Prevention Program (NAEPP) Expert Panel in 2002 discouraged prophylactic antibiotic use for an acute exacerbation of asthma and recommended antibiotic use only in the presence of purulent sputum, pneumonia, or bacterial sinusitis (NAEPP, 2002). Parenteral and oral antibiotics are indicated for acute infections of cystic fibrosis, bronchopulmonary dysplasia (BPD), and bronchiectasis. The inhaled form of antibiotics is playing a larger role during both acute treatment and chronic management of respiratory infections.

A safe and effective means of preventing respiratory infections is to ensure patients receive scheduled and recommended vaccinations. Current Centers for Disease Control and Prevention (CDC) recommendations for the prevention of the flu virus and associated complications is administration of the influenza vaccine to high-risk populations, including persons 2 to 64 years with comorbid conditions, persons 65 and older, and residents of long-term care facilities every fall (CDC, 2005). The CDC recommendation for pneumococcal vaccine is a one-time vaccination. Revaccination is reserved for those 65 and older when the first vaccine was received before the age of 65, or those in high-risk populations 5 years after the original vaccine (CDC, 1997).

Hydration. Amounts of fluid that are adequate to replace fluid losses, maintain hydration, and keep mucous membranes moist facilitate the mobilization of secretions. It is not necessary to force fluids because excess fluid is excreted and does not affect the composition of respiratory secretions, and excess fluids aggravate comorbid conditions, such as heart failure. Caffeinated coffee and tea act as diuretics and are avoided or

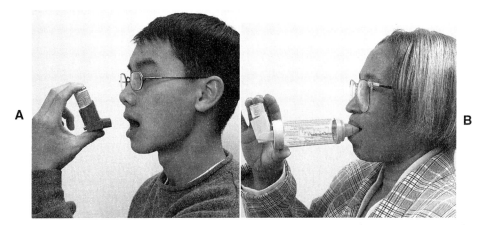

Figure 17-3 Correct use of a metered dose inhaler (MDI). **A,** Open mouth technique holding MDI 1½ to 2 inches in front of mouth. **B,** Mouth closed around spacer device attached to MDI. (From Perry, A., & Potter, P. [2004]. *Clinical nursing skills & techniques* [6th ed.]. St. Louis, MO: Mosby.)

not included in daily fluid intake. However, some patients may find drinking warm fluids facilitates the coughing up of secretions and promotes hydration of mucous membranes. Monitoring fluid status includes assessing mucous membranes, skin turgor, and thirst and evaluating the urine.

All *environmental humidifiers* used during cold weather must be cleaned regularly to prevent growth of bacteria and fungi, and the home should be assessed for excess humidity to decrease mold growth. For patients with a tracheostomy, the heat and moisture exchanger (HME) connects directly to the tracheostomy tube. It warms and humidifies inspired gases by recovering humidity from expired gases. Adult and pediatric sizes are available for inpatient and home use with or without mechanical ventilation. The HME is not used continuously for more than 24 hours. When a patient coughs up secretions or needs suctioning, the HME is disconnected from the tracheostomy tube. If secretions or mucus adhere to the mesh inside the unit, it is replaced immediately. Therefore caution should be used in those with copious secretions or with a cognitive deficit. Only patients or caregivers who can independently remove the humidifier when the mesh becomes obstructed with secretions should use the HME at home.

Nebulization. Nebulization delivers water vapor or medication in fine mist droplets that travel through the respiratory system and penetrate deep within the lungs. Various methods produce droplets of varying sizes; generally the smaller the particle, the deeper the penetration into the respiratory tract. Particles of 1 to 5 mm penetrate to the periphery, particles of 5 to 10 mm are deposited in the bronchi, and particles larger than 10 mm are deposited in the upper airway passages.

Aerosols are bland or medicated. A bland aerosol contains water or saline solution from a reservoir container and is delivered either at room temperature or heated. Medicated aerosols can be administered through metered-dose inhalers or nebulizers. Scientific evidence does not support the use of inhalation of bland aerosolized water or saline via mask or mouthpiece (ATS, 1995). The small amount of aerosolized water droplets that reach the lower airways does not aid in liquefying secretions, except in the case of a patient with a tracheostomy when bland aerosols are necessary to prevent thickening of airway secretions. Hazards associated with nebulization include overhydration, airway irritation, and risk of pneumonia. Special precautions in the administration of aerosol mists include educating patients on proper cleaning to prevent infection. One method of disinfecting nebulizers is to soak immersible parts (not the tubing) in a weak vinegar solution, rinsing each part three to four times. This should be done 2 to 3 times a week.

Cough Techniques. Coughing is an important physiological mechanism for the removal of secretions from the respiratory tract. Maximal effect from coughing can be achieved through controlled coughing or a forced-expiratory technique called huff coughing (Frownfelter & Dean, 2006). This technique can help control coughing and remove mucus more easily. Using timing to control coughing on exhalation and while simultaneously using the arms to push on the abdomen is less tiring for the patient and more productive. Although these techniques are beneficial in patients with COPD and CF, they are difficult with patients who have dyspnea. Individuals with COPD or neuromuscular disorders may not be able to perform these techniques effectively because of collapsed airways. The cough technique is selected according to patients' needs (Frownfelter & Dean, 2006). A discussion of cough techniques follows.

- **Controlled cough.** A *controlled cough* consists of a slow maximal inspiration followed by holding one's breath for several seconds and then by two or three coughs.
- **Huff cough.** *Huff coughing* ("open glottis coughing") is a form of controlled cough designed to clear the airways while conserving energy. Patients cross their arms just below the rib cage, take a deep breath while leaning forward with arms crossed over a pillow, and exhale sharply while whispering the word "huff" several times. Whispering the word "huff" prevents closure of the glottis and reduces airway compression during the cough. Continued relaxation takes place with slow diaphragmatic breathing between coughs (Frownfelter & Dean, 2006).
- **Pump cough.** *Pump coughing* is a variation of the huff technique that extends the huff and improves efficiency of the effort. The patient makes three short huffs and follows these with three short, easy coughs at lower lung volumes.
- **Quad cough.** The *quad cough* is used for persons with expiratory muscle weakness secondary to a neuromuscular dysfunction. The technique is also referred to as the *manual cough* or *diaphragmatic push* (Frownfelter & Dean, 2006). The person assisting the patient positions his or her hand below the patient's xiphoid process and pushes quickly on the epigastric area, diagonally inward toward the head, while the patient attempts to cough. Quad-assist coughing is similar to the Heimlich maneuver. This motion should be coordinated with the patient's attempt to exhale forcefully. Some patients can assist themselves by quickly compressing the abdomen. With the feet positioned on the floor or stool, the patient takes a slow, deep breath through the nose and exhales, simultaneously bending forward and pressing a pillow against the abdomen. After several deep breaths and exhalations, the patient coughs several times while exhaling and bending forward. Most patients appreciate privacy during the coughing procedure because they regard sputum production as socially unattractive.
- **Glossopharyngeal breathing.** Patients with neuromuscular disorders with little or no respiratory muscle function can use *glossopharyngeal breathing* (GPB) to increase VC and improve cough force. To perform GPB, also known as "frog" breathing, the patient traps air in the mouth and then pushes it back into the trachea with the tongue. The vocal cords remain closed until the air enters the trachea. Mastery of GPB takes time, but it is useful to assist minimal voluntary ventilation and to provide a ventilator-free time. Since GPB can be fatiguing, patients must be carefully monitored with the

checking of oxygen levels with pulse oximetry (Frownfelter & Dean, 2006).

Deep Breathing Exercises. *Deep breathing exercises* mobilize secretions to facilitate airway clearance. Difficulty with deep breathing can be caused by weak muscles of inspiration, as with neuromuscular disorders, and by pain after surgery or trauma. Maximal deep breathing is obtained in the upright position because gravity helps pull the diaphragm and abdomen downward. In the supine position the abdomen pushes upward on the diaphragm, and FRC and decreased VC reduce the patient's ability to take a deep breath. The patient, sitting in upright position, takes a prolonged deep inspiration through the nose, holds the breath for at least 3 seconds, and then exhales slowly in a relaxed manner while simulating a normal sigh. Patients with COPD are instructed to inhale only until midbreath to avoid air trapping and to prevent dynamic hyperinflation. In this group, exhalation should be through pursed lips and last twice as long as inhalation (Frownfelter & Dean, 2006).

Incentive Spirometry. An *incentive spirometer* can facilitate efforts for lung inflation, cough, and/or secretion clearance. This is not to be confused with a peak flow meter, which measures how much air can be forced out of the lungs in 1 second. Incentive spirometry can be performed 3 to 4 times per day independently by the patient after receiving appropriate instructions (Timby & Smith, 2003).

Chest Physiotherapy. *Chest physiotherapy* is a general term for assistance in moving pooled airway secretions from peripheral airways to more central airways for expectoration and/or suctioning (Dochterman & Bulechek, 2004). The maneuvers include chest percussion, chest vibration, postural drainage techniques, and secretion mobilization devices used independently or in combination to assist in mobilizing secretions. Using bronchodilators, humidity, and effective cough techniques before chest physiotherapy may facilitate airway clearance. In patients with CF the benefits are limited to those who produce at least 25 ml of sputum per day because this modality is effective only for patients with copious sputum production (Celli, 1998). Most of these therapies encourage optimal bronchial hygiene in those with bronchiectasis. Although findings have not been validated, many patients report subjective benefit in dyspnea, cough, and sputum (O'Regan & Berman, 2004).

Chest Percussion. *Chest percussion* is performed by the health care provider, who cups the hands and rhythmically strikes the targeted area of the patient's chest. The cupping creates an air pocket between the hand and chest and produces a hollow, not slapping, sound on percussion. To avoid fatigue the provider's wrists are kept loose with the elbows slightly flexed. Patients are more comfortable when percussion is performed over a thin layer of clothing. This technique requires only 2 to 3 minutes and should cause no discomfort. Chest percussion often is used in conjunction with postural

drainage, chest vibration, and coughing techniques. Percussion is not performed over the sternum, vertebrae, kidneys, or tender areas and is contraindicated for patients with cardiac conditions, osteoporosis, and pleural effusion (Frownfelter & Dean, 2006).

Chest Vibration. *Chest vibration* may follow percussion and is also performed by the health care provider. Chest vibrations transmit through the chest wall while the patient takes a deep breath, then exhales slowly. The provider's arms and shoulders are straight with the hand placed flat over the area of the chest to be drained. An alternate tensing and contracting of the arm and shoulder muscles create vibration that continues for the duration of the patient's expiration so that fine vibratory movements are transmitted to the patient's chest wall. If the patient does not cough spontaneously, encourage a cough after vibration or assisted coughing. Chest vibration can be repeated several times.

Secretion Mobilization Modalities. There are a wide variety of devices that produce external oscillation of airflow to facilitate secretion clearance. The *flutter valve*, held in the mouth and used independently by the patient, has been shown to be beneficial in patients with CF (O'Regan & Berman, 2004). *Positive expiratory pressure (PEP)* adjuncts are also useful for those patients with retained secretions as in CF or COPD. The patient is seated with a mouthpiece or mask over the mouth and nose to which a flow resistance device is attached. A fixed-resistance cap is used to produce expiratory pressures of 10 to 20 cm H_2O pressure during the midpart of expiration. After 10 PEP breaths and minimal expiratory effort by the patient, huff and spontaneous coughing are used to raise secretions mobilized by PEP therapy (Meyer, 2000). Devices such as the *acapella* or *TheraPEP* combine PEP with airway vibrations. This therapy may be used with a mouthpiece or pediatric or adult mask to administer high- or low-flow resistance. Advantages include the ease of self-administration for a patient sitting, standing, or reclining with less time involved than conventional chest physiotherapy.

Postural Drainage. *Postural drainage* uses the principles of gravity to drain pulmonary secretions from the various segments of each lung. It is effective for patients who produce copious amounts of sputum daily (25 ml or more), such as in CF and bronchiectasis (Frownfelter & Dean, 2006). Postural drainage with percussion and vibration is the most effective combination of techniques to manage the significant secretions associated with CF in children. However, the use of postural drainage in patients with chronic bronchitis remains controversial, is contraindicated in conditions that predispose the patient to increased intracranial pressure and hypertension, and has been associated with bronchoconstriction and decreases in arterial oxygenation (Frownfelter & Dean, 2006).

Twelve positions can be used to drain various lobes and bronchopulmonary segments. The nurse examines radiographical reports to determine which lobe(s) require drainage because few require drainage in each position. Several of the positions require the patient's head to be below the trunk and must be modified for patients who cannot tolerate the head-down position. The head-down position is used only when the upper lung segment requires drainage and is never used when increased intracranial pressure is suspected. It is used cautiously when patients are being monitored for hypoxemia, cardiovascular or hemodynamic instability, and marked bronchospasm. Oxygen may be administered or increased, unless contraindicated, in patients with compromised respiratory status.

Postural drainage should not be performed immediately before or after a meal. Before beginning, the nurse explains the procedure and provides the patient with tissues and a sputum cup. Bronchodilating medications given by nebulization, if ordered, are administered approximately 15 minutes before beginning the technique to facilitate drainage through dilated airways. The patient is then assisted into proper position, using extra pillows for support. Loosely fitted clothes facilitate coughing, deep breathing, and position changes. Postural drainage in patients who have spinal cord injury is performed only within the limitations of orthopedic alignment and stabilization, type of immobilization bed in use, and patient tolerance and with continuous monitoring of respiratory status. If the patient complains of respiratory difficulty or demonstrates unstable vital signs, immediately assist the patient to a more upright position and be prepared to provide supplemental oxygen or ventilator support. Auscultation before and after postural drainage determines effectiveness of the procedure.

Percussion and vibration in conjunction with postural drainage may help secretions move into the upper airways for expectoration and suctioning. These measures fatigue patients, especially when many lung segments require therapy. A patient remains in a position for 5 to 10 minutes to drain one segment of the lung. In the home, postural drainage is most effective with another person assisting. Mechanical vibrators are available to help patients who must perform this procedure alone. A recent systematic review of the literature on bronchopulmonary hygiene physical therapy in patients with COPD and bronchiectasis whose conditions are stable revealed that the effect of these techniques on lung function is not clear. No statistically significant effects on pulmonary function measurements or arterial oxygen tension were reported in seven randomized controlled studies (Jones & Rowe, 2000). However, anecdotal reports indicate that secretion mobilization and increased patient comfort after therapy continue to provide a rationale for these therapies.

A schedule for performing chest physiotherapy is based on the patient's needs. The procedure commonly is performed in the morning on arising to remove secretions that have pooled during the night and in the evening before going to bed to allow for optimum ventilation during sleep. A respiratory infection may increase secretions and necessitate therapy more frequently.

Suctioning the Patient. Suctioning removes secretions when the patient is unable to clear their airway by coughing or through a noninvasive therapy. Airway suctioning is most effective when performed after administration of appropriate bronchodilator then mobilizing tracheobronchial secretions by one or more of the interventions previously described for airway clearance. All airway suctioning has the potential for serious complications: hypoxia, atelectasis, bronchoconstriction, hypotension, cardiac arrhythmias, infection, irritation of the mucous membranes, and laryngospasm (Chulay & Burns, 2006).

Suction protocols must be modified according to the patient's need for and response to suctioning. The presence of coughing, audible secretions, tachypnea or labored respirations, coarse rhonchi, or oxygen desaturation *all indicate the need for suctioning. These clinical indicators should be assessed before each suctioning maneuver.*

Nasotracheal suctioning can be uncomfortable and exhausting for a patient but necessary in those with a poor cough effort as in neuromuscular disease. The use of a nasopharyngeal airway, or nasal trumpet, can facilitate suctioning and prevent trauma to the mucous membranes. The nasopharyngeal airway is lubricated with a water-soluble gel then gently inserted into one of the nares. The patient is instructed to take a few deep breaths of oxygen. The sterile, flexible catheter is lubricated with sterile water for easy passage. Suction pressure of 100 to 120 mm Hg for children and 100 to 150 mm Hg for adults is applied as the catheter is slowly withdrawn. The patient takes a few deep breaths of oxygen before additional passes, if needed, are performed (American Association for Respiratory Care [AARC], 2004). The nostril used is rotated every 8 hours to prevent bleeding, sinusitis, or erosion of the mucous membranes. The need for this device should be assessed on a daily basis (Chulay & Burns, 2006).

The presence of an artificial airway, such as a tracheostomy tube or an endotracheal tube, prevents glottic closure and effective coughing. Suctioning removes pulmonary secretions but should only be done when clinically indicated and never on a routine basis. The closed method of suctioning refers to a catheter system device that remains attached to the ventilator circuit. This requires disconnection of the tracheostomy or endotracheal tube from the ventilator and oxygen source each time the patient requires suctioning. In the rehabilitation and home settings, the open suctioning method is more commonly used.

Interventions for Patients With Tracheostomies

Tracheostomy Tubes. For individuals with ineffective airway clearance, a tracheostomy tube (Figure 17-4) may be inserted to (1) relieve airway obstruction, (2) protect the airway from aspiration because of impaired gag reflexes, (3) facilitate the removal of respiratory tract secretions, and (4) provide for mechanical ventilation. Patients often are admitted to rehabilitation facilities with temporary or permanent tracheostomies in place. Patients who cannot be weaned from a ventilator or cannot effectively cough up secretions have permanent tracheostomies.

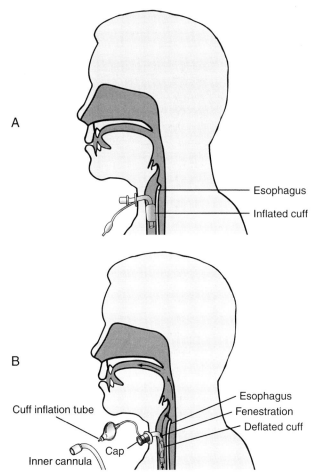

Figure 17-4 A, Placement of tracheostomy tube with inflated cuff. **B,** Fenestrated tracheostomy tube with cuff deflated, inner cannula removed, and tracheostomy tube capped to allow air to pass over the vocal cords. (From Lewis, S. M., Collier, I. C., Heitkemper, M. M., & Dirksen, S. R. [2004]. *Medical-surgical nursing: Assessment and management of clinical problems* [6th ed.]. St. Louis, MO: Mosby.)

Commonly used tracheostomy tubes are described in Table 17-2 and are made of silicone, pliable plastic, or metal. They may have an inner and outer cannula or only one lumen and come with or without a cuff. The cuff is inflated with air when a sealed airway is desired for mechanical ventilation (see Figure 17-4). In long-term care, plastic tubes are common, but metal tubes are more durable. The tracheostomy tube best suited to the patient's needs is chosen. Anatomical changes such as growth, development of granulation tissue, or changes in ventilation require ongoing evaluation.

The soft-cuffed tracheostomy tube is deflated when problems arise or once every 2 to 3 days to check for overinflation. Inflation pressures are kept between 20 and 25 cm H_2O to prevent high-pressure damage to the lateral wall of the trachea. The cuff pressure is monitored 3 times a day with a manometer without deflating the cuff. The oropharynx is suctioned

before deflation to prevent aspiration of pooled secretions above the inflated cuff. Hard cuffs are not recommended because they do not conform to the shape of trachea and therefore require higher pressures to prevent excessive leaking around the cuff. With higher pressures the cuffs press against the lateral wall of the trachea, causing necrosis of the tracheal tissue.

Communication is a problem for patients with a tracheostomy. The fenestrated tube can be used to facilitate verbal communication; alternatively, a tracheostomy tube with no cuff or deflated cuff can be used for patients receiving mechanical ventilation. If the patient is receiving positive pressure ventilation (PPV), the ventilator settings can be adjusted to provide higher airflow, allowing air to flow around the tube toward the vocal cords for speaking. The ability to tolerate this procedure depends on the patient's ventilatory stability, strength, and secretion volume. A number of additional communication aids are available, such as the Passy-Muir tracheostomy speaking valve (Frownfelter & Dean, 2006). This device fits into the tracheostomy tube opening and is a one-way valve, allowing inspiration only and forcing exhalation through the upper airway. Refer to a speech pathologist to evaluate the patient's need for additional communication devices. Children who have a tracheostomy are often taught sign language to facilitate developmental growth. The family and caregivers are also taught sign language. A system must be established in the home for outside communication and contact with designated persons in an emergency.

Tracheal buttons or plugs can be used for ventilatory support for only part of the day. The button is used to occlude the tracheostomy and establish normal airflow through the larynx, oral cavity, and nasal passages, allowing the patient to speak and to cough. The Olympic tracheostomy button can be used as a transition before occlusion of the tracheostomy. This button maintains the stoma should a tracheostomy be needed again.

Tracheostomy Care. Rehabilitation patients with tracheostomies have special care requirements to prevent complications and maintain adequate ventilatory function. Some differences apply to the suctioning principles previously described and must be noted. With tracheostomy suctioning the suction pressure should be reduced to only 60 to 80 mm Hg. The distal tip of the suction catheter is inserted into the tracheostomy until slight resistance is met, with care being taken not to traumatize the airway by pushing forcefully.

With a tracheostomy in place, the humidifying and warming mechanisms of the nose are bypassed. Cold, dry air causes drying of the tracheobronchial mucosa and thickening of secretions and promotes encrustation within the tube. The risk for problems of this nature can be reduced by providing humidity via a tracheostomy collar with a heated jet nebulizer (ATS, 1995).

Cannula and stoma care is performed every 8 hours using a sterile disposable cleaning kit. The inner cannula is soaked in hydrogen peroxide, cleansed with a test tube brush and pipe cleaners, and rinsed with saline solution. Be sure the inner

TABLE 17-2 Tracheostomy Tubes

Types	Indications
Cuffed tube with soft flexible cuff	A soft-cuffed tube is used in mechanically ventilated patients to prevent the leak of air and aspiration of secretions around the tube. Soft cuffs are less likely to cause problems with high pressures on the tracheal wall.
Fenestrated tube	Fenestrated tubes are used during weaning. They have opening(s) or fenestration(s) in the outer cannula so air can flow through the fenestrations to the larynx for speaking (see Figure 17-4, *B*). The fenestrations also allow the patient to cough and expel secretions through the mouth. The cuff should be deflated before inserting the inner cannula.
Uncuffed plastic and metal tubes	Uncuffed tubes frequently are used for long-term care when the patient has a functioning glottis. Metal tubes are rigid and can cause localized tissue irritation and excessive production of mucus.

cannula is locked securely in place on reinsertion. Cleanse the stoma site or area around the tracheostomy tube with a hydrogen peroxide solution to remove secretions. With one hand, hold the tracheostomy tube to lessen its movement and decrease the cough stimulus. Carefully cleanse the area around the stoma site, rinse with saline solution, and replace the tracheostomy dressing. Tracheostomy ties should be changed only with another person assisting to hold the tracheostomy firmly in place. If another person is not available, never remove the soiled ties until the clean ones are tied firmly in place. An extra sterile tracheostomy tube of the same size with its obturator must be immediately available at all times along with a sterile hemostat to hold the stoma open. The physician is notified immediately if tracheostomy reinsertion is needed following accidental decannulation. Generally reinsertion of a tracheostomy tube is not difficult if the tracheostomy is more than 72 hours old.

A tracheostomy tube remains in place only as long as necessary. Complications of delayed removal include tracheal stenosis, tracheoesophageal fistula, and infection. Initiate decannulation procedures as soon as the patient can maintain adequate ventilation and is able to cough and expel secretions. First, the cuff (if present) is deflated; if tolerated, the tracheostomy tube then can gradually be reduced in size. With the cuff deflated, the tube can be intermittently plugged with a tracheal button. As previously noted, the buttons allow ready access for suctioning or ventilation. Monitor the patient closely at this time for respiratory distress. Initially, until "plugging" is well tolerated, the nurse should stay with the patient to encourage proper breathing technique and provide reassurance. This procedure is very stressful for the patient. If tracheostomy tube occlusion is tolerated and the patient is able to cough and expel secretions, the tube can be removed after 24 to 72 hours. The tracheal button may remain in place if there is concern that the patient may require suctioning. Once the tube is removed, place a sterile gauze piece over the stoma, and it will close spontaneously in a few days. Observe the patient closely for any evidence of respiratory distress.

Education for Home Health Care. Patients discharged to home may participate in specialized day care during the week if available in their community. Ultimately, family

members are responsible for some or all of the care necessary to maintain the airway. When family participates in care while the patient is in a health facility, they are more apt to learn in a relaxed and unhurried manner. Inner cannula care, especially, is easier and less anxiety producing for them to learn in the structured, safe setting with the team available.

Equipment for cleaning the inner cannula and stoma includes hydrogen peroxide, dressings, and pipe cleaners or a brush to remove secretions from inside the tracheostomy tube. The primary caregiver must demonstrate competence and comfort with all aspects of care, including accidental decannulation and insertion of a new tracheostomy tube. The patient should be capable of directing someone in proper tracheostomy care, and emergency telephone numbers should be readily available and visible in the home. In addition, emergency agencies should be made aware of the potential need for services such as the emergency medical service (EMS). Proper humidification of the patient's air supply via a mechanical room humidifier or a portable source of humidified air or oxygen is essential; a dressing dampened with sterile water placed over the tracheostomy tube may be sufficient. However, the patient is cautioned to protect the tracheostomy opening from water (careful bathing and planning to shower during times the trach may be "plugged"), inhalation of foreign substances (e.g., powder, aerosol sprays), and dry air. Adequate amounts of fluid help liquefy secretions.

If suctioning will be required after the patient leaves the facility, the caregivers should be instructed in the procedure and potential complications early in the rehabilitation process. A mirror may help the patient to visualize the procedure. Clean rather than sterile technique can be used in the home. Catheters are not discarded but washed in a mild soap solution after each use, rinsed thoroughly, and then boiled for 5 minutes. Wrapped in a clean towel, they are ready for use. A new supply of sterile water or saline is made daily to prevent bacterial contamination: 1 teaspoon of salt per quart of water and stored in a sealed container. Once opened, it is also boiled. Referral to a home health care agency for follow-up care allows the nurse to evaluate how the patient and family are coping and to make any modifications in the care. Agency social services can facilitate purchase or rental of a portable suction machine and other equipment.

Nutritional Therapies. Nutritional assessment and appropriate interventions are essential in the rehabilitation of any patient with chronic lung disease. Nutritional depletion contributes to peripheral skeletal muscle wasting, a decrease in diaphragm muscle mass, impairment of ventilatory drive, and immune dysfunction (Sherk & Grossman, 2000). Weight loss has been shown to be a factor in poor outcomes of acute exacerbations and has been associated with increased morbidity and mortality of COPD (Pouw et al., 2000; Sherk & Grossman, 2000). Patients with COPD have a higher resting energy expenditure from the work of breathing, an increased activity-related energy level, and low dietary intake, all contributing to weight loss and muscle wasting. The low intake is attributed to the dyspnea and oxygen desaturation associated with chewing, swallowing, and alteration in respiratory pattern. Gastric filling may limit diaphragm excursion, reduce functional residual capacity, and increase dyspnea further.

Nutritional evaluation begins with a thorough history of food intake; height and weight measures; routine laboratory values, including albumin and serum ferritin; and total lymphocyte count. Serum albumin value reflects visceral protein stores and signs of chronic malnourishment, and the lymphocyte count is an indicator of cellular immune status. Important clinical indicators for malnutrition are recent weight loss of 10% of body weight, body weight of less than 90% or greater than 120% of ideal body weight, visible muscle wasting, dietary intake changes, gastrointestinal symptoms persisting for more than 2 weeks, decreased functional capacity, and edema or ascites. In-depth nutritional assessments require referral to a dietitian.

Nutritional support goals include both maintaining body weight and preventing protein breakdown. Daily protein intake should include at least 1.5 mg/kg of body weight for optimal protein synthesis (Schols & Wouters, 2000). For patients who are hypercapnic, reduced carbohydrate intake relative to fat intake may improve the metabolic workload and decrease the amount of carbon (removed as CO_2) released through respiration. Interventions include increased consumption of calorie-rich foods, dietary supplements, and vitamins and minerals to meet the recommended daily allowances. Supportive nursing interventions include utilizing a nasal cannula during meals and monitoring oximetry to ensure adequate oxygenation. Offering nutritional supplements between small meals reduces the sensation of gastric fullness to further reduce dyspnea. Encouraging physical activity and exercise can further stimulate the patient's appetite (Gronkiewicz & Borkgren-Okonek, 2004). Overweight patients are also referred to a dietitian for the planning of healthy diets that include macronutrients and vitamins and minerals for good lung health but fewer calories for weight reduction. This is especially significant for children who need calories to grow and should not be on a very low calorie diet plan. Weight instruction should include suggestions for exercise or physical activities reasonable for their disease state. Ongoing monitoring for adherence and encouragement is necessary for either nutrition regimen.

Outcome Criteria

For the patient with airway clearance problems, the following outcome criteria are identified. The patient will demonstrate adequate airway clearance as evidenced by being able to recognize need for airway clearance intervention, demonstrate an effective cough technique, utilize chest physiotherapy technique or secretion mobilization device for secretion clearance, understand the appropriate use of prescribed bronchodilators, and demonstrate proper maintenance of an artificial airway device: cleaning, suctioning, and changing.

IMPAIRED GAS EXCHANGE

Impaired gas exchange is a "disturbance in oxygen or carbon dioxide exchange in the lungs or at the cellular level" (Gordon, 2002). Impaired gas exchange is seen in many patients with chronic lung disease, including COPD, interstitial lung disease, BPD, and acute infections. In pulmonary rehabilitation, patients with impaired gas exchange most commonly have COPD or interstitial lung disease; whereas in general rehabilitation, patients have severe restrictive lung disease associated with spinal cord injury, Guillain-Barré syndrome, and scoliosis. All patients with impaired gas exchange also experience ineffective breathing pattern and ineffective airway clearance.

Alterations in Gas Exchange

Alterations in gas exchange are primarily reflected by hypoxemia (decreased PaO_2). Alveolar hypoventilation and abnormalities of diffusion can cause hypoxemia, but the most common cause of hypoxemia is a mismatch of ventilation and perfusion. Chronic problems with gas exchange are described in the following sections using four clinical examples of chronic lung disease: COPD, interstitial lung disease, BPD, and asthma. Acute problems with gas exchange can also occur with respiratory tract infections.

COPD. COPD is characterized by chronic inflammation throughout the central and peripheral airways, lung parenchyma, and pulmonary vasculature. This inflammation is caused by exposure to inhaled noxious particles and gases, most notably cigarette smoke, which accounts for 85% to 90% of all cases. Genetic factors (such as alpha$_1$-antitrypsin deficiency emphysema), passive smoking, occupational exposure, air pollution, and possibly hyperresponsive airways can also contribute to COPD. This inflammation affects the lungs in a variety of ways. In the central airways, inflammatory cells infiltrate the epithelium where goblet cells cause hypersecretion of mucus. In the peripheral airways, repeated cycles of injury and repair to their walls result in structural remodeling and scar formation. The lumen narrows, causing fixed airway obstruction. Inflammatory cell infiltration of the smooth muscle further causes thickening of the vessel walls. Peripheral airway obstruction, parenchymal destruction, and pulmonary vascular abnormalities reduce the ability for gas exchange (Barnes, 2000).

Ventilatory abnormalities result from airway inflammation, edema, bronchospasm, and increased mucus production. Perfusion abnormalities result from hypoxia-induced constriction of the arterioles, an abnormal respiratory pattern, and respiratory muscle fatigue. Progression of this disease causes hypoxemia and/or hypercapnia. The major cardiovascular complication of COPD is pulmonary hypertension, which often occurs along with cor pulmonale (Barnes, 2000).

Interstitial Lung Disease. Interstitial lung disease refers to a group of lung disorders associated with extensive alterations of the alveolar, airway, and vascular architecture. A large number of occupational and environmental exposures are associated with the development of diffuse parenchymal lung disease: inorganic dust, organic dust, drugs, pets, chemicals, and gases. Many, such as sarcoidosis and idiopathic pulmonary fibrosis (IPF), have no known cause. In all these disorders an initial injury is followed by an influx of inflammatory and immune effector cells. As the initial inflammatory response resolves, pulmonary fibrosis or scarring results. The specific cellular mechanisms involved in the transition from inflammatory response to tissue repair or irreversible fibrosis is unknown (King, 2004).

Most of the interstitial disorders have a restrictive defect seen on pulmonary function tests (PFTs) in the reduced total lung capacity, functional residual capacity, and residual volume. A reduction in the diffusing capacity is common and caused by the mismatch of ventilation and perfusion in the alveoli. Serial assessments of resting and activity gas exchange are the best indicators of disease activity and response to treatment (King, 2004).

Bronchopulmonary dysplasia is discussed in Chapter 31.

Asthma. Asthma is a chronic condition that affects more than 20 million Americans, causing about 5,000 deaths each year. The risk of uncontrolled asthma is significant; asthma can cause life-threatening situations requiring emergency department visits, hospitalization, and even death. African Americans and Puerto Ricans are three to five times more affected by asthma in the United States (Akinbami & Morgenstern, 2006). For patients with asthma, comprehensive care employs many of the principles of pulmonary rehabilitation: disease management programs to decrease utilization of health care resources, education to increase adherence to treatment programs, and instructions on health-enhancing behaviors to improve self-management.

In asthma the bronchi and bronchioles are more sensitive—they become unstable and produce an increase in mucus, which causes irritation and results in cough. The bronchial muscle tightens and contracts, resulting in bronchospasm. The diameter of the bronchus narrows, and the chest feels "tight." The mucosa becomes swollen and inflamed. The bronchial glands produce large amounts of sticky mucus, which forms plugs in the bronchus. This further blocks the flow of air. There is greater pressure needed to push air through the bronchus, necessitating increased use of accessory muscles and resultant sweating, fatigue, and irritability. Vibrations caused by forcing air through narrowed uneven bronchial tubes past mucus and the bronchus itself results in wheezing, squeaking, or whistling sounds with each breath. The mucus caught in the bronchi becomes irritating and results in a persistent cough. As the difficulty of forcing air into and out of the lungs progresses, the lack of oxygenation results in anxiety, inability to speak in sentences, headache, and ultimately loss of consciousness progressing to death.

The goals of therapy for asthma as put forth by the NAEPP 2002 guidelines include minimal or no chronic symptoms day or night; minimal or no exacerbations; no limitation on activities; no school/work missed; maintenance of (near) normal pulmonary function; minimal use of short-acting inhaled beta$_2$-agonist (less than 1 time per day, less than 1 canister per month); minimal or no adverse effects from medications; allowance for child's maximum level of growth and development and normal activities through use of asthma self-management and emergency management plans (action plans), environmental control, medication, using controller and reliever, and education.

Asthma attacks can be "triggered" by many things, including outdoor allergens (pollen, mold), indoor allergens (roaches, dust mites, animals, birds, mold), other allergens (food, stinging insects, medications), irritants (smoking, strong odors, aerosol sprays, pesticides, perfumes, cleaning products, pollution, craft supplies), exercise, viral infections, cold air, changing weather, hot muggy weather, poor air quality days, stress, laughing, and crying.

Assessment

The NANDA (North American Nursing Diagnosis Association) defining characteristics for impaired gas exchange include visual disturbances; decreased carbon dioxide; dyspnea; abnormal arterial blood gas levels; hypoxia; irritability; somnolence, restlessness; hypercapnia; tachycardia; cyanosis abnormal skin color (pale, dusky); hypoxemia; abnormal rate, rhythm, and depth of breathing; diaphoresis, abnormal arterial pH; and nasal flaring (Ackley & Ladwig, 2006). Defining characteristics reported by Carlson-Catalano et al. (1998) are abnormal blood gas levels and expressed fatigue.

Subjective Assessment. Subjective assessment includes a thorough history taking. Smoking behaviors should be detailed as to number of pack years, smoking cessation interventions, and quit date, if applicable. Notes should be made regarding secondhand smoke exposure or family history of lung disease. Environmental risks and occupational exposures should include specific agents and length of exposure. Characteristics of the patient's chief complaint include the length, severity, frequency, and duration of any cough, wheeze, or shortness of breath as well as interventions that relieve or worsen the symptoms. The color, amount, and frequency of sputum produced can be specific to a particular disease state. Any recent respiratory infection or previous occurrence should be noted. Patients may also report feelings of fatigue, anxiety, confusion, irritability, and/or restlessness related to their respiratory complaints. All medications currently and previously used should be taken into consideration.

Objective Assessment. Objective assessment of the patient with impaired gas exchange should include complete physical examination, pulmonary function tests with diffusing capacity, arterial blood gas values, exercise and nocturnal oximetry, chest x-ray examination, complete blood count, electrolytes, and immunoglobulins. Further testing depends on results of the above and the patient's history and clinical presentation. More specific tests are indicated when considering respiratory involvement of a systemic disease.

Goals

The primary nursing goal is for the patient to achieve and maintain adequate oxygenation (see Table 17-1). Patient goals include the following: demonstrate improved ventilation and adequate oxygenation of tissues during rest, exercise, and sleep; display appropriate age-related cognitive abilities; incorporate energy conservation and work simplification into activities of daily living (ADLs) with acceptable level of dyspnea; and understand purpose and correct use of supplemental oxygen therapy.

Interventions for Patients With Impaired Gas Exchange

The underlying causes of impaired gas exchange may be related to ineffective airway clearance and ineffective breathing pattern, as described earlier. In most cases patients will have more than one of the related respiratory problems, and combined approaches are warranted. If secretions are excessive and tenacious, nursing interventions related to ineffective airway clearance are appropriate; when the underlying problem is an ineffective breathing pattern, then interventions are directed at increasing breathing effectiveness.

Positioning. Assisting the patient with leaning forward at a 30- to 40-degree angle with the arms resting on the thighs or an over-the-bed table may relieve breathlessness (ATS, 1995). Because the patient is unable to efficiently use the accessory muscles of respiration, leaning forward improves the upward action of the diaphragm, allowing more complete emptying of the lungs on exhalation. Position influences pulmonary function and is critical for maximum performance in patients with spinal cord injury. In patients with quadriplegia or paraplegia, significant decreases in forced vital capacity (FVC) can occur with changes in posture. Assess the patient's tolerance when moving from supine to upright positions, and alter therapies based on tolerance to the postural changes (Frownfelter & Dean, 2006).

Patients with unilateral lung disease are routinely positioned from side to side because gravity offers dependent areas of the lung a greater proportion of ventilation and perfusion. When the patient is upright, the bases receive a greater proportion of ventilation and perfusion than the apex. When the patient is side-lying, the dependent lung receives the greater proportion. Patients with unilateral lung involvement have the highest arterial oxygen levels when they alternate between the semi-Fowler's position and side-lying with the uninvolved lung down every 60 to 90 minutes (Frownfelter & Dean, 2006). The heart and blood vessels may compress the lung more with the patient lying on the left side. Clinical guidelines recommend uninvolved side down in patients with unilateral lung involvement. The patient with bilateral lung involvement rests with the head elevated and on the right side (Frownfelter & Dean, 2006).

Oxygen Therapy. Oxygen is considered part of the pharmaceutical management of the patient. Oxygen therapy does not treat the underlying cause of hypoxemia but does decrease the cardiopulmonary workload, allows the patient to breathe easier, and reduces the long-term effects of hypoxemia. Oxygen also improves lung mechanics, exercise capacity, mental acuity, and hematological characteristics. Many patients resist the use of oxygen therapy because they feel it symbolizes a worsening of their condition, are concerned about becoming addicted to oxygen, or may consider it inconvenient and restrictive to their lifestyle, Allow the patient early on to adjust to the idea of oxygen use and its potential benefits and to actively participate in selecting the type of oxygen delivery system. Educate patients that oxygen is as important as other medications and is the only therapy shown to be associated with increased survival in COPD patients with chronic hypoxemia.

Long-term oxygen therapy (LTOT) is often prescribed for patients with severe hypoxemic COPD and to treat children who have varying degrees of respiratory insufficiency from multiple causes. Oxygen therapy may allow a patient to return home, prolong life, and improve quality of life. High oxygen concentrations for prolonged periods are associated with toxicity but are uncommon in the rehabilitation setting.

Carbon dioxide retention must be evaluated when a patient receives supplemental oxygen therapy. It is known that carbon dioxide may rise due to a blunted hypercapnic respiratory drive resulting from chronic carbon dioxide retention. The hypoxic drive now becomes more critical. Precautions should be taken with any increase in inspired oxygen to avoid reducing ventilation and increasing CO_2 pressure. Higher levels of inspired oxygen may also increase the amount of wasted perfusion to poorly ventilated lungs, causing greater mismatch of ventilation and perfusion. Thus, when LTOT is prescribed, the arterial blood gases are measured when the patient is both on and off the planned oxygen regimen.

Controlled oxygen therapy is administered when the oxygen saturation is below 89% or the PaO_2 is less than 55 mm Hg on room air at rest, with ambulation, or during sleep. The goal of supplemental oxygen is to raise the PaO_2 value to 60 to 65 mm Hg or achieve an oxygen saturation of at least 90%.

Home Oxygen Therapy. The primary care provider prescribes oxygen based on medical necessity and specific guidelines adopted by Medicare and other insurance companies for reimbursement. If oxygen is ordered, Medicare requires the qualifying data be obtained no more than 2 days before discharge. As in the inpatient setting, oxygen therapy is assessed at rest and with ambulation to document an oxygen saturation below 89% or a PaO_2 less than or equal to 55 mm Hg on room air. With concomitant conditions such as cor pulmonale, pulmonary hypertension, polycythemia, or heart failure, the patient needs a PaO_2 between 55 and 60 mm Hg and one of the following:

1. Dependent edema, which suggests congestive heart failure; cor pulmonale on electrocardiogram (ECG); or erythrocytosis with a hematocrit value greater than 55%
2. PaO_2 level drops to or is less than 55 mm Hg or drops more than 10 mm Hg or the SaO_2 level drops to or is less than 85% or drops more than 5% during sleep
3. PaO_2 level drops to or is less than 55 mm Hg or the SaO_2 level drops to or is less than 85% during exercise

The home oxygen prescription must clearly specify the number of liters per minute, minimal number of hours per day for use, oxygen source, the method of delivery (e.g., nasal prongs), and the need for portable oxygen. The specific respiratory diagnosis and duration of need (e.g., 3 months) should also be included. Because Medicare and insurance companies can change their qualifying guidelines for home oxygen reimbursement at any time, it is the responsibility of the pulmonary rehabilitation team to verify eligibility before discharge.

Oxygen Delivery Systems. There are three methods of oxygen delivery in the home: compressed gas in tanks or cylinders, liquid oxygen in reservoirs, and oxygen concentrators. Refer to Table 17-3 for a more detailed description of these systems. The type of oxygen system chosen should consider the patient's clinical condition, oxygen flow rate, duration of daily use, activity level, need for a portable oxygen unit, and the patient's ability and/or desire to adhere to the therapy. In the home, concentrators and liquid oxygen are the most common systems used. Oxygen concentrators use electrical power to separate oxygen molecules from the air, concentrate them in a reservoir, then deliver oxygen to the patient through a nasal cannula. They can provide 40% oxygen and function as a humidifier. Because they require electrical power, a back-up gas cylinder is always provided. For portability the patient uses smaller, lightweight gas cylinders. Another alternative is liquid

oxygen where the main stationary unit keeps the temperature of oxygen below 29° F. In this form a large amount of oxygen is stored in a small space. As it warms, it converts to the gas form for delivery. The small, compact portable units (referred to as walkers, companions, strollers, or liberators) now weigh only 4 to 7 pounds while providing 2 L/min of oxygen for 7 to 10 hours. The primary drawback to the liquid system is cost of operation; hence it has limited use in the United States and many countries. Gas cylinders are large and heavy yet remain the primary method of providing long-term oxygen worldwide. The portable gas units require adequate storage space and changing of regulators yet provide minimal duration of flow for those patients who desire long times away from home.

The dual-prong nasal cannula is a simple, effective way to administer low to moderate oxygen concentrations for the patient with hypoxemia in stable condition. Each liter per minute of oxygen flow adds about 3% to 4% to the concentration of oxygen in inspired air (FIO_2), but this varies depending on the patient's respiratory rate and tidal volume. An FIO_2 of up to 40% can be achieved with a well-placed cannula at flow rates up to 6 L/min (Meyer, 2000). Humidification is not required when oxygen flow rates are less than 5 L/min. Advantages of nasal cannulas are ease of administration and no interruption of oxygen flow to eat, cough, and perform other activities. Cannulas can cause nasal irritation even when the oxygen is humidified. Small amounts of a water-soluble lubricant applied to the nares can reduce or prevent discomfort.

A simple oxygen mask consists of small ports on each side that allow exhaled gases to exit the mask while providing entrainment of room air during inspiration. At flow rates of 6 to 10 L/min, it can deliver an FIO_2 of 35% to 50% (Meyer, 2000). Care should be taken to fit the mask over the nose and mouth while avoiding skin irritation. Disadvantages with this device are the need to remove the mask for eating and the limited ability to generate the required flow rates on home oxygen systems. When a more precise oxygen percentage is required, usually in those patients with carbon dioxide retention or varied ventilatory patterns, an air entrainment (or Venturi)

TABLE 17-3 Types of Oxygen Systems

Type	Advantages	Disadvantages	Important Information
Compressed gas	Ability to deliver 100% oxygen with accuracy over a wide range of liter-per-minute flow	Large, heavy unit with limited capacity	Back pressure-compensated flowmeter called for when long tubing is used with smaller E tank
Liquid oxygen	Small, light, and portable system (<10 lb)	Expensive; loses small amount of oxygen if not used	Ideal for the active patient: check insurance coverage
Oxygen concentrators	Most economical and efficient system	Not suitable for patients requiring high flow rates; somewhat noisy, and backup gas system is required in case of power outage	Does increase electric bill; most suitable for homebound patients

mask is used. The FIO_2 delivered is controlled by the jet size and entrainment port size on the mask, thus maintaining a precise oxygen percentage at all times (Meyer, 2000). Because this requires a snug-fitting mask, attention should be paid to the patient's skin condition. A nasal cannula can be offered during meals if an adequate oxygen saturation can be maintained for brief periods off the Venturi mask. Although high-flow oxygen masks are available, they are not commonly used in rehabilitation settings or the home.

T-pieces and trach collars or masks are used to deliver continuous oxygen through a tracheostomy tube. Humidification is necessary even at low flow rates because the upper airway passages are bypassed by the tracheostomy.

Alternative Delivery Systems. A number of alternative delivery systems are available to conserve oxygen and permit longer use of a portable unit. The Oxymizer pendant cannula and the Oxymizer mustache cannula provide higher oxygen concentrations because of their reservoir design. The reservoir refills with oxygen as the patient is exhaling. Another noninvasive means to conserve oxygen is with a pulse-dose demand valve device attached to a portable cylinder. Several electronic and pneumatic types are available through CHAD Therapeutics (2006). The valve senses the beginning of inhalation and immediately delivers a bolus but stops flow during the exhalation phase. An oxygen assessment study should be done on the chosen system to ensure adequate oxygenation with its use. Transtracheal oxygen systems deliver supplemental oxygen directly into the trachea via a small plastic cannula that is inserted into the trachea at the base of the neck. These systems are less conspicuous than nasal prongs. A lower flow rate is needed because oxygen is delivered continuously and directly into the trachea throughout inspiration and expiration, bypassing part of the anatomical dead space. Humidification of oxygen is necessary. Advantages of the system are increased portability, mobility, and comfort. Complications of transtracheal oxygen delivery are infrequent and mild, including catheter displacement, subcutaneous emphysema, and infection. The best candidates for transtracheal oxygen delivery are patients who have a strong desire to remain active, are willing to follow the care protocol, have few exacerbations, and can identify a caregiver willing to actively participate in the care (ATS, 1995).

Education and Monitoring. Most patients qualifying for supplemental oxygen in the rehabilitation setting will be using it in the home setting as well. This is an excellent opportunity for the rehabilitation team to educate the patient and family as to its vital purpose and long-term benefits, as well as alleviate any fears regarding "addiction" to oxygen. Reframing the perception of oxygen as a drug to increase functional capacity and improve quality of life helps with acceptance of this treatment modality. The occupational therapist can demonstrate the use of supplemental oxygen while cooking, bathing, or performing home-related chores. The physical therapist encourages its use and prescribed flow rate while walking and during a patient's individual exercise regimen.

As mentioned, oxygen systems and portable units used after discharge are much different than the ones used in the inpatient setting. It is important to involve the patient in the decision-making for the home oxygen system, portable unit, and conserving device. The optimal delivery system chosen should consider the individual's oxygen requirements, finances, lifestyle, and physical capabilities. Many homecare companies are willing to come to the hospital to demonstrate the variety of systems available. After discharge, the oxygen saturation should be periodically checked to confirm the continued need. This includes its use at rest, with activity, and during sleep. A patient's oxygen requirements will always increase following an acute exacerbation of the underlying respiratory disease but is expected to stabilize within 6 weeks.

Travel and Oxygen Therapy. One of the biggest misconceptions regarding supplemental oxygen is the need to be homebound because of its size, weight or bulkiness. With the appropriate system the patient can enjoy many extracurricular activities including travel. For long distance auto or train travel, homecare companies can identify sites for oxygen refills or replacement units. Air travel by individuals using supplemental oxygen is more commonplace today despite poor standardization of in-flight oxygen by the Federal Aviation Administration (FAA) or individual airlines. The oxygen delivery system and flow rates vary considerably by airline, but all carriers offer nasal cannula delivery. Generally airlines require 48- to 72-hour advance notification of oxygen need by the individual's health care provider. Actual charges for in-flight oxygen vary among airlines, but all charge for each leg of the trip. Therefore patients should always be instructed to book direct flights when possible. Individuals are not allowed to carry their own portable oxygen unit on an airplane; however, an FAA-approved portable oxygen concentrator is available. In addition, Seapuffer Cruises offers cruise travel for patients with respiratory diseases. They provide medical assistance and respiratory therapists while on the ship and during shore excursions (www.seapuffers.com). For all travel the patient and family should remember to request wheelchair assistance through airports, place all medications in carry-on luggage, and allow plenty of time for connections between travel sites.

Outcome Criteria

For the patient with impaired gas exchange the following outcome criteria are identified. The patient will demonstrate adequate gas exchange as evidenced by oxygen saturation equal to or greater than 88% at rest, with activity, and during sleep; appropriate cognitive abilities for age and related comorbid illnesses; ability to use supplemental oxygen during activities of daily living; improved level of sleep quality reported; and use of optimal portable oxygen system for needs and lifestyle used.

INEFFECTIVE BREATHING PATTERN

Ineffective breathing pattern is defined as respiration inadequate to maintain sufficient oxygen supply for cellular requirements

(Gordon, 2002). Effective breathing requires normal lung and airway structures; a feedback mechanism involving the nervous system structures that control respiration (peripheral chemoreceptors, central chemoreceptors, and respiratory neurons of the pons and medulla); intact nerve pathways to the muscles of respiration; and an intact structure of the chest wall. Damage in these components results in ventilatory failure when alveolar ventilation is insufficient to accomplish adequate gas exchange.

Dyspnea and fatigue were found to be the defining characteristics of ineffective breathing pattern (Carlson-Catalano et al., 1998). In rehabilitation, nurses most commonly address chronic problems related to ineffective breathing patterns, such as those seen in patients with obstructive lung disease and restrictive lung disease. (Box 17-3 outlines the mechanisms for altered ventilatory patterns in both obstructive and restrictive lung disease.)

Alterations in Ventilation

Alveolar hyperventilation and hypoventilation are clinically defined by the $PaCO_2$ value. Hyperventilation causes the $PaCO_2$ to fall to less than 35 mm Hg, usually in patients who are breathing rapidly for an extended period. Hyperventilation is a normal response to a high-altitude environment, but it also appears in patients who have greatly increased anxiety levels. In contrast, alveolar hypoventilation causes the $PaCO_2$ level to rise above 45 mm Hg. Hypoventilation occurs in individuals with severe lung disease and neuromuscular disease. Ventilatory failure is the extreme form of alveolar hypoventilation, characterized by a $PaCO_2$ level greater than 45 mm Hg and a PaO_2 level less than 60 mm Hg (Frownfelter & Dean, 2006).

Alveolar hypoventilation results from either an inadequate minute ventilation (V_E) and/or an excessive dead space (V_{DS}). Minute ventilation is the sum of alveolar ventilation and dead space. Inadequate V_E can be caused by alterations in respiratory mechanics, inadequate ventilatory drive, and/or respiratory muscle weakness. Excessive V_{DS} can be caused by either the mismatch of ventilation and perfusion or by shallow breathing.

Obstructive Defects. Patients with very severe COPD are more likely to experience chronic alveolar hypoventilation, as evidenced by chronic hypercapnia. Hypercapnia is seen most commonly in patients with COPD having an FEV_1 of less than 1 L. The precise mechanisms for the development of alveolar hypoventilation are not well understood in patients with COPD, but evidence points to blunting of the ventilatory response to chemical stimuli, such as hypoxia and hypercapnia, and/or the development of rapid shallow breathing patterns to reduce the work of breathing and protect against respiratory muscle fatigue (Montes de Oca & Celli, 2000).

In infancy significant areas of vulnerability exist within the respiratory system. Box 17-1 lists the parts of the pediatric respiratory anatomy that differ from the adult respiratory anatomy. In pediatric patients with BPD, hypoventilation and hypercapnia are observed as a result of ineffective ventilation

due to airway damage and obstruction. Characteristic interstitial markings or strand densities are evidenced on the chest radiograph. Pulmonary function is compromised by increased airway resistance, decreased compliance, increased dead space, and increased airway reactivity.

Adult patients with COPD have increased airway resistance, and respiratory muscles must generate higher forces to maintain a given level of ventilation. Hyperinflation of the chest wall places the inspiratory muscles at a mechanical disadvantage to generate the higher forces. Nutritional deficits can impede muscle strength, mass, and efficiency. These patients are predisposed to respiratory muscle fatigue and rapid shallow breathing, which increases the V_{DS}. With severe COPD the mismatch of ventilation and perfusion contributes to alveolar hypoventilation.

Restrictive Defects. Patients with neuromuscular disease develop alveolar hypoventilation secondary to respiratory muscle weakness and decreased compliance of the lungs and chest wall. Weakened inspiratory muscles make them unable to take a deep breath, leading to a decline in V_E. Secondly, the reduced VC leads to microatelectasis and increased stiffness of the chest wall, thereby increasing the work of breathing and further contributing to the decline in V_E.

In the early stages of neuromuscular disease, mild respiratory muscle weakness can exist without clinical consequences if the respiratory muscles are capable of meeting ventilatory demands and generating an effective cough. Respiratory muscle fatigue and ventilatory failure occur when the ventilatory demands exceed the ability of the respiratory muscles.

The extent of respiratory muscle involvement depends on the nature of the pathophysiology and its pattern of progression. In Duchenne's muscular dystrophy, respiratory muscle weakness appears early in the course of the disease and progresses slowly until death. In amyotrophic lateral sclerosis (ALS), respiratory muscle weakness is secondary to denervation atrophy, beginning with the expiratory abdominal muscles and eventually progressing to the inspiratory muscles. In ALS the progression of respiratory muscle weakness is faster than in other neuromuscular diseases. In persons with spinal cord injury the extent of respiratory muscle involvement depends on the level and nature of the injury. Persons with high cervical lesions (above C4) typically require mechanical ventilation; with midcervical lesions (C4 to C8) individuals experience severe expiratory muscle weakness and/or paralysis and mild inspiratory muscle weakness. Many spinal cord injury lesions are oblique, interrupting innervation to one side of the diaphragm and producing severe diaphragmatic weakness on only one side.

Combined Obstructive and Restrictive Defects. Patients with CF have two abnormal copies of a defective CF gene that, in turn, code for a defective or mutant cystic fibrosis transmembrane regulator (CFTR) protein located on chromosome 7. With a mutant CFTR protein, chloride movement is inhibited, and the balance of sodium, chloride, and water is disrupted in affected cells. This imbalance results in classic findings in CF: dehydrated secretions and mucous obstruction in the ducts of exocrine glands (Yankaskas, 2004).

CF affects multiple organ systems to varying degrees in different individuals, but lung disease is the major cause of morbidity and mortality. Generally patients with normal pancreatic function have milder lung disease, possibly related to improved nutritional status. The lung disease in CF results from an ongoing cycle of obstruction, infection, inflammation, and injury, with resultant restrictive elements. Dehydrated secretions block airway passages. These secretions also contain large amounts of uninhibited proteolytic enzymes, which contribute to tissue injury and impaired mucociliary transport. Obstruction leads to endobronchial infection. Two bacteria primarily responsible for infections in the CF lung—*Staphylococcus aureus* and *Pseudomonas aeruginosa*—continue to colonize the CF lung. Antimicrobial therapies that reduce bacterial colony counts offer clinical improvement (Yankaskas, 2004).

Chronic obstruction and infection cause progressive deterioration of lung structure and function. Early changes, more prominent in the upper lobes, include air trapping, airway inflammation, and peribronchial thickening, which contribute to restrictive symptoms. As lung injury continues, changes become more diffuse with evidence of bronchiectasis, fibrosis, and cyst formation. When fibrosis develops in some tissues, restrictive lung disease compounds what began as obstructive lung disease. Box 17-3 contains a summary of mechanisms.

Subjective Assessment

Patients have a subjective feeling that ventilation requirements are not being met, and dyspnea is the chief complaint associated with ineffective breathing patterns. Clinical assessment includes the patient's perception of the frequency, intensity, and contributing factors. Various scales (previously discussed) can be used to quantify the patient's perception of dyspnea. Research suggests that worsening dyspnea is not directly related to changes in lung impairment (Lareau, Meek, Press, Anholm, & Roos, 1999). Perceptions of fatigue, another subjective complaint, are explored as to severity, time of day, and possible underlying causes. Reports of snoring, apneic episodes during sleep, and excessive daytime sleepiness indicate sleep pattern disturbance.

Objective Assessment

On physical examination the nurse should pay particular attention to changes in mental status, use of accessory muscles of respiration, pursed-lip breathing, and paradoxical abdominal breathing—findings that suggest ineffective breathing patterns and ventilatory failure. Investigate signs of airflow obstruction, wheezing during auscultation, a prolonged forced expiratory time, and the need to assume unusual positions to relieve dyspnea.

Pulmonary function testing differentiates between restrictive and obstructive lung disease, but results are more difficult to interpret with mixed restrictive and obstructive disease. In obstructive lung disease the time needed to forcefully exhale after full inspiration is increased as reflected in the low FEV_1/FVC ratio. In restrictive lung disease, air can be expelled rapidly and the FEV_1/FVC ratio is high. Spirometry can measure the volume of air expelled from fully inflated lungs.

Goals

The primary nursing goals for the patient with ineffective breathing pattern are to maximize ventilation and improve airflow (see Table 17-1). Patient goals include the following: ventilation parameters in expected range for specific disease

---

BOX 17-3 Mechanisms for Altered Ventilatory Patterns

Restrictive Lung Disease: Decreased Expansion of the Lungs
Disease states: Degenerative neuromuscular diseases, spinal cord injury, scoliosis, bony deformities of the chest wall, interstitial pulmonary fibrosis
Clinical presentation: With increasing weakness and fatigue of the respiratory muscles, patients may develop uncoordinated breathing and alternate between use of the muscles of the chest wall and the diaphragm to breathe. Paradoxical breathing (inward displacement of the abdomen with inspiration) is seen as the diaphragm weakens. Paradoxical movement of the abdomen on inspiration becomes especially pronounced in the supine position because the diaphragm cannot fall passively. Respiratory impairment can be either unilateral or bilateral, temporary or permanent.

Obstructive Lung Disease: Increased Resistance to Airflow
Disease states: Emphysema, chronic bronchitis, asthma, BPD, some cystic fibrosis
Clinical presentation: During quiet breathing, patients with moderate to severe COPD commonly demonstrate an increased respiratory rate with a normal tidal volume and V_E, even when their lung condition is stable and they are in their best state of health. During an exacerbation and/or during an episode of respiratory failure, the respiratory rate will further increase and the V_E will decrease, producing rapid, shallow breathing. The precise mechanisms for altered breathing patterns in individuals with COPD may include respiratory muscle fatigue with declines in maximum inspiratory force and injury to the airways with subsequent stimulation of irritant receptors.

BPD, Bronchopulmonary dysplasia; *COPD,* chronic obstructive pulmonary disease; V_E, minute ventilation.

process, adequate breathing pattern observed during sleep, minimal or no complaints of dyspnea or breathlessness at rest, increased ability to perform activities of daily living through energy conservation and work simplification, and psychological support for feelings of anxiety, depression, isolation, and insomnia.

Interventions for Patients With Ineffective Breathing Patterns

Nursing management is aimed at maintaining adequate ventilation through breathing retraining, exercise training, energy conservation techniques, ventilatory support devices, mechanical ventilation, and psychological support from a multidisciplinary pulmonary rehabilitation team.

Ventilation Assistance. Persons with ineffective breathing pattern may benefit from breathing retraining techniques such as PLB, abdominal-diaphragmatic breathing, segmental breathing, and GPB. Breathing retraining is designed to assist the patient in controlling breathing patterns, promote ventilation through effective breathing patterns, and relieve symptoms of dyspnea.

Pursed-Lip Breathing. *PLB* is a technique of exhaling slowly through partially closed, or "pursed," lips. By controlling expiration and maximum emptying of the alveoli, PLB reduces respiratory rate, minute ventilation, and carbon dioxide levels and increases tidal volume, arterial oxygen pressure, and oxygen saturation (ATS, 1999). Patients with COPD may gain some control over breathing patterns but are cautioned about increased breathlessness at rest and during exercise. When teaching a patient, the nurse may explain that exhaling with pursed lips increases the resistance to both the outflow and the airway pressure. The small airways remain open longer to allow more air to be exhaled. Exhalation lasts two or three times longer than inhalation to effectively empty the lungs of trapped air.

To perform PLB, instruct the patient to inhale slowly through the nose (with mouth closed) and to pause slightly at the end of inspiration, then exhale slowly while relaxed through pursed lips. Folding the arms across the abdomen while sitting and bending forward while exhaling further aids complete emptying of the lungs. Counting during the technique helps pace exhalation at two or three times as long as inspiration.

Diaphragmatic Breathing. *Diaphragmatic breathing* exercises traditionally have been used in pulmonary rehabilitation to increase efficiency of the respiratory muscles while reducing the ineffective movements of the rib cage. The American Thoracic Society does not recommend routine use of diaphragmatic breathing as a training protocol for persons with COPD in pulmonary rehabilitation because of lack of supporting empirical evidence (ATS, 1999). However, diaphragmatic breathing been shown to strengthen a partially paralyzed diaphragm in persons with spinal cord injury. When a patient is partially paralyzed, placing your hand on the diaphragm helps focus attention on it even though the

patient may not be able to feel your hand (Frownfelter & Dean, 2006).

Glossopharyngeal Breathing. Patients who may benefit from GPB (previously described) include those who are dependent on mechanical ventilation due to respiratory muscle paralysis but who can tolerate short periods without ventilatory support and those patients who have intact mental status and bulbar musculature without any obstructive lung disease. GPB also can increase voice volume for patients not dependent on a ventilator.

Exercise. *Exercise training* is the foundation of pulmonary rehabilitation and may be integrated into a home- or facility-based program. Exercise has positive effects on dyspnea and minimizes the effects of deconditioning. Specific muscle groups can be strengthened with regular training for 20 to 30 minutes, 2 to 5 times per week. Either interval or continuous training at up to 60% of maximal workload may be possible. Patients with respiratory disease usually find interval training easier to tolerate and more enjoyable than continuous bouts of training. Interval training alternates periods of work with periods of rest and elicits training effects similar to continuous training regimens. Controversy exists regarding the optimal training intensity for COPD. Effective training strategies for all patients should include combined strength and endurance training (Make, 2004). The following section describes exercises performed at home or in rehabilitation with supervision.

Upper Extremity Exercise. Patients with severe COPD report a marked increase in the perception of dyspnea with routine tasks that require arm use, especially activities associated with unsupported arm elevation. Merely raising the arm increases the metabolic demand and ventilatory effort for patients with severe COPD, thus making unsupported arm exercise training a way of enhancing endurance. A simple and inexpensive unsupported arm training exercise for patients with COPD is performing lifts with a lightweight dowel rod from waist to shoulder level. Adding weights to the rod will increase resistance as tolerance increases. Providing arm support, such as bracing them on a table, may increase the patient's ability to perform common arm tasks. The current recommendation is to incorporate both supported and unsupported upper extremity training into comprehensive pulmonary rehabilitation programs (Make, 2004).

Lower Extremity Exercise. Numerous studies have documented that pulmonary rehabilitation incorporating aerobic exercise training of the lower extremities improves exercise tolerance (Make, 2004). Many methods have been used to accomplish conditioning of the lower extremities, including treadmill walking, bicycling, stair climbing, walking, and swimming. Declines in oxygen consumption, heart rate, respiratory rate, and minute ventilation and an increase in exercise duration have been observed with steady-state exercise following rehabilitation (Make, 2004). Some experts believe that individuals can improve their condition by walking in corridors and on stairs instead of on treadmills or riding on bicycles because walking has been found to be more enjoyable and more representative of day-to-day activity.

Respiratory Muscle Training. Inspiratory muscle training (IMT) can be used to improve strength and endurance of the respiratory muscles, primarily in patients with COPD. The training requires either an alinear resistive breathing device or a linear resistive breathing device. With either device the patient performs IMT by breathing in and out through the device, generating high airway pressures during inspiration and normal airway pressures during expiration. The patient must work hard during inspiration, whereas expiration is normal and relaxed.

Benefits of respiratory muscle training are not well established, and it is unclear whether results signify improvements in symptoms or disability. Ventilatory muscle training is considered an adjunctive form of therapy to improve exercise capacity and quality of life in selected patients when an adequate training load can be achieved (Make, 2004).

Outcome Assessment of Exercise Training. Pulmonary rehabilitation improves both objectively assessed functional capacity and patient-perceived functional status. A group of standard outcome assessment tools are available to evaluate the effectiveness of techniques and programs. An individual's progress can be measured by incremental and submaximal exercise tests and walking tests. General health status can be evaluated with questionnaires such as St. George's Respiratory Disease Questionnaire, Pulmonary Functional Status Scale (PFSS), the Functional Performance Inventory (FPI), and other functional instruments. Exertional dyspnea can be quantified with the use of a visual analog scale (VAS) rating and the category rating (Borg) during exercise testing. Overall dyspnea may be evaluated with the Medical Research Council Scale (MRC), the Baseline Dyspnea Index (BDI), and the Transitional Dyspnea Index (TDI) (ATS, 1999).

Energy Conservation Techniques. Energy management techniques can facilitate the performance of daily tasks. This includes energy conservation techniques, improving work efficiency, and using proper body mechanics to pace oneself through an activity. By coordinating breathing techniques with specific activities, a patient can take full mechanical advantage of muscle movement to assist breathing during self-care activities. Techniques that reduce dyspnea include the following:

1. Inhaling before bending, then exhaling slowly through pursed lips while bending, and then inhaling again while returning to the upright position
2. Moving the arms forward away from the side, or above the head, which elevates the chest and assists with inspiration
3. Putting the hands on the hips at frequent intervals or moving the arms away from the body on inspiration while performing ADLs, such as bathing or dressing

In addition, specific energy-saving strategies and adaptive equipment assist the patient in maximizing his or her energy use. Suggestions are to wear a terry cloth bathrobe after bathing to reduce the need to towel dry, sit on a stool while

showering, use arm rests and hand bars for support, place items at waist height in the home, sit at counter/table height during meal preparation, and consume foods that can be cooked in a microwave or prepared by other less time-consuming methods. Referral to Meals on Wheels may help the family, especially if the patient requires a special diet. For the child in school it may be helpful to incorporate use of a computer to take notes in the child's individual educational plan (IEP).

Altered Sleep Patterns. Respiratory abnormalities may cause alterations in sleep patterns, including sleep fragmentation, nocturnal oxygenation and heart rate disturbances, and resulting daytime sleepiness. Sleep-disordered breathing is present in 10% to 15% of patients with COPD alone, and those who snore may have obstructive sleep apnea. A formal polysomnography study is needed to appropriately diagnose and treat patients. Patients with COPD who snore have poor sleep quality with nocturnal hypoxemia and heart rate disorders similar to those observed in patients with COPD with severe obstructive sleep apnea. Positive airway pressure treatment including bilevel (BIPAP) or continuous positive airway pressure (CPAP) support by mask can provide relief for patients with these altered sleep patterns. These noninvasive therapies have been shown to be beneficial for patients with a wide range of both restrictive and obstructive pulmonary and neuromuscular disorders (Consensus Conference Report, 1999). For the child with asthma, nighttime cough and wakening often indicate the need for better asthma management.

Ventilatory Support Devices. Noninvasive ventilatory support devices are mechanical means to move the chest wall by manually pushing on the stomach, chest, or back. They do not require an artificial airway, but the chest wall must be capable of effective movement. Noninvasive support devices have proven useful in respiratory muscle paralysis associated with neurological disease or injury but are inappropriate for patients with COPD. The most commonly used ventilatory support devices are rocking beds and pneumobelts.

Rocking Beds. *Rocking beds* assist ventilation by using gravity and the pressure of the abdominal contents to alternately apply and remove pressure on the diaphragm. When the patient's body is tilted with the head up, the abdominal contents fall, and the diaphragm is pulled downward to assist with inhalation. Exhalation is assisted when the body is tilted head-down and the abdominal contents push against the diaphragm for expiration. Rocking beds are simple to operate and maintain and are noninvasive. Unfortunately, many patients cannot tolerate the rocking motion, nor does it control tidal volumes. The bed is best for patients who are bedridden or when used as a nighttime alternative to a ventilator.

Pneumobelts. *Pneumobelts* consist of an inflatable rubber bladder inside a corset worn around the abdomen and are most effective when a person sits upright, as in a wheelchair. As the bladder inflates, it pushes the abdominal contents up against the diaphragm, assisting with expiration. When the bladder deflates, abdominal contents and the diaphragm drop, assisting with inhalation. The pneumobelt connects to a positive pressure generator with 15 to 50 cm H_2O pressure. Some patients find the belt uncomfortable, and it does not control tidal volumes. Patients with a progressive condition may need more extensive assistance; mechanical ventilation is the next step.

Mechanical Ventilation. Although care of patients who receive mechanical ventilation is primarily an acute aspect of respiratory care, some individuals require long-term mechanical ventilatory support. They have chronic, underlying lung disease, such as emphysema, or a neurological impairment resulting from cervical spinal cord injuries. Two commonly used ventilation devices are negative-pressure ventilators (NPVs) and positive-pressure ventilators (PPVs).

Negative-Pressure Ventilators. NPVs that were used during the 1950s and 1960s to provide mechanical ventilation to victims of poliomyelitis have been less popular since PPVs were introduced. Cuirass respirators replaced the "iron lung" as an alternative to the PPVs. Individuals with neuromuscular diseases are candidates for this type of ventilator. The use of an NPV in patients with COPD is not recommended (ATS, 1995). NPVs apply negative pressure around the thorax, creating a pressure gradient inside the thoracic cavity and allowing air to flow into the lungs. Unfortunately, the patient is sealed off in the cumbersome device with markedly restricted mobility, but tracheal intubation is not required.

Positive-Pressure Ventilators. PPV applies positive pressure to the airways to promote inspiration, whereas expiration is passive. An artificial airway usually is necessary to connect the ventilator to the patient, although mouthpieces can be used if only intermittent ventilation is required. The two types of PPV devices are pressure-cycled ventilators and volume-cycled ventilators. *Pressure-cycled ventilators* inflate the lungs until a predetermined pressure is reached, at which point inspiration ends and expiration begins. The volume of air delivered to the patient can vary with each inspiration, depending on the compliance of the airways. For example, an individual experiencing bronchospasm quickly reaches the pressure set on the ventilator so that only a small volume of air is delivered into the lungs. In contrast, *volume-cycled ventilators* deliver a fixed predetermined tidal volume of air into the lungs. The pressure to deliver this volume of air varies depending on the compliance of the lungs and chest wall. A safety valve or pressure-limit device stops the ventilator from continuing the inspiratory cycle at a preset volume, therefore preventing trauma from air being forced into the lungs at too high of a pressure. Volume-cycled ventilators are preferred for hospital and home use because of the consistent volume of air delivered to the lungs. The advantages of PPVs over NPVs are better accessibility to the patient and increased mobility of the patient. Most patients with COPD chose assist-control ventilation, intermittent mandatory ventilation, or pressure-support ventilation (ATS, 1995). Some evidence suggests that adding pressure support ventilation increases comfort, promotes

patient synchrony with the ventilator, and may facilitate weaning for patients with stable COPD and acute respiratory failure who maintain adequate ventilatory drive (Kirton, 1997).

Mechanical Ventilation in the Home. As a rule, ventilators developed for home use are more compact than those used in hospitals. Some self-contained and self-powered ventilators are mounted on motorized wheelchairs. Ventilators used in the home can be powered by electricity, batteries, or gas, but backup systems must be available in case of a power outage. In choosing home ventilator equipment, consideration should be given to the home environment, long-term home health care commitment by the individual and family, financial considerations, and home support services. Every effort should be made to choose and modify ventilatory support devices according to patient and family needs and preferences.

Usually the home physical environment is rearranged to allow room for safe, effective, and efficient operation of the equipment with maximum freedom for the patient. Consider the amount of time a patient spends in an area of the house or outdoors. Evaluate electrical requirements, ability to maneuver the equipment, safety, temperature, and air control. Establish schedules and equipment checks with vendors of supplies and services, as well as with the local pharmacy. A self-inflating resuscitation bag should also be accessible in case the ventilator has a mechanical failure. An emergency call system and telephone numbers allows the patient to summon help when needed. Service agencies, such as emergency medical services, electrical and telephone companies, and fire or rescue departments, are notified when a patient dependent on mechanical ventilation is living in the community.

Home support services may include home health care nurses, home health care aides, and respiratory therapists. Respiratory equipment is maintained by the patient and family along with the company that supplies the ventilator. Individuals discharged from the hospital with volume-cycled ventilators must understand how to operate the equipment and possible mechanical problems. Although third-party payment is available for home ventilator care, the financial arrangements are changing rapidly and can be confusing and frustrating. Referral to a case manager or social worker to assist with arrangements, planning, and reimbursement helps with the complex needs because programs and regulations vary. This process should be initiated early in the rehabilitation process.

Rehabilitation of persons dependent on mechanical ventilation requires a team approach. Mechanical ventilation in the home provides certain individuals with an improved quality of life through familiar surroundings. It can be more cost-effective than institutional care (Frownfelter & Dean, 2006). However, patients with ventilators in the home and their families necessitate frequent evaluation of their physical and psychological management.

Patients requiring long-term mechanical ventilation experience a special nutritional problem. Abdominal distention can occur because of aspiration of air into the stomach, or food may be aspirated into the lungs when a patient is intubated. Cuffed tracheostomy tubes are kept inflated during meals and for 1 to 2 hours after meals to prevent aspiration. Adequate nutritional intake is important. Studies show that semistarvation in patients receiving ventilation therapy can lead to a diminished hypoxic drive, especially in patients with COPD, that can precipitate respiratory failure (Berry & Braunschweig, 1998).

Differences in upper airway mechanics during sleep and wakefulness may affect air leaks around uncuffed tracheostomies. Monitor the status of any patient showing signs of hypoxia and hypercapnia (increased restlessness, confusion, seizures) with oximetry. At night, some patients may require increased levels of ventilation for management.

Weaning. Weaning from mechanical ventilation may be the goal for many patients but not for those with progressive neuromuscular diseases. Although it is not practical to strive for this goal in all cases, periods of freedom from mechanical ventilation may be possible for many patients. Various weaning parameters provide objective criteria to predict patient readiness to sustain spontaneous ventilation with adequate oxygenation. Weaning parameters may include measurements such as inspiratory muscle strength (PImax), airway occlusion pressure, vital capacity, respiratory system compliance, and airway resistance. Although some of these measures are not available in rehabilitation, several integrative indexes have been examined for predictive ability.

One simple index is the Rapid Shallow Breathing Index, which measures the respiratory rate:tidal volume ratio (breaths/min/L) during a 1-minute T-piece trial. The threshold for weaning is 105 breaths/min/L. Patients who have more rapid and shallow breaths are less successful. Traditional weaning predictors have included a fraction of inspired oxygen of less than 50%, vital capacity of 10 ml/kg or more, and PImax (or negative inspiratory force [NIF]) of at least −20 cm H_2O (Burns et al., 1995). Generally the weaning process may be initiated when the patient is free of infection and other pulmonary or medical complications requiring continued respiratory support.

Several modes of ventilation have proven to be helpful during the weaning process. Pressure support, CPAP, and T-piece trials are the most common methods used for testing readiness to wean. Pressure support, a spontaneous mode of ventilation that delivers a high flow of gas early in inspiration until a predetermined pressure level is reached, decreases the work of breathing and decrease oxygen consumption. CPAP is also a continuous level of positive pressure in the airways used during spontaneous breathing that assists the alveoli in remaining open. The T-piece trial is used to provide humidification and oxygen but no ventilatory assistance or positive airway pressure for the patient. There is inconclusive evidence regarding the superiority of CPAP, T-piece, or synchronized intermittent mandatory ventilation (SIMV). The consensus is that all of these methods are equally effective in supporting the weaning process.

Most importantly, with all methods, the patient's status must be monitored closely for signs of respiratory distress throughout the weaning process. The use of accessory muscles, tachycardia, decrease or increase in blood pressure, tachypnea or bradypnea, and somnolence must be regarded as signs of intolerance to the weaning trial. Continuous oximetry to monitor venous oxygen saturation is helpful. The patient should be encouraged to use proper breathing techniques, relaxation strategies to decrease anxiety, and assistive coughing techniques. The weaning process predictably is a time of high anxiety for the patient. Psychological support, biofeedback with oximetry, and the use of relaxation techniques have been found to decrease anxiety. Weaning trials should never follow meals, exercise, or physical/occupational therapy sessions but introduced when the patient is most rested. The goal of the weaning process is complete withdrawal of ventilatory support. However, each patient must be evaluated on an individual basis. Some patients may tolerate breathing without the ventilator only during waking hours, whereas others may tolerate independent breathing indefinitely.

Diaphragmatic Electrophrenic Nerve Pacing. Diaphragmatic electrophrenic nerve pacing provides an alternative for some patients (ventilator dependent) with respiratory paralysis who have normal phrenic nerves, diaphragms, and lungs but require ventilatory assistance during the day. Most often, patients treated with diaphragmatic pacing have had high cervical quadriplegia or central alveolar hypoventilation. Diaphragmatic pacing is accomplished through high-frequency stimulation of the phrenic nerve by radio frequency transmissions from an electrode surgically attached to the phrenic nerve. A receiver implanted subcutaneously and attached to the electrode receives transmission through a battery-operated transmitter.

The major physiological limitation is diaphragmatic muscle fatigue. This can be minimized with gradual conditioning using low-frequency pacing over 3 to 6 months for adults and a longer period for children as prescribed. However, a four-pole stimulation system may shorten the conditioning time, increasing tolerance for diaphragmatic pacing. Initially a patient's regimen is 1 hour on and 1 hour off; gradually tolerance may reach 8 to 12 hours.

Family members must be fully informed about potential mishaps and educated to adhere to a regular medical schedule and follow-up visits for the patient. Pulse oximetry with an alarm and memory capacity is necessary for home monitoring. A readily available alternative method of ventilation must be available in the event of pacer failure due to external or internal components. The batteries in the transmitter are replaced each day. An emergency call system should be available to the patient in the home. Diaphragmatic pacing can offer long-term advantages to a carefully selected population.

Psychosocial Interventions. Patients with chronic lung disease frequently exhibit emotional and psychological concerns. Dyspnea is commonly associated with high levels of anxiety, especially in patients with COPD. Depression is common and may in part be caused by a reduced functional capacity and inability to pursue recreational interests and activities of daily living. These changes in lifestyle can impair patients' quality of life, diminish their role within their family and community, and lead to feelings of isolation and poor self-image.

Social workers, clinical psychologists, and psychiatrists provide psychosocial evaluation and support services within the pulmonary rehabilitation program. This can include group and individual counseling, stress management, relaxation, and support groups (Make, 2004). The peer group support a patient receives from others with chronic respiratory disease is invaluable. It allows patients to feel less isolated and alone in their feelings, and it provides other coping mechanisms for living with chronic lung disease.

A calm and reassuring approach by the rehabilitation team, providing adequate time for therapeutic interventions, and deferring to patient's preferences when feasible can also reduce anxiety. Using taped relaxation messages and muscle relaxation exercises are effective in reducing anxiety associated with dyspnea. Music therapy has been found to be effective in reducing anxiety and promoting relaxation in patients receiving ventilatory assistance (Chlan, 1998).

However, most people will not relax unless provided with a specific technique that they believe is effective. Progressive muscle relaxation is a technique commonly used for pulmonary patients. One portion of this technique alternately tenses and relaxes muscle groups. By doing so, the patient becomes more aware of the differences between tension and relaxation and better able to achieve a relaxed state. Controlled breathing techniques and yoga have also been used to reduce anxiety and dyspnea.

When anxiety or depression becomes an obstacle to achieving the benefits of a pulmonary rehabilitation program or management of an acute exacerbation, pharmacological interventions should be pursued. Buspirone is a mild anxiolytic without respiratory depression effects. The selective serotonin reuptake inhibitors are commonly prescribed to treat both depression and anxiety.

Outcome Criteria

For the patient with ineffective breathing pattern, the following outcome criteria are identified. The patient will demonstrate an effective breathing pattern as evidenced by incorporating breathing retraining techniques to relieve symptoms of dyspnea associated with activities of daily living; participation in an individualized upper and lower extremity exercise program; demonstrating energy conservation techniques at home, during recreation, or at work/school; appropriate use of prescribed ventilatory support devices if indicated; and acceptance of psychosocial support to decrease feelings of anxiety, depression, isolation, and poor self-image.

PATIENT AND FAMILY EDUCATION

Education is essential to any pulmonary rehabilitation program with its most effective role in positive behavior change of

self-management skills. Based on the health beliefs model, patients' and families' perceptions of the disease, complications, benefits of treatment, and barriers to therapy should be assessed (see Chapters 5 and 22). The educational efforts of the pulmonary rehabilitation team can then be used to modify the treatment plan to be more readily acceptable. An initial educational evaluation of the patient's learning level, learning style, native language, and reading level is recommended. Education may be formal or informal throughout the comprehensive pulmonary rehabilitation program and based on the needs of the individual patient (Make, 2004). Areas of teaching include anatomy and physiology; pathophysiology of lung disease; airway management; breathing training strategies; energy conservation and work simplification; medications; self-management skills; benefits of exercise and safety guidelines; oxygen therapy; environmental irritant avoidance; respiratory and chest therapy techniques; symptom management; psychological factors such as coping, panic, control, and stress management; end-of-life planning; smoking cessation; travel/leisure; sexuality; and nutrition (ATS, 1999).

The education should be pertinent to the family's needs and situation. Recommendations should be cost-effective and achievable. Thought should always be given to developing, delivering, and writing culturally sensitive educational materials. Patient learning should be assessed both formally and informally to determine when learning objectives are met.

Addressing Unmet Patient Needs

Smoking Cessation. Many patients with lung disease continue to smoke or be exposed to passive smoke that worsens their lung status. Smoking cessation is the single most effective approach to halt the progression of COPD (Pauwels et al., 2001). Therefore smoking cessation education should be provided both for family members who smoke and for the patient. A five-step intervention approach is outlined for health care providers in the U.S. Public Health Service document *Treating Tobacco Use and Dependence: A Clinical Practice Guideline* (Tobacco Use and Dependence Clinical Practice Guideline Panel, Staff, and Consortium Representatives, 2000). Practical counseling, formal group support treatment, and social support outside a formal smoking cessation program are the most effective nonpharmacological strategies. With any approach the nurse should include basic information about the hazards of smoking and the benefits of cessation. When the patient is willing, set a quit date within 1 to 2 weeks of the counseling session. Behavior modification strategies may include a smoking diary with notations of social cues, cravings, and triggers associated with each cigarette smoked.

Pharmacotherapy with nicotine replacement should be seriously considered because all forms increase long-term smoking abstinence rates (Pauwels et al., 2001). The ideal duration of nicotine replacement therapy has not been established, but most protocols range from 6 to 12 weeks. See Chapter 7 on pharmacology for further information. In addition, other medications have been utilized to minimize symptoms of nicotine withdrawal, including anxiolytics (buspirone or benzodiazepines), antidepressants (bupropion), and the alpha$_2$-agonist clonidine. Combining nicotine replacement therapy with behavioral counseling or other medications results in 6- to 12-month abstinence rates in the 30% to 40% range, compared with only 20% to 25% when using single therapy (Jorenby et al., 1999; Stitzer & Walsh, 1997).

Follow-up is essential in supporting patients and families during smoking cessation programs. Contact within the first 1 to 2 weeks is recommended because relapses occur within this time frame. Relapse within the first 2 weeks of smoking cessation suggests undertreatment of nicotine addiction, and replacement therapy should be adjusted. Additional follow-up 1 to 3 months after the quit date assists patients with coping with longer-term maintenance issues. If relapse occurs, the patient renews the commitment to cessation and sets a new quit date. Assure the patient that many persons achieve stable abstinence after five or six attempts.

Sexuality. Sexual functioning can be altered in patients with chronic respiratory disorders. Dyspnea may limit intercourse, alter relationships with significant others, and lead to a reduced sexual self-image. Education and counseling to address sexual issues are usually included in pulmonary rehabilitation programs.

Pharmacological interventions, such as bronchodilators used shortly before sexual activity, may permit more comfortable breathing and enjoyment. Patients taking medications that depress sexual drive can discuss alternatives with the physician or nurse practitioner. Supplemental oxygen should be used during sexual activity in the same way as prescribed for other exercise. Patients report less fatigue when sexual activities do not immediately follow a meal or airway clearance maneuvers. Energy-conserving positions for sexual activity are recommended for this population. If one partner can avoid placing weight on the chest of the patient or use a side-lying position, this can decrease some associated dyspnea. Ultimately, energy and breathing conservation must guide all activities (Haas & Haas, 2000).

End-of-Life Planning. No predictions for length of life are available, with or without lung disease. Two factors are important in the longevity of a patient with COPD: the age at diagnosis and the FEV$_1$ in relation to the age. Being relatively young at diagnosis and having a smaller FEV$_1$ usually mean that the disease progresses faster (Haas & Haas, 2000). Preparation and decision making for death and dying must be done for everyone, regardless of health status. Advance directives

outlining wishes with regard to mechanical ventilation are especially relevant for those with chronic lung disease. Home health care with respiratory equipment is possible and may be the first choice for many with hospice care as they approach the end of their life. Death without medical intervention may appeal to some, whereas others desire medical intervention to postpone death. The process of deciding a patient's wishes for managing the last phase of life are also discussed with the family, if the patient agrees, so that everyone is informed, clear, and comfortable in respecting the patient's decisions and wishes. Refer to Chapter 3 for additional discussions on ethics, problem resolution, and advance directives.

Community Resources

Support groups and community services can be very helpful in providing information, leisure activities, and networking for patients with chronic pulmonary disease. Rehabilitation facilities or lung associations typically offer patients a place to meet, help with planning programs and finding guest speakers, and a forum to discuss topics of interest or to exchange tips about managing lung disease. The support patients provide and receive from one another is a valuable outcome of pulmonary rehabilitation programs but one often overlooked. There are also support groups for family and friends of patients with lung disease.

In addition to support groups, identification of other community supports is recommended for families. This includes church members, relatives, neighbors, and other social service agencies. Another concern with chronic lung diseases is the ability of families to access health care. This means not only going to a clinic or emergency department but obtaining medications and devices necessary for disease management. One suggestion might be to have the family watch for local health fairs or hospital-sponsored programs providing medical information and supplies such as spacers or peak flowmeters to attendees. For families overwhelmed by caring for a member with chronic lung disease, respite care can provide a temporary and much-needed break from the caregiver role

SUMMARY

Comprehensive pulmonary rehabilitation programs can improve physiological measures of exercise capacity, functional capacity, and quality of life in patients with chronic respiratory disease. Through a multidisciplinary team approach, an individually tailored program can help an individual achieve his or her maximum level of independence and functioning.

Case Study

Mrs. Smith is a 74-year-old former smoker diagnosed with COPD. She smoked one to two packs of cigarettes per day for 40 years but quit 2 years ago. She recently completed an outpatient pulmonary rehabilitation program following her hospitalization and was given a home exercise regimen. Mrs. Smith lives with her daughter, Leslie, and three grandchildren in a single-family home. Mrs. Smith is depressed because she feels she is a burden to her daughter. She previously drove herself places, including the local senior center, but is now embarrassed to be seen wearing her oxygen.

Leslie has smoked for 15 years and would like to quit but feels there is too much stress in her life right now. She recently lost her job because of frequent absenteeism related to caring for her mother. Leslie says her mother is becoming forgetful, her medicines and oxygen equipment are too confusing, and she does not think it is safe for her mother to drive with oxygen. She is overwhelmed with getting her mother to exercise and with the change in her personality since her last hospitalization. Every night Leslie loses sleep worrying about what she should do.

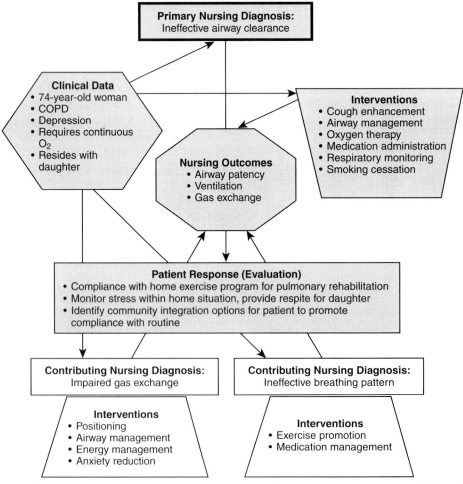

Concept Map. Mrs. Smith's primary problem is that of the ineffective airway clearance. Interventions are needed to address the contributing issues of impaired gas exchange and ineffective breathing pattern. The concept map illustrates the interrelationships between the nursing diagnoses of ineffective airway clearance, impaired gas exchange, and ineffective breathing pattern. The rehabilitation nurse will focus on coordinating interventions to achieve the outcomes of airway patency, anxiety management, and energy conservation.

CRITICAL THINKING

1. Prioritize the needs of both Mrs. Smith and Leslie based on your assessment and goals.
2. What should be considered when educating Leslie about COPD to enable her to better care for her mother?
3. What interventions are necessary to ensure Mrs. Smith's safety while increasing her self-esteem and independence?
4. What and how are the best ways to make referrals for this family?

REFERENCES

Ackley, B. J., & Ladwig, G. B. (2006). *Nursing diagnosis handbook: A guide to planning care.* (7th ed.). St. Louis, MO: Mosby.

Akinbami, L. M., & Morgenstern, H. (2006). Heterogeneity of childhood asthma among Hispanic children: Puerto Rican children bear a disproportionate burden. *Pediatrics, 117*(1), 43-53.

American Association for Respiratory Care. (2004). Nasotracheal suctioning—2004 revision and update. *Respiratory Care, 49*(9), 1080-1084.

American Thoracic Society. (1981). Pulmonary rehabilitation. *American Review of Respiratory Disease, 124,* 663-666.

American Thoracic Society. (1995). Standards for the diagnosis and care of patients with chronic obstructive pulmonary disease. *American Journal of Respiratory and Critical Care Medicine, 152,* S77-S120.

American Thoracic Society. (1999). Pulmonary rehabilitation—1999. *American Journal of Respiratory and Critical Care Medicine, 159,* 1666-1682.

American Thoracic Society. (2002). ATS statement: Guidelines for the six-minute walk test. *American Journal of Respiratory and Critical Care Medicine, 166,* 111-117.

Barnes, P. J. (2000). Chronic obstructive pulmonary disease. *New England Journal of Medicine, 343*(4), 269-278.

Berry, J. K., & Braunschweig, C. A. (1998). Nutritional assessment of the critically ill patient. *Critical Care Nursing Quarterly, 21,* 33-46.

Bickley, L. S. (2004). *Bates' pocket guide to physical examination and history taking* (4th ed.). Philadelphia: Lippincott Williams & Wilkins.

Borg, G. (1998). *Borg's perceived exertion and pain scales.* Champaign, IL: Human Kinetics.

Carlson-Catalano, J., Lunney, M., Paradiso, C., Bruno, J., Kraynyak Luise, B., Martin, T., et al. (1998). Clinical validation of ineffective breathing pattern, ineffective airway clearance, and impaired gas exchange. *Image—The Journal of Nursing Scholarship, 30,* 243-248.

Celli, B. R. (1998). Pulmonary rehabilitation for COPD: A practical approach for improving ventilatory conditioning. *Postgraduate Medicine, 102,* 159-160, 167-168, 173-176.

Centers for Disease Control and Prevention. (2005). Prevention and control of influenza: Recommendations of the Advisory Committee on Immunization Practices (ACIP), *MMWR, 54*(No. RR-8), 1-40.

Centers for Disease Control and Prevention. (1997). Prevention and control of pneumococcal disease: Recommendations of the Advisory Committee on Immunization Practices (ACIP). *MMWR, 46,* 1-24.

CHAD Therapeutics, Inc. (2006). Retrieved June 2006 from www.chadtherapeutics.com.

Chlan, L. (1998). Effectiveness of a music therapy intervention on relaxation and anxiety for patients receiving ventilatory assistance. *Heart and Lung, 27,* 169-176.

Chulay, M., & Burns, S. (2006). *AACN essentials of critical care nursing.* Chicago: McGraw-Hill.

Consensus Conference Report. (1999). Clinical indications for noninvasive positive pressure ventilation in chronic respiratory failure due to restrictive lung disease, COPD, and nocturnal hypoventilation—A consensus conference report. *Chest, 116,* 521-534.

Copstead, L. C., & Banasik, J. (Eds.). (2005). *Pathophysiology* (3rd ed.). Philadelphia: W. B. Saunders.

Dochterman, J. M., & Bulechek, G. M. (2004). *Nursing interventions classification (NIC)* (4th ed.). St. Louis, MO: Mosby

Frownfelter, D., & Dean, E. (Eds.). (2006). *Cardiovascular and pulmonary physical therapy: Evidence in practice* (4th ed.). St. Louis, MO: Mosby.

Global Initiative for Chronic Obstructive Pulmonary Disease (GOLD)—Updated 2005. (Based on April 1998 NHLBI/WHO Workshop, 1-128). Retrieved November 2005 from http://www.goldcopd.com.

Gronkiewicz, C., & Borkgren-Okonek, M. (2004). Acute exacerbation of COPD: Nursing application of evidence-based guidelines. *Critical Care Nursing Quarterly, 27*(4), 336-352.

Haas, F., & Haas, S. S. (2000). *The chronic bronchitis and emphysema handbook* (2nd ed.). New York: John Wiley & Sons.

Johnson, B. D., & Weisman, I. M. (2006). Clinical exercise testing. In J. Crapo, J. Glassroth, J. Karlinsky, & T. E. King (Eds.), *Baum's textbook of pulmonary diseases* (7th ed.). Philadelphia: Lippincott Williams & Wilkins.

Jones, A., & Rowe, B. H. (2000). Bronchopulmonary hygiene physical therapy in bronchiectasis and chronic obstructive pulmonary disease: A systematic review. *Heart and Lung, 29,* 125-135.

Jorenby, D., Leischow, S., Nides, M., Rennard, S., Johnston, J., Hughes, A., et al. (1999). Effect of sustained-release bupropion, a nicotine patch or their combination for smoking cessation. *New England Journal of Medicine, 340,* 685-691.

King, T. E. (2004). Approach to the patient with interstitial lung disease. In J. Crapo, J. Glassroth, J. Karlinsky, & T. E. King (Eds.), *Baum's textbook of pulmonary diseases* (7th ed.). Philadelphia: Lippincott Williams & Wilkins.

Kirton, O. C. (1997). Ventilatory support modes. In J. M. Civetta (Ed.), *Critical care* (3rd ed.). Philadelphia: Lippincott-Raven.

Lareau, S. C., Meek, P. M., Press, D., Anholm, J. D., & Roos, P. J. (1999). Dyspnea in patients with chronic obstructive pulmonary disease: Does dyspnea worsen longitudinally in the presence of declining lung function? *Heart and Lung: Journal of Acute and Critical Care, 28,* 65-73.

Make, B. (2004). Pulmonary rehabilitation. In J. Crapo, J. Glassroth, J. Karlinsky, & T. E. King (Eds.), *Baum's textbook of pulmonary diseases* (7th ed.). Philadelphia: Lippincott Williams & Wilkins.

Meyer, R. (2000). *Master guide for passing the respiratory care credentialing exams* (4th ed.). New Jersey: Prentice Hall Health.

Montes de Oca, M., & Celli, B. (2000). Respiratory muscle recruitment and exercise performance in eucapnic and hypercapnic severe chronic obstructive lung disease. *American Journal of Respiratory and Critical Care Medicine, 161,* 880-885.

NANDA International. (2005). *Nursing diagnoses: Definitions and classification, 2005-2006* (6th ed.). Philadelphia: Author.

National Asthma Education and Prevention Program. (2002, July). *Expert Panel report: Guidelines for the diagnosis and management of asthma—Update on selected topics 2002.* (NIH Publication No. 02-5075). Bethesda, MD: National Institutes of Health; National Heart, Lung and Blood Institute.

O'Regan, A. W., & Berman, J. S. (2004). Bronchiectasis. In J. Crapo, J. Glassroth, J. Karlinsky, & T. E. King (Eds.), *Baum's textbook of pulmonary diseases* (7th ed.). Philadelphia: Lippincott Williams & Wilkins.

Pauwels, R. A., Buist, A. S., Calverley, P. M. A., Jenkins, C. R., & Hurd, S. S. (2001). Global strategy for the diagnosis, management, and prevention of chronic obstructive pulmonary disease. *American Journal of Respiratory and Critical Care Medicine, 163,* 1256-1276.

Pouw, E. M., Ten Velde, G. P. M., Croonen, B. H. P. M., Kester, A. D. M., Schols, A. M. W. J., & Wouters, E. F. M. (2000). Early non-elective readmission for chronic obstructive pulmonary disease is associated with weight loss. *Clinics in Nutrition, 19,* 95-99.

Schols, A. M. W. J., & Wouters, E. F. M. (2000). Nutritional abnormalities and supplementation in chronic obstructive pulmonary disease. *Clinics in Chest Medicine, 21*(4), 753-762.

Seemungal, T. A. R., Donaldson, G. C., Bhowmik, A., Jeffries, D. J., & Wedzicha, J. A. (2000). Time course and recovery of exacerbations in patients with chronic obstructive pulmonary disease. *American Journal of Respiratory and Critical Care Medicine, 161,* 1608-1613.

Sherk, P. A., & Grossman, R. F. (2000). The chronic obstructive disease exacerbation. *Clinics in Chest Medicine, 21*(4), 705-721.

Stitzer, M., & Walsh, S. L. (1997). Psychostimulant abuse: The case for combined behavioral and pharmacological treatments. *Pharmacology and Biochemical Behavior, 57,* 457-470.

Timby, B. K., & Smith, N. E. (2003). *Introductory medical-surgical nursing* (8th ed.). Philadelphia: Lippincott Williams & Wilkins.

Tobacco Use and Dependence Clinical Practice Guideline Panel, Staff, and Consortium Representatives. (2000). A clinical practice guideline for treating tobacco use and dependence. *JAMA, 283,* 244-254.

Yankaskas, J. R. (2004). Cystic fibrosis. In J. Crapo, J. Glassroth, J. Karlinsky, & T. E. King (Eds.), *Baum's textbook of pulmonary diseases* (7th ed.). Philadelphia: Lippincott Williams & Wilkins.

18

Urinary Elimination and Continence

Kathleen A. Stevens, PhD, RN, CRRN

Care of persons with alterations in urinary elimination has long been a priority of rehabilitation nursing practice. The majority of patients who enter a rehabilitation setting are admitted with urinary incontinence or functional impairments that put them at risk for incontinence. In fact, the Functional Independence Measure (FIM) scale (see Figure 11-1) includes sphincter control as one of 18 functional items required to be scored on admission to rehabilitation. Although many persons enter rehabilitation incontinent, the majority have the potential to leave continent. The intervening variables are rehabilitation nursing interventions that address urinary sphincter control and functional deficits associated with urinary incontinence. (See Chapter 8.)

Since 1995 the prevalence of incontinence has been a quality indicator in long-term care settings (Zimmerman & Karon, 1995). The Minimum Data Set (MDS) is used to gather relevant clinical data and screen for urinary incontinence. When urinary incontinence is identified, a more complete assessment using the appropriate Resident Assessment Protocol (RAP) is required and a treatment plan implemented. Research has shown that when properly assessed and treated, urinary incontinence can be corrected in about 30% of nursing facility residents and suitably managed in the rest (Fantl et al., 1996).

National recognition of the scope of the problem of incontinence presents an opportunity for rehabilitation nurses to expand their practice by developing and participating in continence programs. To do this, rehabilitation nurses must bolster their knowledge base to include an understanding of urinary function, common etiologies of urinary incontinence, and appropriate interventions for different types of incontinence.

Alterations in urinary elimination can be associated with impairments in renal function, as well as lower urinary tract dysfunction. This chapter will focus on alterations in urinary elimination associated with lower urinary tract dysfunction. Chapter 36 addresses renal dysfunction.

SCOPE OF THE PROBLEM OF URINARY INCONTINENCE

Urinary incontinence is a symptom associated with lower urinary tract dysfunction. The groundbreaking work in the field of urinary continence was done by the Urinary Incontinence Guideline Panel, convened by the Agency for Health Care Policy and Research (AHCPR) in 1992. The AHCPR (now known as the Agency for Healthcare Research and Quality [AHRQ]) panel defined urinary incontinence as "the involuntary loss of urine which is sufficient to be a problem" (Urinary Incontinence Guideline Panel, 1992a and 1992b). In a revision of the guideline in 1996 the definition was amended to "urinary incontinence is the unintentional loss of urine" (Fantl et al., 1996). Subsequently the International Continence Society, in conjunction with the World Health Organization (WHO), defined urinary incontinence as a symptom or a subjective sign of urinary leakage. These newer definitions emphasize that urinary incontinence or the involuntary loss of urine, whether reported by the individual or observed by others, warrants further diagnostic evaluation by health care professionals.

More than 17 million Americans in community or institutional settings experience urinary incontinence or overactive bladder (Newman, 2002). The prevalence of urinary incontinence in persons younger than 30 years ranges from 14% to 40% in women and 4.6% to 15% in men (Newman, 2002). In the 30- to 60-year age-group the average prevalence rate for women is 29% and for men ranges from 2% to 12% (Hampel, Weinhold, Brekan, Eggersman, & Thuroff, 1997). For community-dwelling persons older than 65 years, the prevalence for elderly women ranges between 12% and 49% (Yarnell, Richards, & Stephenson, 1981) and between 7% and 22% for elderly men (Teasdale, Taffet, Luci, & Adam, 1988). Across the life span women are more likely to be incontinent than men.

Urinary incontinence results in a loss of self-esteem in children and adults and limits an individual's ability to achieve or maintain independence. In children with disabilities, incontinence may limit social interaction with other children of their own age and significantly delay or obstruct their social development and other developmental milestones. Fear of incontinence causes an individual to curtail excursions outside the home, including social interaction with friends and family. Urinary incontinence is generally recognized as one of the major causes of institutionalization of elderly persons (Fantl et al., 1996). Promoting urinary continence can significantly improve the quality of life of those with incontinence, their families, and caregivers.

To provide effective continence care, it is essential to overcome attitudinal barriers posed by individuals, staff, and society. At a symposium, "The State of the Science on Urinary Incontinence," leading experts called for a mass media campaign "to lift the veil of embarrassment about incontinence" (Wyman, 2003). According to symposium recommendations, the media campaign should also target correcting nurses' knowledge deficits related to continence care. Recent public education campaigns and television ads now encourage individuals to report and seek treatment for urinary incontinence.

Rehabilitation nurses work with patients across the life span. Because of this and the intimacy of interactions with patients, rehabilitation nurses are in a unique position to detect unreported bladder dysfunction and to initiate the assessment and intervention needed to offer treatment to persons with urinary incontinence.

ANATOMY AND PHYSIOLOGY

Normal Urinary Function

The urinary tract is composed of the kidneys, ureters, bladder, and urethra. The upper urinary tract, the kidneys and ureters, is responsible for urine production and drainage into the bladder. The kidneys filter waste products from the blood and continuously produce urine. The ureters are bilateral muscular tubes that drain urine from the kidneys to the bladder. The ureters enter the posterior surface of the bladder at an oblique angle, which limits backflow of urine into the upper tract. The lower urinary tract comprises the bladder, the internal and external urinary sphincters, and the urethra. The primary function of the lower tract is bladder filling, storage, and expulsion of the urine.

The lower urinary tract structures play a pivotal role in the micturition or voiding process. The largest structure in the lower urinary tract is the bladder, which serves as a reservoir for urine. It is a hollow muscular organ with two parts. The bladder's body is made up of the detrusor muscle, which consists of layers of intertwining smooth muscle. The other part, the trigone, is a small triangular area at the base of the bladder through which the ureters and urethra pass and is contiguous with the bladder neck. The bladder neck is 2 to 3 cm long and

is part of the posterior urethra. The muscles in this area form the internal sphincter. The urethra is a tube that carries urine from the bladder out of the body. The urethra is notably shorter in females than males; consequently the rate of incontinence is greater in females. The urethra continues through an extension of the deep perineal muscles. This striated muscle is called the rhabdosphincter, which in conjunction with the urogenital diaphragm makes up the external sphincter mechanism (Gray, 2000). Figure 18-1 is a diagram of the anatomy of the lower urinary tract. The external sphincter mechanism is a voluntary skeletal muscle in contrast to the smooth autonomic muscle of the detrusor and bladder neck. The external sphincter mechanism is under voluntary control, thus allowing a person to prevent urination even when involuntary mechanisms are attempting to empty the bladder (Guyton & Hall, 1996).

Other structures that contribute to continence are the pelvic floor muscles and, in males, the prostate gland. Recent advances in continence management have focused on the role of pelvic floor muscles in maintaining continence. The pelvic muscles include the levator ani, pubococcygeus, internal obturator, pyriform, and the superficial and deep perineal muscles that make up the urogenital diaphragm (Figure 18-2). Voluntary contraction of the pelvic muscles results in compressing, lengthening, and elevating the urethra. The pelvic floor musculature is composed primarily of voluntary, striated muscles; thus it can be strengthened with exercise. In men the prostate gland is important in maintaining continence. The urethra, which passes through the prostate gland, contains both smooth and striated muscle (Rathe & Klioze, 2000).

Innervation of the Lower Urinary Tract

The nerve supply of the lower urinary tract includes parasympathetic and sympathetic fibers, as well as somatic nerve fibers. The parasympathetic nerves provide motor stimulation

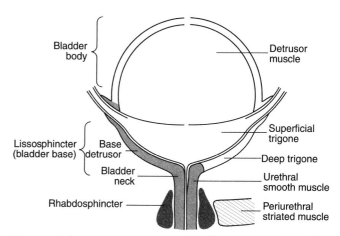

Figure 18-1 Lower urinary tract and bladder anatomy. The bladder can be divided into two regions: fixed base, sometimes called the lissosphincter, and flexible bladder body containing detrusor muscle. (From Doughty, D. B. [2006]. *Urinary and fecal incontinence: Current management concepts* [3rd ed.]. St. Louis, MO: Mosby.)

to the bladder, causing bladder contraction through the pelvic nerve. The pelvic nerve exits the spinal cord at the S2-S4 level. Stimulation of parasympathetic fibers causes the ureters to speed up transport of urine from the kidneys to the bladder, the detrusor muscle to contract, and the internal sphincter to open, resulting in bladder emptying.

The sympathetic nerves mediate the storage of urine in the bladder by stimulating contractions of the bladder neck and proximal urethra. The sympathetic fibers exit the thoracic lumbar cord at the T12-L2 level via the hypogastric nerve. Stimulation of sympathetic fibers causes the ureters to slow the transport of urine from the kidneys to the bladder, the detrusor to relax, and the internal sphincter to constrict, thus facilitating urine storage.

Somatic innervation consists of both efferent (motor) and afferent (sensory) fibers. The efferent fibers of the somatic nervous system originate in the anterior horn of the S2-S4 segments and travel through the pudendal nerve to the external striated sphincter and the muscles of the pelvic floor. Somatic nerves release the neurotransmitter acetylcholine. The external sphincter mechanism normally is contracted, supporting bladder storage by preventing leakage of urine. This mechanism, however, can be relaxed at will, allowing urination.

Afferent fibers originate in the bladder and proceed through the pelvic and hypogastric nerves to the posterior horn of the spinal cord. Sensory fibers of the pelvic nerve are stimulated during bladder filling by mechanoreceptors in the detrusor muscle. Messages travel from the bladder to the sacral micturition center and stimulate the voiding reflex, whereas other messages are transmitted to the brain through the spinothalamic tract. Parasympathetic stimulation promotes bladder emptying. Table 18-1 lists neurotransmitters that mediate micturition.

Normal micturition consists of three phases: filling/storage, contraction, and emptying (Figure 18-3). During the filling phase, bladder or intravesicular pressure rises while the urethral sphincters and the pelvic floor muscles maintain continence. When the bladder volume reaches the micturition threshold, usually 200 to 300 ml as noted on cystometry, the person feels the urge to void as the pressure increases. DeWachter and Wyndale (2003), reporting voiding records of 19 adult females, showed that 65% of the voiding episodes occurred before the micturition threshold recorded on cystometry.

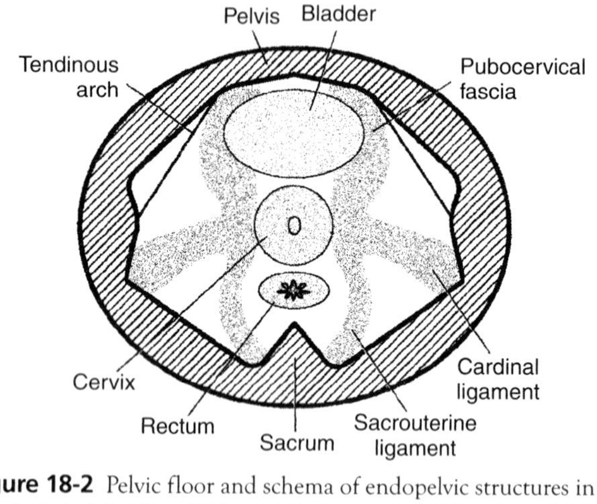

Figure 18-2 Pelvic floor and schema of endopelvic structures in the female. (Modified from Wahle, G. R., Young, G. P. H., & Raz, S. [1996]. Anatomy and physiology of pelvic support. In Raz, S. [Ed.], *Female urology* [2nd ed.]. Philadelphia: W. B. Saunders.)

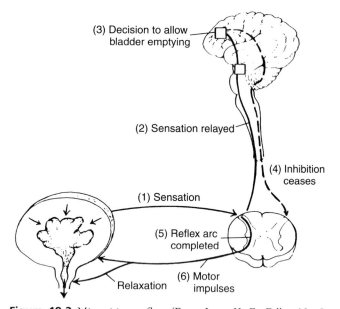

Figure 18-3 Micturition reflex. (From Jeter, K. F., Faller, N., & Norton, C. [1990]. *Nursing for continence.* Philadelphia: W. B. Saunders.)

TABLE 18-1 Neurotransmitters That Mediate Micturition

Neurotransmitter	Innervation	Neuroreceptor	Location of Neuroreceptor	Physiological Effect
Acetylcholine	Somatic	Cholinergic	External sphincter	Bladder storage
Acetylcholine	Parasympathetic	Cholinergic	Bladder base and body	Bladder contraction
Norepinephrine	Sympathetic	Adrenergic	Alpha: bladder base, neck, and proximal urethra	Bladder storage
			Beta: bladder body	Bladder storage

Data from Doughty, D. B. (2006). *Urinary and fecal incontinence: Current management concepts* (3rd ed.). St. Louis, MO: Mosby.

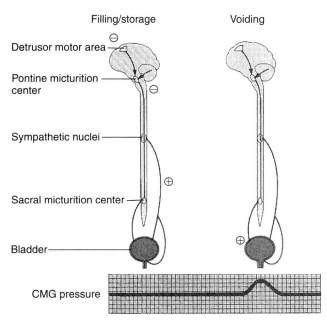

Filling/storage   Voiding

Detrusor motor area

Pontine micturition center

Sympathetic nuclei

Sacral micturition center

Bladder

CMG pressure

Figure 18-4 Schema of neurological control of detrusor during bladder filling and storage and during micturition. (From Gray, M. [1992]. *Genitourinary disorders.* St. Louis, MO: Mosby.)

Perception of bladder fullness and the urge to void found during cystometric bladder filling may not truly reflect normal filling. To remain continent, sympathetic stimulation increases, resulting in contraction of the internal sphincter through α-adrenergic reception, which increases urethral resistance and intraurethral pressure. At the same time the sympathetic stimulation suppresses detrusor activity through β-adrenergic reception. This inhibits bladder contractility (Rathe & Klioze, 2000). Voluntary contraction of the external sphincter mechanism increases by stimulating the pudendal nerve. This reaction is known as the guarding reflex; it further increases urethral resistance (Siroky & Krane, 1982).

Cystometrography studies have demonstrated that bladder distention increases sensory afferent stimulation, leading to voluntary coordinated micturition. The micturition reflex is mediated by a complex reflex arc (Figure 18-4). During the emptying phase, voluntary inhibition of somatic stimulation to the striated external sphincter decreases resistance at the urinary outlet. There is a decrease in sympathetic nerve activity, causing unopposed parasympathetic stimulation. This parasympathetic stimulation opens the bladder neck and facilitates bladder contraction. As the detrusor contracts, bladder pressure increases as the bladder neck relaxes, urethral resistance decreases, and normal voiding occurs (Gray, 2000).

In summary, during the filling phase the intraurethral pressure must exceed the intravesical (bladder) pressure, whereas in the emptying phase the intravesical pressure exceeds intraurethral pressure. Continence is maintained when the intraurethral pressure remains higher than the intravesical pressure (Guerrero & Sinert, 2001).

Cortical Control of Micturition

Continence is achieved when the micturition reflex is aligned with cortical control. During the micturition reflex, sensory messages pass from the bladder into and through the sacral cord to cortical centers in the brainstem and frontal lobe. Recent studies have identified that the regions of the cortex associated with recognition of bladder fullness are distinct from those associated with the perception of bladder filling (Athwal et al., 2001). The detrusor motor area is located bilaterally in the frontal lobe. The cerebral cortex is the key center for "social continence" (Doughty, 2000), which occurs when sensory messages are correctly interpreted and judgment is made to postpone bladder emptying until time and place are socially appropriate for voiding. The anterior and middle cerebral arteries are the primary source of blood flow to the detrusor motor area, so when a stroke occurs in these vessels, damage to the detrusor motor area often occurs. Many patients who have a recent stroke have a neurogenic bladder characterized by detrusor overactivity, frequency, urgency, and urinary leakage (Figure 18-5).

Other centers in the brain such as the thalamus and the basal ganglia play a role in control of micturition. Damage to the basal ganglia is assumed to be the source of the detrusor hyperreflexia in patients with Parkinson's disease.

Brainstem centers, especially the pons, coordinate the relaxation of the urethral sphincter with detrusor contraction. If a person does not want to urinate, the frontal micturition center sends inhibitory messages from the frontal cortex to the pons, down the reticulospinal tract to the sacral micturition center and inhibits the motor messages for detrusor contraction and sphincter relaxation. Continence involves active inhibition of the complex reflex arc (Figure 18-6). There is also direct cortical control of the external sphincter mechanism. Direct corticospinal connections travel from the frontal cortex to the S2-S4 segments, then through the pudendal nerve to provide voluntary contraction and relaxation of the external sphincter mechanism (Gray, 2000).

Age-Related Factors in Voiding

A newborn baby voids by virtue of the complex reflex arc. As the bladder fills, stretch receptors in the detrusor send sensory messages through the S2-S4 segments to the pontine micturition center. When the impulses are strong enough, the reflex arc is completed, motor impulses cause bladder contraction coordinated with urethral sphincter relaxation, and the bladder empties. This filling and emptying cycle is repeated throughout the 24-hour period. At this stage the baby's immature central nervous system cannot consciously appreciate or voluntarily control this cycle. The child is thus incontinent. Between the ages of 2 and 3 years, a child acquires continence from the combination of two processes: societal expectation and maturation of the central nervous system. By the age of 3 years, most children have the mental and neuromuscular capacity to inhibit the reflex arc to prevent voiding and initiate voluntary voiding appropriately during the day. However, it is common for children up to 5 years old to have both periodic

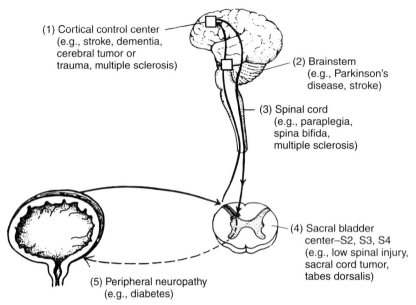

Figure 18-5 Micturition and common sites of neurological damage. (Modified from Jeter, K. F., Faller, N., & Norton, C. [1990]. *Nursing for continence*. Philadelphia: W. B. Saunders.)

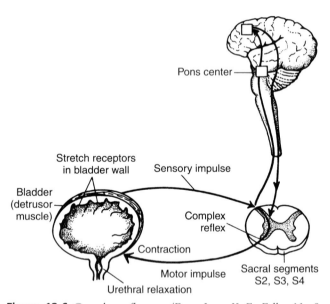

Figure 18-6 Complex reflex arc. (From Jeter, K. F., Faller, N., & Norton, C. [1990]. *Nursing for continence*. Philadelphia: W. B. Saunders.)

incontinence accidents during the day and nocturnal enuresis (Rathe & Klioze, 2000).

At puberty the pelvic genitalia become functional in both boys and girls. In boys the prostate gland grows large enough to assist with ejaculation. The growth of the prostate gland provides support for the pelvic floor and increases urethral resistance. In girls the structures of the pelvic floor mature. The tone of muscles of the pelvic floor and the urethra in women is maintained by stimulating estrogen receptors in

those structures. At puberty the release of estrogen increases muscle tone of the pelvic floor and increases urethral resistance.

Women may experience temporary or permanent distortion or trauma to the pelvic floor and urethral anatomy as a result of childbirth. With normal pregnancy and delivery, postpartum exercises, and return of normal estrogen levels, the tone of the pelvic floor and the integrity of the lower urinary tract usually are restored. Women involved in strenuous physical sports such as marathon running have also been noted to display symptoms associated with pelvic floor dysfunction.

In the adult male the prostate grows slowly until approximately age 45 years, when growth accelerates. With prostate enlargement, there is increased urethral resistance. Depending on the severity of urethral obstruction, the increased contractility needed to overcome the urethral resistance can cause the bladder to hypertrophy or decompensate, leading to urinary retention.

After menopause, women experience a decrease in estrogen levels, causing atrophy of the pelvic floor structures. The urethral mucosa becomes thin and friable, thus decreasing urethral resistance and predisposing to infection. For women who have sustained pelvic floor muscle injury secondary to childbirth or activity, these hormonal changes in the presence of pelvic floor dysfunction can precipitate herniation of the urinary tract through the supporting structures, thereby further decreasing urethral resistance. Postmenopausal women may experience incontinence when bladder pressure surpasses urethral resistance such as during coughing, sneezing, laughing, or exercising.

There are other, less clearly understood, effects of aging on bladder function, but urinary incontinence should not be accepted as a normal part of aging. Older persons experience an increase in the number of involuntary detrusor contractions, sometimes referred to as overactive bladder (OAB), contributing to the symptoms of urgency, frequency, and incontinence. Older persons experience a delayed onset of the desire to void, making it more difficult to further delay voiding. As a result, an increase in the residual urine volume raises potential for urinary tract infections. The decrease in urethral and bladder compliance coupled with lowered maximal urethral closure pressure puts the individual at high risk for incontinence (Resnick & Yalla, 1985). Elderly patients may experience functional changes in vision, mobility, and dexterity, making it difficult to locate and reach the toilet, as well as manage clothing in time to void without being incontinent (Guerrero & Sinert, 2001). All of these problems may be exaggerated by medications such as diuretics, which may increase urgency.

In summary, normal function of the urinary tract and continence are dependent on anatomical integrity of the bladder and urethra, an intact neurological system that provides voluntary control of micturition, the pattern of urine production, and the physical and mental ability and the psychological willingness of the person to perform tasks associated with toileting (Tanagho, 1990). Rehabilitation nurses help individuals affected by chronic illness or physical disability to adapt to their disabilities, achieve their greatest potential, and work toward productive, independent lives (Association of Rehabilitation Nurses [ARN], 2005). Urinary elimination management begins with a symptomatic approach to the assessment that can be used to determine treatment priorities and nursing interventions to improve the quality of life for these individuals (Table 18-2).

ASSESSMENT

History

It is important to remember that incontinence carries a social stigma. Not only are many persons embarrassed and reluctant to report incontinence, but often they define the problem of incontinence differently. Awareness and sensitivity to the emotional issues patients associate with incontinence are crucial. Furthermore, terminology used may need to be pragmatic (Dowling-Castronovo, 2001). Rather than asking, "Are you incontinent?" or "Do you have bladder control difficulties?" it may be more useful to ask, "Do you have trouble making it to the bathroom in time?" or "Have you lost urine (passed water) unexpectedly?" or "Do you wear pads to catch your urine?" (Wyman, 1988). For persons with neurological impairments, important questions include, "Do you know when you have urinated (passed water)?" and "Can you start or stop your urinary stream?"

The history focuses on the characteristics of the urinary elimination before hospitalization, as well as current voiding pattern (Box 18-1). Problems associated with maintaining sphincter control and continence can be a preexisting condition or a new condition secondary to the onset of disability.

Individuals with borderline or marginal voluntary control of the urethral sphincter before the onset of disability may now experience episodes of incontinence secondary to cognitive or mobility deficits associated with orthopedic or neurological injury. Individuals admitted with a recent neurological injury may now demonstrate urinary retention or incontinence secondary to neurogenic bladder dysfunction.

Neurological disorders with lesions in the cortical or subcortical areas, such as stroke, Parkinson's disease, or traumatic brain injury, may lead to uninhibited neurogenic bladder dysfunction, resulting in urge incontinence. Neurological disorders with lesions in the spinal cord, such as multiple sclerosis, spinal cord injury (SCI), or tumors, cause reflex neurogenic bladder dysfunction. Autonomous neurogenic bladder may be caused by pathological conditions in the lower part of the spinal canal, such as disk disease or neurological lesions of the peripheral nerves (cauda equina). (See Appendix 18-A.)

If incontinence is identified as a symptom, then more in-depth questioning is needed to determine the type of incontinence, acute or chronic. The characteristics of onset, duration, frequency, and precipitating circumstances of the urinary incontinence are related to the type of incontinence. For instance, urinary leakage that occurs with sneezing, coughing, lifting, bending, laughing, or exercising is suggestive of stress incontinence, whereas leakage that occurs with hand washing or difficulty reaching the bathroom on time is suggestive of urge incontinence. The amount of urine lost with each episode suggests the type of incontinence. A sudden brief spurt of urine may denote stress incontinence; however, a prolonged steady stream is associated with urge incontinence, and continual dribbling is associated with overflow incontinence (Wyman, 1988).

Timing of the incontinence is another variable to note in the history. Bladder voiding records are helpful supplements to the history for many patients. A voiding record, or bladder diary, is a tool to determine the frequency, timing, amount of voiding, and other factors associated with urinary incontinence (Figure 18-7). The person or the caregiver is instructed to document each occurrence in the voiding diary for several days before the incontinence evaluation. Generally a 3-day record of fluid intake, voiding time, and amount will be sufficient to identify the individual's voiding pattern (Registered Nurses Association of Ontario, 2005). These records may provide clues to deciphering the underlying cause of a patient's urinary incontinence, as well as setting a baseline to evaluate the efficacy of interventions (Guerrero & Sinert, 2001; Registered Nurses Association of Ontario, 2005; Wyman, Choi, Harkins, Wilson, & Fantl, 1988). Usual voiding patterns range from six to eight times during the day and do not exceed two voidings during the night (Abrams, Fenely, & Torrens, 1983).

Other factors to assess include the presence of concomitant fecal incontinence or other alterations in bowel habits, sensation of bladder fullness before or after voiding, ability to delay voiding once the urge is perceived, symptoms of hesitancy or straining to void, dysuria, or hematuria. It also is important to

TABLE 18-2 Nursing Interventions Classification (NIC) Interventions

NIC Intervention	Definition	Common Nursing Activities
Self-care assistance: toileting	Assisting another with elimination	Assist patient to toilet/commode/bedpan Evaluate need for assistive device (commode, clothing loops, bedpan, orthosis) Offer toileting assistance Provide fluids Provide privacy during toileting
Urinary elimination management	Maintenance of an optimum urinary elimination pattern	Assess voiding status using voiding diary Monitor for signs and symptoms of urinary retention Obtain PVR using bladder ultrasound Perform urinary assessment Provide and encourage fluids Assist with toileting as needed
Urinary catheterization	Insertion of a catheter into the bladder for temporary or permanent drainage	Monitor fluid intake Use and teach sterile technique for catheter insertion Secure catheter appropriately Maintain closed urinary drainage system Monitor for signs and symptoms of infection
Urinary catheterization: intermittent	Regular periodic use of a catheter to empty the bladder	Provide regular, consistent fluid intake Perform catheterization according to prescribed schedule and appropriate technique Monitor catheterization volumes Teach self-catheterization before discharge Teach signs and symptoms of urinary tract infection
Urinary bladder training	Improving bladder function for those with urge incontinence by increasing the bladder's ability to hold urine and the patient's ability to suppress urine	Obtain voiding record Assess patient's ability to recognize urge to void Establish toileting schedule and appropriate training method Toilet patient at prescribed intervals and record voiding pattern Discuss continence and daily progress toward continence with patient
Urinary habit training	Establishing a predictable pattern of bladder emptying to prevent incontinence for persons with limited cognitive ability who have urge, stress, or functional incontinence	Obtain 3-day voiding record Establish toileting schedule based on voiding patterns Toilet patient at prescribed intervals Encourage fluids
Urinary incontinence care	Assistance in promoting continence and maintaining perineal skin integrity	Discuss procedure and expected outcome with patient Select appropriate urinary collecting product/device Indicate skin check frequency Provide perineal skin care based on schedule Teach patient to apply/remove device
Urinary retention care	Assistance in relieving bladder distention	Monitor voiding pattern and obtain PVR Catheterize patient as prescribed Use stimulation techniques (running water, stroking thigh, etc.) as appropriate Encourage use of commode or use of urinal in standing position Monitor intake and output Use Coudé catheter when there is difficulty inserting catheter

Modified from Dochterman, J. M., & Bulechek, G. M. (2004). *Nursing interventions classification (NIC)* (4th ed.). St. Louis, MO: Mosby.
PVR, Postvoid residual.

BOX 18-1 Nursing History for Urinary Incontinence

Characteristics of Incontinence
- Onset and duration
- Frequency
- Timing (day, night, or both)
- Precipitating circumstances (cough, sneeze, laugh, exercise, positional changes, hand washing, other)
- Associated urgency
- Amount of leakage
- Type of loss (spurt or stream, or continuous dribbling)
- Use of pads/protective briefs (number of pads or clothing changes per day)

Toileting Patterns
- Diurnal frequency
- Nocturnal frequency

Associated Genitourinary Symptoms
- Awareness of bladder fullness
- Ability to delay voiding
- Sensation of incomplete bladder emptying
- Dribbling after urination
- Obstructive symptoms (hesitancy, slow or interrupted stream, straining)
- Symptoms of urinary tract infection (dysuria, hematuria)

Genitourinary History
- Childbirth
- Surgery (pelvic or lower urinary tract)
- Recurrent urinary tract infections
- Previous incontinence treatment and results (drugs, pelvic floor exercises, surgery, dilatations)

Relevant Medical History
- Acute illness
- Depression
- Diabetes mellitus
- Neurological disease (e.g., cerebrovascular accident, Parkinson's disease, dementia)
- Cardiovascular disease (e.g., hypertension, congestive heart disease)
- Renal disease
- Bowel disorders (constipation, impaction, fecal incontinence)
- Psychological disorders (depression, mental illness)
- Cancer

Medications (Including Nonprescription Drugs)

Patient's/Caregiver's Perceptions of Incontinence
- Perception of cause and severity
- Interference with daily activities
- Expectations for cure

Environmental Factors
- Accessible bathrooms
- Distance to bathrooms
- Use of toileting aids

From Wyman, J. F. (1988). Nursing assessment of the incontinent geriatric outpatient population. *Nursing Clinics of North America, 23*, 178-179.

identify how the person manages the incontinence—for instance, with padding, frequent clothing changes, protective garments, or preventive toileting. Have there been treatments for incontinence? If so, how successful were they? Has the person had any genitourinary surgery? Review current and past medical problems and any medications used, both prescribed and over-the-counter.

Many chronic conditions can predispose the individuals to problems with lower urinary tract dysfunction. In persons with diabetes, incontinence may be a result of polyuria or from a sensory paralytic bladder causing overflow incontinence as when a bladder becomes overly distended owing to a lack of sensation signaling the need to void. Persons using diuretics may experience incontinence due to a combination of increased urine output and their inability to get to the toilet on time.

Perceptions of both patient and caregiver or significant others about incontinence are important assessments in the patient's history. How does incontinence affect each of their daily lives? How has the onset of incontinence impacted their lifestyle and daily activities? What do they expect from the incontinence treatment/management regimen? Are there environmental factors that affect the incontinence, such as accessibility of the commode or bathroom, lighting, availability of someone to assist with toileting, or managing clothing? Assessing social factors is important for persons with functional impairments. Social factors include living arrangements, social contacts, and caregiver availability (Williams & Gaylord, 1990). The Incontinence Impact Questionnaire (IIQ) and the Urogenital Distress Inventory have been used to objectively quantify the degree of impact of urinary incontinence on quality of life (Doughty, 2000). Refer to Chapter 14 regarding activites of daily living.

Physical Examination

The physical examination includes functional physical and cognitive assessments; examination of the abdomen, the genital/pelvic, and rectal areas; and neurological and general examinations (Box 18-2). The functional assessment evaluates a person's mobility and manual dexterity to determine the ability to reach the toilet and to disrobe in time to be continent (Williams & Gaylord, 1990). A functional assessment of the person's cognitive status provides information about the ability to perceive the need to void, to understand how to reach and use the toilet or toilet substitute, and to participate in the treatment regimen. The Folstein Mini Mental State Examination (MMSE) is one tool used in standardizing this portion of the physical examination (Folstein, Folstein, & McHugh, 2007).

The abdominal examination includes inspection of the skin for scars, which may indicate previous surgeries the patient has neglected to report. The abdomen is palpated to identify a distended bladder or suprapubic masses and the presence of any tenderness.

Male genitalia are examined to detect abnormalities of the foreskin, penis, and perineal skin; noting the condition of the skin and any swelling, lesions, nodules, or discharge.

NAME: _____

DATE: _____

INSTRUCTIONS: Place a check in the appropriate column next to the time you urinated in the toilet or when an incontinence episode occurred. Note the reason for the incontinence and describe your liquid intake (for example, coffee, water) and estimate the amount (for example, one cup).

Time interval	Urinated in toilet	Had a small incontinence episode	Had a large incontinence episode	Reason for incontinence episode	Type/amount of liquid intake
6-8 AM					
8-10 AM					
10-noon					
Noon-2 PM					
2-4 PM					
4-6 PM					
6-8 PM					
8-10 PM					
10-midnight					
Overnight					

No. of pads used today: _____   No. of episodes: _____

Comments: _____

_____

_____

Figure 18-7 Voiding record sample. (From Fantl, J. A., Newman, D. K., Colling, J., DeLancey, J., Keeys, C., Loughery, R., et al. [1996, March]. *Urinary incontinence in adults: Acute and chronic management* [AHCPR Publication No. 96-0682, Clinical Practice Guideline No. 2, 1996 Update]. Rockville, MD: U.S. Department of Health and Human Services, Public Health Service, Agency for Health Care Policy and Research.)

For women, external genitalia are inspected noting the condition of the skin and signs of atrophic vaginitis or monilial infection. A simple pelvic examination performed by inserting one or two lubricated gloved fingers into the vagina can detect the presence of masses, pelvic prolapse, tenderness, or discharge. During the vaginal examination ask the woman to squeeze around the examiner's fingers to assess her ability to contract the muscles of the pelvic floor and paravaginal muscle tone.

During the physical examination it is important to ascertain current voiding ability. Patients with neurogenic bladder dysfunction who exhibit areflexia associated with spinal shock will not demonstrate reflex control over micturition; therefore a plan for urinary retention management is the priority for these patients. Stroke can result in urge incontinence associated with neurogenic bladder; however, only in rare instances does stroke result in urinary retention because reflex emptying is still possible (Arena et al., 1992). Kong and Young (2000) found urinary retention post stroke was associated with individuals with severe cognitive impairment, history of diabetes mellitus, aphasia, lower functional admission scores, and urinary tract infection. If an individual is able to demonstrate reflex voiding, the initial nursing priority is evaluating effectiveness of bladder emptying and initiating a toileting assistance program to promote continence.

If the individual is able to void and incontinence has been identified as a symptom, objective testing or provocative stress testing is recommended to assess incontinence type. During provocative stress testing the person is asked to relax and cough vigorously while the examiner observes the urethra for loss of urine. If leakage occurs instantaneously, then stress urinary incontinence is suspected. If leakage is delayed or persists after the cough, then urge incontinence or detrusor overactivity is suspected. Direct observation of a patient's voiding may detect signs of hesitancy or strain or a slow or interrupted urinary stream. Presence of these symptoms may indicate urinary obstruction or problems with bladder emptying.

BOX 18-2 Physical Examination for Urinary Incontinence

Cognitive and Affective Status
- Mental status
- Mood
- Motivation

Mobility Status
- Manual dexterity (ability to disrobe for toileting)
- Gait and balance (walking speed, use of assistive devices)

Neurological Examination
- Focal signs
- Signs of Parkinson's disease

Abdominal Examination
- Scars
- Distended bladder
- Suprapubic tenderness
- Mass

Genital Examination
- Skin condition
- Signs of infection
- Bulbocavernous reflex
- Women—atrophic vaginitis, pelvic relaxation, or other abnormality

Rectal Examination
- Sphincter tone
- Fecal impaction
- Masses
- Men—prostatic size

Stress Test (With Full Bladder)
- Supine and standing

Other
- Signs of congestive heart failure

From Wyman, J. F. (1988). Nursing assessment of the incontinent geriatric outpatient population. *Nursing Clinics of North America, 23,* 178-179.

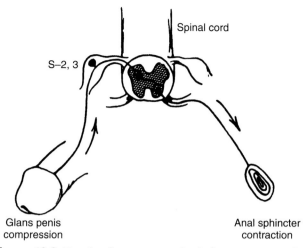

Figure 18-8 Test for the presence of a bulbocavernosus reflex. (Reprinted with permission from Rancho Los Amigos Medical Center, Downey, CA.)

When neurogenic bladder dysfunction is suspected, a rectal examination is conducted to test for perineal sensation, sphincter tone with both resting and with active contraction, rectal masses, or fecal impaction. In men the size, consistency, and contour of the prostate is assessed. A bulbocavernosus reflex is attempted during rectal examination for both men and women to determine the status of the sacral reflex arc. This reflex is elicited by squeezing the glans penis or glans clitoris while the examiner's gloved finger is inserted just inside the anus. The examiner notes whether there is anal contraction around the finger and how brisk the contractual response is to the stimulus (Figure 18-8). A further neurological and general examination may detect conditions such as edema, which may contribute to nocturia, and neurological conditions that may contribute to incontinence.

Diagnostic Testing

Estimation of Postvoid Residual. A postvoid residual (PVR) is a comparison between amount voided and a residual volume in the bladder as measured by straight catheterization or noninvasive bladder scanning. See Box 18-3 for the procedure for obtaining a PVR using BladderScan. Estimation of PVR volume using a noninvasive bladder scanner has become a relatively standard practice in many clinical settings to evaluate urinary retention and bladder emptying (Fantl et al., 1996; Registered Nurses Association of Ontario, 2005; Stevens, 2005). Although PVR has been recommended to evaluate effectiveness of bladder emptying, no clear research is documented in the literature on allowable PVR volumes. The general consensus of the AHCPR Urinary Incontinence Guideline Panel is that a PVR volume less than 50 ml is considered adequate bladder emptying (Fantl et al., 1996). Multiple residuals between 100 and 200 ml generally are an indicator of incomplete emptying, warranting some type of intervention (Fantl et al., 1996).

Urinalysis. Urinalysis is a basic test required to detect conditions that may contribute to urinary incontinence. For instance, hematuria may be a symptom of infection, cancer, or urinary stones; glycosuria and proteinuria indicate further medical workup for diabetes; and pyuria with bacteriuria suggests infection and a specimen for culture. There is no consensus about the relationship of asymptomatic bacteriuria and urinary tract infection in nursing home populations and in those with neurogenic bladder dysfunction. Until clear data are available, urinary infection is treated first, before further diagnostic tests and treatment are initiated or completed (Hooton, 1999; Ouslander, 1989).

BOX 18-3 **Procedure for Obtaining a Postvoid Residual**

Purpose
1. Evaluate voiding adequacy
2. Assess residual volume post voiding

Equipment
1. Urine collecting device with measure (urinal or commode hat)
2. Bladder Scan
   Or
2. Sterile catheter kit (sterile gloves, catheter, povidone-iodine, water soluble lubricant, collecting container)

Procedure
1. Have the individual void into measuring device.
2. Encourage individual to take deep breath and contract pelvic muscles to empty bladder.
3. Record amount voided.
4. Assist individual to bed.
   Within 10 minutes of the void perform bladder scan with Bladder Scan according to manufacturer's instructions
   Or
   perform sterile catheterization to determine residual volume.
5. Record scan volume or catheterized volume as postvoid residual (PVR) volume.
NOTE: Total volume = Voided volume + Postvoid residual volume.

Supplementary Tests. Additional blood or imaging testing may be done in high-risk populations. Blood tests, including determination of blood urea nitrogen (BUN), creatinine, glucose, and calcium, are often performed to evaluate renal function or polyuria. Creatinine levels are performed when outlet obstruction or retention is suspected (Fantl et al., 1996). These tests are often part of the routine follow-up in persons with neurogenic bladder dysfunction. Urine cytologic examination is no longer recommended in the routine evaluation of the incontinent patient (Fantl et al., 1996).

Advanced Testing—Urodynamics. After initial treatment, patients who continue to be incontinent or those who are not appropriate for treatment based on presumptive diagnosis should undergo further evaluation to identify the cause of urinary incontinence. Testing that reproduces leakage can help the provider make a differential diagnosis between causes that have similar symptoms but require different interventions. Specialized diagnostic tests include urodynamic tests, endoscopic tests, and imaging tests of both upper and lower urinary tract with and without voiding.

Urodynamic tests are used to evaluate the anatomical and functional status of the bladder. Uroflowmetry is a visual or electronic measure of the rate of urine flow. When an electronic unit is used, it generates an electric flow curve that displays voiding patterns. Uroflowmetry is used when diagnosing bladder emptying problems but is not useful in

distinguishing between bladder outlet obstruction and detrusor weakness (Urinary Incontinence Guideline Panel, 1992b) or in diagnosing the types of incontinence specific to women (Diokno, Normelle, Brown, & Herzog, 1990).

CMG tests detrusor function. Cystometry can be used to assess bladder sensation, capacity, and compliance and to determine the presence and magnitude of both voluntary and involuntary contractions. Simple cystometry is a test that may become a bladder training procedure as well. It is performed by using a urethral catheter to fill the bladder by gravity until either an involuntary contraction occurs or until bladder capacity is reached. This test can be conducted at the bedside to answer questions about how the bladder fills. Results from simple cystometry also can provide answers to questions about how efficiently the bladder stores urine, whether there is sphincter incompetence or detrusor instability, whether the person accurately perceives the urge to void, and whether the person inhibits the urge to urinate. How adequately the bladder is emptied can be assessed by removing the urinary catheter at the "must" urge, then allowing the person to void, then measuring the PVR volume by catheterization.

A filling CMG measures abdominal and rectal pressure simultaneously, to differentiate involuntary detrusor contraction from an increase in intraabdominal pressure that occurs when a patient strains to void (Pires & Lockart-Pretti, 1992). A voiding CMG or pressure flow study can measure detrusor contractility and detect outlet obstruction when a person is able to void. Another use of the filling CMG is to determine the leak point pressure. That is, the intravesical pressure is measured at the moment fluid leakage begins during urinary straining or involuntary detrusor contraction. This information is useful to determine whether the person has either low or high voiding pressures. Voiding under high pressure may affect the upper urinary tract, especially with reflex neurogenic bladder dysfunction.

Urethral pressure profilometry measures resting and dynamic pressures in the urethra. Passive measurements may be used to help identify intrinsic sphincter deficiency. The relative usefulness of the urethral pressure profilometry versus that of abdominal leak point pressure has not been adequately studied (Fantl et al., 1996).

Electromyography (EMG) is performed on the striated urethral sphincter using needle, wire, or surface electrodes to determine the integrity of and function of its innervation. When CMG and EMG are used together, the results are helpful in diagnosing detrusor-sphincter dyssynergia (DSD), which often is seen in reflex neurogenic bladder dysfunction (Blaivas, 1990) (Table 18-3).

The most useful endoscopic test in evaluating urinary incontinence is cystourethroscopy. This procedure may be helpful in identifying bladder lesions and urethral diverticula, fistulas, strictures, or intrinsic sphincter deficiency. Cystoscopy is not recommended in the basic evaluation of urinary incontinence. However, cystoscopy may be indicated in the further evaluation when the following situations are present: sterile hematuria, pyuria, when urodynamics fail to duplicate symptoms,

TABLE 18-3 Diagnostic Test Options for Urinary Incontinence*

Mechanism	Associated Factors	Diagnostic Test Options
Urge Incontinence		
Unstable bladder or detrusor instability (DI)	No neurological deficit	Simple or multichannel CMG with or without EMG
Detrusor hyperreflexia, detrusor sphincter dyssynergia	With neurological lesion such as stroke, supraspinal cord lesions, multiple sclerosis	Simple cystometry or multichannel
Detrusor hyperactivity with impaired contractility	Elderly, usually also associated with obstructive or stress symptoms	Multichannel CMG with or without EMG Videourodynamics
Stress Incontinence		
Hypermobility of bladder neck (female)	Detachment of bladder neck with concomitant hypermobility of the urethra	Provocative stress test (direct visualization) Tests for bladder neck hypermobility Simple or multichannel CMG (to exclude DI) UPP or leak point pressure Videourodynamics
Intrinsic sphincter deficiency	Postoperative (after prostatectomy or antiincontinence surgery), trauma, aging, radiation, congenital (epispadias)	Same as above
Neurogenic sphincter deficiency	Neurogenic, sacral, or infrasacral lesion (e.g., myelomeningocele)	Same as above EMG
Overflow Incontinence		
Overflow from underactive or acontractile detrusor	Neurogenic (low spinal cord lesion, neuropathy, postradical pelvic surgery), idiopathic detrusor failure	Elevated PVR volume Uroflowmetry Voiding CMG (pressure flow) with EMG Cystourethroscopy
Overflow from outlet obstruction	Male: prostate gland disease, urethral stricture Female: postoperative	Same as above Videourodynamics

From Fantl, J. A., Newman, D. K., Colling, J., DeLancey, J., Keeys, C., Loughery, R., et al. (1996, March). *Urinary incontinence in adults: Acute and chronic management* (AHCPR Publication No. 96-0682, Clinical Practice Guideline No. 2, 1996 Update). Rockville, MD: U.S. Department of Health and Human Services, Public Health Service, Agency for Health Care Policy and Research.
CMG, Cystometrogram; EMG, electromyogram; PVR, postvoid residual; UPP, urethral pressure profilometry.
*The urodynamic tests listed here are not recommended for routine use but are options for patients who require further evaluation.

new onset of irritative voiding symptoms, bladder pain, recurrent cystitis, or suspected foreign body (Fantl et al., 1996).

Imaging Studies

Imaging tests that are sometimes used with persons who have urinary incontinence include upper urinary tract imaging by intravenous pyelogram or, more commonly, ultrasonography of the kidneys. Although these procedures are not routine evaluations of urinary incontinence, they are an important part of routine follow-up in patients with neurogenic bladder dysfunction or those with outlet obstruction who have high bladder pressures. Upper urinary tract imaging can help identify dilation of the ureters and kidney pelvis. Lower urinary tract imaging with and without voiding is helpful for examining the anatomy of the bladder and the urethra. Nonvoiding cystourethrography can identify mobility or fixation of the bladder neck, funneling of the bladder neck and proximal urethra, and degree of cystocele. The voiding component of

the cystourethrogram can identify urethral diverticulum, obstruction, and vesicoureteral reflux (Fantl et al., 1996). Imaging studies or renal ultrasound testing is much more common in outpatient clinics that see patients with neurogenic bladder dysfunction.

NEUROGENIC BLADDER DYSFUNCTION

Urinary retention is a common sequela in patients who have a neurological impairment and associated disability. The priority in care planning and urinary management is to prevent urinary retention.

A Special Concern: Spinal Shock

Immediately after spinal injury the person experiences a temporary condition of flaccid paralysis that is characterized by a loss of all reflex activity below the level of the lesion. This is

TABLE 18-4 Neurogenic Bladder Dysfunction Types and Etiologies

Type	Location of Neural Injury	Possible Etiology	Signs and Symptoms
Uninhibited neurogenic	Cortex, brainstem, pons, and subcortical areas	Newborn infant, stroke, brain injury, brain tumor, multiple sclerosis, encephalopathy, dementia, Alzheimer's disease	Lack of awareness, frequency, urgency, nocturia, decreased bladder capacity with low residual volumes
Reflex neurogenic	Spinal cord above T12-L1 or level of sacral reflex arc	Spinal cord injury (SCI) above T12-S1, multiple sclerosis, spinal cord tumor	Some to no awareness of voiding, unpredictable voiding, voiding occurs in response to reflex—stroking, tapping, pulling at pubic hairs, adequacy of voiding dependent upon degree of detrusor/sphincter dyssynergy, frequently high postvoid residuals
Autonomous (areflexic) bladder	Sacral reflex arc	All SCI during period of spinal shock, SCI damage to sacral arc, polio, vascular occlusion to spinal cord, spina bifida, myelomeningocele, postoperative radical pelvic surgery or radiation, herniated lumbar disk	Absent voiding reflex although may have sensation of fullness, dribbling with abdominal pressure, high residual volumes
Motor paralytic	Anterior horn cells or S2-4 ventral roots	Poliomyelitis, herniated disk, pelvic trauma	Normal sensation with difficulty passing urine, dribbling with abdominal pressure, incomplete emptying with high residual volumes
Sensory paralytic	Damage to dorsal horn at level of sacral arc or damage to dorsal roots S2-4	Childbirth neuropathy secondary to diabetes mellitus, tabes dorsalis, pelvic survey or trauma, peripheral vascular disease	Able to void completely but lacks awareness of need to void, infrequent voiding secondary to lack of sensory awareness, large-volume voids with low residual volume

referred to as spinal shock. The signs of spinal shock related to the urinary tract mirror the signs of autonomous neurogenic bladder—that is, reflexes are absent, perception of fullness is absent, and the bladder becomes overdistended. As spinal shock resolves, it is critical to recognize the signs of resolution in order to correctly determine the type of neurogenic bladder that results, either reflex or autonomous. During this time the nursing management priority is urinary retention management (Nursing Interventions Classification [NIC]). See the expanded Case Study in Chapter 14.

Neurogenic bladder dysfunction is the most common form of bladder impairment seen in rehabilitation settings. Neurogenic lower tract urinary dysfunction is "due to a disturbance of neurological control mechanisms" (Stoher et al., 1999). Neurogenic bladders are classified into five types and are labeled according to the underlying pathological process: (1) uninhibited, (2) reflex or spastic, (3) autonomous or flaccid, (4) sensory paralytic, and (5) motor paralytic neurogenic bladders. Most neurogenic bladders represent a combined motor and sensory impairment. For ease of description, the types of neurogenic bladder are described in Table 18-4 according to the schema proposed by Lapides and Diokno (1976).

Uninhibited Neurogenic Bladder

The uninhibited neurogenic bladder results from a disruption of the corticoregulatory tract or a malfunction of the supraspinal center that regulates voiding. Figure 18-9 illustrates areas of the nervous system where damage may occur.

Frequent uninhibited contractions occur, but the bladder usually empties completely, resulting in no residual urine. The micturition reflex remains intact. Sensation is present as is the bulbocavernosus reflex. A CMG will demonstrate strong, uninhibited contractions as the bladder is filled. The capacity of the bladder is decreased, and involuntary voiding will take place almost as soon as the urge is perceived.

Persons with uninhibited neurogenic bladder frequently complain about the urgency and frequency of urination and nocturia. After the urge is perceived, they cannot inhibit flow. When the external sphincter is voluntarily contracted, partial control of urination, even with strong voiding contractions, is possible. The intravesical pressure, however, remains high because of the force of detrusor contractions. Anticholinergic medication may be recommended to decrease bladder contractility and increase bladder capacity. See Chapter 7 for details on drug actions. These patients may be able to avoid incontinence by voiding before the bladder is full enough to trigger the

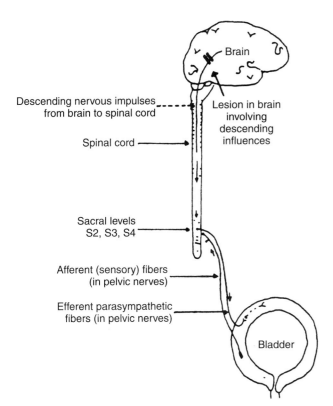

Figure 18-9 Uninhibited neurogenic bladder sites. (From Pires, M., & Lockhart-Pretti, P. A. [1992]. *Nursing management of neurogenic incontinence: An independent study module.* Skokie, IL: Rehabilitation Nursing Foundation.)

micturition reflex. Therefore an important part of nursing intervention is scheduled voiding, habit training, and attention to fluid intake, to anticipate the need to void before the urge becomes too strong. For those patients who can follow three-step commands and volitionally start and stop their urinary stream, bladder training is a nursing intervention that may lead to continence.

Reflex Neurogenic Bladder

The reflex neurogenic bladder is referred to as an upper motor neuron, suprasacral, spastic, or central neurogenic bladder. This type of bladder dysfunction occurs when both the sensory and motor tracts of the spinal cord, which send messages between the bladder and the supraspinal center, are disrupted. Bladder overdistention can also predispose the individual to autonomic dysreflexia, a life-threatening complication (see Appendix 18A).

The reflex arc remains intact, and voiding is involuntary because of the lack of cerebral control and may be incomplete because of uncoordinated bladder contractions. The bulbocavernosus reflex is present and hyperactive. A CMG shows uninhibited contractions with decreased bladder capacity. The detrusor muscle frequently hypertrophies, which can lead to vesicoureteral reflux, hydronephrosis, and permanent renal damage.

The person with reflex neurogenic bladder is unable to sense fullness and is unable to void volitionally; therefore micturition cannot be started or stopped in the normal manner. If the detrusor contraction and external urinary sphincter are coordinated, spontaneous voiding will occur when the micturition reflex arc is stimulated. If the two events are uncoordinated, however, pressure within the bladder wall will increase as the detrusor attempts to contract against the contracted external urinary sphincter. The resulting dysfunction is termed detrusor-sphincter dyssynergia. This pattern causes increased resistance to outflow with high intravesical pressure, high residual urine volumes, and poor bladder emptying (Erickson, 1980).

Drugs such as baclofen (Lioresal) may be valuable in decreasing the spasticity of skeletal muscle, including that of the external sphincter. Recently botulinum toxin type A (Botox) has been used to provide short-term relaxation of the urethral sphincter in patients with SCI and detrusor-sphincter dyssynergia (Petit et al., 1998; Schurch et al., 1996) as well as others with pelvic floor dysfunction (Phelan et al., 2001). Botox injections produce effects similar to those of a sphincterotomy but are short term in nature. Anticholinergic medications used in combination with these antispasmodic medications may reduce the voiding pressures enough to allow low-pressure reflex voiding (40 cm H_2O). This bladder program requires incontinence management (NIC) because these individuals may have intermittent episodes of incontinence associated with reflex voiding. An alternative for those with good hand function is to increase the anticholinergic medications, allowing the person to stay dry and to empty the bladder by intermittent catheterization every 4 to 6 hours (Lloyd, Giroux, & Toth, 1988), in which case the nursing intervention is urinary retention management (NIC).

Autonomous Neurogenic Bladder

The autonomous neurogenic bladder is referred to as a lower motor neuron, flaccid, or areflexic bladder. It is difficult to determine when spinal shock subsides for a patient who has an autonomous neurogenic bladder, because the characteristics are similar. Damage occurs to the conus medullaris or cauda equina (lesions involving the reflex arc), disrupting pathways that carry sensory impulses from the bladder to the spinal cord, motor impulses from the spinal cord to the detrusor muscle, and motor impulses from the spinal cord to the external sphincter. Autonomous neurogenic bladder is the most common neurogenic bladder dysfunction seen in children with congenital disabilities such as spina bifida and myelomeningocele.

Voiding is involuntary and occurs when the bladder overflows. Peripheral reflexes and the bulbocavernosus reflex are absent or hypoactive. Sensation and motor control are absent. Findings from a CMG demonstrate the absence of uninhibited contractions, a bladder capacity above normal (600 to 1000 ml), decreased intravesical pressure, and residual urine.

As with reflex neurogenic bladder, the patient with autonomous neurogenic bladder cannot sense fullness, or cannot void volitionally, and therefore cannot start or stop voiding in a normal manner. The bladder can be partially emptied with manual pressure (Credé's method) and straining (Valsalva maneuver). Two patterns of external sphincter activity may occur: (1) no motor activity or (2) some uncontrollable activity. In both patterns the amount of residual urine depends on how well the individual can expel urine by applying pressure, the tone of smooth muscle and elasticity of the bladder wall, and the amount of muscle resistance offered by the internal and external urinary sphincters (Peschers, Jundt, & Dimpfl, 2000). Recently there has been increasing concern about the safety of Credé's methods because of the potential risk of the complications of high-pressure voiding, vesicoureteral reflux, hydronephrosis, and permanent renal damage (Vickrey et al., 1999). An alternative method of bladder emptying is intermittent catheterization every 4 to 6 hours as the management program. The most appropriate program for children with spina bifida or myelomeningocele takes into account the type of neurogenic bladder, functional and cognitive levels, and the child's developmental level. Typically children as young as 3 to 5 years of age are able to learn and perform intermittent catheterization with adult supervision.

Sensory Paralytic Bladder

The sensory paralytic bladder occurs when the afferent or sensory side of the micturition reflex arc is damaged. This condition is most often seen in persons with diabetes who have sensory neuropathy.

The patient with sensory paralytic bladder is able to void volitionally, but the sensation of bladder fullness and emptiness is absent. Findings from the CMG demonstrate the absence of uninhibited contractions with an increased bladder capacity. Because of the lack of the sensation of emptiness, the presence of residual urine is variable, as is the presence of the bulbocavernosus reflex and perineal sensation.

The patient senses no fullness, pain, or temperature but is able to initiate voiding unless the bladder has become markedly atonic because of prolonged periods of retention and overdistention. A loss of bladder wall tone may develop because of the large volumes of urine that collect in the bladder between voids. This urinary retention can lead to overflow incontinence. Because persons with sensory paralytic bladder retain motor control, they can avoid incontinence by utilizing a timed voiding program (Lloyd et al., 1988).

Motor Paralytic Bladder

The motor paralytic bladder occurs when the efferent or motor side of the micturition reflex arc is damaged. Voluntary control of urination is variable, and sensation is normal. The bulbocavernosus reflex is absent. The CMG demonstrates no uninhibited contractions with increased bladder capacity. Residual urine is markedly increased. Because sensory nerves are intact, the patient will sense fullness and emptiness. Motor loss, however, will be partial or complete. When the onset of a motor paralytic bladder is slow and left untreated, the detrusor muscle may stretch and lose tone, resulting in large residual urine volumes. The patient may complain of difficulties in initiating voiding, decreased force of the urinary stream, and a need to strain to void. These signs and symptoms result from loss of motor function and decreased muscle tone. The person may experience overflow incontinence, but distention may be prevented by intermittent catheterization. Persons with motor paralytic bladder may learn to empty the bladder by using a Valsalva maneuver, Credé's method (if permitted), or intermittent catheterization.

TYPES OF INCONTINENCE

Various authors have used different terms to describe function of the lower urinary tract, thus making it difficult to interpret research findings. For the purpose of this chapter the International Continence Society (ICS) terminology will be used. Incontinence is categorized into two basic types: transient/acute or established/chronic. Transient or acute incontinence has a precipitous onset. It usually is associated with an acute medical or surgical condition and often resolves when the precipitating condition is addressed. Persistent or established incontinence occurs because of chronic, long-term abnormalities of the structure or function of the urinary tract (Guerrero & Sinert, 2001; Newman, 2002; Newman & Palmer, 1999). Overactive bladder (OAB) is a relatively new term that is used to refer to detrusor overactivity, which produces urgency, frequency, and sometimes pain but does not necessarily result in incontinence. Table 18-5 lists management options for each type of established or chronic incontinence (Fantl et al., 1996).

Transient Incontinence

The onset of transient incontinence, especially in older adults, is often associated with factors that are reversible and amenable to treatment if an appropriate urinary assessment is conducted (Tannenbaum, Perrin, DuBeau, & Kuchel, 2001). The mnemonic **DIAPPERS** (Resnick, 1996) (Box 18-4) is frequently used to identify common causes for transient incontinence. Patients subject to these factors need comprehensive diagnostic evaluation that focuses not only on the lower urinary tract but also on the person's general medical condition and functional status (Fantl et al., 1996).

Established Incontinence

Established incontinence cannot be easily reversed; it is usually caused by a pathological condition within the urinary tract or neurological system or by irreversible cognitive impairment (Brandeis, Baumann, Hossain, Morris, & Resnick, 1997). The ICS originally identified four major types of incontinence: stress incontinence, urge incontinence, overflow incontinence, and reflex incontinence (Bates, Bradley, & Glen, 1979). In an updated report functional incontinence was added to these classifications (Fantl et al., 1996; NANDA International, 2005).

Stress Incontinence. Stress incontinence is the involuntary loss of urine when intravesical pressure exceeds the maximum intraurethral pressure in the absence of detrusor

TABLE 18-5 Types of Incontinence and Management Options After Basic Evaluation

Type of Urinary Incontinence	Characteristics	Management Options

Urge	Detrusor instability with normal PVR; no complicating factors	Behavioral techniques:
		    Bladder training
		    Pelvic muscle rehabilitation
		    Other (e.g., fluid management)
		Pharmacological interventions:
		    Anticholinergic medications; tricyclic antidepressants as alternative

Stress	With normal PVR; no complicating factors	Behavioral techniques:
		    Pelvic muscle rehabilitation
		    Bladder training
		Pharmacological interventions:
		    α-adrenergic medications or tricyclic antidepressants
		    Estrogen
		    Combination if needed
		Surgical techniques:
		    Uncomplicated, nonrecurrent SUI resulting from hypermobility

Mixed (urge and stress)	With normal PVR; no complicating factors	Combinations of above, excluding surgical options in most cases

PVR, Postvoid residual; *SUI,* stress urinary incontinence.

BOX 18-4 Reversible (Transient) Causes of Urinary Incontinence

D Delirium, dehydration, dietary irritants
I Infection of urinary tract, symptomatic
A Atrophic urethritis and vaginitis: acute urogenital prolapse
P Pharmaceuticals
P Psychological, especially depression
E Excess urine output (endocrine disorders, congestive heart failure, overhydration, sleep apnea)
R Restricted mobility, retention
S Stool impaction

Modified from Resnick, N. (1996). Geriatric incontinence. *Urologic Clinics of North America 23,* 55-74.

---

contraction (Abrams, Blaivas, Stanton, & Anderson, 1988). Stress incontinence is characterized by sudden loss of small amounts of urine with an increase in intraabdominal pressure during coughing, sneezing, laughing, lifting, or bending (Figure 18-10). Stress incontinence is seen more commonly in women but also may occur in men after prostatectomy.

Urge Incontinence. Urge incontinence is the involuntary loss of urine associated with a strong urge to void. Urge incontinence is divided into motor and sensory urgency. Motor urgency is ascribed to overactive detrusor function—either detrusor contractions or detrusor hyperreflexia. The term *overactive bladder* (OAB) may be used to describe detrusor instability and the associated symptoms of urgency, frequency, and nocturia. Sensory urgency is ascribed to hypersensitivity (Abrams et al., 1988). Urine is lost in moderate to large

amounts, and patients cannot reach the toilet before leakage occurs. They also report symptoms of urinary frequency and nocturia (Guerrero & Sinert, 2001). Urge incontinence is associated with supratentorial central nervous system lesions. When this is the case, it is referred to as uninhibited bladder (see the neurogenic bladder section). When there is no overt neuropathy, the cause usually is referred to as detrusor instability (Figure 18-11). The causes may be local irritation of the bladder or simply idiopathic (Gray, 2000).

Overflow incontinence occurs when urine is lost involuntarily when associated with an overdistended bladder (Abrams et al., 1988). Overflow incontinence is characterized by continuous dribbling of small amounts of urine and frequent voiding of small amounts of urine as a result of an overdistended bladder, either because of outlet obstruction (Figure 18-12) or impaired bladder contractility (Guerrero & Sinert, 2001). The most common nonneurogenic cause of overflow incontinence in men is prostatic hypertrophy because it causes an outlet obstruction. Although outlet obstruction is rare in women, it can occur as a complication of an antiincontinence surgical procedure or because of severe pelvic organ prolapse (Fantl et al., 1996). When the intravesical pressure is significant enough to cause overflow incontinence, the risk for urinary backflow into the ureters also increases. Chronic overflow incontinence can predispose the individual to serious upper urinary tract damage.

Mixed Incontinence. Mixed incontinence shows patterns of both urge and stress incontinence. Further evaluation is often necessary to determine the most appropriate treatment.

Functional Incontinence. Functional incontinence is defined as urine loss caused by a person's inability or unwillingness

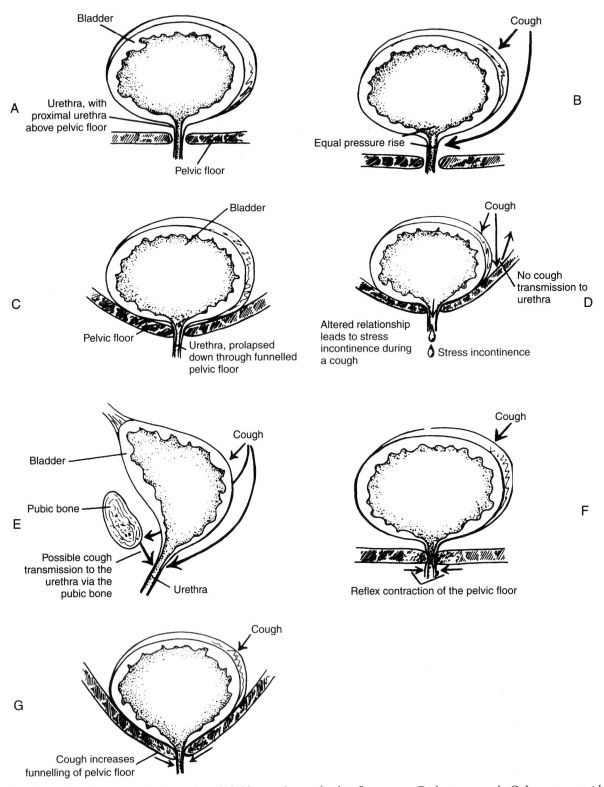

Figure 18-10 A, Normal anatomical relationship of bladder, urethra, and pelvic floor at rest; **B,** during a cough. **C,** In a woman with stress incontinence: at rest; **D,** During a cough. **E,** Possible cough transmission to the urethra by way of the pubic bone. **F,** Normal contraction of the pelvic floor with raised abdominal pressure. **G,** Contraction of the pelvic floor with stress incontinence. (From Jeter, K. F., Faller, N., & Norton, C. [1990]. *Nursing for continence.* Philadelphia: W. B. Saunders.)

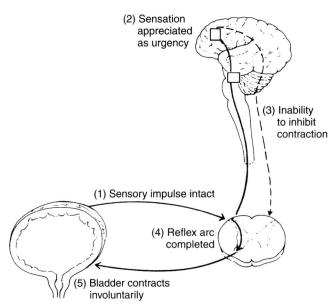

Figure 18-11 Detrusor instability. (From Jeter, K. F., Faller, N., & Norton, C. [1990]. *Nursing for continence.* Philadelphia: W. B. Saunders.)

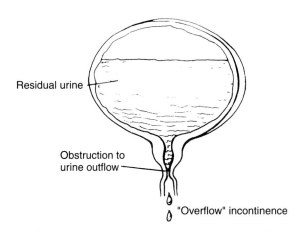

Figure 18-12 Outflow obstruction. (From Jeter, K. F., Faller, N., & Norton, C. [1990]. *Nursing for continence.* Philadelphia: W. B. Saunders.)

to use toilet facilities because of problems outside of the urinary tract such as neurological injury, impaired mobility, or reduced cognitive function (Newman, 2002). The lower urinary tract functions correctly, but problems in other areas affect bladder control. In true functional incontinence, there is normal functioning of the lower urinary tract although cognitive and physical impairment can exacerbate incontinence from other causes.

NURSING DIAGNOSES

Based on the above assessment data, the rehabilitation nurse will make an appropriate nursing diagnosis for the patient with

altered urinary elimination. Potential diagnoses are as follows (NANDA-I, 2005):

- Impaired urinary elimination
- Urinary retention
- Risk for urge urinary incontinence
- Urge urinary incontinence
- Functional urinary incontinence
- Stress urinary incontinence
- Total urinary incontinence
- Reflex urinary incontinence
- Risk for autonomic dysreflexia

NURSING OUTCOMES

Short-term goals are established with the patient and vary according to the type of bladder dysfunction and lifestyle issues. Continence is socially important and a significant factor in quality of life; therefore it is critical to involve the patient and significant other in setting mutually acceptable goals. Goals that may be established are as follows:

- Patient achieves an acceptable level of urinary continence.
- Patient and family follow a bladder management program consistent with lifestyle.
- Patient verbalizes knowledge of medications and their side effects related to bladder management program.
- Patient demonstrates, as applicable, ability to care for indwelling catheter, intermittent catheterization program, external collection device, and perineal/periurethral skin.
- Patient achieves complete bladder emptying by using appropriate bladder management technique.
- Patient verbalizes signs and symptoms of urinary retention and actions to take.
- Patient verbalizes signs and symptoms of urinary tract infection, follows measures to prevent or reduce infection, and what actions to take should it occur (McCourt, 1993).

INTERVENTIONS

Several NIC interventions can be used to outline and direct the process of assessing and managing urinary elimination. See the urinary decision tree (Figure 18-13) for an overview of associated NIC interventions. However, individual preferences must be respected (Fantl et al., 1996). For instance, a person may choose a more invasive treatment for the sake of expediency. When the risks, benefits, and outcomes are understood clearly and the patient provides informed consent, the person's wishes may supersede this general guideline.

Treatment categories, notably behavioral techniques, generally fall within the scope of the independent realm of rehabilitation nursing. Physical therapists may be used as consultants when more advanced pelvic muscle training is needed. Occupational therapists are an excellent resource on assistive devices that can promote independence with toileting or self-catheterization. Pharmacological and surgical treatments require nurses' collaboration with physicians and/or

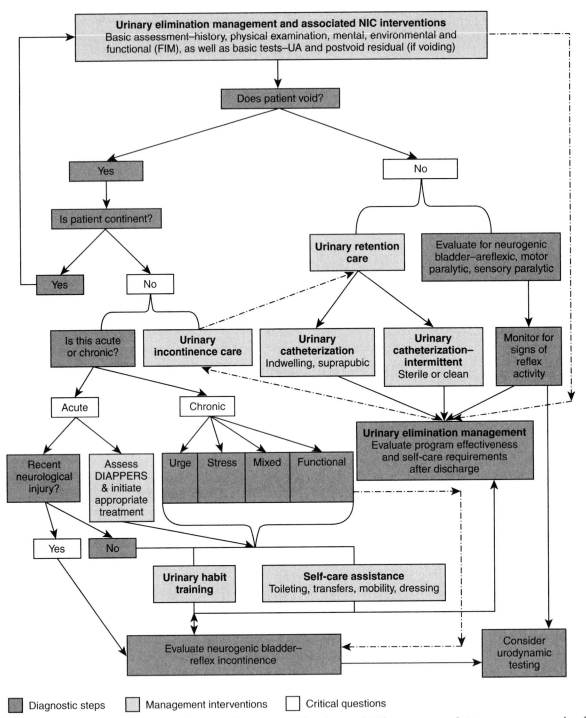

Figure 18-13 Urinary elimination and associated Nursing Interventions Classification (NIC) interventions. It is important to note that diagnosis and management interventions must be implemented concurrently. (Courtesy Kathleen A. Stevens, PhD, RN, CRRN.)

advanced practice nurses and reflect the interdependent and dependent realm of nursing practice.

If patients are voiding yet as a result of their illness or disability are experiencing limitations in mobility that interfere with independence in toileting, the most appropriate nursing intervention would be self-care deficit toileting (NIC). Self-care deficit toileting includes activities such as assisting another person with elimination and providing environmental

modifications that support independence in toileting. Environmental modifications described in Chapter 14 can include a raised toilet seat, grab bars, or use of bedside commode. See Table 18-6 for categories and types of toileting and assistive devices for managing urinary continence. These interventions are most appropriate for individuals who are able to void adequately yet are experiencing limitations in mobility related to illness or disability. Concurrently the intervention

TABLE 18-6 Toileting and Assistive Devices to Manage Continence

Product Category	Product Types
Clothing aids (may be used for toileting or clothing management by individuals on ICP)	Dressing stick Clothing loops Reacher Clothing fasteners Velcro closures in place of zippers/buttons Zipper pulls
Hygiene management (for individuals with limited upper extremity function or ROM these devices are designed to manipulate and secure toilet paper)	Tongs, spring clip, S-shaped hook or small cup-shaped head with recessed serrations may be used to manipulate Bidet
Male external or external occlusive device (used to collect urine when reflex or unconscious voiding occurs)	Self-adhesive external catheters Hydrocolloid strips Retracted penis pouches Condom catheter Reusable external catheter system Pneumatic and electric leg bag openers
Female external occlusive device	Female urinary collecting pouch
Urinary drainage devices	Leg bag Belly Bag Night drainage bag
Urinals	Male urinal Rehabilitation male urinal Female urinal Bedpan Fracture bedpan
Commodes	Over-the-toilet commode Stand-alone commode (bedside commode) Raised toilet seats or risers Grab bars
Absorbent products	Perineal pads Panty liners Guards for men Undergarment Fitted briefs Refastenable underwear Adult briefs (diapers)
Intravaginal supports or pessaries (designed to support bladder neck and prevent bladder prolapse)	Ring Donut Marland Oval Shaatz Gehrung Dish
Penile clamps	
Intermittent catheterization devices	Button hook to hold catheter Standard hair clip mounted in splinting material and attached to universal cuff Bungee cord to assist with clothing management C-handle catheter inserter Labia spreader

ICP, Intermittent catheterization program; *ROM,* range of motion.

urinary elimination management (NIC) may be used to prescribe activities such as fluid management, ongoing monitoring of a bladder management program, and planning for a urinary management program appropriate for home or community discharge.

Constipation may be a major contributing factor to urinary incontinence, and restoring regular bowel elimination often alleviates urinary urgency and lack of control. Therefore it is essential to evaluate the individual's bowel management. An effective method of restoring regular bowel elimination is to remove any impaction, increase intake of fiber and fluids, and promote mobility or exercise. This should be a priority because it is difficult to retrain the bladder until the bowel is adequately retrained (see Chapter 19).

Behavioral Interventions

The behavioral techniques delineated in the AHRQ urinary guidelines are low-risk interventions intended to decrease frequency of urinary incontinence in most individuals when techniques are provided by knowledgeable health care professionals. Behavioral therapies can be divided into caregiver-dependent techniques for patients with cognitive and motor deficits and those requiring active patient participation in rehabilitation and education techniques. Behavioral techniques will be addressed in the order of those requiring passive involvement to those requiring more active patient participation. These behavioral techniques include toileting assistance (scheduled voiding, habit training, prompted voiding), and bladder training.

The term *independent continence* is commonly used in long-term care settings to refer to residents who are able to maintain continence using these techniques without assistance from caregivers or staff. *Dependent continence* refers to programs that produce continence for the resident that are performed solely by caregivers or nursing staff (Newman, 2002).

Toileting assistance intervention (NIC) includes routine or scheduled toileting, habit training, and prompted voiding. The terms *timed voiding, habit training, prompted voiding,* and *bladder training* have at times been used interchangeably when discussing treatment options, yet each refers to a distinctly different type of intervention (Table 18-7). Scheduled toileting or timed voiding is defined as scheduled toileting on a planned basis. It is the practice of toileting a person using a bedpan/urinal, commode, or toilet at regular intervals, such as every 2 or 3 hours. Dependent continence can often be achieved with a well-designed toileting schedule and a consistent caregiver even with patients with significant cognitive impairments (Lyons & Pringle Specht, 2001; Newman, 2002). A successful toileting program requires a dedication and consistency on the part of the caregiver. Although greater success may be achieved in a home setting when an individual has a dedicated caregiver, studies in nursing home settings have shown that a toileting assistance program can result in a reduction in number of incontinent episodes per day in residents (Lekan-Rutledge & Colling, 2003).

TABLE 18-7 Scheduled Voiding Regimens

Intervention	Description	Patient Characteristics
Timed voiding	Toileting on a fixed schedule, typically every 2 hours during waking hours; the interval does not change	Used for stress, urge, mixed incontinence and uninhibited neurological bladder dysfunction in patients with cognitive or physical impairments; also in adults without impairments who have infrequent or irregular voiding patterns
Habit training	Scheduled toileting, voiding intervals adjusted (longer or shorter) based on the individual's voiding pattern	Used for stress, urge, mixed incontinence and uninhibited neurological bladder dysfunction especially in institutionalized or homebound adults with cognitive homebound adults with cognitive or physical impairments; may also be used with patients who have diuretic-induced incontinence or predictable incontinence episodes
Patterned urge response toileting	Habit training that involves the use of an electronic monitoring device to identify timing of incontinence episodes	Used for stress, urge, and mixed incontinence in nursing home and homebound elderly populations
Prompted voiding	Scheduled toiletings in which a caregiver gives prompts to void, typically every 2 hours; patient assisted in toileting only if response is positive; used in conjunction with operant conditioning techniques to reward patient for maintaining continence and appropriate toileting	Used for stress, urge, mixed incontinence and uninhibited neurological bladder dysfunction in patients who are functionally able to use a toilet or toilet substitute, able to feel urge sensation, and able to acknowledge need for toileting assistance appropriately; primarily used in institutional settings or with homebound older adults with available caregiver
Bladder training	Scheduled toiletings with progressive voiding intervals; includes teaching of urge-control strategies using relaxation and distraction techniques, self-monitoring, and reinforcement techniques	Used for stress, urge, mixed incontinence and uninhibited neurological bladder dysfunction in patients who are sufficiently cognitively able to employ urge-control strategies and motivated to comply with toileting program

Modified from Wyman, J. F. (2003). Treatment of urinary incontinence in men and older women. *American Journal of Nursing, 103*(3, Suppl), 26-35.

Urinary habit training (NIC) relies on the caregiver to establish a predictable pattern of bladder emptying to prevent incontinence for persons with incontinence. Timed voiding assistance is provided based on a predesigned time schedule. Timed voiding relies on an external stimulus, the clock, as the determining factor for toileting frequency, whereas habit training relies on an assessment of the individual's pattern to establish toileting frequency. Within a rehabilitation setting a timed voiding program is often the precursor to habit training.

Habit training uses assessment data and bladder voiding records to identify times for toileting. Habit training is recommended for patients once a natural voiding pattern can be determined (Fantl et al., 1996). Habit training is toileting scheduled to match the patient's natural voiding habits. Staff is instructed to toilet the individual according to prescribed times no matter whether the urge to void is present. By having the patient void at a predetermined time, the person is often able to reduce episodes of urinary incontinence. Success often depends on the caregiver, not the person with incontinence (Pires & Lockart-Pretti, 1992).

Prompted voiding is defined as a scheduled voiding program that reinforces the person for remaining dry rather than for wetness. This behavioral intervention requires more interaction between caregiver and patient and is recommended

when the patient can learn to recognize some degree of bladder fullness or the need to void or the patient can ask for assistance or respond when promoted to toilet. Homebound cognitively impaired elders were found to respond to a prompted voiding intervention (Engberg, Sereika, McDowell, Weber, & Brodak, 2002), so it is important to take self-care abilities, caregiver resources, and commitment in consideration with the cognitive ability of the patient when prescribing a toileting assistance program. According to Lyons and Pringle Specht (1999), the best predictor of an individual's response to prompted voiding is his or her success with a prompted voiding trial.

There are three major components of prompted voiding:
- **Monitoring:** The patient is checked by the caregiver on a regular basis and asked if he or she needs to use the toilet or feels bladder fullness. The caregiver is instructed to look for nonverbal behaviors that indicate need for toileting and to report if the patient is wet or dry.
- **Prompting:** The patient is asked (prompted) to try to use the toilet.
- **Praising:** The caregiver provides positive reinforcement, praising the individual for maintaining continence and for trying to toilet (Fantl et al., 1996; Lyons & Pringle Specht, 1999).

Newman (2002) subsequently in her recommendations for a prompted voiding program in long-term care settings added two additional steps, talk and correct. She encourages the caregiver to talk with the individual and ask questions that encourage awareness of the individual's condition. If the individual is dry, he or she is praised. If the individual is wet, then the caregiver should provide corrective feedback in a coaching supportive manner.

If the individual is wet when toileted, then in the correcting step, the caregiver should tell the individual about the wetness and suggest to the individual an action that may be used in the future to reduce potential for incontinence such as, "to stay dry, press your call light as soon as you feel desire to void so staff have time to come and assist you."

The goal is to teach the person responsibility for wetness and toileting behavior. Caregivers learn to give a positive response when the patient voids in the toilet or is dry. Success often depends on staff commitment to the program. Burgio and Burgio (1990) used a staff training program called behavioral supervision model to educate staff on their role in prompted voiding programs and ways to provide staff feedback and reinforcement for proper commitment and program performance. When properly conducted, prompted voiding has been useful for assisting persons with cognitive impairments and those who reside in nursing home settings.

Once an individual is continent, either as a result of staff efforts in cases of dependent continence or as a result of the individual's own control, the next goal may be to upgrade the program by decreasing the frequency of voiding or increasing the time interval between voids. This intervention is most commonly referred to as urinary bladder training (NIC). Urinary bladder training, sometimes termed bladder retraining (Box 18-5), uses distraction or relaxation techniques so a patient is able to learn to consciously inhibit or resist the urge to void. The goals of bladder training are to improve ability to control bladder urgency, decrease episodes of bladder frequency, increase bladder capacity and sphincter control, and promote social continence. Bladder training is strongly recommended for managing urge and mixed incontinence. Bladder training may also be used when managing stress incontinence, overactive bladder, and with patients with urge incontinence post stroke.

Three components to bladder retraining are an education program, scheduled voiding with systematic delay of voiding, and positive reinforcement. The education program contains information about the physiology and pathophysiology of the lower urinary tract and strategies the individual can use to enhance urge control. Ideally, nurses and physical therapists work together with the individual on exercises to increase detrusor contractility and voluntary control of the urinary sphincter. The retraining program begins with a toileting schedule of 2 to 3 hours, with the exception of sleep time. A goal-oriented bladder record helps provide immediate positive feedback to encourage progress to the next interval level. For instance, an initial goal may be to void every 2 hours; using inhibition techniques, the person may progress gradually to 3-hour voiding intervals. Nurses can obtain or create their own relaxation tapes to assist patients who are learning how to relax as a technique for inhibiting the urge to void.

Incontinence can cause individuals to be embarrassed and anxious. At times individuals become so fearful of being incontinent that they demonstrate obsessive toileting needs. These individuals request toileting assistance every 10 to 30 minutes and void minimal amounts, if at all, with each void. Obsessive toileting may also occur in individuals post stroke as a result of damage to the cortical sensory or motor micturition centers. It is important to acknowledge the patient's anxiety and secure their trust and willingness to attempt a bladder training program. Newman (2002) suggests using the bladder scanner to assess bladder volume and provide feedback. If the prevoid volume is less than 100 ml, feedback is given to the individual on bladder volume either verbally or by viewing the scanner screen. The caregiver reinforces that this is a very small volume and suggests strategies that can be used to postpone voiding. The individual is encouraged to postpone voiding and praised for attempt. Program success depends on the individual's willingness to participate and trust in the caregiver to respond to requests for toileting.

Advanced Techniques and Pelvic Muscle Rehabilitation

Advanced behavioral techniques include pelvic floor exercises, which may be enhanced by biofeedback, vaginal cone retention, or electrical stimulation. These are appropriate for individuals with cognitive function and sufficient motor ability to follow through with an exercise program. These techniques are offered to persons who are motivated to avoid use of protective garments, external devices or medications or who shun more invasive treatment methods.

The first step in pelvic muscle reeducation is for the patient to gain an awareness of the pelvic muscles. This requires some concentration but is essential before the next step. Pelvic muscle exercises (PME), also called Kegel exercises, improve urethral resistance through active contraction of the pubococcygeus muscle. Contraction of the pubococcygeal muscle exerts a closing force on the urethra and, over time, improves muscle support to the pelvic structures and strengthens the voluntary periurethral and pelvic musculature. Components of the pelvic muscle exercises are locating and identifying the correct muscles, engaging in active exercise on a regular basis, and using the muscles to control continence (Pires & Lockart-Pretti, 1992).

Kegel exercises (Box 18-6) are performed by holding the muscles in contraction for a count of 10 and then relaxing for a count of 10; repeat for 10 minutes 3 times daily for a total of 30 to 80 exercises per day. An individual can perform these exercises when in any position. The muscle contractions are not visible to anyone else and require no equipment; thus they can be performed in any environment.

Teaching pelvic muscle exercises may prevent urinary incontinence. These exercises strengthen pelvic muscles and may decrease the incidence of urinary incontinence. Pelvic exercises are strongly recommended for women with stress incontinence. Pelvic muscle exercises are also recommended for men and women as an adjunct to bladder training for

BOX 18-5 Procedure for Bladder Retraining

Purpose
1. Improve the patient's pattern of voiding
2. Restore normal bladder function
3. Teach the client how to redevelop control of his/her voiding

Equipment
1. Bladder records
2. Bladder retraining teaching tool

Procedure
1. Send the client's bladder records to complete 1 to 2 weeks before the client's evaluation visit.
2. At the time of evaluation, analyze the client's history, symptoms, and bladder records and determine if bladder retraining will be a part of the treatment regimen.
3. Initiate bladder retraining if the client is mentally and physically capable of toileting as indicated by the nursing assessment and/or a Mini-Mental test and if she has frequency, urgency, urge, or functional incontinence. Frequent toileting would be every 3 hours or more often or a schedule that interferes with and limits a person's lifestyle.
4. Always explain the rationale for the instructions in detail.
5. Teach the client to eliminate or reduce from her diet products containing caffeine or aspartame (NutraSweet).
6. Teach the client to have a daily fluid intake of 48 to 64 oz of caffeine-free liquids.
7. If the client has nighttime frequency, nocturia, or enuresis, teach the client to stop drinking fluids 2 hours before bedtime or to stop after 6 PM.
8. Teach the client relaxation techniques for inhibiting or diverting the urge sensation.
9. Teach these relaxation techniques during the bedside cystometrogram (CMG):
   - When the client gets the first (initial) urge to void, teach the client to take slow, deep breaths through the mouth until the urge sensation lessens or goes away.
   - As the CMG continues, when the client gets the second ("must") urge to void again, instruct the client to take slow, deep breaths until the urge sensation disappears.
10. If a bedside CMG is not performed, teach the client to do the following when a strong urge occurs:
    - Sit and relax.
    - Take slow, deep breaths in and out of the mouth until the urge sensation goes away.
    - Concentrate only on the deep breathing until the urge sensation goes away.
11. Determine the client's average current voiding pattern from the symptoms and the bladder record.
12. Then increase this interval by 15 minutes at a time, teaching the client to use relaxation techniques if the client gets the urge to void sooner.
13. Teach the client not to empty her bladder before she gets the urge to void.
14. Teach the client first to use relaxation techniques at home—when the client is relaxed and knows that the bathroom is readily accessible—so as to avoid anxiety-producing situations.
15. Gradually increase the client's voiding interval as she meets with success.
16. Also, teach the client to use the relaxation technique for diverting the urge to void in common instances when the urge occurs—for example, the "key in the lock" syndrome. Teach the client that if she gets the urge to void when trying to unlock a door, she should stop and use the relaxation technique.
17. Inform the client that at first these techniques may not work but that she should keep attempting to attain the control that these techniques teach.
18. Teach the client never to rush to the bathroom.
19. Have the client keep bladder records to monitor voiding patterns and to record improvement. The client may not notice significant changes in voiding for 6 to 8 weeks.
20. Schedule follow-up visits according to the client's needs and reinforce the bladder retraining teaching.
21. Provide encouragement to the client at each visit and do not allow her to get discouraged by setbacks that can occur during a cold or an acute illness, during a menstrual period, or if she becomes anxious or fatigued.

BOX 18-6 Patient Teaching: Pelvic Muscle (Kegel) Exercises

How to Find the Pelvic Muscle
To find the muscle, imagine you are at a party and the rich food you have just consumed causes you to have gas. The muscle that you use to hold back gas is the one you want to exercise. Some persons find this muscle by voluntarily stopping the stream of urine. If you are a woman, another way to find the muscle is by pulling your rectum, vagina, and urethra up inside. Try to think about the area around the vagina.

Exercising the Muscle
Begin by emptying your bladder, and then try to relax completely. Tighten this muscle and hold it for a count of 10 or 10 seconds; then relax the muscle completely for a count of 10 or 10 seconds. You should feel a sensation of closing between your legs and lifting of the area around the vagina (in women).

When to Exercise
Do 10 exercises in the morning, 10 in the afternoon, and 15 at night—or else you can exercise for 10 minutes, 3 times a day. Set a timer for 10 minutes, 3 times a day. Initially you may not be able to hold this contraction for the complete count of 10; however, you will build slowly to 10-second contractions over time. The muscle may start to tire after 6 or 8 exercises. If this happens, stop and go back to exercising later.

Where to Practice These Exercises
These exercises can be practiced anywhere and anytime. Most persons seem to prefer exercising lying on their bed or sitting in a chair. Women can try doing these exercises during intercourse. Tighten your pelvic muscles to grip your partner's penis and then relax. Your partner should be able to feel an increase in pressure.

Common Mistakes
Never use your stomach, legs, or buttock muscles. To find out if you also are contracting your stomach muscles, place your hand on your abdomen while you squeeze your pelvic muscle. If you feel your abdomen move, then you also are using these muscles. In time you will learn to practice effortlessly. Eventually work these exercises in as part of your lifestyle; tighten the muscle when you walk, when you sneeze, or when you are on the way to the bathroom.

When Will I Notice a Change?
After 4 to 6 weeks of constant daily exercise, you will begin to notice fewer urinary accidents, and after 3 months you will see an even bigger difference.

Can These Exercises Hurt Me?
No! These exercises cannot harm you in any way. Most clients find them relaxing and easy. If you get back pain or stomach pain after you exercise, then you probably are trying too hard and using stomach muscles. Go back and find the pelvic muscle and remember this exercise should feel easy. If you experience headaches, then you also are tensing your chest muscles and probably holding your breath.

Copyright 1986 by Golden Horizons, Inc., St. Davids, PA.

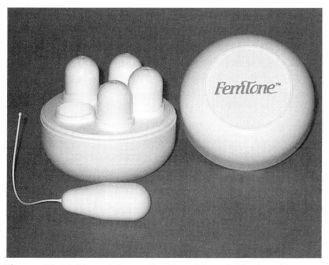

Figure 18-14 Vaginal Cones FemTone Vaginal Weights. (Courtesy Seekwellness.com.)

urge incontinence. Pelvic muscle exercises may benefit men who develop urinary incontinence after prostatectomy (Fantl et al., 1996) or women who have had multiple surgical repairs.

Several techniques assist persons with urinary incontinence in isolating and training the correct pelvic muscles. They include vaginal weight training, biofeedback, and electrical stimulation (Burgio, Locher, Roth, & Goode, 2001).

Vaginal Weight Training. Vaginal weight training uses vaginal cones as an adjunct to pelvic muscle exercises in women (Figure 18-14). The woman is given a set of cones of the same size and shape, that increase in weight from 20 to 100 g. The goal of the program is to retain the weighted cone for 15 minutes, twice a day. The woman starts with the lowest weight and then progresses to the next weight when she can retain the lower-level weight for 15 minutes. The woman must stand and retain the weight for the exercise to be effective (Burgio et al., 2001). The sustained contraction required to retain the weighted cone increases the strength of the pelvic muscles. The weight of the cone is assumed to heighten the proprioceptive feedback to the desired pelvic muscle contraction. Vaginal weight training is recommended for stress urinary incontinence in premenopausal women (Fantl et al., 1996).

Biofeedback. Biofeedback is a group of strategies that use electronic or mechanical instruments to display information to individuals about their neuromuscular activity. The aim of biofeedback is to alter bladder dysfunction by teaching patients to change the physiological responses that affect bladder control (Burgio & Engel, 1990). Methods of biofeedback include surface electrodes and sensors inserted either vaginally or rectally. Auditory or visual display of proper muscle contraction forms the core of biofeedback procedures (Schwartz, 1995). Biofeedback systems range from stationary to portable and include home training devices. Biofeedback is best used in conjunction with other behavioral techniques such as PME and bladder training.

Success of biofeedback is dependent largely on the skill of the health care provider. The provider must have comprehensive knowledge about evaluation techniques, anatomical and physiological relationship of symptoms to types of bladder dysfunction, and behavioral principles that guide the procedure (Fantl et al., 1996). This is an area appropriate for rehabilitation nurses to expand their practice, because a knowledgeable nurse meets and exceeds these criteria. Pelvic muscle rehabilitation and biofeedback therapy are recommended for patients with stress, urge, and mixed urinary incontinence (Fantl et al., 1996). Studies have also demonstrated reductions in urinary incontinence associated with neurological disease and in frail elderly persons when a combination of biofeedback and behavioral techniques are used (McDowell et al., 1999).

Electrical Stimulation. Electrical stimulation of the pelvic floor produces a contraction of the levator ani and the external urethral and anal sphincters, accompanied by reflex inhibition of the detrusor. This activity depends on a preserved reflex arc through the sacral micturition center. Nonimplantable pelvic floor electrical stimulation uses vaginal or anal sensors or surface electrodes (Vodusek, Plevink, Vrtacnik, & Janez, 1998). Minimal adverse side effects occur, with pain and local discomfort being the most prominent reactions. Electrical stimulation has been used to inhibit detrusor overactivity in persons with neurological impairments by modifying the sacral micturition reflex arc (Tanagho, 1990). Pelvic floor electrical stimulation has been shown to decrease incontinence in women with stress urinary incontinence, and it may be effective in men and women with urge and mixed incontinence (Fantl et al., 1996).

Urinary Retention

Urinary retention can result in serious and life-threatening complications, such as upper urinary tract infection, kidney damage, and renal failure, if not properly managed. Urinary retention may occur as a result of spinal shock, post spinal cord injury, neurogenic bladder dysfunction, obstruction from an enlarged prostate gland, or DSD. When the individual demonstrates an inability to void or postvoid residual volumes are repeatedly elevated, the priority is to implement a urinary catheterization program to minimize urinary retention and safely empty the bladder.

Two NIC interventions, urinary catheterization and urinary catheterization intermittent, are commonly used to manage retention. Urinary catheterization describes a program that uses an indwelling catheter placed either via the urethra or a suprapubic ostomy to provide continuous bladder drainage. Common complications associated with indwelling urinary catheterization include urinary tract infection, upper tract damage, and urethral trauma in males. Haley et al. (1981) reported that if a urinary catheter was left in place for 30 days, nearly all patients showed evidence of bacteriuria. Long-term use of an indwelling urinary catheter has been associated with pyelonephritis and renal inflammation (Warren, Muncie, Hebel, & Hall-Craggs, 1994). Several guidelines have been published that describe best practices for care of an indwelling catheter (Society of Urologic Nurses and Associates, 2005) or for prevention of catheter-associated infections (Wong, & Hooton, 1981) (Box 18-7).

Urinary catheterization intermittent (NIC) or an intermittent catheterization program (ICP) is a catheterization program that relies on scheduled insertion and removal of a catheter at prescribed intervals to empty the bladder. Intermittent catheterization is not without risk; however, the risks of bladder infection and urethral trauma are more likely to be limited to the lower urinary tract.

Intermittent catheterization every 4 to 6 hours is the preferred method of management of urinary retention and overflow incontinence resulting from autonomous, sensory, or motor paralytic bladder. The goal of an intermittent catheterization program is to empty the bladder at regular, consistent intervals and maintain catheterization volumes at safe levels. Fluid management and an appropriate catheterization schedule are necessary to maintain safe volumes. Generally patients will start on a schedule of every 4 hours until a pattern is determined, and then the catheterization frequency will be adjusted based on pattern of urinary output. In the hospital the catheterization schedule will generally be managed by the physician; however, before discharge the patient should be educated to adjust his or her catheterization frequency, at home and in the community, based on fluid intake and urinary output patterns.

Sterile technique commonly is practiced when the patient is hospitalized; however, clean technique generally is considered safe in the home. King, Carlson, Mervine, Wu, and Yarkony (1992) demonstrated that a modified clean technique may be safely used in the hospital setting with patients with spinal cord injury when the catheterization interval is less than 6 hours and the catheterization volumes are less than 400 ml (Box 18-8). An individual's willingness to commit and follow through with a catheterization schedule that results in routine emptying and safe volumes is the key to a successful program.

BOX 18-7 Clinical Practice Guidelines: Care of the Patient With an Indwelling Catheter

Guideline for Prevention of Catheter-Associated Urinary Tract Infections (UTIs)
Category I: Strongly Recommended
1. Educate staff on proper catheter insertion/care.
2. Utilize catheter only when necessary.
3. Utilize strict hand-washing principles.
4. Utilize sterile technique with catheter insertion.
5. Secure catheter properly.
6. Maintain closed sterile system.
7. Obtain urine sample aseptically.
8. Maintain free flow to urine (no obstruction).

Category II: Moderately Recommended
1. Reeducate staff periodically.
2. Use smallest size (bore) catheter. Use sterile water for balloon inflation per manufacturer's guidelines.
3. Avoid irrigation unless needed to relieve/prevent obstruction.
4. Do not perform daily meatal care as described in texts (using antibiotic ointments or Betadine). Basic hygiene is sufficient.
5. Do not change catheter at arbitrary fixed intervals. Catheters should be changed as needed based on clinical symptoms: catheter encrustations, leakage, bleeding, catheter-associated UTI.

Category III: Weakly Recommended
1. Consider alternative to indwelling urethral catheters.
2. Replace the collecting system when sterile closed drainage has been compromised.
3. Separate infected from uninfected catheterized patients. That is, being located in same room or sharing adjacent beds. (NOTE: This recommendation is a weak recommendation and studies in rehabilitation and LTC have not shown significant risk for nosocomial infection when good hand-washing practices are used.)
4. Avoid routine bacteriological monitoring. Routine urine cultures are not recommended.

Recommendations for Patient Education
1. Daily skin care is not necessary—basic hygiene or showers are sufficient.
2. Adequate fluid intake is necessary; 30 ml/kg of body weight is currently recommended.
3. Maintain closed drainage system whenever possible.
4. Care of collection bags must be done daily with a commercially available product, a household bleach solution diluted in a 1:10 ratio with tap water. Bags should be rinsed twice and agitated with water. Then fill the bag with 15 ml of "diluted" bleach solution, allowing 30 ml for tubing and spigot. Vigorously agitate, drain, and air dry.
   When using bleach solution, patients need to be cautioned to wear protective gloves and avoid eye contact. Skin irritation can occur.
5. The urinary drainage bag should be emptied when ½-⅔ full or every 3-6 hours.

Modified from Society of Urologic Nurses and Associates. (2005). *Clinical practice guidelines–Care of the patient with an indwelling catheter.* Available from http://www.suna.org/clinicalpracticeguidelines.
LTC, Long-term care.

Individuals with urinary retention associated with neurogenic bladder dysfunction or detrusor-sphincter dyssynergy secondary to spinal cord damage often require a lifelong urinary catheterization program. A decision on the optimal program, intermittent catheterization or indwelling catheter, must involve the individual and take into account the individual's functional skills, lifestyle and goals, and caregiver resources, as well as risks associated with the program. Before discharge the nurse is responsible for educating the individual and caregiver on the program and proper care and maintenance of equipment in the home setting.

Urinary Incontinence Care

Urinary leakage, or the risk of being wet, is anxiety producing to the individual. When urinary incontinence occurs, a variety of interventions can be used to minimize the frequency or volume of urine loss, hopefully reducing embarrassment. These interventions include use of urinary collecting devices and/or clamps, pharmacological treatment, or surgical interventions.

Urinary leakage can also predispose the individual to skin breakdowns such as fungal infections, rashes, or in severe cases pressure ulcers. Urinary incontinence care (NIC) refers to activities to promote continence while maintaining skin integrity. In anticipation of a potential problem, some individuals may want to use a protective device to promote a sense of self-esteem. Other individuals may perceive use of a collecting device as demoralizing or embarrassing. The decision to use a urinary collecting device as a means of incontinence care should be made by the individual.

BOX 18-8 Procedure: Intermittent Catheterization (Clean Technique)

Purpose
To provide complete and regular bladder drainage, to decrease trauma to the bladder and urethra associated with the use of an indwelling catheter.

General Considerations
1. It is possible to significantly decrease the incidence of urinary tract infection by using intermittent catheterization rather than an indwelling catheter. Infection occurs when bacteria enter the bladder during catheterization and multiply because of prolonged intervals between catheterization and bladder emptying.
2. Clean technique may be used if catheterizations occur at an interval of every 6 hours or less.
3. Catheter size and type will vary based on age, size, and special needs (i.e., Coudé tip).
4. Frequency of catheterization and fluid intake is prescribed by the physician.
5. Common complications associated with intermittent catheterization include the following:
   - Bladder overdistention
   - Autonomic dysreflexia
   - Bladder infection
   - Urethral trauma
6. When voiding between catheterizations does not occur, ideally catheterization volume should not exceed 40 ml.
7. Clean technique in the hospital uses a modified clean technique, which requires a new sterile catheter for each catheterization.
8. Maintain privacy during procedure.

Equipment
Red rubber or clear plastic straight catheter.
Drainage container (not needed if urine is drained directly into the toilet)
Water-soluble lubricant (packet or tube)
Soap and water
Washcloth or disposable wipe
Clean gloves (needed only when catheterization is performed by caregiver)

Steps
1. Gather equipment, and provide privacy.
2. Adjust lighting if needed.
3. Wash hands with soap and water or disposable wipe.
4. Lower clothing to expose urinary meatus.
5. If catheterization is performed by caregiver or family—person performing catheterization dons clean gloves.
6. Open lubricant, and squeeze onto catheter tip.
7. Expose the urinary meatus (for males pull back foreskin, for females spread the labia using fingers or labia spreader).
8. Position drainage container if used.
9. Cleanse the urinary meatus with soap and water.
10. Gently insert the catheter (in males insert until resistance is felt, for females insert ½ inch beyond start of urine flow).
11. Drain urine into drainage container or the toilet.
12. As urine flow subsides, if recommended by your physician, gently empty the bladder using Credé's maneuver on the suprapubic area.
13. Once urine flow subsides, gently remove the catheter.
14. Wipe lubricant off, and wash the area with soap and water.
15. For males replace foreskin.
16. Dispose of supplies. Clean and store catheter as appropriate.
17. Wash hands.

Urinary collecting devices come in a wide range of types and sizes, so selecting the right product can be a daunting task. The most common types of urinary collecting devices are pads/inserts, briefs, diapers, or externals with drainage bags. When selecting a device, the nurse must take into account why the device is needed, duration of use, functional level, cost, and maintenance required. The nurse can advise the individual on the benefits and limitations associated with each type. It is beyond the scope of this text to review all product options, so the focus will be on urinary continence care interventions. Once a product is selected, routine patient education should include specifics on application and removal of the device, wearing schedule, skin check method and frequency, product cleaning and maintenance, and information on purchasing supplies post discharge in the community. When functional limitations interfere with the individual's ability to adequately apply or remove the urinary collecting device, the rehabilitation nurse may suggest trial use of an assistive device or consult with the occupational therapist or physical therapist on strategies to promote self-care and independence.

Urinary Clamps. Urinary clamps or inserts have been used successfully in some cases to limit urinary leakage. Clamps, inserts, or pessaries are typically not used with individuals with impaired sensation or motor deficits that prohibit self-insertion or application. Therefore these are rarely used with individuals with urinary incontinence secondary to neurogenic bladder dysfunction. These devices may be an option for individuals with stress incontinence or established incontinence associated with orthopedic impairments.

Pharmacological Treatment of Incontinence

Medications have been beneficial in treating urinary incontinence. They can be categorized into two main groups: medications for incontinence resulting from urethral sphincter insufficiency and medications for incontinence resulting from detrusor overactivity.

Medications used to treat urethral sphincter insufficiency are α-adrenergic agonist agents and estrogen supplementation therapy. α-Adrenergic agonist agents increase urethral resistance by stimulation of urethral smooth muscle acting on α-adrenergic receptors in the urethra. Phenylpropanolamine (PPA) and pseudoephedrine have been the first-line pharmacological therapy for women with stress incontinence; however, recent Food and Drug Administration (FDA) warnings are prompting use of other class drugs or newer agents.

Estrogen replacement in postmenopausal women may restore urethral mucosal coaptation and increase vascularity, tone, and the α-adrenergic response of the urethral muscle, thus increasing bladder outlet resistance and decreasing stress incontinence. Estrogen (oral or vaginal) may be considered as an adjunctive pharmacological agent for postmenopausal women with stress or mixed incontinence. Conjugated estrogen is usually administered either orally (0.3 to 1.25 mg/day) or vaginally (2 g or fraction per day). Progestin (e.g., medroxyprogesterone 2.5 to 10 mg/day) may be given continuously or intermittently. Combined PPA and oral or vaginal estrogen is recommended in the treatment of postmenopausal women with stress incontinence when initial single-medication therapy has proven inadequate. Imipramine is recommended as an alternative pharmacological therapy for stress incontinence when the first-line agents have proven unsatisfactory (Fantl et al., 1996).

Medications used to treat detrusor overactivity are anticholinergic and antispasmodic agents. The purpose of these medications is to relax the bladder and increase bladder capacity. Several new medications have been introduced that provide extended bladder control with less side effects than the traditional anticholinergics. Tricyclic antidepressants include imipramine, doxepin, desipramine, and nortriptyline. Medications not as well documented but considered useful are calcium-channel blocking agents (e.g., terodiline) (Fantl et al., 1996).

Anticholinergic agents are the primary pharmacological therapy for patients with detrusor instability as well as those with uninhibited and reflex neurogenic bladder dysfunction. With many new options coming onto the market, nurses are advised to consult a pharmacist on the benefits and risks associated with medications. Anticholinergics are used to decrease urinary frequency in patients with urge incontinence or uninhibited bladder. In this situation the PVR volume is checked on instituting or adjusting these medications to ensure that emptying has not been compromised. In persons with reflex bladder who void with high pressures or when bladder emptying is incomplete, they may be used as an adjunct to intermittent catheterization with the goals of normalizing bladder pressures and establishing continence between catheterizations.

Surgical Treatment

Surgical treatment of urinary incontinence should be considered only after a comprehensive clinical evaluation, including an estimation of the surgical risk, confirmation of the diagnosis and severity, correlation of anatomic and physiological findings with the surgery planned, and an estimation of the impact of the surgical procedure on the quality of the person's life (Fantl et al., 1996).

In addition to the surgeries listed in Table 18-8 several surgical procedures are available for the care of neurogenic bladder dysfunction. Most often these surgeries are indicated in persons with reflex neurogenic bladder when conservative bladder management has failed to maintain a low-pressure, nonrefluxing system. They include transurethral sphincterotomy, placement of a sphincter stint, augmentation enterocystoplasty, continent diversion, and neurostimulators.

Transurethral sphincterotomy is a surgery that has been useful in managing DSD in males when medications to reduce spasticity of the bladder neck and sphincter have been ineffective and bladder outlet obstruction contributes to high bladder pressures. The indications for transurethral sphincterotomy include detrusor-sphincter dyssynergia, bladder wall

TABLE 18-8 Surgical Management of Urinary Incontience

Type of Urinary Incontinence	Cause	Treatment
Stress	Hypermobility	Retropubic suspension, needle endoscopic suspension
Stress	Intrinsic sphincter deficiency	Sling (mostly female), artificial sphincter, urethral bulking
Urge	Refractory detrusor instability	Augmentation cystoplasty
Overflow	Obstruction Nonobstructive	Relieve obstruction Intermittent catheterization, other

trabeculations, persistent high voiding pressure, hydronephrosis, repeated urinary tract infections, vesicoureteral reflux, urolithiasis, and severe autonomic dysreflexia.

The procedure consists of visualizing the posterior urethra and making an incision at the 12 o'clock position. This procedure permanently opens the sphincter so men will void reflexively with low bladder pressures but will require an external condom collection device to manage leakage (Perkash, 1993). A newer procedure uses a wire mesh stent placed at the external sphincter and bulbous urethra to drain the bladder at safe pressures (Revas, Abdill, & Chancellor, 1996).

In augmentation enterocystoplasty, a short section of small intestine is removed and sutured into place over the bladder (detubularized), which has been bivalved in the sagittal plane, creating a large, low-pressure urinary reservoir. If limited hand function prevents independent urethral catheterization, a continent stoma can be created by bringing an intussuscepted limb of bowel through the anterior abdominal wall and creating a continent stoma, which can be catheterized more easily. Continent diversions generally are reserved for those persons who have undergone prior cystectomy or those with severe urethral dysfunction (Bennett & Bennett, 1993).

There are many subtypes of continent diversions. Most consist of creating a neobladder from detubularized small intestine and creating an efferent nipple valve to form the continent stoma, as previously described, and creating

an afferent nipple valve to form a nonrefluxing attachment for the ureters to pass into the neobladder (Bennett & Bennett, 1993).

New developments in neurourology that are generating excitement are neuromodulation and neurostimulation. Several types of neuroprosthesis are in use or under investigation, including external stimulators that restore micturition. These spinal nerve stimulators consist of an electrical pulse generator with electrodes placed either intradurally or extradurally at the S2-S3 spinal segments. The next frontier of neuroprosthetics is the application of myoplasty, transposed skeletal muscle, coupled with neurostimulation to restore function to dysfunctional smooth muscle structures of the bladder and sphincters (Chancellor & Revas, 1996).

SUMMARY

Managing bladder elimination problems is an integral component of rehabilitation nursing practice. As described in this chapter, rehabilitation nurses use a number of interventions to promote continence or reduce frequency of incontinence. Many of the treatments fall within the independent realm of nursing practice. Other treatments require collaboration with physicians and are within the interdependent scope of nursing practice; however, nursing care is essential to the successful outcomes of the treatments.

Case Study

A parish nurse is doing grief counseling with the oldest daughter of an elderly couple. The father has just died, and the daughter is worried about her mother. "With Dad gone, I am not sure what will happen with my mother. I would love to have her home with me. My husband is very supportive and loves my mother, but I know he just couldn't deal with her urinary incontinence. I wish there were something I could do. She gets so embarrassed and feels so bad." The parish nurse asks, "Has your mother ever been evaluated for her incontinence?" The daughter replies, "No, I don't think so; we all thought it was just something that happens when a woman gets older." The parish nurse answers, "Actually, there is a lot that can be done to treat urinary incontinence. A friend of mine is a rehabilitation nurse who has her own continence practice. If you would like, I can give you her number and you can make an appointment for your mother." The daughter responds, "Oh, that would be great! It would be such a blessing if Mom could get help for this problem. It would make the difference between having to think about a nursing home and living with us."

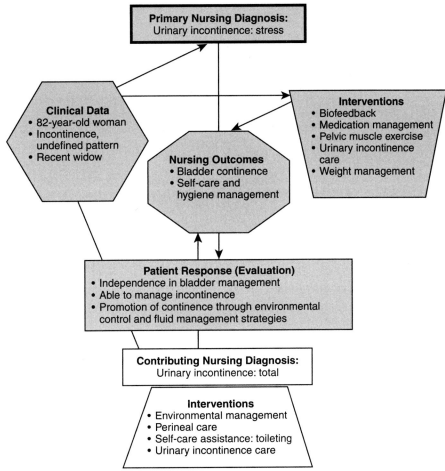

Concept Map. Mrs. Jones' problem with urinary incontinence has not been assessed. It is likely a problem with stress incontinence, but could be more complex, as a total incontinence pattern. Interventions should be directed at assessment with identification of strategies that match the cause and pattern of incontinence. The rehabilitation nurse will focus on coordinating interventions to achieve the outcomes of incontinence management.

CRITICAL THINKING

1. The daughter brings her mother to your outpatient clinic for evaluation. As a rehabilitation nurse, list key questions and assessments you would consider for this patient.

2. Your patient has more cognitive deficits than functional deficits. How would you instruct the daughter to document the patient's current voiding pattern?

3. List a goal for this patient and a urinary continence program you would recommend to your patient and her daughter.

REFERENCES

Abrams, P., Blaivas, J. G., Stanton, S. L., & Andersen, J. T. (1988). The standardization of terminology of lower urinary tract function. *Scandinavian Journal of Urology and Nephrology, 114*, 5-9.

Abrams, P., Fenely, R., & Torrens, M. (1983). *Urodynamics*. New York: Springer-Verlag.

Arcudi, L., Ruello, C., Maqaudda, A., & Medieri, M. (1992) Voiding disorders in patients with cerebrovascular disease. *Functional Neurology, 7*, 47-49.

Association of Rehabilitation Nurses. (2005). *Definition of rehabilitation nursing*. Retrieved August 27, 2006, from http://rehabnurse.org/about/definition.html.

Athwal, B. S., Berkley, K. J., Hussain, I., Brennan, A., Craggs, M., Sakakibara, R., et al. (2001). Brain responses to changes in bladder volume and urge to void in healthy men. *Brain, 124*, 369-377.

Barat, M. (1998). Botulinum A toxin treatment for detrusor-sphincter dyssynergia in spinal cord disease. *Spinal Cord, 36*, 91-94.

Bates, P., Bradley, W. E., & Glen, E. (1979). The standardization of terminology of lower urinary tract function. *Journal of Urology, 121*, 551-554.

Bennett, C. J., & Bennett, J. K. (1993). Augmentation cystoplasty and urinary diversion in patients with spinal cord injury. *Physical Medicine and Rehabilitation Clinics of North America, 4*, 377-389.

Blaivas, J. G. (1990). Diagnostic evaluation of incontinence in patients with neurogenic disorders. *Journal of the American Geriatrics Society, 38*, 306-310.

Brandeis, G. H., Baumann, M. M., Hossain, M., Morris, J. N., & Resnick, N. M. (1997). The prevalence of potentially remediable urinary incontinence in frail older people: A study using the Minimum Data Set. *Journal of the American Geriatrics Society, 45*, 179-184.

Burgio, K., Locher, J., Roth, D., & Goode, P. (2001). Psychological improvements associated with behavioral and drug treatment of urge incontinence in older women. *Journal of Gerontological, Behavioral, Psychological Science and Sociology Science, 56*(1), 46-51.

Burgio, K. L., & Engel, B. T. (1990). Biofeedback-assisted behavioral training for elderly men and women. *Journal of the American Geriatrics Society, 38*, 338-340.

Burgio, L. D., & Burgio, K. L. (1990). Institutional staff training and management: A review of the literature and a model for geriatric, long-term-care facilities. *International Journal of Aging and Human Development, 4*, 287-302.

Chancellor, M. B., & Revas, D. A. (1996). Neuromodulation and neurostimulation in urology. *Topics in Spinal Cord Injury Rehabilitation, 1*(5), 18-35.

Consortium for Spinal Cord Medicine. (2001). *Acute management of autonomic dysreflexia.* Washington, D.C.: Paralyzed Veterans of America. Available from http://www.NCSCIMS.org/home.

DeWachter, S. D., & Wyndale, J. (2003) Frequency-volume charts: A tool to evaluate bladder sensation. *Neurourology and Urodynamics, 22,* 638-642.

Diokno, A. C., Normelle, O. P., Brown, M. B., & Herzog, A. R. (1990). Urodynamic tests for female geriatric urinary incontinence. *Urology, 36,* 431-439.

Dochterman, J. M., & Bulechek, G. M. (2004). *Nursing interventions classification (NIC)* (4th ed.). St. Louis, MO: Mosby.

Doughty, D. B. (Ed.). (2006). *Urinary and fecal incontinence: Nursing management* (3rd ed.). St. Louis, MO: Mosby.

Dowling-Castronovo, A. (2001). *Urinary continence assessment. Try this: Best practices in nursing care to older adults.* Hartford, CT: The Hartford Institute for Geriatric Nursing.

Engberg, S., Sereika, S. M., McDowell, B. J., Weber, E., & Brodak, I. (2002). Effectiveness of prompted voiding in treating urinary incontinence in cognitively impaired homebound older adults. *Journal of wound, ostomy, and continence nursing, 29,* 252-265.

Erickson, R. P. (1980). Autonomic dysreflexia: Pathophysiology and medical management. *Archives of Physical Medicine and Rehabilitation, 61,* 431-440.

Fantl, J. A., Newman, D. K., Colling, J., DeLancey, J., Keeys, C., Loughery, R., et al. (1996, March). *Urinary incontinence in adults: Acute and chronic management* (AHCPR Publication No. 96-0682, Clinical Practice Guideline No. 2, 1996 Update). Rockville, MD: U.S. Department of Health and Human Services, Public Health Service, Agency for Health Care Policy and Research.

Folstein, M., Folstein, S., & McHugh, P. (2007). The Mini Mental State Examination. Psychological Assessment Resources, Inc., Lutz, FL.

Gray, M. I. (1992). *Genitourinary disorders.* St. Louis, MO: Mosby.

Gray, M. I. (2000). Physiology of voiding. In D.B. Doughty (Ed.), *Urinary and fecal incontinence: Nursing management* (2nd ed., pp. 1-27). St. Louis, MO: Mosby.

Grimby, A., Milsom, I., Molander, U., Wiklund, I., & Ekelund, P. (1993). The influence of urinary incontinence on the quality of life of elderly women. *Age and Ageing, 22,* 82-89.

Guerrero, P., & Sinert, R. (2001). Urinary incontinence. *Emergency medicine/genitourinary,* eMedicine.com inc. Available from http://www.knowledge.emedicine.com.

Guyton, A. C., & Hall, J. E. (1996). *Textbook of medical physiology* (9th ed., pp. 405-421). Philadelphia: W. B. Saunders.

Haley, R. W., Hooton, T. M., Culver, D. H., Stanley, R. C., Emori, T. G., Hardison, C. D., et al. (1981). Nosocomial infections in U.S. hospitals, 1975-1976: Estimated frequency by selected characteristics of patients. *American Journal of Medicine, 70,* 947-959.

Hampel, C., Weinhold, D., Brekan, N., Eggersman, C., & Thuroff, J. W. (1997). Prevalence of overactive bladder and epidemiology of urinary incontinence. *Urology, 50* (Suppl. 6A), 4-14.

Hooton, T. (1999). Uncomplicating urinary tract infections. In: *Program and abstracts of the 39th Interscience Conference on Antimicrobial Agents and Chemotherapy.* Washington, D.C.: American Society for Microbiology.

Jeter, K. F., Faller, N., & Norton, C. (1990). *Nursing for continence.* Philadelphia: W. B. Saunders.

Kane, R., Ouslander, J., & Abrass, I. (1994) *Essentials of clinical geriatrics* (3rd ed.). New York: McGraw-Hill.

King, R. B., Carlson, C. E., Mervine, J., Wu, Y., & Yarkony, G. (1992). Clean and sterile intermittent catheterization methods in hospitalized patients with spinal cord injury. *Archives of Physical Medicine and Rehabilitation, 73,* 798-802.

Kong, K. H., & Young, S. (2000). Incidence and outcome of post-stroke urinary retention: A prospective study. *Archives of Physical Medicine and Rehabilitation, 81,* 1464-1467.

Kuric, J., & Hixon, A. K. (1996). *Clinical practice guideline: Autonomic dysreflexia.* Jackson Heights, NY: Eastern Paralyzed Veterans Association.

Kurnick, N. B. (1956). Autonomic hyperreflexia and its control in patients with spinal cord lesions. *Annals of Internal Medicine, 44,* 678-686.

Lapides, J., & Diokno, A. C. (1976). Urine transport, storage, and micturition. In J. Lapides (Ed.), *Fundamentals of urology.* Philadelphia: W. B. Saunders.

Lekan-Rutledge, D., & Colling, J. (2003). Urinary incontinence in the frail elderly. *American Journal of Nursing, 103,* 36-46.

Lloyd, E. E., Giroux, J., & Toth. L. (1988). Alterations in bladder elimination. In P. H. Mitchell, L. C. Hodges, M. Muwaswe, & S. C. A. Wallack (Eds.), *AANN's neuroscience nursing phenomena and practice.* Norwalk, CT: Appleton & Lange.

Lyons, S. S., & Pringle Specht, J. K. (1999). *Evidence based protocol, prompted voiding for persons with urinary incontinence.* Iowa City, IA: The University of Iowa Nursing Interventions Research Center Research Dissemination Core.

McCourt, A. (1993). *The specialty practice of rehabilitation nursing: A core curriculum* (3rd. ed., pp. 104-107). Skokie, IL: Rehabilitation Nursing Foundation.

McDowell, B. J., Engberg, S., Sereika, S., Donovan, N., Jubeck, M. E., Weber, E., et al. (1999). Effectiveness of behavioral therapy to treat incontinence in homebound older adults. *Journal of the American Geriatrics Society, 47*(3), 309-318.

NANDA International. (2005). *Nursing diagnoses: Definitions and classification, 2005-2006* (6th ed.). Philadelphia: Author.

Newman, D. K. (2002). *Managing and treating urinary incontinence.* Baltimore, MD: Health Professions Press.

Newman, D. K., & Palmer, M. H. (1999). Incontinence and PPS: New era. *Ostomy/Wound Management, 45,* 12, 32-50.

Nygaard, I. E., Thompson, F. L., Svengalis, S. L., & Albright, J. P. (1994). Urinary incontinence in elite nulliparous athletes. *Obstetrics and Gynecology, 84,* 183-187.

Ouslander, J. G. (1989). A symptomatic bacteriuria and incontinence [Letter]. *Journal of the American Geriatrics Society, 37,* 197-198.

Perkash, I. (1993). Long-term urologic management of the patient with spinal cord injury. *Urologic Clinics of North America, 20,* 423-434.

Peschers, U., Jundt, K., & Dimpfl, T. (2000). Differences between cough and Valsalva leak-point pressure in stress incontinent women. *Neurological Urodynamics, 19*(6), 677-681.

Petit, H., Wiart, L., Gaujard, E., Le Breton, F., Ferriere, J. M., Lagueny, A., et al. (1998). Botulinum A toxin treatment for detrusor-sphincter dyssynergia in spinal cord disease. *Spinal Cord, 36*(2), 91-94.

Phelan, M. W., Franks, M., Somogyi, G. T., Yokoyama, T., Fraser, M., Lavelle, J., et al. (2001). Botulinum toxin urethral sphincter injection to restore bladder emptying in men and women with voiding dysfunction. *The Journal of Urology, 165,* 1107-1110.

Pires, M., & Lockhart-Pretti, P. A. (1992). *Nursing management of neurogenic incontinence: An independent study module.* Skokie, IL: Rehabilitation Nursing Foundation.

Rathe, R., & Klioze, A. (2000). Basic clinical skills. *Integrated medical curriculum.* Gainesville: University of Florida.

Registered Nurses Association of Ontario. (2005). *Promoting continence using prompted voiding.* Toronto, Canada: Registered Nurses Association of Ontario. Available from http://www.rnao.org/bestpractices/pdf/bpg_continence.pdf.

Resnick, N. (1996). Geriatric incontinence. *Urologic Clinics of North America 23,* 55-74.

Resnick, N. M., & Yalla, S. V. (1985). Management of urinary incontinence in the elderly. *New England Journal of Medicine, 313,* 800-805.

Revas, D. A., Abdill, C. K., & Chancellor, M. B. (1996). Current management of detrusor sphincter dyssynergia. *Topics in Spinal Cord Injury Rehabilitation, 1*(5), 18-35.

Schurch, B., Hauri, D., Rodic, B., Curt, A., Meyer, M., Rossier, A. B. (1996). Botulinum-A toxin as a treatment of detrusor-sphincter dyssynergia: A prospective study in 24 spinal cord injury patients. *Journal of Urology, 155,* 1023-1029.

Schwartz, M. S. (1995). *Biofeedback: A practitioner's guide.* New York: Guilford Press.

Siroky, M. B., & Krane, R. J. (1982). Neurologic aspects of detrusor-sphincter dyssynergia, with reference to the guarding reflex. *Journal of Urology, 127,* 953-957.

Society of Urologic Nurses and Associates. (2005). *Clinical practice guidelines–Care of the patient with an indwelling catheter.* Available from http://www.suna.org/clinicalpracticeguidelines.

Stevens, E. (2005). Bladder ultrasound: Avoiding unnecessary catheterizations. *Medsurg Nursing, 14,* 249-253.

Stoher, M., Oepel, M., Kondo, A., Kramer, G. M., Madersbacher, H., Millard, R., et al. (1999). The standardization of terminology in neurogenic lower tract dysfunction. *Neurourology and Urodynamics, 18,* 139-158.

Tanagho, E. A. (1990). Electrical stimulation. *Journal of the American Geriatrics Society, 38,* 352-355.

Tannenbaum, C., Perrin, L., DuBeau, C. E., & Kuchel, G. A. (2001). Diagnosis and management of urinary incontinence in the older patient. *Archives of Physical Medicine and Rehabilitation, 82,* 134-138.

Teasdale, T., Taffet, G., Luchi, R., & Adam, E. (1988). Urinary incontinence in a community-residing elderly population. *Journal of the American Geriatrics Society, 36,* 600-606.

Urinary Incontinence Guideline Panel. (1992a). *Urinary incontinence in adults: Quick reference guide for clinicians* (AHCPR Publication No. 92-0041).

Rockville, MD: Agency for Health Care Policy and Research, Public Health Service, U.S. Department of Health and Human Services.

Urinary Incontinence Guideline Panel. (1992b). *Urinary incontinence in adults: Clinical practice guidelines* (AHCPR Publication No. 92-0038). Rockville, MD: Agency for Health Care Policy and Research, Public Health Service, U.S. Department of Health and Human Services.

Vickrey, B. G., Shekelle, P., Morton S. Clark, K., Pathak, M., & Kamberg C. (1999). *Prevention and management of urinary tract infections in paralyzed persons.* (Evidence Report/Technology Assessment No. 6, Prepared by Southern California Evidence-Based Practice Center RAND under Contract No. 290-97-0001, AHCPR Publication No. 99-E008). Rockville, MD: Agency for Health Care Policy and Research.

Vodusek, D. B., Plevnik, S., Vrtacnik, P., & Janez, J. (1998). Detrusor inhibition on selective pudendal nerve stimulation in the perineum. *Neurology Urodynamics, 6,* 389-393.

Warren, J. W., Muncie, H. L., Jr., Hebel, J. R., & Hall-Craggs, M. (1994). Long-term urethral catheterization increases risk of chronic pyelonephritis and renal inflammation. *Journal of the American Geriatrics Society, 42,* 1286-1290.

Wheeler, J. S., Niceestro, R. M., & Goggin, C. (1988). Urinary incontinence: Diagnosing the problem. *Journal of Enterostomal Therapy, 15*(6), 240.

Williams, M. E., & Gaylord, S. A. (1990). Role of functional assessment in the evaluation of urinary incontinence: National Institutes of Health Consensus Development Conference on Urinary Incontinence in Adults. Bethesda, MD, October 3-5, 1988. *Journal of the American Geriatrics Society, 38,* 296-299.

Wong, E., & Hooton, T. M. (1981). *Guideline for the prevention of catheter-associated urinary tract infections.* Retrieved August 2006 from http://www.cdc.gov/ncidod/dhqp/gl_catheter_assoc.html.

Wyman, J. F. (1988). Nursing assessment of the incontinent geriatric outpatient population. *Nursing Clinics of North America, 23,* 169-187.

Wyman, J. F. (2003) Treatment of urinary incontinence in men and older women. *American Journal of Nursing, 103*(3, Suppl.), 26-35.

Wyman, J. F., Choi, S. C., Harkins, S. W., Wilson, M. S., & Fantl, J. A. (1988). The urinary diary in evaluation of incontinent women: A test-retest analysis. *Obstetrics and Gynecology, 71,* 812-817.

Yarnell, J., Richards, C., & Stephenson, T. (1981). The prevalence and severity of urinary incontinence in women. *Journal of Epidemiology and Community Health, 35,* 71-74.

Zimmerman, D. R., & Karon, S. L. (1995) Development and testing of nursing home quality indicators. *Health Care Financing Review, 16,* 107.

APPENDIX 18A: AUTONOMIC DYSREFLEXIA*

Pathophysiology of Autonomic Dysreflexia (AD)

Autonomic dysreflexia occurs after the phase of spinal shock in which reflexes return. Individuals with injuries above the major splanchnic outflow have the potential of developing autonomic dysreflexia.

The major splanchnic outflow is T6 through L2 (the level of the second lumbar vertebra). Intact sensory nerves below the level of the injury transmit impulses to the spinal cord, which ascend in the spinothalamic and posterior columns. Sympathetic neurons in the intermediolateral gray matter are stimulated by these ascending impulses. Sympathetic inhibitory impulses that originate above T6 are blocked as a result of the injury. Therefore, below the injury, there is a relatively unopposed sympathetic outflow (T6 through L2) with a release of norepinephrine, dopamine-beta-hydroxylase, and dopamine.

The release of these chemicals may cause piloerection, skin pallor, and severe vasoconstriction in the arterial vasculature, which can cause a sudden elevation in blood pressure. The elevated blood pressure may cause a headache. Intact carotid and aortic baroreceptors detect the hypertension.

Normally two vasomotor brainstem reflexes occur in an attempt to lower the blood pressure. (Parasympathetic activity originating from the dorsal motor nucleus of the vagus nerve—cranial nerve X—continues following a spinal cord injury.) The first compensatory mechanism is to increase parasympathetic stimulation to the heart via the vagus nerve to cause bradycardia. However, this bradycardia cannot compensate for the severe vasoconstriction. According to Poiseuille's formula, pressure in a tube is affected to the fourth power by change in radius (vasoconstriction) and only linearly by change in the flow rate (bradycardia). The second compensatory reflex is an increase in sympathetic inhibitory outflow from vasomotor centers above the spinal cord injury. However, the inhibitory impulses are unable to pass below the injury, and above the level of injury there may be profuse sweating and vasodilation with skin flushing (Erickson, 1980; Kurnick, 1956).

Signs and Symptoms

An individual may have one or more of the following signs or symptoms when he or she is having an episode of autonomic dysreflexia. Symptoms may be minimal or even absent, despite an elevated blood pressure. Some of the more common symptoms are:

- Elevation of systolic blood pressure more that 15 to 20 mm Hg above baseline in adolescents with SCI or more that 15 mm Hg above baseline in children with SCI may be a sign of AD.
- A sudden and significant increase in both the systolic and diastolic blood pressure above their usual levels, usually associated with bradycardia. **An individual with SCI above T6 often has a normal systolic blood pressure in the 90 to 110 mm Hg range.** Therefore a blood pressure of 20 mm to 40 mm Hg above baseline may be a sign of autonomic dysreflexia.
- Pounding headache.
- Profuse sweating above the level of the lesion, especially in the face, neck, and shoulders, or possibly below the level of the lesion.
- Goose bumps above or possibly below the level of the lesion.
- Flushing of the skin above the level of the lesion, especially in the face, neck, and shoulders, or possibly below the level of lesion.
- Blurred vision.
- Appearance of spots in the patient's visual fields.
- Nasal congestion.
- Feelings of apprehension or anxiety over an impending physical problem.
- Minimal or no symptoms, despite an elevated blood pressure.
- Cardiac arrhythmias, atrial fibrillation, ventricular contractions, and atrioventricular conduction abnormalities.

---

*From Consortium for Spinal Cord Medicine. (2001) Acute management of autonomic dysreflexia. Clinical practice guidelines. Washington, D.C.: Paralyzed Veterans of America. Reprinted with permission.

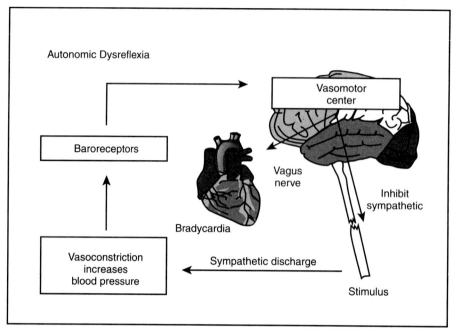

From Consortium for Spinal Cord Medicine. (2001). *Acute management of autonomic dysreflexia: Clinical practice guidelines*. Washington, D.C.: Paralyzed Veterans of America. Reprinted with permission. Available at http://www.pva.org.

Causes

Autonomic dysreflexia has many potential causes. It is essential that the specific cause be identified and treated in order to resolve an episode of autonomic dysreflexia. Following are some of the more common causes (Kuric & Hixon, 1996):

- Bladder distention
- Urinary tract infection
- Bladder or kidney stones
- Cystoscopy, urodynamics, or detrusor sphincter dyssynergia
- Epididymitis or scrotal compression
- Bowel distention
- Bowel impaction
- Gallstones
- Gastric ulcers or gastritis
- Invasive testing
- Hemorrhoids
- Gastrocolic irritation
- Appendicitis or another abdominal pathology or trauma
- Menstruation
- Boosting (an episode of AD intentionally caused by an athlete with SCI in an attempt to enhance physical performances).
- Pregnancy, especially labor and delivery
- Vaginitis
- Sexual intercourse

- Sexually transmitted diseases (STDs)
- Ejaculation
- Epididymitis
- Scrotal compression
- Electroejaculation and vibratory stimulation to induce an ejaculation
- Deep vein thrombosis
- Pulmonary emboli
- Pressure ulcers
- Ingrown toenail
- Burns or sunburn
- Blisters
- Insect bites
- Contact with hard or sharp objects
- Constrictive clothing, shoes, or appliances
- Heterotopic bone
- Fractures or other trauma
- Surgical or diagnostic procedures
- Pain
- Temperature fluctuations
- Any painful or irritating stimuli below the level of injury
- Substance abuse
- Excessive caffeine or other diuretic intake
- Excessive alcohol intake

Summary of Treatment Recommendations for Autonomic Dysfunction

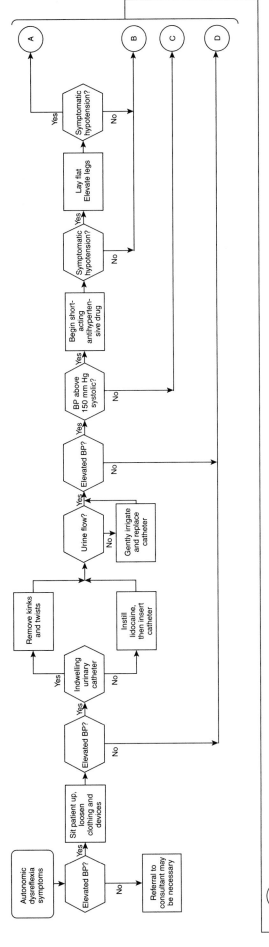

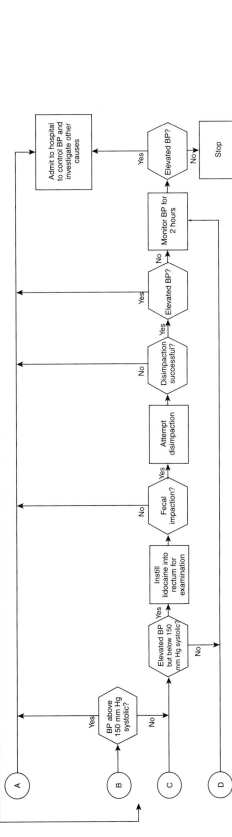

From Consortium for Spinal Cord Medicine. (2001). *Acute management of autonomic dysreflexia: Clinical practice guidelines.* Washington, D.C.: Paralyzed Veterans of America. Reprinted with permission. Available at http://www.pva.org.

Treatment Recommendations

NOTE: Pregnant women should be referred to an appropriate consultant.

1. Check the individual's blood pressure.
2. If the blood pressure is not elevated, refer the individual to a consultant, if necessary.
3. If the blood pressure is elevated and the individual is supine, immediately sit the person up.
4. Loosen any clothing or constrictive devices.
5. Monitor the blood pressure and pulse frequently.
6. Quickly survey the individual for the instigating causes, beginning with the urinary system.
7. If an indwelling urinary catheter is not in place, catheterize the individual.
8. Before inserting the catheter, instill 2% lidocaine jelly (if readily available) into the urethra and wait several minutes.
9. If the individual has an indwelling urinary catheter, check the system along its entire length for kinks, folds, constrictions, or obstructions and for correct placement of the indwelling catheter. If a problem is found, correct it immediately.
10. If the catheter appears to be blocked, gently irrigate the bladder with a small amount of fluid (10 to 15 cc), such as normal saline at body temperature. Irrigation should be 5 to 10 ml for children under 2 years of age and 10 to 15 ml in older children and adolescents. Avoid manually compressing or tapping on the bladder.
11. If the catheter is draining and the blood pressure remains elevated, proceed with step 16.
12. If the catheter is not draining and the blood pressure remains elevated, remove and replace the catheter.
13. Prior to replacing the catheter, instill 2% lidocaine jelly (if readily available) into the urethra and wait several minutes.
14. If the catheter cannot be replaced, consider attempting to pass a coudé catheter, or consult a urologist.
15. Monitor the individual's blood pressure during bladder drainage.
16. If acute symptoms of autonomic dysreflexia persist, including a sustained elevated blood pressure, suspect fecal impaction.
17. If the elevated blood pressure is at or above 150 mm Hg systolic, consider pharmacologic management to reduce the systolic blood pressure without causing hypotension before checking for fecal impaction. If the blood pressure remains elevated but is less than 150 mm Hg systolic, proceed to step 20.
18. Use an antihypertensive agent with rapid onset and short duration while the causes of autonomic dysreflexia are being investigated.
19. Monitor the individual for symptomatic hypotension.
20. If fecal impaction is suspected, and the elevated blood pressure is less than 150 mm Hg systolic, check the rectum for stool, using the following procedure: With a gloved hand, instill a topical anesthetic agent such as 2% lidocaine jelly generously into the rectum. Wait 2 minutes for sensation in the area to decrease. Then, with a gloved hand, insert a lubricated finger into the rectum and check for the presence of stool. If present, gently remove, if possible. If autonomic dysreflexia becomes worse, stop the manual evacuation. Instill additional topical anesthetic and recheck the rectum for the presence of stool after approximately 20 minutes.
21. Monitor the individual's symptoms and blood pressure for at least 2 hours after resolution of the autonomic dysreflexia episode to make sure that it does not recur.
22. If there is poor response to the treatment specified above or if the cause of the dysreflexia has not been identified, strongly consider admitting the individual to the hospital to be monitored, to maintain pharmacologic control of the blood pressure, and to investigate other causes of the dysreflexia.
23. Document the episode in the individual's medical record. This record should include the presenting signs and symptoms and their course, treatment instituted, recordings of blood pressure and pulse, and response to treatment. The effectiveness of the treatment may be evaluated according to the level of outcome criteria reached:
    - The cause of the autonomic dysreflexia episode has been identified.
    - The blood pressure has been restored to normal limits for the individual (usually 90 to 110 mm Hg systolic for a tetraplegic person in the sitting position).
    - The pulse rate has been restored to normal limits.
    - The individual is comfortable, with no signs or symptoms of autonomic dysreflexia, of increased intracranial pressure, or of heart failure.
24. After the individual with spinal cord injury has been stabilized, review the precipitating cause with the individual, members of the individual's family, significant others, and care givers. This process entails adjusting the treatment plan to ensure that future episodes are recognized and treated to prevent a medical crisis or, ideally, are avoided altogether. The process also entails discussion of autonomic dysreflexia in the spinal cord injury individual's education program, so that he or she will be able to recognize early onset and obtain help as quickly as possible. It is recommended that an individual with a spinal cord injury be given a written description of treatment for autonomic dysreflexia at the time of discharge that can be referred to in an emergency.

19

Bowel Elimination and Regulation

Aloma R. Gender, MSN, RN, CRRN

Fecal incontinence affects many persons with disabilities and chronic illness. A humiliating and devastating condition, fecal incontinence can lead to social isolation and low self-esteem. Many elderly persons are placed in long-term care facilities prematurely because of the burden of caring for an incontinent adult at home.

Other persons with disabilities limit their activities outside of the home for fear of incontinence (Stiens, Bergman, & Goetz, 1997). In a study of 115 persons with spinal cord injury (SCI), researchers found that for 54%, bowel management was a source of emotional upset because of the frequency of fecal incontinence and the time needed for toileting (Glickman & Kamm, 1996). Disorders of regularity, such as constipation or diarrhea, also cause considerable difficulties for many; the estimated prevalence of constipation ranges from 2% to 34% of the population (Cheskin, Kamal, Crowell, Schuster, & Whitehead, 1995).

Managing altered bowel elimination is a key responsibility for a rehabilitation nurse. Effective bowel training programs can control incontinence and prevent constipation and diarrhea. The goal of this chapter is to enable the reader to develop effective bowel programs through knowledge of normal and altered bowel physiology, an in-depth assessment of bowel function, and accurate identification of causative and contributing factors (Doughty, 2006).

LIFE SPAN ISSUES ASSOCIATED WITH ALTERED BOWEL ELIMINATION PATTERNS

Control of bowel function is a basic human need that is the subject of varying levels of concern throughout a person's life. Children learn early that successful control of bowel function gains them praise and signifies that they are maturing. They learn that control of elimination is valued and that lack of control can be humiliating. Patterns of elimination change throughout the life span. Infants from birth to 1 year of age lack neuromuscular maturity to control their bowels; toddlers are physically ready for bowel control at 18 to 24 months, although cognitive and psychosocial readiness may be achieved later. Daytime control usually occurs at 30 months. Constipation can be common among preschool and school-age children because of fevers, dietary changes, or emotional and environmental changes. A characteristic individual elimination pattern usually is established at this time. As children mature into adolescence and then young and middle-age adulthood, other developmental tasks become primary and bowel function receives little thought. Bowel patterns vary with dietary intake, lifestyle, exercise, and emotional state. Irregular meals, changing schedules, and increased stress all affect elimination.

Bowel function reemerges as a concern for some elders who believe a regular or routine bowel habit is essential to maintain health. Belief in a daily bowel movement stems from the theory of autointoxication, developed in the early 1900s by Sir Arbuthnot Lane (Ross, 1993). This theory postulated that fluids in the colon were in a constant interchange with the blood current and that without regular elimination, a person could contract self-poisoning and a variety of diseases and illnesses. Many people raised during this era were led to believe that regular catharsis, such as laxatives, was necessary for good health (Brocklehurst, 1980). Today advertisements continue to promote products that prevent constipation and imply benefits from a daily bowel movement. Despite the heightened awareness of bowel function and habits, most people decline to think or talk about the subject until faced with a problem in controlling or regulating function.

ANATOMY AND PHYSIOLOGY

Normal Bowel Function

Bowel elimination is the process by which the body excretes waste products. Undigested dietary matter passes through the gastrointestinal (GI) tract after nutrients and water have been extracted for use by the body. The alimentary tract (Figure 19-1) provides the body with a continual supply of water, electrolytes, and nutrients through digestion and absorption. Digestion of food occurs in the stomach, duodenum, jejunum, and ileum; absorption occurs in the small intestine and the proximal half of the colon. A myriad of autoregulatory processes keeps food moving along the GI tract at an appropriate pace for digestion and absorption and to provide the body with nutrients. Defecation of undigested or unabsorbed food involves complex integration of voluntary regulation by the central nervous system, as well as involuntary intrinsic reflex mechanisms (Heitkemper, 2000). Any interruption of these mechanisms may result in impaired bowel function. In this section, normal function of the GI tract is discussed in relation to those functions that affect bowel elimination: secretion, innervation, functional movements, and defecation (Guyton & Hall, 2006).

Secretion. Secretory glands located throughout the GI tract serve two primary functions. First, digestive enzymes are produced from the mouth to the end of the ileum. The appropriate amount of enzymes and electrolytes are formed and secreted in response to food in the alimentary tract for proper digestion. Second, glands located from the mouth to the anus produce mucus to protect and lubricate the walls of the tract and to ease the passage of food and partially digested products.

Innervation. The GI tract is composed of several layers of smooth muscle fibers, which are arranged in bundles. In the longitudinal muscle layer (Figure 19-2) the bundles extend longitudinally down the intestinal tract, and the circular muscle layer bundles extend around the gut. The muscle fibers within each bundle are electrically connected so signals can transmit from one fiber to the next.

Electrical Activity. The smooth muscle undergoes almost continual but slow electrical activity with two types of electrical waves: (1) slow waves and (2) spikes. Slow waves produce rhythmic contractions. Spike waves produce tonic contractions, as may also hormones or the entry of calcium ions into the interior of the cell. Tonic contractions maintain a steady pressure on the contents of the GI tract, whereas rhythmic contractions regulate phasic functions, such as mixing of food and peristalsis (Guyton & Hall, 2006). The internal anal sphincter, a circular smooth muscle (Figure 19-3), maintains a state of tonic contraction and safeguards against small amounts of fecal material escaping into the anal canal.

Intrinsic Neural Control. The GI tract has its own enteric nervous system that lies entirely in the wall of the gut, beginning in the esophagus and extending to the anus. This system is important in controlling gastrointestinal movements and secretion. The enteric nervous system is composed of two plexuses: (1) the outer or myenteric (motor) plexus, located between the longitudinal and circular muscle layers, and (2) the inner plexus, which is called Meissner's plexus or submucosal (sensory) plexus, that lies in the submucosa (see Figure 19-2). The myenteric plexus is far more extensive and controls GI movements; the submucosal plexus controls gastrointestinal secretion and local blood flow. The enteric nervous system allows the gut to continue to function in isolation from its extrinsic nerve supply; however, stimulation by the parasympathetic and sympathetic systems can greatly enhance or inhibit GI functions (Guyton & Hall, 2006).

Extrinsic Neural Control. Although the primary mediator for peristaltic activity is the intrinsic, or enteric, nervous system, the extrinsic innervation plays an important modulating role (Heitkemper, 2000). Extrinsic innervation includes both parasympathetic and sympathetic activity of the autonomic nervous system that may alter the overall activity of the gut or specific parts.

The parasympathetic cranial supply is transmitted almost entirely by the vagus nerve and provides extensive innervation to the esophagus, stomach, pancreas, and somewhat less to the intestines down through the first half of the large bowel. The parasympathetic sacral fibers originate in S2, S3, and S4 segments of the spinal cord and pass through the pelvic nerves to the distal half of the large intestine and all the way to

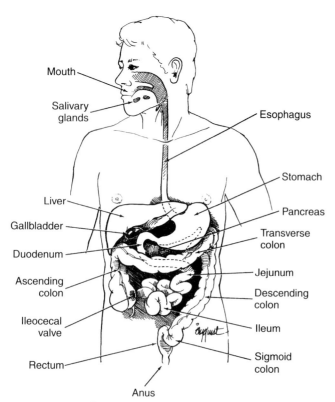

Figure 19-1 The alimentary tract.

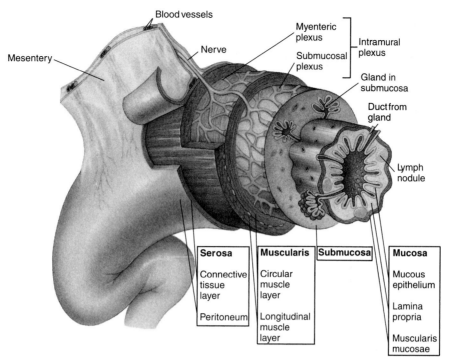

Figure 19-2 Wall of the gastrointestinal tract. (From Thibodeau, G. A., & Patton, K. T. [2007]. *Anatomy & physiology* [6th ed.]. St. Louis, MO: Mosby.)

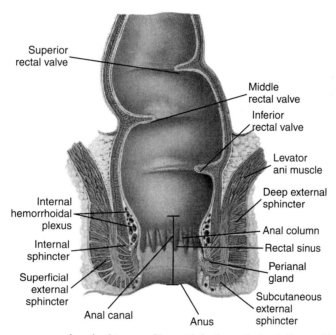

Figure 19-3 Anatomy of rectum, anus, and anal sphincters. (From Thibodeau, G. A., & Patton, K. T. [2007]. *Anatomy & physiology* [6th ed.]. St. Louis, MO: Mosby.)

the anus (Figure 19-4). The sigmoid, rectal, and anal regions of the large intestine are abundantly supplied with parasympathetic fibers that function to facilitate the defecation reflexes. The postganglionic neurons of the parasympathetic system are located in the myenteric and submucosal plexuses. Stimulation of these parasympathetic nerves causes increased activity of the entire enteric nervous system (Guyton & Hall, 2006).

The sympathetic fibers to the GI tract originate in the spinal cord between spinal cord segments T5 and L2 and innervate essentially the entire GI tract. The sympathetic nerve endings secrete mainly norepinephrine, but also small

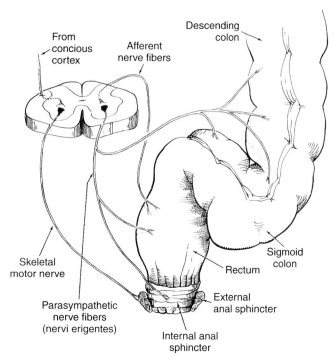

Figure 19-4 Afferent and efferent pathways of the parasympathetic mechanism for defecation reflex. (From Guyton, A. C., & Hall, J. E. [2006]. *Textbook of medical physiology* [11th ed.]. Philadelphia: W. B. Saunders.)

amounts of epinephrine. Stimulation of the sympathetic nervous system generally results in decreased activity of the GI tract, with effects opposite to parasympathetic stimulation. Strong stimulation can totally halt movement of food through the GI tract (Guyton & Hall, 2006).

The enteric nervous system and its connections with the sympathetic and parasympathetic systems support three types of reflexes that are important to GI control:

1. Reflexes that control GI secretion, peristalsis, mixing contractions, etc.
2. Gastrocolic reflex from the stomach that causes evacuation of the colon
3. Defecation reflexes that travel from the colon and rectum to the spinal cord and back (Guyton & Hall, 2006)

Functional Movements of the Gastrointestinal Tract.
Two basic types of movement occur in the GI tract: (1) mixing movements, which keep the intestinal contents blended thoroughly by contracting small segments of the gut wall, and (2) propulsive movements or peristalsis, which causes food to move along the GI tract at an appropriate rate for digestion and absorption. The usual stimulus for peristalsis is distention of the gut as with a collection of food. The stretching of the gut wall stimulates the enteric nervous system to contract the intestinal wall 2 to 3 cm behind this point. A contractile ring then forms and spreads along the gut tube, initiating peristalsis. Some mixing and propulsion occur simultaneously (Guyton & Hall, 2006).

The Oral Cavity. The ingestion of food begins with proper chewing of food for digestion because digestive enzymes act only on the surfaces of the food particles. The rate of digestion is highly dependent on the total surface area exposed to intestinal secretions. Grinding food into a fine consistency prevents excoriation of the GI tract and increases the ease with which food is emptied from the stomach into the small intestine and all succeeding segments of the gut (Guyton & Hall, 2006).

The Stomach. The stomach has three motor functions: (1) mixing of food with gastric secretions until it forms chyme, which is a semifluid mixture; (2) storage of large quantities of food until it can be accommodated by the lower portion of the GI tract; and (3) slow emptying of chyme into the small intestine at a rate suitable for proper digestion and absorption by the small intestine (Guyton & Hall, 2006).

The Small Intestine. The mixing contractions of the small intestine occur when chyme is present. The chyme elicits localized, concentric ringlike contractions spaced at intervals along the intestine, appearing as a chain of sausage. As one set of contractions subsides, another occurs at a different point along the small intestine, chopping and progressively mixing intestinal contents with secretions. Chyme is propelled through the small intestine by peristaltic activity or a series of waves caused by distention and excitation of the stretch receptors in the gut wall.

Passage of chyme from the pylorus to the ileocecal valve, between the small and large intestine, normally requires 3 to 5 hours. After meals this peristaltic activity is greatly increased because of the distention of the stomach and duodenum from chyme, which causes gastrocolic and duodenal reflexes (Beddar, Holder-Bennett, & McCormick, 1997). These reflexes stimulate the myenteric plexus to increase peristalsis and secretions in the small intestine. Hormones can also enhance intestinal motility, such as gastrin, insulin, motilin, and serotonin. These hormones are secreted during the phases of food processing (Guyton & Hall, 2006).

Although peristalsis in the small intestine is normally weak, intense irritation such as with infectious diarrhea, can cause a powerful peristalsis called a peristaltic rush. The waves travel the entire length of the small intestine quickly and can sweep contents of the small bowel into the colon within a few minutes, thus relieving irritation or distention (Guyton & Hall, 2006).

The ileocecal valve (see Figure 19-1) has the principal function of preventing backflow of fecal contents from the colon into the small intestine. The ileocecal sphincter remains mildly constricted at all times and slows the emptying of small intestine contents into the cecum except after meals, when the gastrocolic reflex intensifies peristalsis. This resistance to emptying prolongs retention of intestinal contents to facilitate digestion and absorption. Normally only 1500 ml to 2000 ml of chyme empty from the ileum into the cecum every day (Guyton & Hall, 2006).

The Large Intestine. The colon is 5 feet of tubular muscle lined with mucous membrane extending from the ileum to the anal canal. It is divided into the cecum; ascending, transverse, and descending colon; sigmoid colon; and rectum and anus (see Figure 19-1). The colon functions to absorb water and electrolytes from the intestinal contents and to store fecal material until expulsion. The colon is normally sluggish (Guyton & Hall, 2006).

Colonic mucus protects the lining of the colon from excoriation, provides a barrier to prevent acids formed in the feces from attacking the intestinal wall, and binds fecal matter (Guyton & Hall, 2006). A patient's extreme emotional reaction may overstimulate the parasympathetic nerves, causing overproduction of stringy mucoid stools with little or no feces. The colon absorbs large quantities of water (as much as 2.5 L) and up to 55 mEq of sodium and 23 mEq of chloride daily (Berger & Williams, 1992).

Fecal elimination is accomplished by moving the chyme along the colon and into the rectum and anal canal by muscular actions called haustrations and by propulsive or "mass movements." Large circular constrictions occur in the large intestine in the same way that segmentation movements occur in the small intestine. These contractions of muscle cause the unstimulated portion of the large intestine to bulge outward into baglike sacs called haustrations. The fecal material is therefore slowly dug into and rolled over and moved forward in the colon. It requires 8 to 15 hours to move the chyme from the ileocecal valve through the colon (Guyton & Hall, 2006).

Peristalsis in the colon occurs in mass movements 1 to 3 times per day about 15 minutes to 1 hour after a meal, facilitated by gastrocolic and duodenocolic reflexes. These movements can be strongest after the first meal of the day. A distended or irritated portion of the colon, most often the transverse or descending colon, constricts, forcing the fecal material en masse down the colon to the rectum, where the person feels an urge to defecate. Stimulation of the gastrocolic and duodenocolic reflexes occurs when the stomach and duodenum are distended through the myenteric plexus. These mass movements usually last for 10 to 30 minutes. When they stop, they may return a half day later. Irritation in the colon can also initiate mass movements. For example, a person with ulcerative colitis has mass movements most of the time; others may have them after ingesting hot or cold liquids (Guyton & Hall, 2006).

Sigmoid Colon, Rectum, and Anal Canal. The adult rectum is 4 to 6 inches long; the distal anal canal is 1½ inches long. The anal canal contains an internal and external sphincter (see Figure 19-3). The internal sphincter is inside the anus and is a continuation of the circular smooth muscle layer. The external sphincter surrounds the internal sphincter and is made up of striated voluntary muscle. The external sphincter is controlled by the pudendal nerve, which is part of the somatic nervous system and under voluntary control. The rectum is empty of feces most of the time. When a mass movement forces feces into the rectum, the need for defecation occurs (Guyton & Hall, 2006).

Defecation. Defecation reflexes (intrinsic and parasympathetic) initiate defecation. When feces enter the rectum, the rectal wall distends and sends afferent signals through the myenteric plexus to initiate peristaltic waves in the descending colon, sigmoid, and rectum. As the peristaltic waves approach the anus, the internal anal sphincter relaxes. This reflex is relatively weak. In order to be effective for defecation, it must be fortified by the parasympathetic defecation reflex. This occurs when nerve endings in the rectum are stimulated, transmitting signals into the sacral portion (S2-4) of the spinal cord and reflexively back to the descending colon, sigmoid, rectum, and anus via parasympathetic nerve fibers in the pelvic nerves. The defecation signals entering the spinal cord initiate other concurrent activities associated with defecation such as taking a deep breath, closing the glottis, the Valsalva maneuver, and raising the levator muscles around the rectum. These activities aid in defecation, as does a squat position that straightens the anorectal angle (Guyton & Hall, 2006; Heitkemper, 2000).

Somatic control also is necessary for voluntary defecation because the conscious mind controls the external sphincter by inhibiting its action to defecate or further contract if inconvenient. Maintained voluntary inhibition can disrupt the defecation mechanism until more feces enter the rectum. Repeatedly ignoring the urge to defecate can result in constipation (Guyton & Hall, 2006).

Altered Bowel Elimination

Incontinence. When motor and sensory pathways of the autonomic nervous system or somatic nervous system are compromised, voluntary bowel control is altered. Impairment of cerebral control, anal sphincter control, or sensation results in fecal incontinence. Damage to the central nervous system (CNS) interrupts nervous pathways between the brain, spinal cord, and GI system, causing neurogenic bowel. Three of the five categories of neurogenic bowel dysfunction are seen commonly in rehabilitation practice: uninhibited, reflex, and autonomous neurogenic bowel; less often, motor paralytic and sensory paralytic neurogenic bowel are seen.

Motor and Sensory Tests. Motor and sensory tests can classify the bowel dysfunction and determine the appropriate bowel program:

1. Saddle sensation is a perianal sensation elicited in response to a pinprick or light touch. Sensation indicates intact sensory function at the sacral spinal cord level; this awareness of the urge to defecate helps establish bowel control.

2. The bulbocavernosus reflex test is used for patients with spinal cord injuries to determine whether an intact reflex arc is present at the level where the bowel, bladder, and genitalia are innervated. Positive results indicate an upper motor neuron (UMN) (above T12) or reflexic injury with reflex activity in these areas. With a lower motor neuron (LMN) (T12 or below) or areflexic injury, reflex activity in the bladder, bowel, or genitalia is improbable. A person generally will not have a positive bulbocavernosus reflex while in spinal shock, but this reflex may appear before spinal shock fully subsides (Zejdlik, 1992). Spinal shock is a transient condition

with decreased synaptic excitability of neurons, lasting from hours to weeks, and is manifested by absence of somatic reflex activity and flaccid paralysis below the level of damage. Hypotension, bladder paralysis, and interference with defecation may occur because of autonomic nervous system involvement, especially in higher-level lesions. Reflex activity may return earlier with incomplete lesions.

3. The bulbocavernosus reflex is elicited by inserting a gloved, lubricated finger into the patient's rectum while gently squeezing the clitoris or glans penis. The nurse observes for a visible contraction of the external anal sphincter and a palpable contraction of the bulbocavernosus and ischiocavernosus muscles. A positive response will be immediate and brisk or slow and weak; no contraction is a negative result. The test is performed weekly until positive or until a permanent areflexic injury is confirmed.

4. The anal "wink" reflex is similar to the bulbocavernosus test. It is elicited by a pinprick to the skin adjacent to the external anal sphincter. A visible "wink" contraction of the sphincter is a positive response.

Uninhibited Neurogenic Bowel. In cortical and subcortical lesions above the C1 vertebral level, as seen in stroke, multiple sclerosis, and certain types of brain trauma and tumors, bowel function is classified as uninhibited (Figure 19-5). There is damage to the upper motor neurons located in the

cerebral cortex, internal capsule, brainstem, or spinal cord, with sparing of lower motor neurons located in the anterior gray matter throughout the entire length of the spinal cord. Bowel sensation is intact, as is saddle sensation, and the bulbocavernosus reflex and anal reflex are intact or increased. Sensory impulses travel through the sacral reflex arc to the brain, but the brain is unable to interpret the impulses to defecate. As a result of decreased cerebral awareness of the urge to defecate, there is decreased voluntary control of the anal sphincter. Involuntary elimination occurs when the sacral defecation reflex is activated. Because sensation is not impaired, the incontinence is accompanied by a sense of urgency and often occurs in close proximity with the gastrocolic reflex (Beddar et al., 1997).

Reflex Neurogenic Bowel. Reflex neurogenic (automatic) bowel function (Figure 19-6) occurs with spinal cord lesions above the T12 to L1 vertebral level that involve the upper motor neurons and sensory tracts but spare the lower motor neurons. Tetraplegia, high thoracic paraplegia, and multiple sclerosis are associated disorders. Other causes include tumor, vascular disease, syringomyelia, and pernicious anemia. In most instances bowel sensation and saddle sensation are diminished or absent. The bulbocavernosus reflex and anal reflex are increased.

Interruptions of the nerve pathways between the brain and spinal cord may be complete or incomplete. In a complete lesion, and many incomplete, the person has no voluntary

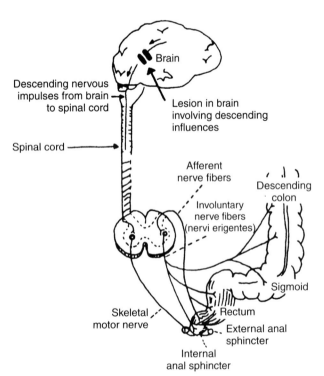

Figure 19-5 Uninhibited neurogenic bowel. (From Pires, M., & Lockhart-Pretti, P. [1992]. *Nursing management of neurogenic incontinence.* Glenview, IL: Association of Rehabilitation Nurses.)

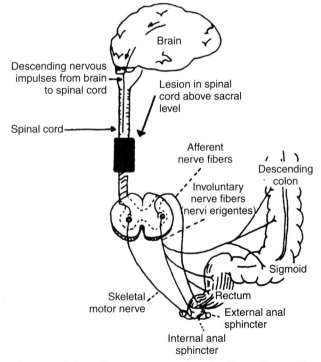

Figure 19-6 Reflex neurogenic bowel. (From Pires, M., & Lockhart-Pretti, P. [1992]. *Nursing management of neurogenic incontinence.* Glenview, IL: Association of Rehabilitation Nurses.)

control of defection or of the anal sphincter and fecal incontinence occurs without warning from a mass reflex. The sacral nerve segments of S2-4 are intact, so it is possible for a patient to develop a stimulus-response type of bowel control using the mass reflex. Because the intact spinal reflex arc functions when feces accumulate in the rectum and create distention, the bowel can empty by reflex. The parasympathetic innervation through the sacral segments of the spinal cord maintains anal sphincter tone so that fecal incontinence between mass reflex emptying is not a problem.

Autonomous Neurogenic Bowel. Autonomous (flaccid or nonreflex) bowel function (Figure 19-7) occurs with spinal cord lesions at or below the T12 to L1 vertebral level. Lesions in this area affect the lower motor neurons and usually are associated with paraplegia, spina bifida, tumor, and intervertebral disk disease. Sensation is diminished to absent, as are the bulbocavernosus and anal reflexes. Although nerve pathways between the brain and spinal cord are interrupted, the extent of neural compromise depends on whether the injury is complete or incomplete. As with reflex bowel function, the person has neither cerebral control of defecation nor voluntary control of the anal sphincter. Unlike reflex bowel function, however, the lesion directly involves the S2-4 segments and the activity of the spinal reflex arc is destroyed or unable to be accessed. No reflex emptying of the bowel occurs. Both the internal and external anal sphincters lack tone, offering little or no resistance in the rectum, resulting in frequent fecal incontinence with oozing stool. Performing the Valsalva maneuver, such as may occur during transfers, can also result in fecal leakage (Lynch, Antony, Dobbs, & Frizelle, 2001).

Motor Paralytic Bowel. A motor paralytic bowel occurs with damage to the anterior horn cells of S2, S3, and S4 ventral roots, such as with poliomyelitis, intervertebral disk disease, trauma or tumor (Figure 19-8). Saddle sensation is intact, but the bulbocavernosus reflex and anal reflex are absent. Incontinence is rare except in widespread disease (Cannon, 1981).

Sensory Paralytic Bowel. Damage to the dorsal roots of S2, S3, and S4 or dorsal horns of the spinal cord results in a sensory paralytic bowel (Figure 19-9); diabetes mellitus and tabes dorsalis can cause this damage. Saddle sensation is diminished or absent. The bulbocavernosus reflex and anal reflex may be normal, decreased, or absent. Incontinence is rare except in advanced stages (Cannon, 1981).

Other Factors Contributing to Incontinence. Diseases of peripheral nerves supplying the external anal sphincter may result in fecal incontinence. Bowel problems also may arise from disease of the anal sphincter or weakness of the diaphragm, the abdominal muscles, or muscles of the pelvic floor, or as a result of a surgical ostomy after cancer, trauma, or other diseases. Two types of bowel diversion ostomies are ileostomy and colostomy (Figure 19-10). The stoma site determines the consistency of the stool. Ileostomies result in frequent, liquid stools because almost no water has been absorbed. Ascending colostomies also have liquid stools, but transverse colostomies have more solid, formed feces, as do descending and sigmoid colostomies (Berger & Williams, 1992).

Constipation. Constipation is a slowing of the transit time of feces through the large intestine, which leads to more water being removed, resulting in large quantities of hard, dry feces (Guyton & Hall, 2006). Constipation is present if two or more of the following criteria are present for at least 12 weeks in the preceding 12 months (Thompson et al., 1999):
- Straining at defecation more than 25% of the time
- Lumpy or hard stools at least 25% of the time
- Feeling of incomplete evacuation of feces at least 25% of the time
- Manual maneuvers (i.e., digital evacuations) needed to facilitate defecation more than 25% of the time
- Less than three defecations per week

Transit time through the colon can be measured clinically by the radiopaque colonic transit time study. The patient swallows small capsules containing radiopaque markers followed with either direct radiographic examination of the abdomen or radiographs of the feces on successive days. A person with normal bowel motility passes 80% of the swallowed markers within 5 days, whereas constipated individuals experience

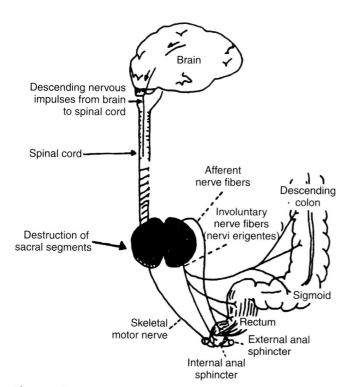

Figure 19-7 Autonomous (nonreflex) bowel. (From Pires, M., & Lockhart-Pretti, P. [1992]. *Nursing management of neurogenic incontinence.* Glenview, IL: Association of Rehabilitation Nurses.)

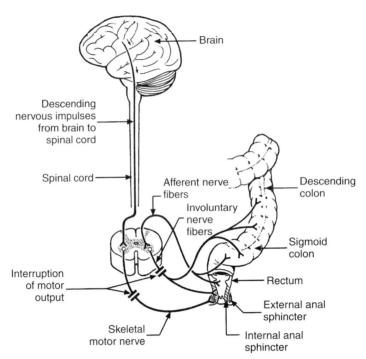

Figure 19-8 Motor paralytic bowel. (From Pires, M., & Lockhart-Pretti, P. [1992]. *Nursing management of neurogenic incontinence.* Glenview, IL: Association of Rehabilitation Nurses.)

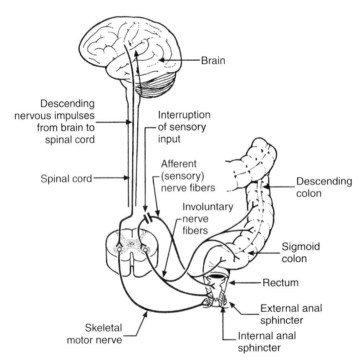

Figure 19-9 Sensory paralytic bowel. (From Pires, M., & Lockhart-Pretti, P. [1992]. *Nursing management of neurogenic incontinence.* Glenview, IL: Association of Rehabilitation Nurses.)

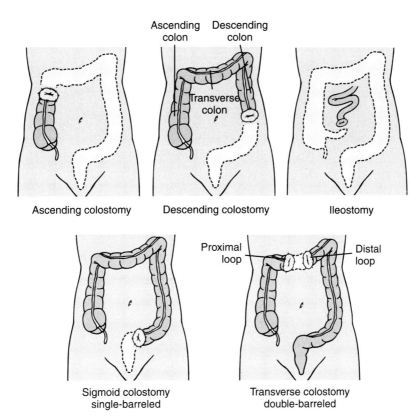

Ascending
colon   Descending
colon

Transverse
colon

Ascending colostomy   Descending colostomy   Ileostomy

Proximal
loop   Distal
loop

Sigmoid colostomy
single-barreled   Transverse colostomy
double-barreled

Figure 19-10 Ostomy types. (From Lewis, S. L., Collier, I. C., Heitkemper, M. M., & Dirksen, S. R. [2004]. *Medical-surgical nursing: Assessment and management of clinical problems* [6th ed.]. St. Louis, MO: Mosby.)

delayed transit time of the markers through the colon (Abyad & Mourad, 1996).

Etiology. A variety of factors contribute to constipation, including those intrinsic to an existing physiological disorder and those extrinsic or environmental. Intrinsic factors may be neuropathic or myopathic in origin. Neuropathic disorders affect nerve pathways and cause motility problems and disordered defecation, which leads to constipation. Major neurological disorders that affect GI function are diabetic neuropathy, stroke, spinal cord lesions, Parkinson's disease, multiple sclerosis, or cerebral palsy. In diabetes mellitus, damage to the efferent autonomic nerves leads to diminished intestinal motility and weak smooth muscle contraction (Waldrop & Doughty, 2000). In Parkinson's disease there is degeneration within the autonomic nervous system, and outlet obstruction with paradoxical puborectalis contraction may occur during straining. This prevents normal straightening of the anorectal angles, accentuating the flap valve action and preventing onward passage of feces (Edwards, Quigley, & Pfeiffer, 1992), and possibly delaying colonic transit time (Edwards, Quigley, Hofman, & Pfeiffer, 1993). Myopathic or specific muscle disorders, such as muscular dystrophy, may also affect GI motility (Waldrop & Doughty, 2000). Depression and anxiety may also slow the transit time and reduce appetite (Eberhardie, 2003).

Extrinsic factors that may cause constipation include reduced fiber and fluid intake, decreased activity and mobility, toileting habits, and pharmacological agents. Insufficient fiber intake decreases the amount of water, resulting in small, hard stools that fail to stimulate the enteric nervous system sufficiently to elicit strong peristaltic contractions. Transit time is thus prolonged, and more water is absorbed from the stool. Inadequate oral fluid intake will cause more reabsorption of water from the stool and cause constipation. Poor toileting habits or suppressing the normal defecation reflex prolongs exposure of the stool to the rectal mucosa and causes further dehydration of the feces. Children, too busy playing, may ignore the urge to defecate and become constipated (Waldrop & Doughty, 2000). Lack of privacy or difficulty getting to a toilet due to degenerative changes with aging or other conditions may lead to constipation (Eberhardie, 2003). Many medications adversely affect intestinal motility through stimulation of the sympathetic nervous system, inhibition of the parasympathetic nervous system, or direct effect on absorption or secretion within the GI tract. Box 19-1 lists various medications that may contribute to constipation.

Diarrhea. Diarrhea occurs when fecal matter moves rapidly through the large intestine (Guyton & Hall, 2006). The greatest hazard of diarrhea is the loss of water and electrolytes needed for normal cell function. Severe dehydration and electrolyte imbalance can cause cardiac arrhythmias, severe hypotension, renal failure, and death, especially in infants, very young children, elderly persons, and those debilitated by

From Doughty, D. (2000). *Urinary and fecal incontinence: Nursing management* (2nd ed.). St. Louis, MO: Mosby.

extreme illness. Otherwise, diarrhea is not severe or life-threatening, although it may be chronic, recurring, or an acute symptom lasting for a short time. It does signal that something has disrupted normal function of the GI tract.

Etiology. Diarrhea may be classified as acute (lasting less than 2 to 4 weeks) (Tobillo & Schwartz, 1998) or chronic. Several pathological processes may cause diarrhea. Common causes are infectious agents of bacteria or a virus in the GI tract, usually at the terminal ileum or large intestine. The mucosa of the bowel becomes irritated wherever the infection is present and increases the rate of secretion. Bowel motility is also increased. The large amounts of fluid are intended to flush the infectious agent towards the anus, and the peristalsis moves the fluid forward. Diarrhea can be an important mechanism for ridding the intestinal tract of debilitating infections (Guyton & Hall, 2006).

Disorders that reduce absorption of water and electrolytes into the intestinal epithelial cells directly increase the volume of stool and its liquidity. Common causes include ingestion of sorbitol and other hyperosmolar medications and fat malabsorption syndromes. Lactose intolerance (Waldrop & Doughty, 2000), often a response to milk products and chocolate, is more common among African Americans and Asians (Doughty, 1992).

Motility disorders within the bowel are a third cause of diarrhea. Increased motility may occur with ulcerative colitis, diabetes mellitus, and irritable bowel syndrome. Decreased motility of the bowel may lead to constipation with seepage of liquid stool that may be misinterpreted as diarrhea (Waldrop & Doughty, 2000). Nervous tension can cause excessive stimulation of the parasympathetic nervous system, which excretes excess mucus and increases motility. These two effects can also lead to diarrhea (Guyton & Hall, 2006).

Finally, diarrhea may result from mixed disorders caused by alterations in secretion or absorption in addition to disordered motility. Examples are laxative abuse, which increases intestinal motility and reduces absorption, infection with *Clostridium difficile* after antibiotic therapy, and acquired immunodeficiency syndrome–related diarrhea (Waldrop & Doughty, 2000).

NURSING PROCESS

A patient's individualized bowel program must be built from a comprehensive nursing assessment combined with knowledge of normal and impaired bowel function. This is the foundation for successful management.

History

The history elicits a detailed description of the present illness, the perceived bowel problem, bowel function between the time of injury and the present, past bowel routine, dietary factors, medication usage, beliefs about bowel function, and lifestyle goals.

Current Elimination Pattern. The patient, or family member if patient is unable, should be asked to describe, in his or her own words, the bowel elimination pattern since the injury or illness. Data include frequency, level of continence, volume and consistency of stool (Doughty, 1992), and time of last bowel movement. If the disability is not recent in onset, patients can describe their bowel care techniques and factors associated with bowel incontinence, such as time of day, frequency, and relationship to eating (Stiens et al., 1997). For persons with cancer the current history of bowel patterns is more important (Bisanz, 1997). A patient's sensory awareness of rectal filling and the ability to delay and control defecation should be ascertained (Doughty, 1992).

Past Bowel Routine. Questions about former bowel habits include time of day of evacuation, frequency, volume and consistency of stool, the time needed to complete bowel care (Stiens et al., 1997), and personal habits to stimulate defecation. Note reliance on laxatives or enemas, as well as the premorbid pattern, and any incidence of diarrhea or constipation (Lincoln & Roberts, 1989). In most cases premorbid bowel function and patterns will lay the groundwork for developing a workable rehabilitation bowel regimen (Stiens et al., 1997).

Dietary Factors. The patient's diet and appetite should receive careful attention. Assessment of preonset habits should include food preferences, usual meal routine, amount and type of fluid intake, cultural practices, and number of servings of fiber per day (raw fruits, vegetables, whole grains, bran) (Doughty, 1992). Foods that caused diarrhea, excessive flatus, or constipation before the onset of disability are likely to cause the same response now.

Medication Usage. Patients take many medications that may have undesirable side effects. Antibiotics destroy normal bowel flora and may result in diarrhea. Propantheline (Pro-Banthine) and oxybutynin chloride (Ditropan), used in the management of urinary incontinence, can cause constipation. Previous and current use of laxatives, stool softeners, suppositories, or enemas are part of the nursing history.

Relevant Medical History. A premorbid bowel disorder, such as irritable bowel syndrome, can complicate a postinjury program. Laxative dependency may prolong transit time and decrease responsiveness of the gut to bowel medications (Stiens et al., 1997). Any historical report of sphincter disturbances, ulcerative colitis, diverticulitis, spastic colon, diabetes, prolapse, or hemorrhoids should be noted and explored.

Lifestyle Goals and Beliefs About Bowel Function. Patients can identify their bowel management goals in light of their schedules for work or school, available assistance after discharge, and the time to complete a bowel care regimen when at home (Stiens et al., 1997). If the disability is not recent, ask patients to describe the effect of their bowel program on their current lifestyle and any changes they would like made (Doughty, 1992). Beliefs about bowel management can be ascertained throughout the history-taking process.

Physical Examination

The overall physical condition of the patient must be assessed with special notation made of the cause of the disability, the neurological status, and any other factors that might affect bowel function or ability to participate. The three common neurogenic bowel dysfunctions discussed previously have specific interventions that are described in more detail later in this chapter. The level of neural dysfunction of the bowel is assessed using the motor and sensory tests described earlier. Inspect the abdomen for distention, visible peristalsis, masses, or bulges. Auscultate for normal, hyperactive, or hypoactive bowel sounds, and percuss any unexpected dullness, such as over the lower quadrant, which may indicate a mass of feces (Beddar et al., 1997). Abdominal palpation notes muscle tone, contractility (Doughty, 1992), tenderness, and impacted stool (Bisanz, 1997). A rectal examination assesses sphincter tone, strength of the anal sphincter (Beddar et al., 1997), presence and consistency of stool in the rectum (Hogstel & Nelson, 1992), and any rectal excoriations or lesions. Cognitive and communication abilities influence

whether a patient understands the staff when questioned about the need to toilet. Patients who need assistance to reach or correctly use call buttons or signals, such as patients with speech, language, visual, or auditory impairments, may not be able to notify staff or participate fully in a bowel program.

Persons with a stroke or brain injury may suffer from dysphagia, which makes chewing and swallowing difficult. Individuals with facial paralysis or who have lost a great deal of weight after their disability may be left with ill-fitting dentures that now affect their ability to chew food properly. The patient's endurance level is considered because those who tire easily may require small, frequent meals rather than struggle to complete a large meal.

Patients' abilities to turn in the bed and ambulate or transfer from bed to toilet or commode may require them to make adaptations, such as bedside rails to pull up on, so they can perform the bowel program with the greatest degree of independence. Hand dexterity for inserting suppositories, performing digital stimulation (Doughty, 1992), or completing personal hygiene should be noted.

Environmental Assessment

A new, unfamiliar environment may affect a person's ability to call for help or use the toilet or commode. Use of restraints or pain can also be a factor (Beddar et al., 1997). Assess family and social support because family members or attendants may need to help a person with tetraplegia, for example, whereas a person with paraplegia may require only assistive devices and equipment. An elderly patient may find degenerative joint disease makes getting to the toilet difficult. A couple may decide that an attendant rather than the spouse will provide assistance.

Nursing Diagnoses

From the assessment data the rehabilitation nurse makes appropriate nursing diagnoses for the patient with altered bowel elimination. Potential diagnoses are listed in Table 19-1.

Bowel incontinence may be related to environmental factors (e.g., inaccessible bathroom), incomplete emptying of bowel, cognitive impairment, abnormally high abdominal or intestinal pressure (from gas), laxative abuse, dietary habits, immobility, general decline in muscle tone (e.g., abdominal, perineal, bowel sphincter), impaction, incomplete emptying of bowel (NANDA-I, 2005). The following are classifications of bowel impairment (McCourt, 1993):
- Uninhibited
- Reflex neurogenic
- Autonomous neurogenic
- Motor paralytic
- Sensory paralytic

Constipation may be related to habitual denial/ignoring of urge to defecate, inadequate toileting (timeliness, positioning for defecation, privacy; irregular defecation habits), insufficient physical activity, abdominal muscle weakness, mental confusion, emotional stress, depression, obesity, hemorrhoids, medication, poor eating habits, insufficient fiber

TABLE 19-1 Nursing Diagnoses, Interventions, and Outcomes Applicable to Bowel Elimination NIC/NOC

Nursing Diagnosis	Nursing Interventions	Nursing Outcomes
Bowel incontinence	Bowel incontinence care Bowel management Bowel training	Bowel continence Bowel elimination Tissue integrity: skin & mucous membranes
Constipation	Constipation/impaction management Fluid management Nutrition management	Bowel elimination Hydration Symptom control
Perceived constipation	Bowel management Counseling Fluid management Teaching: individual	Bowel elimination Health beliefs Knowledge: health behavior
Risk for constipation	Constipation/impaction management Bowel management Bowel training Fluid management Nutrition management Medication management	Bowel elimination Hydration Mobility Appetite Knowledge: medication Nutritional status: food & fluid intake
Diarrhea	Diarrhea management Medication management Bowel management Fluid/electrolyte management Perineal care Skin surveillance	Bowel continence Bowel elimination Electrolyte & acid/base balance Fluid balance

Data from Moorhead, S., Johnson, M., & Maas, M. (Eds.). (2004). *Nursing outcomes classification (NOC)* (3rd ed.). St. Louis, MO: Mosby; Dochterman, J. M., & Bulechek, G. M. (2004). *Nursing interventions classification (NIC)* (4th ed.). St. Louis, MO: Mosby.; and NANDA International. (2005). *Nursing diagnoses: Definitions and classification, 2005-2006* (6th ed.). Philadelphia: Author.

or fluid intake, decreased motility of GI tract (NANDA-I, 2005).

Perceived constipation may be related to cultural or family health beliefs, faulty appraisal, impaired thought processes (NANDA-I, 2005).

Risk for constipation may be related to dietary factors (dehydration, insufficient fiber intake, poor eating habits, change in usual foods and eating patterns, decreased motility of GI tract, inadequate dentition or oral hygiene, insufficient fluid intake), functional factors (insufficient physical activity, inadequate toileting, positioning for defecation, privacy, irregular defecation habits, abdominal muscle weakness, habitual denial or ignoring of urge to defecate, recent environmental changes), psychological factors (depression, emotional stress, mental confusion), pharmacological factors (NANDA-I, 2005).

Diarrhea may be related to laxative abuse, tube feedings, travel (e.g., bacteria in food and water), alcohol abuse, high stress or anxiety (NANDA-I, 2005).

Nursing Outcomes

Outcomes are established with the patient and vary according to disability, type of bowel dysfunction, and lifestyle. Table 19-1 displays relevant outcomes for the identified bowel elimination diagnoses. The following are specific short-term goals that may be established:

1. Achieve control on a regular basis (a bowel movement every 1 to 3 days) at a planned time and place without the need for laxatives or enemas
2. Establish a bowel program that permits evacuation in the least amount of time possible with no incontinent episodes after the program (Steins et al., 1997)
3. Normalize stool consistency (Doughty, 1992)
4. Eliminate or minimize involuntary bowel movements
5. Plan a diet that includes the appropriate amount of fluid and fiber
6. Incorporate exercise into daily program
7. Help the patient to achieve the highest level of independence possible with the program
8. Assist patient with problem solving when the bowel program does not perform as planned and with choosing appropriate interventions to achieve goal
9. Help the patient with an uninhibited neurogenic bowel to plan and regulate bowel elimination at a time when there is likely to be a response
10. Help the patient with a reflex neurogenic bowel to stimulate reflex activity that moves feces into the rectum for predictable elimination

11. Assist the patient with an autonomous neurogenic bowel with maintaining firm stool consistency and keeping the distal colon empty

12. Avoid complications of diarrhea, constipation, and impaction by maintaining adequate nutrition, hydration, and activity (McCourt, 1993)

Long-term goals must minimize associated impairments, disabilities, and handicaps, considering instead the person's life goals and role expectations, particularly cultural, sexual, and vocational roles. The entire process requires knowledge of the individual and derivation of his or her person-centered goals (Stiens et al., 1997).

Interventions

Basic Components of a Bowel Program

A "Clean" Bowel. The bowel must be free from impacted feces. Manual disimpaction, cleansing enemas, or laxatives may be used to free the bowel from an impaction. Laxatives are given 8 to 12 hours before results. Examples of laxatives or enemas that may be used are milk of magnesia, milk of magnesia with cascara, magnesium citrate, Fleet's Enema, oil retention enema, or bisacodyl enema. Patients with loss of sphincter function are not able to retain enemas (Doughty, 1992), and those with pelvic floor dystonia, such as in Parkinson's disease, will not have effective results from laxatives or enemas (Edwards et al., 1992). For children with myelomeningocele who have impacted feces, Coffman (1986) recommends a cleansing enema of lactated Ringer's solution. Persons with cancer benefit from oil retention or milk and molasses enemas because these types ease the stool removal in a nonirritating, noncaustic way, unlike a soapsuds or tap water enema (Bisanz, 1997).

Because laxatives increase the motility of the small bowel and colon, routine use produces unpredictable results and can create bowel dependence (Doughty, 1992). Enemas are not used routinely because they stretch the colon walls and result in loss of elasticity; continued use causes the bowel to respond poorly to reflex stimulation and become dependent. Therefore, after impacted feces have been removed and the bowel training program started, no laxatives or enemas are given except in the following instances:

1. The patient becomes impacted or severely constipated.

2. There is medical necessity, such as bowel preparation for tests or surgery. (Patients with spinal cord injury have their routine bowel program the night before with manual removal in the morning, rather than the usual preparation.)

3. Recommendations based on evaluations are that this is the best program for the patient.

Timing. Scheduling the time of day for a bowel program is important for effectiveness. Timing also accommodates the patient's previous or preferred routine to fit with discharge plans and his or her future lifestyle. Venn, Taft, Carpentier, and Applebaugh (1992) conducted a research study of 46 stroke patients and discovered that when their premorbid time for elimination was used as the scheduled time of day for their bowel training program, a significantly higher number were able to establish effective bowel regimens. For children and adolescents a regular routine for toileting needs to be planned around school times (Coffman, 1986); for an adult, around work hours. For example, defecation may be attempted every morning but evaluated and modified according to the patient's physical condition and response. Some find an every-other-day routine satisfactory; others manage good evacuation with a 3-day routine.

A key is a consistent time habit for elimination. Clinical experience has demonstrated that for prompt bowel response to stimulation (a bowel movement within 30 minutes), the stimulation method must take place at the same hour every time. The gastrocolic reflex also aids the bowel routine, ideally after any meal, but a hot cup of coffee or tea or an evening snack may produce the gastrocolic reflex at a more convenient time.

Diet and Fluid Intake. The patient's preonset dietary habits are evaluated before implementing a bowel program. Physical condition and personal preferences are incorporated as much as possible into a diet high in nutrients and containing a variety of foods. High fiber is important because dietary fiber traverses the small intestine without being digested by the endogenous secretions. Fiber functions by binding water in the intestine in the form of a gel to prevent overabsorption from the large bowel. This action ensures that the fecal content is both bulky and soft and also that its passage through the intestine is not delayed. Delayed transit time of the fecal contents generally results in constipation. Dietary fiber is beneficial in the management of both constipation and diarrhea. Its bulking action helps alleviate diarrhea, and its softening action helps prevent constipation.

The chief sources of dietary fiber are whole-grain cereals and breads, leafy vegetables, legumes, nuts, and fruits with skins. By simply replacing white bread with whole grain bread, the fiber content of the diet can be increased greatly. A diet that includes 2½ cups of vegetables and 2 cups of fruits a day is recommended (U.S. Department of Agriculture Center for Nutrition Policy and Promotion, 2005). Granola, bran, and wheat germ are excellent sources of fiber and easily added to soups, cereals, meat loaf, baked goods, and other foods. Fiber is introduced into the diet gradually to allow the GI tract time to adapt. Too rapid an increase in fiber may produce distressing side effects such as flatulence, distention, or diarrhea.

Unless fluid intake is restricted for medical reasons, patients should drink 2 to 3 quarts of liquid daily to maintain soft stool consistency. Drinking hot coffee, hot water, or prune juice every morning for breakfast is helpful to some who are initiating a bowel movement. Prunes and prune juice stimulate intestinal motility and therefore act as natural laxatives. Large quantities of prune or other fruit juices, however, may result in loose stools. Setting the table with two or more types of fluid at each meal may increase total intake. Popsicles or ice also may help (Smith, 1988).

Exercise. Physical activity is vital to a successful bowel program. Prolonged bed rest has an adverse effect on bowel motility and tends to cause fecal retention. The patient who can be out of bed and involved in physical activities increases muscle tone and has return of bowel function more quickly. In a study of stroke patients, Munchiando and Kendall (1993) discovered that as the number of hours spent in bed increased, the number of days needed to establish a bowel program also increased.

Physical status and type of disability determine exercise capabilities. Encouraging the patient to perform activities of daily living (ADLs) with minimum assistance from others helps compensate for the decreased activity level as a result of physical disability. Exercise tapes may be used to guide activities that can be performed while the patient is in a wheelchair (Smith, 1988). When subjected to extended periods of bed rest for medical reasons, the patient must be urged to continue to carry out as many activities as possible. Turning in bed, lifting the hips, bathing, performing range-of-joint-motion exercises, and carrying out other self-care activities aid in preventing decreased bowel motility and constipation.

Privacy. The act of elimination in most cultures is performed in private. Privacy and modesty are particularly important to patients who are of Mexican American or Native American heritage (Hoeman, 1989). Privacy facilitates relaxation, which in turn facilitates the act of defecation. Privacy also ensures that others will not detect embarrassing sounds or notice odors. Patients in any institution have little privacy; the more dependent the patient, the less the privacy. Patients benefit psychologically when privacy is incorporated into the bowel program. Whenever possible, the nurse should assist the patient out of bed and onto a toilet where the bathroom door may be closed. If a portable commode must be used, safely roll it into a bathroom or other secluded area.

Positioning. Whenever possible, the patient should assume an upright sitting position to defecate. This normal physiological position allows gravity to assist in peristalsis and stool expulsion. A squat position with the knees slightly higher than the hips and feet flat on the floor helps to increase abdominal pressure and thus facilitate stool passage. It also straightens the angle between the rectum and anal canal to promote rectal emptying (Heitkemper, 2000). This position is especially important for persons with Parkinson's disease because of their difficulty with voluntary contraction and dystonia of the pelvic floor and anal sphincter muscles (Edwards et al., 1992). If balance is a problem, use armrests and a back support (Wald, 1991).

For those persons with weak abdominal muscles, an abdominal binder increases abdominal pressure as the person bends at the waist to push out the stool (Hogstel & Nelson, 1992). Abdominal massage also may stimulate and hasten the defecation process. Persons with all types of disabilities and ages find it helpful to massage the abdomen in the direction of the bowel from right groin upward, across, and down to the left groin. Breathing techniques can increase intraabdominal pressure. Slow, deep breaths with each inspiration are held for 5 seconds and then combined with abdominal muscle contractions to bear down or perform a Valsalva maneuver. Children can be taught this maneuver by having

them blow up a balloon (Doughty, 1992), cough, or blow bubbles (Smith, 1990).

Unless absolutely necessary, avoid bedpans, and never use them with a patient who does not have sensation in the buttocks or sacral area. If a bedpan is unavoidable, position the patient carefully to limit the sacral pressure exerted by the bedpan. Elevate the head of the bed, support the back and legs with pillows, and bridge the hips and legs, as necessary. To avoid excessive pressure and potential skin breakdown, never allow anyone to remain on the bedpan or sit on a toilet or commode for longer than 25 minutes (Hogstel & Nelson, 1992). As soon as the patient receives medical approval to get out of bed, bedpans should be abandoned.

Patients with impaired skin integrity involving the buttocks or who do not have buttock or sacral sensation (i.e., patients with SCIs) may evacuate on an incontinence pad in bed. Positioning the patient on the left side after inserting a suppository or for manual removal aids elimination because gravity assists evacuation of the descending colon in that position.

Suppositories and Medications. The rehabilitation nurse develops protocols in collaboration with the physician, nurse practitioner, or physician assistant that specify ranges and guidelines for suppositories and medications so the nurse can make adjustments according to the individual patient's response. Suppositories are used to initiate reflex emptying of the bowel. To have an optimum effect, the suppository must come in contact with the bowel wall. Before a suppository is inserted, the rectum should be checked for stool. If stool is present, enough should be removed to ensure proper placement of the suppository against the bowel wall. The suppository should be stored at room temperature before insertion, because refrigeration delays action and temperatures higher than 90° F (32.2° C) cause the suppository to melt. Table 19-2 summarizes the three types of suppositories commonly used in rehabilitation settings.

Minienemas, such as the Therevac SB, which is a 4-ml solution of docusate and glycerin, may be used to soften and lubricate the stool and initiate evacuation (Dunn & Galka, 1994). Stool softeners and bulk formers are often prescribed to aid in the establishment of a bowel program. For example, dioctyl sodium sulfosuccinate (Colace), 100 mg 2 to 3 times per day, may be used initially and the dosage adjusted according to the consistency of the stool. When hard stools accompanied by constipation or frequent soft, pasty stools are a problem, bulk-forming laxatives can be given to alter the consistency by making stools soft and bulky. Whenever a mild laxative is needed, senna tablets and granules assist in moving the stool to the lower bowel so that a suppository or digital stimulation can completely empty the bowel.

The nurse should remember that for most diagnoses the terminal goal of any bowel program is continence and control without the need for medication. Should medication be needed, consideration must be given to providing medications that will be covered by the patient's insurance carriers on an outpatient basis.

TABLE 19-2 Suppositories

Suppository (Strength)	Action	Time When Results Expected	Disadvantages
Glycerin	Draws fluid from the bowel, creating a volume that distends the bowel and initiates reflex peristalsis	Approximately 30 minutes	Abdominal cramping possible
Sodium bicarbonate and potassium bitartrate (CEO-Two)	Activated in water before insertion; suppository releases carbon dioxide, which distends bowel and initiates reflex peristalsis	30-45 minutes	Use of petroleum lubricants negates effectiveness of suppository Abdominal cramping possible
Bisacodyl (Dulcolax)	Contact suppository that stimulates sensory nerve endings in colon and results in reflex peristalsis	15-60 minutes	Abdominal cramping possible

One suppository is the usual dose. Suppositories are given within a half hour after a meal or after a hot drink.

Digital Stimulation. Digital stimulation is a technique used to induce reflex contraction of the colon and relaxation of the anal sphincter muscle (Munchiando & Kendell, 1993), resulting in elimination. To perform digital stimulation, the index finger is gloved, lubricated, and gently inserted ½ to 1 inch into the rectum. To stimulate the inner sphincter to relax, the finger is gently rotated in a clockwise motion against the anal sphincter wall. It may take from 30 seconds to 2 minutes for relaxation of the sphincter to occur. While feces pass, the rectal wall is moved gently to one side. When no more stool is expelled, digital stimulation is resumed and the process repeated until the bowel is evacuated. The patient should be instructed to take slow, deep breaths during this process.

In successful bowel programs, digital stimulation may replace the suppository after a reflex-response defecation pattern is established. However, digital stimulation also may be used to trigger a bowel movement if a suppository has been less than successful or to ensure complete emptying of the colon after a bowel movement. In persons with SCI who are susceptible to dysreflexia, dibucaine hydrochloride (Nupercainal) lubricant can lower the incidence of dysreflexia during stimulation. The rehabilitation nurse should be aware that children may be unwilling to use a digital stimulation technique for their bowel program (Doughty, 1992).

Education. The details of patient education should parallel the individualized bowel program. Education should begin early during hospitalization to give the patient sufficient time and opportunity to discover and clarify problems or concerns. Teaching should include an explanation of the disability and how it affects bowel control, including basic anatomy and physiology of the GI tract. The rationale behind a routine bowel program and importance of diet, fluid intake, exercise, timing, and positioning are other educational elements. If medication is used for the program, explain the purpose, precautions, and techniques of suppository insertion or digital stimulation. Decide where the bowel program will take place when the patient is at home, and ensure that patient and caregiver practice safe and proper positioning. Discussion of potential problems encountered with a bowel program

includes the patient and family's explaining the steps they would take if diarrhea, constipation, or an accident occurred. They also verbalize their rationale for adjustments in the program and when they would consult with their physician or rehabilitation nurse. Cultural or familial beliefs regarding bowel movements or diet are important, and adaptations in the program are made to meet their needs. During the educational experience the patient and family need encouragement, reassurance, and emotional support, as well as information.

Bowel Incontinence. The primary nursing intervention for a patient with a diagnosis of bowel incontinence is to establish a bowel training program (Dochterman & Bulechek, 2004). Any changes in a bowel program should not be made before at least a 5- to 7-day trial, and then only one change at a time. Daily changes in a program result in modifying a program blindly without any learning about the response to the previous bowel program. Accurate documentation of the results of any bowel program is vital to evaluating effectiveness of the program (Figure 19-11).

Uninhibited Neurogenic Bowel. Studies on fecal incontinence in stroke patients have revealed that full or partial incontinence is present in 31% to 56% of patients on admission (Baztan, Domenech, & Gonzalez, 2003; Brocklehurst, Andrews, Richards, & Laycock, 1986; Nakayama, Jorgensen, Pederson, Raaschou, & Olsen, 1997). By discharge, Nakayama et al. (1997) noted that only 18% were still incontinent. Brocklehurst et al. (1986) found that almost all of their 42 subjects were continent at discharge, and Baztan et al. (2003) found that 21.1% were incontinent at discharge. Six months later, the incontinence rate was 9% to 22.1% (Baztan et al., 2003; Nakayama, et al., 1997). The conclusion by Brocklehurst et al. (1986) is that fecal incontinence is a common but transient phenomenon in stroke patients. Those who continue to be incontinent 6 months to a year or more later have more impairment of consciousness, greater functional damage leading to increased immobility and need for assistance to use the toilet (Brocklehurst et al., 1986; Harari, Coshall, Rudd, & Wolfe, 2003).

Date:		
Suppository = / Type		
Time		
Inserted by:		
Digital stim Time		
Manual removal Time		
Evacuation Time		
Stool Amt.		
Consistency		
Place		
Initials		
Normal evacuation Time		
Amt.		
Consistency		
Place		
Initials		
Accidents Time		
(Chart in red) Place		
Consistency		
Initials		
Accidents Time		
(Chart in red) Place		
Consistency		
Initials		
Enema Time & initials		
Initials R.N., L.V.N.		

Figure 19-11 Bowel record. (Courtesy San Diego Rehabilitation Institute, San Diego, CA.)

In general, the following measures should be taken in establishing a bowel program for a patient with an uninhibited neurogenic bowel:

1. Select the time of day for the bowel program according to past habits and for future convenience.
2. Follow a consistent schedule. Assist patient to toilet 30 minutes after meals to take advantage of the gastrocolic reflex. Start with a daily program, and progress to every other day (Munchiando & Kendall, 1993).
3. Provide a nutritious diet with adequate fiber.
4. Give fluids adequate to stimulate reflex activity and to promote soft stool (2000 to 2400 ml/24 hr unless contraindicated).
5. Begin the program with an empty colon.
6. Obtain a physician's order for stool softeners in the early stages of the program if needed.
7. Give a daily suppository if needed to initiate the defecation reflex. The research study by Venn et al. (1992) suggests that if a spontaneous bowel movement occurs within 4 hours before the scheduled time, the suppository may be held back for that day. Table 19-2 provides more detail about suppositories.

Usually the effects of softeners will not be seen for 3 days. Stool softeners, if needed, should be used on a routine rather than an as-needed basis. Softeners that may be used include the following:

1. Docusate sodium (Dialose; usually one 2 times daily)
2. Docusate calcium (Surfak; usually one 2 times daily; good to use if sodium intake is restricted)
3. Dioctyl sodium sulfosuccinate (Colace; usually one 2 times daily; available in liquid form)
4. Dioctyl sodium sulfosuccinate (Doxinate; usually one 2 times daily).

Softeners with a laxative component may be used when additional softening or peristaltic stimulus is needed. They should be given approximately 12 hours before desired results and also used on a routine basis. Those that may be used include the following:

1. Docusate sodium and phenolphthalein (Dialose Plus; usually one to two every day)
2. Casanthranol and docusate sodium (Peri-Colace; usually one to two every day)
3. Standardized senna concentrate (Senokot; usually one to two every day)

If combining softeners and softener/laxatives, it is preferable to combine like products (i.e., Dialose with Dialose Plus, Colace with Peri-Colace). Bisacodyl tablets may be used if all other measures are unsuccessful in preventing constipation or impaction. A maximum of two tablets may be given at one time approximately 12 hours before desired results.

Bulk producers may be used for the patient who lacks bowel tone, who needs additional softening of the stool, or who has small, infrequent stools. They are not appropriate for the impacted patient. They may be used to "form up" stools if the patient is on a liquid or tube feeding diet or has an "irritable bowel." Bulk producers that may be used include the following:

1. Psyllium hydrophilic mucilloid (Metamucil) or psyllium and senna (Perdiem): 1 teaspoon mixed in 200 ml of water or juice and followed by a glass of water
2. "Organic" bulk products of the patient's choice, such as alfalfa tablets
3. Calcium polycarbophil (Mitrolan): one to two tablets chewed 1 to 4 times per day

When the patient's condition improves so that the diet, fluid intake, and physical activity are well tolerated, these medications may be unnecessary. Harari, Norton, Lockwood, and Swift (2004) found that poststroke patients benefit from altering diet and fluid intake to control bowel problems. Rectal outlet delays can lead to constipation, and therefore suppositories, rather than laxatives, are recommended. Bulking agents, rather than stool softeners, can be used for weak anal sphincters in order to avoid leakage. Because patients with uninhibited bowel function have intact sensation, digital stimulation may be painful.

Accurate documentation is critical because, depending on the patient's condition, it may take a week or longer to establish a satisfactory pattern. Verbal and nonverbal efforts by the patient to communicate the need to eliminate are important in those with absence of functional speech. Educate and alert all staff to notice behaviors—something as subtle as a patient's restlessness may indicate awareness of rectal sensation. Munchiando and Kendall (1993) discovered that it took longer to establish a bowel program in patients with right-sided hemiplegia, probably as a result of expressive aphasia and difficulty communicating the urge to defecate. Evaluate program effectiveness daily and weekly with only one change at a time. Gradually increase patient and family participation in the program and decision making. Guidelines for changes in the program to every other day or every third day include the following:

1. Patient has small or no results every other day.
2. Patient's stool is not hard on daily program.
3. Patient is well controlled on every day program (i.e., results within 1 hour, no constipation or accidents for at least a week).

By complying with the basic components of a bowel program, continence and control can be achieved by the time of discharge and suppositories and medications discontinued.

Reflex Neurogenic Bowel. An upper motor neuron or reflex neurogenic bowel is characterized by fecal retention and requires a scheduled evacuation plan to avoid incontinence and impaction (Lynch, Anthony, Dobbs, & Frizelle, 2000). Fecal continence requires internal anal sphincter tone and external anal sphincter contraction in response to increased intraabdominal pressure, rectal distention, and rectal contraction. Although these responses might still be intact following a spinal cord injury, they are no longer modulated by cortical input (Lynch et al., 2000). The altered central or peripheral nervous system results in delayed gastric emptying, prolongation of intestinal transit time, and poor colonic motility (Correa & Rotter, 2000). Studies have shown that many patients with traumatic SCI have GI problems after their rehabilitation program that result in severe constipation, difficult evacuation, pain with defecation, urgency with incontinence (Han, Kim, & Kwon, 1998), or distention (Harari & Minaker, 2000). Harari and Minaker (2000), in a study of 128 Veterans Administration patients, discovered that patients 10 years out from their SCI and age 50 or older were at higher risk for megacolon. Megacolon occurs in incidences where constipation is so severe that bowel movements occur only once every several days or once a week. Due to the large accumulation of fecal matter, the colon distends to a diameter of 3 to 5 inches, hence the name megacolon (Guyton & Hall, 2006). Lynch et al. (2000) discovered that SCI patients have fewer bowel movements per week on average than non-SCI persons (6.6/week versus 9.3/week).

Lengthy programs that last longer than 3 hours have also been reported (Stiens, 1995). In a study of 42 SCI patients (22 with UMN and 20 with LMN), the required time for evacuation for UMN patients was 57.36 minutes per defecation. Lower motor neuron injuries required 28.98 minutes per defecation (Pryor & Jannings, 2004). Korsten et al. (2004) conducted a study of 14 SCI patients, both UMN and LMN,

and found that there was a significant decrease in colon motility during sleep, which could contribute to a prolonged colon transit time for stool in SCI patients. All of these problems lead to a decreased quality of life and altered ADL functioning. Given these findings, it is imperative that the rehabilitation nurse take responsibility for designing an appropriate bowel program with adequate education (Han et al., 1998; Yim, Yoon, Lee, Rah, & Moon, 2001).

During the acute stage of SCI, spinal shock is responsible for tonic paralysis of the GI tract and flaccid tone of the anal sphincter. Manual removal may be used until spinal shock subsides. In general, the following measures should be taken to establish a bowel program for a patient with a reflex neurogenic bowel:

1. After bowel sounds are present, physical activity increases, and oral fluid and food, including high fiber of 15 g/day to 30 g/day (Stiens et al., 1997), is tolerated, administer a suppository daily to trigger reflex elimination. Administration time should be consistent with the establishment of preonset habits and anticipated future lifestyle. The suppository is inserted 15 to 30 minutes ahead of the planned evacuation time (Venn et al., 1992). Following a regular schedule is important even if stool elimination does not occur each time. Missed bowel care sessions can contribute to excessive buildup of stool in the colon. The stool then becomes less plastic and more difficult to eliminate. Distention of the colon can occur with a decrease in effectiveness of peristalsis (Stiens et al., 1997). If a bisacodyl suppository is chosen, rehabilitation nurses should be aware that it is prepared with either a vegetable oil base or a polyethylene glycol polymer base. Glycol bases have been reported to produce quicker elimination (Stiens, 1995). A clinically significant research study by Stiens with a single subject T2 SCI patient 10 years after injury showed that using a glycol-based bisacodyl suppository reduced total bowel program time to 46 minutes as compared with 86 minutes for the oil-based suppository. Total bowel program time included insertion of the suppository until transferring off of the toilet. Dunn and Galka (1994) found that the Therevac SB minienema cut the time needed for bowel care by as much as an hour or more when compared with bisacodyl suppositories.
2. After a reliable bowel pattern is observed, suppository administration may be decreased to every other day or every third day as long as the stool consistency remains soft. Be alert for signs of fecal impaction or constipation that may develop with infrequent elimination.
3. Have patient evacuate on the toilet if possible and bear down if abdominal muscles are strong. The patient should lean forward and massage the abdomen in a clockwise manner (Zejdlik, 1992). Digital stimulation may be used alone or in addition to a suppository when the suppository has not produced results within 15 to 20 minutes.
4. Stool softeners, bulk agents, and stimulant laxatives may be necessary to assist elimination when abdominal muscles are weak or paralyzed. Oral senna agents are stimulant

laxatives that may facilitate movements in 6 to 8 hours (Stiens et al., 1997). Harsh cathartics must be avoided. The need for medications should decrease as activity increases.

5. Documentation of progress remains important to detect reliable patterns of elimination and to initiate appropriate changes.

For individuals with spinal cord lesions above the T6 vertebral level (above the splanchnic outflow), autonomic dysreflexia is a potential problem. Autonomic dysreflexia (hyperreflexia) is an abnormal hyperactive reflex activity as a result of an interrupted spinal cord. It is set off most often by stimuli arising from a distended bladder, but rectal distention, stimulation, and passage of feces also may precipitate this sympathetic response. This syndrome constitutes a medical emergency that can result in death if not treated promptly. Chapter 18, Appendix 18-A contains specific information regarding autonomic dysreflexia. Nupercainal ointment applied to the rectum 10 minutes before suppository insertion or digital stimulation is helpful in preventing symptoms in susceptible individuals.

Autonomous Neurogenic Bowel. Management of autonomous neurogenic bowel is difficult. Lower motor neuron loss results in absence of the spinal reflex activity. An atonic bowel with diminished propulsive forces and tone results. A program of suppositories and manual removal can be effective in evacuating stools (Zejdlik, 1992). In general, the following measures should be taken in establishing a bowel program for the patient with an autonomous neurogenic bowel:

1. Develop a stool consistency that is firm yet not hard by providing dietary fiber and using bulk-forming agents such as Metamucil and Citrucel.

2. Have the patient evacuate on a toilet and perform the Valsalva maneuver (see the discussion on defecation). Massaging the abdomen and leaning forward will augment the effectiveness of the bowel program.

3. If these measures are not successful, manual removal of the stool with a generously lubricated gloved finger can be performed.

4. After removal of stool from the lower rectum, administer a suppository as high as possible against the rectal wall. This stimulates the colon to empty stool into the rectum for manual removal. When a patient is active, any stool in the rectum may be expelled when intraabdominal pressure is increased. Therefore a daily program is recommended (Zejdlik, 1992). Yim et al. (2001) found that 20 LMN patients in his study evacuated twice a day to avoid accidents. Despite this, the average accidents were 2.61 per month.

5. Assess stool consistency. Loose stools will leak through a flaccid sphincter. Hard stools are difficult to remove manually and can lead to impaction and atony of the colon over time (Rauen & Aubert, 1992).

Children with neurogenic bowels should follow the same routine as adults. Incontinence occurs because of the inability to control the external sphincter. By maintaining the bowel in an empty or near-empty state, continence can be achieved (Gleeson, 1990). The goal for a person born with myelomeningocele, for example, is a soft, formed stool on a daily basis at the same time each day. This can be achieved through a high-fiber diet, adequate water intake, and habit training (Rauen & Aubert, 1992). Stool softeners, suppositories, and digital stimulation also may be needed (Smith, 1990). When suppositories are used, children with neurogenic bowels may need to have the buttocks closed with paper tape after suppository insertion to facilitate absorption (Gleeson, 1990).

In infants with neurogenic bowels, stool consistency must be monitored for signs of constipation. If constipation is present, dietary regulation is the first step before decreasing milk and dairy products and increasing fluids, vegetables, and fruits. Senna concentrate syrup may be added if stool continues to be hard. Bowel continence in children may take months to establish; therefore parents need encouragement and support. Illnesses, changes in medication, and emotional changes can lead to irregular bowel patterns. Patterns may also alter after the child reaches adolescence (Gleeson, 1990).

Table 19-3 provides a summary overview of the types of neurogenic bowel dysfunctions previously discussed. A successful bowel routine for the patient with incontinence resulting from any type of neurological bowel dysfunction requires effort and consistency for the patient and the nurse.

Ostomies. A bowel program cannot be established with an ileostomy or ascending colostomy. A bag or pouch must therefore be worn at all times. With regular irrigation a person with a descending and sigmoid colostomy and sometimes a transverse colostomy can regain a regular bowel pattern. Regulating the diet with selected foods at specific times can also lead to a predictable elimination pattern.

The rehabilitation nurse usually collaborates with an enterostomal therapist to establish a routine program including supplies, skin care, and education of the patient. Members of the United Ostomy Association are instrumental in visiting patients and explaining how to live with an ostomy (Berger & Williams, 1992).

Constipation. Constipation is one of the most common complications in persons with neurogenic bowel dysfunction. The definition of constipation is slow movement of feces through the large intestine (Guyton & Hall, 2006). Slow transit time causes more water to be removed, resulting in hard stool (Eberhardie, 2003). Constipation is also common in patients with cancer as a result of using opioids for pain relief (Bisanz, 1997). Opioids decrease motility and secretion in the GI tract (Mancini & Bruera, 1998). Other diseases that affect constipation are diabetes, Parkinson's disease, and hypothyroidism (Mancini & Bruera, 1998). Patients with diabetes have impaired GI motility, particularly of the colon, and a delayed or absent gastrocolic reflex (Haines, 1995). Infants are seldom constipated, but as children get older and learn to control defecation, they may inhibit the natural defecation reflexes. The colon can become atonic if defecation reflexes are ignored over time or if overuse of laxatives occur (Guyton & Hall, 2006).

TABLE 19-3 Neurogenic Bowel Dysfunction

Diagnosis	Level of Lesion	High-Risk Populations	Pattern of Incontinence	Bowel Program
Uninhibited	Brain	Cerebrovascular accident, multiple sclerosis, brain injury	Urgency: poor awareness of desire to defecate	Consistent habit and time according to premorbid history; physical exercise; high fluid intake; high-fiber foods; stool softener, suppository as needed
Reflex	Spinal cord above T12 to L1 vertebral level	Trauma, tumor, vascular disease, syringomyelia, multiple sclerosis	Infrequent, sudden, unexpected	Consistent habit and time; physical exercise; high fluid intake; high-fiber foods; suppository program, digital stimulation, stool softener as needed
Autonomous	Spinal cord at or below T12 to L1 vertebral level	Trauma, tumor, spina bifida, intervertebral disk	Frequent; may be continuous or induced by exercise or stress	Consistent habit and time; physical exercise; high fluid intake; high-fiber foods and bulk agents as necessary for firm stool consistency; suppository program, Valsalva maneuver, manual removal

To assist the patient with constipation with achieving elimination of soft bulky stools on a regular basis, the rehabilitation nurse develops a program of constipation/impaction management (Dochterman & Bulechek, 2004) incorporating diet, fluid intake, exercise, timing, and medication.

Diet and Fluid Intake. The most important dietary factor when considering constipation is the amount of fiber ingested. The recommended amount is 28 to 30 g/day (Doughty, 2006).

In adding fiber to the diet, the rehabilitation nurse must be cognizant of the person's likes and dislikes and especially of ability to chew because many high-fiber foods require adequate mastication. This consideration is extremely important with persons whose residual deficits affect either the innervation or muscle function of the face, mouth, and throat. If the person is unable to handle high-fiber foods adequately, then supplementing the diet with unprocessed bran or adding bran to cooked vegetables and fruit should be considered. As stated previously, fiber binds water in the intestine in the form of a gel. This prevents the overabsorption of water in the large intestine and ensures that the feces are bulky and soft. Fiber also adds weight to the stool, speeds up slow passage, and slows down rapid transit.

The highest source of fiber is minimally processed cereal. Other sources of fiber are legumes such as peas, beans, and millet; root vegetables such as potatoes, parsnips, and carrots; and fruits and leafy vegetables. Bran is one of the most concentrated sources of natural food fiber available. It is the outer layer or covering of the wheat kernel. Miller's bran is the richest source of fiber available, containing 44% dietary fiber (Brunton, 1990). Recipes for adding fiber to the diet are shown in Box 19-2.

Fiber should be introduced gradually into the diet to avoid untoward effects such as abdominal discomfort, flatulence, and diarrhea (Brunton, 1990). Bran is considered superior to other bulk laxatives because it is most effective in increasing

---

BOX 19-2 Fiber Supplement Recipes

Power Pudding*
½ cup prune juice
½ cup applesauce
½ cup wheat bran flakes
½ cup canned or stewed prunes
¼ to 1 cup per day for desired results

Bran Formula
1 cup unprocessed miller's bran
1 cup applesauce
¼ cup prune juice
1 tablespoon per day and increase daily dose by 1 tablespoon each week until desired results

*From Neal, L. J. (1995). Power-pudding: Natural laxative therapy for the elderly who are homebound. *Home Healthcare Nurse, 13*(3), 66-71.

---

fecal weight (Iseminger & Hardy, 1982). Bran, however, can bind orally with and reduce the intestinal absorption of many drugs such as cardiac glycosides, salicylates, nitrofurantoin, and coumarin derivatives and should therefore be taken separately from them (Brunton, 1990).

Adequate fluids are essential to avoid and manage constipation. It is often necessary for the nurse to be creative in assisting the patient with meeting the necessary fluid intake. The nurse also must be fully aware of all aspects of the patient's rehabilitation plan, including bladder rehabilitation and therapy schedules, so as not to jeopardize but rather to enhance and facilitate the comprehensive plan for rehabilitation.

Exercise. Diet alone is not sufficient to alleviate constipation. Physical activity is essential and can be accomplished easily in rehabilitation settings by incorporating therapy sessions as a means of achieving needed exercise. The activity of physical movement or even ambulating a short distance can be sufficient to stimulate defecation.

Timing. The timing of the bowel program should be considered when establishing the therapy schedule. Ignoring the urge to defecate is a major cause of constipation, and the individual should not be given the impression that defecating is less important than any other part of the rehabilitation plan. For diabetics a daily toileting time in the morning, when colonic activity is maximal, may help avoid constipation (Haines, 1995).

Medications. Although laxatives are beneficial for treating acute constipation, they are not recommended for chronic problems. An exception would be cancer patients who are taking narcotics. They may need to add a senna derivative, such as Senokot S, plus a stool softener, to their plan to offset the opiate effect on the GI tract. As narcotic doses increase, so should the amount of senna or stool softener to prevent constipation (Bisanz, 1997).

Diarrhea. When a patient experiences diarrhea, an investigation for impacted feces is conducted before other action. If the bowel is impacted, then the basic components of bowel management should be explained and the nursing interventions for the patient with constipation should be instituted. If diarrhea is treated without assessing for impaction, then a more complex problem could arise—namely, bowel obstruction.

Diarrhea management (Dochterman & Bulechek, 2004) is most easily obtained by treating or eliminating the cause. If it is the result of disease, then the pathological condition should be managed. As stated previously, if antibiotics are the cause, then other antibiotics should be tried. Yogurt can be beneficial in managing the diarrhea. Foods may also cause diarrhea, and offending foods can be discovered and eliminated. Some foods help treat diarrhea in children, such as bananas, rice, milk products, or applesauce. Monitor nutritional content in the process of juggling the diet.

Electrolyte imbalance is a potentially serious problem when diarrhea occurs. The patient should drink 2 to 3 quarts of fluid a day and also supplement for fluid lost. Excessive use or an excessive dosage of laxatives or the initial phase of dietary supplementation with bran can lead to diarrhea. The following medications may cause diarrhea as a side effect:

1. Broad-spectrum antibiotics
2. Adrenergic neuron-blocking agents (reserpine)
3. Bile acids
4. Quinidine
5. Cholinergic agents and cholinesterase inhibitors
6. Prokinetic agents

Whenever diarrhea or incontinence occurs, the potential for skin breakdown exists. Meticulous perianal hygiene, thorough yet gentle, is essential after each episode. Commercial spray cleansers, such as Peri-Wash or Hollister Skin Cleanser, contain substances that emulsify the stool and aid in its removal. The skin also needs protection from exposure to stool.

If the skin is denuded, protective powder such as Stomahesive may be applied and then a petroleum-based protective ointment. If a candida infection has caused redness and itching, a medicated antifungal powder or ointment can be prescribed (Lincoln & Roberts, 1989).

Collaboration With the Health Care Team and Community Resources. Although the rehabilitation nurse is the primary team member involved in planning and implementing a successful bowel program with the patient and family, other members of the interdisciplinary team may offer important input for the successful management of impaired bowel elimination. The physician, dietitian, occupational, physical, or recreational therapist, speech pathologist, psychologist, pharmacist, and social worker or case manager collaborate with the nurse to plan interventions based on individual needs.

The physician prescribes treatments and medications and attends to any active medical problems. The dietitian assists the rehabilitation team in meeting the nutritional and fiber needs of the patient. The physical therapist assists the patient with an appropriate exercise program and transfer techniques. The occupational therapist designs adaptive devices to help the individual in managing the bowel program. Also, the occupational therapist and physical therapist may perform a home evaluation to determine if any bathroom modifications or adaptive equipment are needed to carry out the bowel program at home. The speech pathologist assists with helping patients communicate their needs and, along with the nurse and occupational therapist, assists with feeding and swallowing if a problem is present.

Recreational therapists, or activity coordinators in long-term care settings, assist with toileting goals during activities and community outings. The psychologist assists with any self-esteem or body image issues related to incontinence. The pharmacist is a resource on medication effectiveness, side effects, and interactions. The social worker or case manager assists with discharge planning and discusses with the family any care needs that may be necessary regarding implementing a bowel program at home.

The rehabilitation nurse, along with the case manager, plays a major role in coordinating the discharge plan and community referrals. Supplies and equipment needs related to the patient's bowel program must be considered and arranged well in advance. A bedside commode, raised toilet seat, or grab bars may need to be ordered for the home and can be coordinated with the appropriate therapy department. (See Chapter 14 for details.) Patients with SCI may require an assistive suppository inserter to be independent in their program. Gloves and lubricant as well as prescriptions for medications need to be arranged. Each patient's needs are different and require different community services. However, there are basic considerations when any patient with impaired bowel elimination is discharged. The nurse should give attention to the following items:

1. Cost and availability of supplies and equipment needed at home

2. Location of supplier and availability and cost of delivery service
3. Availability of support groups
4. Location of the bathroom in the home
5. Family or agency assistance needed at home to carry out the bowel program

IMPLICATIONS FOR BOWEL REGULATION AND ELIMINATION

Return to Work, Education, Community, Independence

Regulation of bowel elimination and prevention of incontinence, diarrhea, and constipation are key to achieving a high quality of life for persons with chronic illness and disability. Incontinence limits a person's social activities and may lead to premature placement in long-term care facilities. Incontinence "accidents" and lengthy sessions for managing bowel programs will affect a person's desire to attend school or ability to maintain a job. Self-esteem and body image suffer when bowel programs are unsuccessful.

Implications for Practice, Research, Administration, and Professional Education

Control of bowel incontinence and prevention of constipation and diarrhea have been under the purview of the rehabilitation nurse for years. Rehabilitation nurses are now practicing in a variety of settings where this same knowledge base can be used, such as home health care, outpatient clinics, assisted living, day hospitals, long-term acute care hospitals, specialized day care programs, subacute rehabilitation, and long-term care, as well as the traditional comprehensive inpatient rehabilitation unit or hospital. Nurses in all settings should receive education on the management of bowel elimination problems.

Research Needs. There is still a need for more research on bowel training methods. Early research on bowel elimination began in the 1960s. It focused primarily on the effects of enemas versus suppositories in achieving control and decreasing nursing time and hospital costs. These studies demonstrated the superiority of suppositories in terms of patient comfort and control.

Studies that followed focused on the effects of dietary fiber in preventing constipation and on studying the transit time of food in the GI tract. Recent research on bowel management has been conducted on comparing various bowel training methods for effectiveness and timeliness. More research is needed in this area. The nurse is in the best position to initiate future studies to validate rehabilitation nursing practice in the area of bowel elimination.

Case Study

Norma Smith is an 80-year-old woman with a right hemisphere stroke. She is a widow and has been living with her 50-year-old daughter. Her daughter works as a high school teacher full time.

Upon Norma Smith's admission to the rehabilitation unit, the RN notices weakness in both left upper and lower extremities. Ms. Smith is alert and oriented with some slurred speech. An in-depth history is taken. Ms. Smith denies any past bowel problems except for occasional constipation, for which she took milk of magnesia. She usually empties her bowels daily or every other day at 9 PM. Her last regular bowel movement was the day before admission. Since her stroke, 4 days ago, she has experienced fecal incontinence and felt a sense of urgency.

Upon physical examination, the nurse noted no abdominal distention, visible peristalsis, masses, or bulges. Normal bowel sounds were auscultated. Percussion and abdominal palpation were normal.

A rectal examination revealed a small amount of soft stool. A strong anal reflex was present, as was sensation. No rectal excoriations or lesions were present.

Ms. Smith has full dentures. A bedside swallowing examination conducted by the speech pathologist was normal. A history of prior dietary patterns revealed that Ms. Smith usually had tea, cereal, and fruit for breakfast; a sandwich with whole grain bread and fruit for lunch; and a full dinner of salad, meat, potatoes, and vegetables. Less than three glasses of fluid, other than tea, were usually consumed in a day.

Ms. Smith stated that she wanted to be as independent as possible because she would be home alone when her daughter was working. She expressed that she did not want to be a burden on her daughter. Current medications revealed none that would cause a problem with either constipation or diarrhea.

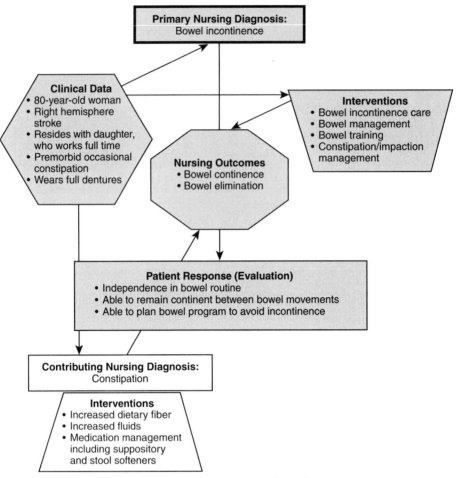

Concept Map. Mrs. Smith's primary problem related to bowel management is that of incontinence. Interventions are needed to address the contributing issues of diet and fluid balance. The concept map illustrates the interrelationships between the nursing diagnoses of bowel incontinence and constipation. To promote independence for Mrs. Smith, the rehabilitation nurse will focus on coordinating interventions to achieve the a good fluid balance, increase fiber in the diet, and work with Mrs. Smith on timing of bowel movements to ensure a period of continence between bowel movements.

CRITICAL THINKING

1. Identify the appropriate nursing diagnosis and outcomes for this patient.
2. List the interventions the RN would initiate to establish a bowel program.
3. Develop a teaching plan for the patient and her daughter.

REFERENCES

Abyad, A., & Mourad, F. (1996). Constipation: Common sense-care of the older patient. *Geriatrics, 51,* 28-36.

Baztan, J. J., Domenech, J. R. & Gonzalez, M. (2003). New-onset fecal incontinence after stroke: Risk factor on consequence of poor outcomes after rehabilitation? *Stroke, 34,* e101-e102.

Beddar, S. A. M., Holder-Bennett, L., & McCormick, A. M. (1997). Development and evaluation of a protocol to manage fecal incontinence in the patient with cancer. *Journal of Palliative Care, 13,* 27-38.

Berger, K. J., & Williams, M. B. (Eds.). (1992). *Fundamentals of nursing collaborating for optimal health.* Norwalk, CT: Appleton & Lange.

Bisanz, A. (1997). Managing bowel elimination problems in patients with cancer. *Oncology Nursing Forum, 24,* 679-686.

Brocklehurst, J. C. (1980). Disorders of the lower bowel in old age. *Geriatrics, 35,* 47-54.

Brocklehurst, J. C., Andrews, K., Richards, B., & Laycock, P. J. (1986). Incidence and correlates of incontinence in stroke patients. *Journal of the American Geriatrics Society, 33*(8), 540-542.

Brunton, L. L. (1990). Agents affecting gastrointestinal water flux and motility, digestants, and bile acids. In A. G. Gilman, T. W. Rall, A. S. Nies, & P. Taylor (Eds.), *The pharmacological basis of therapeutics* (8th ed.). New York: Pergamon Press.

Cannon, B. (1981). Bowel function. In N. Martin, N. Holt, & D. Hicks (Eds.), *Comprehensive rehabilitation nursing.* New York: McGraw-Hill.

Cheskin, L. J., Kamal, N., Crowell, M. D., Schuster, M. M., & Whitehead, W. E. (1995). Mechanisms of constipation in older persons and effects of fiber compared with placebo. *Journal of American Geriatric Society, 43,* 666-669.

Coffman, S. (1986). Description of a nursing diagnosis: Alteration in bowel elimination related to neurogenic bowel in children with myelomeningocele. *Issues in Comprehensive Pediatric Nursing, 9,* 179-191.

Correa, G. I., & Rotter, K. P. (2000). Clinical evaluation and management of neurogenic bowel after spinal cord injury. *Spinal Cord, 38,* 301-308.

Dochterman, J. M., & Bulechek, G. M. (2004). *Nursing interventions classification (NIC)* (4th ed.). St. Louis, MO: Mosby.

Doughty, D. (1992). A step-by-step approach to bowel training. *Progressions, 4,* 12-23.

Doughty, D. B. (2006). *Urinary & fecal incontinence: Current management concepts* (3rd ed.). St. Louis, MO: Mosby.

Dunn, K. L., & Galka, M. L. (1994). A comparison of the effectiveness of Therevac SB and bisacodyl suppositories in SCI patients' bowel programs. *Rehabilitation Nursing, 22,* 32-35.

Eberhardie, C. (2003). Constipation: Identifying the problem. *Nursing Older People, 15*(9), 22-26.

Edwards, L., Quigley, M. M., Hofman, R., & Pfeiffer, R. F. (1993). Gastrointestinal symptoms in Parkinson disease: 18-month follow-up study. *Movement Disorders, 8,* 83-86.

Edwards, L. L., Quigley, E. M. M., & Pfeiffer, R. F. (1992). Gastrointestinal dysfunction in Parkinson's disease: Frequency and pathophysiology. *Neurology, 42,* 726-732.

Gleeson, R. M. (1990). Bowel continence for the child with a neurogenic bowel. *Rehabilitation Nursing, 15,* 319-321.

Glickman, S., & Kamm, M. A. (1996, June 15). Bowel dysfunction in spinal-cord-injury patients. *The Lancet, 347,* 1651-1653.

Guyton, A. C., & Hall, J. E. (2006). *Textbook of medical physiology* (11th ed.). Philadelphia: W. B. Saunders.

Haines, S. T. (1995). Treating constipation in the patient with diabetes. *The Diabetes Educator, 21,* 223-232.

Han, T. R., Kim, J. H., & Kwon, B. S. (1998). Chronic gastrointestinal problems and bowel dysfunction in patients with spinal cord injury. *Spinal Cord, 36,* 485-490.

Harari, D., Coshall, C., Rudd, A., & Wolfe, C. (2003). New-onset fecal incontinence after stroke: Prevalence, natural history, risk factors and impact. *Stroke, 34,* 144-150.

Harari, D., & Minaker, K. L. (2000). Megacolon in patients with chronic spinal cord injury. *Spinal Cord, 38,* 331-339.

Harari, D., Norton, C., Lockwood, L., & Swift, C. (2004, November). Treatment of constipation and fecal incontinence in stroke patients: Randomized controlled trial. *Stroke, 35,* 2549-2555.

Heitkemper, M. M. (2000). Physiology of defecation. In D. B. Doughty (Ed.), *Urinary & fecal incontinence: Nursing management* (2nd ed., pp. 313-323). St. Louis, MO: Mosby.

Hoeman, S. P. (1989). Cultural assessment in rehabilitation nursing practice. *Nursing Clinics of North America, 24,* 277-289.

Hogstel, M. O., & Nelson, M. (1992). Anticipation and early detection can reduce bowel elimination complications. *Geriatric Nursing, 13,* 28-33.

Iseminger, M., & Hardy, P. (1982). Bran works! *Geriatric Nursing, 3,* 402-404.

Korsten, M. A., Fajardo, N. R., Rosman, A. S., Creasey, G. H., Spungen, A. M. & Bauman, W. A. (2004). Difficulty with evacuation after spinal cord injury: Colonic motility during sleep and effects of abdominal wall stimulation. *Journal of Rehabilitation Research and Development, 41*(1), 95-100.

Lincoln, R., & Roberts, R. (1989). Continence issues in acute care. *Nursing Clinics of North America, 24,* 741-754.

Lynch, A. C., Antony, A., Dobbs, B. R., & Frizelle, F. A. (2000). Anorectal physiology following spinal cord injury. *Spinal Cord, 38,* 573-580.

Lynch, A. C., Antony, A., Dobbs, B. R., & Frizelle, F. A. (2001). Bowel dysfunction following spinal cord injury. *Spinal Cord, 39,* 193-203.

Lynch, A. C., Wong, C., Anthony, A., Dobbs, B. R., & Frizelle, F. A. (2000). Bowel dysfunction following spinal cord injury: A description of bowel function in a spinal cord-injured population and comparison with age and gender matched controls. *Spinal Cord, 38,* 717-723.

Mancini, I., & Bruera, E. (1998). Constipation in advanced cancer patients. *Support Care Cancer, 6,* 356-364.

McCourt, A. E. (Ed.). (1993). *The specialty practice of rehabilitation nursing; A core curriculum* (3rd ed.). Skokie, IL: Rehabilitation Nursing Foundation.

Moorhead, S., Johnson, M., & Maas, M. (2004). *Nursing outcomes classification (NOC)* (3rd ed.). St. Louis, MO: Mosby.

Munchiando, J. F., & Kendall, K. (1993). Comparison of the effectiveness of two bowel programs for CVA patients. *Rehabilitation Nursing, 18,* 168-172.

Nakayama, H., Jorgensen, H. S., Pederson, P. M., Raaschou, H. O. & Olsen, T. S. (1997). Prevalence and risk factors of incontinence after stroke. *Stroke, 28,* 58-62.

NANDA International. (2005). *Nursing diagnoses: Definitions & classifications 2005-2006.* Philadelphia: Author.

Pryor, J., & Jannings, W. (2004). Preparing patients to self-manage faecal continence following spinal cord injury. *International Journal of Therapy and Rehabilitation, 11*(2), 79-82.

Rauen, K. K., & Aubert, E. J. (1992). A brighter future for adults who have myelomeningocele—one form of spina bifida: A comprehensive overview of this complex disease. *Orthopaedic Nursing, 11,* 16-27.

Ross, D. G. (1993). Subjective data related to altered bowel elimination patterns among hospitalized elder and middle-aged persons. *Orthopedic Nursing, 12,* 25-32.

Smith, D. A. (1988). Continence restoration in the homebound patient. *Nursing Clinics of North America, 23,* 207-218.

Smith, K. A. (1990). Bowel and bladder management of the child with myelomeningocele in the school setting. *Journal of Pediatric Healthcare, 4,* 175-180.

Stiens, S. (1995). Reduction in bowel program duration with polyethylene glycol based bisacodyl suppositories. *Archives of Physical Medicine and Rehabilitation, 76,* 674-677.

Stiens, S. A., Bergman, S. B., & Goetz, L. L. (1997). Neurogenic bowel dysfunction after spinal cord injury: Clinical evaluation and rehabilitative management. *Archives of Physical Medicine and Rehabilitation, 78,* 86-101.

Thompson, W. G., Longstreth, G. F., Drossman, D. A., Heaton, K. W., Irvine, E. J., & Muller-Lisaner, S. A. (1999). Functional bowel disorders and functional abdominal pain. *Gut, 45*(suppl. 2), II43-II47.

Tobillo, E. T., & Schwartz, S. M. (1998, October). Acute diarrhea. *Advance for Nurse Practitioners,* 39-76.

U.S. Department of Agriculture Center for Nutrition Policy and Promotion. (2005, April). *My Pyramid: Steps to a healthier you.* Retrieved August 11, 2005, from http://www.mypyramid.gov/guidelines/index.html.

Venn, M. R., Taft, L., Carpentier, I. B., & Applebaugh, A. (1992). The influence of timing and suppository use on efficiency and effectiveness of bowel training after a stroke. *Rehabilitation Nursing, 17,* 116-121.

Wald, A. (1991). Approach to the patient with constipation. In T. Yamada (Ed.), *Textbook of gastroenterology* (Vol. 1). New York: J. B. Lippincott.

Waldrop, J., & Doughty D. B. (2000). Pathophysiology of bowel dysfunction and fecal incontinence. In D. B. Doughty (Ed.), *Urinary & fecal incontinence: Nursing management* (2nd ed., pp. 325-352). St. Louis, MO: Mosby.

Yim, S. Y., Yoon, S. H., Lee, I. Y., Rah, E. W., & Moon, H. W. (2001). A comparison of bowel care patterns in patients with spinal cord injury: Upper motor neuron bowel versus lower motor neuron bowel. *Spinal Cord, 39,* 204-207.

Zejdlik, C. P. (1992). *Management of spinal cord injury.* Boston: Jones and Bartlett.

20

Muscle and Skeletal Function

Rhonda S. Olson, MS, RN, CRRN

As the young parents watch, their toddler takes his first clumsy steps into their hopeful, outstretched arms. They laugh and the child giggles with the pleasure of accomplishing something he was programmed at birth to achieve. Some 80 years later, the child, having grown and raised his own children, suffers a stroke and enters a rehabilitation unit. His family, the therapists, and nurses watch with hope, as he again takes his first hesitant steps through the use of a Lite Gait device. The staff members and his family cheer loudly—because this time he has regained an ability that was thought forever lost.

Regaining motor function is a key element of rehabilitation. This chapter contains information to guide rehabilitation nurses through the nursing process to develop plans of care with patients who have musculoskeletal injuries, conditions, or disorders. Whether the problem is one of weakness, fatigue, pain, or immobility and atrophy, the goal for rehabilitation is to enable patients to regain optimal function, coordination, strength, endurance, and comfort.

MUSCULOSKELETAL FUNCTION

Anatomy and Physiology

Bone Structure and Function. The human body comprises 206 bones, which give form, provide structure, ensure protection, and allow movement. In addition, bones are integral to hemopoiesis through cell formation within the marrow and to mineral homeostasis through regulation of calcium, magnesium, phosphate, and carbonate levels. The three basic types of bone cells are osteoblasts (bone-forming cells), osteocytes (which maintain bone), and osteoclasts (which reabsorb bone cells). These cells work to achieve a balance required for life. In young children the osteoblasts are active in forming new cells for growth. Postmenopausal women experience bone loss as bone cells are reabsorbed at rates that may exceed replacement.

Bones are made of two types of tissue. Compact or cortical bone tissue is strong, highly organized, and solid and constitutes 85% of the skeleton. Spongy or cancellous bone constitutes

the remaining 15%. All bones contain a portion of compact and spongy bone tissue. Approximately 14% of the body's weight is attributed to the skeleton, which may be subdivided into the axial skeleton (the 80 bones of the skull, thorax, and vertebral column) and the appendicular skeleton (the 126 bones of the extremities and pelvis).

Bone integrity is maintained through remodeling and repair. Remodeling includes laying of new bone tissue, for example, in response to a physical stressor such as exercise or a drug such as a bisphosphonate. Approximately 3 to 4 months are required for completion of the remodeling process. Repair occurs when a bone is damaged, for example, through a fracture or surgical wound. The time required for repair of bone is significantly longer and may take up to 4 years for severe injuries.

Joint Structure and Function. Joints exist where two bones meet, and they provide stability and mobility. Based on degree of movement and connecting tissue, joints may be classified as synarthrosis, amphiarthrosis, and diarthrosis. Synarthrodial joints, such as cranial sutures, are connections of bone to bone through a fibrous connective tissue and are immovable. Amphiarthrodial joints, such as the symphysis connecting the vertebrae, are slightly movable.

Diarthrodial joints, or synovial joints, such as the wrists, are freely movable. These joints are composed of a joint capsule or connective tissue that covers the end of each bone and is lined with the synovial membrane. Between the two bones in a diarthrodial joint is an enclosed synovial cavity filled with superfiltrated plasma or synovial fluid, which protects the articular cartilage. This structure provides a supportive cushion for the joint to absorb weight and stress with movement and activity. Rehabilitation nurses should be familiar with the movements of synovial or diarthrodial joints described in Table 20-1.

Muscle Structure and Function. Skeletal muscles are 40% of the body weight of an average adult. They are composed of water (75%), protein (20%), and other compounds (5%). A third of the protein stores within the body are found within muscles and are used for metabolism.

TABLE 20-1 Synovial or Diarthrodial Joint Movement

Movement	Description	Joint Example
Circumduction	Circular movement	Wrist
Extension	Straighten muscle	Elbow
Supination	Turn palm up	Wrist
Pronation	Turn palm down	Wrist
Adduction	Bring extremity into body	Arm
Abduction	Move extremity away from body	Arm
Flexion	Bend joint	Knee
Hyperextension	Extend joint beyond neutral point	Vertebrae (backbend)
Hyperflexion	Flex joint beyond neutral point	Neck (flex head forward)
Rotation	Turn head from side to side	Neck
Dorsiflexion	Lift foot up with heel down	Ankle
Plantar flexion	Lower toes below heel	Ankle
Eversion	Turn foot outward	Metatarsal joints
Inversion	Turn foot inward	Metatarsal joints

The motor unit is the functional unit of the muscle. It includes the anterior horn cell (lower motor neuron) of the spinal cord, the motor nerve axons, and the muscle fibers. Muscle fibers include sensory receptors that transmit impulses to the spinal cord to allow response to and identification of pain, injury, or fatigue. Muscles are designed to allow movement through contraction. Isometric contractions are static or holding, in which the muscle contracts but the limb does not move, for example, when pushing against a wall. Isotonic contractions are lengthening or shortening contractions and occur when the tension of the muscle is constant, for example, when lifting a weight or running. Muscles move in groups, with some fibers acting as agonists and others as antagonists. As the elbow is flexed, the biceps relaxes (shortens, antagonist), and the triceps lengthens and becomes firm (agonist). Chapter 14 contains details on muscles and their innervation and more about vertebral stuctures. (See Figure 14-5.)

Aging, injuries, and disease impact the musculoskeletal system and disrupt function permanently, temporarily, or sporadically. Although degenerative changes in bone mass, muscle strength, and joint structures are natural responses to the aging process, injuries and chronic diseases occur at any age. Many congenital conditions are precursors to musculoskeletal problems later in life.

CLINICAL PROBLEMS RELATED TO MUSCULOSKELETAL DYSFUNCTION

Rehabilitation nurses encounter patients with musculoskeletal disorders ranging from acute fractures and multiple traumas to chronic disorders, such as rheumatoid arthritis (RA) and fibromyalgia. Because many problems are complex and have potential for complications, patients benefit from the combined expertise of the rehabilitation team approach.

Scope of Problems in Musculoskeletal Dysfunction

Arthritis affects more than 45.7 million persons in the United States at a cost of $15 billion annually and is the leading cause of disability (Healthy People 2010, 2005; National Center for Health Statistics, 2003). The financial impact is calculated at $86.2 billion (1997 data, Centers for Disease Control and Prevention [CDC], 2004). An estimated 10 to 15 million persons have osteoporosis, associated with 1.5 million fractures every year (Iqbal, 2000; National Osteoporosis Foundation, 2005). Osteoporotic fractures of the hip, spine, and forearm are often related to falls. Hip fractures cause most problems and deaths. Fractures cost more than $17 billion annually; hip fractures alone account for $9 billion (Theodorou, Theodorou, & Sartoris, 2003).

With an aging population, the increased personal and economic tolls of arthritis and related conditions have a tremendous impact on public health and quality of life. Health-related quality-of-life measures for persons with arthritis and rheumatic diseases are determined by (1) healthy days in the past 30 days, (2) days without severe pain, (3) ability days without activity limitations, and (4) difficulty in performing personal care activities (Healthy People 2010, 2005).

The National Arthritis Action Plan (NAAP) connects public health and arthritis organizations with other interest groups at national, state, and local levels and sponsors a network of professionals and trained volunteers. The overall program goal is to improve the quality of life among people affected by arthritis. In 1998 the NAAP developed three key strategies to reduce the burden of arthritis: (1) surveillance, epidemiology, and prevention research; (2) communications and education; and (3) programs, policies, and systems (National Center for Chronic Disease Prevention and Health Promotion, 2005).

Classification of Arthritic Disorders

More than 100 types of arthritis have been identified and may be categorized as degenerative, inflammatory, or metabolic in nature (Arthritis Foundation, 2005b) (Figure 20-1). The categories of arthritis are described in more detail in the following section.

Arthritis Resulting in Degenerative Joint Disorders.
Osteoarthritis (OA) or degenerative joint disease (DJD) affects synovial joints, causing degeneration and destruction of hyaline cartilage (Osiri et al., 2005). Primary osteoarthritis (idiopathic) is most common and occurs throughout the central and peripheral joints. Previously intact joints are involved, in particular the hands, knees, hips, and spine. The etiology of primary DJD is unknown; incidence increases with age, and diagnosis is based on clinical and radiological evidence (Stacy & Basu, 2006).

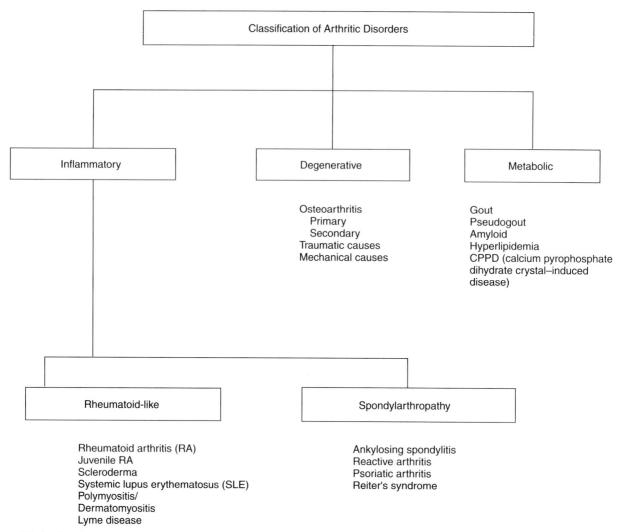

Figure 20-1 Classification of arthritic disorders. (From National Association of Orthopaedic Nurses. [1996]. *Core curriculum for orthopaedic nursing* [3rd ed.]. Pitman, NJ: National Association of Orthopaedic Nurses.)

Osteoarthritis is an active anabolic and catabolic process. Characteristic pathological changes are eroding of articular cartilage, thickening of underlying subchondral bone, and formation of osteophytes (bone spurs). Symptoms present a slow, uneven, and variable course involving mild to severe flare-ups. Joint involvement is generally unilateral, and systemic symptoms are rare. Pain and disability result from secondary effects, which include synovitis, joint capsule distention, bony proliferation, and damage to surrounding articular structures. Crepitus, palpable grating, swelling, mild inflammation (e.g., cool effusion), deformity, pain, limited mobility, weakness, and instability of the involved joint, such as hips and knees, are frequent complaints.

Secondary osteoarthritis is attributed to earlier trauma to the involved joint and to long-term mechanical stressors (Phipps, Monahan, Sands, Marek, & Neighbors, 2003). It is usually limited to the specific joints that were subjected to stressors. Mechanical stressors are wide ranging and include obesity, athletics, repetitive tasks, infection, endocrine disorders

such as acromegaly or hyperparathyroidism, neurological disorders associated with pain, skeletal deformities, and hemophilia (bleeding at the joints).

Arthritis Inflammatory Classifications. Arthritis inflammatory classifications encompass rheumatoid-like arthritis and spondylarthropathies. The symptoms of RA, juvenile rheumatoid arthritis (JRA), and osteoarthritis differ in ways that ultimately determine a patient's functional activity, long-term goals, and quality of life (Table 20-2).

Rheumatoid Arthritis. RA is a systemic autoimmune disease causing widespread inflammation of joint synovial tissues; it can affect organs. The specific etiology of RA is unknown; genes, viruses, and bacteria may play a role. Inflammatory and destructive aspects are due largely to activities of several cytokines (biologically active proteins produced by cells), especially interleukin (IL)-1, IL-6, and tumor necrosis factor alpha (TNF-α) (Bruce & Peck, 2005; Moreland, 2005). Presentation is variable and nonspecific, making early

TABLE 20-2 Three Types of Arthritis

	Osteoarthritis	Rheumatoid Arthritis	Juvenile Rheumatoid Arthritis
Onset	Females >40	Any age, but usually females 20-50	<16 years
Types of disease	Degenerative; localized	Inflammatory, systemic	Inflammatory, systemic
Signs/symptoms	Morning stiffness less than 1 hour / Stiffness at end of day	Morning stiffness longer than 1 hour; improves with activity	Decreased activity level; joint pain and stiffness
Joints affected	Weight-bearing; lower extremities	Multiple joints; symmetrical involvement	One or more joints; large joints
Treatment	Mobilization of joints; moderate exercise	Immobilization of joints in acute flare-ups; functional splints to maintain function	Rest periods and self-pacing; use of casting controversial; recommend no longer than 48 hours
Medications	NSAIDs, hyaluronan, Hylan G-F, intraarticular steroid injections	Steroids, NSAIDs; DMARDs (MTX, Plaquenil); BRMs (Remicade, Enbrel)	NSAIDs and DMARDs (MTX); BRMs (Remicade, Enbrel)

Modified from Krug, B. (1997, September/October). Rheumatoid arthritis and osteoarthritis: A basic comparison. *Orthopedic Nursing, 16,* 73-76; Driscoll, S., Noll, S., & Koch, B. (1994, November). Juvenile rheumatoid arthritis. *Physical Medicine and Rehabilitation Clinics of North America, 5,* 763-783; and Moorthy, L. N., & Onel, K. B. (2004). Juvenile idiopathic arthritis: The pharmaceutical treatments. *Journal of Musculoskeletal Medicine, 21*(12), 634-636, 638-639.
BRM, Biological response modifier; *DMARD,* disease-modifying antirheumatic drug; *NSAID,* nonsteroidal antiinflammatory agent.

identification a challenge. RA can rapidly and permanently destroy joint structures; therefore early diagnosis and aggressive treatment are desirable. Currently no diagnostic tests conclusively confirm RA, leaving confirmation to ongoing clinical analysis. The test for rheumatoid factor is nonspecific and has poor validity. Anemia may occur with active RA, and the erythrocyte sedimentation rate (ESR), the platelet count, and C-reactive protein may be elevated in the acute phase (Bruce & Peck, 2005). The basic symptoms of RA are symmetrical involvement, prolonged morning stiffness, and gelling (a period of increased stiffness when immobilized for a period of time, as if the joints had jelled). The swollen, painful joints may be quite warm and have restricted range of motion (ROM) and function. Patients often have constitutional symptoms, such as fatigue or weight loss.

The inflammation of RA is a progressive cycle that begins in the joint synovial membrane; the inflamed tissues cause edema, which produces stiffness. Continued inflammation leads to thickening of the synovium, particularly where it joins the articular cartilage. Pannus (granulation tissue) forms at these junctures, invades subchondral bone, and interferes with normal nutrition of the articular cartilage, causing necrosis. The pannus leads to adhesions between the joint surfaces, and fibrous or bony union (ankylosis) develops with loss of joint motion. Secondary atrophy of the surrounding muscles follows rapidly, making the joint unstable.

The hands are affected early, progressing to the classic fusiform tapering of the fingers and ulnar deviation. The wrist, ankle, elbow, and knee joints often are involved; shoulder and hip problems occur later. If unarrested, eventually RA may affect all joints and severely limit function. For example, temporomandibular joint (TMJ) involvement may hinder opening the mouth, or subluxation or dislocation of cervical

vertebra due to RA may result in paralysis or death (Phipps et al., 2003).

Although joint involvement is the most obvious problem, the inflammatory process of RA affects all connective tissue. Manifestations can appear within the pulmonary, cardiac, vascular, ophthalmological, and hematological systems. The unpredictable course and severity are marked by periods of exacerbation and remission. Physiological and psychological stressors can contribute to exacerbations. A few patients may have *malignant rheumatic disease,* marked by rapid progression, unremitting joint destruction, and diffuse vasculitis.

Juvenile Rheumatoid Arthritis. JRA is a common chronic disease in children, recently termed juvenile idiopathic arthritis. It is defined by joint inflammation and stiffness lasting more than 6 weeks for a child of 16 years of age or less; 1 in 1000 children are affected. The three classifications are pauciarticular (affecting four or fewer joints), polyarticular (affecting five or more joints), and systemic (affecting joints and internal organs). Genetic and environmental triggers, such as a virus, are possible etiologic factors (National Institute of Arthritis and Musculoskeletal and Skin Diseases [NIAMS], 2001).

Symptoms of systemic JRA include persistent joint swelling, pain, and stiffness; a high fever; and light skin rash. Laboratory tests that aid in establishing the diagnosis include elevated white blood cell count, low hemoglobin, positive antinuclear antibody (ANA) test (positive in 40% of cases), positive rheumatoid factor (RF) (positive in 10% to 15% of cases), and elevated ESR (sedimentation rate >100). An effective interdisciplinary treatment plan must address the special considerations required when managing the child's rehabilitation program. For example, JRA and other chronic conditions may contribute to delays in growth and development and interfere with education. One complication includes the tendency for these children to tighten their joints into positions of comfort, resulting in compensatory contractures and more marked functional loss (Cakmak & Bolukbas, 2005). Family members, teachers, and health providers are challenged to cope with the demands of the illness (Arthritis Foundation, 2005c).

Systemic Sclerosis. Systemic sclerosis (SSc) or scleroderma is a complex, multisystem connective tissue disease that affects the skin and internal organs, mainly the lungs and gastrointestinal tract. SSc is an inflammatory disease characterized by skin thickening (scleroderma) and deposition of excessive connective tissue and, eventually, severe fibrosis. Widespread vascular involvement is a prominent feature of SSc. Most patients have significant muscle and joint involvement, including arthralgias, myalgia, and fibrosis of the tendons; contractures may develop because of fibrotic changes in the skin (Black & Hawks, 2005).

Systemic lupus erythematosus (SLE) is a multisystem, autoimmune, inflammatory disorder with unknown etiology, although genetic, hormonal, viral, and environmental factors are under investigation (Trethewey, 2004). Women constitute 90% of SLE cases; 80% occur during the childbearing years (Lamont, 2005). Diagnosis is based on history and clinical symptoms.

Systemic Lupus Erythematosus. Initially SLE is manifested as a transient arthritis that responds to treatment. Joint deformity and contractures may develop. Remissions and exacerbations occur when multiple systems are involved and lead to a myriad of manifestations ranging from the characteristic butterfly facial rash, low-grade fever, weakness, and fatigue to clinical glomerulonephritis and pericarditis (Lamont, 2005).

Lyme Disease. Lyme disease, caused by the bacterium *Borrelia burgdorferi*, is transmitted to humans by the bite of blacklegged ticks (CDC, 2005). Serological testing supports the diagnosis, although the antibodies may not be detected until 4 to 6 weeks after the initial infection (Knisley & Johnson, 2004). Treatment is initiated based on a history of living or visiting areas in which Lyme disease is endemic. Lyme disease can be cured in most cases when treated in the early stages. Oral antibiotics, such as doxycycline, amoxicillin, and cefuroxime axetil, are effective first-line agents that require a 14- to 28-day treatment course. Manifestations of Lyme disease are classified into three poorly differentiated stages. In the early localized stage a patient may have flulike symptoms; the differential diagnosis is a "bull's-eye"-shaped rash (erythema migrans). Stage 2, early disseminated Lyme disease, may present numbness and pain in extremities, paralysis of facial muscles, meningitis, abnormal heart rate, and mild myocarditis (rare). When Lyme disease is resistant to treatment, undiagnosed, or reemerging, it produces chronic Lyme arthritis (especially in the knees), neurocognitive difficulties, fatigue, chronic muscle pain, and/or sleep disturbances. This third stage, late (or chronic) Lyme disease, may last for years (American College of Physicians, 2005).

Spondylarthropathies. Spondylarthropathies (SPAs) (spinal arthritis) are a cluster of interrelated chronic inflammatory arthropathies (see Figure 20-1). Although the etiology is unknown, they are genetically predisposed and triggered by environmental factors. Symptoms include inflammatory arthritis involving the back, an increase of a specific human leukocyte antigen (HLA) (HLA-B27), frequent inflammation of tendon-ligament insertion, and extraarticular manifestations, such as iritis or skin lesions. Diagnosis is more elusive than for osteoarthritis or rheumatoid arthritis. SPAs are seronegative spondyloarthropathies because the rheumatoid factor is uniformly absent (Khan, 2002)

Ankylosing Spondylitis. Ankylosing spondylitis, the most typical and common SPA, usually begins during the teenage years as a dull aching and stiffness in the back. It progresses to increased pain and restricted movement in the back, ribcage, and neck. Later postural abnormalities develop, such as flexion of the neck and back and flexion contracture of the hips. Severity determines impairment. Although new bone is formed, the ankylosis makes the spine osteoporotic with increased risk of spinal fracture; joint replacement may be indicated when the hips are affected severely. Advanced ankylosis may cause lower extremity weakness (cauda equina syndrome) and bowel and bladder dysfunction. Diagnostic symptoms are palpation tenderness to the sacroiliac joints, reduced chest expansion, calcifications (syndesmophytes) between vertebrae, and fusion of sacroiliac joints; radiological evidence is sacroiliitis ("bamboo" spine). Laboratory tests may show an elevated ESR or mild anemia but may be unspecific.

Reiter's Syndrome. Reiter's syndrome is a type of reactive arthritis that causes a triad of arthritis, conjunctivitis, and urethritis (Khan, 2004). It is the most common type of arthritis affecting young men between the ages of 20 and 40. Symptoms appear 1 to 3 weeks after an infection in either the genitourinary (GU) or gastrointestinal (GI) tract. GU tract infection, generally transmitted through sexual intercourse, is associated with *Chlamydia trachomatis*. GI tract Reiter's syndrome is associated with *Salmonella*, *Shigella*, *Yersinia*, and *Campylobacter*. About 80% of people with Reiter's syndrome have a predisposing genetic factor (HLA-B27) (Medical College of Wisconsin, 2005).

Reiter's syndrome can affect many body areas. Most typical are the GI tract, joints, and the eyes; less common symptoms are mouth ulcers, skin rashes, and heart-valve problems. An associated arthritis may affect the knees, ankles, and feet causing inflammation where the tendon attaches to the bone (enthesopathy). Spondylitis and sacroiliitis may occur when joints in the back become involved.

Arthritis Metabolic Disorders. Metabolic disorders, such as gout, may lead to arthritic problems. Gout is a clinical syndrome caused by the deposition of urate crystals in the synovial fluid, joints, or articular cartilage. Men older than 30 years of age constitute 95% of the 20 million persons in the United States with gout (Francis and Ranatunga, 2006). Risk factors include obesity, high-purine diet (e.g., organ meats or sardines), excessive alcohol consumption, hyperlipidemia, hypertension, renal insufficiency, diuretic therapy, and lead exposure (Choi & Curhan, 2005; Phipps et al., 2003).

Clinical manifestations of gout develop in stages (Table 20-3). More than 50% of the initial symptoms are in the great toe.

TABLE 20-3 Manifestations of Gout by Stage

Stage	Manifestation
Acute	Sudden-onset exquisite pain, swelling, and redness of the joint. Great toe is most common site. Often develops overnight.
Intercritical	Asymptomatic hyperuricemia (>7 mg/dl).
Chronic tophaceous	Development of solid urate deposits (tophi) in connective tissues, which leads to destructive arthropathy. Involves predominantly the upper extremity.

Modified from Black, J. M., & Hawks, J. H. (2005). *Medical-surgical nursing: Clinical management for positive outcomes* (7th ed). St. Louis, MO: Elsevier/Saunders; and Ene-Stroescu, D., & Gorbien, M. J. (2005). Gouty arthritis: A primer on late-onset gout. *Geriatrics, 60*(7), 24-31.

Patients experience acute attacks of gout as severe joint pain, edema in the affected extremity, and difficulty walking to the extent of making modifications in their lifestyle. As gout progresses to chronic symptoms, joint are painful and may become deformed. Patients may need to modify activities of daily living (ADLs) and their work environment. Complications include thrombosis, hypertension, and chronic pain, which can disrupt normal living patterns, family-related activities, or employment, creating financial burdens. Hospitalization may be required for episodes of renal dysfunction, cardiovascular lesions, or tophic monosodium urate crystal deposit–related infection. Persistent hyperuricemia and clinical manifestations are diagnostic (Black & Hawks, 2005). Rapid diagnosis and interventions, including education about dietary factors that contribute to gout, may reduce patient and family stressors.

Gout in the elderly differs from that found in middle-age males and has a more equal gender distribution. The elderly have polyarticular symptoms involving upper extremity joints and fewer acute gouty episodes but a more chronic clinical course and an increased incidence of tophi. Long-term use of diuretics, low-dose aspirin regimens, alcohol consumption, and renal insufficiency contribute to elevated uric acid levels and thus to gout (Ene-Stroescu & Gorbien, 2005).

Other Related Conditions

Fibromyalgia. Fibromyalgia syndrome (FMS) is a complex syndrome that affects approximately 2% to 4% of the general U.S. population; 80% to 90% are women. Characterized by fatigue and widespread pain throughout the musculoskeletal system, FMS is sometimes mistaken as a form of arthritis (Peterson, 2005). Since 1990 the American College of Rheumatology (ACR) has defined FMS as a chronic, painful, noninflammatory syndrome involving muscles, rather than joints. The ACR diagnosis depends on two key criteria: a history of widespread pain for at least 3 months and pain in 11 of 18 specific tender bilateral point sites (Wolfe et al., 1990). FMS symptoms are muscle pain at specific points on the body

(pain is elicited with gentle palpation), in broad muscle groups, and from trigger points (very sore points throughout the body that feel like ropy bands in some persons) (Peterson, 2005). A wide array of individualized symptoms range from fatigue, sleep disturbances, chronic low back pain, irritable bowel syndrome, restless leg syndrome, and chronic headache, to problems with memory or cognitive functioning. Diagnosis is based on history, largely subjective symptoms, and the ACR criteria; no serological tests detect it. The time between onset of FMS symptoms until diagnosis and treatment may take months to years, a source of frustration for the patient (Peterson, 2005).

Although the etiology of FMS is not completely understood, most researchers agree that it is a disorder of central processing with neuroendocrine/neurotransmitter dysregulation; there may be a genetic predisposition (National Fibromyalgia Association, 2005). The pain, fatigue, and anxiety exhibited by most patients with FMS often have been attributed to depression or a psychological disorder; stress, medical illness, and pain conditions may play a role in some patients (Mease, 2005). Self-help groups and resources, such as the Fibromyalgia Network and the National Fibromyalgia Association, provide information and education, research data, and offer help with coping strategies to patients, families, and providers.

Spinal Stenosis. Spinal stenosis, a narrowing of the vertebral canal at any level, creates pressure on spinal nerves or nerve roots, leading to neurological symptoms. Degenerative lumbar stenosis is common in elderly adults; bony overgrowth and ligament enlargement into the spinal canal, intervertebral disk herniation, or vertebral slippage (spondylolisthesis) may be responsible for nerve compression. The compression results in low back pain, leg fatigue and pain, numbness and paresthesias in the thighs and legs, and reduced tolerance for physical activity. Symptoms are aggravated by prolonged walking or standing and relieved with sitting or lying down. When severe, walking is greatly restricted and patients may have urinary incontinence (Snyder, Doggett, & Turkelson, 2004; Yuan & Albert, 2004). Smoking, sedentary lifestyle, and extensive motor vehicle driving are risk factors (Phipps et al., 2003).

Traumatic Injuries. Traumatic injuries may be acute and short term, or create long-term impairment, especially without appropriate rehabilitation. Most orthopedic trauma occurs in conjunction with falls, motor vehicle accidents, or crushing injuries. Musculoskeletal injuries range from simple bone fractures, dislocations, and sprains to complex and multiple traumas. Falls, crushing injuries, motor vehicle accidents, and gunshot wounds, especially those causing injury to the brain or spinal cord, are complex traumas. Multiple fractures and internal bleeding may be fatal.

Fractures. The highest incidence of trauma-related fractures occur in young men between 15 and 24 years of age and from osteoporosis-related falls in elderly females; 95% of pelvic fractures occur in persons older than 50 years. A severe blow to the body can cause a fracture, as well as minimal injury to weakened bones, as with osteoporosis or metastatic cancer (Phipps et al., 2003). Lack of weight-bearing activity and calcium leaving the bone matrix cause the pelvis to become porous and at risk for fractures. In the elderly the pelvis, wrist, and vertebrae are the most common sites; pelvic fractures may be complicated by hemorrhage, hypotension, or coagulation. Fractures represent a source of long-standing pain, functional impairment, disability, and death among the elderly and have devastating effects on their quality of life. In 1999, 338,000 people were hospitalized with pelvic fractures (Popovic, 2001); 50% of older adults did not return home or live independently after hospitalization for pelvic fractures (CDC, 2000).

Osteoporosis and falls are primary risk factors in older adults. For example, a person with osteoporosis who is unable to rise from a chair without using the arms was found to have the most significant risk factor for incurring a pelvic fracture (Bensen et al., 2005). Other factors, such as aging, inactivity, poor nutrition, smoking, excess use of alcohol, diseases, medications, cognitive impairments, functional impairments, and disabilities contribute to the primary risk factors (Kannus, Uusi-Rasi, Palvanen & Parkkari, 2005). Prevention and attention to risk factors, safety, activity limitations, environmental modifications, history of falls, and evaluations of cognitive status are interventions that involve the interdisciplinary team. Chapter 10 discusses patient safety in detail. Restraint-free environments preserve the patient's dignity, rights, and respect.

Simple fractures, knee and ankle ligament damage, and meniscus tears may occur after a fall, sports injury, or motor vehicle accident. Minor injuries are treated as outpatient surgery or in clinics with primary care follow-up visits. Short-term therapy to restore range of motion and function may be part of a home health care plan.

Amputations

An estimated 1.2 million persons in the United States have experienced loss of a limb (Amputation coalition of America, 2007). Malignancy, birth defects, and traumatic injury are other reasons for amputations. The objective of an amputation is to preserve healthy tissue with sufficient blood flow, maintain functional length of the extremity, and remove infected or ischemic tissue. Types of amputations based on their body location are defined in Box 20-1.

A last resort in severe cases of peripheral vascular disease, amputation of a limb is performed to alleviate pain, eliminate infection (necrotic tissue or gangrene), and restore function. Older adults with diabetes mellitus have risks that are aggravated by obesity, hyperglycemia, and even minor injury to the foot, and they may experience complications such as impaired vision, neuropathy, delayed wound healing, and renal insufficiency. Lower extremity angioplasty (preferably with stenting) or bypass surgery affects outcomes for patients with advanced lower extremity vascular disease. However, amputation is

---

> **BOX 20-1** **Types of Amputations**
>
> Below-the-knee amputation (BKA)
> Above-the-knee amputation (AKA)
> Amputation of the foot and ankle (Syme's)
> Amputation of the foot between metatarsus and tarsus (Hey's or Lisfranc's)
> Hip disarticulation—removal of the limb from the hip joint
> Hemicorporectomy—removal of half of the body from the pelvis and lumbar areas
> Amputation of hand or partial (specific digits)
> Amputation of arm—above the elbow or below the elbow (A/E or B/E)
> Shoulder disarticulation—removal of the limb from the shoulder joint

Modified from Phipps, W. J., Monahan, F. D., Sands, J. K., Marek, J. F., & Neighbors, M. (2003). *Medical-surgical nursing: Health and illness perspectives* (7th ed.). St. Louis, MO: Mosby.

performed if tissue loss has progressed beyond the point of salvage or if functional limitations diminish the benefit of limb salvage (Aronow, 2005).

Comorbid conditions and their degree of complexity influence how a patient adapts to amputation and the prosthesis. Impaired eyesight can make multiple medication administration, including insulin and blood glucose monitoring, difficult and potentially unsafe. Neuropathy can impair sensation of fingers necessary for preparing injections and manipulating oral medications. Preexisting cardiac and respiratory conditions may limit endurance. Pressure areas may be ignored owing to poor eyesight and lack of sensation. Delayed healing limits mobility and increases the risk for complications, such as urinary tract infections, pressure areas, and respiratory infections. The residual limb may not heal properly and delay preparation of the limb for the prosthesis; it may eliminate the patient as a candidate for any prosthesis.

Experiencing an amputation can have a devastating effect on a patient's quality of life and lead to social isolation and depression, especially when the person has to manage other medical conditions. Community reentry may be to assisted living housing. Although any amputation affects function and body image, young persons and those with upper extremity amputations tend to adjust more easily. Patients are more likely to use their prostheses when they regain function and accept the cosmetic design; new prosthetic devices appear very natural. Chapter 14 contains additional information about mobility and prostheses.

Trauma-Related Amputation. Amputations due to trauma often involve adolescents and young adults because they occur with motorcycle or pedestrian accidents, firearm injuries (4%), or blasts, such as in military conflict (Ramalingam, Pathak, & Barker, 2005). A quarter of those with lower limb amputation following a traumatic event report severe residual limb pain, phantom limb pain, and wounds at the closure site. Length of the residual limb and level of amputation greatly affect quality of life, ambulation with a prosthesis, and return to work (Pezzin, Dillingham, & MacKenzie, 2000).

Postoperatively the traditional soft dressing (elastic bandage) helps to shape the residual limb and reduce edema; then "shrinkers" further shape the limb in preparation for a temporary prosthesis. Following surgical amputation, the residual limb initially is wrapped with elastic bandages using the figure-eight technique (Figure 20-2). The bandages help control edema and conform the shape of the distal site for future prosthetic application. Rigid dressings, removable rigid dressings, and immediate postoperative prostheses (IPOPs) were introduced in the 1970s (Choudhury et al., 2001). These plaster cast sockets have been reported to reduce pain and healing time, prevent knee flexion contractures, and expedite early ambulation when compared with conventional dressings. Similar techniques are effective with above-the-knee amputation. Shortened hospital stays reduce cost, and mobility lessens complications.

Total hip disarticulation is a radical form of surgery in which the entire femur is removed; this is performed only when alternatives fail. The prosthetic limb of choice since 1957 is the Canadian hip disarticulation version, refined as the Otto modular endoskeletal version (Foort, 1957; Zaffer, Braddom, Conti, Goff, & Bokma, 1999). It has the advantage of lighter weight, improved cosmetic appearance, and flexibility. The prosthesis design has total contact suction suspension and an auxiliary custom-shaped pelvic belt offering independent ambulation, improved function overall, and optimal cosmetic appearance. Recently, total femur replacement in select patients with bone tumors has been successful in place of total hip disarticulation (Katrak, O'Connor, & Woodgate, 2003; Mankin, Hornicek, & Harris, 2005).

Successful ambulation using a prosthetic device depends on multiple factors. The residual limb tissue must be able to support the body weight, and the person must be able to balance and adjust to the gait pattern. Cardiac function, metabolic requirements, and energy consumption are components that give younger persons more success, especially with lower limb amputations. An aggressive inpatient rehabilitation program, followed by an outpatient clinic program, provides support, training, and education and helps with motivation for patients who are capable of achieving

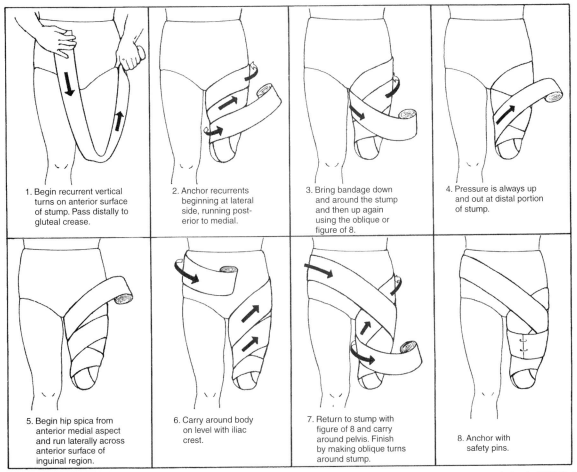

1. Begin recurrent vertical turns on anterior surface of stump. Pass distally to gluteal crease.

2. Anchor recurrents beginning at lateral side, running posterior to medial.

3. Bring bandage down and around the stump and then up again using the oblique or figure of 8.

4. Pressure is always up and out at distal portion of stump.

5. Begin hip spica from anterior medial aspect and run laterally across anterior surface of inguinal region.

6. Carry around body on level with iliac crest.

7. Return to stump with figure of 8 and carry around pelvis. Finish by making oblique turns around stump.

8. Anchor with safety pins.

Figure 20-2 Method of wrapping to help shape the residual limb after above-the-knee amputation. (From Mourad, L. A. [1991]. *Orthopedic disorders*. St. Louis, MO: Mosby.)

independent function and return to employment. Elderly persons benefit from intensive therapies and nursing interventions in hospitals paced to their endurance or from gait training as an outpatient. Goals may be modified to wheelchair mobility only when ambulation is unsafe or falls have occurred. Criteria for using a prosthesis and techniques for transfers, positioning, and ambulation following an amputation are featured in Chapter 14.

Muscular Dystrophies

Muscular dystrophy (MD) encompasses a group of nine inherited disorders characterized by muscle weakness arising from a mutation in a gene that codes for a protein necessary for muscle fiber integrity. Myotonic is the most common type of MD present in adults; Duchenne MD (DMD) is most common in children (Metules, 2002). DMD affects 1 in 3500 males at birth (Roland, 2000), and survival is rare beyond the early 30s (Muscular Dystrophy Association, 2005); advances in respiratory care have increased the life expectancy in recent years. Table 20-4 illustrates selected muscular dystrophies.

The genetic abnormality in MD causes a defect of the intracellular metabolism of the muscle fibers; muscle cells exhibit phagocytosis and necrosis with breaking of myofilaments. Altered striation of muscle fibers leads to hypertrophy or atrophy. Eventually, muscle fibers are replaced with fat and connective tissue, causing fatty infiltration and fibrosis. Diagnosis is based on history and physical examination, muscle biopsy, electromyography, and serum muscle enzyme levels. Creatine kinase levels are elevated during infancy but may elude detection in children who have limited symptoms without onset of muscle weakness (Phipps et al., 2003).

TABLE 20-4 Muscular Dystrophies

Onset	Symptoms	Progression	Inheritance
Duchenne Muscular Dystrophy (DMD)			
Early childhood—about 2 to 6 years	Generalized weakness and muscle wasting affecting limb and trunk muscles first; calves often enlarged	Disease progresses slowly but will affect all voluntary muscles; survival rare beyond late 20s	X-linked recessive (females are carriers)
Becker Muscular Dystrophy (BMD)			
Adolescence or adulthood	Almost identical to Duchenne but often much less severe; can be significant heart involvements	Slower and more variable than Duchenne with survival well into mid to late adulthood	X-linked recessive (females are carriers)
Emery-Dreifuss Muscular Dystrophy (EDMD)			
Childhood to early teens	Weakness and wasting of shoulder, upper arm, and shin muscles; joint deformities are common	Disease usually progresses slowly; frequent cardiac complications are common	X-linked recessive (females are carriers)
Facioscapulohumeral Muscular Dystrophy (FSH or FSHD)			
Childhood to early adulthood	Facial muscle weakness, with weakness and wasting of shoulders and upper arms initially	Slow progression with some periods of rapid deterioration; may span many decades	Autosomal dominant
Myotonic Muscular Dystrophy (MMD)			
Childhood to middle age	Generalized weakness and muscle wasting first affecting the face, feet, hands, and neck; delayed relaxation of muscles after contraction; congenital form more severe	Slow progression, sometimes spanning 50 to 60 years	Autosomal dominant
Distal Muscular Dystrophy (DD)			
40-60 years	Weakness and wasting of muscles of the hands, forearms, and lower legs	Slow progression but not life-threatening	Autosomal dominant

Modified from Muscular Distrophy Association (2006). Neuromuscular diseases in the MDA program (On-line). Available from http://www.mdausa.org/disease/40list.html.

Postpolio Syndrome

Another chronic disorder of the musculoskeletal system, postpolio syndrome (PPS) is a collection of symptoms that emerge in 28.5% to 64% of persons who experienced acute poliomyelitis (Khan, 2004). Of undetermined origin, PPS appears after an average of 35 years of functional stability, and incidence increases with aging. It is widely accepted that degeneration of the motor units, most likely caused by overuse, is responsible for new muscle weakness. This new weakness occurs only in muscles originally affected by the poliovirus (Halbritter, 2001). The mechanism of nerve degeneration has several possible explanations. It may be the result of excessive long-term metabolic stress on motor neurons. New nerve terminals, and eventually the motor neurons themselves, are lost. Inflammation of the spinal cord is found frequently on autopsy, possibly the result of an immunological or inflammatory event (Halbritter, 2001). It is important to allay patient anxiety by noting that there is no reactivation of the original poliomyelitis virus or reinfection (Khan, 2004).

Symptoms of PPS include generalized fatigue, lack of energy occurring with minimal activity (the "polio wall"), difficulty concentrating, muscle or joint pain, and muscle atrophy. The weakness is usually gradual, asymmetrical, and can be proximal, distal, or patchy. Deterioration is more rapid than in normal aging. Strength of several muscle groups declines, notably in the upper and lower extremity flexor muscles of shoulders, elbows, wrists, hips, or knees, but not in the extensor muscle groups used in weight bearing (Khan, 2004; Klein, Whyte, Keenan, Esquenazi, & Polansky, 2000). Other possible symptoms include cold intolerance and bulbar symptoms (swallow, speech, and respiratory symptoms).

Repetitive Motion Injuries

Injuries associated with repetitive motion can occur from an acute incident or overuse during recreational activities, exercise, and job-related tasks. Muscle strain, actually a tearing of muscle fibers, may present with tenderness, edema, or discoloration of the skin. With continued use, muscle fibers continue to tear and add to less-elastic scar tissue that tends to tighten. Excessive stretching before elasticity is restored may cause reinjury, turning a minor injury into a chronic problem, such as contractures. Electrolyte imbalance may occur during any aggressive exercise or recreation without adequate nutrition and fluid intake, causing muscle cramps.

Exercise Injuries. Several types of musculoskeletal injuries are associated with exercise. When bones are subjected to repeated stressors or forces in excess of normal activities, they initially thicken at the cortex. When stress ends, the thickening gradually disappears and returns to normal, without residual effect. Repeated contact with hard surfaces can cause lower extremity injuries; over time impact and shock may cause stress fractures.

Sports Injuries. Participation in sports activities, whether for fitness, recreation, or competition, is associated with health benefits. However, it also brings an inherent risk of injury; repetitive activity and overuse are common causes (Pink & Tibone, 2000); running is an example.

Running, an activity enjoyed by nearly 10.5 million persons in the United States (American Sports Data, 2005), results in lower extremity injuries for 70% of runners annually (Flinke, 2005). The primary cause is overuse resulting from training errors, such as running too far, too fast, and too soon. Common injuries from running include patellofemoral pain syndrome with dull aching behind or around the knee, calf and Achilles tendon injury, stress fractures, medial tibial stress syndrome (shin splints), ilio-tibial band syndrome, plantar fasciitis (burning heel pain), and sesamoid injury (injury to the sesamoid bones, which cushion the great toe) (Joy & Campbell, 2005; Pribut, 2004). Stress fractures are of particular concern because they may cause long-term morbidity if not treated appropriately. Although many running injuries can be prevented, walking may be an alternative with low risk for musculoskeletal injury (Colbert, Hootman, & Macera, 2000). Proper footwear and stretching, especially the Achilles tendon, may prevent or alleviate plantar fascitis.

Injuries differ across the life span and with gender. The musculoskeletal system of children and adolescents grows actively; their level of skill and conditioning differing from that of adults (Hutchinson & Nasser, 2000). For older persons, age-related changes in strength, flexibility, and coordination play a role in increased risk for injury, severity of injury, and subsequent rehabilitation time (Lindsay, Horton, & Vandervoort, 2000). Women may be more likely than men to sustain athletic injury, particularly in jumping and cutting action sports, such as basketball, soccer, and volleyball. Increased risk of serious knee injuries, such as to the anterior cruciate ligament, may have relationships with anatomical or hormonal differences and with knee instability, knee proprioceptive and neuromuscular control, or length of sports participation (Dugan, 2005; Hewett, 2000).

As Ferrara and Peterson (2000) state, "participation in sports activities for people with disabilities continues to gain in popularity." However, injury rates and problems appear to be similar for athletes regardless of their disabilities. Lower extremity injuries are more common among athletes who are ambulatory (e.g., with amputations, visual impairments, or cerebral palsy), whereas upper extremity injuries and carpal tunnel syndrome are found more among athletes who use a wheelchair in sports (Dec, Sparrow, & McKeag, 2000; Ferrara & Peterson, 2000).

Sports or exercise programs that include training for strength and flexibility, as well as promote gradual increases in activity, tend to prevent injuries. Early treatment is important. Rehabilitation nurses play a role in preventing injury and long-term disability or dysfunction. Simply educating athletes and coaches about the difference between soreness and pain may help minimize damage and facilitate return to the sport. Nonetheless, complications from an injury may develop later. For instance, athletes who had a knee injury earlier in life have an increased incidence of osteoarthritis of the knee later (Roos, 2005). Leisure and sports activities are discussed further in Chapter 28.

Job-Related Musculoskeletal Injuries. Although the incidence of injuries overall has declined since 1995, over 1.3 million occurrences of nonfatal illness and injury resulted in lost workdays in 2003; one third involved musculoskeletal disorders (MSDs) (C. Clarke, personal communication, October 17, 2005). In 2002 the U.S. Department of Labor initiated comprehensive industry and task-specific ergonomic guidelines to reduce workforce injuries. Developed by the Occupational Safely and Health Administration (OSHA), the guidelines are advisory only and intended to provide evidence-based information to help employers establish programs and protocols to prevent employee injuries (Nathenson, 2004). As Nathenson (2004) suggests, the ergonomic guidelines established for nursing homes may be adapted to inpatient rehabilitation facilities. In 2005 Texas passed the first state legislation requiring hospitals and nursing homes to implement a safe patient handling and movement program; a number of other states continue working toward legislative protection of health care workers against preventable injury from manual patient lifting (American Nurses Association Nursing World, 2005).

Carpal tunnel syndrome is three times more common in women (Viera, 2003). Repeated trauma, metabolic changes, or edema within the carpal tunnel compresses a median nerve, producing numbness and tingling in its distribution. A weakened abductor pollicis brevis muscle lessens thumb abduction. Gradual muscle wasting impairs functional independence.

Ganglion cysts can develop as a result of light repetitive motion activities such as writing, typing, and knitting or as a sudden onset due to extreme pulling or pushing of heavy objects. The cyst emerges gradually (it can enlarge rapidly) and may limit movement and cause pain during certain activities. Surgical removal may be required to restore function.

Secondary Complications

Several primary diagnoses may have secondary musculoskeletal complications. Shoulder pain and complications after a stroke and spinal cord injury (SCI), and steroid myopathy are discussed.

Musculoskeletal Problems Associated With Stroke

Pain. A variety of musculoskeletal problems may occur following a stroke. Upper extremity pain associated with hemiplegia may be due to glenohumeral joint subluxation, adhesive capsulitis, spasticity of shoulder muscles, nerve impingement related to improper positioning, soft tissue trauma, complex regional pain syndrome (CRPS), rotator cuff tears, and shoulder-hand syndrome (Aras, Gokkaya, Comert, Kaya, & Cakci, 2004; Lo et al., 2003). Precipitating factors include immobilization of the upper extremity, trauma to the joint, rotator cuff tears, spasticity of the shoulder muscle, and glenohumeral joint subluxation causing injury to central or peripheral neural tissue (Dursun, Dursun, Eksi Ural, & Cakci, 2000).

Hemiplegic Shoulder Subluxation. Shoulder subluxation (glenohumeral subluxation) results from the loss of normal muscle tone in the supraspinatus and deltoid muscles, allowing downward scapular rotation as the humerus slides down the slope of the glenoid fossa. There is extensive variation reported in literature regarding the incidence of shoulder subluxation. Because the integrity of the muscle and capsuloligamentous structures of the shoulder become compromised with the loss of muscle tone and function following a stroke, it is likely that most patients experience a degree of shoulder subluxation (Paci, Nannetti, & Rinaldi, 2005). Assessment of subluxation is done through an x-ray examination and through palpation. As the patient sits with the shoulder unsupported, palpation reveals a gap greater than one finger's breadth between the inferior aspect of the acromion and the superior aspect of the humeral head. Symptoms include pain with limited range of motion, impaired performance of ADLs, and reduced recovery of function in the arm.

A patient who has weakened shoulder musculature and needs moderate to maximal assistance in transfers is at risk for glenohumeral joint subluxation. If the patient is incorrectly transferred, such as being pulled under the axilla of the arms, the humeral head may displace inferiorly in the absence of muscular support. Shoulder subluxation, a devastating and painful complication of stroke, is preventable through good range of motion, proper positioning, and support of the shoulder and affected arm (Seneviratne, Then, & Reimer, 2005).

Complex Regional Pain Syndrome. CRPS (previously reflex sympathetic dystrophy or shoulder-hand syndrome with post-stroke upper extremity hemiplegia) (Quisel, Gill, & Witherell, 2005a) is a multisymptom syndrome usually affecting one or more extremities. The key symptom is continuous, intense pain out of proportion to the severity of the injury, which worsens over time. "Burning" pain; increased skin sensitivity; changes in skin color, temperature, and texture; swelling and stiffness; and motor disability are typical (National Institute of Neurological Disorders and Stroke, 2005). Evidence-based medical management includes pharmacological agents (topical analgesic creams, intravenous bisphosphonates, corticosteroids, calcitonin), physical therapy, epidural clonidine injection, regional sympathetic block (bretylium), and spinal cord stimulation (Quisel, Gill, & Witherell, 2005b). A national nonprofit organization, the Reflex Sympathetic Dystrophy Syndrome Association, provides information to patients and family members.

Conditions such as hemiparesis with an unstable knee or preexisting osteoarthritis may aggravate affected degenerative joints and limit range of motion during neurological recovery. Altered gait patterns predispose patients to falls. Patients who walk in a flexed, rotated posture and sit in a flexed position for extended periods may develop lower back pain, possibly lumbosacral radiculopathy (nerve root damage). Improper positioning eventually creates thoracic kyphosis and kyphoscoliosis, and patients ambulating with a cane or a hemiwalker may develop carpal tunnel syndrome in the unaffected upper extremity (Liss & Liss, 2000).

Musculoskeletal Problems Associated With Spinal Cord Injury. Secondary complications after SCI include muscle spasticity, contractures, and overuse syndrome in the upper extremities with functional limitations, including altered joint range of motion. Complications, such as knee flexion contractures and footdrop, are preventable. Hypercalcemia, more common in younger patients with SCI, causes calcium to leave the body through the urinary tract, producing increased risk of renal calculi and imbalance in bone remodeling. Heterotopic ossification (HO), deposit of new bone in soft tissue surrounding a joint that does not normally ossify, may follow SCI or traumatic brain injury. The buildup of bone deposits can cause contractures and limit range of motion, further impaired by pain. Range-of-motion and weight-bearing exercises help prevent HO, and patients who can tolerate weight bearing, even in a standing frame, benefit from doing so. SCI is discussed in detail in Chapter 14.

Muscle spasticity is more prevalent at higher levels of SCI involvement. These sudden involuntary movements may raise safety concerns for injury to the patient or caregiver during transfers or during treatments such as intermittent catheterization. Spasms may be severe enough to cause tissue trauma, bone contusions, and fractures or lead to contractures. Spasticity management clinics in rehabilitation facilities provide services to prevent complications of severe muscle spasms, including contractures. Approaches to the management are based on early mobilization and minimizing problems associated with disuse. Intrathecal baclofen pumps and other antispasticity medications such as Botox injections are used.

Overuse Syndrome. Overuse syndrome of the shoulders can occur after several years of using a wheelchair (Dec et al., 2000). Important activities, such as weight shifts and other position changes that protect skin integrity, transfer techniques requiring extreme stress on the shoulder joints, and adaptations for independent functioning of ADLs, can produce secondary shoulder injuries. Obesity, insufficient muscle strength, and neurological impairment associated with SCI may contribute to shoulder dysfunction. Problems appear when a patient is no longer able to perform activities and maintain quality of life owing to new limitations of shoulder overuse.

Steroid Myopathy. Steroid myopathy is a secondary complication of glucocorticoid treatment for systemic autoimmune diseases, such as SLE and RA. Corticosteroid use remains controversial and is restricted to relief of acutely inflamed joints with close monitoring for muscle deterioration. Although useful, many toxic effects occur. Muscular atrophy and weakness with the use of adrenocorticosteroids (glucocorticoid) therapy is well documented; side effects are less likely with low doses. Early signs of proximal muscle weakness, as with hip and thigh muscle atrophy, appear when the patient begins to have difficulty getting out of a low chair or climbing stairs (Black & Hawks, 2005). Muscle function studies are essential for the patient at risk for steroid myopathy, especially if symptoms of decline emerge.

FACTORS RELATED TO MUSCULOSKELETAL DYSFUNCTION

Osteoporosis

Osteoporosis, skeletal deformities, age, gender, and ethnic background may influence musculoskeletal dysfunction and affect rehabilitation negatively. The normal aging process, along with obesity, previous trauma, and genetics can increase the likelihood of complications.

Osteoporosis, as well as low bone mass (osteopenia), is becoming a major health problem. An estimated 15 million Americans have osteoporosis. More effectively prevented than treated, it is four times more common in women, especially when postmenopausal with decreased estrogen. Contrary to common belief, men are not immune to osteoporosis (Parsons, 2005). One and one-half million osteoporotic fractures occur every year; the disease is often "silent" until a fracture occurs. Osteoporosis results when bone resorption (osteoclasts) exceeds bone formation (osteoblasts), an imbalance often begun when peak bone mass is not achieved during adolescence. Risk factors include age, white race, family history, smoking, female gender, low body weight (less than 127 pounds), excess alcohol, low calcium intake, estrogen deficiency, and physical inactivity. Immobility results in decreased muscle action and diminished weight-bearing activities and leads to bone loss and disuse osteoporosis. Certain medications increase the risk of osteoporosis; glucocorticoids are the most common (Parsons, 2005; Whyte & Peraud, 2005).

Other Musculoskeletal Problems

Vertebral compression fractures (Figure 20-3), a complication of osteoporosis, are painful and may lead to progressive deformity with function limitations. The fractures are diagnosed through x-ray examination or computed tomography (CT). Thoracic lumbar sacral orthosis may be used to support the spinal column and maintain proper positioning for optimal healing; rigid bracing should be avoided, because complete immobilization results in bone loss. Kyphoplasty and percutaneous vertebroplasty are two new, minimally invasive procedures that stabilize vertebral compression fractures and reduce pain. Kyphoplasty may partially restore lost vertebral height and spinal alignment (Lieberman, 2005).

Other common musculoskeletal difficulties include scoliosis, kyphosis, lordosis, genu varum (bowing of the knees), and genu valgum ("knock-knees") (Figure 20-4). Lordotic (concave) extreme curvature of the spine and kyphotic (convex) excessive curve of the thoracic spine can cause impairments in cardiovascular function, respiratory status, anemia, and altered ambulatory ability. Muscle mass deformities, asymmetries, and masses may be evident.

ASSESSMENT

Comprehensive Assessment

Comprehensive assessment includes physiological and biopsychosocial data, such as the person's perception of the situation, current lifestyle, and support system. Chapter 14 details more about integrating musculoskeletal and neuromuscular assessment. Rehabilitation nurses initially examine baseline functional capacities, a specific dysfunction, or generalized complaints of pain and stiffness. Musculoskeletal assessment can be challenging; some diagnoses are formed entirely by subjective data or by exclusion, as with fibromyalgia. Function may be impaired apart from a patient having a painful or limiting condition.

History of trauma, strain, muscle weakness, limitation of joint movement, crunching, creaking, or giving way of weight-bearing joints accompanied by pain and stiffness are indicators of a musculoskeletal disorder (Mangini, 1998). Rheumatic fever and Lyme disease manifest with joint pain, fever, rashes and skin changes, eye symptoms, sleep disorders, or fatigue; generalized aches of the joints and muscles may signal acute viral infections. Any evidence of previous trauma may be indicative of reinjury, rather than a new onset of an acute injury, information pertinent in work-related injuries. Limitations in performing ADLs that affect social function, finances, and psychological or spiritual health are important initial assessments.

Psychological assessment includes adjustment to changes in body image, self-concept, and relationships with family members, friends, and co-workers. Assess the patient and family roles and functions before and after the disability and any role changes. Depression can be recognized and treated early. Chapter 22 discusses roles, responsibilities, and effective means of coping in detail. Additional resources may assist with financial management and other home or maintenance functions.

Establish a baseline through observation of a patient's gait, stance, height, posture, and proportions, and screen for abnormalities. When muscular weakness is evident, details of the problem and the evaluation are important to understanding the source. Weakness may be acute or chronic and may fluctuate with activity or result from fatigue; it may limit movement to perform ADLs, such as combing hair or brushing teeth. Numbness or tingling in the affected area is investigated to determine the presence of peripheral nerve damage. Distal weakness is often the result of neuropathy leading to difficulty with fine motor actions, such as clothing management or altering gait pattern. Flaccid paralysis results from denervated muscles and may present with visible atrophy, as in stroke or spinal cord injury. Limited joint range of motion frequently is accompanied by pain and joint stiffness; Heberden's nodes and Bouchard's nodes appear with osteoarthritis, whereas subcutaneous nodules and ulnar drift are present in RA (Figure 20-5). In RA, morning stiffness lasts more than an hour or does not improve much after moving around. In contrast, morning stiffness in OA eases after about 30 minutes of moving around; however, joint pain may worsen with overactivity (Bruce & Peck, 2005; Oliver & Ryan, 2004).

Postsurgical Assessment

After surgery for musculoskeletal problems, patients have a postoperative stay and then transfer either to a rehabilitation unit, a "fast track" unit for joint replacement, or skilled facility.

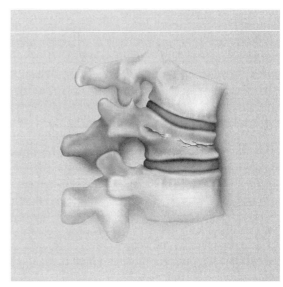

Figure 20-3 Vertebral compression fracture. (Courtesy Kyphon Inc., Sunnyvale, CA.)

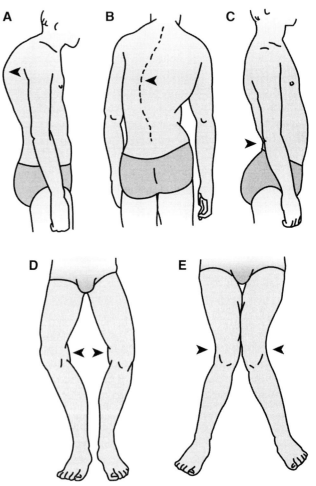

Figure 20-4 Common musculoskeletal deformities. **A,** Kyphosis. **B,** Scoliosis. **C,** Lordosis. **D,** Genu varum. **E,** Genu valgum. (From Black, J. M., & Hawks, J. H. [2005]. Medical-surgical nursing: Clinical management for positive outcomes [7th ed.]. St. Louis, MO: Saunders.)

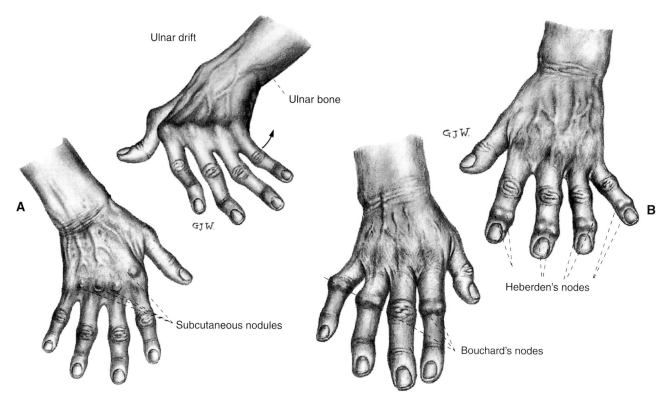

Figure 20-5 A, Joint involvement with rheumatoid arthritis. **B,** Osteoarthritis. Heberden's nodes and Bouchard's nodes. (From Mourad, L. A. [1991]. *Orthopedic disorders*. St. Louis, MO: Mosby.)

Some may go directly home. A rehabilitation nursing assessment is essential at all levels of care to prevent complications. The surgical site must be monitored continually for circulation, sensation, and movement (CSM). Specifically, observe, evaluate, and document skin color, temperature, and sensation, level of pain, pulses, and swelling. CSM is standard for monitoring the extremities when patients have casts, splints, and elastic dressings. Drains usually are removed from the surgical site in the acute hospital. The site is assessed for increased edema, firmness on palpation, or evidence of bleeding. Decreased blood pressure, increased pulse, and anxiety are early signs of postoperative hemorrhage.

Compartment syndrome, a result of trauma, occurs when pressure from bleeding or edema within a limited anatomical space compromises circulation, viability, and function of the enclosed tissues. It may arise from external pressure of a cast or tight dressing, especially in the lower legs, forearm, and hand. Undetected, this syndrome can cause loss of function, deformity, and possible amputation. Any new immobilization device, including a cast or splint, may press on a bony prominence to irritate the skin or form blisters, which may become infected. With skin breakdown patients experience delayed healing, complications, and have more hospital stays and costs.

When severe anemia occurs following musculoskeletal surgery, myocardial ischemia and cardiopulmonary complications are risks during acute care rehabilitation (Diamond, 2000). Episodes of oxygen desaturation and cardiopulmonary responses may compromise self-care and therapy sessions. Low endurance and poor exercise tolerance limit progress in

therapy, lead to extended hospital stays, and elevate risks for complications.

Fat embolism syndrome (FES) is a rare, but potentially fatal complication in which fat globules released into the bloodstream from the bone marrow and surrounding tissue travel to the lungs and block the capillaries and arterioles. Risk occurs with fractures of the pelvis, femur, and tibia or multiple trauma, or after total hip replacement or total knee arthroplasty. Symptoms of FES include hypoxia, tachypnea, tachycardia, petechiae, fever, lipuria, and chest pain; neurological symptoms are altered mental status with restlessness, confusion, and lethargy. Arterial partial pressure of oxygen, infiltrates found on chest x-ray film, arterial blood gases, and lowered hemoglobin and platelet counts are diagnostic.

Laboratory Tests and Diagnostic Studies

Blood studies provide useful data about musculoskeletal problems in several ways. Red blood cell count reflects the actual number of formed cells and the specific volume of blood; when abnormal, the body is responding or lacks response to certain processes, such as postoperative anemia after hip replacement in elderly persons. White blood cell count and differential detect inflammation and infection. Culture and sensitivity identify the source of infections in surgical wounds, urine, blood, or respiratory secretions.

C-reactive protein is used to support the diagnosis of RA and may also correlate directly with the presence of atherosclerosis in patients with RA (who are at a greater risk of developing cardiovascular events than individuals without RA)

(Gonzalez-Gay et al., 2005). The ESR is elevated with RA and other types of inflammation. RF and other proteins coat the erythrocytes and make them heavier; rapid settling of red blood cells is the result of the level of fibrinogen (Phipps et al., 2003).

Immunoglobulins (gamma globulins) are inflammatory proteins that possess known antibody activity. Immunoglobulin G and immunoglobulin M antibodies are significant in inflammatory and infectious diseases such as hepatitis and rubella. Chronic hepatitis is associated with an array of rheumatic manifestations, including arthritis and arthralgias (Vassilopoulos & Calabrese, 2003).

Electrolyte levels are significant in musculoskeletal dysfunction and monitored throughout the entire postoperative phase of recovery, especially for elderly patients. Calcium levels affect musculoskeletal conditions. Hypercalcemia occurs with immobilization, lack of weight bearing, and conditions such as metastatic bone disease when bone calcium is lost. Hypocalcemia often occurs in conjunction with hyperkalemia.

Blood urea nitrogen (BUN) and serum creatinine are two renal function studies that detect levels of dehydration, increased protein metabolism, and renal impairment. In the case of renal insufficiency, the BUN and creatinine elevate together in a 10:1 ratio.

Alkaline phosphatase (ALP) and creatine kinase (CK) are significant in bone disease and muscular damage. Increases in ALP indicate new bone formation and healing fractures. Healthy carriers of X-linked Duchenne muscular dystrophy also have elevated CK levels. Uric acid levels, when persistently elevated in men older than 30 years who have recurrent monoarthritis, may indicate gout. Joint aspiration fluid of urate crystals is the definitive diagnosis.

Dual-energy x-ray absorptiometry (DXA) is an accurate, sensitive, and painless measure of bone mineral density (BMD). It is the gold standard in testing for osteoporosis (Small, 2005). Central (hip and spine) DXA is preferred over peripheral (wrist and heel) DXA; peripheral DXA is less sensitive and less specific (Whyte & Peraud, 2005).

Diskography is used to evaluate the integrity of intervertebral disk space and determine specific levels of vertebral involvement. This test is more uncomfortable because it requires contrast medium and saline to be injected into the disk space to reproduce the back or leg pain associated with the pathological condition.

Scintigraphy, such as bone scan, determines uptake of radionuclide in areas called "hot spots" of osteoblastic and osteolytic processes in the bones. Analysis of joint fluids can be beneficial in the diagnosis of gout and infectious arthritis. Aspirated fluid is analyzed for Gram stain, white blood cell count with differential, urate crystals, culture, and sensitivity.

Pediatric Assessment

Infants, young children, and adolescents experience musculoskeletal conditions, such as muscular dystrophy, JRA, and fractures, as well as sequelae from congenital conditions of myelomeningocele and cerebral palsy. Pediatric assessment differs greatly because of the need for age and developmentally

appropriate techniques and subjective data gathered from parents. Observation, including play and pediatric pain assessment, may replace extensive hands-on assessment. Observing a child's body posture, facial expression, and vocalizations of discomfort while at rest or during movement may provide information about pain. Chapter 23 provides details about pain, and Chapter 31 contains information specific to pediatric rehabilitation.

Assessment of muscular dystrophy in children follows the same age-appropriate techniques as for JRA. Specific assessment involves observation of posture, respiratory function, cardiac status, ability to ambulate with or without specific devices, and functional level in the home, school, and at play.

NURSING DIAGNOSES

After conducting a thorough assessment of the patient with a musculoskeletal disorder, the rehabilitation nurse identifies nursing diagnoses. Table 20-5 lists nursing diagnoses common to the rehabilitation of patients with musculoskeletal disorders.

GOALS

Goals of patients with musculoskeletal conditions are to achieve and maintain maximum independence and function, comfort, and safety. A young man with a below-the-knee amputation may set a realistic, long-term goal of independently performing all tasks of daily living and functioning at work or school with his prosthesis. A woman with PPS may set goals to coordinate tasks of a caregiver and be independent using a power wheelchair. A child with JRA who has minimal pain and stiffness may desire to participate actively in school and play. Related outcome goals are to maintain joint function and prevent complications, to manage energy and promote strength and endurance, control pain, and practice effective coping against depression.

Health Promotion and Prevention

Rehabilitation nurses incorporate the national goals of health promotion and prevention into care within all practice settings. *Healthy People 2010* (2005) lists more than 16 goals for persons with musculoskeletal disorders as highlighted in Table 20-6. Health promotion and prevention plans support ergonomic work environments, healthy body weight, and moderate physical exercise. Sample programs that promote these goals are the Arthritis Foundation Self-Help Courses, Arthritis Aquatics, and PACE Land Exercise Program (People With Arthritis Can Exercise) (Arthritis Foundation, 2005a). The self-help courses are a 6-week health promotion program designed to help those with arthritis to better understand the disease, become active in their arthritis care, and cope with chronic pain. Such programs are opportunities for rehabilitation nurses to become involved in community action and are referral resources for patients.

TABLE 20-5 Nursing Diagnoses, Interventions, and Outcomes Applicable to Musculoskeletal Disorders   **NIC/NOC**

Nursing Diagnosis	Nursing Interventions	Nursing Outcomes
Pain, acute and chronic	Pain management	Pain control
Activity intolerance (pain and fatigue)	Energy management	Energy conservation
Self-care deficit	Self-care assistance	Self-care: ADL Self-care: IADL
Impaired physical mobility	Exercise therapy: Joint mobility Exercise promotion: Strength training Exercise therapy: Ambulation	Joint movement: Active muscle function Ambulation: Walking Ambulation: Wheelchair
Disturbed body image	Body image enhancement	Adjustment to changes in physical appearance and body function

Possible associated nursing diagnoses:
- Reactive depression
- Anxiety
- Social isolation
- Deficient knowledge
- Impaired skin integrity
- Ineffective sexuality pattern

Data from Moorhead, S., Johnson, M., & Maas, M. (Eds.). (2004). *Nursing outcomes classification (NOC)* (3rd ed.). St. Louis, MO: Mosby; Dochterman, J. M., & Bulechek, G. M. (2004). *Nursing interventions classification (NIC)* (4th ed.). St. Louis, MO: Mosby; and NANDA International. (2005). *Nursing diagnoses: Definitions and classification, 2005-2006* (6th ed.). Philadelphia: Author.

TABLE 20-6 *Healthy People 2010* Objectives

Goal	Baseline	Current Progress
• Increase the mean number of days without severe pain among adults who have chronic joint symptoms	Developmental	N/A
• Reduce the proportion of adults with chronic joint symptoms who experience a limitation in activity due to arthritis by 22%	27% (1997)	No significant trend (2000)
• Increase the employment rate among adults with arthritis in working-age population by 16%	67% (1997)	No significant trend (2000)
• Reduce the proportion of adults with osteoporosis by 20%	10% (1988-94)	No data available
• Reduce the proportion of adults who are hospitalized for vertebral fractures associated with osteoporosis by 20%	17.5 per 10,000 population (1998)	No significant trend (1999)
• Reduce activity limitation due to chronic back conditions by 22%	32 per 1,000 population (1997)	Decline to 26 per 1,000 population (2000)
• Reduce the rate of lower extremity amputation in persons with diabetes by 55%	4.1 per 1,000 population (1997)	Increase to 4.8 per 1,000 population (1998-2000)
• Reduce hip fractures among older adults by 60% in females, 20% in males	1,056 (women); 593 (men) per 100,000 population	Favorable trend (2000)
• Reduce work-related injuries resulting in medical treatment, lost time from work, or restricted work activity by 30%	6.2 per 100 full-time workers (1998)	Decline to 5 per 100 full-time workers
• Reduce the rate of injury and illness cases involving days away from work due to overexertion or repetitive motion by 50%	675 per 100,000 full time workers (1997)	No data reported

Modified from *Healthy People 2010*. (2005). Available from http://www.healthypeople.gov; and *Healthy People 2010 Progress Review*. (2005). Available from http://www.healthypeople.gov/data/PROGRVW/.

REHABILITATION NURSING INTERVENTIONS

Rehabilitation nurses use traditional and creative interventions when working with patients challenged by musculoskeletal disorders and meeting mutually established goals. Box 20-2 provides goals and health promotion and prevention interventions specific to musculoskeletal situations.

Surgical Interventions

Surgical interventions may relieve pain, stabilize joints, and correct deformities. More than 200,000 persons in the United States undergo total hip replacement (THR) annually (Phipps et al., 2003), a number that has increased steadily since 1990 (Kurtz et al., 2005). THR improves quality of life and functional recovery for many healthy adults (Ethgen, Bruyere, Richy, Dardennes, & Reginster, 2004). Diagnoses that indicate a THR include osteoarthritis, RA, traumatic arthritis, avascular necrosis, hip fractures, benign and malignant bone tumors, arthritis associated with Paget's disease, and ankylosing spondylitis, or JRA.

Choices of surgical techniques, rehabilitation approaches, prosthetic designs, and materials for specific patient groups vary among physicians. Surgical repair techniques are based on the location of the fracture, bone quality, displacement, and type (simple or comminuted). Femoral neck fractures are treated by either internal fixation using screws or pins or by prosthetic replacement. Intertrochanteric fractures are treated using internal fixation such as screws. Prosthetic replacement is used for older patients with displaced fractures to minimize complications. Total hip arthroplasty replaces both the acetabular cup and the femoral head with prostheses, whereas a hemiarthroplasty replaces only the femoral head. New, minimally invasive techniques for hip replacement are under development and may reduce postoperative pain and recovery time significantly; similar innovations are being developed in robotically aided surgery. Prosthetic devices are either cemented in place or may be press-fitted or porous-coated to allow the bone to grow into the prosthesis, or a combination of both (hybrid) (Phipps et al., 2003). Figure 20-6 illustrates cemented and cementless hip prosthetic devices.

Persons who have weight-bearing and hip precautions need close monitoring after hip surgery. Although weight bearing is restricted to reduce the distraction force on the prosthesis, those patients with cemented prostheses usually are allowed to bear weight as tolerated. Walkers and canes allow patients to

---

BOX 20-2 Goals for Specific Musculoskeletal Situations

1. Decreasing Osteoporotic Fractures

Short-term goals:	Decrease falls; prevent fractures
Prevention:	Healthy dietary habits; calcium and vitamin D supplements; exercise to maintain muscle strength and balance

2. Decreasing Rate of Amputations

Short-term goal:	Safe management of blood glucose levels
Prevention:	Lower Extremity Amputation Prevention Program* (standardized foot sensation screening); education—avoid trauma, foot inspection; early intervention with podiatrists; tight control of blood glucose levels early in disease course

3. Reducing Pain With Arthritis and Other Rheumatic Conditions

Short-term goals:	Reduce pain and discomfort; reduce limitations in activity; maintain joint ROM, strength, and overall mobility
Long-term goals:	Minimize effects of pain and joint stiffness; prevent complications or further disability; self-paced regimen of exercise and rest periods

4. Decreasing Injury Rates Due to Overexertion, repetitive Motion

Short-term goals:	Maximize function; plan for efficient energy expenditure; appropriate use of assistive devices
Long-term goals:	Maintain active lifestyle; maintain optimal level of wellness; avoid overexertion

5. Prevention of Workplace Injuries

Short-term goals:	Proper body mechanics when lifting; recognize and control ergonomic hazards; early detection and treatment of musculoskeletal injuries
Long-term goals:	Institute ergonomic approaches in design stage of work processes; prevent disability; increase public awareness and education about interventions

*LEAP Program. (2005). *Bureau of Primary Health Care Lower Extremity Amputation Prevention Program* [Online]. Retrieved October 19, 2005, from http://www.bphc.hrsa.gov/leap/.

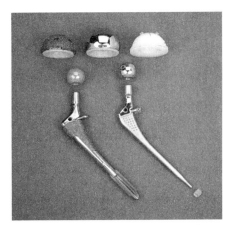

Figure 20-6 Hip prostheses. *Left,* Porous ingrowth acetabular cup and femoral stem, ceramic femoral head; *middle,* bipolar head for hemiarthroplasty (component fits on top of femoral head component), used with either cemented or uncemented femoral stems; *right,* cemented femoral stem and cemented acetabular cup. (Courtesy Zimmer, Inc., Warsaw, IN.)

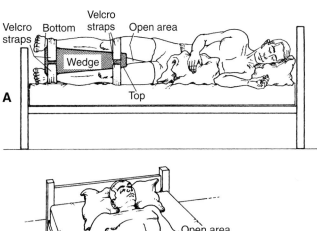

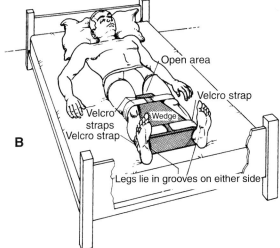

Figure 20-7 A, A patient who has a hip fracture or hip replacement surgery is positioned on his uninvolved side. His affected hip is slightly flexed. A foam wedge (or pillows) is used to keep his legs apart and abduct the hip joints. Note the 90-degree angle limit of flexion at the hip. **B,** The same patient viewed from the front illustrates the use of the foam wedge (or pillows) between his knees and legs. These supports keep the hip joints abducted. The top or affected knee must be supported firmly and steadily. It must not fall off of the wedge. His knees must not be allowed to touch one another. (From Hoeman, S. P. [1990]. *Rehabilitative/restorative care.* St. Louis, MO: Mosby.)

apply part of their weight on their upper extremities and maintain proper balance and posture. Hip flexion, adduction, or rotation must be avoided after total hip arthroplasty; flexion is limited to 90 degrees for 2 to 3 months. Pillows or abduction splints are used whenever a patient is in supine or side-lying position until the hip capsule is healed to prevent adduction of the operative limb (Figure 20-7). Positioning the patient on the operative side is usually avoided to prevent adduction of the operative limb.

Another potential complication from hip replacement surgery is infection at the incision site. It is characterized by a dull ache or unusual or persistent pain. Early signs include fever, redness, swelling, or drainage at the surgical site and increased pain. Infections may be treated with intravenous antibiotic administration and sterile wound care techniques. Because more than half of the infections occur at least 3 months after joint replacement and more than 2 years postoperatively, discharge instructions must include ways to avoid infection, symptoms, and the necessity of antibiotic treatment if infection occurs. Instances of systemic bacterial infections have been documented.

Prophylactic antibiotics before dental procedures, previously recommended for 2 years following all total joint replacements, are no longer routinely indicated in this population. However, premedication is appropriate for patients at risk of experiencing hematogenous total joint infection, such as those with immunocompromised status (e.g., RA, SLE) and those with comorbidities (e.g., previous prosthetic joint infections, malnourishment, hemophilia, human immunodeficiency virus [HIV] infection, type 1 diabetes, and malignancy) (American Dental Association, 2003).

Patient education programs may help prevent postoperative complications, reduce pain levels, and promote recovery for progress during therapy (Sedlak, Doheny, & Jones, 2000).

However, a systematic review of studies found little evidence that use of preoperative education over and above standard care improved postoperative outcomes, especially with respect to pain, functioning, and length of hospital stay (McDonald, Green, & Hetrick, 2005). Patients, families, and the rehabilitation team are responsible for adhering to precautions and being aware of the time span they require.

Total knee replacement often is bilateral and completed during a single surgical event. The bilateral knee x-ray films shown in Figure 20-8 demonstrate the condition of the joints before *(A)* and after *(B)* surgery with internal prosthetic implants. Mobilization may be more challenging, but improved ambulatory function in these weight-bearing joints can improve quality of life in a short period. Continuous passive motion (CPM) machines sometimes are used in the immediate postoperative phase of total knee replacement surgery, but they do not replace joint-range-of-motion exercises or ambulation

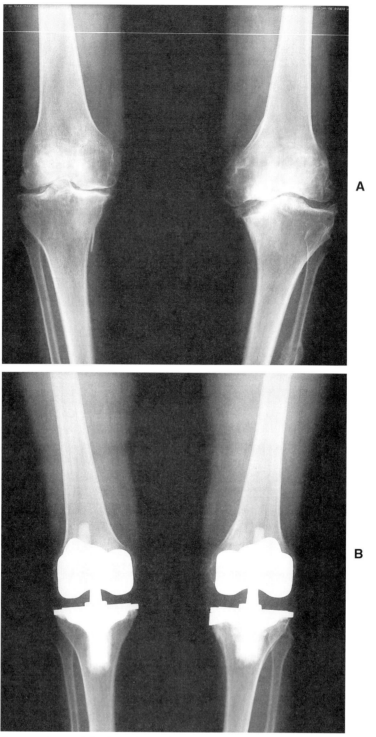

Figure 20-8 A, Radiograph of osteoarthritis of the knee. **B,** Radiograph of Duracon PS Total Knee System implants. (Courtesy Stryker Howmedica Osteonics, Allendale, NJ.)

during therapy. The CPM machine is complementary to therapy programs to increase the degree of movement. Findings from studies of surgeries for various types of DJD will be beneficial in weighing the risks versus benefits for patients at greater risk owing to their comorbid or coexisting conditions.

An intraarticular metallic spacer, the UniSpacer Knee System, is being evaluated. It is proposed that this implant can improve knee function, maintain ROM, and provide pain relief in patients with unicompartmental OA. This procedure is conservative and easily revised, if necessary, to any type of arthroplasty in the future. Although study results are mixed, early findings suggest that the UniSpacer is a viable treatment option for OA in the younger patient (Hallock & Fell, 2003; Scott, 2003).

Some surgical procedures may be performed for fractures and tumors or in attempts to relieve pain or correct deformities. For example, fusion of bony joints may be a last resort for severe pain and deformity. Total disk replacement and cervical anterior decompression is currently being investigated in patients with symptomatic cervical spondylosis. Preliminary results with the ProDisc-C arthroplasty indicate significant improvement in pain and functional outcome scores (Bertagnoli et al., 2005).

Phipps et al. (2003) provide the following definitions:

- *Laminectomy:* Removal of a portion of the lamina, the posterior arch of the vertebra to access the disk and spinal canal
- *Discectomy:* Removal of all or part of a herniated intervertebral disk
- *Foraminotomy:* Widening of the intervertebral foramen to allow free passage of the spinal nerve
- *Spinal fusion:* Stabilization of two or more vertebrae by inserting bone grafts, with or without hardware to gain vertebral stability
- *Decompression:* Release of pressure or impingement on spinal nerve roots by removal of osteophytes, bone, or soft tissue

Patient and family education, including discussions about pharmacological and nonpharmacological agents, occurs before interventions. The rehabilitation nurse encourages patients to have dialogues about previous pain management strategies and activities that may aggravate pain. Patients may take analgesics before exercise or with certain activities that increase discomfort during therapy, so they can manage the pain, reduce anxiety, and participate fully. Fusion after trauma to the spine may be an emergency procedure to prevent complications of cord compression. As part of informed consent, details are explained about the intended results, side effects, precautions, and possible complications or risk of paralysis for patients. It also weighs the potential benefits of increased function and decreased pain. Education and full information build trust in relationships and increase possibilities for improved outcomes.

Activity Intolerance

The nursing diagnosis of activity intolerance is defined as abnormal responses to energy-consuming body movements involved in required or desired daily activities (Gordon, 2000). Activity intolerance may be related to pain, discomfort, or muscle weakness; energy management, relaxation techniques, and stress reduction may increase a patient's tolerance for activities.

Energy Management. Energy management means regulating energy use to treat or prevent fatigue and optimize function (Dochterman & Bulechek, 2004). After assessing a patient's physical limitations, perceptions of fatigue, and feelings about the situation, the rehabilitation nurse seeks potential sources of fatigue. Chronic and disabling conditions can cause pain and fatigue; medication regimen, nutritional intake, and sleep patterns may contribute. Patients with reduced independence in ADLs may need assistance from a caregiver and use adapted or assistive devices to conserve energy. Even those who are able to walk independently at home may use a wheelchair to combat fatigue when out in the community.

Patients who experience variations in energy and pain levels or extreme fatigue work with the rehabilitation nurse to schedule their physical activities and find other ways to reduce demands for oxygen supply to vital body functions. Planning for rest paces a patient until activities can be relearned in steps and better endured. Performing activities when the patient has the most energy and arranging commonly used items in convenient places on shelves and in kitchen cabinets helps conserve strength. Table 20-7 explains several energy conservation techniques recommended for those patients who have conditions that produce variations in energy and pain levels.

Treatment recommendations regarding energy management specifically for PPS have changed over the years (Table 20-8). After the polio epidemic of the 1950s, patients were told to exert maximal energy by training hard, being as active as possible, trying to blend into society, making the best of their situation, and managing in society. Society considered institutionalization appropriate because the patients were not viewed as peers (Ahlstrom & Karlsson, 2000). Some patients responded by overly achieving, trying to fit in, and minimizing the impairments created by polio. In the current culture, persons with PPS are accepted and included in society and encouraged to conserve or improve existing muscle strength to help maintain independence (Black & Hawks, 2005; Klein et al., 2000). Rehabilitation methods and equipment can improve function, namely orthotic devices made of lightweight material, alterations to the home, ergonomic modifications to work settings, appropriate levels of exercise, and selected physical therapy activities (Gandevia, Allen, & Middleton, 2000; Halbritter, 2001).

Patient and Family Education. Support groups specific to a problem can help patients share concerns and solutions for energy conservation because ideas come from those who have dealt with obstacles of pain and fatigue in their own lives. Likewise, rehabilitation nurses can share information gained

TABLE 20-7 Energy Conservation Techniques

Technique	Example
1. Take your time	Plan ahead; stay with schedule
2. Rest breaks	Rest 10 minutes for every hour of activity; 30-45 minutes after meals
3. Sit down	Adapt activities to perform from sitting position
4. Avoid extreme temperatures	Do outdoor activities on cool days; use a fan when cooking or ironing; keep water and juices in the refrigerator; use an electric blanket
5. Avoid extra movements	Plan ahead all items needed for an activity; make bed while still in it; put clothing in easy to reach locations; put underwear inside pants to put on together
6. Keep frequently used items in easy reach	Avoid bending, reaching, and stooping; keep items at arm level
7. Ask for help	If an activity is exhausting, get assistance with the task
8. Analyze your activities	Watch for stress signals (chest pain, shortness of breath, sweating, fatigue); start small and build up; use a rolling cart and work in a circle
9. Use good posture	Sit and stand straight; do not cross your legs
10. Use correct body mechanics	Use two hands; use smooth movements that flow; slide or roll objects; push objects instead of pulling on them

Modified from Romanik, K. (1994). *Around the clock with C.O.P.D.: Helpful hints for respiratory (chronic obstructive pulmonary disease) patients.* Washington, DC: American Lung Association.

TABLE 20-8 Treatments for Postpolio Syndrome

Symptoms	Treatments
Generalized fatigue	Energy conservation; weight-loss program; lower extremity orthoses
Muscle weakness	Strengthening exercises; physical activity pacing with rest periods; avoid overuse of weakened muscles
Bulbar muscle weakness (respiratory failure and dysphagia)	Noninvasive positive-pressure ventilation at night and as needed; tracheostomy and permanent ventilation may be necessary; instruct on swallowing techniques
Pain and joint instability	Reduce stress on joints and muscles through lifestyle changes; weight loss; avoid overworking muscles; return to use of assisted devices; antiinflammatory medications
Cardiopulmonary conditioning	Upper extremity exercise program; aquatic exercise

Modified from Jubelt, B., & Agre, J. (2000, July 26). Characteristics and management of postpolio syndrome. *JAMA, 284,* 412-414.

through their knowledge and experiences and during formal or informal educational sessions with patients and caregivers.

Self-Care Deficit

Self-care activities to carry out tasks of daily living include personal hygiene, grooming, dressing, eating, and toileting. The level of participation in self-care activity is dependent upon the patient's strengths, abilities, and readiness to learn, and the level of assistance must correlate with the extent of injury, degree of impairment (including muscle stiffness and weakness or pain), and time since onset of the disorder. Sensitivity to the patient's lifestyle, beliefs, and preferences helps to individualize self-care goals. Alternative approaches often appeal to patients with chronic pain and musculoskeletal disorders. Chapter 14 discusses self care and ADLs in more detail.

An array of assistive devices aid patients in performing tasks safely and independently. For instance, after THR, an elevated commode seat helps patients avoid hip flexion past 90 degrees, and a long-handled, lightweight reacher grasps items without bending or flexing the hip joint. Other assistive devices help patients to conserve energy during self-care while adhering to precautions (Figures 20-9 and 20-10). Patients with limited joint range of motion learn dressing and self-care with modifications, such as large buttons or zippers with loop pull tabs. Elastic shoelaces, Velcro fasteners, and long-handled shoehorns enable patients to put on socks and shoes despite limited fine motor coordination or dexterity. Assistive devices also aid in donning and doffing prostheses.

Various adaptive devices are introduced to the patient and family members as recovery progresses to include independent self-care. The Utah Arm, an example of a motor-driven upper extremity prosthesis, allows greater independence in self-care and work skills (Figure 20-11). The Boston Digital Arm System is a variation on a prosthesis that features control of up to four other prosthetic devices, such as hands, grippers, wrist rotators, etc., in addition to the elbow itself (Liberating Technologies, Inc., 2005). The therapist and rehabilitation nurse evaluate a patient's readiness to learn, cognitive ability,

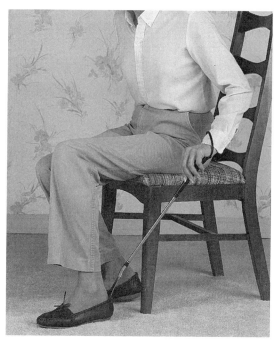

Figure 20-9 Long-handled shoehorn. (Courtesy Sammons Preston, Bolingbrook, IL.)

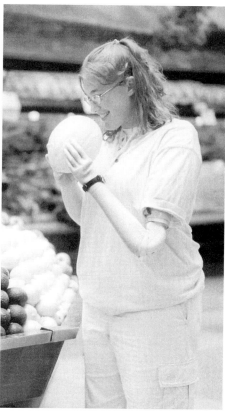

Figure 20-11 The Utah Arm 2 is a myoelectric elbow and hand system developed to enable patients with above-elbow amputations to function independently and with high levels of skill in their daily activities and work. The Utah myoelectric Arm 2 features proportional control. (Reproduced with permission of Motion Control, a subsidiary of Fillauer, Inc., Salt Lake City, UT.)

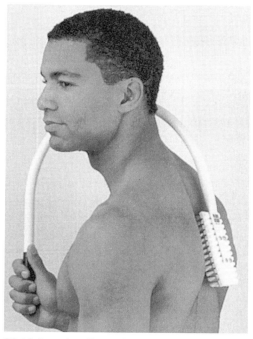

Figure 20-10 Long handles on brushes enable patients to perform their own bathing activities. (Courtesy Sammons Preston, Bolingbrook, IL.)

and strength and endurance when selecting devices or practicing new techniques. Patients initially may reject assistive devices; they may need time to adjust to an altered body image. A willingness to perform self-care tasks may signal the patient's acceptance and readiness to master self-care and

employ assistive devices. Chapter 14 discusses more about assistive devices and adapted equipment.

Impaired Physical Mobility

Impaired physical mobility may be related to muscle weakness, joint swelling or pain, and degeneration of bone or muscle, or absence of an extremity. The impairment may be temporary, as following a fracture or meniscus tear, or long-term, as with osteoarthritis. Rehabilitation is of paramount importance at all levels of care. For example, short-term rehabilitation after a fracture—a tertiary intervention—is really primary prevention in that it is an intervention to prevent complications and long-term mobility problems. The rehabilitation nurse assesses extremities, performs site care, promotes wound healing, ensures safety and maintenance of external fixation devices, and encourages optimal mobility for patients during healing.

Various types of traction allow a patient to move while a musculoskeletal injury heals or following reconstructive surgery. Skeletal traction paraphernalia can be attached to a trapeze device on a hospital-style bed or affixed to the patient. Halo traction applied to the head stabilizes the bony structure and promotes correct positioning (Figure 20-12).

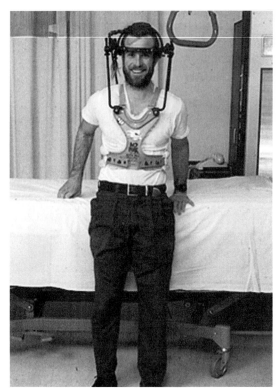

Figure 20-12 Halo vest. Note the rigid shoulder straps and encompassing vest. Various vest sizes are available prefabricated. The halo ring, superstructure, and vest are magnetic resonance imaging (MRI) compatible. (Courtesy Acromed Corp., Cleveland, OH.)

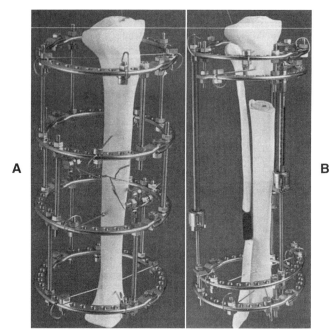

Figure 20-13 A, Ilizarov device in place to treat comminuted fracture. **B,** Ilizarov device assembly for lengthening of tibia. (Courtesy Smith & Nephew, Memphis, TN.)

The Ilizarov device is a form of external traction shown in Figure 20-13. This external fixation device lengthens the distance between the proximal ends of a bone by separating them in traction, simultaneously fixing them in alignment as they grow back together.

Skeletal pin site care has been standardized by the National Association of Orthopaedic Nurses (Holmes, Brown, & Pin Site Care Expert Panel, 2005) and accepted as a guideline by the National Guideline Clearinghouse (www.guideline.gov). At a minimum, skeletal pin site care should include daily pin site care for the first 48 to 72 hours followed by weekly pin site care with chlorhexidine cleansing.

Exercise Promotion and Therapy. Exercise regimens tailored to patients' specific conditions offer opportunities for them to participate in altering the course of their disease, such as by maintaining muscle strength and mobility. An individualized treatment plan targets relief of pain, control of inflammation, maintenance of joint integrity, and maximization of function (Fitzgerald & Oatis, 2004); goals must be realistic and acceptable to the patient. See Chapter 14 for more information on therapeutic exercise.

Joint protection, important during all activities, is augmented through muscle conditioning and controlled movement (Box 20-3). Aids to ambulation, such as canes, crutches, and

---

BOX 20-3 Principles of Joint Protection

1. Respect pain (fear of pain can lead to inactivity; ignoring pain can lead to joint damage).
2. Balance work and rest.
3. Reduce effort to joints.
4. Avoid positions of stress on joints.
5. Use larger/stronger joints.
6. Use joints in most stable positions.
7. Avoid remaining in one position.
8. Avoid activities that cannot be stopped.

Modified from Black, J. M., & Hawks, J. H. (2005). *Medical-surgical nursing: Clinical management for positive outcomes* (7th ed.). St. Louis, MO: Elsevier/Saunders.

---

walkers, alleviate stress to weight-bearing joints. Patients can prevent high-impact shock to the joints by wearing good-quality shoes with crepe soles, selecting soft walking surfaces, such as grass or cinder rather than cement, and choosing low-impact exercises. Proper joint alignment protects joints from extra pressure; bracing and orthotic shoe inserts with a heel wedge relieve pain and pressure (Medical Multimedia Group, 2005).

Redesigning daily activities also limits strain on joints. Recommendations include limited standing or stair climbing, frequent rest periods, parking close to destinations, and using assistive devices such as elevated beds, chairs, and commodes. The Americans With Disabilities Act contains provisions to improve access in the community, such as special permits to park in reserved locations. Patients, families, and the interdisciplinary team collaborate to identify and activate creative interventions that match mutually acceptable goals and patients' abilities, lifestyle, and preferences.

Ambulation Techniques. Safety is an important goal for any patient with a musculoskeletal disorder, whether a simple ankle sprain, a gouty great toe, or an above-the-knee amputation. Altered gait patterns require the interdisciplinary team to assess mobility and develop a plan to retrain and strengthen muscles, ligaments, and tendons. However, a patient's health status, financial situation, acceptance of adaptive and assistive devices, home environment, and available caregivers directly influence the plan for care.

An accessible environment is essential to optimal function in ambulation and requires a detailed home and community assessment. Chapters 12 and 21 contain more information. Family and caregivers assist in preparing a safe environment. For instance, safety devices, such as a Lifeline call-response system, notify selected family or community responders should a patient fall or have another problem. Walkers, crutches, and canes assist patients with ambulating during the initial phase of rehabilitation after hip and knee surgery (Figure 20-14 and Table 20-9); some will advance to walking independently by hospital discharge.

Ambulation in the community is a challenge after hospitalization. Caregivers need training to assist patients who use wheelchairs or assistive devices with ambulating, performing safe transfers, and moving about the home. They need information about proper use and measurement of assistive devices and basic wheelchair maintenance (see Chapter 14). Many community resources are available for transportation or services. Manual wheelchairs and motorized carts are available in some shopping malls, airports, and theaters, but gaining access to events using a wheelchair or scooter requires making phone calls and planning in advance. Successful social experiences promote self-confidence and life satisfaction.

Children with muscular dystrophy may be able to maintain functional ambulation after lower limb musculotendinous releases, which allow for ambulation without bracing and less physical therapy. Use of long leg braces has declined in recent years, possibly as a result of earlier surgical interventions or increased costs of orthoses (Bach & Chaudhry, 2000).

Persons with amputations have benefited from advances in technology and prosthesis choices, such as ultralightweight components of titanium and carbon fiber composites, improved cosmetic appearance, and functional flexibility, enabling some patients to set realistic goals to walk without assistive devices (Figure 20-15) (Esquenazi, 2004; Habel, 2005).

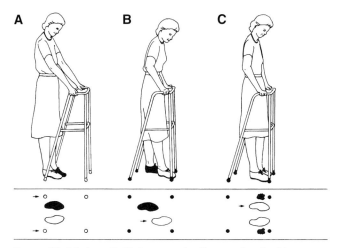

Figure 20-14 A to **C,** Technique of walking with a double-support device. (From Hoeman, S. P. [1990]. *Rehabilitative and restorative care in the community.* St. Louis, MO: Mosby.)

Patient and Family Education for Improving Mobility. Goals for exercise, therapy, and ambulation are set mutually among the patient and team from the time of admission to final discharge from the acute rehabilitation unit; they also depend on the patient's readiness to learn and

TABLE 20-9 Techniques of Walking With Ambulatory Aids

Device	Gait
Single-support device (cane, quad cane, single crutch)	Device is held in the hand opposite the involved leg Device and involved leg are advanced first, followed by the uninvolved leg
Double-support device (walker)	Walker is advanced first, followed by the involved extremity and then the uninvolved extremity
Crutches	2-Point gait: Both crutches, both legs (one leg may be non–weight bearing) 3-Point gait: Crutches are advanced, followed by the involved leg and then the uninvolved leg 4-Point gait: One crutch is advanced, followed by the involved leg, the opposite crutch is advanced, followed by the uninvolved leg

NOTE: Climbing stairs is accomplished by moving the uninvolved leg first, then the device and the involved leg; to descend stairs, the involved leg and the device are moved first, then the uninvolved leg. *The device and the involved leg always move together.*

From Phipps, W., Sands, J., & Marek, J. (1999). *Medical-surgical nursing: Concepts and clinical practice* (6th ed.). St. Louis, MO: Mosby. Copyright 1999 by Mosby. Reprinted by permission.

family participation. Education about various external fixation devices focuses on preventing complications of infection (Holmes et al., 2005). Preventive care for braces and casts emphasizes maintaining skin integrity, sensation, and circulation. A community rehabilitation nurse or therapist may visit the home when a patient uses assistive or immobilizing devices.

Body Image Disturbance

Negative feelings or perceptions about characteristics, functions, or limits of body or body parts create a disturbance in body image (Gordon, 2000). Common problems associated with musculoskeletal disorders include altered gait patterns, use of assistive devices or wheelchairs, deformities, rheumatoid nodules, loss of height or osteoporosis, easy bruising, or loss of an extremity. All may affect a patient's body image.

Body image enhancement requires improving patients' conscious and unconscious perceptions and attitudes toward their bodies (Dochterman & Bulechek, 2004). Rehabilitation nurses conduct ongoing assessments of patients' expectations of body image based on their developmental stage and intervene with anticipatory guidance for predictable changes.

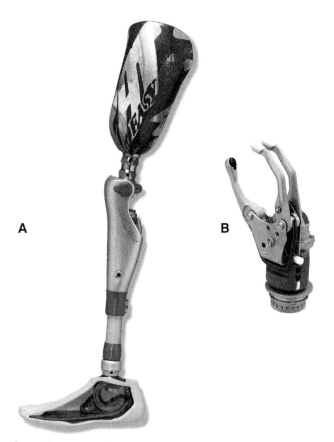

Figure 20-15 A, The 3C100 C-Leg has a microprocessor-controlled hydraulic knee with a stance control feature that adjusts to slopes, stairs, and other uneven surfaces. **B,** The SensorHand has an automatic grasping feature that senses when an object is about to slip and makes necessary adjustments. (Copyrighted photographs used with permission of Otto Bock Health Care, Minneapolis, MN.)

Body image is directly related to a person's functional ability. The impact of changes may be reduced by having patients view pictures of persons using assistive devices in daily activities or recreation or handling tools that will enhance their appearance and improve function. Timing is important, and adjustment is influenced by premorbid function, personal and cultural attitudes of the patient, family, and community, and the degree or severity of changes. The rapidity of body image–changing events after a spinal cord injury may be more traumatic than a gradual change in muscle mass resulting from PPS or RA.

Additional interventions for persons with altered body image include involvement in peer support groups to encourage interactions with others when appropriate; some patients benefit from meeting someone with a similar experience in a private situation. Professional counseling that focuses on the needs, problems, and feelings of the patient and family or significant others to enhance and support coping, problem solving, and interpersonal relationships may be indicated (Dochterman & Bulechek, 2004).

Pharmaceutical Management of Selected Musculoskeletal Disorders

Advances in pharmacological therapy slow the progression or alleviate symptoms of musculoskeletal disorders. Medications used to manage osteoporosis are discussed in the following section.

Osteoporosis. Medications utilized for osteoporosis management include selective estrogen receptor modulators (SERMs), bisphosphonates, and calcitonin-salmon. SERMs include raloxifene (Evista) and tamoxifen (Nolvadex). These drugs work by selectively binding with estrogen receptors to strengthen bones, reduce breast cancer risk, and decrease low-density lipoprotein (LDL) cholesterol. Adverse effects include uterine cancer risk and coagulopathy. Raloxifene is a drug of choice in the treatment of osteoporosis but does not reduce the risk of noninvasive breast cancer, as tamoxifen does (National Cancer Institute, 2006). However, tamoxifen is less effective in strengthening bones and is not recommended for osteoporosis.

Another category of medications used to treat osteoporosis is the bisphosphonates, including Fosamax. Bisphosphonates are currently considered standard treatment for severe osteoporosis, because they have the greatest effect on the spine; beneficial effects typically are seen within a year (Whyte & Peraud, 2005). Bisphosphonates are available in several formulations and for daily, weekly, and monthly dosing regimens. Esophagitis and osteonecrosis are potential side effects of the bisphosphonates; precautions are listed in Box 20-4.

The SERMS and bisphosphonates are approved for prevention and treatment, whereas calcitonin-salmon is approved only for treatment of osteoporosis. In contrast to the above therapies that inhibit bone resorption, teriparatide (Forteo) is a bone formation agent, used for short-term treatment in patients at high risk for fractures.

BOX 20-4 Bisphosphonates Guidelines for Administration

- Take first thing in the morning each day (or weekly or monthly) as ordered.
- Drink one full glass (8 ounces) of water with medication.
- Be sure to take with water only.
- Do not eat or drink anything for 30 minutes to 1 hour after taking medication.
- Stay in an upright position during this period to minimize esophageal irritation.
- Do not lie down until after eating a meal following the 1-hour waiting period.

Modified from Herndon, R., & Mohandas, N. (2000, June). Osteoporosis in multiple sclerosis: A frequent, serious, and under-recognized problem. *International Journal of Multiple Sclerosis Care*, 2, 1-9. Available from www.mscare.com.

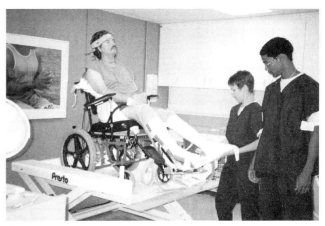

Figure 20-16 Use of a height-adjustable platform creates an ergonomic workstation for rehabilitation staff doing frequent casting. (Courtesy The Institute for Rehabilitation and Research [TIRR], Houston, TX.)

Hormone replacement therapy (HRT) was found to increase the risk of breast cancer and cardiovascular disease in the Women's Health Initiative study. The authors do not recommend HRT unless the fracture risk benefit is greater than the risk of the adverse conditions (Writing Group for the Women's Health Initiative Investigators, 2002); currently Food and Drug Administration (FDA) recommendations align with the conclusions (Greenblatt, 2005).

HEALTH PROMOTION AND PREVENTION

Primary prevention and interventions (i.e., health promotion, early intervention, and prevention) are essential components of rehabilitation in all settings. They range from primary prevention, as with osteoporosis, to tertiary prevention of complications, such as avoiding shoulder subluxation with hemiplegia, or involve modifying or changing the environment and patients' lifestyle choices. Rehabilitation nurses may teach self-care and mobility skills to patients who are using crutches or have an upper extremity cast or are recovering from surgery. They educate families and communities about strategies for primary prevention of traumatic injuries. Topics might include the importance of using everyday safety devices, such as seat belts, car seats, and air bags; or safety in sports, such as helmets and other gear, safe activities in play, and diving precautions. Home safety and fall prevention contrasted with information about a restraint-free environment, including medications, or raising awareness of violence in the home or community, including abuse or neglect, are other examples.

Wellness programs promote weight-bearing exercise and healthy choices in nutrition and adequate intake of calcium with vitamin D to prevent bone density loss. When osteoporosis has developed, secondary interventions include redesigning activities to reduce physical demands of job tasks and using ergonomic principles in a variety of settings to prevent or reduce risks for fractures or injury. Ergonomic principles are used in conjunction with programs for physical conditioning, maintaining ideal body weight, training for body mechanics, and eliminating medications, notably steroids. If fracture occurs, the accompanying deconditioning and immobility during healing perpetuates bone loss.

Identifying these risks enables the rehabilitation nurse to promote strategies, such as low-impact exercises, nutritional supplements, and environmental modifications for safe ambulation. Education alone has not motivated patients to change their behavior. Lifestyle changes are more likely when a patient is experiencing an acute episode, such as a fracture, a functional decline, or altered body image. Understanding the losses and fears associated with musculoskeletal dysfunction helps rehabilitation nurses provide meaningful and compassionate care.

Prevention Through Ergonomics. Ergonomics is a study of the work or home environment that results in adaptations or modifications for safe, effective, and accessible activity. The underlying principle is that by "fitting the job" to the worker by actions such as adjusting the workstation, rotating between tasks, or using mechanical assists, stress on the musculoskeletal system can be reduced and ultimately eliminated (Ergonomics Society, 2005). Many work environments promote healthy living through ergonomic workstation assessment, educational programs, and incentives for participation in health facilities. An important component of the work environmental analysis involves education about positioning, proper body mechanics, periodic rest and stretch breaks, and stress reduction techniques all designed to prevent injuries. The adjustable-height lift device pictured in Figure 20-16 illustrates how therapists who perform serial casting may use it to prevent back strain during these lengthy procedures. Many nursing interventions and techniques can be modified

TABLE 20-10 Nursing Outcomes for Patients With Musculoskeletal Disabilities

Pain control	• Patient uses nonanalgesic pain relief measures • Patient uses analgesic relief measures • Patient reports pain controlled sufficiently to allow participation in ADLs
Energy conservation	• Patient balances activity and rest • Patient adapts lifestyle to energy level • Patient uses energy conservation techniques
Self-care deficit: activities of daily living (ADLs)	• Patient performs ADLs at maximum level of independence
Mobility level	• Patient safely performs mobility skills at maximum level of independence
Body image	• Patient will adjust to changes in physical appearance • Patient will adjust to changes in body function • Patient will use strategies to enhance appearance and function

Modified from Moorhead, S., Johnson, M., & Maas, M. (Eds.). (2004). *Nursing outcomes classification (NOC)* (3rd ed.). St. Louis, MO: Mosby.

to prevent repetitive motion injuries. Creative problem solving is a role for rehabilitation nurses in evaluating work sites, modifying repetitive tasks, adapting routines or procedures, and educating patients during discharge planning, and incorporating ergonomic principles when teaching staff and others.

Promoting a Healthy Lifestyle. Healthy lifestyle patterns often have roots in a family's social, cultural, or economic models. Those who practice a healthy lifestyle may have more motivation in related areas, such as accepting responsibility for self-care and adhering to therapeutic regimens. Healthy living is not compartmentalized; it occurs in the home, workplace, and with others in the community. Family modeling of regular exercise and activities, healthy choices in diet, maintaining proper weight, and avoiding alcohol and other substances during a child's life can have a lasting behavioral effect on wellness. Persons with physical impairments may require adjustments in the mode of exercise, activities, or special diets, but overall they can lead a healthy lifestyle to enhance wellness and prevent complications or further disability. Industries can support the concept of healthy lifestyles by offering employee fitness centers on site or discounts for private clubs, gyms, or community organizations, such as the YMCA. Stress management workshops, along with employee assistance programs promote conflict resolution and resource management that convey the message of health promotion and wellness. Many musculoskeletal problems result from or are exacerbated by stressors. A proactive approach to employee wellness communicates that the organization values its employees and offers solutions and resources to resolve problems encountered in everyday life. The benefit of these services lies in the prevention of lost hours, a positive work climate, and a constructive and positive environment that nurtures the individual, regardless of a person's acute or chronic impairment.

Chapter 12 discusses more about vocation and the community, and Chapter 14 contains additional information about safety and movement.

OUTCOMES

The broad outcome for patients with musculoskeletal dysfunction is the ability to manage pain and energy, to promote maximum independence in ADLs and instrumental ADLs (IADLs), and to prevent complications and further disability. Samples of measurable outcome criteria are listed in Table 20-10.

Preventing Complications. In the community, nurses conduct health promotion programs and screening activities at a variety of locations, such as at health fairs, shopping malls, churches, or senior centers. Rehabilitation nurses contribute to the overall health of the community by providing education about restorative care and prevention in these settings. Examples of other venues are speaking at local organizations, such as Rotary Club meetings, writing columns for the newspaper, or providing continuing education about rehabilitation principles or restorative care for colleagues in community health agencies. Health promotion and prevention of complications improve outcomes. For example, lifetime increased calcium intake and preventive medication (raloxifene or bisphosphonates) by persons unable to participate in weight-bearing activities contribute to decreased incidence of osteoporotic fractures. Similarly, foot care and control of blood glucose levels decrease amputations associated with diabetes mellitus.

Implications. Quality of life is one of the most important factors to consider when assisting individuals with musculoskeletal dysfunction. Whether patients experience an acute injury or have a chronic, slowly progressing degenerative illness, their commonly held goal is to attain meaning and satisfaction in their lives. A positive self-concept is related to a person's attitudes and outlook, combined with that of the family, significant others, and the rehabilitation team. An effective nurse-patient relationship must include trust and close collaboration to help the patient become independent of the health care system. Nurses contribute by conducting ongoing and comprehensive assessments, developing appropriate nursing diagnoses and setting realistic goals with patients, and evaluating a patient's progress toward achieving the highest possible level of wellness. Rehabilitation nurses are advocates who learn about available resources, evaluate their worth, educate patients about their operations, and understand how to access their services to help patients meet their goals within the health care continuum.

One function of a healthy community is to encourage agencies and groups to collaborate in promoting wellness and preventing musculoskeletal dysfunction in its members. The economic benefit impacts the national and worldwide economy. Rehabilitation nurses are crossing socioeconomic, ethnic, cultural, and religious barriers to collaborate in research and present information at international conferences. They share ideas and information on the World Wide Web and travel to rehabilitation facilities or programs across the world. They share interventions, collaborate on their knowledge, and learn to appreciate the challenges experienced by others. Many nurses provide rehabilitation services—such as during mission trips sponsored by international voluntary organizations—including technology, equipment, and education. Developing countries and persons living in remote areas have great needs for medications, wheelchairs, braces, and many other treatment modalities for managing with musculoskeletal problems. They also need education about preventing problems and promoting health that is specific to their environment and situation. Rehabilitation nurses have an important role in the international scope of practice in the twenty-first century.

Research directions are to uncover the causes of diseases such as RA, to determine the effectiveness of alternate therapies and treatment modalities, such as for fibromyalgia, and to identify methods for preventing complications involving musculoskeletal disorders. Many new medications and dietary supplements are being evaluated, such as biological response modifiers, glucosamine, and chondroitin. Rehabilitation nurses are in positions where they can investigate ways to promote behavioral changes that encourage patients to enhance their wellness and test clinical practices concerning musculoskeletal impairments.

Case Study

Ms. Thorpe, a rehabilitation nurse, developed severe steroid-dependent asthma at 31 years of age. She presents to the acute rehabilitation unit following a fracture and pinning of her right hip.

History

Ms. Thorpe has developed numerous stress/minimal injury fractures, including fractures of the left knee, left ankle, right foot, pelvis, ribs, and a flail chest secondary to cardiopulmonary resuscitation. Vertebral compression fractures, T5 through L5, have resulted in a 5-inch loss of height. Before the development of complications from chronic steroid use, Ms. Thorpe had been a triathlete and avid bicyclist. She is admitted to acute care following a stress fracture sustained while walking in a mall. A right hemiarthroplasty is performed, and a brief, intensive course of therapy is planned.

Current Assessment

Ms. Thorpe is a small-framed white woman, appearing chronically ill with cushingoid features, multiple bruises, and skin tears. ADLs are performed independently; 2½ hours are required for bathing and dressing due to frequent rest breaks. She has difficulty with buttons and zippers. She is unable to lift more than 10 pounds, grip strength is poor, and she reports numbness and tingling in her hands secondary to diabetic neuropathy.

Ms. Thorpe reports that "pain is a daily companion," with morning stiffness, aching in joints, and sharp pain in the back after sitting for 3 to 4 hours. Pain is relieved with rest, heat, and Lortab 7.5 mg qid. Nonsteroidal antiinflammatory drugs (NSAIDs) are contraindicated as a result of a GI bleed.

Ms. Thorpe lives alone in a third-floor apartment with an elevator. Her family lives out of state but is very supportive, as is a close network of friends. She is on permanent physical disability and does volunteer work, writing, and occasional teaching. She has unsuccessfully tried returning to work. She states, "I used to be a strong, physically fit triathlete; now I am a weakling who has been in a wheelchair since I was 37. I guess I am in a different chapter of my life."

Nursing Diagnoses

- Chronic pain
- Activity intolerance (pain and fatigue)
- Impaired physical mobility
- Risk for injury (muscle weakness, history of falls, history of fractures, balance difficulties)
- Disturbed body image

Interventions and Evaluation

Ms. Thorpe is motivated and readily able to employ many of the necessary interventions. However, the entire rehabilitation team has been essential in securing positive outcomes in this complex case. Interventions focus on pain control with the analgesic and nonpharmacological treatments. She is able to perform ADLs and most IADLs with manageable discomfort; assistance of friends is required for heavy cleaning and laundry. Pacing activities, using energy conservation techniques, and frequent rest periods allow her to remain active.

Over time Ms. Thorpe has adjusted to her changed physical appearance and body function. She sees the wheelchair as her "freedom wheels," allowing her to travel and participate in many community activities. She no longer covers her bruises and skin tears with long-sleeved clothing and long pants. Although conscious of her

Continued

Case Study—cont'd

moon face, Ms. Thorpe knows she must continue on oral steroids. The 5-inch loss of height has resulted in several adaptations, such as keeping frequently used items in lower cupboards, using a reacher, and needing a power driver's seat to see over the steering wheel in her automobile. She realizes that revisions of the hip arthroplasties to THRs may be necessary as the pain increases and that the UniSpacer may also need to be replaced; anticipatory guidance is helpful. Ms. Thorpe also reports that the mental toughness learned from endurance racing has helped her to cope and adjust to the changes in her life, as has inner spiritual strength and social support.

Outcomes

The outcomes targeted are pain control, energy conservation, independent performance of ADLs and mobility skills, and adjustment to body image changes with Ms. Thorpe continuing to set goals for an active life and functional progress.

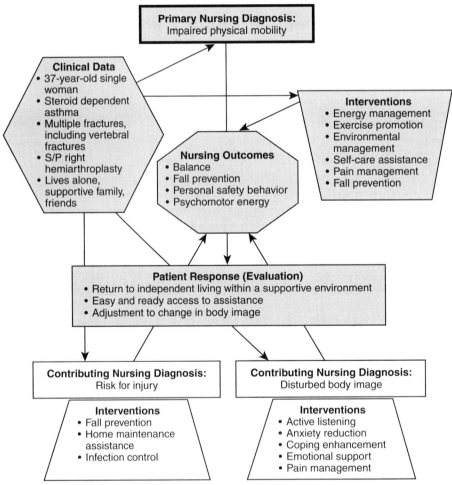

Concept MAP. Ms. Thorpe's situation is very complex, and the concept map is helpful in organizing her many concerns. Her primary problem is that of mobility, with risk for additional injury due to balance and falls. Interventions are needed to address the contributing issues of risk for falls and body image disturbance. The following concept map illustrates the interrelationships between the nursing diagnoses of impaired mobility, body image disturbance and risk for injury from falls. The rehabilitation nurse will focus on coordinating interventions to achieve the outcomes of balance, fall prevention, psychomotor energy and personal safety behaviour, which, given Ms. Thorpe's level of independence, should be the outcomes necessary for a successful return to home.

CRITICAL THINKING

1. NSAIDs are contraindicated for Ms. Thorpe, and pain control is a significant issue, limiting her progress in therapy. What strategies do you recommend she try to control pain?
2. Additional fractures are a strong potential for Ms. Thorpe. What strategies would you recommend to prevent fractures?
3. Ms. Thorpe would like to return to work. Given her background and experience as a rehabilitation nurse, and her physical limitations, what do you recommend she consider?

REFERENCES

Ahlstrom, G., & Karlsson, U. (1999). Disability and quality of life in individuals with postpolio syndrome. *Disability and Rehabilitation, 22,* 416-422.

American College of Physicians. (2005). *Lyme disease: A patient's guide* [Online]. Retrieved September 5, 2005, from www.acponline.org/lyme/patient/diagnosis.htm.

American College of Rheumatology. (2005). *Fibromyalgia* [Online]. Retrieved October 24, 2005, from http:www.rheumatology.org/public/factsheets/fibromya_new.asp?.

American Dental Association. (2003). Antibiotic prophylaxis for dental patients with total joint replacements. *Journal of the American Dental Association, 134*(7), 895-899, 901-904 [Online]. Retrieved October 24, 2005, from http://www.ada.org/prof/resources/pubs/jada/reports/report_prophy_statement.pdf.

American Nurses Association Nursing World. (2005). *Handle with care: Texas passes safe lifting law for hospitals, nursing homes* [Online]. Retrieved October 14, 2005, from http://www.nursingworld.org/handle with care/txleg.htm.

American Sports Data. (2005). *Running USA-RRIC* [Online]. Retrieved September 12, 2005, from http://www.runningusa.org/cgi/trends.pl.

Amputee Coalition of America (1999/2000). *Limb loss research and statistics program update* [Online]. Available at http://www.amputee-coalition.org/IIrsp/IIrsp update.html.

Aras, M. D., Gokkaya, N. K., Comert, D., Kaya, A., & Cakci, A. (2004). Shoulder pain in hemiplegia: Results from a national rehabilitation hospital in Turkey. *American Journal of Physical Medicine and Rehabilitation, 83*(9), 713-719.

Aronow, W. S. (2005). Management of peripheral arterial disease. *Cardiology Review, 13*(2), 61-68.

Arthritis Foundation. (2005a). *Arthritis Foundation programs and services* [Online]. Retrieved October 19, 2005, from http://www.arthritisfoundation.org/webprograms&service.doc.

Arthritis Foundation. (2005b). *The facts about arthritis* [Online]. Retrieved August 25, 2005, from http://arthritis.org/resources/gettingstarted/default.asp.

Arthritis Foundation. (2005c). *Juvenile rheumatoid arthritis: Quality of life issues* [Online]. Retrieved October 16, 2005, from http://www.arthritis.org/conditions/DiseaseCenter/JRA/qol.asp.

Bensen, R., Adachi, J. D., Papaioannou, A., Ioannidis, G., Olszynski, W. P., Sebalt, R., et al. (2005, September 5). Evaluation of easily measured risk factors in the prediction of osteoporotic fractures [Online]. *BioMedCentral Musculoskeletal Disorders, 6,* 47. Retrieved April 2, 2006, from http://www.pubmedcentral.gov/articlerender.fcgi?tool=pubmed&pubmedid=16143046.

Bertagnoli, R., Yue, J. J., Pheiffer, F., Fenk-Mayer, A., Lawrence, J. P., Kershaw, T., & Nanieva, R. (2005). Early results after ProDisc-C cervical disc replacement. *Journal of Neurosurgical Spine, 2*(4), 403-10.

Black, J. M., & Hawks, J. H. (2005). *Medical-surgical nursing: Clinical management for positive outcomes,* (7th ed.). St. Louis, MO: Saunders.

Bruce, M. L., & Peck, B. (2005). New rheumatoid arthritis treatments. *Nurse Practitioner. 30*(4), 28-39.

Cakmak, A., & Bolukbas, N. (2005). Juvenile rheumatoid arthritis: Physical therapy and rehabilitation. *Southern Medical Journal, 98*(2), 212-216.

Calabrese, L., Zein, N., Vassilopoulos, D. (2004). Safety of antitumour necrosis factor (anti-TNF) therapy in patients with chronic viral infections: hepatitis C, hepatitis B, and HIV infection. *Annals of Rheumatic Disorders. 63*(Suppl 2), ii18-ii24.

Centers for Disease Control and Prevention. (2000). Recommendations regarding selected conditions affecting woman's health [Online].

Morbidity and Mortality Weekly Report, 49(RR-2), 1-12. Retrieved September 14, 2005, from http://www.cdc.gov/mmwr/PDF/RR/RR4902.pdf.

Centers for Disease Control and Prevention (2004). Update: Direct and Indirect Costs of Arthritis and Other Rheumatic Conditions—United States, 1997. *Morbidity and Mortality Weekly Report, 53*(18), 388-389.

Centers for Disease Control and Prevention. (2005). *Lyme disease prevention and control* [Online]. Retrieved October 25, 2005, from http://www.cdc.gov/ncidod/dvbid/lyme/ld_prevent.htm.

Choi, H. K., & Curhan, G. (2005). Gout: Epidemiology and lifestyle choices. *Current Opinions in Rheumatology, 17*(3), 341-345.

Choudhury, S. R., Reiber, G. E., Pecoraro, J. A., Czerniecki, J. M., Smith, D. G., & Sangeorzan, B. J. (2001). *Postoperative management of transtibial amputations in VA hospitals* [Online]. Retrieved October 13, 2005, from http://www.vard.org/jour/01/38/3/choud383.htm.

Colbert, L. H., Hootman, J. M., & Macera, C. A. (2000). Physical activity-related injuries in walkers and runners in the aerobics center longitudinal study. *Clinical Journal of Sports Medicine, 10,* 259-263.

Dec, K. L., Sparrow, K. J., & McKeag, D. B. (2000). The physically-challenged athlete. *Sports Medicine, 29,* 245-258.

Diamond, P. (2000). Severe anemia: Implications for functional recovery during rehabilitation. Rehabilitation in practice. *Disability and Rehabilitation, 22,* 574-576.

Dochterman, J. M., & Bulechek, G. M. (2004). *Nursing interventions classification (NIC)* (4th ed.). St. Louis, MO: Mosby.

Dugan, S. A. (2005). Sports-related knee injuries in female athletes: What gives? *American Journal of Physical Medicine and Rehabilitation, 84*(2), 122-130.

Dursun, E., Dursun, N., Eksi Ural, C., & Cakci, A. (2000). Glenohumeral joint subluxation and reflex sympathetic dystrophy in hemiplegic patients. *Archives of Physical Medicine and Rehabilitation. 81*(7), 944-946.

Ene-Stroescu, D., & Gorbien, M. J. (2005). Gouty arthritis: A primer on late-onset gout. *Geriatrics, 60*(7), 24-31.

Ergonomics Society. (2005). *Ergonomics: Definition.* [Online]. Available at http://www.ergonomics.org.uk/ergonomics/definition.htm

Esquenazi, A. (2004). Amputation rehabilitation and prosthetic restoration: From surgery to community reintegration. *Disability and Rehabilitation, 26*(14/15), 831-836.

Ethgen, O., Bruyere, O., Richy, F., Dardennes, C., & Reginster, J. (2004). Health-related quality of life in total hip and total knee arthroplasty: A qualitative and systematic review of the literature. *Journal of Bone and Joint Surgery, 86A*(5), 963-974.

Ferrara, M. S., & Peterson, C. L. (2000). Injuries to athletes with disabilities: Identifying injury patterns. *Sports Medicine, 30,* 137-143.

Fitzgerald, G. K., & Oatis, C. (2004). Role of physical therapy in the management of knee osteoarthritis. *Current Opinion in Rheumatology, 16*(2), 143-147.

Flinke, W. (2005). Early detection and treatment of running injuries [Online]. *Team Oregon.* Retrieved August 31, 2006, from http://www.teamoregon.com/publications/injuries.html.

Foort, J. (1957). Construction and fitting of the Canadian type hip disarticulation prosthesis. *Artificial Limbs, 4*(2), 39-51.

Francis, M., & Ranatunga, S. (2006). Gout. eMedicine. Retrieved April 12, 2006, from http://www.emedicine.com/med/topic924.htm.

Gandevia, S., Allen, G., & Middleton, J. (2000). Post-polio syndrome: assessments, pathophysiology and progression. *Disability Rehabilitation, 22,* 38-42.

Gonzalez-Gay, M. A., Gonzalez-Juanatey, C., Pineiro, A., Garcia-Porrua, C., Testa, A., & Llorca, J. (2005). High-grade C-Reactive protein elevation correlates with accelerated atherogenesis in patients with rheumatoid arthritis. *Journal of Rheumatology, 32*(7), 1219-23.

Gordon, M. (2000). *Manual of nursing diagnosis* (9th ed.). St. Louis, MO: Mosby.

Greenblatt, D. (2005). Treatment of postmenopausal osteoporosis. *Pharmacotherapy, 25*(4), 574-584.

Habel, M. (2005). *Artificial limbs: Hope for the future* [Online]. Retrieved September 12, 2005, from http://www2.nurseweek.com/ce/self-study_modules/tools/print.html?ID=345.

Halbritter, T. (2001). Management of a patient with post-polio syndrome. *Journal of the American Academy of Nurse Practitioners, 13*(12), 555-559.

Hallock, R. H., & Fell, B. M. (2003). Unicompartmental tibial hemiarthroplasty: Early results of the UniSpacer™ knee. *Clinical Orthopaedics and Related Research, 416,* 154-163.

Herndon, R., & Mohandas, N. (2000, June). Osteoporosis in multiple sclerosis: A frequent serious and under-recognized problem. *International Journal of Multiple Sclerosis Care, 2,* 1-9. Available from www.mscare.com.

Hewett, T. E. (2000). Neuromuscular and hormonal factors associated with knee injuries in female athletes: Strategies for intervention. *Sports Medicine, 29,* 313-327.

Holmes, S. B., Brown, S. J., & Pin Site Care Expert Panel. (2005). Skeletal pin site care: National Association of Orthopaedic Nurses guidelines for orthopaedic nursing. *Orthopaedic Nursing, 24*(2), 99-107.

Hutchinson, M. R., & Nasser, R. (2000). *Common sports injuries in children and adolescents* [Online]. Available at http://www.medscape.com/medscape/ OrthoSportsMed/journal/2000/vo4.no4/mos4420.hutc/mos4420. hutc-01.html.

Iqbal, M. M. (2000). Osteoporosis: Epidemiology, diagnosis, and treatment. *Southern Medical Journal, 93*(1), 2-18.

Joy, E. A., & Campbell, D. (2005). Stress fractures in the female athlete. *Current Sports Medicine Reports,* 4(6), 323–328.

Kannus, P., Uusi-Rasi, K., Palvanen, M., & Parkkari, J. (2005). Non-pharmacological means to prevent fractures among older adults. *Annals of Medicine, 37*(4), 303-310.

Katrak, P., O'Connor, B., & Woodgate, I. (2003). Rehabilitation after total femur replacement: A report of two cases. *Archives of Physical Medicine and Rehabilitation, 84*(7), 1080-1084.

Khan, F. (2004). Rehabilitation for postpolio sequelae. *Australian Family Physician, 33*(8), 621-624.

Klein, M., Whyte, J., Keenan, M., Esquenazi, A., & Polansky, M. (2000). Changes in strength over time among polio survivors. *Archives of Physical Medicine and Rehabilitation, 81,* 1059-1064.

Klein, P. J., & Adams, W. D. (2004). Comprehensive therapeutic benefits of Taji: A critical review. *American Journal of Physical Medicine and Rehabilitation, 83*(9), 735-745.

Knisley, J., & Johnson, M. (2004). Lyme disease: Knowledge is the best prevention. *Nurse Practitioner, 29*(8), 34–43.

Kurtz, S., Mowat, F., Ong, K., Chan, N., Lau, E., & Halpern, M. (2005). Prevalence of primary and revision total hip and knee arthroplasty in the United States from 1990 through 2002. *Journal of Bone and Joint Surgery,* 87-A(7), 1487–1497.

Lamont, D. W. (2005). *Systemic lupus erythematosus* [Online]. Retrieved September 5, 2005, from http://www.emedicine.com/emery/topic564.htm.

LEAP Program. (2005). *Bureau of Primary Health Care Lower Extremity Amputation Prevention Program* [Online]. Retrieved October 19, 2005, from http://www.bphc.hrsa.gov/leap/.

Liberating Technologies, Inc. (2005). *Products: LTI Boston Arm systems* [Online]. Retrieved October 24, 2005, from http://www.liberatingtech.com/products/ LTI_Boston_Arm_Systems.asp.

Lieberman, I. H. (2005). *Spine specialists on-call: Osteoporotic vertebral compression fractures–restoring spinal stability and quality of life* [Online]. Available from http://www.spineuniverse.com/print.php/article2134.html.

Lindsay, D. M., Horton, J. F., & Vandervoort, A. A. (2000). A review of injury characteristics, aging factors and prevention programs for the older golfer. *Sports Medicine, 30,* 89-103.

Liss, H., & Liss, D. (2000). *Musculoskeletal sequelae of cerebrovascular accidents* [Online]. Retrieved October 19, 2000, from http://www. rehabmed.net/ documents/cva.htm.

Lo, S. F., Chen, S. Y., Lin, H. C., Jim, Y. F., Meng, N. H., Kao, M. J. (2003). Arthrographic and clinical findings in patients with hemiplegic shoulder pain. *Archives of Physical Medicine and Rehabilitation, 84*(12), 1786-1791.

Mangini, M. (1998). Physical assessment of the musculoskeletal system. *Nursing Clinics of North America, 33,* 643-653.

Mankin, H. J., Hornicek, F. J., & Harris, M. (2005, September). Total femur replacement procedures in tumor treatment. *Clinical Orthopaedics & Related Research, 438,* 60-64.

McDonald, S., Green, S. E., & Hetrick, S. (2005). Pre-operative education for hip or knee replacement. *The Cochrane Database of Systematic Reviews, 2005*(3), ID#CD003526. In the Cochrane Library (Oxford).

Medical College of Wisconsin. (2005). *Healthlink: Reiter's syndrome* [Online]. Retrieved September 6, 2005, from http://www.healthlink.mcw.edu/article/ 926056398.html.

Medical Multimedia Group. (2005). *A patient's guide to rehabilitation for arthritis* [Online]. Retrieved October 24, 2005, from http://www.eorthopod.com/ eorthopodv2/index.php/fuseaction/topics.detail/ID/79791a8f7dd9f446 b38653cbcab9a955/TopicID/34ba1fbf4ad6deeacd678793e3e84ff8/area/1.

Metules, T. (2002). A new age for childhood diseases: Duchenne muscular dystrophy. *RN, 65*(10), 39-44, 47-48.

Mease, P. (2005). Fibromyalgia syndrome: Review of clinical presentation, pathogenesis, outcome measures, and treatment. *Journal of Rheumatology, 75*(Suppl.), 6-21.

Moorhead, S., Johnson, M., & Maas, M. (Eds.). (2004). *Nursing outcomes classification (NOC)* (3rd ed.). St. Louis, MO: Mosby.

Moreland, L. (2005). Unmet needs in rheumatoid arthritis. *Arthritis Research and Therapy,* 7(Suppl. 3), S2-S8.

Muscular Dystrophy Association. (1999). *Neuromuscular diseases in the MDA program* [Online]. Available from http://www/mdausa.org/disease/ 40list.html.

Muscular Dystrophy Association. (2005). *Duchenne muscular dystrophy* [Online]. Retrieved September 11, 2005, from http://www.mdausa.org/disease/ dmd.cfm.

Nathenson, P. (2004). Adapting OSHA ergonomic guidelines to the rehabilitation setting. *Rehabilitation Nursing, 29*(4), 127-130.

National Center for Chronic Disease Prevention and Health Promotion. (2005). *Arthritis Program Information* [Online]. Retrieved August 25, 2005, from http://www.cdc.gov/arthritis/about_us.htm.

National Center for Health Statistics. (2003). *Summary health statistics for adults National Health Interview Survey 2003,* Series 10, (225). Hyattsville, MD: Author.

National Fibromyalgia Association. (2005). *Fibromyalgia* [Online]. Retrieved August 8, 2005, from http://www.fmaware.org/fibromyalgia/general information.pdf.

National Institute of Arthritis and Musculoskeletal and Skin Diseases. (2001). *Questions and answers about juvenile rheumatoid arthritis* [Online]. Retrieved October 16, 2005, from http://www.niams.nih.gov/hi/topics/juvenile_ arthritis/juvarthr.htm.

National Institute of Neurological Disorders and Stroke. (2005). *Reflex sympathetic dystrophy syndrome fact sheet* [Online]. Retrieved October 14, 2005, from http://www.ninds.nih.gov/disorders/reflex_sympathetic_dystrophy/ detail_reflex_sympathetic_dystrophy.htm#30753282.

National Osteoporosis Foundation. (2005). *Fast Facts* [Online]. Retrieved August 25, 2005, from http://www.nof.org/osteoporosis/diseasefacts.htm.

Oliver, S., & Ryan, S. (2004). Effective pain management for patients with arthritis. *Nursing Standard, 18*(50), 43–52, 54, 56.

Osiri, M., Welch, V., Brasseau, L., Shea, B., McGowen, J., Tugwell, P., et al. (2005). Transcutaneous electrical nerve stimulation for knee osteoarthritis. *The Cochrane Database of Systematic Reviews, 2005*(3), ID#CD002823. In the Cochrane Library (Oxford).

Paci, M., Nannetti, L., Taiti, P., Baccini, M., Pasquini, J., Rinaldi, L. (2006). Shoulder subluxation after stroke: Relationships with pain and motor recovery. *Physiotherapy Research International.* 12(2), 95–104.

Parsons, L. C. (2005). Osteoporosis: Incidence, prevention and treatment of the silent killer. *Nursing Clinics of North America, 40*(1), 119-133.

Peterson, J. (2005). Understanding fibromyalgia and its treatment options. *Nurse Practitioner, 30*(1), 48-55.

Pezzin, L., Dillingham, T., & Mackenzie, E. (2000). Rehabilitation and the long-term outcomes of persons with trauma-related amputations. *Archives of Physical Medicine and Rehabilitation, 81,* 292-300.

Phipps, W. J., Monahan, F. D., Sands, J. K., Marek, J. F., & Neighbors, M. (2003). *Medical-surgical nursing: Health and illness perspectives* (7th ed.). St. Louis, MO: Mosby.

Pink, M. M., & Tibone, J. E. (2000). The painful shoulder in the swimming athlete. *Orthopedic Clinics of North America.* 31, 247–261.

Popovic, J. R. (2001). 1999 National Hospital Discharge Survey: Annual summary with detailed diagnosis and procedure data. *Vital Health Statistics, 13*(151), 23, 154.

Pribut, S. M. (2004). A quick look at running injuries. *Podiatry Management* [Online]. Retrieved August 31, 2006, from http://www.drpribut.com/sports/ pributruna.pdf.

Quisel, A., Gill, J. M., & Witherell, P. (2005). Complex regional pain syndrome underdiagnosed. *Journal of Family Practice, 54*(6), 524-532.

Quisel, A., Gill, J. M., & Witherell, P. (2005b). Complex regional pain syndrome: Which treatments show promise? *Journal of Family Practice, 54*(7), 599-603.

Ramalingam, T., Pathak, G., Barker, P. (2005). A method of determining the rate of major limb amputations in battle casualities: Experiences of a British Field Hospital in Iraq, 2003, *Annals in the Royal College of Surgeons, England.* 87(2), 113–116.

Roland, E. H. (2000). Muscular dystrophy. *Pediatric Review, 21*(7), 233-237, 238.

Romanik, K. (1994). *Around the clock with C.O.P.D.: Helpful hints for respiratory (chronic obstructive pulmonary disease) patients.* Washington, DC: American Lung Association.

Roos, E. M. (2005). Joint injury causes knee osteoarthritis in young adults. *Current Opinion in Rheumatology, 17*(2), 195-200.

Ryan, T. (2000). *The therapeutic effects of Tai Chi* (2000, October 11-14). Association of Rehabilitation Nurses 26th Annual Educational Conference, Reno, NV.

Scott, R. D. (2003, November). UniSpacer ™: Insufficient data to support its widespread use. *Clinical Orthopaedics and Related Research, 416,* 164-166.

Sedlak, C., Doheny, M., & Jones, S. (2000). Osteoporosis education programs: Changing knowledge and behaviors. *Public Health Nursing,* 17, 398-402.

Small, R. E. (2005). *Uses and limitations of bone mineral density measurements in the management of osteoporosis* [Online]. Retrieved May 20, 2005, from http://www.medscape.com/viewarticle/503801_print.

Snyder, D. L., Doggett, D., & Turkelson, C. (2004). Treatment of degenerative lumbar spinal stenosis. *American Family Physician, 70*(3), 517-520; 437-439, 602 passim.

Stacy, G., Basu, P. (2007). Osteoarthritis, Primary. *eMedicine.* Retrieved January 24, 2007 from http://www.emedicine.com/radio/topic492.htm.

Theodorou, S. J., Theodorou, D. J., & Sartoris, D. J. (2003). Osteoporosis and fractures: The size of the problem. *Hospital Medicine, 64*(2), 87-91.

Trethewey, P. (2004). Systemic lupus erythematosus. *Dimensions of Critical Care Nursing, 23*(3), 111-115.

Tsao, B. (2000). Lupus susceptibility genes on human chromosome 1. *International Review of Immunology, 19*, 319-334.

U.S Department of Health and Human Services. (2001). *Healthy people 2010* (Vol. 1) (2nd ed.). [Online]. Retrieved July 10, 2005 from http://www.healthypeople.gov/Document/html/volume1/02Arthritis.htm.

Viera, A. (2003). Management of carpal tunnel syndrome. *American Family Physician, 68*(2), 265-272.

Whyte, J. J., & Peraud, P. (2005). Osteoporosis: Diagnosis and treatment. *Type 1 Continuing Education for Texas Nurses 2005.* Sacramento, CA: CME Resource.

Wolfe, F., Smythe, H. A., Yunus, M. B., Bennett, R. M., Bombardier, C., Goldenberg, D. L., et al. (1990). The American College of Rheumatology 1990 criteria for the classification of fibromyalgia: Report of the multicenter criteria committee. *Arthritis Rheumatology, 33*(2), 160-172.

Writing Group for Women's Health Initiative Investigators. (2002). Risks and benefits of estrogen plus progestin in healthy postmenopausal women. *Journal of the American Medical Association, 288*(3), 321-333.

Yuan, P. S., & Albert, T. J. (2004). Managing degenerative lumbar spinal stenosis. *Journal of Musculoskeletal Medicine, 21*(12), 640-642, 644, 645-648.

Zaffer, S., Braddom, R., Conti, A., Goff, J., Bokma, D. (1999). Total hip disarticulation prosthesis with suction socket: Report of two cases. *American Journal of Physical Medicine and Rehabilitation. 78*(2), 160-162.

21

Neuromuscular Disorders

Leslie Neal Boylan, PhD, RN, CRRN, FNP-C

This chapter discusses several neuromuscular disorders—Huntington's disease (HD), Parkinson's disease (PD), multiple sclerosis (MS), Guillain-Barré syndrome (GBS), myasthenia gravis (MG), and amyotrophic lateral sclerosis (ALS)—that have a significant impact on the patient, family, and caregiver. Spinal cord injury is discussed in Chapter 14. With the exception of GBS, these diseases are only manageable, not curable. Rehabilitation nurses play a key role in assisting patients, families, and caregivers with adjusting to the lifestyle and functional changes and promoting everyone's successful adaptation to these alterations.

Because the diseases discussed in this chapter share many common traits, parts of the discussion are grouped, and tables are used throughout the chapter to list information specific to a particular disease. Issues related to each disease, including statistical information, such as the prevalence and incidence of each disease, are discussed specific to each disease.

ANATOMY AND PHYSIOLOGY RELEVANT TO NEUROMUSCULAR DISORDERS

The nervous system is divided into the peripheral nervous system and the central nervous system (CNS). The CNS includes the brain and the spinal cord, whereas the peripheral nervous system includes the autonomic nervous system (ANS) and the spinal and cranial nerves. The CNS, peripheral nervous system, and ANS function together in an integrated way.

The spinal nerves consist of 31 pairs. The pairs include 8 cervical nerves, 12 thoracic spinal nerves, 5 lumbar, 5 sacral, and 1 coccygeal spinal nerve. These nerves each consist of a posterior branch that carries sensory stimuli along the afferent pathway to the spinal cord and brain and an anterior branch that carries motor impulses along the efferent pathway to the muscle tissue. Spinal nerves have designated areas of the body for which they are responsible. These areas approximate the segments of the dermatomes. Dermatomes innervate the skin and process sensory stimulation from the spinal nerves. Depending on which spinal nerves are injured or impaired,

various areas of the body will exhibit sensory deficits consistent with the corresponding dermatome (Figure 21-1).

There are 12 cranial nerves. Four of these nerves have both sensory and motor components. See Box 21-1 for a list of cranial nerves and their functions. See Table 23-1 for assessment of cranial nerves.

The somatic nervous system and the ANS make up the functional component of the peripheral nervous system. The somatic system regulates voluntary motor ability, whereas the autonomic system controls the internal environment of the body through involuntary regulatory mechanisms. The ANS comprises the sympathetic and the parasympathetic nervous systems (PNS) (McCance & Huether, 2006).

The sympathetic nervous system (SNS) is activated along chains of ganglia on either side of the spinal cord. These chains transmit impulses as spinal nerves are stimulated. In response to stimulation, the heart beats faster, glucose is released for energy, and blood flow to the kidney is restricted. Blood vessels in the musculature dilate to push peripheral blood flow toward the brain and heart. In addition, the thyroid is overstimulated and diaphoresis occurs. A consequence of these mechanisms is that blood pressure and fluid volume increase. The SNS is vital for responding in emergency situations or when blood pressure drops.

The cells for both the SNS and PNS are located in the gray matter. Those involved with the SNS are located along the thoracolumbar section of the spinal cord, whereas the cells involved in the PNS are located from S2 to S4. Cranial nerves III, VII, IX, and X are involved to some extent as well in the PNS. In many ways the PNS responds in opposite ways when compared to the SNS. The PNS is responsible for directing the ANS during nonstressful periods. SNS stimulation occurs in response to alterations in homeostasis that require adjustment for the organism to survive. Table 21-1 compares the effects of the SNS and the PNS.

The CNS consists of the brain and spinal cord. Ascending pathways carry impulses to the CNS, and efferent pathways carry impulses away from the CNS. Efferent pathways stimulate skeletal muscle and effector organs (McCance & Huether, 2006). The spinal cord facilitates the transmission of impulses

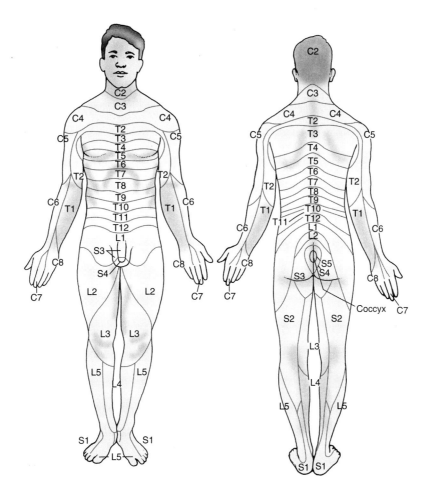

Figure 21-1 Dermatomes (cutaneous innervation of spinal nerves). (From Ignatavicius, D. D., & Workman, M. L. [2006]. *Medical-surgical nursing: Critical thinking for collaborative care* [5th ed.]. St. Louis, MO: W.B. Saunders.)

between the brain and spinal nerves that innervate organs and muscles. Spinal reflexes regulate responses to pain, muscle tone, and urination. Gray matter in the spinal cord is involved in the integration and processing of impulses and responses, whereas the white matter consists of myelinated axons that transmit impulses. The ventral roots of the spinal cord contain motor neurons that travel to the skeletal muscles. The dorsal roots of the spinal cord convey sensory information.

Mature nerve cells in the CNS are not capable of dividing (although recent research indicates that this theory may not be completely true), so when injury occurs, it is typically accompanied by permanent loss of function. Myelinated nerves in the PNS may regenerate after injury depending on the location, type, and severity of the injury (McCance & Huether, 2002).

Nervous tissue is made up of two basic types of cells: neurons and supporting cells (neuroglia in the CNS; Schwann cells in the PNS). Neurons detect threats to homeostasis and initiate change to maintain the steady state. Each neuron is specialized in its function. Glucose fuels neurons. Neurons are composed of a body, dendrites, and an axon. The axon of the neuron

may or may not be covered with a membrane called a *myelin sheath*. This sheath insulates the axon and allows neural transmission to occur rapidly (McCance & Huether, 2006).

A system of neurons called the basal ganglia is located at the base of the brain and works with the cerebellum and cerebral cortex to stimulate and carry out motor activity. Stimulation of the basal ganglia inhibits muscle tone and refines voluntary muscle movements with the assistance of dopamine and acetylcholine, two neurotransmitters.

Neurotransmitters are chemicals that transmit impulses from one cell to another. Among them are acetylcholine, dopamine, norepinephrine, serotonin, and histamine. Deficiencies or excesses in neurotransmitters contribute to pathologic conditions (McCance & Huether, 2006). Table 21-2 lists sites and functions of the neurotransmitters. See Chapter 14 for additional neurological information.

LIFE SPAN ISSUES

During the third week of embryonic development the nervous system begins to develop. Beginning at this time, neurons

BOX 21-1 Origins, Types, and Functions of Cranial Nerves

Cranial Nerve	Origin	Type	Function
I: Olfactory	Olfactory bulb	Sensory	Smell
II: Optic	Retina	Sensory	Vision
III: Oculomotor	Midbrain	Motor to eye muscles	Eye movement via medial and lateral rectus and inferior oblique and superior rectus muscles; lid elevation via the levator muscle
		Parasympathetic-motor	Pupil constriction; ciliary muscles
IV: Trochlear	Lower midbrain	Motor	Eye movement via superior oblique muscles
V: Trigeminal	Pons	Sensory	Sensation from skin of face and scalp and mucous membranes of mouth and nose
		Motor	Muscles of mastication (chewing)
VI: Abducens	Inferior pons	Motor	Eye movement via lateral rectus muscles
VII: Facial	Inferior pons	Sensory	Pain and temperature from ear area; deep sensations from the face; taste from anterior two thirds of the tongue
		Motor	Muscles of the face and scalp
		Parasympathetic-motor	Lacrimal, submandibular, and sublingual salivary glands
VIII: Vestibulocochlear	Pons-medulla junction	Sensory	Hearing and equilibrium
IX: Glossopharyngeal	Medulla	Sensory	Pain and temperature from ear; taste and sensation from posterior one third of tongue and pharynx
		Motor	Skeletal muscles of the throat
		Parasympathetic-motor	Parotid glands
X: Vagus	Medulla	Sensory	Pain and temperature from ear; sensations from pharynx, larynx, thoracic and abdominal viscera
		Motor	Muscles of the soft palate, larynx, and pharynx
		Parasympathetic-motor	Thoracic and abdominal viscera; cells of secretory glands; cardiac and smooth muscle innervation to the level of the splenic flexure.
XI: Accessory	Medulla (anterior gray horn of the cervical spine)	Motor	Skeletal muscles of the pharynx and larynx and sternocleidomastoid and trapezius muscles
XII: Hypoglossal	Medulla	Motor	Skeletal muscles of the tongue

Modified from Ignatavicius, D. D., & Workman, M. L. [2006]. *Medical-surgical nursing: Critical thinking for collaborative care* [5th ed.]. St. Louis, MO: W. B. Saunders.

multiply quickly and begin to make synaptic connections. Stimulation appears to cause division of neurons specific to a particular function. The size of the brain increases until puberty and then remains steady until middle adulthood. Neurons are lost gradually as adults age, without significant loss of function within a typical life span. However, older age is directly correlated to neurological impairment and excessive neuronal loss, and degeneration is associated with dementia. The secretion and metabolism of neurotransmitters are also altered by age. Dopamine and norepinephrine decrease in particular. In addition, nerve fibers in the ANS decline in quantity, and motor nerve fibers and the myelin sheath in the PNS degenerate.

Changes in posture and fluidity of movement occur with age. Bradykinesia, rigidity, and tremor may be signs of age or of PD (discussed later in this chapter). Visual changes, such as decreased acuity and pupillary response time, may occur. These changes combined with hearing loss may lead to confusion and disorientation.

In addition, elderly persons may be more sensitive to cold temperatures than to heat and less sensitive to pain. Sensitivity to taste, smell, and tactile sensation also tends to diminish. Changes in mental status should be carefully evaluated as to their source because medications, dehydration, depression, and changes in the ability to hear and see may account for confusion; it may not be related to a disease process.

ASSESSMENT

Nursing assessment of the patient with a neurological impairment includes the health history, review of systems, physical

TABLE 21-1 Autonomic Effects on Various Organs of the Body

Organ	Effect of Sympathetic Stimulation	Effect of Parasympathetic Stimulation
Eye		
Pupil	Dilated	Constricted
Ciliary muscle	Slight relaxation (far vision)	Constricted (near vision)
Glands	Vasoconstriction and slight secretion	Stimulation of copious (except pancreas) secretion (containing many enzymes for enzyme-secreting glands)
Nasal		
Lacrimal		
Parotid		
Submandibular		
Gastric		
Pancreatic		
Sweat glands	Copious sweating (cholinergic)	Sweating of the palms of the hands
Apocrine glands	Thick, odoriferous secretion	None
Heart		
Muscle	Increased rate	Slowed rate
	Increased force of contraction	Decreased force of contraction
Coronary arteries	Dilated (beta$_2$); constricted (alpha)	Dilated
Lungs		
Bronchi	Dilated	Constricted
Blood vessels	Mildly constricted	? Dilated
Gut		
Lumen	Decreased peristalsis and tone	Increased peristalsis and tone
Sphincter	Increased tone (most times)	Relaxed (most times)
Liver	Glucose released	Contracted
Gallbladder and bile ducts	Relaxed	Slight glycogen synthesis
Kidney	Decreased output and renin secretion	None
Bladder		
Detrusor	Relaxed (slight)	Contracted
Trigone	Contracted	Relaxed
Penis	Ejaculation	Erection
Systemic arterioles		
Abdominal viscera	Constricted	None
Muscle	Constricted (alpha-adrenergic)	None
	Dilated (beta$_2$-adrenergic)	None
	Dilated (cholinergic)	
Skin	Constricted	
Blood		
Coagulation	Increased	None
Glucose	Increased	None
Lipids	Increased	None
Basal metabolism	Increased up to 100%	None
Adrenal medullary secretion	Increased	None
Mental activity	Increased	None
Piloerector muscles	Contracted	None
Skeletal muscles	Increased glycogenolysis	None
	Increased strength	None
Fat cells	Lipolysis	None

From Gyton, A. C., & Hall, J. E. (2006). *Textbook of medical physiology* (11th ed.). Philadelphia: W. B. Saunders.

examination, selected tests and procedures, and environmental assessment. The neurological assessment begins when the examiner first encounters the patient because the level of consciousness, physical appearance, behavior, affect, facial expression, and ability to communicate can all be noted during the greeting phase of the encounter. Should the patient be an unreliable source for the information to be elicited during the health history, this first encounter will signal the nurse to consider exploring the history with a reliable family member and proceeding directly to the objective phases of the assessment.

Health History

Neurological dysfunction may be a primary complaint or may be secondary to other problems. Thyroid disease, diabetes

TABLE 21-2 Sites, Functions, and Actions of Transmitters, Probable Transmitters, and Neuromodulators

Transmitter Substance	Site	Function/Comments	Action
Acetylcholine	Brain, brain stem, basal ganglia, autonomic nervous system	Nerve and muscle transmission Parasympathetic and preganglionic sympathetic system	Excitatory, but some inhibitory
Serotonin	Medial brain stem, hypothalamus, dorsal horn of spinal cord	Possible onset of sleep, mood control; pain pathway inhibitor in spinal cord	Inhibitory
Catecholamines			
Dopamine	Substantia nigra to basal ganglia	Complex movements, emotional response regulation, attention	Usually inhibitory
Norepinephrine (epinephrine parallels)	Hypothalamus, brain stem, reticular formation, cerebellum, sympathetic nervous system	Maintenance of arousal, reward system, dreaming sleep, mood regulation	Mainly excitatory
Amino Acids			
Aspartate	Brain, spinal cord interneurons	Sensation	Excitatory
γ-Aminobutyric acid (GABA)	Brain, brain stem, basal ganglia, autonomic nervous system	Nerve and muscle transmission Possibly one third of neurons	Inhibitory
Glutamate	Sensory pathways	Sensation	Excitatory
Glycine	Spinal cord interneurons	Muscle control	Inhibitory
Peptides*			
Substance P	Brains, neurons in spinal cord	Pain transmission	Excitatory
Endorphins, enkephalins	Thalamus, hypothalamus, spinal cord, pituitary	Pleasure sensation, reward system, analgesia (inhibits release of substance P), released with ACTH (corticotrophin) during stress	Probably excitatory
Gases			
Nitric acid	Neurons	Not stored in specific site; made by enzymes as needed; released by diffusion	Excitatory
Carbon monoxide	Neurons	Function not well understood	Questionable

From Ignatavicius, D. D., Workman, M. L. (2006). *Medical-surgical nursing: Critical thinking for collaborative care* (5th ed.). Philadelphia: W. B. Saunders.
*Other peptides under investigation as probable transmitters are vasopressin (ADH), gastrin, cholecystokinin, glucagons, insulin, somatostatin, angiotensin, melanocyte-stimulating hormone (MSH), luteinizing hormone-releasing hormones (LH-RH), and thyrotropin-releasing hormone (TRH). Prostaglandins, also under investigation, are thought to be modulators.

mellitus, cancer, infection, pernicious anemia, hypertension, and substance abuse may contribute to neurological dysfunction. In addition, hospitalizations and surgeries will offer clues to whether the patient has a history of neurological impairment.

A thorough medication history is integral to any health assessment. Mood elevators, tranquilizers, narcotics, and sedatives are particularly influential in causing neurological symptoms such as dizziness and drowsiness. In addition, medications are a cue to health status. Patients receiving antiepileptic medication or antispasmodics are likely to have neurological dysfunction. The patient should be questioned regarding the use of over-the-counter medications as well as prescription drugs because ephedrine has recently been implicated in brain attacks.

Exposure during the perinatal period to toxic substances, including alcohol, viruses, drugs, tobacco, and radiation, can adversely affect embryonic neurological development. Alterations from the norm of success at developmental tasks during growth may indicate neurological dysfunction. Exposure to these elements from birth may also contribute to neurological dysfunction. A family history of stroke, seizures, and brain or spinal tumors is also worth documenting for future reference during the assessment.

It is important that the nurse ask key questions related to health patterns while obtaining the patient's history. Box 21-2 contains possible alterations in health patterns related to neurological impairment or dysfunction.

Risk factors associated with neurological disease include increasing age, sex (male), heredity, hypertension, cigarette smoking, diabetes mellitus, carotid artery disease, heart disease, and polycythemia. In addition, use of drugs and alcohol and certain climactic conditions and socioeconomic factors may contribute to brain attacks and injury.

BOX 21-2 Health Patterns and Neurological Dysfunction

Health Perception–Health Management Pattern
- Daily activities
- Drug use
- Safety practices
- Previous hospitalizations

Nutrition-Metabolic Pattern
- Diet recall
- Difficulty chewing, swallowing

Elimination Pattern
- Incontinence
- Constipation
- Hesitancy, urgency, retention

Activity-Exercise Pattern
- Weakness
- Poor coordination
- Reduced independence

Sleep-Rest Pattern
- Problems sleeping
- Use of sleep-inducing medications

Cognitive-Perceptual Pattern
- Changes in memory
- Vertigo

- Temperature insensitivity
- Numbness, tingling, pain
- Difficulty communicating

Self-Perception–Self-Concept Pattern
- Effect of neurological problem on self-concept

Role-Relationship Pattern
- Changes related to neurological dysfunction

Sexuality-Reproductive Pattern
- Satisfaction
- Dysfunction
- Need for counseling
- Alternative methods

Coping–Stress Tolerance Pattern
- Coping pattern
- Needs being met

Value-Belief Pattern
- Culturally specific beliefs, perceptions that may influence treatment

Modified from Neal, L. J. (2004). Neuromuscular disorders. In L. J. Neal & S. E. Guillett (Eds.). *Care of the adult with a chronic illness or disability: A team approach* (pp. 378-392). St. Louis, MO: Mosby.

BOX 21-3 Is Anybody Home?

I: Intellect, including thought processes and reasoning, judgment, and simple calculations
S: Sensation, including touch, pain, temperature
A: Appearance, appropriateness, affect
N: Nerves, cranial
Y: Yak, yak; communication and use of language
B: Balance
O: Orientation
D: Deep tendon reflexes
Y: Yesterday; short- and long-term memory
H: Health history
O: Observe for alterations between assessments
M: Muscle strength and motor ability
E: Energy level and emotional state

From Neal, L. J. (1997). Is anybody home? *Home Healthcare Nurse,* *15*(3), 158-167.

Any changes in function noted by the patient or others should be investigated. Any history of neurological disease, trauma, or chronic disease should also be explored in depth.

Physical Examination

A simple but thorough tool can be used to guide the neurological assessment (Neal, 1997). The tool consists of a mnemonic device ("Is anybody home?") that helps the clinician to remember to include the many parts of the neurological assessment (Box 21-3).

The clinician uses a variety of instruments while conducting the neurological assessment. However, perhaps the most important instrument the clinician uses is the power of observation. Looking at the patient while observing for alterations in affect, appearance, and appropriateness will provide clues to neurological dysfunction that may be substantiated as the assessment continues.

Diagnostic Tests and Procedures

A number of tests and procedures can be performed to determine and evaluate neurological function. Table 21-3 includes a brief description of these tests and procedures.

Environmental Assessment

The environmental assessment is particularly crucial in patients with a neuromuscular disorders related to safety issues. The environmental assessment includes the tangible environment, such as the home or other setting in which the patient lives. However, the environment also refers to the patient's support system and the patient's ability to obtain resources, such as food, medicine, and equipment. The setting in which the patient resides should be assessed for clear pathways; cleanliness; adequate light and stair railings; and accommodations for bathing, eating, and sleeping.

TABLE 21-3 Neurological Tests and Procedures

Test/Procedure	Rationale/Purpose
Computed tomography	X-ray beam scans head in layers to provide images of the brain; distinguishes differences in densities
Positron emission tomography	Computer imaging of organ function; allows measurement of blood flow, brain metabolism, and tissue composition
Magnetic resonance imaging	Uses a magnetic field to show images; gives information about intracellular chemical changes
Single photon emission computed tomography	Three-dimensional imaging; contrasts normal and abnormal tissue
Cerebral angiography	X-ray film of cerebral circulation using contrast dye
Electromyography	Needle electrodes in skeletal muscles measure changes in electrical potentials
Nerve conduction studies	Stimulation of a peripheral nerve to record muscle action potential or sensory action potential
Lumbar puncture and cerebrospinal fluid examination	Spinal tap to remove cerebrospinal fluid for analysis

Modified from Neal, L. J. (2004). Neuromuscular disorders. In L. J. Neal & S. E. Guillett (Eds.). *Care of the adult with a chronic illness or disability: A team approach* (pp. 378-392). St. Louis, MO: Mosby.

Whether the patient with a neuromuscular disease has a solid support system and a caregiver must be assessed carefully. There may be members of his or her religious congregation who can visit to bring food or clean the home on a short-term basis. On a long-term basis, these persons may be able to provide social interaction rather than continued food and services. Family members may be very young, elderly, or frail and unable to provide the physically demanding services needed by the patient with a neuromuscular disease. Again, in the short term, family members may be able to assume the burden of personal care services but may find themselves worn down and debilitated by the time and attention required. Family dynamics may also preclude comfortable interaction between the patient and family caregivers.

Financial status may present another barrier to obtaining the environmental support needed by the patient. If family members work outside the home, a full-time hired caregiver might be necessary. In addition, expenditures for food, medicine, equipment, and supplies may not be reimbursed by insurance.

The patient's environment consists of both tangible and intangible elements that require assessment. Box 21-4 lists some of these tangible and intangible elements.

PATHOPHYSIOLOGY OF SELECTED NEUROMUSCULAR DISEASES

It is important to have background knowledge of the pathophysiology of the neuromuscular diseases to be discussed in this chapter before beginning to design realistic goals and plans for patients with these diseases. The diseases are described in an order that should help the reader logically understand the differences and similarities among the diseases and begin to comprehend why these diseases share many goals, interventions, and outcomes.

BOX 21-4 Tangible and Intangible Environmental elements

Tangible Elements
- Safety
- Functional navigability
- Ability to perform activities of daily living and instrumental activities of daily living
- Availability and ability of a caregiver to provide satisfactory care
- Availability and accessibility of telephone service
- Availability and accessibility of equipment and assistive devices
- Access to transportation and community facilities
- Presence and strength of a social support network
- Cleanliness of environment
- Presence of pets or others that need care

Intangible Elements
- Dynamics of the family or support network
- Financial support
- Informal support networks such as neighbors and religious congregation members (Neal, 2002)

Huntington's Disease

HD is a degenerative neuromuscular disease. Its prevalence is 5 per 100,000 persons, and it is not race or gender specific (McCance & Huether, 2006). It is genetically acquired but typically does not present itself until approximately 40 years of age. The gene abnormality has been isolated to chromosome 4. Children of a parent with HD have a 50% chance of acquiring the disease. Once the disease is diagnosed, patients usually survive for 10 to 15 years and may die of infection, choking, falls, pneumonia, or heart failure (Neal, 2004).

Glutamine, used in protein synthesis, builds up to abnormal levels in the brain and destroys brain cells. The degeneration

BOX 21-5 Diagnostics Related to Huntington's Disease

- Clinical presentation of symptoms
- Family history
- Neurological examination
- Ruling out other causes of symptoms
- Imaging studies
- Magnetic resonance imaging (MRI) scan
- Computed tomography (CT) scan: shrinkage of brain in some cases
- Genetic marker: 28 or fewer CAG repeats

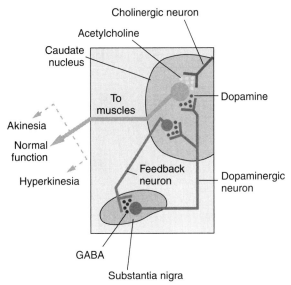

Figure 21-2 Dopaminergic synaptic activity is mediated by dopamine. Cholinergic synaptic activity is mediated by acetylcholine. A balance between the two kinds of activity produces normal motor function. A relative excess of cholinergic activity produces akinesia and rigidity. A relative excess of dopaminergic activity produces involuntary movements. Neurons in the caudate nucleus contain γ-aminobutyric acid (GABA) and possibly control dopaminergic neurons in the substantia nigra through a feedback pathway. (From Huether, S. E., & McCance, K. L. [2004]. *Understanding pathophysiology* [3rd ed.]. St. Louis, MO: Mosby.)

occurs in the basal ganglia and in the cerebral cortex. The basal ganglia normally control movement, and the cerebral cortex is involved with thought, judgment, perception, and memory. The cerebellum is also affected, and consequently balance and coordination are disrupted. The neurotransmitters acetylcholine and γ-aminobutyric acid (GABA) are lost, and this contributes to dysfunction in motor and mental capability. An excess of dopamine also occurs relative to the deficiency of GABA and acetylcholine, and this contributes to chorea, or nonfluid, writhing, twisting, involuntary movements (McCance & Huether, 2006). Chorea and dementia characterize the manifestations of the disease. Dopamine is an inhibitory neurotransmitter, whereas acetylcholine is an excitatory neurotransmitter. Consequently an excess of dopamine relative to acetylcholine deficiency results in involuntary and abnormal movement.

Purposeful movement is lost as the disease progresses. All of the muscles in the body are involved in involuntary movement. Speech, chewing, swallowing, and gait become disorganized and difficult. Eventually the person displays dementia but will also be irritable and may act out violently. Hallucinations, paranoia, and impaired judgment evolve with the disease, whereas emotional changes such as impatience, anger, and suicidal tendencies tend to decrease later on. Box 21-5 lists diagnostics related to HD.

Parkinson's Disease

PD also affects the basal ganglia and is related to a deficiency rather than an excess of the neurotransmitter dopamine. It affects approximately 1% of Americans (130 to 150 per 100,000 [McCance & Huether, 2006]) and like HD usually presents in persons older than 40 years. PD occurs in both sexes and in persons of all races (it is slightly more likely in men [McCance & Huether, 2006]). PD may be idiopathic in that the cause is unknown, or it may occur as a consequence of infection, trauma, or drug or other toxicity.

Enzymes required to metabolize dopamine are deficient in the basal ganglia. Consequently, dopamine levels are reduced, and the classic triad of symptoms, rigidity, tremor, and bradykinesia, appears (Figure 21-2). A fourth symptom has been added to this classic triad: impaired postural righting reflexes (Imke, 2000). Interestingly the brains of some patients

with PD present on autopsy with amyloid plaques and neurofibrillary tangles characteristic of Alzheimer's disease. However, the dementia that occurs in PD (30% to 50% of all cases) may occur in patients with or without the plaques or tangles (McCance & Huether, 2006).

The deficiency of dopamine results in a relative excess of acetylcholine, the opposite of what occurs in HD. This deficiency of dopamine allows acetylcholine to contribute to sustained, excitable activity and is manifested in the classic triad mentioned above. In addition, patients with PD typically display dysarthria, dysphagia, and postural disturbance. Reduced arm swing, foot drag, a hoarse voice, and a flat affect are also characteristic (Figure 21-3). Initially one side of the body is affected, but eventually both sides are involved. Imke (2000) reports that patients often remark that their handwriting has become illegible (micrographia), an important clue to the clinical diagnosis.

One current theory regarding the pathophysiology of PD is that free radicals add to the damage done to neurons. Reduced levels of ferritin in patients with PD support this theory because ferritin is normally used to protect neurons from free radicals. Another theory is that PD is genetic. This is supported by the fact that 15% to 20% of persons with PD have a relative who demonstrates parkinsonian symptoms. This theory is currently the focus of intensive study. In addition, it is thought that certain persons may experience accelerated aging of dopaminergic neurons, which causes the disease (NINDS, 2004).

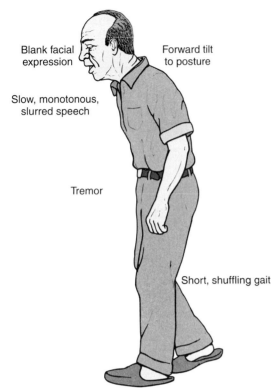

Blank facial expression

Forward tilt to posture

Slow, monotonous, slurred speech

Tremor

Short, shuffling gait

Figure 21-3 Characteristic shuffling gait of a patient with Parkinson's disease. (From Lewis, S. M., Heitkemper, M. M., & Dirksen, S. R. [2004]. *Medical-surgical nursing: Assessment and management of clinical problems* [6th ed.]. St. Louis, MO: Mosby.)

> **BOX 21-6 Diagnostics Related to Parkinson's Disease**
>
> - History
> - Medication review
> - Neurological examination
> - Review of systems
> - Positron emission tomography (PET) scan
> - Two of the three classic symptoms: bradykinesia, rigidity, and tremor

The onset of PD is insidious, and medications and treatments may contribute to the patient's safety risk (McCance & Huether, 2006). Box 21-6 lists diagnostics related to PD.

Myasthenia Gravis

MG is a disease of impaired transmission of acetylcholine across the neuromuscular junction. It affects people of both genders, all races, and all ages. However, women between the ages of 20 and 30 years are most commonly affected. According to the Myasthenia Gravis Foundation of America, 20 of every 100,000 Americans acquire the disease (MGFA, 2007). Thymomas are fairly common among people, especially the elderly, with MG (Adis International Limited, 2001).

MG is a chronic autoimmune disease and is associated with other autoimmune diseases. Acetylcholine receptors cease to be recognized as "self"; thus autoantibodies (immunoglobulin G) are produced against the acetylcholine receptors and block the binding of acetylcholine. This immune response eventually destroys receptor sites for acetylcholine and results in diminished nerve transmission (McCance & Huether, 2006). Muscle weakness and fatigability result.

There are three types of MG: ocular (more prevalent in men, and muscle weakness is restricted to the eyes), generalized (typically includes the proximal muscles with occasional remissions), and bulbar (includes muscles innervated by cranial nerves IX, X, XI, and XII). Generalized and bulbar MG

may be rapidly progressive or fulminating. However, generalized MG may also be slowly progressive.

The onset of MG is usually insidious, and the patient presents with fatigue. A history of frequent upper respiratory tract infections is also common. The symptoms of muscle weakness manifest in ptosis, speech slurring, dysphagia, and facial droop. Neck, shoulder, and hip flexor muscles may also be affected. Eventually all muscles are affected, and ventilatory support is needed (McCance & Huether, 2006).

Profound muscle weakness occurs with myasthenic crisis and causes quadriparesis or quadriplegia. This is a condition requiring emergency respiratory support. A cholinergic crisis occurs related to toxicity from the administration of anticholinesterase drugs used to treat MG (Table 21-4). Smooth-muscle hyperactivity occurs related to an accumulation of acetylcholine and excessive parasympathetic nerve activity. Clinically the crisis resembles myasthenic crisis with added parasympathetic nerve–like symptoms (McCance & Huether, 2006). Diagnostics related to MG for the person who presents with a drooping eyelid or ptosis are listed in Box 21-7.

Multiple Sclerosis

MS is an immune-mediated demyelinating disease of the CNS (Kalb, 2004). Onset presents between the ages of 20 and 50 years and is twice as prevalent in women as in men. It is most common in whites, and 500,000 persons in the United States and Canada are estimated to have MS.

The cause of MS remains largely unclear. A hypersensitivity response to a slow-growing virus followed by recurring inflammatory reactions may be responsible. Another prevailing theory is that an autoimmune response against myelin causes the disease (Kalb, 2004). A particular genetic marker has been found in more people with MS than in those without MS (National Multiple Sclerosis Society, 2004).

There appear to be myriad risk factors for MS, including environmental and infectious agents and immune system and genetic factors. Prevalence appears to increase with increased distance from the equator. In the United States MS is more common in northern states than in southern states. If an individual lives closer to the equator in the first 15 years of life than in the years after age 15, the individual appears to be less likely to acquire MS. The converse is true for regions farther from the equator.

TABLE 21-4 Comparison of Myasthenic Crisis and Cholinergic Crisis

	Myasthenic Crisis	Cholinergic Crisis
Causes	Exacerbation of myasthenia following precipitating factors or failure to take medication as prescribed or dose of medication too low	Overdose of anticholinesterase drugs resulting in increased acetylcholine at the receptor sites, remission (spontaneous or after thymectomy)
Differential diagnosis	Improved strength after intravenous administration of anticholinesterase drugs; increased weakness of skeletal muscles manifesting as ptosis, bulbar signs (e.g., difficulty in swallowing, difficulty in articulating words), or dyspnea	Weakness within 1 hour after ingestion of anticholinesterase; increased weakness of skeletal muscles manifesting as ptosis, bulbar signs, dyspnea; effects on smooth muscle include pupillary miosis, salivation, diarrhea, nausea or vomiting, abdominal cramps, increased bronchial secretions, sweating, or lacrimation

Modified from Shpritz, D. W. (2002). Interventions for clients with problems of the peripheral nervous system. In D. D. Ignatavicius & M. L. Workman (Eds.), *Medical-surgical nursing* (4th ed.). St. Louis, MO: W. B. Saunders.

BOX 21-7 Diagnostics for Myasthenia Gravis

- Tensilon test: administration of Tensilon immediately improves muscle strength
- Electrophysiology to evaluate nerve conduction
- Serological tests to check antiacetylcholine receptor antibody titers
- History
- Neurological examination
- Computed tomography (CT) scan to check if there is an enlarged thymus (Armstrong & Schumann, 2003)

Random repeated inflammatory responses (exacerbations) leave behind plaques and lesions in the myelin, and nerve transmission is disrupted. The body's immune system appears to stimulate these attacks. Some researchers contend that axonal loss may begin earlier and be more profound than previously thought (Peterson, 2001). Recent magnetic resonance imaging evidence suggests that atrophy in the brain and spinal cord may occur earlier and with a milder presentation of the disease than is commonly recognized (Hardmeier et al., 2003).

The subsequent demyelination or destruction of the myelin sheath of axons in the CNS most frequently affects the optic and oculomotor cranial nerves and the cerebellar, corticospinal, and posterior column systems (Figure 21-4). Consequently, clinical manifestations, although typically individualized, include abnormalities of vision and eye movement, motor skills, coordination, and gait, as well as spasticity and sensory disturbances, such as pain and paresthesia (Kalb, 2004).

Fatigue is the symptom most commonly identified by individuals with MS followed in order by ambulation difficulties, bowel and bladder problems, visual disturbances, cognitive dysfunction, tremor, and problems with arm movement (Kalb, 2004). Dysphagia and dysarthria are other common symptoms. In 1996 (Lublin & Reingold, 1996) a new classification system for MS was devised. These categories

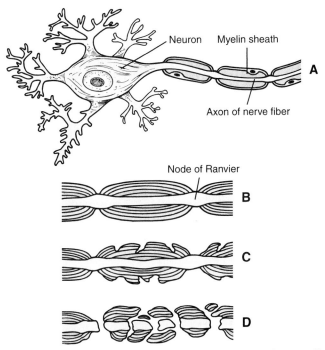

Figure 21-4 Pathogenesis of multiple sclerosis. **A,** Normal nerve cell with myelin sheath. **B,** Normal axon. **C,** Myelin breakdown. **D,** Myelin totally disrupted; axon not functioning. (From Lewis, S. M., Heitkemper, M. M., & Dirksen, S. R. [2004]. *Medical-surgical nursing: Assessment and management of clinical problems* [6th ed.]. St. Louis, MO: Mosby.)

include relapsing-remitting MS (RRMS), primary-progressive MS (PPMS), secondary-progressive MS (SPMS), and progressive-relapsing MS (PRMS) (Kalb, 2004). The categories are not intended to be used to rate a person's disease but to help to describe it and to assist in the performance of research studies on MS. Table 21-5 differentiates the forms of MS.

Most patients are initially diagnosed with relapsing-remitting MS. Clinical manifestations relate to the portion of the CNS that is affected. Fifty percent of those persons who begin with the relapsing-remitting form of the disease will

TABLE 21-5 Classifications of Multiple Sclerosis

Category	Definition
Relapsing remitting	No disease progression between exacerbations*
Primary progressive	Progressive functional decline without distinct relapses*
Secondary progressive	Starts with relapsing remitting and becomes progressive
Progressive relapsing	Progressive disease, acute exacerbations with progression

*Exacerbation: Relapse or "an episode of new or worsening MS symptoms that lasts more than 24 hours and is not related to metabolic changes or steroid withdrawal" (Kalb, 2004).

progress to secondary-progressive MS within 10 years. Ninety-five percent of the group that started with RRMS will progress to SPMS in 25 years (Kalb, 2004).

Many persons develop cognitive disturbances or psychosocial problems related to MS (McCance & Huether, 2006). Furthermore, complications from MS may be debilitating and include bowel and bladder management difficulties, impaired skin integrity, and contractures.

Gulick's 10-year longitudinal study of patients with MS (1998) found that over time there is "a slow but significant increase in three symptom complexes: motor (extremity weakness, tremors, balance difficulties, spasms, falling, and knee locking), brain stem (double vision, dysphagia, blurred vision, and forgetfulness), and elimination (urinary frequency and difficulty reaching the toilet during the daytime and nighttime) and an overall downward trajectory in all ADL functions: fine and gross motor (eating, bathing, transfer, dressing, travel, walking), socializing/recreation (indoor and outdoor activities), communication (writing, phoning, reading), and intimacy." Subjects ranked the symptoms.

Previously it was believed that damage to the axons was less significant than damage to the myelin sheath. Research has shown, however, that axons can become damaged irreversibly as a result of the attacks of the immune system on the myelin and the inflammation that occurs during a relapse. Early intervention is now recommended because irreversible loss of axon function can result in neurological deficits early in the disease (Kalb, 2004) (Figure 21-5). Box 21-8 lists diagnostics related to MS.

Guillain-Barré Syndrome

GBS, or acute infectious polyradiculoneuritis, affects the PNS. It is an inflammatory disease that affects approximately 1 person per 100,000 in the world (Pritchard & Hughes, 2004). It appears to affect more men than women and occurs at all ages with a peak in late adolescence and young adulthood (Kuwabara, 2004).

The inflammatory reaction that occurs in GBS is an autoimmune response that may be triggered by a viral or bacterial infection. Pathogens that are typically implicated in the etiology of GBS include *Campylobacter jejuni*, cytomegalovirus, Epstein-Barr virus, and *Mycoplasma pneumoniae*. A link

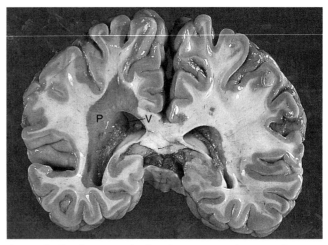

Figure 21-5 Chronic multiple sclerosis. Demyelination plaque *(P)* at gray-white junction and adjacent partially remyelinated shadow plaque *(V)*. (From Lewis, S. M., Heitkemper, M. M., & Dirksen, S. R. [2004]. *Medical-surgical nursing: assessment and management of clinical problems* [6th ed.]. St. Louis, MO: Mosby.)

BOX 21-8 Diagnostics Related to Multiple Sclerosis

- History, including sexual history
- Neurological examination
- "Evidence of lesions or plaques in two distinct areas of the central nervous system
  Evidence that plaques occurred at discrete points in time
  No explanation other than MS for the plaques in the white matter of the CNS" (Kalb, 2004)
- On magnetic resonance imaging (MRI) the brain appears abnormal in 95% of cases
- Lumbar puncture to rule out other diagnoses
- Evoked potential studies to rule out other diagnoses

---

between vaccination and GBS has been suggested but has not been sufficiently demonstrated by research. Rabies, swine-flu, and poliovirus vaccinations have been most frequently associated with the disease (Kuwabara, 2004).

Although MS affects the myelin of the nerves in the CNS, GBS affects the myelin of the nerves of the peripheral nervous system, the Schwann cells. An antimyelin antibody has been identified as the cause of an antimyelinating process that occurs in the segmental peripheral nerves and the anterior and posterior spinal nerve roots. Sensitized leukocytes destroy the myelin. The inflammatory response further contributes to nerve degeneration and demyelination (Pritchard & Hughes, 2004).

Persons with GBS may or may not present with paresthesias and numbness. The most common symptom is muscle weakness that evolves over days to weeks in a more or less symmetrical fashion (Kuwabara, 2004). Sympathetic and parasympathetic nervous system dysfunction results in blood pressure changes (orthostatic hypotension or hypertension), bradycardia, bowel and bladder problems, and diaphoresis. Most patients with GBS recover spontaneously with or

---

BOX 21-9 Diagnostics for Guillain-Barré Syndrome

- History to rule out other causes
- Neurological examination
- Electrodiagnostic and pathological studies that show demyelination within the Schwann cell surface or the myelin
- Lymphocytic infiltration of the peripheral nerve: myelin sheath and Schwann cells
- Electrodiagnostic studies of nerve conduction that show demyelination in two or more motor nerves (Kuwabara, 2004)

BOX 21-10 Diagnostics for Amyotrophic Lateral Sclerosis

- History
- Physical examination
- Electrodiagnostic studies for fasciculation potentials
- Nerve conduction studies
- Transcranial magnetic stimulation (considered experimental at this time)
- Neuroimaging studies to rule out other causes: MRI of the brain
- Laboratory tests: routine laboratory work to assess general health: CBC, ESR, chemistries, endocrine, immunology, Lyme titer; test for venereal disease, HIV if risk factors are present
- Superoxide dismutase (SOD 1) (Han et al., 2003)

MRI, Magnetic resonance imaging; *CBC,* complete blood count; *ESR,* erythrocyte sedimentation rate; *HIV,* human immunodeficiency virus.

---

without residual disability. In some cases, weakness progresses to total paralysis and death occurs from respiratory failure (Kuwabara, 2004). Acute inflammatory demyelinating polyneuropathy is the most common subtype of GBS. Box 21-9 lists diagnostics of GBS.

Amyotrophic Lateral Sclerosis

ALS affects approximately 1.2 of every 100,000 persons each year (Bradbury, 2003). It is more common in men than in women (although after menopause, the incidence equalizes) and usually occurs after the age of 40 years. It occurs all over the world and involves the upper and lower motor neurons (McCance & Huether, 2002; Neal, 2004).

The disease primarily involves the brain stem, spinal cord, and cerebral cortex and specifically affects the motor neurons in these areas. Progressive muscle weakness and wasting lead to death within 3 to 5 years after diagnosis. New research indicates that two haplotypes in the sequences of the gene for vascular endothelial growth factor (VEGF) increase the risk of acquiring ALS. Individuals with ALS who are homozygous for either of the two haplotypes have reduced VEGF. Researchers have discovered that VEGF protects mice from motor neuron loss following ischemia of the spinal cord (Bradbury, 2003).

Most patients present with upper body weakness and wasting, whereas some present with symptoms in the lower extremities. Dysarthria and dysphagia occur, eventually followed by altered respiratory function (Neal, 2004). The ability to move the eyes and maintain continence usually remains until late, and muscle involvement is typically asymmetrical. Fasciculations of the tongue, hands, and upper extremities are early signs of brain stem involvement. Bulbar palsy, or paralysis or paresis of muscles innervated by the cranial nerves, may be of either the flaccid or spastic type. Neuronal involvement is typically confined to motor function, whereas sensation and intellectual function remain intact (Neal, 2004). Box 21-10 includes diagnostics for ALS.

NURSING DIAGNOSES

The neuromuscular diseases discussed in this chapter share several common characteristics (Box 21-11). Therefore many of the same nursing diagnoses, nursing interventions, and desired outcomes apply (Table 21-6).

BOX 21-11 Shared Characteristics of Degenerative Neuromuscular Diseases

- Usually progressive
- Etiology typically unknown
- Brain degeneration (some cases)
- Neuromuscular changes with regard to the following:
  - Coordination
  - Speech
  - Swallowing
  - Ambulation
  - Cognition
  - Fatigue
  - Weakness
  - Tremors
  - Self-care agency
  - Bowel and bladder management
  - Respiration
- Diagnosis is typically made after ruling out other possibilities
- Usually no known cure
- Palliative measures:
  - Provide comfort
  - Maintain function
  - Teach self-care
  - Support patient/family
  - Administer medication
- Consider hospice care
- Suggest genetic counseling
- Prevent rehospitalization
- Obtain adaptive equipment and durable medical equipment
- Refer to dietitian or physical, occupational, or speech therapist

---

GOALS

The goals for *Healthy People 2010* (USDHHS, 2000) are relevant to a discussion of neuromuscular disease and include the following:

- To increase quality and years of healthy life
- To eliminate health disparities

TABLE 21-6 Nursing Diagnoses, Interventions, and Outcomes Applicable to Degenerative Neuromuscular Diseases

NIC/NOC

Nursing Diagnosis	Nursing Interventions	Nursing Outcomes
Ineffective breathing pattern	Respiratory monitoring	Normal breathing pattern Arterial blood gases within normal range Lungs clear to auscultation No respiratory distress Normal chest x-ray
Risk for aspiration	Aspiration precautions	No aspiration
Impaired swallowing	Aspiration precautions, swallowing therapy	No aspiration Maintenance of adequate body weight
Chronic pain/disturbed sensory perception	Pain management	Comfort
Risk for injury	Surveillance: safety	Safety No injury
Activity intolerance	Energy management	Energy conservation
Fatigue	Energy management	Activity tolerance
Imbalanced nutrition: less than body requirements	Nutrition management	Nutritional status
Disturbed thought processes	Cognitive stimulation, emotional support	Cognitive orientation
Impaired verbal communication	Active listening	Communication
Grieving	Counseling	Quality of life
Chronic sorrow	Emotional support	Hope
Fear	Active listening	Mood equilibrium
Anxiety	Touch	Fear control
Risk for constipation	Constipation/impaction management	Bowel elimination
Bowel incontinence	Bowel incontinence care, bowel training Urinary catheterization: intermittent	Bowel management
Urinary incontinence: urge, urinary incontinence: reflex, urinary incontinence: retention	Urinary incontinence care, bladder training	Bladder management, urinary continence, urinary elimination
Impaired physical mobility	Exercise therapy, positioning	Mobility
Risk for impaired skin integrity	Skin surveillance	Intact skin
Sexual dysfunction	Sexual counseling	Sexual function
Self-care deficit: all ADLs	Self-care assistance	Self-care
Caregiver role strain	Caregiver support	Caregiver well-being

Data from Moorhead, S., Johnson, M., & Maas, M. (Eds.). (2004). *Nursing outcomes classification (NOC)* (3rd ed.). St. Louis, MO: Mosby; Dochterman, J. M., & Bulechek, G. M. (2004). *Nursing interventions classification (NIC)* (4th ed.). St. Louis, MO: Mosby; and NANDA International. (2005). *Nursing diagnoses: Definitions and classification, 2005-2006* (6th ed.). Philadelphia: Author.
ADLs, Activities of daily living.

The ideal goal for the patient with a neuromuscular disease is to enhance the quality and length of life as much as possible. These patients and their caregivers cope with disability and an altered lifestyle, so interventions are always guided by the goal of enhancing quality of life and prolonging health to the maximum extent possible.

Health disparities are evident in the incidence and prevalence of these diseases. It is unknown whether increased prevalence by ethnicity, geographical location, or gender are related more to genetic differences or to disparities in the health of groups and individuals because of the inability to obtain adequate food, nutrition, or health care.

More specifically the primary goals of nursing for patients with neuromuscular disease pertain to comfort measures and to maintaining maximum function. Other than the possibility of a functional recovery with GBS, there is no known cure for any of the other diseases. Each disease involves functional loss that is typically progressive. Self-care to the patient's maximum ability, reduced caregiver strain, patient comfort, and safety are key goals.

PLANNING

Breathing

The risk for aspiration and respiratory failure inherent in these diseases requires long-term planning. Assessment of breathing patterns and swallowing should be incorporated into every assessment of the patient. The additions to the interdisciplinary team of a respiratory therapist, should ventilatory support be required, and of a speech pathologist for the evaluation and treatment of dysphagia should be anticipated.

Pain

Planning for the patient with pain or paresthesias should include short- and long-term alternatives. The nature of pain and paresthesias related to neuromuscular disease, although chronic, is often intermittent. A thorough and ongoing assessment of pain will provide the data necessary to plan interventions and to keep interventions effective.

Injury

The risk of injury is high for all patients with neuromuscular disorders because of alterations in mobility, muscular strength, balance, and cognition. The site of care must be a safe environment, and careful consideration must be given to appropriate equipment to enhance mobility and reduce the risk of injury.

Activity Intolerance

Patients with neuromuscular disease are typically easily fatigued and unable to negotiate previous levels of activity without frequent rest periods. Rest periods need to be built into planning for these patients, as do methods for participating in ADLs while conserving energy. A qualitative study of patients with MS discovered five themes associated with the experience of patients with fatigue (Stuifbergen & Rogers, 1997):

* Fatigue as an ever-present, ongoing experience
* The pervasive impact of fatigue on life
* The exacerbation of symptoms with increasing fatigue
* Fatigue as a paralyzing force
* The "undertow effect" of severe fatigue

According to researchers, self-care strategies need to be directed to reducing the impact of fatigue on the lives of patients. Nurses should recognize that managing chronic fatigue is different from managing acute fatigue.

Altered Nutrition

Despite decreased levels of activity, patients may not be consuming enough food and fluids to meet the demands of the body. Energy with which to eat may be compromised. Dysphagia and the risk of aspiration often require feeding tube placement to ensure that patients receive sufficient calories for energy. A dietitian should provide input during the planning phase of the nursing process and should be included as needed as the patient's condition deteriorates.

Altered Thought Processes

Long-term planning for the potential eventuality of altered thought processes should be considered by the interdisciplinary team. Patients with MS, HD, or PD may develop cognitive changes. All patients with HD develop dementia.

Communication

Impaired verbal communication related to muscular weakness and paralysis reduces the patient's ability to participate in his or her own care. Planning should include the input of a speech pathologist and adaptive equipment to enhance and maintain whatever form of communication is possible for the patient.

Psychosocial Status

Patients with neuromuscular disease are likely to experience changes in the opportunities for social interaction, in roles, and in relationships. Whether patients can continue to be employed and for how long they can work in an office or at home may be significant to their views of themselves. Loss of hope and feelings of helplessness may contribute to higher than normal rates of suicide compared with the general population.

Patients may be fearful and anxious, confused, and in a state of denial about the disease. The fact that these diseases are incurable may precipitate feelings of grief and loss among patients. Limits on mobility and energy are likely to restrict activities and may contribute to the exclusion of the patient from previously enjoyable pastimes. Considerations related to fertility and the effects of the disease on pregnancy and childbearing may be devastating.

Planning regarding psychosocial issues should pervade all communication among interdisciplinary team members. Interventions related to any of the other problem areas are likely to affect or be affected by patients' perceptions of themselves and their situation. Considerations about how each intervention will be received by patients in the context of their views about their care and their goals are vital to the nursing process.

Bowel and Bladder Management

Patients with neuromuscular diseases may be at risk for constipation and/or may become incontinent of bowel and bladder. Some patients, such as those with MS, may retain urine at times. Behavioral techniques may be appropriate to incorporate early in planning. However, medications and procedures, such as intermittent catheterization for patients with MS, will likely be added later. The urologist and the enterostomal nurse may be added to the team at any point from initiation of the plan because they can help guide short- and long-term care planning.

Mobility

Muscular weakness, paresis, and paralysis are characteristic features of all of the diseases discussed in this chapter. Physical therapy is an integral component of the care plan because the goals are to maintain and optimize patient mobility. The rehabilitation nurse and the other team members, including the caregiver, follow the plan of the physical therapist and recommend alterations to the plan as needed.

Skin Integrity

Frequent assessments of the patient's skin must be incorporated into the plan of care. Careful positioning is vital to the maintenance of skin integrity, and arrangements must be included for the caregiver to provide this properly and frequently. The caregiver's sleep time and daily activities must be considered because outside assistance may be needed to help with positioning when the caregiver is unavailable.

Self-Care Deficit

It is important that maximal participation in self-care activities be made possible for each patient with a neuromuscular disease.

However minimal that participation may be, it is crucial to assisting patients with maintaining some control over their care during a time when others are so involved in their lives. Caregivers and family members must be included in planning regarding how to help the patient participate, and nurses are obliged to teach them why patient self-care is necessary.

Sexual Dysfunction

Sexual dysfunction may be an early sign of disease in many patients. After careful assessment of the extent of the problem, planning to either include suggestions for improved function or include a sex therapist on the team must take place. The nature of the problem may convince some professionals that sexual dysfunction is a low priority for planning. However, patients may consider it very important, and therefore it is the patient's perception of the problem that determines the order of the problem among the priorities.

Caregiver Role Strain

Because neuromuscular diseases tend to be progressive and degenerative, tremendous stress, both physical and emotional, is placed on the caregiver. Planning should incorporate time to instruct caregivers regarding strategies for maintaining their emotional and physical health and for locating acceptable respite care for the patient.

The possible genetic component of some of the diseases discussed in this chapter (MS, ALS, HD) supports the need for lifelong planning by patients and their families (Aubeeluck, 2005). Consideration of the likelihood of a genetic component may reduce the incidence of these diseases, particularly HD. Long-term planning may also include the need for institutionalization, such as nursing home placement, or full-time home health care.

Short-term planning often includes the need for reliable support systems of skilled and support professionals, as well as durable medical equipment and adaptive equipment. A realistic assessment of the caregiver's capabilities both in the short and long term will help the nurse, patient, and family to design a realistic plan. The interdisciplinary team must be involved in the planning and should also include the physician; physical, occupational, and if needed, speech therapists; dietitian; and community resources as appropriate.

The environment to which the patient will be discharged must be considered in planning. Goals or the planning designed to achieve the goals may be unrealistic depending on the site of care. The home setting may be more or less adaptable to the plan, as might be the economic resources of the patient and caregiver to carry out the planning.

INTERVENTIONS

The neuromuscular diseases discussed in this chapter share many of the same interventions. All of the interventions discussed are only as effective as the strength and collaborative capacity of the interdisciplinary team that plans and performs them. Always, the director of the team is the patient

and/or the family, and their needs as individuals and as a group must be considered when designing interventions that meet the patient's needs. The planning phase of the patient's care should include the setting for care so that interventions can be performed and adapted to the site of care. In addition, community resources such as support groups for both the patient and the caregiver and organizations that provide services and equipment might be included during the planning and interventions stages. Representatives of community resources can be invited to participate in care planning and conferencing because their input enhances the ability of each team member to view care in realistic terms. Interventions common to the diseases described in this chapter will be discussed. See Table 21-7 for disease-specific interventions.

Airway Management

Maintenance of an effective airway is the most important of all nursing interventions. A thorough and ongoing assessment of breathing patterns and factors that could disrupt them is integral to timely and appropriate intervention. Proper management of the dysphagia and muscular weakness associated with these diseases will help prevent or forestall respiratory complications.

The nurse monitors the patient's vital signs for changes in respiratory function. Oxygen therapy and positioning may be needed to assist breathing as early interventions. Eventually, many of these patients may require mechanical ventilation to assist or assume respiratory function. Interventions specific to patients with difficulty breathing include the following:

- Maintaining a patent airway
- Assessing respiration frequently
- Monitoring arterial blood gas levels
- Providing chest physiotherapy as needed
- Referring to the respiratory therapist
- Assisting with mechanical ventilation if needed
- Offering emotional support
- Assessing cough
- Suctioning as needed

Swallowing and Nutrition

Dysphagia places the patient with neuromuscular disease at increased risk of aspiration. Initially positioning and alterations of the consistency of foods may suffice. Later, placement of an enteral feeding tube may become appropriate.

A diet that promotes energy is high in calories. Small, frequent meals allow the patient to conserve energy while consuming the calories and nutrients needed to meet metabolic demands. Adequate fluid intake to prevent dehydration may be oral initially and may require alternative methods as the disease progresses. Water administered through the patient's enteral feeding tube will ensure adequate fluid intake. Interventions specific to patients with dysphagia and altered nutrition (less than body requirements) are listed below. Many drugs may contribute to dysphagia by causing dry mouth. A saliva substitute or sips of water before and after meals can help. A barium swallow can help diagnose and assess swallowing problems. Behavioral therapies, such as sensory enhancement and postural techniques, can be effective interventions. Other interventions specific to dysphagia and altered nutrition include the following:

- Assessing for gag reflex
- Noting drooling and difficulty controlling secretions
- Monitoring fluid and electrolytes
- Providing a balanced diet that can be chewed and swallowed easily
- Referring to a dietitian
- Providing thick liquids or semisolid food
- Maintaining an upright position during meals
- Massaging the neck and facial muscles before eating
- Monitoring calorie count and weekly weights
- Scheduling medications so peak action minimizes chewing difficulty
- Referring to a speech pathologist

Injury

The key to preventing injury in a patient with a neuromuscular disease is surveillance. This includes not only the patient's physical environment for safety hazards but also the patient's cognitive ability related to the identification of potential hazards and his or her understanding of the existence of real hazards in the environment. Patients may be in denial about the disease or be unrealistic about their ability to negotiate potential safety hazards. In addition, caregivers may overestimate the patient's ability to recognize a safety hazard and be able to avoid it.

Teaching the patient and the caregiver about the potential for injury to the patient is the primary intervention. The plan for teaching will need to be modified as care continues and as the patient's awareness or mobility declines. The following list provides interventions specific to risk for injury related to sensory deficit and inadequate self-protective abilities:

- Assess environment for safety hazards.
- Teach patient and caregiver how to avoid injury.
- Provide supportive devices such as padded side rails if ordered and if permitted in care setting.

Activity Intolerance/Impaired Physical Mobility

Energy conservation measures, physical and occupational therapy, strength training, and pain control all serve to enhance activity tolerance and physical mobility. The patient's ability to breathe without difficulty also contributes to active participation in activities. Participation in activities requiring energy should occur when energy levels are highest. Scheduled rest periods can be helpful to conserve energy.

Because these neuromuscular diseases are incurable (although GBS may be curable, recovery may be prolonged), therapeutic exercises are important to maintaining and maximizing strength, to preventing muscle atrophy, and to decreasing the risk of complications related to immobility, such as deep venous thrombosis. Exercise is recommended for patients with MS and PD. However, it is stressed that moderation should be practiced because overdoing exercise can further compromise the muscular system, increase pain,

and contribute to overwork and stress. Endurance programs, aerobic and aquatic exercise, and inpatient rehabilitation programs have been shown to be effective with MS patients. Multiple Sclerosis Society chapters often offer exercise groups.

The physician and the physical therapist should be consulted to help determine the best exercises for the individual, the appropriate intensity, and the duration of the workout. It is recommended that patients exercise in a safe environment, use grab bars to stabilize balance, and proceed slowly. MS patients in particular should avoid exercising during the heat of the day and should be aware of the outside temperature and their body temperature.

Patients with HD are also encouraged to maintain fitness as much as possible. Walking is recommended even if the patient's coordination is poor. Padding, assistive devices, and sturdy shoes can help prolong the ability to walk for as long as possible.

The following interventions are specific to patients with activity intolerance and impaired physical mobility (Figure 21-6):

- Assess sensory and motor status regularly.
- Ensure good pulmonary function.
- Perform range of motion frequently.
- Use assistive devices as needed to minimize fatigue and to prevent contractures.
- Assist with ambulation if possible.
- Teach and assist with therapeutic exercises.
- Teach ways to assist with mobility.
- Assess tremor if appropriate.
- Position properly.
- Administer medication to enhance motor function.
- Refer to physical and/or occupational therapist.

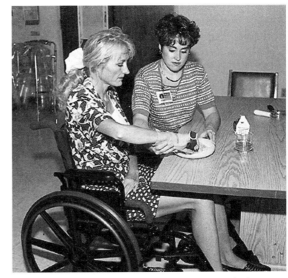

Figure 21-6 Patient participating in occupational therapy using mobile arm supports and upper extremity orthotics. (From Lewis, S. M., Collier, I. C., Heitkemper, M. M., & Dirksen, S. R. [2000]. *Medical-surgical nursing: Assessment and management of clinical problems* [5th ed.]. St. Louis, MO: Mosby.)

Communication

Difficulties with verbal communication provide another valid reason to refer to the speech pathologist. These specialists are trained to conduct thorough assessments of communication problems and to recommend and implement strategies to improve communication. Specific interventions for patients with impaired verbal communication follow:

- Provide opportunity for the patient to communicate without pressure.
- Instruct the patient to take deep breaths before speaking.
- Use assistive devices to enhance communication: flash cards, pictures, computer technology.
- Massage neck and facial muscles to enhance relaxation.
- Refer to the speech pathologist.

Psychosocial Issues

It is important that the nurse acknowledge to the patient that psychosocial issues may arise. The patient and family may be reluctant to voice concerns for fear that their feelings are unusual or unjustified. Patients and their significant others might benefit from speaking to the nurse in private and as a group. However, the nurse will find that a thorough assessment of the patient alone should occur initially because confidentiality is paramount. Some specific interventions for patients with psychosocial concerns follow:

- Provide information about the anticipated pattern of illness.
- Provide information about treatments as they become available and appropriate.
- Affirm patient's symptoms and concerns.
- Encourage patient and family to express concerns.
- Recruit community resources as appropriate.
- Recruit neighbors and congregation members to provide support.
- Recommend support groups and associations/societies.
- Provide pain relief.
- Provide interventions for sufficient rest.

Bowel and Bladder

Alterations in neurological function, dysphagia, altered nutrition, and decreased mobility contribute to bowel and bladder problems among patients with neuromuscular diseases. Behavioral techniques and medications can supplement interventions related to motor and sensory loss, reduced bulk in the diet, inadequate fluid intake, and decreased gastric motility. Interventions specific to bowel and bladder management follow.

Constipation

- Encourage mobility to increase peristalsis.
- Maintain adequate fluid intake.
- Provide high-fiber foods.
- Consider advising the patient to use Power Pudding (Neal, 1995).
- Administers tool softeners as ordered.
- Instruct patient and caregiver in regular bowel program.

Urinary Retention (MS)

- Administer medications as ordered.
- Teach patient/caregiver intermittent catheterization techniques.
- Use reflex stimulation as an alternative method.
- Maintain adequate fluid intake.
- Instruct patient/caregiver in signs/symptoms of urinary tract infection.

Urinary Incontinence

- Administer medications as ordered.
- Instruct patient/caregiver in prompted/timed voiding.
- Maintain fluid intake.
- Consider intermittent or continuous catheter urinary drainage.

Skin Integrity

Impaired mobility and altered nutrition, as well as a susceptibility to infection related to the disease process, interact to alter the integrity of the skin. Preventing pressure ulcers from developing is key because healing of wounds once they occur is also compromised by the aforementioned alterations in health status. Interventions related to the prevention and care of the skin follow:

- Inspect skin frequently for signs of breakdown.
- Position and turn patient frequently.
- Provide optimal nutritional (protein and fluids) intake.
- Keep skin clean and well moisturized.

Self-Care Deficit

A guiding principle of rehabilitation nursing is that patients will be taught and encouraged to participate to the best of their ability in self-care management. Often it is deemed easier by the caregiver to perform ADLs for the patient, and caregivers may not recognize that participation in self-care is therapeutic. Very debilitated patients can assist with self-care in some form even if their participation is limited to communicating choices about how someone else will perform their care.

Instruction of patients and caregivers and the use of assistive devices to maximize self-care ability are the key interventions. Assistive or adaptive devices such as special eating utensils, dicem, and plates with guards can significantly increase patients' abilities to feed themselves.

Rehabilitation nurses play a vital role in helping patients with chronic diseases and disabilities to adjust to their illnesses. Nurses can best assist these patients by complying with the following:

- Assess patient for psychological and adjustment problems.
- Encourage patients to express feelings.
- Do not make promises or give false assurances.
- Communicate empathy for the patient's feelings.
- Be aware of cultural differences in the way patients cope.
- Inform patients about the disability and the treatment.
- Encourage a positive body image.
- Encourage the use of role modeling and mentoring.
- Build a network of support.
- Promote the use of a variety of coping techniques.
- Guide toward seeking employment.
- Cultivate a positive and realistic outlook on life.

Sexual Dysfunction

Patients with sexual dysfunction frequently require the service of a trained sex counselor. It is best to provide the patient and significant other a safe and confidential environment in which to express their concerns, explain that these concerns are not unexpected in light of the patient's condition, and provide resources for seeking counseling. Special aids, pain medications, lubricants, and prosthetics may enhance comfort and confidence.

Caregiver Role Strain

The stress and strain on caregivers of patients with neuromuscular diseases is great. Permission giving allows the caregiver to express frustration and stress without guilt or fear of betrayal. Some caregivers may require professional counseling if stress is impairing their ability to provide safe care for the patient. Specific suggestions for obtaining rest and respite are most helpful to caregivers and include, but are not limited to, the following:

- Requesting the assistance of neighbors or members of the caregiver's congregation
- Hiring a companion or aide to sit with the patient for brief periods or care for the patient at night
- Reserving respite space at a local nursing home so the caregiver can take a vacation

Disease-Specific Interventions

In addition to the aforementioned interventions, Table 21-7 lists interventions and research specific to the neuromuscular diseases discussed in this chapter.

TABLE 21-7 Disease Specific Interventions: Current and Under Investigation

Clinical Diagnosis	Interventions
Guillain-Barré syndrome (Kuwabara, 2004)	• Immunomodulating treatments: plasma exchange, high-dose immunoglobulin • Supportive treatment: respiratory support, continuous monitoring of blood pressure and heart rate, prevention of deep venous thrombosis and pulmonary embolism, prevention of respiratory infection, pain control • Cerebrospinal fluid filtration; interferon-β; COX-2 inhibitors
Amyotrophic lateral sclerosis (Han et al., 2003)	• Baclofen, dantrolene or tizanidine for spasticity • Robinul or transdermal scopolamine for drying up secretions • Neurontin for neuropathic pain; fentanyl or morphine for pain • Glutamate antagonists in clinical trials • Myotrophin (insulin-like growth factor-I) in trials to enhance motor neuron survival • Topiramate in clinical trials to reduce glutamate • Calcium channel blockers in clinical trials
Myasthenia gravis (Adis International Limited, 2001; Armstrong & Schumann, 2003)	• Pyridostigmine • Azathioprine • Cyclosporine if azathioprine is contraindicated • Cyclophosphamide and mycophenolate in refractory cases • Plasmapheresis • Intravenous immunoglobulin • Thymectomy
Parkinson's disease (Hauser & Lyons, 2004)	• Levodopa • Carbidopa • Acetylcholinesterase inhibitors for dementia • Apomorphine as rescue therapy for "off" episodes • Rotigotine constant delivery system for consistent symptom control • Ropinirole controlled-release formula for consistent symptom control • Zydis selegiline to reduce "off" time • Rasagiline to improve motor fluctuations • Istradefylline to enhance symptom control without worsening dyskinesias • NS-2330 to block uptake of dopamine, serotonin, and norepinephrine
Multiple sclerosis (MS) (Hess & Hughes, 2005)	• Interferon beta 1-α (Avonex) for the treatment of relapsing forms of MS to slow disability • Interferon beta 1-β (Betaseron) for the treatment of relapsing forms of MS to reduce the frequency or exacerbations • Glatiramer acetate for the treatment of relapsing-remitting MS • Mitoxantrone for progressive forms of MS • Rebif • Tysabri

NOTE: Some of these drugs have not yet been approved by the Food and Drug Administration.

Pharmaceutical Management

According to the National Multiple Sclerosis Society (NMSS) (2002), there are several considerations when medicating patients with MS. These considerations appear to apply to all of the patients discussed in this chapter:

- Determine contraindications.
- Instruct patients in anticipated outcomes and adverse or side effects of drug therapy.
- Encourage patients to attend follow-up visits so that the effectiveness and tolerance of treatments can be evaluated.

Table 21-8 lists medications currently used to treat the neuromuscular diseases discussed in this chapter.

OUTCOMES

To achieve the desired outcomes for patients with neuromuscular disease, careful planning, appropriate intervention, and the continued involvement of all pertinent interdisciplinary team members are necessary. As the goals of care are set with the patient and/or caregiver and evaluated as realistic and

TABLE 21-8 Drugs Commonly Used to Manage Neuromuscular Diseases

Drug Class	Use	Chronic Condition
Corticosteroids	Treat exacerbations	Multiple sclerosis Myasthenia gravis
Immunomodulators	Treat exacerbations	Multiple sclerosis Myasthenia gravis
Cholinergics	Treat urinary retention	Multiple sclerosis
Anticholinergics	Treat urinary frequency Reduce tremor	Multiple sclerosis Parkinson's disease
Muscle relaxants	Reduce spasticity	Multiple sclerosis Spinal cord injury
Antispasmodics	Treat urinary retention	Multiple sclerosis Spinal cord injury
Dopaminergic agents	Treat bradykinesia, tremor, rigidity, maintain mean arterial pressure	Parkinson's disease Spinal cord injury
Antihistamines	Treat tremor, rigidity	Parkinson's disease
MAO inhibitors	Treat bradykinesia, tremor, rigidity	Parkinson's disease
Anticholinesterase agents	Prolong action of acetylcholine	Myasthenia gravis
Antipsychotics, antichorea agents	Reduce psychosis, chorea	Huntington's disease
Antidepressants	Reduce depression	Amyotrophic lateral sclerosis Guillain-Barré syndrome Huntington's disease Myasthenia gravis Multiple sclerosis Parkinson's disease Spinal cord injury
Methylprednisolone	Improve blood flow, reduce edema	Spinal cord injury
Catechol O-methyltransferase (COMT)	Inhibit breakdown of levodopa	Parkinson's disease
Antioxidants	Slow disease progression	Parkinson's disease
Methotrexate	Provide immunosuppression	Multiple sclerosis
T-cell receptor peptides	Inhibit immune system attack	Multiple sclerosis
Monoclonal antibodies	Suppress abnormal immune response	Multiple sclerosis
Stool softeners	Prevent constipation	Amyotrophic lateral sclerosis Guillain-Barré syndrome Huntington's disease Myasthenia gravis Multiple sclerosis Parkinson's disease Spinal cord injury
β-Agonist/γ-aminobutyric acid (GABA) antagonist	Treat spasticity	Multiple sclerosis
Riluzole (Rilutek)	Reduce release of glutamate from cells	Amyotrophic lateral sclerosis
G_{M1} ganglioside	Increase functional recovery	Spinal cord injury

Modified from Neal, L. J., & Guillett, S. E. (Eds.). (2004). *Care of the adult with a chronic illness or disability: A team approach.* St. Louis, MO: Mosby.
MAO, Monoamine oxidase.

attainable by all involved, outcomes should reflect successful achievement of these goals. It is difficult to predict outcomes related to a population of patients. It is preferable to design goals and measure outcomes on the basis of the individual's clinical presentation and disease process. Table 21-6 lists the desired outcomes for the goals and interventions that have been discussed in this chapter.

EVALUATION

The outcomes listed in Table 21-6 are ideal. As stated earlier, the patient, caregiver, and interdisciplinary team design goals that are realistic for the patient in the context of his or her environment and resources. Satisfactory achievement of these goals as outlined and agreed on by the team constitutes a successful outcome. Ongoing modification of the plan and the goals is necessary so that efforts to accomplish goals remain realistic.

SUMMARY

During early stages of disease, many patients will be able to continue work and their normal activities. All patients with neuromuscular disease need to plan for the long term. The ability to work, attend school, participate in the community, and be independent will depend largely on the patient's motivation and emotional resources; support system, both professional and nonprofessional; and adaptive and assistive equipment. Many persons with disabilities currently remain in work settings that are adapted to meet their needs. Others work from home. However, the ability to continue these activities changes as the patient's condition deteriorates.

Care planning must be ongoing, and goals and interventions must be modified as the patient's status changes. Goals and desired outcomes should remain realistic to avoid frustration and hopelessness.

The prevalence of neuromuscular disease has implications for research because recent studies indicate correlations with climatic conditions, geographical regions, sex, and genetics. Clinical research that investigates the relationships between and among these variables will certainly impact prevention, treatment, and recovery. Research that explores the quality of life of patients and caregivers may help persons cope with and better understand these diseases and how to adapt to them. Studies of various interventions and their effects will undoubtedly contribute to improved outcomes and may influence increased length of life after diagnosis. Pharmacological research studies continue to result in improved medications to help persons manage symptoms and prevent complications. Much work remains to be done toward eventual eradication of these diseases or at least improved management of them. Rehabilitation nurses are in a unique position to participate as principal investigators and as members of research teams to explore the possibilities.

Case Study

Mr. Jenkins is a 75-year-old man diagnosed with Parkinson's disease 24 years ago. When he was no longer able to operate his watch repair shop because of his hand tremors, he and his wife sold the business and lived on business profits, payments from a preexisting disability insurance policy, and their investments. Within 2 years he developed increased tremors of the hands and tongue, "pill rolling" with his fingers, and a shuffling gait. He refused medication, embarking instead on his own regimen of nutrition; vitamins; herbal remedies; and a tonic of honey, water, and cider vinegar. Always self-disciplined, he performed daily exercise. His wife prepared his diet and joined him in activities to "keep mentally alert." Although he had difficulty walking and experienced slurred speech, little changed for 6 more years. The Jenkinses traveled and met with friends, and Mr. Jenkins continued to drive their car.

At 62 years of age, Mr. Jenkins began levodopa concurrent with his own regimen. Mr. Jenkins used a cane, a wheelchair, or an Amigo cart in public. The Jenkinses moved to a one-level ranch-style house accessible for Mr. Jenkins' wheelchair; he walked "on good days." After his urinary frequency, difficulty turning in bed, and nightmares began interrupting sleep for both Mr. and Mrs. Jenkins, he slept in a separate bedroom. Larger and more frequent doses of levodopa did not control periods of bradykinesia, cogwheeling, and rigidity. "Freezing," which impaired self-care with ADLs and drooling caused him

embarrassment and anxiety. He contacted a physician who would prescribe anti-PD drugs in combinations and newly released medications.

At 70 years of age Mr. Jenkins took a "drug holiday," a decision not supported by his wife or physician, both of whom described Mr. Jenkins as "demanding and stubborn" concerning his health regimen. He was rushed to the hospital after experiencing dyskinesia, hypotension, pain, confusion, nausea, and incontinence. Mrs. Jenkins was depressed and anxious about how she would continue to care for him. He returned home unable to perform bathing or dressing but able to walk "on good days." Although he could feed himself, everything was slowed, including his speech. His overall health status was excellent, except for dental care needs because he had not visited a dentist for 15 years. He played games for stimulation, but fewer friends came to visit, and Mrs. Jenkins became his main contact. Ironically Mr. Jenkins drove the car to his biweekly physical therapy sessions.

Mrs. Jenkins continued care for her husband until he fell during the night several times. Unable to assist him off the floor, she called 911 for help. The Jenkinses refused visiting nurse services as "charity care," so Mrs. Jenkins hired the first of three "helpers" who were to assist Mr. Jenkins with his personal care, meals, and exercises 3 times a week. When the third helper left, Mrs. Jenkins, who had experienced a mild stroke earlier the same year, decided that her husband should move to a nursing home. Their long-term care policy covered

Continued

Case Study—cont'd

most costs. Mrs. Jenkins would visit regularly, and Mr. Jenkins would receive therapy, medical supervision, and assistance with ADLs. Reluctantly Mr. Jenkins agreed to a trial stay in the nursing home, provided he came home on Saturdays.

After a month at the nursing home, Mr. Jenkins was functioning at a higher level: walking more, sleeping through the night, and experiencing fewer speech problems. Mrs. Jenkins began to attend local social activities and rejoined her bridge and garden clubs. Mr. Jenkins came home on Saturdays but increasingly objected to returning to the nursing home on Saturday nights. He began to complain about the nursing home food and being lonely for his own home. When Mrs. Jenkins stated she could not take care of him at home, he accused

her of "putting him away." However, both Mr. and Mrs. Jenkins are reluctant to have help in the home, especially live-in help. They state they want privacy and are fearful and distrustful of outsiders.

Recently, at age 75, Mr. Jenkins informed his wife that he was coming home. He arranged a driving assessment and planned to resume driving. Although he had difficulty with ambulation, he insisted that the reflexes required for driving were intact. Mrs. Jenkins sought advice from a cousin whose husband lived at home after a stroke and as a result hired an independent rehabilitation nurse as case manager. Eventually the Jenkinses worked with the nurse to write a health contract identifying their goals and responsibilities based on the following nursing diagnoses and process.

TABLE 21-9 Nursing Diagnoses, Interventions, and Outcomes Applicable to Mr. Jenkins **NIC/NOC**

Nursing Diagnosis	Assessment	Nursing Interventions	Nursing Outcomes
Ineffective coping due to denial and anger	Inability to adjust to changes; unrealistic expectations from self and others; lack of control over disease process; lack of problem solving; fear of abandonment by spouse	Write health contract, elicit Mr. Jenkins' perception and appraisal, then institute reframing and decision-making techniques; discuss methods for coping with loss and change; remove barriers to self-care; evaluate marriage relationship	Adherence to written contract, empowerment for decision making, and improved interpersonal relationships
Deficient knowledge	Stress from rejection or denial of disease process and drug therapy; lack of acknowledgement of wife's health condition	Empower patient by educating about disease trajectory; inform of local PD support groups; educate regarding wife's health condition; educate about medications and drug holidays, assistive devices, speech therapy, and relaxation techniques	Revise regimen; recognize wife's role and responsibilities; use assistive devices and techniques to reduce stressors; verbally describe treatment program (see Chapter 5 for discussion of education and teaching)
Caregiver role strain; potential for breakdown of trust in the marriage relationship	Caregiver has history of stroke, restricted socialization, primary responsibility for patient's care and safety	Arrange respite care when Mr. Jenkins returns home; educate about services and support groups; teach relaxation techniques and interpersonal skills; ensure safety in home; inform community emergency services; evaluate relationship	Reduced stress from daily responsibilities; resumption of club activities; use of personal relaxation techniques; monitoring of health status
Ineffective health maintenence (dental)	Regular checkups and overall excellent health status apart from signs and symptoms of PD, except for dental caries, reddened gums with bleeding, chipped teeth, and malocclusion resulting in damage to lips and oral mucosa	Provide information about dentist skilled in working with patients who have conditions such as PD	Dental appointments for preventive and restorative care
Impaired urinary elimination; frequency, incontinence	(See Chapter 18 for discussion of bladder elimination)		

Case Study—cont'd

Table 21-9 Nursing Diagnoses, Interventions, and Outcomes Applicable to Mr. Jenkins—cont'd

NIC/NOC

Nursing Diagnosis	Assessment	Nursing Interventions Classification (NIC)	Nursing Outcomes Classification (NOC)
Impaired physical mobility; risk for impaired skin integrity	Reduced ability to initiate movements voluntarily or to move from bed to chair or commode; rigidity, tremor bradykinesia, cogwheeling, "pill rolling," and shuffling gait; potential for injury, falls, damage to skin	Teach ROM exercises; teach exercises specific for coping with immobility due to PD (e.g., position "nose over toes" to rise from chair, stepping over imaginary mark to initiate walking, or rocking side to side to move legs); evaluate need for special mattress and trapeze bar in bed; observe for edema; consider occupational and/or physical therapy consultations for ambulation, fine motor movements (see Chapter 20 for discussion of mobility)	Prevent complications or further immobility; maximize comfort and sense of control; adherence to regimen
Insomnia; safety issues	Inability to sleep through the night; nightmares, falls	Negotiate use of side rails or other devices, bedside urinal; relaxation and ROM before bedtime; medications as ordered	Establish rest and sleep patterns with minimal interruptions (refer to Chapter 26 for discussion of sleep and rest)
Social isolation; potential for reduced satisfaction with quality of life	Physical, social, and spiritual isolation; reduced stimulation and access to information or contact with others; caregiver has responsibility for all interactions	Institute community programs such as day care centers, senior center, van transportation, attendant services, church programs, Meals on Wheels, partners for "thinking games," support groups, exercise or therapy programs; respite for wife; obtain realistic evaluation of ability to drive	Encourage maximum stimulation and independence in social interaction; reduced stressors in marriage relationship; improved quality of life

Data from Moorhead, S., Johnson, M., & Maas, M. (Eds.). (2004). *Nursing outcomes classification (NOC)* (3rd ed.). St. Louis, MO: Mosby; Dochterman, J. M., & Bulechek, G. M. (2004). *Nursing interventions classification (NIC)* (4th ed.). St. Louis, MO: Mosby; and NANDA International. (2005). *Nursing diagnoses: Definitions and classification, 2005-2006* (6th ed.). Philadelphia: Author.

Other problems for nursing diagnosis and process related to neuromuscular diseases include (1) Impaired verbal communication, slurred speech; (2) self-care deficit, ADLs; (3) threats to community reentry, driving, refusing attendant services; (4) potential for altered nutritional status, family dysfunction, financial problems, and chronic condition for caregiver; (5) disturbed body image; (6) risk for social isolation; (7) insomnia; (8) ineffective role performance.

ADLs, Activities of daily living; *PD,* parkinson's disease; *ROM,* range of motion.

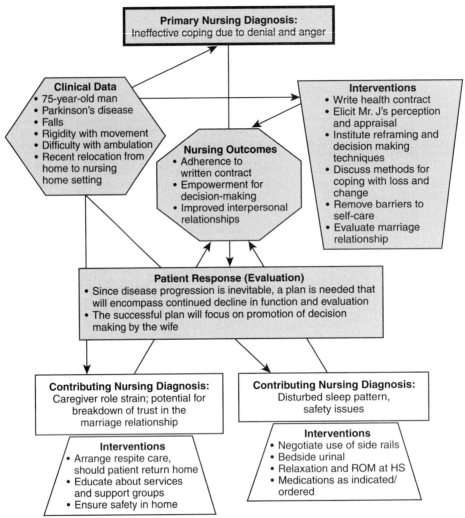

Concept Map. Mr. Jenkin's primary problem related to the progression of Parkinson's disease is that of ineffective coping due to denial and anger. Although it may be unrealistic to change his denial, perhaps related to Lewy body dementia associated with Parkinson's, the rehabilitation nurse will focus on safety and interpersonal relationships. Interventions targeted to ensuring continued support for the patient and his wife, while promoting choice and independence, are essential.

CRITICAL THINKING QUESTIONS

1. How should the nurse prioritize care for Mr. Jenkins and his wife?
2. What recommendations should the nurse make regarding environmental issues related to Mr. Jenkins' disease?
3. What should the nurse advise patients regarding the use of herbal and over-the-counter remedies?

WEBSITE RESOURCES

Amyotrophic lateral sclerosis: www.lougehrigsdisease.net.
Huntington's disease: www.hdsa.org.
Multiple sclerosis: www.nmss.org.
Myasthenia gravis: www.myasthenia.org.
Parkinson's disease: www.pdf.org.
Spinal cord injury: www.aascin.org, www.alsa.org, and www.fscip.org.

REFERENCES

Adis International Limited. (2001). Treatment alternatives in the successful management of myasthenia gravis. *Drugs & Therapy Perspectives: For National Drug Selection and Use, 17*(21), 12-15.

Armstrong, S. M., & Schumann, L. (2003). Myasthenia gravis: Diagnosis and treatment. *Journal of the American Academy of Nurse Practitioners, 15*(2), 72-78.

Aubeeluck, A. (2005). Caring for the carers: Quality of life in Huntington's disease. *British Journal of Nursing, 14*(8), 452-454.

Bradbury, J. (2003). New clue found to amyotrophic lateral sclerosis. *The Lancet, 362,* 136.

Dochterman, J. M., & Bulechek, G. M. (2004). *Nursing interventions classification (NIC)* (4th ed.). St. Louis, MO: Mosby.

Gulick, E. E. (1998). Symptom and activities of daily living trajectory in multiple sclerosis: A 10-year study. *Nursing Research, 47*(3), 137-146.

Han, J. J., Carter, G. T., Hecht, T. W., Schuman, N. E., Weiss, M. D., & Krivickas, L. S. (2003). The amyotrophic lateral sclerosis center: A model of multidisciplinary management. *Critical Reviews in Physical and Rehabilitation Medicine, 15*(1), 21-40.

Hardmeier, M., Wagrupfeil, S., Freitag, P., et al. (2003). Atrophy is detectable within 3-months period in untreated patients with active relapsing remitting multiple sclerosis. *Archives of Neurology, 60*, 1736-1739.

Hauser, R. A., & Lyons, K. E. (2004). Future therapies for Parkinson's disease. *Neurological Clinics, 22*(3 Suppl.), S149-S166.

Hess, D. C, & Hughes, M. D. (2005, September 1). Multiple sclerosis: New help, new hope. *Consultant*, 1144-1148.

Imke, S. (2000). Parkinson's: A medical management update. *The Parkinson Report, 19*(3), 1-7.

Kalb, R. (Ed.). (2004). *Multiple sclerosis: The nursing perspective*. New York: National Multiple Sclerosis Society.

Kuwabara, S. (2004). Guillain-Barré syndrome. *Drugs, 64*(6), 597-610.

Lublin, F. D., & Reingold, S. C. (1996). Defining the clinical course of multiple sclerosis: Results of an international survey. *Neurology, 46*, 907-911.

McCance, K. L., & Huether, S. E. (Eds.). (2006). *Pathophysiology: The biologic basis for disease in adults and children*, (4th ed.). St. Louis, MO: Mosby.

Moorhead, S., Johnson, M., & Maas, M. (Eds.). (2004). *Nursing outcomes classification (NOC)* (3rd ed.). St. Louis, MO: Mosby.

Myasthenia Gravis Foundation of America. (2007). What is myasthenia gravis? Available at http://www.myasthenia.org/amg_whatismg.cfm.

NANDA International. (2005). *Nursing diagnoses: Definitions and classification, 2005-2006* (6th ed.). Philadelphia: Author.

National Multiple Sclerosis Society. (2004). Multiple sclerosis: Definition and much more. Available at http://www.answers.com/topic/multiplesclerosis.

National Institute of Neurological Disorders and Stroke (2004). Parkinson's disease: challenges, progress, and promise, Available at http://www.NINDS.nih.gov/disorders/parkinsons_disease.htm.

Neal, L. J. (1995). Power pudding: Natural laxative therapy to the elderly who are homebound. *Home Healthcare Nurse, 13*(3), 66-71.

Neal, L. J. (1997). Is anybody home? *Home Healthcare Nurse, 15*(3), 158-167.

Neal, L. J. (2002). Rehabilitation in the home. In I. M. Martinson, A. G. Widmer, & C. J. Portillo (Eds.), *Home health care nursing* (2nd ed., pp. 127-139). Philadelphia: W. B. Saunders.

Neal, L. J. (2004). Neuromuscular disorders. In L. J. Neal & S. E. Guillett (Eds.), *Care of the adult with a chronic illness or disability: A team approach* (pp. 378-392). St. Louis, MO: Mosby.

Peterson, J. W., Bö, L., Mörk, S., Chang, A., & Trapp, B. D. (2001). Transected neuritis, apoptotic neurons, and reduced inflammation in cortical multiple sclerosis lesions. *Annals of Neurology, 50*, 389-400.

Pritchard, J., & Hughes, R. A. (2004). Guillain-Barré syndrome. *The Lancet, 363*, 2186-2188.

Stuifbergen, A. K., & Rogers, S. (1997). The experience of fatigue and strategies of self-care among persons with multiple sclerosis. *Applied Nursing Research, 10*(1), 2-10.

U.S. Department of Health and Human Services. (2000). *Healthy People 2010*. Available at http://www.health.gov/healthypeople.

22

Patient and Family Coping

Julie Pryor, RN, RM, BA, MN, PhD

Coping is central to the experience of being human. It is a process that is entered into in response to the everyday experiences of individuals striving to maximize their quality of life and satisfaction with life. When wellness required for optimal quality of life is disrupted by an episode of illness, the immediate effects and the life consequences are central to nursing.

A rehabilitation nurse who would optimize health processes and outcomes for patients and families must understand the body of knowledge related to coping. This chapter introduces concepts and theories relating to how patients and their families cope, especially with interruptions in health. These theories are applied to rehabilitation nursing practice by relating the nursing process to the coping–stress-tolerance functional health pattern with the aim of developing an understanding of how nurses can support individuals to cope effectively.

CONCEPTS AND THEORIES

Foundation Concepts

Several concepts are foundational to understanding how persons cope with interruptions in health. These are listed in Box 22-1 and discussed in this section.

Biography. Like all other life experiences, the experience of disability and rehabilitation is best understood as part of the flow of a person's life story or biography rather than a biographical disruption (Faircloth, Boylstein, Rittman, Young, & Gubrium, 2004). Ville (2005) explains coping as the biographical work a person does in response to an interruption to one's well-being, personal integrity, or comfort. Survivors of hematological malignancies reported this work as "a secular spiritual journey" (McGrath, 2004).

Wellness. Wellness is "a state of harmony, energy, positive productivity, and well-being in an individual's mind, body, emotions and spirit" (Jones & Kilpatrick, 1996). Wellness is about person-in-environment functioning, including relationships with family, the community, society as a whole, and the physical environment. Although illness can disrupt wellness, even persons who have a chronic, disabling, or developmental disorder can achieve wellness (Zemper, et al., 2003).

Personal Integrity. Personal integrity is a sense of being whole and having control over one's life. It is "characterized by feelings of effectiveness and [of] connectedness" to others (Leidy & Haase, 1999) and is synonymous with wisdom, ability, will, and courage (Hornsten, Norberg, & Lundman, 2002). Persons actively strive to maintain personal integrity in the face of acute and chronic illness (Morse, 1997).

Comfort. Comfort is the state of having met basic human needs for ease ("a state of calm or contentment"), relief ("the experience of a patient who has had a specific need met"), and transcendence ("the state in which one rises above problem or pain") (Kolcaba, 1991). Comfort, however, is always relative. "Comfort has no meaning without discomfort, nor comfortable without uncomfortable" (Morse, Bottorff, & Hutchinson, 1995). There are physical, social, psychospiritual, and environmental contexts of patient comfort (Dowd, Kilcaba, & Steiner, 2006); it can be given and received. Kolcaba (1995) concludes, "comfort is holistic, complex, individualized, dynamic, immediate, and measurable."

Vulnerability. Vulnerability means being susceptible to hurt, harm, or injury (Irurita, 2000). When vulnerable, persons are less able to preserve their personal integrity. This is especially true for many persons who are hospitalized or disabled. For example, in a study by Hagren, Petersen, Severinsson, Lutzen, and Clyne (2005), hemodialysis patients (n = 41) reported feeling vulnerable as a consequence of the disease and their dependence upon others.

Stress. Our understanding of stress began with the physical body (Cannon, 1914, 1935; Selye, 1976) but is now related to the total person. Lazarus and Folkman (1984) were instrumental in extending the concept of stress, taking into account the roles of personal characteristics and the environment in creating a stressful situation. "Psychological stress is neither

---

BOX 22-1 Foundation Concepts

- Biography
- Wellness
- Personal integrity
- Comfort
- Vulnerability
- Stress
- Enduring and suffering
- Chronic sorrow
- Transition

BOX 22-2 Unbearable Aspects of Illness

Intrapersonal
- Pain for which the person is unprepared or that is unanticipated, unexplained, or irretractable
- Physical damage associated with a loss of former self
- Recurrence of symptoms after cure is believed to have happened
- Loss of function and dependency
- Loss of control
- Isolation
- Confronting reality
- Uncertainty

Interpersonal
- Not believed or listened to by caregivers
- Being treated as an object
- Being made to feel a burden
- Caregiver insensitivity
- Disregard from significant others
- Burdening significant others
- Causing grief to significant others

Data from Dewar, A. L., & Morse, J. M. (1995). Unbearable incidents: Failure to endure the experience of illness. *Journal of Advanced Nursing, 22,* 957-964.

---

solely in the environment itself nor just the result of personality characteristics, but depends on a particular kind of person-environment relationship" (Lazarus, 1999). Lazarus distinguishes three types of psychological stress: harm/loss, threat, and challenge. Harm/loss relates to something that has already happened; threat relates to harm or loss that is yet to happen; and challenge relates to difficulties that can be overcome.

Stressors associated with life events are discrete, observable events followed by a well-defined set of subevents and an end point. Chronic stressors may start slowly, continue, and be open ended. Forms of chronic stress include threats, demands, structural constraints, complexity, uncertainty, conflict, restriction of choice, underreward, and resource deprivation (Wheaton, 1997).

Enduring and Suffering.

Enduring and suffering exist on a continuum in the response to illness or injury but differ in nature and purpose. Enduring is about holding on: "It is a condition in which the individual expends extraordinary amounts of energy 'holding oneself together.' When enduring, the individual is relatively devoid of emotion [and] is focused on the immediate present" (Dewar & Morse, 1995). Individuals usually do not have a choice about the situations they have to endure (Morse & Carter, 1995) (Box 22-2).

Suffering, on the other hand, "refers to the emotional response to the loss. Suffering requires reflection, a looking back, an evaluation of the immensity of loss. Suffering is work, an all-consuming endeavor that one must experience to work through the event" (Morse & Carter, 1995). For example, in a study by Lohne and Severinsson (2005) patients (n = 10) reported suffering as feelings of loneliness, impatience, disappointment, bitterness, and dependency during the first year following spinal cord injury.

Chronic Sorrow.

Chronic sorrow, a concept developed by Olshansky (1966) while counseling families with mentally retarded children, refers to recurrent sorrow for the potential person. It is a loss that is continually redefined as new situations arise and is a trigger for sadness across the life span (Hobdell, 2004). Persons with chronic conditions and their caregivers, as well as the elderly, may experience chronic sorrow.

Transition.

Transition refers to movement or change from one state of being to another. The three distinct phases are separating from the previously known (endings), being neither part of the old nor the new (neutral zone), and becoming accepted as a new status (new beginnings) (O'Connor, 2004). Transitions are experienced throughout life, but they are especially challenging when associated with acquired disability. Attitudinal resources needed for successful transitions include "the sense of determination, inner strength, belief in the self, energy and focus" (Harms, 2004). Kralik (2002) found midlife women with chronic conditions to transition through cyclical periods of ordinariness and extraordinariness in response to changes in their conditions.

How Persons Cope

Coping is defined as "constantly changing cognitive and behavioral efforts to manage specific external and/or internal demands that are appraised as taxing or exceeding the resources of the person" (Lazarus & Folkman, 1984). Coping is a process, with an emphasis being placed on *efforts to manage* rather than *outcomes and mastery* (Lazarus & Folkman, 1984), and "coping is a powerful mediator of the emotional outcome of a stressful encounter" (Lazarus, 1999).

Psychological stress cannot be adequately explained by simply focusing on either the nature or the relative size of the stimulus or stressor or on the characteristics that make one person more vulnerable than another to a particular stimulus. The cognitive appraisal process—"the meaning constructed by a person about what is happening" (Lazarus, 1999)—differs among persons and groups. To understand variations "we must take into account the cognitive processes that intervene

---

BOX 22-3 Types of Cognitive Appraisal

Primary Appraisal
- Judgment of an encounter as irrelevant, benign-positive, or stressful
- Stressful appraisals may pose harm/loss, threat, challenge, or benefit
  - Harm/loss refers to damage already sustained
  - Threat refers to anticipated losses or harms
  - Challenges are events that are possible to master
  - Benefit may be gained from the encounter

Secondary Appraisal
- Judgment of what might and can be done
- Considers options and evaluates the consequences of each option

Reappraisal
- A changed appraisal in response to new information

Data from Lazarus, R. S., & Folkman, S. (1984). *Stress, appraisal, and coping.* New York: Springer; and Lazarus, R. (1999). *Stress and emotion: A new synthesis.* New York: Springer.

BOX 22-4 Environmental Variables

Demands
- Pressure to behave a certain way
- Pressure to possess socially correct attitudes

Constraints
- Pressure not to do certain things
- May be associated with punishment

Opportunity
- Arises from fortunate timing
- May depend on wisdom to see the opportunity

Culture
- Cultural differences have potential to affect stress, coping, and emotion in individuals
- Reality of multiethnic and multicultural societies challenges previous generalizations about culture

Data from Lazarus, R. (1999). *Stress and emotion: A new synthesis.* New York: Springer.

---

between the encounter and the reaction, and the factors that affect the nature of this mediation."

Lazarus and Folkman (1984) described three types of cognitive appraisal: primary, secondary, and reappraisal. In later work Lazarus (1999) added gaining a benefit from the encounter as another dimension to primary appraisal. The nature of each type of cognitive appraisal is outlined in Box 22-3.

Appraising is an active process that can be accomplished by deliberate and largely conscious or intuitive, automatic, and unconscious evaluating "whether or not what is happening is relevant to one's values, beliefs about self and world, and situational intentions" (Lazarus, 1999). Goal commitment, the strongest influence, "implies that a person will strive hard to attain the goal, despite discouragement or adversity."

Acknowledging that appraisal takes place within a context, Lazarus (1999) discusses environmental and personal variables that will influence a person's reaction through the appraisal process. Environmental variables consist of demands, constraints, opportunity, and culture (Box 22-4). The personal variables are goal and goal hierarchies, beliefs about self and the world, and personal resources (Box 22-5).

The process of coping described by Lazarus and Folkman (1984) has three main features: observation and assessment of what the person actually thinks or does, examination of the context, and coping as a process that shifts as the relationship of the person to his or her environment changes. These changes trigger reappraisal and subsequent coping efforts. Lazarus (1999) notes that *no universally effective or ineffective coping strategy exists,* and the study of what the person thinks and does at each stage of the coping process must also include examination of the context in which it takes place.

BOX 22-5 Personal Variables

Goals and Goal Hierarchies
- Goals provide motivation
- Emotions result from evaluation of the fate of one's goals
- Relative value of the goal and the probability and cost of attainment determine choice of goal and emotions

Beliefs About Self and World
- Shape our expectations about what might happen and what we hope for

Personal Resources
- Include intelligence, money, social skills, education, supportive family and friends, physical attractiveness, health and energy, and optimism

Data from Lazarus, R. (1999). *Stress and emotion: A new synthesis.* New York: Springer.

The function of coping is related to the purpose of a particular strategy. Thus emotion-focused coping aims to reduce the emotional distress, or conversely, to temporarily increase emotional distress for a particular purpose. Examples of emotion-focused coping are cognitive reappraisal of the situation to be less significant, selective attention or avoidance, and distraction. Self-deception is a potential risk associated with this type of coping (Lazarus & Folkman, 1984).

Problem-focused forms of coping are similar to, but broader than, strategies used for problem solving. They are "often directed at defining the problem, generating alternative solutions, weighing the alternatives in terms of their costs and benefits, choosing among them, and acting" (Lazarus & Folkman, 1984). Problem-focused forms may be directed

---

BOX 22-6 Ways of Coping

- Confrontive coping
- Distancing
- Self-controlling
- Seeking social support
- Accepting responsibility
- Escape-avoidance
- Planful problem solving
- Positive reappraisal

Data from Folkman, S., & Lazarus, R. (1988). *Ways of coping questionnaire, sampler set manual, test booklet, scoring key.* Palo Alto, CA: Mind Garden.

---

at the self as well as the environment and may occur with emotion-focused coping. Box 22-6 lists the ways of coping identified by Folkman and Lazarus (1988).

Despite many claims that emotion-focused strategies, in particular avoidance, are not effective (for example, Lowit & van Teijlingen, 2005), Austenfeld and Stanton (2004) draw attention to Lazarus and Folkman's claim (1984) that "both sets of coping strategies have adaptive potential." They also put forward a convincing argument for greater recognition of the role of emotions in effective coping.

Meaning-Making as Coping. Persons seek to maintain a sense that life is meaningful (Thompson, 1991). When meaning is lost, it may be a source of stress. The work of Park and Folkman (1997) highlights the importance of reappraisal, which follows primary and secondary appraisal.

Building on an understanding of meaning as a perception of significance, Park and Folkman (1997) explain two types of meaning—global and situational. "Global meaning encompasses a person's enduring beliefs and valued goals." Situational meaning "is formed in the interaction between a person's global meaning and the circumstances of the particular person-environment transaction."

Global meaning includes beliefs about order, as well as the person's life goals and purpose. The notion of order includes beliefs about the world, beliefs about self, and beliefs about the self in the world. Global meaning is built through experiences across the person's life span and is reported as possessing three attributes: stability, optimistic bias, and personal relevance.

Situational meaning is reported as having three major components (Park & Folkman, 1997): appraisal of meaning, search for meaning, and meaning as outcome. These are explained in Box 22-7.

Situational meaning, the search for meaning, and meaning as outcome were common themes in Folkman's (1997) longitudinal study of caregivers of partners who are dying, with 99.5% of the 1794 persons interviewed reporting positive meaningful events during their experiences of caregiving or bereavement. On the basis of these findings,

---

BOX 22-7 Situational Meaning

Appraisal of Meaning
- Primary appraisal
- Secondary appraisal
- Comparison of appraised meaning with global meaning

Search for Meaning
- Reappraisal of meaning
- Functions of reappraisal
  - To transform the appraised meaning
  - To modify the appraised meaning
  - To modify relevant beliefs and goals
  - To decrease threat of the event
- Changing appraised meaning
  - Changing appraised meaning of attributes (e.g., reasons why it happened, why it happened to me, responsibility)
  - Perception of benefits
- Changing global meaning
  - Revising beliefs
  - Revising goals

Meaning as Outcome
- Enduring changes in global meaning (e.g., changes in philosophical or religious beliefs)
- Personal growth
- Not all meaning-related outcomes are positive

Data from Park, C. L., & Folkman, S. (1997). Meaning in the context of stress and coping. *Review of General Psychology, 1*(2), 115-144.

Folkman (1997) supported an alternative outcome of coping (i.e., positive emotion).

Stress, Appraisal, and Emotions. Stress, emotion, and coping form one conceptual unit: when there is stress, there is emotion (Lazarus, 1999). Folkman's model (1997) demonstrates that emotions flow from our appraisal of what is happening. Our evaluation of what is happening (based on what is known, competing goals, and hierarchy of goals) determines our emotional reaction to it.

Thus it is extremely difficult to understand others' evaluation of a situation or event. Their response may appear irrational to others, but rational for that person based on what is known or able to be known. Lazarus (1999) attributes failure of reason to four common causes of erroneous judgments:
- Having a disorder that involves damage to the brain
- Lacking knowledge
- Not paying attention to the right things
- Experiencing denial

Lazarus (1999) proposes a cognitive-motivational-relational theory of emotions as a propositional understanding of how emotions work, listing 15 emotions (Box 22-8), each with a different appraisal process and a core relational theme. For example, the core relational theme for anger is "a demeaning offence against me and mine" (Lazarus, 1991).

BOX 22-8 Emotions

- Anger
- Anxiety
- Fright
- Guilt
- Shame
- Sadness
- Envy
- Jealousy
- Disgust
- Happiness
- Pride
- Relief
- Hope
- Love
- Compassion

Data from Lazarus, R. (1991). *Emotion and adaptation.* New York: Oxford University Press.

BOX 22-9 Factors Influencing the Coping Process

- Sense of coherence
- Self-efficacy
- Locus of control
- Hardiness
- Learned resourcefulness
- Optimism
- Hope
- Uncertainty
- Social support
- Age
- Gender
- Education
- Ethnicity
- Comorbidities
- Time since injury or onset of illness

Factors Influencing the Coping Process

Some persons cope better than others. Both personal and environmental factors influence appraisal of an event or situation and the response to that appraisal.

With a chronic, disabling, or developmental disorder, the physical, social, temporal, and economic environment in which the event takes place influence how the person and others associated with the person are affected, either directly or through the consequences of the event. According to Livneh and Antonak (1997), there are four classes of variables associated with psychosocial adaptation:

Class 1: Variables associated with the disability itself
Class 2: Variables associated with sociodemographic characteristics of the individual
Class 3: Variables associated with personality attributes of the individual
Class 4: Variables associated with characteristics of the physical and social environment

These classes fit with the World Health Organization's understanding (2001) of a person's functioning and disability being the result of interaction between a health condition and personal and environmental factors. Box 22-9 summarizes the factors influencing the coping process discussed in this section.

The closeness of the relationship between many of these characteristics and spirituality is highlighted in recent work by Villagomeza (2005), who situates "inner strength and energy" as one of "seven constructs of a person's sense of spirituality."

Sense of Coherence. Sense of coherence (SOC), the core concept of Antonovsky's (1972, 1979) salutogenic model of health, refers to "a generalized orientation towards the world which perceives it, on a continuum, as comprehensible, manageable and meaningful" (Antonovsky, 1996). This concept is not about being in control; it is perceptual, having both cognitive and affective components. Antonovsky (1979) outlines psychological, social-structural, and cultural-historical sources of SOC.

When confronted with a stressor, the person with a strong SOC will (1) wish to or be motivated to cope (meaningfulness), (2) believe that the challenge is understood (comprehensibility),

and (3) believe that resources to cope are available (manageability) (Antonovsky, 1996).

Life experiences shape SOC, and as a concept SOC is gaining international interest. The relevance of SOC for rehabilitation nursing practice has been demonstrated in several studies. For example, Berglund, Mattiasson, and Nordstrom (2003) found that higher SOC was associated with greater acceptance of disability and better functional status in 18- to 70-year-olds (n = 77) with Ehlers-Danlos syndrome. Conversely, low SOC has been associated with higher burnout in family caregivers of adults with stroke (Nilsson, Axelsson, Gustafson, Lundman, & Norberg, 2001) and dementia sufferers (Andren & Elmstahl, 2005).

Self-Efficacy. Self-efficacy refers to "beliefs in one's capabilities to organize and execute the course of action required to produce given attainments" (Bandura, 1997). It differs from self-concept and self-esteem in that *self-concept* is a composite view of self and *self-esteem* relates to self-worth. Self-concept is the cognitive view of self, self-esteem is the affective view (Seigley, 1999).

Self-efficacy is a major basis for action. Persons who believe they are capable of effective coping with particular situations or stressors have a sense of control; the reverse is also true. The beliefs of a group about their shared capabilities for action (Bandura's collective efficacy [1997]) is applicable to family units.

A central aspect of rehabilitation nursing is to promote the development of self-efficacy in individuals and families. For example, nurse-initiated phone follow-up was effective in increasing self-efficacy in relation to the management of dyspnea for patients with chronic obstructive pulmonary disease (Wong, Wong, & Chan, 2005).

Of concern, however, is Geanellos' study (2005) of how nurse unfriendliness, characterized by "frostiness, officiousness and apathy," undermines patient self-efficacy and well-being.

Locus of Control. The significance of locus of control for rehabilitation in evidenced in various studies. For example, Tak and Laffrey (2003) found that in female osteoarthritis sufferers (n = 107) higher internal locus of control was related to greater perceived social support whereas higher external locus of control was associated with less perceived support and less life satisfaction. Shaw, McColl, and Bond (2003) found that following surgery for fractured neck of femur greater internal locus of control was associated with greater independence in older women (n = 112).

Hardiness. Hardiness, a constellation of stress-resistant tendencies, has been debated as a mediator between stress and adjustments. A long-standing view held hardiness to have three key dimensions: commitment, control, and challenge. Persons who exhibited commitment were actively involved in their own lives and expressed a sense of purpose or direction. Those who believed they could influence, perhaps not prevent, the way events in their life progressed were seen as having control, rather than feeling powerless. Similar to an internal locus of control, they viewed challenge as stimulating and necessary and as opportunity for personal growth or skills development (Kobasa, Maddi, & Kahn, 1982; Kobasa, Maddi, & Zola, 1983).

What is termed *hardiness* may influence how events are cognitively appraised and how coping occurs, thus enabling a person to effectively resist health threats arising from stressors. It would follow that persons with hardiness predictably resist illness, whereas persons who are vulnerable (i.e., have low hardiness) may have lowered resistance to stressors and increased health problems (Pollock, 1986, 1989).

Hardiness is a motivating factor for individuals who exhibit strong psychosocial adjustment and problem-solving skills. Three themes in family life combine to breed hardiness in children: (1) children who receive interest, encouragement, and acceptance from the parents "come to view self and the world as interesting and worthwhile"; (2) children sense they can influence their environments when they have mastered tasks with moderate difficulty; and (3) children learn to appraise change as challenge, not chaos, when their parents see change as "interesting and developmentally valuable" and communicate this to their children (Maddi & Kobasa, 1991). Not related to socioeconomic status, once hardiness has developed, children take it into their adult lives.

Groups also seem to have the ability to develop hardiness. For example, Svavarsdottir, Rayens, and McCubbin (2005) found family hardiness to predict family adaptation in families with young children with chronic asthma.

Resilience, an ability to defuse a potential stressor into a nonstressor event, may be due in part to an ability to recover rapidly, or "bounce back." Those who view change as opportunity while valuing commitment and enjoying challenge, along with a sense of humor, tend to "bounce back" from loss or failure (Kobasa, 1979; Kobasa et al., 1983). They seek change and thrive on it (Orr & Westman, 1990). In a study of nondisabled community-dwelling older persons (n = 546,

age 70+ years), Hardy, Concato, and Gill (2004) found that high resilience was associated with functional (such as independence in instrumental activities of daily living) and psychological (such as few depressive symptoms) factors.

Learned Resourcefulness. Learned resourcefulness is a personality repertoire consisting of beliefs as well as self-control skills and behaviors that make a positive contribution to a person's health (Rosenbaum, 1990). This effect is twofold: "(a) coping with the physical discomforts that are caused either by illness or by painful medical procedures and (b) adoption of and adherence to health behaviors."

Persons who are highly resourceful use self-control strategies to cope with physical discomfort and to guide behavior change (e.g., smoking cessation, diet modification, and maintenance of an exercise program).

Optimism. Optimism is associated with the expectation of a good outcome because optimists make the best of whatever situation. They are more likely to use problem-focused coping strategies because they expect a positive change. Pessimists, preoccupied with their emotions, try to deny the reality of the stressor and may give up (Scheier & Carver, 1987). The self-reports of optimism in 35% of 96 cancer patients with an estimated life expectancy of less than 3 months (van der Lee, Swarte, van der Bom, van den Bout, & Heintz, 2005) supports the belief that optimism is more a trait than a response to one's appraisal of a situation or event.

Hope. Rees and Joslyn (1998) explain that hope can be generalized to mean that things will improve, or it can be a specific patient goal (e.g., being able to walk again). The opposite of despair, hope can be a coping strategy, an emotion, a feeling, a conviction or experience, or a personal attribute.

Hope has been associated with better patient adjustment following a range of acquired disabilities. For example, in the first 3 months following spinal cord injury, hope was central to the experience of all 10 participants in a study by Lohne and Severinsson (2004). While they struggled with disappointments, hope that they would recover and walk again was stimulated by improvements. However, as a consequence of setbacks they were sometimes fearful of hoping.

The relevance of hope for families has also been studied. In a study of 40 families of stroke survivors, Bluvol and Ford-Gilboe (2004) found stroke survivors and their spouses who were more hopeful "perceived their quality of life to be fairly high, despite living with disability."

Felder's finding (2004) that cancer patients (n = 183), 71% of whom had advanced metastatic or recurrent disease, maintained a high level of hope alludes to the ability of a person to be hopeful as being more a trait than a response to one's appraisal of a situation or event. That they found a statistically significant positive relationship between overall level of hope and coping effectiveness indicates the importance of rehabilitation nurses' actively fostering hope in their patients. Hope is discussed further in Chapter 29.

Uncertainty. Uncertainty, the inability to determine the meaning of illness-related events, occurs in situations where the decision maker is unable to assign definite values to objects and events and/or is unable to accurately predict outcomes because sufficient cues are lacking (Mishel, 1990).

Certainty and predictability are valued in Western cultures where persons are uncomfortable with not knowing what to expect and with not knowing how to influence what is expected. Preferred thinking is linear, organized, controlled, and precise. Valued traits are self-efficacy, control, goal direction, and time management, whereas not knowing when or how is less acceptable. Thus, when patients face chronic, disabling, or developmental disorders that have uncertain outcomes, they initially want to know how to cure the problem to counteract system breakdown. When there is no cure, uncertainty about progress and outcome is a familiar concept in rehabilitation.

Uncertainty about the future was central to the experience of juvenile chronic arthritis in the study by Sallfors, Fasth, and Hallberg (2002) of 6- to 17-year-olds (n = 22). In this qualitative study the subcategories of uncertainty were "powerlessness, frustration, distress, being left out, hopelessness, sadness and aggression." That the children were found to have no management strategy or way out when they were suffering as a result of this chaos indicates the importance of understanding and support from rehabilitation nurses at these times.

Uncertainty is also a problem for families. As Mitchell, Courtney, and Coyer (2003) explain, because critical illness allows little time to adapt, families experience difficulty coping. For this reason, they say families of patients recently transferred out of intensive care units need additional support from rehabilitation nurses. Our understanding of the development of effective coping strategies as a process that often begins with chaos, is aided by a study of nine parents of children with asthma by Trollvik and Severinsson (2004). Uncertainty about what could happen when their child was unable to breathe filled parents in this study with fear that returned each time their child became ill. In another study Mu (2005) found uncertainty was negatively associated with coping and positively associated with depression in fathers (n = 210) of children with epilepsy.

Findings of a study by Wonghongkul, Moore, Musil, Schneider, and Deimling (2000) suggest that following successful treatment for cancer, hope may increase and uncertainty decrease in the passage of time and absence of reoccurrence. They found low levels of uncertainty in female survivors of breast cancer with a mean time since diagnosis of 12.3 years (n = 71). These women had high levels of hope, and their most common method of coping was planful problem solving, followed by positive reappraisal, self-controlling, seeking social support and distancing, indicating that they were coping effectively.

Social Support. There is an increasing interest in the influence of social support on the way individuals and families cope with disability, with Langford, Bowsher, Maloney,

and Lillis (1997) identifying four types of social support: emotional, instrumental, informational, and appraisal. Several studies have revealed that individuals with newly acquired disabilities actively seek social support. Studies of trauma patients, for example, spinal cord injury (n = 24; mean time since injury 3.83 months) (Belciug, 2001) and acute hand trauma (n = 20; 8 to 20 days since injury) (Gustafsson, Persson, & Amilon, 2002), found that these patients actively sought various types of social support, including emotional, instrumental, and informational support.

Social support has also been found to play an important part in the overall well-being of family caregivers and the way they cope. In a study of families with a child with congenital heart disease, Tak and McCubbin (2002) found perceived social support to be a predictor of family coping. In another study, a longitudinal randomized controlled trial of a nurse-led support and education program for spouses of stroke patients by Larson et al. (2005), the group who participated in the program five to six times over 6 months "had a significant decrease in negative well-being and increased quality of life over time, while the group attending fewer times had a significant decrease in positive well-being and health state, similar to the control group." Rehabilitation nurses have a particular role in the provision of support in the form of predischarge information and training, as well as postdischarge follow-up.

The right kind and the right amount of support, however, is not always provided. Elderly female caregivers of stroke survivors in a study by Sit, Wong, Clinton, Li, and Fong (2004) found the extent of tangible support and information support to be inadequate. That after 12 weeks in the role of caregiver nearly half of these women were experiencing "somatic symptoms and fatigue to the extent that they needed to see a doctor" indicates the importance of support for family caregivers.

Peer support (Adamsen, Rasmussen, & Pedersen, 2001; Clark, Barbour, White, & MacIntyre, 2004; MacPherson, Joseph, & Sullivan, 2004) and self-help group participation (Adamsen, 2002) are emerging as effective forms of social support that help people cope with health breakdown. A study by Dewar (2001) indicates that sufferers of catastrophic illnesses and injuries (n = 28) can also contribute to the welfare of their significant others by actively seeking to reduce the burden of care they create. Over time, participants in this study developed strategies that put boundaries around their suffering. This involved protecting the significant other by minimizing their workloads and distress.

A small number of studies have highlighted that social support does not always need to be in the form of direct interpersonal contact. Angell et al. (2003) report on a psychosocial intervention for rural women with breast cancer. Women who used the interactive workbook-journal reported increased fighting spirit and decreasing helplessness/hopelessness. Promising results of studies of computer-based support initiatives (for example, Chambers & Connor, 2002; Gustafson, et al., 2001) have also been reported.

Although the provision of social support can be provided as an intervention, existing friendships and networks should not be overlooked as a valuable source of social support. Rehabilitation nurses can contribute to this by making our patients' friends welcome, recognizing their need for information and support, negotiating their involvement with patients, and facilitating that involvement.

Other Factors. Findings of recent studies draw our attention to how a range of other factors might influence the coping process for individuals and families. These include age (Derks, DeLeeuw, Hordijk, & Winnubst, 2005; Link, Mancuso, & Charlson, 2004; Tomberg, et al., 2001); gender (Fortune, Richards, Main, & Griffiths, 2002; Hjorleifsdottir, Hallberg, Bolmsjo, & Gunardsdottir, 2005; Kristofferzon, Lofmark, & Carlsson, 2003; Martin & Bat-Chava, 2003; Tomberg, et al., 2001); education (Richardson, Adner, & Nordstrom, 2001); ethnicity (Roberts, et al., 2003; Tan, Jensen, Thornby, & Anderson, 2005); comorbidities (Garralda & Rangel, 2004; Pagano et al., 2004; St-Louis & Robichaud-Ekstrand, 2003); and time since injury, onset of illness, or diagnosis (Fosberg et al., 2002; Han, 2003; McCausland, 2001; Welch & Austin, 2001; Wonghongkul et al., 2000).

How Persons Cope With Interruptions in Health

In relation to interruptions to health, the coping process begins with the identification of specific demands as stressors, followed by the appraisal of stressors and responses to manage those demands.

Stressors Associated With Interruptions in Health. A variety of specific demands associated with interruptions in health have been identified as stressors. For example, the most common illness-related stressors for persons with rheumatoid arthritis (n = 48) were physical limitations, lack of control/independence, and pain (Melanson & Downe-Wamboldt, 2003). Patients with non–small cell lung cancer were troubled by physical (mostly fatigue, loss of appetite, and weight loss) and psychological (mostly fatigue-inertia, confusion-bewilderment, and depression-dejection) symptoms during the therapeutic period (Kuo & Ma, 2002). Sufferers with multiple sclerosis contended with the "bodily experiences of becoming a chronically ill person … changing relationships, changing identities and challenges in their physical environment" (Driedger, Crooks, & Bennett, 2004).

Physical consequences of chronic illness are recognized more readily than psychosocial consequences such as self-identity. Charmaz (1983) has noted that Western health care systems treat acute illness, whereas chronic illness "results in spiraling consequences such as loss of productive function, financial crises, family strain, stigma, and a restricted existence." She explains that sources of suffering are complex: for example, being discredited may lead to a more restricted life and consequently limited opportunities to construct a valued self. The values of individualism and independence discredit a restricted and often homebound life focused on the illness. Recurrent discrediting leads the chronically ill to perceive themselves as permanent failures and as burdens.

Family members and caregivers of persons experiencing interruptions in health have also identified a variety of specific demands as stressors. Primary caregivers of children with disabilities in a study by Kelso, French, and Fernandez (2005) identified these as the impact of the intensity of care on family functioning, the process of getting a diagnosis, concerns about the appropriateness of schooling options, professionals that do not listen to them, finding out what resources are available, own personal well-being, isolation, and community responses to their child's specific problems and/or their management of those problems. Stressors identified in other studies of caregivers include lifestyle changes, changes in personal identity, giving up paid work, career interruption or early termination, loss of income, relationship change with the loved one, social isolation (Sawatzy & Fowler-Kerry, 2003), financial problems, sleep disruption (Rogers & Hogan, 2003), and physical and mental fatigue (Bergs, 2002).

Appraisal of Interruptions in Health. Although many studies describe how persons cope with interruptions in health, few report on how these events are appraised in terms of harm, threat, challenge, or benefit. In a study by Wonghongkul et al. (2000) survivors of breast cancer with a mean time since diagnosis of 12.3 years most frequently appraised living without recurrence for a minimum of 5 years as a challenge. Relatively low levels of threat and harm were found. In another study (Melanson & Downe-Wamboldt, 2003), living with rheumatoid arthritis (at a mean time of 18 years since diagnosis) was most commonly appraised as harm, followed by threat then challenge. Very few reported having this condition as a benefit.

An appraisal of harm is suggested by reports that "negative definitions" of their situation as "catastrophe" by parents with a child with intellectual disability is "the single most important predictor of parental stress" in a study by Saloviita, Italinna, and Leinonen (2003).

Responses to Interruptions in Health. Many authors (for example, Ahlstrom & Wenneberg, 2002; Carter, 2003; McConaghy & Caltabiano, 2005; Sherwood et al., 2004) have used the work of Lazarus and Folkman (1984), in particular their ways of coping (Folkman & Lazarus, 1988), to guide their studies of coping with interruptions in health. Nevertheless, knowledge of a range of theories about, and interpretations of, how persons cope with interruptions in health enriches nurses' abilities to understand the experiences of their patients and families.

The Sick Role

Parsons (1951) introduced the notion of "being sick" as constituting a social role rather than just a natural phenomenon that happened to individuals. He also alluded to acceptable and unacceptable motives of those who adopt or choose to stay in the sick role. For him coping with interruptions in health was at both an individual and a social system level. Although Parson's work is not relevant when health breakdown is chronic, some patients and families may uphold the expectations associated with Parson's sick role.

Loss of Self in Chronic Illness

In their struggle for identity, chronically ill patients have been found to prefer to construct their lives to find motivation apart from their illnesses. On the basis of data from 85 in-depth interviews with chronically ill persons, Charmaz (1987) created a hierarchy of identities listed in Box 22-10. The concept of identity is related to the person's vision of future self; failure to regain a valued identity is viewed as a failure of self.

Subsequently, Charmaz (1995) conducted 115 intensive interviews with 55 adults with serious, intrusive chronic illnesses and found that adapting (accommodating the physical losses by altering self and life) is one mode of living with loss of bodily function or impairment. Not everyone adapts; adaptation may be a recurring theme down through the levels of identity.

Three major stages were found in adapting to impairment: (1) experiencing an altered body; (2) assessing one's altered body, appearance to self and others, and the context of life; and (3) surrendering to the sick body (Charmaz, 1995). "Other ways of living with illness include ignoring it, minimizing it, struggling against it, reconciling self to it, and embracing it"; differing from resigning to it, being overtaken by the illness, or giving up, surrender is about a new unity between the self and the body.

Reactions to Disability

Antonak and Livneh (1991) analyzed the responses of 118 persons with acquired disability to the Reactions to Impairments and Disability Inventory (RIDI) and found sets of adapted and nonadapted psychosocial reactions to disability.

BOX 22-10 Characteristics of Identity Levels

The supernormal self assumes:
- Success values
- Social acceleration
- Struggle in a competitive world
  The restored self assumes:
- Return to former life
- Current situation is normal after serious illness

A contingent personal identity is:
- Defined as questionable
- Perhaps possible in the future
- Associated with possible failure

A salvaged self:
- Attempts to see self as positive
- Attempts to present self to others most favorably
- Is associated with adverse circumstances
- Holds little hope of realizing typical adult identities

Data from Charmaz, K. (1987). Struggling for a self: Identity levels of the chronically ill. *Sociology of Health Care, 6*, 283-321.

Acknowledgment is about the person's "intellectual recognition of the permanency of the condition and its future implications. *Adjustment* entails further assimilation, affectively and behaviorally, of the ramifications of the disability" (Antonak & Livneh, 1991). They suggest that depression, internalized anger, anxiety, and externalized anger are prerequisites to adaptation; however, these reactions do not occur in any particular sequence and are independent of each other. To this they add, "experiencing shock is apparently prerequisite to experiencing depression and internalized anger" and that shock, anxiety, and externalized anger appear to be experienced concurrently. Denial was an independent reaction.

Responding to Threats to Self

Morse (1997) presented a comprehensive theory that incorporates human responses to acute illness, chronic illness, and injury. Despite differences in the onset and prognosis, "the pattern of responses to a threat to the integrity of the self has remarkable commonalities." The model provides valuable insights into strategies patients employ as they move through each of the five stages: maintaining vigilance, enduring to survive, enduring to live, striving to restore self, and learning to live with the altered self.

Enduring and suffering differ in nature and purpose. Enduring, associated with physical pain after injury or illness, continues once the physiological crisis passes. Enduring for survival shifts to enduring to live; suffering focuses on the implications of the event.

When patients' conditions improve to the point of acknowledging the illness or injury and recognizing the effects, the struggle of mourning what was lost and an altered future begins from release of fixation on the present and permits anticipation of a future. Patients may experience sudden, overwhelming emotion as they work to heal, resolve suffering, and make sense of the experience (Morse, 1997).

Suffering is work, an all-consuming endeavor that one must experience to work through the event. Furthermore, suffering demands that horror be relived again and again, for in this process of reviewing the horror is recontextualized, revalued, resorted, and eventually resolved (Morse & Carter, 1995).

Coping Strategies Used to Manage Demands Associated With Interruptions in Health. The literature reports a wide range of coping strategies used by individuals in response to interruptions in their health. Table 22-1 presents findings of several of these studies highlighting specific demands encountered and strategies used by individuals at various stages of the life span. The use of inductive methods and a variety of tools and scales in quantitative studies make comparison of the findings impossible, suggesting that further research is required in this area.

Family members commonly become involved in providing support and care for individuals experiencing interruptions in health. Recent research illuminates the variety of roles that family caregivers may assume. The findings of two studies are presented in Boxes 22-11 and 22-12. The tacit definitions

TABLE 22-1 Examples of Coping Strategies Used in Response to Specific Demands Associated With Interruptions in Health

	Specific Demand(s)	Coping Strategies Used	Source
Children and Adolescents			
24 children (mean age 15 years) with chronic fatigue syndrome	Ilness-related problems: Symptoms of illness (66%) Limitations caused by illness (4%) Treatment (4%) Worries about return to school (25%) Fear of discrimination because of illness (4%) Disability-related problems: Sports/physical activities (75%) Socializing with friends (10%) Attending school (5%) Activities of daily living (15%)	• Social withdrawal (37%) • Self-criticism (42%) • Emotional regulation (87%) • Social support (92%) • Resignation (71%) • Social withdrawal (43%) • Self-criticism (26%) • Problem solving (65%) • Emotional regulation (91%) • Resignation (83%)	Garralda & Rangel, 2004
65 children age 8-18 years living with Crohn's disease	Living with active Crohn's disease Living with Crohn's disease in remission	Most frequently used coping strategies: • Distraction • Cognitive restructuring • Problem solving • Emotion regulation • Seeking social support • Resignation Most frequently used coping strategies: • Distraction • Cognitive restructuring • Problem solving • Seeking social support	Chotard, Caplan, & Seidman, 2005
Adolescents and Young Adults			
14 (8 females and 6 males) adolescents and young adults; 10 age 16-19 years and 4 age 20-22 years	Living with cancer (thyroid 14%; lymphatic system 37%; sarcoma 14%; leukemia 14%; ovarian 7%; brain 7%; granulocytomatous tumor 7%)—14% had disease for <2 years; 57% for 2-5 years; 29% for >5 years	• Emotional and material support from family members, friends, health care providers and other cancer patients • Searching for information about cancer themselves • Knowledge of cancer patients' group • Belief in God • Hope for recovery • Positive attitude toward life, belief in one's own resources • Returning to one's normal lifestyle as soon as possible and not giving in to cancer	Kyngas et al., 2001
31 adults age 18-40 years with cystic fibrosis (CF); 17 females (mean age 29) and 14 males (mean age 32)	Living as an adult with CF—90% diagnosed by the age of 5 and 10% diagnosed between 5 and 22 years of age	• Comparing oneself to others without CF to maintain perceptions of self as normal • Maintaining a positive attitude by viewing CF as beneficial to overall quality of life and expressing a positive approach towards it (majority) • Acknowledging and minimizing the loss of spontaneity that having CF entailed and adapting social life and daily activities accordingly • Denial of CF (9.7%)	Lowton & Gabe, 2003

Continued

TABLE 22-1 Examples of Coping Strategies Used in Response to Specific Demands Associated With Interruptions in Health—cont'd

	Specific Demand(s)	Coping Strategies Used	Source
24 (17 males and 7 females) persons with spinal cord injury; 5 with tetraplegia and 19 with paraplegia; mean age 34.4 years	Recent spinal cord injury—mean time since injury 3.83 months	In comparison to a normative group, members of this group were: Average in their use of logical analysis Somewhat below average in their use of positive reappraisal Somewhat average in their reliance on seeking guidance and support Somewhat average in their reliance on problem solving Well above average in their use of cognitive avoidance Average in their use of acceptance and resignation Well above average in their reliance on seeking alternative rewards Considerably above average in their reliance on emotional discharge	Belciug, 2001

Midlife Adults

	Specific Demand(s)	Coping Strategies Used	Source
250 adults (132 males and 118 females) attending a psoriasis clinic; median age 43 years (IQR 35-51 years); 56% with a family history of psoriasis	Living with psoriasis—median duration of psoriasis 18 years (IQR 11-28 years);	Coping strategies from most to least commonly used: • Acceptance • Active coping • Planning • Positive reinterpretation • Practical social support • Venting emotions • Suppressions of competing activities • Mental disengagement • Humor • Behavioral disengagement • Religion • Denial • Alcohol and drug use	Fortune et al., 2002
44 adults (25 females and 19 males); age 42-78 (mean 57) years	Diagnosed with cancer 6-24 months ago	41% used strategies to take control of their cancer or situation; 25% did not; 34% were ambivalent The group that used strategies to take control used more proactive strategies aimed at optimizing one's well-being than the other two groups The group that did not use strategies to take control used more reactive strategies aimed at maintaining well-being than the other two groups	Link et al., 2004

Adults of Various Ages

	Specific Demand(s)	Coping Strategies Used	Source
79 (42 males and 37 females) survivors of road trauma; age 22-85 (mean 49) years	Surviving road trauma—3-4 years post trauma	Recovery involved: Finding a new fit Private suffering Anticipatory coping (tapping into high levels of optimism and expectations of future coping) Survivor pride	Harms, 2004

TABLE 22-1 Examples of Coping Strategies Used in Response to Specific Demands Associated With Interruptions in Health—cont'd

	Specific Demand(s)	Coping Strategies Used	Source
20 adults (19 males and 1 female) age 25-71 years	8-20 days post acute hand trauma	• Comparing with something worse • Positive thinking • Relying on personal capacity • Distancing • Distracting attention • Accepting the situation • Seeking social support • Maintaining control • Solving practice problems by oneself • Pain-relieving strategies • Active processing of the trauma experience	Gustafsson et al., 2002
Older Persons			
40 adults (21 females and 19 males) undertaking treatment for cancer; age 18-25 to over 71 years (majority 51-70 years)	Problems associated with cancer and its treatment	Coping strategies from most to least commonly used: • Distancing • Cognitive escape-avoidance • Seeking and using social support • Focusing on the positive • Behavioral escape-avoidance	Hjorleifsdottir et al., 2005
48 older persons (39 females and 9 males); mean age 75 years	Stress associated with rheumatoid arthritis—mean time since diagnosis of rheumatoid arthritis 18 years	Coping strategies used most: • Confrontive (problem-focused) strategies • Palliative strategies Coping strategies used least: • Emotive strategies • Optimistic strategies • Evasive strategies	Melanson & Downe-Wamboldt, 2003

BOX 22-11 Tacit Definitions of Caregiving

Engaged caregivers:
• Play an active role
• Learn how to deliver the care needed
• Become skilful in providing care, including emotional care, hands-on care, clinical care, high-tech nursing, and health care advocacy
• Anticipate person's needs
Conflicted caregivers:
• Urge and/or support their partners to be responsible for their own care and health care decisions
• Deliver care on an as-needed basis
• Do not prepare themselves for the escalating levels of care
• Are concerned about challenges to their own physical and psychological needs
Distanced caregivers:
• Make a priority of keeping their partners in control of their own care and health care decisions
• Work at developing the "skill" of distance to support their partner's independence
• Feel effective when they self-manage their emotions

Data from Wrubel, J., Richards, T. A., Folkman, S., & Acree, M. C. (2001). Tacit definitions of informal caregiving, *Journal of Advanced Nursing*, 33(2), 175-181.

BOX 22-12 Roles Assumed by Spouses

Participative role involves:
• Taking a practical part if lifestyle changes
• Communicating empathetically
• Being positive about changes
Regulative role involves:
• Being either positive or negative about changes
• Giving practical or cognitive support in order to control partner's behavior
• Communicating authoritatively
Observational role involves:
• Being passive
• Complying with suggestions
• Communicating empathetically
Incapacitated role involves:
• Having a positive attitude toward change
• Communicating without making demands
• But unable to provide support because of personal problems
Dissociative role involves:
• Being negative about changes
• Authoritatively declaring a reluctance to be involved in partner's lifestyle changes

Data from Karner, A., Dahlgren, M. A., & Bergdahl, B. (2004). Rehabilitation after coronary heart disease: Spouses' views of support. *Journal of Advanced Nursing*, 46(2), 204-211.

of caregiving in Box 22-11 were identified in a study of 60 men who were caregivers of men with AIDS. Of the 60 men, 33 (55%) were found to be engaged caregivers, 13 (22%) were conflicted caregivers, and 14 (23%) were distanced caregivers (Wrubel, Richards, Folkman, & Acree, 2001).

The roles assumed by spouses in Box 22-12 were reported in a study of 8 male and 17 female spouses of persons in the rehabilitation phase of coronary heart disease.

A variety of family members provide care to persons with disability, including children as young as 3 (Lackey & Gates, 2001). Providing care as a child is not always considered a negative experience; most of the 51 adults who were recounting their experiences of providing care as children indicated "they would permit their own children to assist with care as long as the youngster was not the sole caregiver. Youngsters need to be informed about the illness and caregiving tasks, have adequate support systems, and have some time to 'still be a child.'"

Table 22-2 presents findings of several studies of family caregivers highlighting the coping strategies they used in response to a family member's experiencing an interruption in health. Chapters 29 and 31 discuss more about spirituality and coping during specific developmental stages of childhood.

APPLICATION OF THEORY TO REHABILITATION NURSING PRACTICE

Assessment

Assessment relative to coping with chronic, disabling, or developmental disorders determines the patient's and family members' needs and directs the nursing response. Many and varied needs require nurses to monitor the patient and family, plan nursing interventions, refer to the team or community resources, and form mutual creative solutions.

Triage is appropriate when certain aspects of a patient's situation are clearly associated with unbearable distress. Prioritizing interventions to facilitate patients' comfort (physical, social, psychospiritual, or environmental) may enable them to participate in the rehabilitation program and life in general.

Assessment of effectiveness in coping is a complex, multidimensional process that encompasses cognitive, affective, and psychomotor domains. Developing rapport and trust with the patient and family who are experiencing times of great vulnerability takes time. A comprehensive database for each patient includes and values information about preferences, goals and hopes, frustrations and fears. Especially important for patients with cognitive and communication impairments,

TABLE 22-2 Examples of Coping Strategies Used by Family Caregivers

	Specific Demand(s)	Coping Strategies	Source
Children and Adolescents			

11 children (7 boys and 4 girls) age 7-12 years	A parent with cancer	• Going in and out (literally and emotionally) of the situation in order to:
		  • Face illness intermittently
		  • Displace illness for a while
		  • Collect positive experiences
		• Covering up difficulties
		• Balancing information
			Helseth & Ulfsaet, 2003

83 children (46 girls and 37 boys) age 7-18 (mean 11) years	Sibling diagnosed with a malignant tumor for no more than 4 weeks	• The coping strategy "predictive control" (maintaining positive expectations regarding illness) positively predicted siblings' quality of life • Reliance on "interpretative control" (trying to understand the illness) was associated with fewer positive emotions	Houtzager, Grootenhuis, Hoekstra-Weebers, & Last, 2005
Midlife Adults			

39 males (age 39-58 years)	Partner treated with chemotherapy for breast cancer within past 2 years and one or more children living at home	• Focusing on their wives' illness and care by:
		  • Being there (physically and emotionally)
		  • Relying on health care professionals
		  • Being informed and contributing to decision making
		• Focusing on the family to keep life going by:
		  • Trying to keep patterns normal
		  • Helping out and relying on others to undertake household and child care activities
		  • Trying to be positive
			Hilton, Crawford, & Tarko, 2000

TABLE 22-2 Examples of Coping Strategies Used by Family Caregivers—cont'd

	Specific Demand(s)	Coping Strategies	Source
		• Putting [their] self on hold • Adapting work life • Managing finances	

Older Persons

	Specific Demand(s)	Coping Strategies	Source
290 persons (198 females and 92 males); 78% 50 years and older	Caring for older family members (90% over 80 years)	Most helpful coping strategies: • Establishing one's priorities and concentrating on them (86%) • Believing in oneself and one's ability to handle the situation (85%) • Taking life 1 day at a time (85%) • Looking for the positive things in each situation (83%) • Relying on one's expertise and the experience one has built up (80%) • Accepting the situation as it is (79%) • Keeping the person one cares for as active as possible (78%) • Taking one's mind off things in some way (e.g., reading, watching TV) (75%) • Altering one's home environment to make things as easy as possible (73%) • Keeping one step ahead of things by planning in advance (72%)	Kuuppelomaki, Saski, Yamanda, Asakawa, & Shimanouchi, 2004
246 mothers (mean age 66.6 years) of adults with intellectual disability and 74 mother (mean age 66 years) of adults with mental illness	Adults with intellectual disability (mean age 34.1 years) and adults with mental illness (mean age 35 years)	For both groups an increase in emotion-focused coping led to declining levels of well-being For mothers of adults with intellectual disability, an increase in problem-focused coping resulted in a reduction in distress and an improvement in the quality of the relationship with the adult child For mothers of adults with mental illness, an increase in problem-focused coping only led to an improved relationship with the adult child	Kim, Greenberg, Seltzer, & Krauss, 2003

Adults of Various Ages

	Specific Demand(s)	Coping Strategies	Source
51 parents/caregivers (mainly mothers and grandmothers)	Children with intellectual, visual, or physical disabilities	• Seeking a cure • Support (social and physical/material support) • Beliefs (God's will; witchcraft or spirits; concurrent knowledge of medical causes) • Attitudes (acceptance; inclusion; overcompensation/protection)	Hartley, Ojwang, Baguwemu, Ddamulira, & Chavuta, 2005
37 caregivers (21 spouses; 13 adult children; 3 close relatives); age 23-86 (mean 55.7) years	Caring for stroke survivors aged 50-91 (mean 69.8) years	• Remaining positive • Adapting to change • Comparison of situation with others who were worse off • Changing employment status • Humor • Switching off • Using family support	O'Connell & Baker, 2004
50 family members (82% female and 18% male) over 16 years of age; 14% husband; 48% wife; 28% parent; 4% child; 4% sister; 2% cousin	Caring for family member with brain injury	• Acceptance • Rationalization • Planning activities • Actively looking for solution • Seeking support and encouragement • Directing attention to other activities • Use of social resources	Man, 2002

life before the current situation has purposes in relation to the functional health pattern of coping-stress tolerance. Knowledge of the patient's previous lifestyle does the following:

- Tells us about the patient's likes, dislikes, and preferred activities
- Helps us consider the possible consequences of the current situation for the patient's life
- Alludes to concerns the patient may have but is not verbalizing
- Uncovers details of unresolved conflicts of concern to the patient
- Provides information about important roles, activities, events, persons, or pets that can be used by the nurse to establish links for patients about what is happening now and for the rest of their lives
- Provides valuable cues to be used when exploring the consequences of the current situation and planning for discharge and the future

The history of the current situation may provide insight into the patient's knowledge about the condition, prognosis, and management, whereas details of the acute situation and its management may explain patient or family responses. Assessment incorporates the primary and secondary appraisals:

- Has the patient appraised the event/situation as a harm or loss, a threat, a challenge, or a benefit?
- What has the patient decided might or can be done about the event/situation?
- What personal and environmental variables are relevant?
- What meanings have been assigned to the situation by the patient?
- What emotion(s) is the patient experiencing?
- What problem-focused coping strategies has the patient put in place?
- What emotion-focused coping strategies has the patient put in place?
- Does the patient believe he or she is capable of coping with the current situation?
- Does the patient evaluate his or her coping strategies as effective?

For us to understand how the current situation came about, the patient or family member needs to tell us. Reliving the event may itself be stressful for the patient or family member. This should not necessarily be viewed as a negative experience, in light of Park and Folkman's work (1997) on reappraisal and meaning-making. Persons seek to make sense of what is happening and search for meaning by reappraising the situation and its significance. Providing an opportunity for the patient and family to tell their stories may be therapeutic.

Using a variety of sources (e.g., eyewitness accounts, newspaper articles, and medical reports) to reconstruct the event will enhance the completeness and accuracy and assist the patient or family with gaining a more complete understanding of the event.

The assessment of coping needs to be informed by an accurate interpretation of the emotions experienced by the individual. Lazarus' core relational themes (1991) for each emotion can be used as a framework to interpret emotions from the stories of patients and their families.

The needs of individuals and groups will be many and varied. To meet these, rehabilitation nurses need to approach their role with a genuine desire to understand individual perspectives and experiences and a commitment to respect the individuals. Listen to everything you are told, and interpret what you see. Every piece of information helps to piece together a picture of the complex situation faced by a patient and/or family and to identify the coping strategies used in response to that situation.

Assessment of Coping Effectiveness in the Individual

History and Subjective Data. A history is used to assess a patient's effectiveness in coping, including insight into the patient's appraisal of stressors, underlying meanings, emotions, and ways of coping. The following section contains suggestions and sample queries for eliciting subjective data about coping effectiveness during the course of therapeutic conversation between nurse and patient or family.

Suggestions
- An interview may include questions to elicit a patient's descriptions of beliefs about health and illness, potential causes of the condition, remedies that have been tried, what will help, who can or should help improve things, and how long before relief is expected.
- Parents or significant caregivers may report data for infants or persons with impaired communication or cognition. However, ascertain reliability of the person's report, and validate with other assessment data from the individual, family, or social system.
- Ask patients about their perceptions of what are personal stressors, what strategies they use in coping, and what emotions they are experiencing.
- What is the developmental stage, both individual and family? Draw a health and social genogram to depict family patterns, identify resources, or pinpoint difficulties with adjustments during life transitions, events, or happenings.

Sample Queries
- What has changed specifically due to this loss or event? For example, ask about changes in lifestyle, role relationships, health, and self-perception, including body image, occupation, functional independence, social system, quality of life, behavioral patterns, financial status, attitude or world view, and vocation or education.
- If you could change three things now, what would they be and why were these selected? What do they mean to you?
- What do you think will happen as a result of this stress or this event? What are your major concerns other than this stressor?
- Do you have a lot of daily hassles? How do you respond to annoyances? What is most important to you at this time?
- Why do you think this event happened? Are you or someone else able to control what is happening, or is there anything that can be done to change things? What kind of control do you believe you have over what happens?

- How have you and/or your family managed? What have you tried? Who or what is helpful to you? What do you think will be helpful to you now? Are there things you believe you should not do or things you must do?
- What will be the greatest difficulty for you since this stress or event has occurred? Are you concerned about how others will view or respond to you, who may reject you, or what others may say about you?
- Will you be able to follow the medical and health care plan? Can you perform or direct your own care? Do you have a caregiver or attendant? Do you have questions about your condition or care plan? What do you envision for your future (next day, week, or year, as appropriate)?
- What are your specific strengths and resources? Examples include family, pets, sense of humor, sense of control and self-determination, religious faith, education, income or employment, living arrangement, assistive devices or equipment, interests or hobbies, service agency supports, an acceptable caregiver, other social supports, and personal goals with hope.

Objective Data. Objective data obtained by examination, observation, inspection, and direct report are correlated with subjective, psychosocial data.

- Verify medications, health products, or therapeutic items.
- Elicit the person's description and definition, or denial, of the stressor event. Note whether the person is able to describe concerns, use proactive approaches, or verbalize need for assistance. Assess whether the person is able to depict the situation and roles of self and others accurately.
- Observe affect; alertness and mood; or nonverbal signs such as crying, lack of eye contact (unless culturally inappropriate), withdrawal responses, irritability or anger, inappropriate behavior, nervous manifestations (e.g., picking, twitching, or tapping), or signs of socioemotional deprivation. A child may sleep, suck the hands or toys, avoid response, or engage self in play; attempt several observations apart from clinical examination, such as in the playroom or with other children while in the waiting area. For older patients ensure that they are not tired or hungry from traveling, waiting, or needing medications before assessment.
- Inspect physical appearance for poor grooming or hygiene, bruises, cuts, hair pulling, or other nervous self-inflicted injuries; assess for abuse or neglect by others. Observe gums and mucosa for biting lesions.
- Assess self-destructive manifestations such as weight gain or loss, eating disorders, substance abuse, changes in health maintenance, or self-reported actions.
- Measure weight, vital signs, and blood pressure.
- Conduct a review of systems. Physical signs and symptoms have been associated with ineffective coping responses, as discussed in the next section. All signs or symptoms are evaluated in the context of the whole person and family. This list is not exhaustive.

Physical Signs and Symptoms and Coping. Possible physical manifestations of stressors are racing pulse, palpitations, dizziness or fainting, shortness of breath, hyperventilation, nausea, indigestion, "burping," refluxlike symptoms, burning sensations, changes in tongue or mucosa, difficulty swallowing, constipation, diarrhea, irritable bowel signs, urinary frequency, localized itching, headache, pain, "nervous twitches," fatigue, neck ache, posture, grinding or clenching teeth, or skin eruptions. Other somatic responses or problems may occur.

Acute episodes such as strep throat have been found to follow stressful events; chronic conditions such as arthritis or lupus may be exacerbated with stress.

Evaluate sensory manifestations such as ability to concentrate, memory loss, confusion, changes in speech patterns, changes in communication style or amount, depressive reactions, pain or discomfort, altered hearing, or visual disturbances. Compare assessment with data about location, severity, duration, and type of injury or impairment.

Inspect injured area, altered or impaired body part, or functional disability. Concurrently assess the patient's perception of body image and whether the patient looks at his or her body or withdraws, verbal comments, and destructive or inappropriate mood swings.

Assessment of Coping Effectiveness in Family Systems. An early assessment of the family is essential to effective coping, growth, and future goal setting. Family genograms with psychosocial entries, assessment of open versus closed boundaries, identified problems or concerns, and recent loss or change provide important family data. Although rehabilitation nurses commonly work one-on-one with a patient, the nursing process and outcome must be based on each person as a part of a family, social network, and community system. All family members experience some degree of risk when the system is threatened by illness or disability. This is especially critical when the patient is a child.

Most families experience multiple stressors from various sectors of their lives. Stressors may occur simultaneously; family members develop at different stages, hold unique appraisals, and have personal response times and coping styles. Few families analyze their management style, patterns of communication or action, or coping strategies in preparation for a crisis event. In fact, it may be difficult for a family under great stress to identify and mobilize their resources and strengths. Families may be overwhelmed by the situation. Criteria indicating a family system has maladjusted coping behaviors include regular neglect (even denial) of patient's care, family duties, or responsibilities. Communication among family members may exhibit irritability, resentment, criticism, and frequent arguments. Physical symptoms, anxiety, emotional responses, and feelings of being overwhelmed may occur for any family member.

Many adults return to the community after a stay in a hospital or rehabilitation facility with functional or cognitive impairments that require them to live with family members. Family systems may become strained when family members become caregivers for a family member who has a disability or chronic condition and are overburdened with responsibility or lack caring warmth. They may lack knowledge about the patient's care, condition, or resources. Some caregivers may deny their own health needs or delay seeking care. Unresolved conflicts may emerge, overshadowing care decisions and excluding the patient from decision making. Ideally, rehabilitation nurses will forge collegial relationships with community health nurses or serve as consultants in the community. In these roles nurses can use results of home assessments and family system evaluations as a basis for working with patients to develop preventive interventions and plans to improve outcomes for patients and families.

Other signals may alert a nurse that an individual family member (or system) may collapse or is breaking down. Several or many of the indicators listed in Box 22-13 may appear.

Caregiver Coping. The role of caregiver may be a chronic stressor. The demands are typically repetitive, persistent, and long-term. In addition, the caregiver is commonly in a close relationship with the recipient of care and may be experiencing chronic sorrow. To make their situation manageable, caregivers must use effective coping strategies.

When the role of caregiver was first undertaken, the long-term nature of the role may not have been predicted, anticipated, or believed. Coping strategies that were chosen for their short-term effectiveness may quickly become ineffective as time passes. The process of coping is a cycle of repetitions of cognitive and/or behavioral efforts followed by reappraisal. Gignac and Gottlieb (1997) highlight the importance of ongoing coping appraisal by the caregiver. These appraisals may alter the coping process, their perception of the situation, or their perception about their own ability as a caregiver. Reappraisal becomes the trigger for the choice of alternative coping strategies, especially as the long-term and demanding nature of the role becomes apparent.

Warning. The nursing assessment assumes that the appropriateness and effectiveness of coping undertaken by individuals, families, or communities can actually be assessed

by a person other than the individual. Accurate assessment may not always be possible.

The particular problem-focused or emotion-focused strategies are assessed to determine whether they have been used to achieve the function for which they were chosen: that is, aimed at managing harms, threats, and challenges (problem focused); or managing the emotional reaction to the harm or threat (emotion focused).

The three types of outcomes of coping that have been identified are long-term in nature—"functioning in work and social living, morale or life satisfaction, and somatic health" (Lazarus & Folkman 1984). During assessment the rehabilitation nurse interprets a person's coping history based on the identified long-term outcomes of coping and evaluates the person's responses to the current stress or stressors (associated with the chronic, disabling, or developmental disorder). These data determine the appropriate nursing diagnoses and response.

Development of Assessment Skills. Working with patients and their families as they experience chronic, disabling, or developmental disorders, nurses develop a generic understanding of the impact of these disorders on their lives. Many differences exist in the extent to which individuals appraise a situation as taxing in relation to their resources. An equally wide range of human responses to stress and adversity are governed by expectations related to sex, age, religion, ethnicity, or culture. Many are simply individual differences.

To help nurses gain a deeper appreciation of these differences, a number of alternative sources complement scientific writings. For instance, reading biographical and autobiographical accounts of experiences of disability and illness (written from the perspective of persons living with them) helps in understanding human responses to chronic, disabling, or developmental disorders.

Nursing Diagnoses

Nursing diagnoses are identified after interpretation of the assessment data that may take additional time to collect for a comprehensive database. This is particularly relevant in the coping-stress tolerance functional health pattern, where the time-intensive processes of developing rapport and trust are key to information sharing.

The NANDA International nursing diagnoses chosen are those relevant to the functional health pattern of coping-stress tolerance. Nursing diagnoses relevant to the patient, family, and community are outlined in Box 22-14.

Once the nursing diagnoses have been identified, appropriate nursing outcomes and the interventions required to achieve those outcomes need to be selected. A selection of the NANDA International nursing diagnoses for the coping-stress tolerance health pattern have been matched to the nursing outcomes and nursing interventions presented by Moorhead, Johnson, and Maas (2004) and Dochterman and Bulechek (2004). These are presented in Table 22-3. Goal setting is an important next step in the nursing response.

BOX 22-13 Indicators of Potential Individual Breakdown

- Chronic fatigue
- Anger leading to cynical, sarcastic, or irritable behavior
- Impatience and exhaustion
- Anxiety and fears bordering on paranoia
- Disturbed sleep and rest patterns
- Distress in role relationships
- Illness and accidents or injuries
- Maladaptive behaviors such as depression, substance abuse, avoidance or isolation, inattention to personal care, or eating disorder
- Potential for suicide
- Depleted or inaccessible resources
- Perception of few options

BOX 22-14 Nursing Diagnoses

Relevant for the Patient
- Risk-prone health behavior
- Anxiety
- Fear
- Ineffective coping
- Readiness for enhanced coping
- Defensive coping
- Ineffective denial
- Risk for post-trauma syndrome
- Post-trauma syndrome
- Social isolation
- Impaired social interaction
- Grieving (anticipatory)
- Complicated grieving
- Risk for complicated grieving
- Hopelessness
- Disturbed personal identity
- Risk for loneliness
- Powerlessness
- Risk for powerlessness
- Readiness for enhanced self-concept
- Chronic low self-esteem
- Situational low self-esteem
- Risk for situational low self-esteem

Relevant for the Family
- Interrupted family processes
- Readiness for enhanced family processes
- Compromised family coping
- Fear
- Powerlessness
- Risk for powerlessness
- Disabled family coping
- Readiness for enhanced family coping
- Chronic sorrow
- Grieving
- Complicated grieving
- Risk for complicated grieving
- Caregiver role strain
- Risk for caregiver role strain

Relevant for the Community
- Ineffective community coping
- Readiness for enhanced community coping

Goal Setting

Mutual goal setting is a foundation stone of successful rehabilitation. The purpose of goals is to guide the rehabilitation process. Rehabilitation is a process experienced and owned by patients (Pryor, 1999a), and when patients own their rehabilitation goals, they are much more likely to perceive that they have the capabilities to achieve those goals and strive toward them.

Patient participation in the rehabilitation process should be facilitated through the establishment of a partnership between the rehabilitation nurse and the patient. Goal setting is an ideal vehicle for the establishment of that partnership. The goals must be relevant to the patient as well as the domains of expertise of the rehabilitation professionals.

Broad goals that may enhance goal setting and guide rehabilitation nursing practice include maximizing self-determination, restoring function, and optimizing lifestyle choices (Pryor, 1999b).

Patients' goals are usually linked to what matters to them. Lambert (1999) tells how a young man clearly articulated his need to deal with his loss following an above-knee amputation before he learned amputation care. In a review of the literature on patients' experiences of stroke, Hafsteinsdottir and Grypdonck (1997) concluded that "the stroke patient often has clear goals for himself in relation to functional abilities, against which he measures all success and forward progress in his rehabilitation." Rehabilitation nurses need to clearly relate the steps on the way with the patient's personal goals, especially because the steps on the way are often the health provider's focus. Mutual goal setting may provide opportunity to explain the roles of rehabilitation team members and how each contributes toward achieving the patient's goals.

All the patient's goals may influence the effectiveness of the chosen coping strategies. Rehabilitation goals must be achievable; those the patient perceives as unrealistic may act as deterrents to patient participation and become stressors. Goal setting may be a vehicle for fostering hope and harnessing motivation. Recall that self-efficacy is considered to have a positive effect on a person's ability to cope with stressors (Lazarus, 1999). When patients perceive they have a good chance of achieving their goals, they are more likely to achieve them.

The importance of the relationship between rehabilitation nurses and their patients cannot be overstressed because goal setting is about negotiation (Jones, O'Neill, Waterman, & Webb, 1997). Community nurses in one study demonstrated that goal setting is "a matter of balancing the realistic with the desired, the professional view with the lay view, and the objective plan with subjective motivation" (Lawler, Dowswell, Hearn, Forster, & Young, 1999).

TABLE 22-3 Nursing Diagnoses, Interventions, and Outcomes Applicable to Coping　　**NIC/NOC**

Nursing Diagnosis	Nursing Interventions	Nursing Outcomes
Hopelessness	Complex relationship building Decision making support Hope instillation Presence Reminiscence therapy Support group	Depression self control Hope Mood equilibrium Quality of life Will to live
Ineffective coping	Anger control assistance Calming techniques Coping enhancement Decision-making support Emotional support Meditation facilitation Self-esteem enhancement Support system enhancement	Acceptance: Health status Adaptation to physical disability Coping Decision-making Impulse self-control Knowledge: Health resources Role performance Self-esteem
Defensive coping	Complex relationship building Coping enhancement Patient contracting Self-awareness enhancement Socialization enhancement	Acceptance of health status Adaptation to physical disability Coping Grief resolution Self-esteem Social interaction skills
Impaired social interaction	Milieu therapy Normalization promotion Resiliency promotion Self-awareness enhancement Self-esteem enhancement Values clarification	Family social climate Leisure participation Play participation Social interaction skills Social involvement
Chronic sorrow	Grief work facilitation Hope instillation Support group	Grief resolution Hope Mood equilibrium
Caregiver role strain	Abuse protection support: Child, 　domestic partner, elder Caregiver support Parenting promotion Respite care	Caregiver emotional health Caregiver-patient relationship Family resilience Role performance

Data from Moorhead, S., Johnson, M., & Maas, M. (Eds.). (2004). *Nursing outcomes classification (NOC)* (3rd ed.). St. Louis, MO: Mosby; Dochterman, J. M., & Bulechek, G. M. (2004). *Nursing interventions classification (NIC)* (4th ed.). St. Louis, MO: Mosby; and NANDA International. (2007). *NANDA-I nursing diagnoses: Definitions & classification 2007-2008*. Philadelphia: Author.

NOTE: Highlighted interventions are priority interventions, those most likely to resolve the nursing diagnosis.

Goals should facilitate the ability of families or individuals to do the following:

- Activate strengths and resources
- Remove barriers to effective coping
- Establish health maintenance and safety programs
- Identify and resolve issues
- Gain access or referral to resources, services, and activities that promote independence
- Prevent further disability or complications
- Rectify knowledge deficits and enhance capabilities
- Be involved and empowered in planning and decision-making processes
- Use culturally, developmentally, and personally appropriate strategies

- Develop coping responses/behaviors that lead to improved health outcomes

Nursing Outcomes

The ongoing work of the Iowa Outcomes Project is evidence that rehabilitation nurses must continue to demonstrate that they make a difference to the process and outcome of rehabilitation for patients and their families. The identification of desired outcomes helps us clarify our goals and focus our efforts.

Outcomes from Moorhead et al. (2004) that are relevant for the coping-stress tolerance functional health pattern are many and varied. For the individual the relevant outcomes include psychological well-being, psychosocial adaptation, self-control, and social interaction. For the family, relevant outcomes relate to family caregiver performance, family member health status, family well-being and parenting under the domain of family health. The domain of community health is also relevant for rehabilitation nursing. Table 22-3 includes a selection of nursing outcomes related to coping.

Nursing Interventions

Nursing inventions in the coping-stress tolerance functional health pattern have two purposes: the promotion of effective appraisal and coping and the prevention of ineffective appraisal and coping. These are relevant to most of the 28 focal areas in the United States *Healthy People 2010* initiative that established national goals for health (Healthy People 2010, 2005).

Rehabilitation nurses are in an ideal position in their everyday patient-nurse interactions to promote physical activity and fitness; a healthy diet; mental health; the safe use of food and drugs; and the reduction of unintentional injury, suicide, and violence. When health has been interrupted and patients are expending efforts toward rehabilitation, it is an opportune time to raise all aspects of health promotion. When focused on their current health breakdown, most patients appreciate the time taken to explain how they can contribute to their future health status. Rehabilitation nurses can address issues relevant to reducing the risk factors of many diseases, for example, diabetes, heart disease, and stroke.

Prevention and Monitoring of Stress and Coping.
Prevention of health breakdown in general and ineffective coping in particular are integral components of the nursing response relating to the coping-stress tolerance functional health pattern. Although nursing diagnoses are useful in the identification of problems, relying solely on nursing diagnoses may mean that the rehabilitation nurse's vital contribution to prevention is overlooked.

Accurate identification of the environment or resources needed by patients to support their coping efforts enables the rehabilitation nurse to support the patient through considerations such as the following:
- The number of patients in one room
- Choice of roommates
- Choice of preferred recreational, leisure, or social activities
- Peer support programs
- Family participation in therapy program
- Availability of quiet rooms as well as noisy social areas

Ongoing monitoring of the responses of the patient and family members to the current situation will aid the early identification of increasing or overwhelming stress and appropriate interventions. In addition, when patients and their families know someone is monitoring their progress, their ability to cope may be enhanced.

Promotion of Effective Appraisal and Coping. The
nursing interventions identified in this section have been drawn from the Iowa Interventions Project (Dochterman & Bulechek, 2004). They are suggestive of some of the nursing

interventions that may be chosen in response to a comprehensive assessment and the nursing diagnoses identified for an individual patient or family member, family unit, or community. Individual nursing interventions commonly work to both prevent and promote.

Interventions for the coping-stress tolerance functional health pattern could include behavior therapy, cognitive therapy, communication enhancement, coping assistance, patient education, psychological comfort promotion, crisis management, and risk management for the patient. Many of these interventions will also be relevant for members of the patient's family. In addition, life span care particularly targets the family. The community is targeted under community health promotion and community risk management. Table 22-3 includes a selection of nursing interventions relevant to coping.

Nursing interventions for coping enhancement, hope instillation, complex relationship building, support system enhancement, and milieu therapy are discussed below. In Chapters 6 and 29, spirituality and complementary therapies also are related.

Coping Enhancement. Coping enhancement is defined as "assisting a patient to adapt to perceived stressors, changes, or threats that interfere with meeting life demands and roles" (Dochterman & Bulechek, 2004).

Nursing initiatives aimed at coping enhancement can be applied at the single patient or family level and at a program level. At the patient level, nurses can assist patients with processing what has happened to them by encouraging them to tell their story (Nochi, 2000; Woodgate, 2005). By actively listening the nurse will pick up indicators of the person's appraisal of the significance of specific life events and what the person believes can be done about the situation. This provides opportunities for nurses to increase the patient's self-awareness.

A review of the literature by Lucas and Fleming (2005) revealed a range of interventions for improving self-awareness. Restorative/facilitative strategies include education, feedback, behavioral therapy, individual and group counseling/support and psychotherapy, strength-and-weakness lists, and rating task performance. They concluded that much of the work was pioneering and further research is required, especially when seeking effective interventions for increasing self-awareness in persons with brain injury.

Increased self-awareness can provide opportunities for enhancing self-efficacy. Nurses are ideally positioned to positively influence patients' self-perceptions of their ability to manage and cope effectively with interruptions in health. For example, nurse-initiated telephone follow-up increased self-efficacy in managing dyspnea in persons with chronic obstructive pulmonary disease (Wong et al., 2005).

Self-awareness and self-efficacy are precursors to taking charge of one's own life, an important aspect of effective coping. In a study by Kralik, Koch, Price, and Howard (2004) persons with chronic illness created order in their lives by recognizing and monitoring boundaries, mobilizing resources, managing the shift in self-identify, balancing, pacing, planning, and prioritizing. Nurses can facilitate patients' taking charge of their lives, which incorporates self-management, autonomy, and self-direction (McPherson, Brander, Taylor, & McNaughton, 2001).

At the program level, nurses have introduced a variety of initiatives demonstrated to enhance coping. When former rehabilitation patients continued to seek support from the inpatient rehabilitation team through ongoing phone contact, a formal nurse-managed follow-up program was begun. Using a randomized control trial, Rawl, Esaton, Kwiatkowski, Zemen, and Burczyk (1998) implemented a follow-up program consisting of visits and telephone consultations. Although on discharge the anxiety scores of the two groups were similar, 4 months after discharge the 49 patients in the treatment group experienced significantly less anxiety.

The effectiveness of coping effectiveness training for 21- to 60-year-old men living with human immunodeficiency virus (HIV) (n = 128) was studied in a randomized controlled trial by Chesney, Chambers, Taylor, Johnson, and Folkman (2003). After a 3-month intervention phase the men had significantly higher coping self-efficacy and significantly less stress and burnout. The coping effectiveness training included content and practice in problem- and emotion-focused coping strategies, negotiation skills, social support, coping sabotage, hope, and regoaling.

Family coping was enhanced in a study by Kirsch, Brandt, and Lewis (2003) by the use of a home-based patient education program aimed at supporting women with breast cancer in their role as parents helping their children cope. The program provided the mothers with concrete strategies and materials that assisted both parents with talking to their children about their mother's illness and with enhancing their children's ability to cope.

Hope Instillation. Hope instillation is defined as "facilitation of the development of a positive outlook in a given situation" (Dochterman & Bulechek, 2004).

Rehabilitation nurses interact with patients who experience feelings of fear, uncertainty, and loss of body control on a daily basis. Nurses contribute to the development of a positive outlook in a variety of ways. Connelly (2005) explains how nurses can influence parents' perceptions of their child's quality of life by providing "relevant information, reinforcing disease-specific knowledge, and encouraging them to express their feelings and concerns regarding their child's illness with each other and with the nursing and medical staff."

Hope instillation needs to address the individual situation of the patient. Rees and Joslyn (1998) noted that nurses can improve a patient's level of hope by encouraging small successes, emphasizing potential rather than limitations, and providing encouragement to develop a sense of the possible. These findings are supported by a study of Australian rehabilitation nurses (Pryor & Smith, 2002). Empowerment can also be an important mechanism for instilling hope.

Uncertainty is a form of chronic stress that needs to be addressed to develop a positive outlook. In a study by Close and Procter (1999) uncertainty was expressed by both patients

and their caregivers after stroke. These patients "proactively, without explicit guidance, [built] supportive relationships and gain[ed] knowledge and information from those around" to counteract the uncertainty. These findings clearly demonstrate patient self-assessment and motivation to meet identified needs. Furthermore, patients and their families are not passive recipients of care awaiting their fate. Rehabilitation nurses must encourage patient participation in rehabilitation.

Our objectives in providing encouragement are "to help individuals identify consequences of their decisions, define purpose, spur vitality, overcome free-floating anxiety, and try new ways of living, rather than those that would otherwise maintain dependency" (Beck, 1994). Encouraging patients in care of self (i.e., care that goes beyond physical care) is an essential component of rehabilitation nursing (Singleton, 2000). The nurses in Singleton's study used the development of patient-nurse relationships as a vehicle to provide encouragement, and they manipulated their time to facilitate more communication with their patients.

Complex Relationship Building. Complex relationship building is defined as "establishing a therapeutic relationship with a patient who has difficulty interacting with others" (Dochterman & Bulechek, 2004).

The patient who appears isolated and alone is not an unusual phenomenon. Many patients feel no one can understand their situation. Emotions take over, and the ability to develop rapport with others is compromised by the overwhelming nature of the stressors. These patients are sometimes labeled difficult or unpopular.

Several studies have demonstrated the importance of the patient-nurse relationship. Young adults with cancer in a study by Kyngas et al. (2001) valued safe and permanent relationship with health care professionals that enabled them to discuss their disease, its treatment, and coping strategies. Being told of their diagnosis over the phone was particularly distressing. Being believed by health care professionals assisted children age 6 to 17 years in another study (Sallfors et al., 2002) with coping with juvenile chronic arthritis. Lack of understanding caused the children to experience despair.

The literature exposes a concern about patients who do not follow the advice of health professionals and health promotion campaigns, but further exploration of an individual's coping processes may reveal the complexity of the lived experience of compliance or adherence. Wichowski and Kubsch (1997) suggest that by not following recommended regimens, some adults may be able to avoid acknowledging their chronic illnesses. On the other hand, children who have had their disorders since birth or a young age are more likely to accept their health status as normal.

Denial, Lazarus (1999) points out, may be an effective coping strategy in some circumstances. "When nothing can be done to alter the illness or prevent further harm, denial may be beneficial." One teenager used denial effectively to avoid the reality of having paraplegia by deciding to stay in bed for a day. In bed his deficits were not so visible. To the observer, he did not appear to have paraplegia.

Complex relationship building may be a slow process. Nurses must begin by ensuring realistic self-awareness of their own attitudes towards the patient and proceed to develop rapport and trust by listening in a nonjudgmental and unhurried manner. The enhancement of other support systems is essential to minimize patient dependence upon nurses as their sole source of support.

Support System Enhancement. Support system enhancement is defined as "facilitation of support to patient by family, friends and community" (Dochterman & Bulechek, 2004). The findings of many studies highlight the contribution of social support to effective coping, and rehabilitation nurses are ideally situated to assist patients with tapping into the support of their family, friends, and community networks.

When patients are actively seeking social support, nurses can enable family and friends to participate in the patient's rehabilitation (Gustafsson et al., 2002). This may entail a direct approach from the nurse or a welcoming response to approaches from family and friends. Providing information about the injury or illness is often the first step.

Maintaining friendship networks for patients with cognitive impairments is a particular challenge nurses can embrace. Shortly after injury while the person is still in the hospital setting is the time to start. Ask the family to bring in photos of friends, and suggest they contact friends and ask them to visit. By paying particular attention to the need of friends to have the patient's impairments and behaviors explained during those visits, nurses can allay anxieties. Encourage small groups of friends to visit together to create a social atmosphere where the patient can be immersed in peer conversations, jokes, and stories. Asking friends to designate the time they will visit next helps ensure the visit takes place and helps nurses ensure the patient is ready for the visit.

There is growing awareness of the effectiveness of peer support, particularly support from peers with a similar condition or in a similar circumstance. Stewart, Davidson, Meade, Hirth, and Weld-Viscount (2001) found a support group for couples coping with a cardiac condition cofacilitated by a peer and a health care professional was evaluated well by the group participants (n = 28). MacPherson et al. (2004) report on a buddy system for persons with diabetes that was beneficial for patients and their buddies. Important points to remember are that buddies themselves need ongoing support and monitoring especially because not all patient/buddy combinations work well.

The effectiveness of self-help groups has also been studied. Adamsen (2002) reports that persons with life-threatening disease found self-help groups provided them friendship and understanding as they navigated the journey "from victim to agent." The groups provided opportunities "to rebuild their self-confidence, their self-esteem and to build the mental strength that will later make it possible for them to face the world outside the group." Increasingly, the Internet is proving to be an effective medium for accessing peer and social support (Chambers & Connor, 2002; Scharer, 2005).

Milieu Therapy. Milieu therapy is defined as "use of people, resources, and events in the patient's immediate environment to promote optimal psychosocial functioning" (Dochterman & Bulechek, 2004).

The creation of a physical and social environment that is rehabilitative for a particular individual is a complex undertaking in the inpatient setting. The creation of a rehabilitative milieu has been discussed by Pryor (2000) as a mechanism by which rehabilitation nurses can enhance the rehabilitation process for their patients. This will have a positive flow-on for the psychosocial well-being of patients and their families. The main ingredients that contribute to the rehabilitation process were identified as factors associated with the participants, the activities, and the setting. Many of these, in particular ward routines, can be manipulated to enhance their effectiveness. Most importantly, the preservation of an individual patient's identity has been identified as an important aspect of the rehabilitation process.

Kirkevold (1997) notes that nurses need to provide a context conducive to rehabilitation. She describes the integrative function of nursing, which is an important aspect of ensuring that rehabilitation is extended beyond the input of therapists. Ward atmosphere, a subset of the rehabilitative milieu, is heavily influenced by nurses (Waters, 1986). Patients notice that the rehabilitation setting has a different atmosphere from acute care settings. Patients value humor and encouragement in their interactions with rehabilitation nurses.

The resources available for the continuation of rehabilitation by patients and their families play a significant part in milieu therapy. Newall, Wood, Hewer, and Tinson (1997) report a kitchen, computer room, and coffee shop were provided as initiatives to increase patient participation in the activities of daily living beyond the therapy areas. An accessible cafe and breakfast buffet were used similarly in another rehabilitation facility (Weeks & Feuer, 1998).

Music, noise, and human voice in the nurse-patient environment are the focus of work by Pope (1995). Beyond the formal music therapy interventions advocated by Wiens, Riemer, and Guyn (1999), Pope notes that it is each individual's perception of sound that matters. Rehabilitation nurses themselves create sound, as well as intentionally introducing sound in the form of music to their patients' environments. This can be done more therapeutically if nurses learn to interpret patient's responses to sound in its various forms. One patient's therapy may be another patient's torment.

Jenny is a 30-year-old woman who had been a healthy, active woman, a wife, and mother of 2-year-old Tess until 2 weeks before we met, when she suddenly collapsed at home following an intracranial hemorrhage.

On admission to the rehabilitation service, Jenny was dependent on nursing staff for all her personal care needs and activities of daily living. Unable to turn over in the bed, she was incontinent of urine and feces, had difficulty communicating, was unable to swallow safely, and she experienced a right-sided hemiplegia.

Reading Jenny's history revealed a tragic story. Jenny was overseas with her husband, Tran, at the time of her collapse. Tran had taken the overseas posting to extend his experience in the company and increase his chances of a promotion. Jenny was pregnant with her second child when she suffered the hemorrhage. The baby died in utero and was delivered by cesarean section. The baby was of 6 months' gestation and was yet to be buried when Jenny was admitted to the rehabilitation facility. The funeral and burial had been delayed to allow Jenny time to recover sufficiently to attend.

Jenny's rehabilitation commenced with planning her baby's funeral. While Tran made all the arrangements, the rehabilitation nurses worked with Jenny to ensure her wishes were understood by those involved.

As Jenny's communication improved, her anger became apparent to all who came near her. She was extremely frustrated by her deficits and commonly lashed out physically at the nurses. Her verbalizations included swearing and abuse. Jenny did not talk about the baby she had lost or about her family. She expressed anger about her situation and a determination to fight.

All efforts to comfort Jenny were repelled. Jenny did not want to be touched. She would tolerate instrumental touch (for example, assistance with hygiene), but affective touch was unacceptable. She did not want to celebrate her successes, and she did not want to socialize. She wanted to regain her independence and get out of the hospital.

Appearance was important to Jenny, but in her current situation a satisfactory body image was unattainable. She gave up. She started to eat junk food, gain weight, and smoke.

Once Jenny had relearned her self-care skills, she began to relearn the skills she would need to resume her role as primary caregiver of her young daughter. With enormous determination and self-efficacy, Jenny learned how to dress and groom Tess. She also renegotiated her parenting role with Tran.

Jenny demonstrated a degree of hardiness and determination seldom seen. She battled on against enormous adversity and periods of intense loneliness and despair. I never connected with Jenny, but she taught me many things about rehabilitation nursing. The most painful was my experience as spectator of extreme human suffering—forbidden to touch and comfort. The most privileged was the role of learner as Jenny showed us all how she confronted her unbearable situation with determination and honesty.

The nursing diagnoses, desired outcomes, and nursing interventions for the stress-coping tolerance functional health pattern for Jenny and her family are outlined below.

TABLE 22-4 Nursing Diagnoses, Interventions, and Outcomes Applicable to Jenny   NIC/NOC

Cues	Nursing Diagnosis	Nursing Interventions	Desired Outcomes
No risk factors or warning signs of hemorrhage	Ineffective coping (individual)	Grief work facilitation	Jenny sustains a will to live
No opportunity to prepare for stressor		Cognitive restructuring	Jenny maintains hope
Stressors appraised as harm and loss		Coping enhancement	Jenny copes with her stressors effectively
No previous experience with major stressors in life		Active listening	Jenny achieves mood equilibrium
Impaired communication		Hope instillation	Jenny regains a positive body image
Self-care deficit		Body image enhancement	Jenny commences the journey of grief resolution
Inability to meet role expectations as mother and wife		Role enhancement	Jenny develops appropriate and effective social interaction skills
Angry verbal outbursts associated with dependence on nursing staff		Emotional support	Jenny increases her social involvement with family and friends
Abuse of chemical agents		Self-esteem enhancement	Jenny controls her own abusive behaviors
Perception of no control		Mutual goal setting	Jenny's suffering and anguish reduce over time
		Complex relationship building	Jenny experiences increasing levels of psychological comfort
		Health education	
		Learning readiness facilitation	
		Learning facilitation	
		Socialization enhancement	
Primary support unable to provide sufficient, effective support and comfort	Compromised family coping	Active listening	Family uses effective coping strategies
Limited interaction between Jenny and her family		Grief work facilitation	Family is able to meet Jenny's support needs
Tran expresses little insight into Jenny's psychosocial needs		Role enhancement	Family integrity is maintained
		Emotional support	Family participates in decision making and provision of care
		Caregiver support	
		Family integrity promotion	
		Family involvement promotion	

Case Study—cont'd

TABLE 22-4 Nursing Diagnoses, Interventions and Outcomes Applicable to Jenny—cont'd

NIC/NOC

Cues	Nursing Diagnosis	Nursing Interventions	Desired Outcomes
Jenny's mother has chronic health problems that prevent her from visiting frequently and caring for Tess		Family process maintenance Family support Hope instillation Health education	Tran maintains a satisfactory level of well-being Tran positively appraises own abilities as caregiver Tran and Jenny develop a positive relationship in the roles of caregiver and care recipient

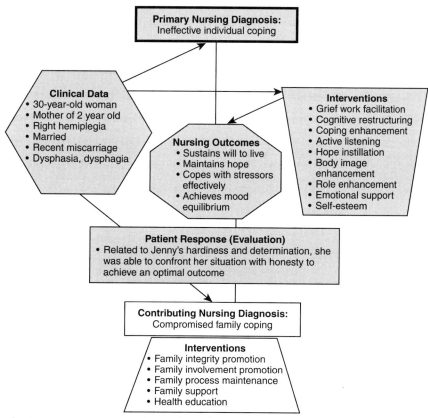

Concept Map. Jenny's situation is quite complex and involves many functional concerns in addition to the psychosocial issues and coping concerns. Focusing on coping strategies is the most logical priority since techniques used should provider Jenny with self-care and self-improvement strategies that will fit within her lifestyle and be most likely to meet with success for her family.

CRITICAL THINKING

1. Review Box 22-2 to identify the many unbearable aspects of Jenny's situation. Discuss how you could enable a patient with newly acquired communication impairments to tell his or her story to ensure an accurate coping-stress tolerance assessment is recorded.

2. Review the types of cognitive appraisal in Box 22-3, and discuss the primary and secondary appraisals that Jenny may have made and then the reappraisals. Identify other patients who have made similar appraisals, and explore similarities and difference between their biographies.

3. Identify and analyze nursing interventions that you could use to help Jenny reappraise her self-image more positively and reappraise what might and could be done to enhance her self-image. In particular, consider how you would include Jenny's family.

4. Jenny was very angry about what had happened to her. Discuss how Jenny and other patients use anger to facilitate effective coping and how as rehabilitation nurses we can enable patients to harness the energy of their anger and use it therapeutically.

REFERENCES

Adamsen, L. (2002). 'From victim to agent': The clinical and social significance of self-help group participation for people with life-threatening diseases. *Scandinavian Journal of Caring Sciences, 16,* 224-231.

Adamsen, L., Rasmussen, J. M., & Pedersen, L. S. (2001). 'Brothers in arms': How men with cancer experience a sense of comradeship through group intervention which combines physical activity with information relay. *Journal of Clinical Nursing, 10,* 528-537.

Ahlstrom, G., & Wenneberg, S. (2002). Coping with illness-related problems in persons with progressive muscular diseases: The Swedish version of the ways of coping questionnaire. *Scandinavian Journal of Caring Sciences, 16,* 368-375.

Andren, S., & Elmstahl, S. (2005). Family caregivers' subjective experiences of satisfaction in dementia care: Aspects of burden, subjective health and sense of coherence. *Scandinavian Journal of Caring Sciences, 19,* 157-168.

Angell, K. L., Kreshka, M. A., McCoy, R., Donnelly, P., Turner-Cobb, J. M., Graddy, K., et al. (2003). Psychosocial intervention for rural women with breast cancer. *Journal of General Internal Medicine, 18,* 499-507.

Antonak, R. F., & Livneh, H. (1991). A hierarchy of reactions to disability. *International Journal of Rehabilitation Research, 14,* 13-24.

Antonovsky, A. (1972). Breakdown: A needed fourth step in the conceptual armamentarium of modern medicine. *Social Science and Medicine, 6,* 537-544.

Antonovsky, A. (1979). *Health, stress and coping.* San Francisco: Jossey-Bass.

Antonovsky, A. (1996). The salutogenic model as a theory to guide health promotion. *Health Promotion International, 11*(1), 11-18.

Austenfeld, J. L., & Stanton, A. L. (2004). Coping through emotional approach: A new look at emotion, coping, and health-related outcomes. *Journal of Personality, 72*(6), 1335-1363.

Babrow, A. S., Kasch, C. R., & Ford, L. A. (1998). The many meanings of uncertainty in illness: Towards a systematic accounting. *Health Communication, 10*(1), 1-23.

Bandura, A. (1997). *Self-efficacy: The exercise of control.* New York: W. H. Freeman.

Beck, R. J. (1994, July/August/September). Encouragement as a vehicle to empowerment in counseling: An existential perspective. *Journal of Rehabilitation,* 6-11.

Belciug, M. P. (2001). Coping responses in patients with spinal cord injury and adjustment difficulties. *International Journal of Rehabilitation Research, 24*(2), 157-159.

Berglund, B., Mattiasson, A-C., & Nordstrom, G. (2003). Acceptance of disability and sense of coherence in individuals with Ehlers-Danlos syndrome. *Journal of Clinical Nursing, 12,* 770-777.

Bergs, D. (2002). 'The Hidden Client'—women caring for husbands with COPD: Their experience of quality of life. *Journal of Clinical Nursing, 11,* 613-621.

Bluvol, A., & Ford-Gilboe, M. (2004). Hope, health work and quality of life in families of stroke survivors. *Journal of Advanced Nursing, 48*(4), 322-332.

Cannon, W. B. (1914). The interrelations of emotions as suggested by recent physiological researches. *American Journal of Psychology, 25,* 256-282.

Cannon, W. B. (1935). Stresses and strains of homeostasis. *The American Journal of the Medical Sciences, 189*(1), 1-14.

Carter, P. A. (2003). Family caregivers' sleep loss and depression over time. *Cancer Nursing, 26*(4), 253-259.

Chambers, M., & Connor, S. L (2002). User-friendly technology to help family care givers cope. *Journal of Advanced Nursing, 40*(5), 568-577.

Charmaz, K. (1983). Loss of self: A fundamental form of suffering in the chronically ill. *Sociology of Health and Illness, 5*(2), 168-195.

Charmaz, K. (1987). Struggling for a self: Identity levels of the chronically ill. *Sociology of Health Care, 6,* 283-321.

Charmaz, K. (1995). The body, identity and self: Adapting to impairment. *The Sociology Quarterly, 36*(4), 657-680.

Chesney, M. A., Chambers, D. B., Taylor, J. M., Johnson, L. M., & Folkman, S. (2003). Coping effectiveness training for men living with HIV: Results from a randomized clinical trial testing a group-based intervention. *Psychosomatic Medicine, 65,* 1038-1046.

Chotard, V., Caplan, A., & Seidman, E. G. (2004). Coping and resilience in pediatric Crohn's disease. *Journal of Pediatric Gastroenterology and Nutrition, 39*(Suppl. 1), S332.

Clark, A. M., Barbour, R. S., White, M., & MacIntyre, P. D. (2004). Promoting participation in cardiac rehabilitation: Patient choices and experiences. *Journal of Advanced Nursing, 47*(1), 5-14.

Close, H., & Procter, S. (1999). Coping strategies used by hospitalized stroke patients: Implications for continuity and management of care. *Journal of Advanced Nursing, 29*(1), 138-144.

Connelly, T. W. (2005). Family functioning and hope in children with juvenile rheumatoid arthritis. *Journal of Maternal and Child Nursing, 30*(4), 245-250.

Derks, W., DeLeeuw, J. R. J., Hordijk, G. J., & Winnubst, J. A. M. (2005). Differences in coping style and locus of control between older and younger patients with head and neck cancer. *Clinical Otolaryngology, 30,* 186-192.

Dewar, A. (2001). Protecting strategies used by sufferers of catastrophic illnesses and injuries. *Journal of Clinical Nursing, 10,* 600-608.

Dewar, A. L., & Morse, J. M. (1995). Unbearable incidents: Failure to endure the experience of illness. *Journal of Advanced Nursing, 22,* 957-964.

Dochterman, J. M., & Bulechek, G. M. (2004). *Nursing interventions classification (NIC)* (4th ed.). St. Louis, MO: Mosby.

Dowd, T., Kolcaba, C., & Steiner, R. (2006). Development of the healing touch comfort questionnaire. *Holistic Nursing Practice, 20*(3), 122-129.

Driedger, S. M., Crooks, V. A., & Bennett D. (2004). Engaging in the disablement process over space and time: Narratives of persons with multiple sclerosis in Ottawa, Canada. *The Canadian Geographer, 48*(2), 119-136.

Easton, K. L., Rawl, S. M., Zemen, D., Kwiatkowski, S., & Burczyk, B. (1995). The effects of nursing follow-up on the coping strategies used by rehabilitation patients after discharge. *Rehabilitation Nursing Research, 4*(4), 119-127.

Faircloth, C. A., Boylstein, C., Rittman, M., Young, M. E., & Gubrium, J. (2004). Sudden illness and biographical flow in narratives of stroke recovery. *Sociology of Health & Illness, 26*(2), 242-261.

Felder, B. (2004). Hope and coping in patients with cancer diagnoses. *Cancer Nursing, 27*(4), 320-324.

Folkman, S. (1997). Positive psychological states and coping with severe stress. *Social Science Medicine, 45*(8), 1207-1221.

Folkman, S., & Lazarus, R. S. (1988). *Ways of Coping Questionnaire sampler set manual, test booklet, scoring key.* Palo Alto, CA: Mind Garden.

Fortune, D. G., Richards, H. L., Main, C. J., & Griffiths, C. E. M. (2002). Patients' strategies for coping with psoriasis. *Clinical and Experimental Dermatology, 27,* 177-184.

Fosberg, A., Backman, L., & Svensson, E. (2002). Liver transplant recipients' ability to cope during the first 12 months after transplantation: A prospective study. *Scandanavian Journal of Caring Sciences. 16,* 345-352.

Garralda, M. E., & Rangel, L. (2004). Impairment and coping in children and adolescents with chronic fatigue syndrome: A comparative study with other paediatric disorders. *Journal of Child Psychology and Psychiatry, 45*(3), 543-552.

Geanellos, R. (2005). Undermining self-efficacy: The consequence of nurse unfriendliness on client wellbeing. *Collegian, 12*(4), 9-14.

Gignac, M. A. M., & Gottlieb, B. H. (1997). Changes in coping with chronic stress: The role of caregivers' appraisals of coping efficacy. In B. H. Gottlieb (Ed.), *Coping with chronic stress* (pp. 245-267). New York: Plenum Press.

Gustafson, D. H., Hawkins, R., Pingree, S., McTavish, F., Arora, N. K., Mendenhall, J., et al. (2001). Effect of computer support on younger women with breast cancer. *Journal of General Internal Medicine, 16,* 435-445.

Gustafsson, M., Persson, L-O., & Amilon, A. (2002). A qualitative study of coping in the early stage of acute traumatic hand injury. *Journal of Clinical Nursing, 11,* 594-602.

Hafsteinsdottir, T. B., & Grypdonck, M. (1997). Being a stroke patient: A review of the literature. *Journal of Advanced Nursing, 26,* 580-588.

Hagren, B., Pettersen, I-M., Severinsson, E., Lutzen, K., & Clyne, N. (2005). Maintenance haemodialysis: Patients' experiences of their life situation. *Journal of Clinical Nursing, 14,* 294-300.

Han, H-R. (2003). Korean mothers' psychosocial adjustment to their children's cancer. *Journal of Advanced Nursing, 44*(5), 499-506.

Hardy, S. E., Concato, J., & Gill, T. (2004). Resilience of community-dwelling older persons. *Journal of the American Geriatrics Society, 52,* 257-262.

Harms, L. (2004). After the accident: Survivors' perceptions of recovery following road trauma. *Australian Social Work, 57*(2), 161-174.

Hartley, S., Ojwang, P., Baguwemu, A., Ddamulira, M., & Chavuta, A. (2005). How do carers of disabled children cope? The Ugandan perspective. *Child: Care, Health & Development, 31*(2), 167-180.

Healthy People 2010. (2005). Available from http://www.health.gov/healthypeople/.

Helseth, S., & Ulfsæt, N. (2003). Having a parent with cancer. *Cancer Nursing, 26*(5), 355-362.

Hilton, B. A., Crawford, J. A., & Tarko, M. A. (2000) Men's perspectives on individual and family coping with their wives' breast cancer and chemotherapy. *Western Journal of Nursing Research, 22,* 438-459.

Hjorleifsdottir, E., Hallberg, I. R., Bolmsjo, L. A., & Gunnardsdottir, E. D. (2005). Distress and coping in cancer patients: Feasibility of the Icelandic version of BSI 18 and the WOC_CA questionnaires. *European Journal of Cancer Care,* 1-10.

Hobdell, E. (2004). Chronic sorrow and depression in parents of children with neural tube defects. *Journal of Neuroscience Nursing, 36*(2), 82-88, 94.

Hornsten, A., Norberg, A., & Lundman, B. (2002). Psychosocial maturity among people with diabetes mellitus. *Journal of Clinical Nursing, 11*, 777-784.

Houtzager, B. A., Grootenhuis, M. A., Hoekstra-Weebers, J. E. H. M., & Last, B. F. (2005). One month after diagnosis: Quality of life, coping and previous functioning in siblings of children with cancer. *Child: Care, Health & Development, 31*(1), 75-87.

Irurita, V. (2000). Preserving integrity. In J. Greenwood (Ed.), *Nursing theory in Australia* (pp. 274-309). Frenchs Forest NSW: Pearson Education Australia.

Jones, G. C., & Kilpatrick, A. C. (1996). Wellness theory: A discussion and application to clients with disabilities. *Families in Society: The Journal of Contemporary Human Services, 77*(5), 259-268.

Jones, M., O'Neill, P., Waterman, H., & Webb, C. (1997). Building a relationship: Communication and relationships between staff and stroke patients on a rehabilitation ward. *Journal of Advanced Nursing, 26*, 101-110.

Karner, A. M., Dahlgren, M. A., & Bergdahl, B. (2004). Rehabilitation after coronary heart disease: Spouses' views of support. *Journal of Advanced Nursing, 46*(2), 204-211.

Kelso, T., French, D., & Fernandez, M. (2005). Stress and coping in primary caregivers of children with a disability: A qualitative study using the Lazarus and Folkman Process Model of Coping. *Journal of Research in Special Educational Needs, 5*(1), 3-10.

Kim, H. W., Greenberg, J. S., Seltzer, M. M., & Krauss, M. W. (2003). The role of coping in maintaining the well-being of mothers of adults with intellectual disability and mental illness. *Journal of Intellectual Disability Research, 47*(4/5), 313-327.

Kirkevold, M. (1997). The role of nursing in the rehabilitation of acute stroke patients: Towards a unified theoretical perspective. *Advances in Nursing Science, 19*(4), 55-64.

Kirsch, S. E. D., Brandt, P. A., & Lewis, F. M. (2003). Making the most of the moment. *Cancer Nursing, 26*(1), 47-54.

Kobasa, S. C. (1979). Stressful life events, personality, and health: An inquiry into hardiness. *Journal of Personality and Social Psychology, 37*, 1-11.

Kobasa, S. C., Maddi, S. R., & Kahn, S. (1982). Hardiness and health: A prospective study. *Journal of Personality and Social Psychology, 42*, 168-172.

Kobasa, S. C., Maddi, S. R., & Zola, M. A. (1983). Type A and hardiness. *Journal of Behavioral Medicine, 6*, 41-51.

Kolcaba, K. Y. (1991). A taxonomic structure for the concept of comfort. *Image—Journal of Nursing Scholarship, 23*(4), 237-240.

Kolcaba, K.Y. (1995). Comfort as process and product, merged in holistic nursing art. *Journal of Holistic Nursing, 13*(2), 117-131.

Kralik, D. (2002). The quest for ordinariness: Transition experienced by midlife women living with chronic illness. *Journal of Advanced Nursing, 39*(2), 146-154.

Kralik, D., Koch., T., Price, K., & Howard, N. (2004). Chronic illness self-management: Taking action to create order. *Journal of Clinical Nursing, 13*, 259-267.

Kristofferzon, M-L., Lofmark, R., & Carlsson, M. (2003). Myocardial infarction: Gender differences in coping and social support. *Journal of Advanced Nursing, 44*(4), 360-374.

Kuo, T-T., & Ma, F-C. (2002). Symptom distresses and coping strategies in patients with non-small cell lung cancer. *Cancer Nursing, 25*(4), 309-317.

Kuuppelomaki, M., Saski, A., Yamanda, K., Asakawa, N., & Shimanouchi, S. (2004). Coping strategies of family carers for older relatives in Finland. *Journal of Clinical Nursing, 13*, 697-706.

Kyngas, H., Mikkonen, R., Nousiainen, E-M., Rytilahti, M., Seppanen, P., Vaattovaara, R., et al. (2001). Coping with the onset of cancer: Coping strategies and resources of young people with cancer. *European Journal of Cancer Care, 10*, 6-11.

Lackey, N. R., & Gates, M. F. (2001). Adults' recollections of their experiences as young caregivers of family members with chronic physical illnesses. *Journal of Advanced Nursing, 34*(3), 320-328.

Lambert, J. (1999). Meeting the emotional needs of a patient. *Rehabilitation Nursing, 24*(4), 141-142.

Langford, C. P. H., Bowsher, J., Maloney, J. P., & Lillis, P. P. (1997). Social support: A conceptual analysis. *Journal of Advanced Nursing, 25*, 95-100.

Larson, J., Franzen-Dahlin, A., Billing, E., Von Arbin, M., Murray, V., & Wredling, R. (2005). The impact of a nurse-led support and education programme for spouses of stroke patients: A randomized controlled trial. *Journal of Clinical Nursing, 14*, 995-1003.

Lau-Walker, M. (2004a). Cardiac rehabilitation: The importance of patient expectations—a practitioner survey. *Journal of Clinical Nursing, 13*, 177-184.

Lau-Walker, M. (2004b). Relationship between illness representation and self-efficacy. *Journal of Advanced Nursing, 48*(3), 216-225.

Lawler, J., Dowswell, G., Hearn, J., Forster, A., & Young, J. (1999). Recovering from stroke: A qualitative investigation of the role of goal setting in late stroke recovery. *Journal of Advanced Nursing, 30*(2), 401-409.

Lazarus, R. (1991). *Emotion and adaptation.* New York: Oxford University Press.

Lazarus, R. (1999). *Stress and emotion: A new synthesis.* New York: Springer.

Lazarus, R. S., & Folkman, S. (1984). *Stress, appraisal, and coping.* New York: Springer.

Leidy, N., & Haase, J. (1999). Functional status from the patient's perspective: The challenge of preserving personal integrity. *Research in Nursing & Health, 22*, 67-77.

Link, L. B., Mancuso, C. A., & Charlson, M. E. (2004). How do cancer patients who try to take control of their disease differ from those who do not? *European Journal of Cancer Care, 13*, 219-226.

Livneh, H., & Antonak, R. F. (1997). *Psychosocial adaptation to chronic illness and disability.* Gaithersburg, MD: Aspen.

Lohne, V., & Severinsson, E. (2004). Hope during the first months after acute spinal cord injury. *Journal of Advanced Nursing, 47*(3), 279-286.

Lohne, V., & Severinsson E., (2005). Patients' experiences of hope and suffering during the first year following acute spinal cord injury. *Journal of Clinical Nursing, 14*, 285-293.

Lowit, A., & van Teijlingen, E. R. (2005). Avoidance as a strategy of (not) coping: Qualitative interviews with carers of Huntington's disease patients. *BioMed Central Family Practice, 6*(38), 1-9.

Lowton, K., & Gabe, J. (2003). Life on a slippery slope: Perceptions of health in adults with cystic fibrosis. *Sociology of Health & Illness, 25*(4), 289-319.

Lucas, S. E., & Fleming, J. M. (2005). Interventions for improving self-awareness following acquired brain injury. *Australian Occupational Therapy Journal, 52*, 160-170.

MacPherson, S. L., Joseph, D., & Sullivan, E. (2004). The benefits of peer support with diabetes. *Nursing Forum, 39*(4), 5-12.

Maddi, S. R., & Kobasa, S. C. (1991). The development of hardiness. In A. Monat & R. S. Lazarus (Eds.), *Stress and coping: An anthology* (pp. 245-257). New York: Columbia University Press.

Man, D. W. K. (2002). Hong Kong family caregivers' stress and coping for people with brain injury. *International Journal of Rehabilitation Research, 25*(4), 287-295

Martin, D., & Bat-Chava, Y. (2003). Negotiating deaf-hearing friendships: Coping strategies of deaf boys and girls in mainstream schools. *Child: Care, Health & Development, 29*(6), 511-521.

McCausland, J. (2001). Experiences of well spouses after lung transplantation. *Journal of Advanced Nursing, 34*(4), 493-500.

McConaghy, R., & Caltabiano, M. L. (2005). Caring for a person with dementia: Exploring relationships between perceived burden, depression, coping and well-being. *Nursing and Health Sciences, 7*, 81-91.

McGrath, P. (2004). Reflections on serious illness as spiritual journey by survivors of haematological malignancies. *European Journal of Cancer Care, 13*, 227-237.

McPherson, K.M., Brander, P., Taylor, W. J., & McNaughton, H. K. (2001). Living with arthritis—what is important? *Disability and Rehabilitation, 23*(16), 706-721.

Melanson, P. M., & Downe-Wamboldt, B. (2003). Confronting life with rheumatoid arthritis. *Journal of Advanced Nursing, 42*(2), 125-133.

Mishel, M. H. (1990). Reconceptualization of the uncertainty in illness theory. *Image—Journal of Nursing Scholarship, 22*(4), 256-262.

Mitchell, M., Courtney, M., & Coyer, F. (2003). Understanding uncertainty and minimizing families' anxiety at the time of transfer from intensive care. *Nursing and Health Sciences, 5*, 207-217.

Moorhead, S., Johnson, M., & Maas, M. (Eds.). (2004). *Nursing outcomes classification (NOC)* (3rd ed.). St. Louis, MO: Mosby.

Morse, J. M. (1997). Responding to threats to integrity of self. *Advances in Nursing Science, 19*(4), 21-36.

Morse, J. M., Bottorff, J. L., & Hutchinson, S. (1995). The paradox of comfort. *Nursing Research, 44*(1), 14-19.

Morse, J. M., & Carter, B. J. (1995). Strategies of enduring and the suffering of loss: Modes of comfort used by a resilient survivor. *Holistic Nursing Practice, 9*(3), 38-52.

Mu, P-F. (2005). Paternal reactions to a child with epilepsy: Uncertainty, coping strategies, and depression. *Journal of Advanced Nursing, 49*(4), 367-376.

NANDA International. (2007). *NANDA-I nursing diagnoses: Definitions & classification 2007-2008.* Philadelphia: Author.

Newall, J. T., Wood, V. A., Hewer, R. L., & Tinson, D. J. (1997). Development of a neurological rehabilitation environment: An observational study. *Clinical Rehabilitation, 11*, 146-155.

Nilsson, I., Axelsson, K., Gustafson, Y., Lundman, B., & Norberg, A. (2001). Well-being, sense of coherence, and burnout in stroke victims and spouses during the first few months after stroke. *Scandinavian Journal of Caring Sciences, 15,* 203-214.

Nochi, M. (2000). Reconstructing self-narratives in coping with traumatic brain injury. *Social Science & Medicine, 51,* 1795-1804.

O'Connell, B., & Baker, L. (2004). Managing as carers of stroke survivors: Strategies from the field. *International Journal of Nursing Practice, 10,* 121-126.

O'Connor, M. (2004). Transitions in status from wellness to illness, illness to wellness. In S. Payne, J. Seymour, & C. Ingleton (Eds.), *Palliative care nursing principles & evidence for practice* (pp. 126-141). Berkshire U.K.: Open University Press.

Olshansky, S. (1966). Parent responses to a mentally defective child. *Mental Retardation, 5*(4), 21-23.

Orr, E., & Westman, M. (1990). Does hardiness moderate stress, and how? A review. In M. Rosenbaum (Ed.), *Learned resourcefulness: On coping, self-control, and adaptive behavior* (pp. 64-94). New York: Springer.

Pagano, M. E., Skokol, A. E., Stout, R. L., Shea, M. T., Yen, S., Grilo, C. M., et al. (2004). Stressful life events as predictors of functioning: Findings from the Collaborative Longitudinal Personality Disorders Study. *Acta Psychiatrica Scandinavica, 110,* 421-429.

Park, C. L., & Folkman, S. (1997). Meaning in the context of stress and coping. *Review of General Psychology, 1*(2), 115-144.

Parsons, T. (1951). *The social system.* New York: The Free Press.

Pollock, S. (1986). Human responses to chronic illness: Physiologic and psychological adaptation. *Nursing Research, 35,* 90-95.

Pollock, S. E. (1989). The hardiness characteristic: A motivating factor in adaptation. *Advances in Nursing Science, 11,* 53-62.

Pope, D. S. (1995). Music, noise, and the human voice in the nurse-patient environment. *Image–Journal of Nursing Scholarship, 27*(4), 291-296.

Pryor, J. (1999a). Nursing and rehabilitation. In J. Pryor (Ed.), *Rehabilitation: A vital nursing function* (pp. 1-13). Deakin, ACT, Australia: Royal College of Nursing Australia.

Pryor, J. (1999b). Goals and focus. In J. Pryor (Ed.), *Rehabilitation: A vital nursing function* (pp. 79-96). Deakin, ACT, Australia: Royal College of Nursing Australia.

Pryor, J. (2000). Creating a rehabilitative milieu. *Rehabilitation Nursing, 25*(4), 141-144.

Pryor, J., & Smith C. (2002). A framework for the role of registered nurses in the specialty practice of rehabilitation nursing in Australia. *Journal of Advanced Nursing, 39*(2), 249-257.

Rawl, S. M., Easton, K. L., Kwiatkowski, S., Zemen, D., & Burczyk, B. (1998). Effectiveness of a nurse-managed follow-up program for rehabilitation patients after discharge. *Rehabilitation Nursing, 23*(4), 204-209.

Rees, C., & Joslyn, S. (1998). The importance of hope. *Nursing Standard, 12*(41), 34-35.

Richardson, A., Adner, N., & Nordstrom, G. (2001). Persons with insulin-dependent diabetes mellitus: Acceptance and coping ability. *Journal of Advanced Nursing, 33*(6), 758-763.

Roberts, J. S., Connell, C. M., Cisewski, D., Hipps, Y. G., Demissie, S., & Green., R.C. (2003). Differences between African Americans and whites in their perceptions of Alzheimer disease. *Alzheimer Disease and Associated Disorders, 17*(1), 19-26.

Rogers, M. L., & Hogan, D. P. (2003). Family life with children with disabilities: The key role of rehabilitation. *Journal of Marriage and Family, 65,* 818-833.

Rosenbaum, M. (1990). The role of learned resourcefulness in the self-control of health behavior. In M. Rosenbaum (Ed.), *Learned resourcefulness: On coping skills, self-control, and adaptive behavior* (pp. 3-30). New York: Springer.

Sallfors, C., Fasth, A., & Hallberg, L. R-M. (2002). Oscillating between hope and despair—a qualitative study. *Child: Care, Health & Development, 28*(6), 495-505.

Saloviita, T., Italinna, M., & Leinonen, E. (2003). Explaining the parental stress of fathers and mothers caring for a child with intellectual disability: A double ABCX model. *Journal of Intellectual Disability Research, 47,* 300-312.

Sawatay, J. E., & Fowler-Kerry, S. (2003). Impact of caregiving: Listening to the voice of informal caregivers. *Journal of psychiatric and Mental Health Nursing, 10,* 277-286.

Scharer, K. (2005). Internet social support for parents: The state of the science. *Journal of Child and Adolescent Psychiatric Nursing, 18*(1), 26-35.

Scheier, M. F., & Carver, C. S. (1987). Dispositional optimism and physical well-being: The influence of generalized outcomes expectancies on health. *Journal of Personality, 55*(2), 169-210.

Seigley, L. A. (1999). Self-esteem and health behavior: Theoretical and empirical links. *Nursing Outlook, 47*(2), 74-77.

Selye, H. (1976). *The stress of life.* New York: McGraw-Hill.

Shaw, C., McColl, E., & Bond, S. (2003). The relationship of perceived control to outcomes in older women undergoing surgery for fractured neck of femur. *Journal of Clinical Nursing, 12,* 117-123.

Sherwood, P., Given, B., Given, C., Schiffman, R., Murman, D., & Lovely, M. (2004). Caregivers of persons with a brain tumor: A conceptual model. *Nursing Inquiry, 11*(1), 43-53.

Singleton, J. K. (2000). Nurses' perspectives of encouraging clients' care-of-self in a short-term rehabilitation unit within a long-term care facility. *Rehabilitation Nursing, 25*(1), 23-30, 35.

Sit, J. W. H., Wong, T. K. S., Clinton, M., Li, L. S. W., & Fong, Y-M. (2004). Stroke care in the home: The impact of social support on the general health of family caregivers. *Journal of Clinical Nursing, 13,* 816-824.

Stewart, M., Davidson, K., Meade, D., Hirth, A., & Weld-Viscount, P. (2001). Group support for couples with a cardiac condition. *Journal of Advanced Nursing, 33*(2), 190-199.

St-Louis, L., & Robichaud-Ekstrand, S. (2003). Knowledge level and coping strategies according to coagulation levels in older persons with atrial fibrillation. *Nursing and Health Sciences, 5,* 67-75.

Svavarsdottir, E. K., Rayens, M. K. & McCubbin, M. (2005). Predictors of adaptation in Icelandic and American families of young children with chronic asthma. *Family & Community Health, 28*(4), 338-350.

Tak, S. H., & Laffrey S. C. (2003). Life satisfaction and its correlates in older women with osteoarthritis. *Orthopaedic Nursing, 22*(3), 182-189.

Tak, Y. R., & McCubbin, M. (2002). Family stress, perceived social support and coping following the diagnosis of a child's congenital heart disease. *Journal of Advanced Nursing, 39*(2), 190-198.

Tan, G., Jensen, M. P., Thornby, J., & Anderson, K. O. (2005). Ethnicity, control appraisal, coping and adjustment to chronic pain among black and white Americans. *American Academy of Pain Medicine, 6*(1), 18-28.

Thompson, S. C. (1991). The search for meaning following stroke. *Basic and Applied Psychology, 12*(1), 81-96.

Tomberg, T., Orasson, A., Linnamagi, U., Toomela, A., Pulver, A., & Asser, T. (2001). Coping strategies in patients following subarachnoid haemorrhage. *Acta Neurological Scandinavia, 104,* 148-155.

Trollvik, A., & Severinsson, E. (2004). Parents' experiences of asthma: Process from chaos to coping. *Nursing and Health Sciences, 6,* 93-99.

Van Der Lee, M. L., Swarte, N. B., Van Der Bom, J. G., Van Den Bout, J., & Heintz, A. P. M. (2005). Positive feelings among terminally ill cancer patients. *European Journal of Cancer Care, 1-5.*

Villagomeza, L. R. (2005, November/December). Spiritual distress in adult cancer patients. *Holistic Nursing Practice, 285-294.*

Ville, I. (2005). Biographical work and returning to employment following a spinal cord injury. *Sociology of Health & Illness, 27*(3), 324-350.

Waters, K. (1986). The role of nursing in rehabilitation. *CARE-Science and Practice, 5*(3), 17-21.

Weeks, S. K., & Feuer, T. E. (1998). The rehab cafe and breakfast buffet. *Rehabilitation Nursing, 23*(1), 46.

Welch, J. L., & Austin, J. K. (2001). Stressors, coping and depression in haemodialysis patients. *Journal of Advanced Nursing, 33*(2), 200-207.

Wheaton, B. (1997). The nature of chronic stress. In B. H. Gottlieb (Ed.), *Coping with chronic stress.* (pp. 43-74). New York: Plenum Press.

Wichowski, H. C., & Kubsch, S. M. (1997). The relationship of self-perception of illness and compliance with health regimens. *Journal of Advanced Nursing, 25,* 548-553.

Wiens, M. E., Reimer, M. A. & Guyn, H. L. (1999). Music therapy as a treatment method for improving respiratory muscle strength in patients with advanced multiple sclerosis: A pilot study. *Rehabilitation Nursing, 24*(2), 74-80.

Wong, K. W., Wong, F. K. Y., & Chan, M. F. (2005). Effects of nurse-initiated telephone follow-up on self-efficacy among patients with chronic obstructive pulmonary disease. *Journal of Advanced Nursing, 49*(2), 210-222.

Wonghongkul, T., Moore, S. M., Musil, C., Schneider, S., & Deimling G. (2000). The influence of uncertainty in illness, stress appraisal, and hope on coping in survivors of breast cancer. *Cancer Nursing, 23*(6), 422-429.

Woodgate, R. L. (2005). Life is never the same: Childhood cancer narratives. *European Journal of Cancer Care, 1-11.*

World Health Organisation. (2001). *International Classification of Functioning, Disability and Health.* Geneva: World Health Organisation.

Wrubel, J., Richards, T. A., Folkman, S., & Acree, M. C. (2001). Tacit definitions of informal caregiving. *Journal of Advanced Nursing, 33*(2), 175-181.

Zemper, E. D., Tate, D. G., Roller, S., Forchheimer, M., Chiodo, A., Nelson, V. S., et al. (2003). Assessment of a holistic wellness program for persons with spinal cord injury. *American Journal of Physical Medicine & Rehabilitation, 82*(12), 957-968.

23

Rehabilitation Involving the Senses, Sensation, Perception, and Pain

Pamela M. Duchene, DNSc, RN, CNAA

THE SENSES

The primary method through which we understand, interpret, and respond to the world around us is through the senses: vision, hearing, taste, smell, and touch. Interpretation of the environment requires that each of the senses be intact. Loss of one or more of the senses places the individual at risk. For example, older persons who experience loss of olfactory acuity cannot smell the characteristic sulfur odor that emanates from a gas stove leak. For safety they can compensate by using an electric stove. Similarly the visual system requires function of the eyes and their associated systems in conjunction with the cerebrum in order to make sense of the world. Individuals with a loss of vision may compensate through assistive devices, seeing-eye dogs and the use of Braille. In this chapter each of the senses, including the sensation of pain, will be reviewed. Common impairments, nursing interventions and outcomes, as well as rehabilitation strategies and advocacy programs are identified.

Cranial Nerves

Understanding of the structure and function of sensation logically begins with a discussion of the cranial nerves. A full review of cranial nerves is included in Chapter 21. There are 12 pairs of cranial nerves, which exit and enter the cranium. Cranial nerves associated with motor function are efferent fibers, transmitting impulses from the brain to muscle fibers, for control of eye movements (CN III, IV, VI), face (CN VII), pharynx and palate (CN IX, X), tongue (CN XII), and shoulders (CN XI). The cranial nerves associated with sensory function are afferent fibers, transmitting impulses from tissue to the brain, and include smell (CN I), visual acuity (CN II), pupillary actions (CN II, III), face (CN V), hearing (CN VIII),

and pharynx and palate (CN IX, X). A brief assessment of the cranial nerves is presented in Table 23-1.

Vision

Healthy People 2010 (U.S. Department of Health and Human Services [USDHHS], 2000) targets a reduction of blindness and visual impairment in those younger than 17 years from 25 in 1000 to less than 20 in 1000. According to the Centers for Disease Control and Prevention (2004), vision impairment is considered to be self-reported blindness in either or both eyes.

Anatomy and Physiology. The eye has three layers, the fibrous tunic, the vascular tunic, and the nervous tunic. The fibrous tunic, including the cornea (Figure 23-1) and the sclera, functions as a protective barrier to the more fragile components of the eye. This layer causes tearing and blinking in response to foreign bodies and prevents microorganisms and chemicals from penetrating the eye.

The middle layer of the eye is the vascular tunic, which includes the iris, the ciliary body, and the choroid. Through constriction and expansion of the iris, the pupil dilates (iris sphincter contraction) and constricts (iris dilator extension). The ciliary body contains the ciliary muscle, which changes the shape of the lens and allows accommodation. The choroid provides vascular nourishment and removal of wastes from the outer half of the retina.

The inner layer of the eye is the nervous tunic, which contains the retina, rods, and cones, which communicate light stimulation to the optic nerve fibers. The cones recognize colors and are responsible for fine discrimination and daylight vision. The rods respond to dim light and are responsible for peripheral vision.

TABLE 23-1 Brief Assessment of Cranial Nerves

	Cranial Nerve	Type	Assessment
CN I	Olfactory	Sensory	Have the patient close the eyes and occlude one naris. Test recognition of common scents such as coffee, lemon, or cinnamon.
CN II	Optic	Sensory	Using a Snellen chart, assess visual acuity. Check peripheral vision by confrontation. While facing the patient, hold arms out at sides, wiggle fingers and bring fingers centrally until patient is able to see them without moving the head.
CN III	Oculomotor	Motor	Examine pupils for size (normal is 3-5 mm), symmetry, and response to light. Assess extraocular movements within the six fields of gaze (up right and left; right; left; down right and left).
CN IV	Trochlear	Motor	Assess extraocular movements within the six fields of gaze (up right and left; right; left; down right and left).
CN V	Trigeminal	Motor	Check for corneal reflex by passing wisp of cotton near cornea. Check for strength of temporal and masseter muscles by having patient clench teeth.
		Sensory	Alternating a toothpick with a brief touch, check sensation of forehead, cheek, and jaw.
CN VI	Abducens	Motor	Assess extraocular movements within the lateral fields of gaze (up right and left; right; left; down right and left).
CN VII	Facial	Motor	Request that patient raise eyebrows, smile, puff out cheeks, close eyes.
		Sensory	Test taste of anterior portion of tongue with cotton swabs dipped in salt, sugar, and lemon.
CN VIII	Acoustic	Sensory	Test hearing through rubbing strands of patient's hair next to each ear. Check hearing of whispered voice from a 2-foot distance.
CN IX and CN X	Glossopharyngeal and vagus	Motor	Request that the patient open mouth and say "ah." Check for a rising palate.
		Sensory	Check gag reflex with a cotton swab.
CN XI	Spinal accessory	Motor	Try to push down on patient's shoulders while the patient is raising them.
CN XII	Hypoglossal	Motor	Have the patient stick out the tongue and move from one side to another.

Data from Wright, W. (2005). *Physical assessment and health history for the adult examination* (4th ed.). North Andover, MA: Fitzgerald Health Education Associates, Inc.; and Bickley, L., & Szilagyi, P. (2003). *Bates' guide to physical examination and history taking* (8th ed.). Philadelphia: Lippincott Williams & Wilkins.

The supporting and accessory structures of the eye include the eyelids, conjunctiva, lens, anterior and posterior eye cavities, and the lacrimal apparatus. The eyelids protect the eye from foreign objects. The conjunctiva is a mucous membrane that lines each lid and covers the eyeball surface. The lens is primarily composed of water. Changes in the lens shape occur with changes in the ciliary body. The lens bulges for near vision and flattens for far vision. The anterior cavity of the eye contains aqueous humor, which maintains intraocular pressure and nourishes the iris and posterior aspect of the cornea. The posterior cavity is filled with vitreous humor, which creates stable pressure. The lacrimal apparatus includes the lacrimal glands, lacrimal canals, lacrimal sacs, and nasolacrimal ducts and is responsible for tears.

The iris controls the amount of light entering the eye through the pupil. Light rays travel to the retina, which records images. The chemical and physical changes that take place in the retina create electrical impulses that are conducted along the optic nerve fibers to the occipital lobe of the cortex, where the impulses are interpreted (Figure 23-2).

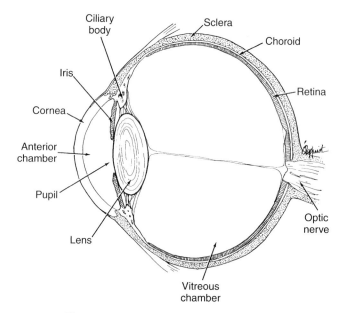

Figure 23-1 Cross-section of the human eye.

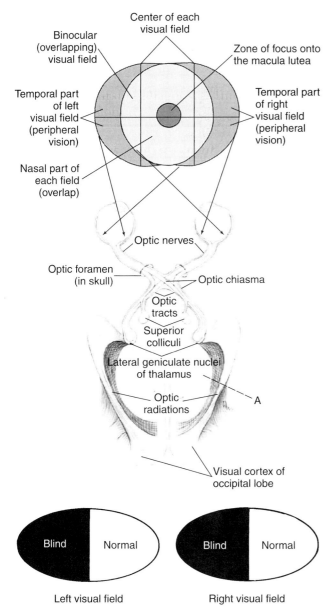

Figure 23-2 Visual fields and neuronal pathways of the eye. Note the structures that make up each pathway: optic nerve, optic chiasma, lateral geniculate body of the thalamus, optic radiations, and visual cortex of the occipital lobe. Fibers from the nasal portion of each retina cross over to the opposite side at the optic chiasma and terminate in the lateral geniculate nuclei. Location of a lesion in the visual pathway determines the resulting visual defect. Damage at point A, for example, would cause blindness in the right nasal and left temporal visual fields, as the ovals indicate. (From Thibodeau, G. A., & Patton, K. T. (2007). *Anatomy & physiology* [6th ed.]. St. Louis, MO: Mosby.)

Assessment of Vision. The initial assessment of vision includes a history, examination of all eye components, and questions about any specific problems, including symptoms, pain, redness, discharge, and visual acuity changes.

Visual Acuity. Visual acuity is assessed through use of a Snellen or other type of eye chart. The patient stands 20 feet (6 m) away from the chart. If the patient usually wears eyeglasses, the test should be administered with glasses in place. Each eye is assessed separately. A Snellen reading of 20/30 (metric 6/9) means that what someone with normal vision can read at 30 feet (9 m), the patient can read at 20 feet (6 m). The glasses should be assessed for cleanliness, scratches, comfort, and the type of problem they are correcting.

Visual Fields. Visual fields are assessed by having the patient hold his head still and follow a pen held by the examiner with his eyes. The examiner assesses any limitations in eye movement, including nystagmus. Limitation of both eyes is reflective of a central lesion, whereas a unilateral problem is indicative of a peripheral disruption of cranial nerve III, IV, or VI or of the neuromuscular junction.

Inspection. The eyelids are assessed for lesions, inflammation, foreign bodies, or other problems. The conjunctiva and sclera are assessed for color and characteristics of the blood vessels. Yellowish conjunctiva may be due to jaundice or fat deposits associated with aging. In children the conjunctiva may appear bluish because it is thinner and allows the pigmentation of underlying structures to be apparent. Reddened conjunctiva and sclera are indicative of conjunctivitis, which requires further investigation. The pupil is examined for size, shape, and equality. Normal pupil size is between 3 and 5 mm.

Pupil Reaction. To assess equal reaction to light, the nurse uses a penlight. The light is moved from the temporal to nasal side of the patient's eye while the patient focuses ahead. The nurse assesses whether the pupils constrict at an equal speed. Pupillary reaction to accommodation is tested while the patient looks into the distance and then at the nurse's finger, which is held 5 to 10 cm from the bridge of the patient's nose. The pupils should converge and constrict symmetrically, with a slightly slower response in older than in younger persons.

Palpation. The area around the lacrimal sacs should be palpated to identify any possible obstructions. Eversion of the eyelids is completed to identify problems with foreign bodies, inflammation, or other issues.

Nursing Diagnosis: Disturbed Sensory Perception (Visual). Loss of vision, compensated or uncompensated, may occur because of a variety of factors, which will be discussed in the following section.

Refractive Error. Refractive error is a defect of the refracting media of the eye. The most common visual impairment, it occurs when light rays fail to converge into a single focus on the retina, resulting in blurred vision and discomfort. Regardless of the cause of the refractive error, most cases may be corrected by corrective lenses.

Hemianopsia. Hemianopsia is defective vision or blindness of half of the visual field due to brain injury from cerebrovascular disorders, trauma, or tumors. It is not a disorder of the eyes but of the cerebrum. Hemianopsia is classified as homonymous, bitemporal, or attitudinal. *Homonymous hemianopsia* refers to the loss of vision in the temporal field of one eye and the nasal field of the other (Figure 23-3). Left homonymous hemianopsia sometimes

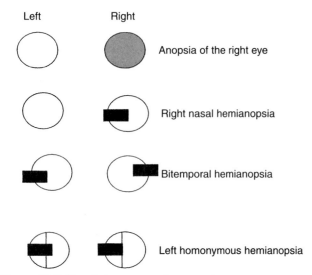

Figure 23-3 Visual alterations with various hemianopsia.

occurs after a right-sided brain lesion. It is not unusual for persons with left homonymous hemianopsia not to recognize the deficit until it is diagnosed during rehabilitation. This syndrome will be discussed further in the section of this chapter on perception.

Intraocular Disease. Intraocular disease may present with cataracts, glaucoma, or retinal detachment. Cataracts are an opacity or clouding of the lens that blocks the passage of light needed for vision. Cataracts develop slowly with age and may cause blurred vision, obliteration of parts of images, double images, decreased perception of color, or distorted images. The only treatment for cataracts is removal. Intraocular lens implantation is an effective method of visual rehabilitation for persons with cataracts (Belluci, 2005). The replacement lens is not able to provide accommodation for distance or near viewing, so individuals continue to require glasses. Mutifocal lens have been developed, but with limited success (Stork, Kreiner, & Rentsch, 2002).

Glaucoma. Glaucoma, the third leading cause of blindness, occurs when a buildup of intraocular pressure (due to a blockage of aqueous humor) gradually destroys the optic nerve. There may be no symptoms or awareness of the problem, thus vision is lost slowly and painlessly. Open-angle glaucoma is due to a reduction in the outflow of aqueous humor and is treated with eyedrops such as pilocarpine and timolol maleate. If eyedrops are ineffective, surgery may be an option. Closed-angle glaucoma presents with acute eye pain and nausea. The iris is displaced in the periphery of the anterior chamber, and the aqueous filtration network is blocked, causing the intraocular pressure to rise quickly, resulting in a surgical emergency.

Retinal Detachment. Retinal detachment is a serious situation occurring when the retina separates from the choroid. The person may report a "shade lowering" over the visual field or may experience blurry vision and light flashes. The rods and cones atrophy and become damaged. Surgical intervention, such as a vitrectomy, is usually required.

Blindness and Low Vision. An estimated 937,000 (0.78%) American adults are blind. There are an additional 2.4 million (2%) who have low vision (Eye Diseases Prevalence Research Group, 2004). The term *legally blind* is used to indicate a corrected visual acuity in the corrected stronger eye of 20/200 (metric 6/60) or less. *Functional blindness* indicates total blindness or a minimum of light perception or projection. *Low vision* refers to corrected visual acuity of 20/40 (metric 6/12). Causes of low vision vary between races. Macular degeneration is the most common cause of blindness and low vision for whites. For African Americans, cataracts and glaucoma are frequent causes of vision loss and blindness (Congdon, et al., 2004).

The number of individuals impacted by vision loss and blindness will increase with the rise in older adults. By 2020 a 70% increase in the number of Americans with blindness and low vision is expected. Among residents of long-term care facilities, the prevalence of vision loss is estimated at 37% (Friedman, et al., 2004).

A global initiative, Vision 2020, has been established to work to resolve treatable and preventable causes of vision loss. By 2020, if action is not taken, there could be 76 million individuals in the world who are blind (Pizzarello et al., 2004). Strategies identified by Vision 2020 include cataract removal, trachoma treatment, ivermectin distribution for onchocerciasis, affordable glasses, and education of health providers and the public regarding treatment of glaucoma and diabetes.

The most common reasons for vision loss present in strikingly different manners. Macular degeneration presents with a loss of central vision. Although peripheral vision remains intact, the characteristics of peripheral vision are different than central vision. Correction for reading with central vision loss is not as simple as magnification, reduction of eye movement, or print modification (Battista, Kalloniatis, & Metha, 2005). Cataracts result in overall dimming of vision, and diabetic retinopathy results in losses of portions of the visual field.

When surgery, medical treatments, or correctional eyeglasses will not fully correct the problem, the rehabilitation strategies listed in Table 23-2 are useful. Rehabilitation efforts revolve around increasing the functional ability of persons with blindness and decreasing the environmental barriers that may be experienced. Of the activities of daily living, individuals with vision loss find the highest limitations reading print, work, leisure, and mobility (Lamoureux, Hassell, & Keeffe, 2004). Access to printed materials for patients with visual deficits has improved through computerized screen-reading programs, such as JAWS (http://www.freedomscientific.com/fs_products/software_jaws.asp) and Window-Eyes (http://www.gwmicro.com/). JAWS enables persons with visual impairments to navigate the Windows environment of the computer system for word processing or any computer text-based program, as well as e-mail and the Internet. Anything presented on the screen is read aloud by the screen-reading programs. Both programs use shortcut keys to eliminate the need to use a mouse with the computer.

Two programs that convert printed documents into speech are OpenBook and Kurzweil 1000 (Wehberg, Kendrick,

TABLE 23-2 Low Vision Rehabilitation Strategies

Device/Strategy	Use and Comments
Magnifying glass	Hand-held magnifying glass with a strong convex lens may be useful for short focal distances, for close vision, and for reading and writing Must be held, thus limiting its practicality in situations requiring both hands (such as crafts, needlepoint, woodworking, and item assembly)
Telescope	Binoculars and field glasses may be used for magnification of items at a distance Require use of the hands, thereby limiting their use in situations requiring both hands
Light filters	Light filters are used over glasses to limit glare Require application and removal with changes in lighting or when entering or leaving sunlight
Tinted lenses	Used to reduce glare Not removable from the glasses and may limit vision in some lighting situations
Prisms	Glass devices used to change images to a different part of the retina and to promote vision through such redirection Require use of the hands
Microscopes	Similar in use to a telescope but for nearby items Require use of the hands and do not assist with peripheral vision
Reading rectangle	Used to limit the number of words on which the reader is focusing at a single time Must be moved as the reader completes reading a section; assists with focus but requires use of the hands; best suited for reading texts and documents
Large type	Many books, magazines, and documents are available in large type Increases the visibility of the text without requiring the use of magnifying glasses or microscopes; increases the size and weight of magazines and books because more pages are required for the printed information

---

BOX 23-1 Guidelines to Reduce Barriers for Individuals With Visual Impairment

1. Present verbal instructions clearly and succinctly, and use touch and other senses to compensate for lack of vision.
2. When teaching, break down tasks into smaller component steps and teach one at a time.
3. Orient the person to the surroundings, and remind staff members and visitors to introduce themselves.
4. Maintain personal items such as combs, brushes, and room furniture in the same place and arrangement; do not move equipment or furniture in the room without discussing the new arrangement with the patient.
5. When speaking with the patient, speak directly to him or her using a natural tone of voice; do not assume the person has poor hearing in addition to a visual impairment.
6. Encourage involvement of the patient in problem solving.
7. Assist the person in organizing the life space (e.g., hanging clothing by color, type, or style).
8. Attach or sew tactile symbols to clothing and personal items to help identify color and contents.
9. Assist the person in localizing and discriminating sounds.
10. Assist the person in learning to detect temperatures and to manipulate objects safely; for example, when pouring a hot beverage, teach the person to wrap the fingers around the upper third of the cup to identify when the beverage is at that level.
11. Instruct the person to visualize the meal plate as a clock to assist in communication of the location of the food or other items.
12. When assisting a visually impaired person in walking, walk about a half step ahead and have the person grasp your arm lightly but firmly just above the elbow so that the thumb is on the outside and the fingers are on the inside of the arm; both of you should hold your upper arms close to the body so that your movements can alert the individual to curbs, turns, and stops.

& Leventhal, 2004). Both programs not only scan printed documents and identify currency, but download books and journals and convert files from a variety of formats. The latest advancements in these programs provide access to written material equivalent to that available for individuals without visual impairment.

Methods of reducing barriers to mobility for persons with functional blindness include the standard white cane or guide dog. Canes are about 0.5 inch in diameter and made of lightweight fiberglass or aluminum. Individuals use the cane by moving it in front of them from side to side in an arc to extend the sense of touch by letting them know whether obstacles lie in their path. Guide dogs work with individuals as part of a team, with the dog serving as the individual's eyes. Strategies for reducing barriers for persons with visual impairment are listed in Box 23-1.

Implications for Rehabilitation. A critical aspect of rehabilitation nursing is the ability to visualize potentials for persons recovering from or coping with devastating disabilities and chronic illnesses. This characteristic of rehabilitation is true with visual deficits as with other physical disabilities. Although rehabilitation programs typically focus on physical function, progress will be limited if attention to the need for visual considerations is overlooked. Use of visual aids, for example, for patients with low vision can be key toward their attainment of rehabilitation goals. Rehabilitation nurses should be aware of adaptive equipment and technology that may be of use for patients with visual impairment.

Hearing

Hearing is a complex phenomenon that requires the integration between the external and internal ear and the cerebrum.

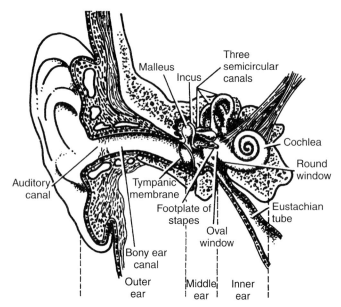

Figure 23-4 The anatomy of the ear has three main areas: the external auditory area, the middle ear, and the inner ear. Obstructions, including earwax, in the auditory canal or fluid in the eustachian tube may reduce hearing. The middle ear contains three small bones (the incus, malleus, and stapes) that vibrate to assist in the transmission of sound during normal hearing. The bones may become stabilized by calcified deposits and produce conductive hearing losses. Inner ear deficits often involve sensorineural losses. These may affect a patient's balance and produce ringing in the ears, as well as hearing loss. (From Hoeman, S. P. [1990]. *Rehabilitative and restorative care in the community.* St. Louis, MO: Mosby.)

Hearing alone does not ensure the person will process and remember what is heard.

Healthy People 2010 (USDHHS, 2000) identified an objective for newborns to be screened for hearing loss by 1 month, referred for audiological evaluation by 3 months, and involved in appropriate intervention by 6 months of age. *Healthy People 2010* also recommends a hearing examination every decade after the age of 18 years.

Anatomy and Physiology. Figure 23-4 illustrates the major anatomical structures of the ear.

External Ear. The external ear forms the passageway for sounds and contains mechanisms to protect the hearing organ from penetration by microorganisms and foreign objects.

The auditory canal extends approximately 2.5 cm to the tympanic membrane. Sebaceous and other glands in the outer half of the canal secrete cerumen, which has a protective function. Hair follicles are also found in the outer half of the canal. The tympanic membrane receives sound waves from the external ear and canal. Normally the tympanic membrane appears cone shaped, shiny, translucent, and pearl gray.

The middle ear cavity is filled with air and transfers airborne sound pressure fluctuations in the external canal to pressure variations in the fluid-filled inner ear. The sound that vibrates the tympanic membrane is transmitted to the cochlea by the malleus, incus (anvil), and stapes bones. The middle

ear also contains the eustachian tube, which opens into the nasopharynx and provides equalization of air pressure between the middle ear and the pharynx. The eustachian tube is usually closed but may open during yawning, swallowing, or chewing. Cranial nerve VII, responsible for control of facial movement, is located within the middle ear.

Inner Ear. As sound vibrations pass through the middle ear, they cause waves of pressure that correspond to incoming sound waves, which transfer the vibrations to the cochlea, which is part of the inner ear. A second function of the inner ear is in maintenance of balance and equilibrium.

The inner ear is a maze formed by a bony labyrinth (vestibule, cochlea, and semicircular canals) and a membranous labyrinth (utricle and saccule). The vestibule, or organ of balance, is the central portion of the bony labyrinth and is bathed in endolymph fluid. The cochlea contains the organ of Corti, the sense organ of hearing, which is composed of 24,000 hair cells bathed in perilymph. The hair cells become distorted and mechanically bent when sound waves enter the cochlea. As hair cells are displaced along the length of the cochlea, they are transformed into neural activity. Neural impulses travel along to the eighth cranial nerve to the brain to produce the sensation and recognition of sound. The three semicircular canals enlarge into ampullae, which contain receptors from cranial nerve VIII (the acoustic nerve).

Perception of Sound. Sound is carried in waves caught in the outer ear and travels as vibrations to the inner ear canal, causing the tympanic membrane to vibrate and initiate movement of the bones in the middle ear. Vibration of the last and smallest bone, the stapes, passes through the oval window to the inner ear. Perilymph fluid vibrates in harmony with incoming sound waves. These waves communicate vibration to the cochlea, where the hair cells bend and activate nerve impulses, which stimulate the auditory nerve. The auditory nerve conveys the impulse to the auditory cortex in the brain, where the vibration is recognized and sound is perceived.

Assessment of Hearing. Hearing assessment is a part of any rehabilitation nursing admission or initial assessment. Given the essential need for communication during rehabilitation, information on the ability of the individual to hear is critical for therapeutic teaching and adherence. The environment in which the hearing assessment is completed should be free from distractions and extraneous noise to the extent possible.

External Inspection and Palpation. External inspection of the ears includes examining for any deviations, redness or swelling. Use an otoscope to visualize the ear canal, and note redness, drainage, accumulated cerumen, or any abnormalities of the tympanic membrane. Palpate the ears and mastoid, noting any pain or tenderness experienced by the patient.

Hearing Acuity. Hearing acuity is a complex phenomenon and requires a multidimensional assessment. The assessment includes differentiation of conductive and sensorineural hearing loss and speech reception and discrimination. Common methods for testing hearing acuity are summarized in Table 23-3.

TABLE 23-3 Methods for Testing Hearing Acuity

Hearing Test Method	Description	Purpose, Comments
Self-assessment	Many questionnaires are available for individuals to identify whether a hearing problem exists; one such method is available through the Miracle Ear website: www.miracle-ear.com/hearing_n_hearing_loss/hearing_assessment_questionnaire.htm	Allows individuals to self-test for possible symptoms of hearing loss; tests are free to administer and can be done at home
Air conduction testing	Acoustic stimulus is presented through earphones to the individual	Detects defects in hearing due to problems in the ear canal, middle ear, inner ear, central auditory pathways, or acoustic nerve (CN VIII)
Tuning fork	Tests for bone conduction of sound through the vibration of the tuning fork tongs	Provides direct stimulation to the inner ear, bypassing the external and middle parts of the ear
Weber's test	After the tuning fork is struck, the vibrating end is placed on the head midline; patient identifies the ear in which the sound is the loudest	Differentiates sensorineural loss from conductive loss: unilateral conductive loss presents as a stronger signal in the affected ear, and unilateral sensorineural loss presents as a stronger signal in the unaffected ear
Rinne's test	Vibrating tuning fork is used by placing it on the mastoid process and then near the pinna; patient is asked to identify the strongest sound	Normally sound is heard by air conduction more loudly than by bone conduction; sensorineural loss presents as a decrease in both air and bone conduction, with air slightly louder; conduction loss presents with air heard less than bone conduction
Audiometry	Audiometer is used to present acoustic stimuli for specific tone frequencies	Allows identification of the hearing threshold for specific frequencies
Speech audiometry	Specific two-syllable words are spoken in conversational English; percentage of words noted correctly is recorded	Assesses speech reception threshold and is an index of the individual's ability to hear under optimal conditions; a score of 90% to 100% is normal
Tympanometry	Sound source probe with a microphone is placed in the ear canal to measure the amount of acoustic energy absorbed by the middle ear	Measures possible hearing impairment resulting from otitis media
Acoustic reflex testing	Tones of various intensities are presented to each ear, and the patient is monitored for a reflex contraction of the stapedius muscle (acoustic reflex)	In neural hearing loss, this reflex decays or adapts
Auditory brainstem response (ABR)	Acoustic stimulation is presented, and electric waveforms are monitored as generated from the brainstem, CN VIII, and other regions	Lesions will present as lost waveforms; testing allows differentiation between sensory and neural hearing loss
Otoacoustic emissions (OAEs)	Sound source is presented in the ear canal, and a microphone records the response	Tests the sounds generated by the outer hair cells within the cochlea; commonly used for hearing testing in infants

Data from Merck. (2000). *The Merck manual of diagnosis and therapy.* Whitehouse Station, NJ: Author.
CN, Central nerve.

Nursing Diagnosis: Disturbed Sensory Perception (Auditory). The percentage of Americans with hearing loss is 9% to 10% (Meador & Zazove, 2005). Hearing deficits increase in frequency with age, with 25% to 40% of those over 65 years experiencing a significant loss of hearing. Hearing loss increases in frequency with age, with a prevalence rate of 80% of those over 85 years experiencing deficits (Yueh, Shapiro, MacLean, & Shekelle, 2003). The prevalence of hearing loss within the population is expected to increase at a rate disproportionate to the increase in age because noise pollution.

Conductive Hearing Loss. Conductive losses are the most common type of hearing deficits and are usually due to frequent or severe otitis media. Risk factors for otitis media include immune deficiencies, day care placement, exposure to tobacco smoke, or craniofacial abnormalities such as a cleft palate. The exposure to smoking is a significant risk factor for conductive hearing loss (Uchida, Nakashimat, Ando, Niino, & Shimokata, 2003). In a study of the impact of smoking on hearing loss, a deterioration at 4000 Hz was noted in individuals not exposed to other causative factors, such as noise. The effect of smoking on hearing loss was noted by the researchers to be dose related. This is a causative factor for hearing loss that can be reduced or eliminated through smoking cessation (Kurata, 2006).

Sensorineural Hearing Loss. Sensory (hair cell) and neural (spiral ganglion cell) factors result in sensorineural hearing loss. Such losses may occur prenatally. According to *Healthy People 2010* (USDHHS, 2000), 1 in 1000 children is born deaf, making hearing loss the most common congenital defect. The inability to hear during infancy affects the development of normal speech and language skills and may adversely affect social, emotional, cognitive, and academic development. It is significant to note that some within the deaf community perceive deafness to be a difference in lifestyle rather than a disability. These individuals would disagree with the perspective that deafness has an adverse impact on development (Breivek, 2005; Ladd, 2005) but instead view the vulnerability (of deafness) as strength.

Despite such perceptions from those affected by deafness, the Joint Committee on Infant Hearing (Connolly, Carron, & Roark, 2005) developed a consensus statement on the need for early identification of hearing impairment in young children. Given that the first 3 years of life are the most crucial in speech and language development and given that most cases of congenital deafness are not diagnosed until after 3 years of age, it is essential that testing be done at a younger age. Universal hearing screening for newborns is done in most hospitals in the United States. The goal of such screening is early intervention for infants with hearing deficits (Hyde, 2005). Recommended testing of newborns is through the auditory brainstem response (ABR) or otoacoustic emissions (OAEs) (see Table 23-3).

Sensorineural hearing loss may be acquired as a result of autoimmune disorders or exposure to ototoxic substances (aminoglycosides, cisplatin, aspirin). It may also be caused by bacterial meningitis, viral infections (congenital rubella, cytomegalovirus, mumps), or bacterial endotoxins and exotoxins. In addition, sensorineural hearing loss may occur as a result of sound trauma from firearms, engine noise, loud toys, loud music, or head trauma. Another cause of sensorineural hearing loss is otosclerosis, which is due to ankylosis of the stapes caused by the growth of immature bone through the vascular channels of the ear. Otosclerosis may affect the stapes, inner ear, or both (Holt, 2003). Cochlear otosclerosis occurs with the spread of otosclerosis to the inner ear and results in sensorineural hearing loss and balance impairment. If the otosclerosis extends to the stapes, surgery may be recommended. Hearing aids may be of benefit.

Sensorineural hearing loss with balance disturbance may be seen with acoustic neuroma (Ishikawa, Wang, Wong, Shibata, & Itasaka, 2004). The tumor is benign and grows on cranial nerve VIII, affecting hearing and balance. Acoustic neuromas grow slowly and cause symptoms that increase in severity with time. Symptoms include unilateral hearing loss, tinnitus, dysphagia, facial numbness, weakness or paralysis, ataxia, headaches, visual loss, and death if untreated. Diagnosis is through symptom presentation and through the ABR test (see Table 23-3). According to researchers, persons presenting with unilateral audiovestibular symptoms should be evaluated for acoustic neuroma. Surgical removal is the usual and recommended treatment, with one study demonstrating significant long-term preservation of hearing following surgery for

---

BOX 23-2 Guidelines for Communication With Persons With Hearing Deficits

1. Gain the listener's attention before speaking, and wait until the person is ready to listen.
2. Face the person.
3. Talk clearly and distinctly, but do not shout.
4. Stand or sit close to the person.
5. Repeat once and then rephrase.
6. Identify the topic, and make it clear when the subject changes.
7. Use your hands to gesture.
8. Confirm comprehension.
9. Avoid background noise and distractions.
10. Use visual aids, if necessary.

---

acoustic neuroma (Inoue, Ogawa, & Kanzaki, 2001). Most surgeries, however, result in permanent hearing loss.

Resources and Technology for Persons With Hearing Loss. Primary concerns for rehabilitation involving persons with hearing losses are communication and safety within the environment. Box 23-2 contains recommended strategies for communicating with persons with hearing impairment. Growth in computer technology has led to a dazzling, confusing, and sometimes misleading array of devices, equipment, and software. These are summarized in Table 23-4.

Despite the advances made during the last decade in resources for persons with hearing loss, artificial acoustic devices or aids are not equivalent to an intact auditory system. Box 23-3 contains information written by consumers on the advantages and disadvantages of different hearing aid systems. Rehabilitation nurses need to be familiar with the variety, benefits, and disadvantages of resources for persons with hearing loss. No single system or method will work for all persons requiring assistance with hearing; therefore the more options there are, the more likely individuals will be to find one that meets their needs and lifestyle. Box 23-4 lists high-quality, consumer advocacy-based websites to provide rehabilitation nurses with insights and direction on resources available for those with limited or no hearing.

Cochlear Implants. About 20 years ago, cochlear implants made headlines as a breakthrough for persons with profound hearing impairment. The cochlear implant is considered a prosthetic device used to replace the function of the cochlea. Part of the device is surgically implanted behind the ear to bypass the cochlea. The remainder of the device is external. It is battery operated and contains a microphone, a speech processor, and connecting cables. The device, implant surgery, and speech therapy are costly, but many of the devices are covered through health care insurance. The cochlear implant offers miracles for some but not without significant effort and adjustment. Earlier implantation (around age 2 years) is associated with improved outcomes (Geers, 2004).

Sign Language. Sign language has been a part of American culture since the time of the Pilgrims' landing.

TABLE 23-4 Resources for Individuals With Hearing Loss

Resource	Description	Comments
Alerting devices	Smoke alarms	Must be visual or vibrating
	Wireless X-10 systems for doorbells, telephone, baby alarms, telephone	Provides remote activation of alarm devices through a visual indicator such as a light
Assistive listening devices	Microphones, pickups, headphones, earphones	All enable user to focus on a single desired signal and filter other noises; intent is to allow one signal to be amplified in comparison with the sounds from the remaining environment
Personal assistive listening devices	Pocket talker	Uses a microphone and headphones connected through a small amplifier
	Personal FM system	Similar to the pocket talker but wireless; speaker is given a transmitter and microphone, and listener receives the acoustic equivalent to the electronic signal; ideal for lectures, church, or concerts
	Wireless headphones	Use an input plug into an audio device, such as the television
Group assistive listening devices	Infrared systems	Depend on a clear line of sight between transmitter and receiver, portable
	FM systems	Signals are more versatile and portable
	Loop systems	Permanently installed in a room
Hearing aids	Acoustic aid	Amplifies sound and sends the amplified acoustic energy to the eardrum
	Conduction aid	Transmits sound to the inner ear using the bones of the skull
	Implantable hearing aid	Experimental treatment, with the first device implanted in December 1999
Automatic speech recognition (ASR)	Dragon System's Naturally Speaking, IBM's Via Voice, Lernout & Hauspie's Voice Xpress, Philips Dictation System's Free Speech	Application for individuals with hearing loss is to have the microphone pick up the speech of one individual and type the spoken words on a computer screen, providing immediate translation of the spoken word; all have difficulty and depend on the clarity and speed of speech; a goal for this technology is use for situations that require interpreting, including business meetings or classrooms
Telephones	Speech-Adjust-A-Tone	Connects to the telephone; can be adjusted to the level of amplification needed
	Cellular phones	Only the Nokia 51-61 series is compatible with hearing aids that use telecoils
TTYs or TDDs	Text telephones, telecommunications devices for the deaf	Assist those with hearing loss to communicate using standard telephone lines; through the TTY or TDD and Telecommunication Relay Service, communication is possible with persons who use standard voice telephones
Two-way pager	ReachNet, RIM Interactive pager by WyndTell	Provide individuals with hearing loss the ability to communicate anywhere at anytime with anyone, are interactive, and provide a visual typed message
Visual communications	Visual intercom	In experimental stages at present but have a significant potential to augment emergency verbal messages in large, crowded environments, such as airports and amusement parks
Relay service		All require use of either a TTY or TDD and connection to a relay access number for the state. All state relay numbers are toll free and can be obtained at the website: http://www.hearinglossweb.com
	Standard relay call	TDD user types in the message, which is interpreted by the state relay operator, who types the response of the person called back to the TDD user

TABLE 23-4 **Resources for Individuals With Hearing Loss—cont'd**

Resource	Description	Comments
	Voice carryover call	TDD user speaks directly, and the state relay operator types the response of the person called; faster than the standard system
	Two-line voice carryover call	TDD user is able to hear the response of the person called, and the state relay operator types in the response to fill in any gaps; requires the cost of a 3-way call

---

BOX 23-3 **Hearing Aid Consumer Tips**

Before Buying a Hearing Aid
- Check with a physician and an audiologist for easily correctable causes to hearing impairment

After the Decision to Purchase a Hearing Aid Has Been Made, Consider the Following Points Before Making a Purchase
- Digital technology offers improvements over standard hearing aids but is costly; consumer should make sure the added quality is worth the added cost.
- Although hearing aids that seem invisible in the ear tend to be visually appealing, they are often more fragile, with a shorter life expectancy and a lower degree of quality than traditional behind-the-ear models.
- The hearing aid selected should include strong, preamplified telecoils, positioned for loop and telephone use.
- Three aids should be tried before making a selection.
- Expect a 90-day return policy, and accept no less than 60 days for return.
- Determine the refund policy; expect that the audiogram and earmold will not be refunded.
- Expect a manufacturer warranty of no less than 2 years.

After Fitting the Aid but Before Leaving the Store
- Use the distributor's phone to check for quality and function of the device.

After Buying the Device
- The aid should be worn continuously.
- Signs that the hearing aid is not fitted well include feedback; causes of an ill-fitted hearing aid are cracked tubing, loose earmold, or loose fitting.
- Every problem and irritation should be recorded.
- At the end of 1 week, the consumer should return to the distributor and review any concerns noted.

If a Return of the Hearing Aid Is Necessary
- Expect return of the audiogram because this is a medical record and belongs to the person for whom it was recorded.

BOX 23-4 **Websites for Consumers With Hearing Impairment**

http://www.hearinglossweb.com: Provides extensive information and links to other sites for resources for those with hearing loss
http://www.deafworks.com: DEAFWORKS organization manufactures technology for those with deafness
http://www.wynd.net: Wynd Communication is a deaf person–owned company specializing in providing accessible communication for persons with hearing loss
http://www.saywhatclub.com: The SayWhatClub provides a listing of resources for those with hearing loss

---

were taught signing from the crib. In this setting deafness was not seen as a handicap (http://www.marthasdirect.com/deafness/community.html). A number of universities recognize sign language as an alternative for foreign language credits.

In several of the states, American Sign Language is recognized as an official foreign language for which academic credit may be given. The first academic program to promote American Sign Language was at Gallaudet University in Washington, D.C. Gallaudet University has served as the hub of education for deaf persons since 1856. At Gallaudet, sign language has served as a major form of communication and a competitive advantage—because it was sign language between Gallaudet's football team members that led to the concept of the football huddle. Rehabilitation nurses who are not bilingual in sign must be able to access translators.

Computerization and the Internet. Perhaps the most significant opportunity to reduce accessibility barriers for persons with significant hearing loss is through the use of computers and the Internet. The use of company e-mail, for example, can minimize or even eliminate the need for voice communication. The Internet makes it possible for those within the deaf community to communicate in chat rooms, web pages, and e-mail, widening communication pathways with every technological advance.

Implications for Rehabilitation. Because hearing deficits are an invisible limitation, they are sometimes overlooked or not included in the overall plan of care. Patients who are deaf or have hearing loss often have difficulty communicating with the health care team. They are most susceptible to misunderstandings about treatment recommendations and plans. Unfortunately, team members sometimes mistake a

Jonathan Lambert, a deaf man originating from the Weald parish in Kent county, moved to Martha's Vineyard. He and his wife had seven children, of whom two were deaf. Given the isolation of Martha's Vineyard, for two centuries the deaf community on the island grew to the point where infants

nod or a shake of the head as comprehension, when it may not be so. Hearing loss is linked with an increase in depressive symptoms. In addition to assessing the presence of hearing deficits, the nurse should identify the degree of deficit, the age of onset, psychological issues linked with the loss, and preferred language (asking about American Sign Language in addition to other languages).

According to Helen Keller, "The problems of deafness are deeper and more complex, if not more important, than those of blindness. Deafness is a much worse misfortune. For it means the loss of the most vital stimulus—the sound of the voice that brings language, sets thoughts astir and keeps us in the intellectual company of man" (Keller, 2005). Her astute comments clearly apply to rehabilitation patients. Patients who are deaf are part of the non–English-speaking minority at highest risk for failures in physician-patient communication (Meador & Zazove, 2005). The following steps should be considered when communicating with those who are deaf or who have a significant hearing deficit:

1. A professional interpreter in American Sign Language should be used for communication regarding the treatment plan, if this is the language preferred by the patient.
2. A clear visual field should be maintained when speaking with the patient. For example, the nurse should not stand in front of a sunny window.
3. The nurse should face the patient directly, avoiding overenunciation (which impedes speech reading).
4. The patient should be faced directly, even if an interpreter is present, because the nurse is communicating with the patient—and the interpreter is able to hear and provide interpretation to the patient.

Taste

Taste is a cellular reaction caused by the mixture of food and drink with saliva, triggering nerve impulses. Substances are recognized as sweet, sour, salty, or bitter by the taste centers in the thalamus and cortex (*Mosby's Dictionary of Medicine, Nursing, & Health Professions,* 2006). Although not a critical sense for survival, taste is a complex sense, and it is influential in nutritional intake. Individuals tend to have a craving or attraction to nutrients in which their bodies are deficient. There is no evidence to indicate that loss of taste or enhanced taste is linked with variations in satiety (Pasquet, Monneuse, Simmen, Marez, & Hladik, 2006).

Anatomy and Physiology. Taste cells are located within the mouth and throat. Clusters of 50 taste cells form taste buds, which are located around the tongue's papillae. Taste buds function through convergence of synapses, with many of the receptors within taste buds synapsing to a single interneuron. Stimulations of the taste receptors within the taste buds travel through the interneuron by the vagus, glossopharyngeal, and facial nerves to the ventral posterior nucleus (thalamus). From the thalamus the signals are transferred to the ipsilateral gustatory cortex of the cerebrum. Taste receptors are specific to the four basic sensations of taste. The posterior central aspect of the tongue is sensitive to bitter tastes. The lateral portions of the tongue are sensitive to sour tastes. Salty tastes are noted by the lateral aspects adjacent to the end of the tongue. In the anterior tip of the tongue, sweet tastes are identified (Figure 23-5). Olfactory sensors in combination with gustatory sensors are responsible for the ability to identify specific flavors.

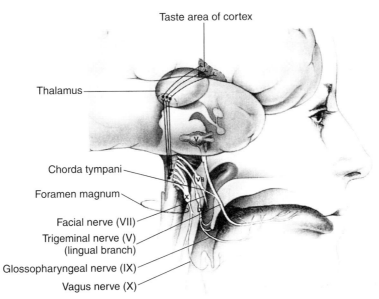

Figure 23-5 Central nervous system pathways for taste from the facial nerve (anterior two thirds of the tongue), glossopharyngeal nerve (posterior one third of the tongue), and vagus nerve (root of the tongue). The trigeminal nerve is also shown. It carries tactile sensations from the anterior two thirds of the tongue. The chorda tympani from the facial nerve (carrying taste input) joins the trigeminal nerve. Nerves carrying taste impulses synapse in the ganglion of each nerve, in the nucleus of the tractus solitarius, and in the thalamus, before terminating in the taste area of the cortex. (From Seely, R. R., Stephens, T. D., & Tate, P. P. [1991]. *Essentials of anatomy and physiology.* St. Louis, MO: Mosby.)

Assessment of Taste. Assessment of taste sensation is a significant portion of the nursing assessment but is typically not completed as a routine inpatient or outpatient admission assessment. Rather, it is a key assessment when indicators are noted that a problem might exist, for example, if the patient reports that all foods taste the same or if the patient demonstrates a decreased or depressed appetite. Assessment is completed by preparing four distinct taste sensations in liquid forms (salt water, sugar water, lemon juice, and coffee). One at a time, cotton swabs are soaked in each liquid and placed individually on the patient's tongue. The patient is asked to identify the category of taste sensation for each one. Assessment includes visualization of the tongue and oral cavity for asymmetrical spots or plaques.

Nursing Diagnosis: Disturbed Sensory Perception (Gustatory). Taste may be impaired by a variety of problems, including heavy smoking, desquamation of the tongue, oral infection, cerebrovascular accident, aging, and radiation of the head or neck. Intake of amitriptyline or vincristine may alter taste. In some cases zinc supplementation has been demonstrated to correct problems with taste. Testing, in addition to a focused history and physical and examination, should be sufficient to identify the problem.

Implications for Rehabilitation. Although impairments in taste may not be life threatening, they do interfere with the quality of life and may impede adequate nutritional intake. If possible, the cause of the problem should be eliminated. If the cause cannot be alleviated, food flavor and appearance should be enhanced. Older persons may be tempted to add large quantities of sugar and salt to achieve flavor. Rehabilitation nurses should work with patients to encourage the addition of seasonings instead. The taste of foods may be enhanced through smoking cessation, tongue cleaning, and adequate nutrition.

Smell

The sense of smell is complex and involves the detection and perception of different odors. Olfactory accuracy peaks between 30 and 60 years of age. Olfactory stimulation through aromatherapy is a key aspect of complementary medicine. Controversy exists on the validity of aromatherapy for treatment of clinical conditions; however, its significance is evident in the mind-body connection (Dunning, 2005). Many nursing interventions have been initiated around the use of aroma therapy, including to promote relaxation and sleep, to decrease anxiety, and to increase satisfaction.

Anatomy and Physiology. Olfactory receptors located in the cilia of the nasal passageways are stimulated through the conversion of odors to chemicals that dissolve in the epithelium of the nose. They are transferred through the cilia to the axon, then to the olfactory bulb and on to the olfactory tract, which leads the signal to the olfactory cortex, amygdala, hippocampus, hypothalamus, and pyriform cortex.

Olfactory information is relayed directly to the cerebral cortex without traveling through the thalamus. The olfactory pathway divides in the amygdala-pyriform area, with one pathway projecting through the medial dorsal nuclei to the orbitofrontal cortex and the second pathway projecting to the limbic system. The first pathway is linked with perception of odor and smell, and the second is associated with memory and the emotional response to smells (see Figure 23-6).

Assessment of Olfactory Sensation. As with gustatory assessment, olfactory assessment is a significant portion of the nursing assessment but is typically not completed as a routine inpatient or outpatient admission assessment. The nurse can assess olfactory acuity through a simple, readily available test using coffee, peppermint oil, and lemon juice. The patient is asked to close the eyes, and each item is held under the nose for a brief time, during which the nurse asks the patient to identify the substance. Examination of olfaction also requires assessment of the upper respiratory tract.

Nursing Diagnosis: Disturbed Sensory Perception (Olfactory). The most common cause of the loss of smell or olfactory acuity is aging, with an estimated 62.5% of those older than 80 years experiencing moderate to severe loss of smell (Murphy et al., 2002). Loss of smell is associated with cognitive impairment and may be one of the earliest signs of mild cognitive impairment (Eibenstein et al., 2005). Other causes of olfactory impairment include sinus infections, allergies, medications, vitamin deficiencies, chemical exposure, radiation, smoking, and cerebrovascular injury. In young adults anosmia (loss of olfaction) may occur after head injury (de Kruijk et al., 2003).

Implications for Rehabilitation. As with geriatric patients with disorders of taste, the rehabilitation nurse should encourage patients with anosmia to use seasonings for flavor instead of salt and sugar. Calorie counts for persons with disorders of olfaction should be monitored to ensure adequate intake of nutrients. Routine assessment of weight should be completed because weight gain or loss may by linked with olfactory impairment. Assessment of the home environment is important to rehabilitation for persons with olfactory disturbance who may not detect a gas leak, something burning, or spoiled foods.

Touch and Sensation

The concept of therapeutic touch and that of Reiki imply that energy transfer is possible without physical contact. In physiological reality, however, the sense of touch relies on physical contact.

Anatomy and Physiology. Touch, pressure, and vibration are components of the somatosensory system. As mechanical stimuli place a force on the skin, the mechanoreceptors located within the skin and subcutaneous tissues are activated. The quality of sensation perceived is a factor of the adequacy of the stimulus, one's threshold for

TABLE 23-5 Types and Function of Sensory Receptors

Receptor Type	Function	Comments
Mechanoreceptors	Touch, flutter, pressure, vibration	Meissner's corpuscle and Merkel's receptors: important for fine discrimination, graphesthesia, stereognosis Ruffini's corpuscle: responds to pressure Pacinian corpuscle: responds to vibration Hair receptors Free nerve endings
Proprioceptors	Position sense	Essential for sense of body schema, limb position, movement, force, or effort
Thermoreceptors	Thermal sense	Identify hot and cold substances
Nociceptors	Pain	Respond to tissue damage or injury
Chemoreceptor	Chemical reactions	Receptors for taste; smell; arterial oxygen; and blood levels of glucose, amino acids, fatty acids, and carbon dioxide
Photic receptors	Vision receptors	Receptors for light; include rods and cones

stimulation, the pattern of discharge, and the adaptation rate. There are six types of sensory receptors, which are summarized in Table 23-5.

The receptors change energy from a stimulus to an electrical signal. The signal must be strong enough to evoke action in the afferent fibers. The stimulus is transmitted through afferent fibers to the spinal cord and brain. The anterolateral spinothalamic tract contains pathways for nondiscriminative sensations such as touch, tickle, itch, pain, and temperature. The information relayed is not specific to intensity and location of the triggering signal. The signal is carried through the spinal cord on the contralateral side of the cord to the thalamus and lower brainstem (Figure 23-6).

The dorsal column medial lemniscal system conveys impulses that are specific with respect to intensity and localization. Information relayed through the dorsal column system includes barognosis, kinesthesia, proprioception, vibration, stereognosis, discriminative touch, tactile pressure, two-point discrimination, and graphesthesia. The impulses are carried through large, rapidly conducting fibers to the dorsal column of the spinal cord, where the impulse crosses over to the opposite side and continues to the thalamus through the medial lemnisci and the sensory cortex (Figure 23-7).

Assessment of Sensation. In a routine assessment, sensory functions would not be reviewed by the nurse. If, however, issues are noted in pain, paresthesias, or motor deficits, a full sensory examination should be completed. Methods of sensory assessment are identified in Box 23-5.

Nursing Diagnosis: Disturbed Sensory Perception (Tactile). Many neurological problems affect sensation. A stroke or cerebrovascular accident resulting in hemiplegia results in impaired sensation to one side of the body. Multiple sclerosis may result in paresthesias to affected body areas. Aging may lead to sensory loss. Diabetic neuropathy is a common cause of paresthesias and loss of sensation in the lower extremities.

Implications for Rehabilitation. The rehabilitation nurse must expect that any patient with neurological impairment may experience sensory losses and impaired sensation and identify risks for the patient. Because the sensory system provides the body with warnings for excessive pressure, potential tissue injury, and location of the body in space, impairment of sensation places the patient at risk for injury. Patients are taught safety in the environment and how to use environmental clues to compensate for the lack of sensory perception. For example, if proprioceptive and tactile sensation is deficient in the left arm and leg, the patient is taught to visually assess the location and safety of the left arm and leg.

Perception

The ability to make sense of the environment through the identification, integration, and interpretation of incoming stimuli is perception. It is difficult to consider perception apart from sensation because perception is the way one interprets sensations, making perception and sensation interrelated phenomena.

Anatomy and Physiology. Perception occurs primarily in the parietal lobes of the cerebral cortex. The right and left parietal lobes tend to process different aspects of perception. Verbal input, through writing and reading, and right/left discrimination are usually processed in the left parietal lobe. Information on space, texture, geography, construction, and body schema is processed in the right parietal lobe.

Perceptual ability is essential for learning and must be present for successful rehabilitation of individuals with or without disabilities. Perception of stimuli is a highly individualized process, influenced by past experiences, age, culture, beliefs, education, attitudes, goals, and expectations. In addition, perception can be modified through feedback from others.

Assessment of Perception. The rehabilitation nurse will assess perception related to specific issues identified in routine assessment from other health care providers. For example,

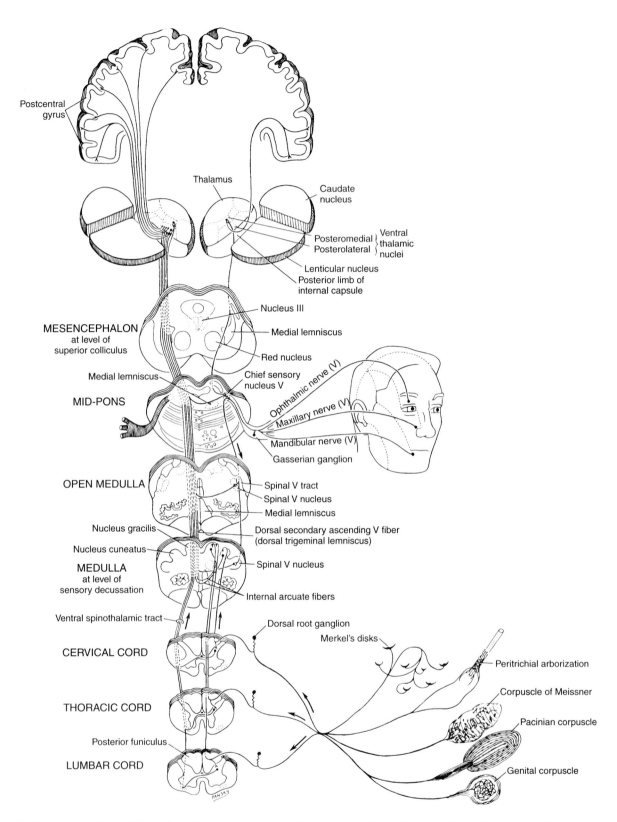

Figure 23-6 Sensory pathways. The pathway for the transmission of light touch is shown. Note that input from the peripheral nerves serving the head and face is at the brainstem level. Touch sensory fibers from the trunk, arms, and legs travel upward in the posterior funiculus and join head and face fibers in the brainstem in the medial lemniscus.

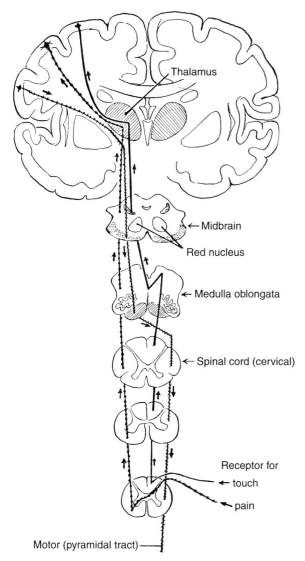

Figure 23-7 Diagram of the main motor and sensory pathways. The perceptions of touch, passive motion, position, and vibration are transmitted through the posterior tract in the spinal cord through the medial lemniscus in the brainstem to the thalamus and through the internal capsule to the cortex (this pathway is represented by the *solid line*). Pain and temperature sensations are transmitted through the anterolateral tract and lateral lemniscus to the thalamus and then through the internal capsule to the cortex (*dotted lines*). (Courtesy John Muhm, EdD.)

a person with left hemiplegia should be assessed for left-sided neglect and homonymous hemianopsia because both are common deficits associated with right cerebrovascular accidents. Assessment of specific perceptual problems is discussed in conjunction with common neurological problems identified in the next portion of this chapter. Motor pathways are discussed in Chapter 14.

Nursing Diagnosis: Unilateral Neglect. Many neurological problems affect cognitive-perceptual patterns. Perceptual problems are often experienced by persons with brain injuries or lesions. There are numerous variations of perception that may present, many of which are discussed next.

> ### BOX 23-5 Sensory Assessment Methods
>
> **Pain discrimination:** a safety pin is opened and placed against the skin; patient is asked to identify the location of the stimulus and to describe it and note if it is sharp or dull
> **Two-point discrimination:** with the patient's eyes closed, two sharp points (toothpicks) are used to lightly prick the skin; patient is assessed to determine the minimum distance at which he or she is able to identify two points
> **Proprioception:** with the patient's eyes closed, a single toe or finger is moved by the nurse, and the patient is asked to identify the location of the phalange and whether it is up or down
> **Vibratory sense:** with the patient's eyes closed, a tuning fork is struck and placed end down on the patient's extremity; patient is asked to report whether any sensation is felt and to describe it; if the patient identifies the vibration, he or she is asked to tell when vibration is no longer perceived
> **Temperature sense:** cold water is placed in one glass container and warm in another; patient is asked to identify the temperature (warm or cold) of each item when placed against the skin
> **Tactile sense:** patient's eyes are kept closed; nurse uses a cotton swab to gently touch the patient's skin in symmetric points, and patient is asked to identify when the touch is felt; results are identified as normal, hypesthetic, anesthetic, or hyperesthetic

Body Image or Schema Problems. These types of problems may result after brain injury because the ability to integrate and make sense of tactile and proprioceptive input may be impaired. Somatognosia is one type of body image problem in which there is an unawareness of one's body structure and body parts. It typically occurs with lesions of the dominant parietal lobe and often is associated with right-sided hemiplegia. The patient may have difficulty imitating movements and following directions such as "move your left leg." The patient may have less difficulty responding to simple gestures and instructions identifying specific body parts.

Right and left discrimination is a type of body image or schema deficit that may occur after damage to either parietal lobe. With this deficit the person is unable to determine the right or left side of his or her own body and will not be able to follow verbal commands that include references to right and left. Rehabilitation nurses should avoid mention of right or left in directions. Correction for the deficit is best done through the use of environmental cues (other than left and right) or pointing.

Another type of body image or schema is visual spatial neglect, which usually occurs after a parietal lobe lesion of the nondominant hemisphere and usually affects awareness of the left side of the body. The person may be unaware of any stimuli on the affected side, including tactile and environmental stimuli. This disorder creates the potential for serious safety hazards because the person is not aware of objects to the left within the environment. Although the person is being taught how to correct the problem, the rehabilitation nurse should provide modifications to the surroundings to create a safe environment. Therapy revolves around increasing the person's awareness of the left side of the environment and of his or her body. The use of auditory and olfactory stimulation on the left side of the body or environment may help provide cues for the person to scan the environment to the left. Placing a radio or tape player on the left side can provide an auditory cue to check that area of the environment. Applying hand cream or perfumed lotions to the left arm can also provide tactile stimulation and olfactory stimulation that can cue the person to remember the left side.

Finger agnosia and anosognosia are two additional types of body image or schema disorders. With finger agnosia, the person is unable to identify specific fingers bilaterally. The problem usually results after a lesion to the parietal lobe of the dominant hemisphere and is linked with aphasia. Anosognosia is a serious problem in which individuals deny the presence of paralysis. Usually the parietal lobe of the dominant side is affected. The condition is linked with a poor prognosis because it is difficult to teach individuals to correct deficits that they do not perceive. Treatment may involve discriminative touch and pressure to cue the individual in to the fingers. The rehabilitation nurse should focus on preventive ways to ensure a safe environment.

Spatial Relation Disorders. These types of perceptual deficits may occur after damage to the nondominant hemisphere of the brain and are usually seen in conjunction with left-sided hemiplegia. Spatial relation deficits entail problems in identifying items' distance and relationship in space. Figure-ground discrimination is the inability to distinguish an item from the background, which creates problems in all activities of daily living. For example, it is necessary to be able to distinguish a towel from the wall and a bar of soap from the sink in order to wash the face, and it is necessary to be able to distinguish a slice of bread from a plate in order to eat. Persons with this deficit tend to have less difficulty with items that are clearly defined and are contrasted by color from the background.

Form constancy is a type of spatial relation problem in which persons have difficulty identifying similarly shaped but distinct objects from one another. For example, a person with spatial relations problems may not be able to distinguish between a glass and a vase sitting side by side. Likewise, a toothbrush lying near a pencil may be confused. Problems with this deficit can be minimized by controlling the environment and encouraging the person to feel the objects and inspect them closely. Persons with spatial relations problems may show deficits in other visual spatial areas requiring judgment, for example, with direction, depth, and distance. These persons, when mobilized with a wheelchair, have difficulty not running into the wall and getting through doorways due to the inability to gauge distance and depth. When using the stairs or ambulating, they need consistent and constant reminders to learn to compensate for the deficit.

Agnosia. Persons with agnosia are unable to identify familiar items with one sense, although the use of an alternative sense may help them recognize the object. For example,

a woman may not be able to find her mirror when looking on a table until she actually feels the mirror with her hands. The fork and spoon may be confused until the person picks up each and recalls the differences. This deficit is corrected by encouraging patients to use more than a single sense in locating and identifying objects. However, correction is not as easy for individuals with agnosias involving other senses. For example, with auditory agnosia, the person may not recognize familiar nonspeech sounds such as bells, whistles, and car horns and the difference between the telephone ringing and the doorbell.

Apraxia. Persons with apraxia cannot remember movements they once knew. Although they have sufficient strength, coordination, and attention to perform the action, they are unable to do so. For example, a patient with ideational apraxia may be capable of shaving, but if he is told to do so, he may not be able to comprehend or conceptualize the task. If the person has ideomotor apraxia, he may be able to pick up the shaver and shave out of habit. However, if a nurse or therapist tells him to shave, he may not be able to formulate a plan of action. Refer to Table 14-2 for information about dyspraxias and apraxias.

Implications for Rehabilitation. Perceptual deficits often are viewed by family members as indicators of dementia. It is essential that they be assisted in understanding the nature of such problems. Through careful assessment of the patterns of behavior and deficits, treatment plans can be designed to correct many of the problems. General approaches to perceptual programs are presented in the following section.

Transfer of Training. The transfer of training approach is based on the belief that learning a skill for one application will carry over to other applications. For example, the practice of scanning for pieces while completing a puzzle can help the patient remember to scan the dinner table during meals.

Sensorimotor Approach. With the sensorimotor approach, motor output is controlled and specific sensory stimulation is offered to influence cerebral sensory organization and processing. Adaptive motor reactions are required in response to carefully controlled sensory stimuli. For instance, the patient could be assisted into a standing table for proprioceptive input.

Functional Approach. Probably one of the most common approaches to sensory and perceptual problems, the functional approach is based on the concept that practicing functional tasks will result in relearning and independence. Methods of compensation and adaptation are incorporated in functional teaching. For example, repeatedly buttoning a shirt with a buttonhook is an example of a functional approach to relearning the skill of buttoning.

Safety Concerns. While the patient is relearning functional skills and abilities, the environment must be as safe as possible. For example, the environment around persons with neglect and homonymous hemianopsia must have essential bedside needs (e.g., telephone, call light, and tissues) on the uninvolved side. While the patient is learning scanning techniques, colored tape may be used to attract attention to items.

Pain

Physical pain is a normal sensation that indicates the presence of tissue damage. Pain impulses are transmitted from tissues and organs to the substantia gelatinosa within the lateral spinothalamic tract of the spinal cord. The impulses ascend to the thalamus of the brain and to the cerebral cortex. Simultaneously, descending fibers from the cerebral cortex moderate the way pain is perceived.

Anatomy and Physiology. According to Melzack (2002), a noted Canadian research psychologist, the substantia gelatinosa of the spinal cord is the "gate" of the pain experience. According to the gate-control theory of pain, pain impulses are transmitted via small α-delta afferent fibers to the substantia gelatinosa of the spinal cord. Large fibers transmit touch, temperature, and pressure and travel a similar route to the spinal cord. The gate theory holds that if the large fibers are stimulated simultaneously with the small fibers, the pain impulse will be weakened and perceived to a lesser degree. Likewise, if one is experiencing pain, the pain perception may be decreased by stimulating the large fibers through touch, temperature change, or pressure. Simultaneously, the descending fibers from the cerebral cortex can decrease the pain perception through distraction and relaxation (Figure 23-8).

Assessment of Pain. Although pain is a common experience, there are a variety of widely held myths regarding pain perception. It seems that few have objective opinions about another's pain experience. There are a variety of myths about the pain experience, all of which affect the assessment of pain (Brown & Richardson, 2006).

Myths. One myth relates to the need for a physical explanation or reason for pain. If none is apparent, it is believed by many that the pain is of a psychological or emotional nature. This is untrue because in some cases the physical reason for pain is undetermined but may become clear at a later date and time. A second myth holds that malingering is common and that individuals will lie about the existence of pain to receive narcotics or sympathy. There is no clinical evidence in support of this myth, although oligoanalgesia is a common problem in emergency departments based on the belief that many individuals are drug seeking (Fosnocht, Swanson, & Barton, 2005). Although some persons may malinger, it is not common. In fact, more patients understate their pain than overstate it. Another commonly held myth about pain is that persons in pain always show visible signs of pain that verify the existence of the pain, including restlessness, apprehension, and a drawn expression. As with the other myths, this is also unfounded. Individuals respond differently to pain.

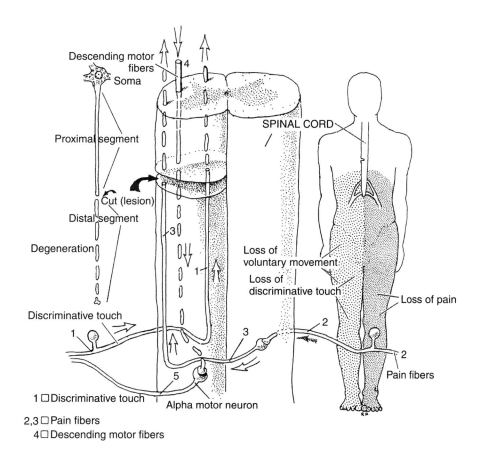

Figure 23-8 Effect of a spinal cord lesion on ascending or descending tracts. Degeneration of ascending tracts occurs above the lesion; descending tracts will degenerate below the lesion.

It is not unusual for persons who have been in pain for long periods of time to fail to show any emotion, let alone the strong emotion expected to be seen with pain. This failure to demonstrate strong emotion with pain is particularly evident with chronically ill children (Scharff et al., 2005).

Until the past two decades, the topic of pain in infancy and childhood was conspicuously absent from the literature or supported by a set of myths. A prevailing notion was that infants and young children with immature neurological systems could not distinguish pain or realized lesser degrees of pain than did adults. "Growing pains" were just to be outgrown. These ideas, coupled with concern that exposure to pain medication would lead children into addiction, contributed to poor pain management for children. Nurse researchers are credited with instituting many of the changes in this area. However, early studies have centered on acute pain, whereas many children in rehabilitation experience chronic or recurring pain (Hoeman, 1990).

A final myth is that health care professionals are the experts about a patient's pain experience. It is imperative that rehabilitation nurses and all health care professionals realize that pain is whatever the experiencing person says it is and exists whenever the person says is does (Pasero & McCaffery, 2005). No one is an expert in describing or identifying another's pain perception.

Cultural Implications. The pain experience is highly individualized. Persons respond to pain based on their culture, their background, and prior ordeals with pain (Work Loss Data Institute, 2004). Culture affects the way individuals respond to pain. A belief in U.S. Western medicine is that pain is unnecessary and should be treated. Persons who report having a headache will be asked if they have taken anything for it. If they respond that they have not taken anything, others will assume that they deserve to suffer for not having done anything to help themselves. Another Western expectation of the pain experience is that the affected individual will deal with the pain in a quiet, controlled manner. That is, it is not appropriate for a person in pain to lose control and yell or cry incessantly. The person in pain should not talk about the pain frequently. In contrast, some cultures, such as some Hispanic groups, consider it proper to display strong emotion with pain. Other groups, such as Scandinavians, consider pain to be a character-building experience.

Prior Pain Experiences and Other Influences on Pain Perception. A person's knowledge about pain can also temper the pain response. One clear example of this is childbirth. The daughter who hears her mother describe a 40-hour labor involving intolerable pain will dread the onset of labor, anticipating that she will also suffer intolerable pain. An additional way in which the pain experience is modified is through prior pain experiences. The individual who experiences migraine headaches, for example, often recognizes the preceding signs and symptoms and anticipates that the pain experience will equate or surpass prior episodes. Part of the pain experienced with migraines may be due to the fear of impending pain.

Assessment Tools. Because there is little correlation between one's physical appearance or facial expressions and the degree of pain experienced, assessment of pain depends primarily on subjective reporting. The nurse records the patient's pain history, including the maximum, minimum, and typical amount of pain experienced. The nurse assesses what the patient reports exacerbates the pain and what alleviates the pain. A standardized scale for pain assessment should be used, such as the visual analog scale (Figure 23-9) or the McGill-Melzack pain questionnaire. In addition, with chronic nonmalignant pain, the nurse assesses the patient's premorbid and postmorbid lifestyle and the impact the patient perceives pain has made on his or her lifestyle.

A number of assessment tools are available that are designed specifically for assessing pain in children. The Wong-Baker Faces scale is used for both children and adults (Figure 23-10). The Wong-Baker scale has the advantage of clear visual identification of pain ratings across age, language, and comprehension continuums. Children may benefit from art, play, or music therapy as both assessment and intervention techniques. All approaches with children consider the total family system and family participation in child-centered goals. The FLACC scale (Face, Legs, Activity, Crying and Consolability Scale), is a 0 to 10 scale used by the nurse to assess pain in someone unable to communicate or under 3 years of age.

Assessment and Management Mnemonics. Regardless of the specific pain assessment scale used, the rehabilitation nurse should use a system to ensure that all parameters of

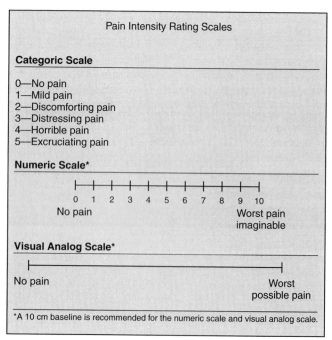

Figure 23-9 Pain intensity rating scales. (From Monahan, F. D, Sands, J. K., Neighbors, M., Marek, J. F., & Green, C. J. [2007]. *Phipps' medical-surgical nursing: Health & illness perspectives* [8th ed.]. St. Louis, MO: Mosby.)

Figure 23-10 Faces pain rating scale. To use, explain to the child that each face is for a person who either feels happy because there is no pain (hurt) or feels sad because there is some or a lot of pain. Face 0 is very happy because there is no hurt. Face 1 hurts just a little bit. Face 2 hurts a little more. Face 3 hurts even more. Face 4 hurts a whole lot, but face 5 hurts as much as you can imagine, although you do not have to be crying to feel this bad. Ask the child to choose the face that best describes his or her own pain. Record the number under the chosen face on a pain assessment record. (From Wong, D. L., Hockenberry-Eaton, M., Wilson, D., & Winkelstein, M. L. [2003]. *Wong's nursing care of infants and children* [7th ed.]. St. Louis, MO: Mosby.)

pain are assessed. A common mnemonic for pain assessment is the following:

P: What *p*rovokes/*p*alliates the pain?

Q: How does the patient describe the *q*uality of the pain? (e.g., burning, sharp, stabbing, aching)

R: Does the pain *r*adiate anywhere, what *r*egion is affected?

S: How *s*evere is the pain? Rate on the 0 to 10 scale with 10 being the worst possible pain.

T: What is the *t*iming of the pain? When does it occur?

Nursing Diagnosis: Acute or Chronic Pain. Pain may be classified as chronic nonmalignant, acute, or chronic malignant (Melzack, 2001). Acute and chronic malignant pain problems tend to follow a predictable course, whereas chronic nonmalignant pain follows an ill-defined clinical course with an uncertain therapeutic outcome.

Chronic Nonmalignant Pain. Although pain is a normal sensation, most persons believe they would be better off without it. Just the opposite is true, however, as demonstrated by the devastation of Hansen's disease, or leprosy. One of the key characteristics of Hansen's disease is the destruction of pain receptors, resulting in anesthesia. The problem, of course, is that persons with Hansen's disease fail to recognize tissue damage in time to prevent serious injury. Yancey (1977) described a patient with Hansen's disease becoming blind because the eye surface did not detect irritation and the patient did not perceive the need to blink, resulting in drying of the eyes. However, just as a complete absence of pain is life threatening, the unceasing presence of pain also is intolerable. Such is the case with chronic nonmalignant pain syndrome.

Chronic nonmalignant pain is a disorder of sensation that affects every aspect of a person's life: family, friends, work, and play. Although there is a wealth of literature on the syndrome, there is no consensus as to why some persons develop chronic nonmalignant pain syndrome and others with equivalent or even more physically severe injuries do not. One hypothesis is that a pain cycle develops and results in chronic nonmalignant pain syndrome. In response to injury, the person protects and immobilizes the injured area, such as a joint. The immobilization of the area leads to the development of scar tissue around the site and a reduction in synovial fluid production. The joint becomes stiff and difficult to move, leading to increased pain, inflammation, and tendonitis. The person guards and immobilizes the joint to an even greater degree, with resulting weakness and loss of function. To continue guarding the area, the person develops compensatory mechanisms to protect the joint, such as limping and altering the gait. These compensatory mechanisms do not act in the body's favor, and the altered gait leads to back pain, resulting in more extensive guarding of multiple areas. The result is chronic presence of pain without a clear link to a pathophysiological problem.

Chronic nonmalignant pain interferes with vocational and avocational aspects of life. Absence from work due to therapy and medical appointments, illness, and loss of function results in poor attendance and difficulty maintaining a job. Complaints about the amount of pain experienced and restrictions of avocational activities lead to limited family and community involvement. Reductions in activity result in weight gain and decreased energy and endurance levels. As more and more money is spent looking for cures, causes, and relief, finances become exhausted. As the pain continues with no relief in sight, depression becomes a way of life. Persons with chronic nonmalignant pain have little reason to look forward to days filled with more and more pain; less and less function; and constant work, family, and financial problems. Such persons experience difficulties coping with their pain and may develop addictions to alcohol and narcotics. Eventually they reach the end of the medical therapeutic gamut and are depressed, financially drained, with employment and family problems, and still in constant pain.

Given the pervasiveness of the problem of chronic nonmalignant pain, it is unlikely that any single modality of intervention will be effective in providing relief from the syndrome. Therefore programs having the greatest success provide a variety of interventions and use a comprehensive and multifaceted approach. Comprehensive programs for chronic nonmalignant pain usually involve a variety of disciplines, including but not limited to nursing, physical therapy, medicine, occupational therapy, vocational counseling, therapeutic recreation, and psychology.

Just as in other areas of rehabilitation, patient education is a cornerstone of treatment for chronic nonmalignant pain. Self-application of local therapies such as ultrasound, transcutaneous electrical stimulation, and hot or cold packs may be of benefit and should be included in patient education programs. A second component of patient education for chronic nonmalignant pain is instruction in the use of behavioral methods of pain relief such as biofeedback, relaxation, and self-hypnosis. Patients should be taught the use of work simplification and energy conservation methods but need to be encouraged to increase activity level gradually. The patient should receive instructions in posture, body mechanics, and positioning. The program should include an assessment of workplace design and ergonomics.

Chronic Nonmalignant Pain Across the Life Span. Persons in two age groups, the very young and the very old, tend to experience subtle discrimination with respect to chronic nonmalignant pain. Although more than 50 million children in the United States experience chronic nonmalignant pain, there is a paucity of health care resources for them. Health care professionals often underestimate the amount of pain experienced by children, and because many children are hesitant to talk to physicians and nurses, their pain may be underreported. The second age-group undertreated for chronic nonmalignant pain is the geriatric group. Many older persons experience chronic nonmalignant pain due to chronic illness and disability, and they assume that it is a normal part of the aging process. Although few children or elderly persons require the comprehensiveness of a chronic nonmalignant pain management program, they will benefit from an open-minded approach toward alleviation and moderation of the pain experienced.

Common conditions for chronic nonmalignant pain in childhood include juvenile rheumatoid arthritis, sickle cell crises, recurrent headaches, recurrent abdominal pain from a variety of conditions, reflex sympathetic dystrophy syndrome, malignancies, and pain after multiple traumas or amputation. The impact of a child's pain on the family is part of the assessment.

Children with chronic, disabling, or developmental disorders must be assessed within the context of their developmental stage. Two variables contribute to difficulty in assessing pain in children: the expression of pain and the experience of pain. A child's experience and expression of pain will differ with the developmental stage, but more importantly, these cannot be equated with adult behaviors or judged using adult terms. A child who has prolonged chronic nonmalignant pain or whose pain worsens gradually may not be able to distinguish changes in pain intensity or determine duration and location of pain. Children may play or sleep through pain as ways of coping with discomfort. In fact, children may not refer to the pain as pain. A child's self-report of having no pain may not be reliable for a variety of reasons. For instance, some children may not be able to associate pain relief measures with improved comfort; others may assign themselves personal responsibility for the pain or believe they deserve punishment.

For these reasons, it often is beneficial to ask a child who or what causes the pain and to describe and explain pain using the child's own words (Hoeman, 1990).

Older persons may try to ignore or bear their pain or conversely may complain about pain. Those who are cognitively intact may not require any adaptations for pain assessment. However, impaired or altered sensory function, such as vision or hearing, and reduced sensation and perception may alter the pain experience. An older person may deny pain but guard movement or positioning, change patterns of ambulation, pace level of activity, or avoid painful activities without reporting pain. The pain threshold increases with aging, and older persons accept pain as a consequence of aging (Lautenbacher, Kunz, Strate, Nielsen, & Arendt-Nielsen, 2005). Those with cognitive or communication impairments may become frustrated, angry, or contentious because they cannot express or explain their pain. In addition, the elderly patient may experience chronic but transient pain and describe it as discomfort, aches, or by such colloquial names as "old friend" or "rheumatiz," thus avoiding the nature of the pain. Older persons are at risk for undertreatment of pain due to their tendency to understate the amount of pain experienced or the appearance of tolerating pain well (Harrison, Kim, Silverberg, & Paget, 2005). Management of pain experienced by older persons should include involving the patient and family and providing them with control over the pain management tools and options selected.

Pain is a multidimensional phenomenon. Even with the use of a comprehensive approach to pain management, the prognosis for persons with chronic nonmalignant pain is a long and hard fight for functional recovery, without any guarantees that pain will cease.

Malignant Pain. Pain from cancer may occur due to nerve compression, infection, and release of prostaglandins. Unlike chronic nonmalignant pain, the cornerstone of treatment for malignant pain is pharmacological. The guiding principles of narcotic use for malignant pain are matching dose to patient response and giving the medication on a regular and consistent basis rather than on an as-needed basis. The World Health Organization's ladder for pharmacological pain management provides a guideline for appropriate steps for managing increasing pain (Meldrum, 2005). The ladder progresses as noted in Figure 23-11.

Nonmalignant, Intermittent Pain. Pain that occurs on an irregular but severe basis, such as with sickle cell disease, typically is treated as acute pain. Nonpharmacological pain relief methods may be of benefit, but the primary mode of treatment is the use of medications to manage acute episodes.

Another type of nonmalignant pain is phantom limb pain, a natural consequence after the loss of a body part. Typically it does not present problems with therapeutic management, although on occasion individuals experience extreme phantom limb pain. Treatment for severe phantom limb problems usually follows the comprehensive approach used for management of chronic nonmalignant pain.

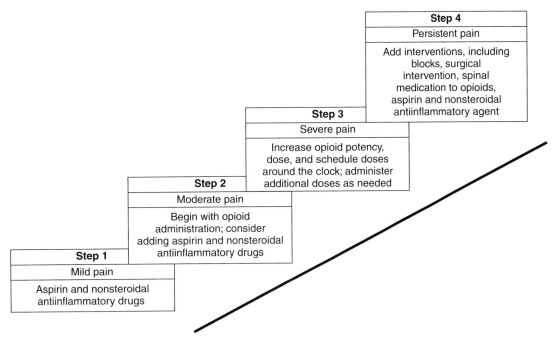

Figure 23-11 Modified, four-step pain ladder. (Modified from the World Health Organization. [1996]. *Cancer pain relief* [2nd ed.]. Geneva: Author.)

TABLE 23-6 Nonpharmacological Pain Management Tools

Method	Comments and Applications
Heat	Use caution in application of heat to prevent burns or tissue injury; temperature of the warm compress should be tested before application, and the site should be reassessed frequently
Cold	Flexible ice packs tend to work well and may assist in decreasing inflammation or swelling, cold treatments should not be applied for longer than 15 minutes and should not be used when peripheral vascular disease is present
Repositioning	Tendency to "fluff and puff" pillows can work well to assist an individual in pain in gaining a position of comfort
Exercise	Avoid exercise during acute pain, with the exception of range of motion; exercise may restore mobilization, coordination, and balance
Massage, pressure, and vibration	Provide physical stimulation and enhance relaxation
Relaxation and imagery	Used to augment other methods of pain relief or during procedures; may provide assistance during times of anxiety and fatigue
Cognitive distraction	Use of music, television, visiting, reading, or a focal point may reduce the focus on pain and provide relief for a limited time
Hypnosis	Used in conjunction with relaxation and visual imagery techniques; most effective when used with individuals whose concentration and motivation are strong
Transcutaneous electrical nerve stimulation	Low-voltage electrical impulse is relayed to peripheral muscle fibers through a device controlled by the person in pain; impulse is believed to function by "closing the gate" and blocking the pain impulse transmission
Acupuncture	Small needles are inserted, and electrical current may be used to block pain impulses; placement of the needles is designed through Eastern vital energy flow theory
Therapeutic touch	Whether through massage or a system such as Reiki, can be beneficial in promoting relaxation and through stimulating large afferent fibers that may block transmission of pain impulses
Biofeedback	Tool through which electrical impulses or skin temperature is assessed as an index of relaxation; can be of benefit in educating patients how to relax
Aromatherapy	May be effective for pain reduction through stimulating descending pathways and providing distraction while enhancing relaxation
Herbal medicines	Many varieties; it is imperative that rehabilitation nurses educate patients that such medications do not go through FDA approval and may have harmful or no effects

FDA, Food and Drug Administration.

Implications for Rehabilitation. Because pain is a unique experience for all individuals, it is unlikely that any single solution will be effective for all. Therefore it makes sense that there should be variety of tools available for those experiencing pain. Table 23-6 contains a listing of nonpharmacological tools for pain management. Although many of these nonpharmacological pain management methods work for some individuals, it is important to note that there is a lack of evidence-based practice to validate the methods. However, it is important for persons in pain to have choices, and it is critical that rehabilitation nurses provide educated options for their patients in pain. It is also important for the nurse to assess what nonpharmacological pain management strategies worked for them in the past.

The response to pain is both automatic and learned. Children who touch a hot stove will remove their fingers automatically and will learn not to touch hot stoves. A similar learned response to perception of other sensations occurs.

In addition, individuals learn how to organize and process sensory input. Because we are constantly bombarded with sensory stimulation, we must select which stimuli we will respond to. Individuals adapt to different environments and learn alternative methods of organizing and processing sensory input in those environments. For example, the smell of smoke outside on a fall day is processed as an insignificant and pleasant olfactory stimulation. The same smoke smell indoors triggers quite a different response. Consider a hospital setting, with all its associated noises, sights, and smells (e.g., paging, footsteps, medication, food carts, alcohol, and cleansers). Although such an environment is not novel to health care professionals, it is novel to the patients we serve. Even patients with intact neurological systems may have difficulty organizing and processing the sensory input associated with a hospital setting. When patients have impaired sensation and perception, their ability to organize and make sense of their environment may be limited severely.

Case Study

Mike, age 43, is a long-haul trucker. To increase his profits on transporting, he unloads his own trucks. This allows a faster delivery time, and he saves the expense of hiring someone to assist with unloading. Long-haul trucking is not conducive to healthy eating, exercise routines, or sleep. As a result, Mike is about 50 pounds overweight and has developed a significant problem with low back pain.

He uses ibuprofen to control the pain and uses alcohol to help him sleep at night. During a recent trip the pain became so severe that Mike was unable to walk following the trip. He saw a physician, who advised him to lose weight, establish an exercise plan, and start physical therapy. Mike filed a worker's compensation claim and remained out of work while attending physical therapy. His weight increased, because he found the pain to be incapacitating. He was not able to exercise due to the pain and spent most days on the couch in his home.

Mike's physician ordered a computed tomography (CT) scan of the spine, which showed degenerative disk disease, with narrowing of the L4 and L5 spaces. He continued physical therapy and ordered OxyContin CR 5 mg every 4 hours for pain in an effort to allow Mike to increase activity while lowering the pain. Mike felt better with the new medication and found that when he combined the OxyContin with two beers, he was able to sleep.

Although Mike received workers' compensation, money was much tighter, and he experienced some financial issues. His wife struggled with his illness. She was used to Mike's frequent and lengthy road trips. Since his injury Mike was home all the time but not able to be involved in activities. She complained that he did nothing but lie on the couch all day and night. Mike and his wife did not have a strong or happy marriage before his illness. Following the injury, Mike and his wife began arguing frequently about money and other stressors.

Mike developed a significant depression and questioned his worth. His weight continued to increase, and he became more deconditioned. Mike was referred to a psychiatrist for depression. The psychiatrist prescribed escitalopram oxalate (Lexapro) 10 mg daily for depression and

lorazepam (Ativan) 1 mg at bedtime for sleep. He referred Mike and his wife to a marriage counselor.

After 9 months Mike was unable to climb a flight of stairs without feeling short of breath. The pain was no better, and his use of and need for medications increased. His physician referred him to a neurologist, who completed electromyogram (EMG) studies, which show some impingement of the sciatic nerve. Mike was referred to a neurosurgeon, who recommended a laminectomy. One year following his last work trip, Mike had a laminectomy for the sciatic nerve compression. He started physical therapy after surgery and made slow progress.

Although the surgery had proceeded smoothly and his recovery was uneventful, Mike continued to experience pain. His dose of OxyContin CR increased to 20 mg every 4 hours. His physician started him on a Duragesic (fentanyl) patch of 25 mcg/hr. Mike continued to drink, with his alcohol consumption up to one to two packs of beer per day. He frequently missed therapy appointments. His wife decided to leave him and filed for divorce.

His trucking firm hired a private investigator who followed Mike around, trying to prove that his injury was not as limiting as Mike claimed. Financial pressures increased, because the company began refusing to pay claims. Mike was forced to hire an attorney to defend his rights for continued benefits. After almost 2 years of health care treatment for his low back injury and pain, Mike continued to experience a decline in health, energy, and endurance. His pain was as bad as ever. He was at the end of the medical therapeutic gamut—and no closer to returning to work or to a productive lifestyle.

Mike was referred to an interdisciplinary pain management program. He agreed to participate in the program, and his wife consented to assist and support him in the process.

Mike was placed on a gradual withdrawal from his medications and alcohol. Related to the amount of narcotics and alcohol he was regularly consuming, Mike was admitted for a short stay at a detoxification program. Following a 3-day stay, Mike entered into a daily

Case Study—cont'd

physical therapy program. Each day he exercised with the therapist and then worked with the rehabilitation nurse in learning and practicing relaxation and guided imagery. A psychologist met with Mike and his wife on a weekly basis to assess progress in the program. He joined AA, and maintained his diet.

Meetings were held with his employers, and a desk position in the company was identified that Mike had the skills to perform.

He returned to work within 6 months of entering the pain management rehabilitation program, initially working half days, and then extending to full time.

When asked to what he attributed the improvement in his health status and his ability to return to work, Mike stated that he believed the full team was needed, because he had tried to do things on his own unsuccessfully for more than 2 years.

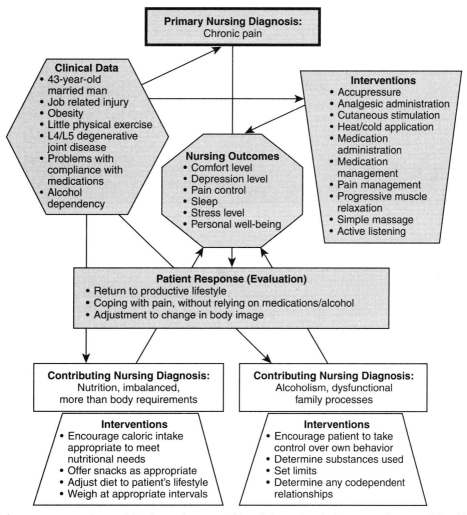

Concept Map. Mike's return to a productive lifestyle revolves around his ability to break the pain cycle. He will be able to do that through the support of the comprehensive pain program in which he is participating. The rehabilitation nurse needs to focus interventions on pain relief, in addition to encouraging a balance of nutrition and assisting Mike through the withdrawl of substances while increasing physical activity and endurance.

CRITICAL THINKING

1. In the case study Mike returns to work. Many individuals with chronic pain resulting from a work-related injury do not return to their prior position or employment status. What factors in Mike's story contributed to the successful outcome?

2. Mike was placed on opioids for control of the pain. He developed tolerance to the medication and combined the drugs with alcohol for added effect. Although the combination with alcohol is ill advised, were opioids appropriate for Mike? Why or why not?

3. Family members are integrally involved when one member develops a chronic pain problem. What are early steps to take, while mindful of private health information, to ensure the family is engaged in care.

REFERENCES

American Speech-Language-Hearing Association. (2000). *Newborn and infant hearing screening action center*. Rockville, MD: Author.

Battista, J., Kalloniatis, M., & Metha, A. (2005). Visual function: The problem with eccentricity. *Clinical and Experimental Optometry, 88*(5), 313-321.

Belluci, R. (2005). Multifocal intraocular lenses. *Current Opinions in Ophthalmology, 16*(1), 33-37.

Bickley, L., & Szilagyi, P. (2003). *Bates' guide to physical examination and history taking* (8th ed.). Philadelphia: Lippincott Williams & Wilkins.

Breivek, J. (2005). Vulnerable but strong: Deaf people challenge established understandings of deafness. *Scandinavian Journal of Public Health Supplement, 66*, 18-23.

Bromley, S. (2000). Smell and taste disorders: A primary care approach. *American Family Physician, 61*(2), 427-436.

Brown, C., & Richardson, C. (2006). Nurses in the multiprofessional pain team: A study of attitudes, beliefs, and treatment endorsements. *European Journal of Pain, 10*(1), 13-22.

Centers for Disease Control and Prevention. (2004). *Vision impairment*. Atlanta, GA: Centers for Disease Control and Prevention. Retrieved October 21, 2006, from http://www.cdc.gov/ncbddd/dd/vision2.htm.

Congdon, N., O'Colmain, B., Klaver, C., Klein, R., Munoz, B., Friedman, D., et al. (2004). Causes and prevalence of visual impairment among adults in the United States. *Archives of Ophthalmology, 122*(4), 477-485.

Connolly, J., Carron, J., & Roark, S. (2005). Universal newborn hearing screening: Are we accomplishing the Joint Committee on Infant Hearing (JCIH) objectives? *Laryngoscope, 115*(2), 232-236.

de Kruijk, J., Leffers, P., Menheere, P., Meerhoff, S., Rutten, J., & Twijnstra, A. (2003). Olfactory functioning after mild traumatic brain injury. *Brain Injury, 17*(1), 73-80.

Dunning, T. (2005). Applying a quality use of medicines framework to using essential oils in nursing practice. *Complementary Therapies in Clinical Practice, 11*(3), 172-181.

Eibenstein, A., Fioretti, A., Simaskou, M., Sucapane, P., Mearelli, S., Mina, C., et al. (2005). Olfactory screening test in mild cognitive impairment. *Neurological Sciences, 26*(3), 156-160.

Fosnocht, D., Swanson, E., & Barton, E. (2005). Changing attitudes about pain and pain control in emergency medicine. *Emergency Medicine Clinics of North America, 23*(2), 297-306.

Freedom Scientific. (2005). http://www.freedomscientific.com/fs_products/software_jaws.asp.

Friedman, J., West, S., Munoz, B., Park, W., Deremeik, J., Massof, R., et al. (2004). Racial variations in causes of vision loss in nursing homes. *Archives of Ophthalmology, 122*, 1019-1024.

Geers, A. (2004). Speech, language and reading skills after early cochlear implantation. *Archives of Otolaryngology–Head & Neck Surgery, 130*(5), 634-648.

Gordon, M. (2000). *Manual of nursing diagnosis* (9th ed.). St. Louis, MO: Mosby.

GW Micro. (2005). http://www.gwmicro.com/.

Harrison, M., Kim, C., Silverberg, M., & Paget, S. (2005). Does age bias the aggressive treatment of elderly patients with rheumatoid arthritis. *Journal of Rheumatology, 3*(7), 1243-1248.

Hoeman, S. P. (1990, October 5). Chronic pain in childhood. *Keynote presentation of Caring for Persons in Pain Workshop*. Reading, PA: Alvernia College.

Holt, J. (2003). Cholesteatoma and otosclerosis: Two slowly progressive causes of hearing loss treatable through corrective surgery. *Clinical Medical Research, 1*(2), 151-154.

Hyde, M. (2005). Newborn hearing screening programs: An overview. *Journal of Otolaryngology, 34*(Suppl. 2), S70-S78.

Inoue, Y., Ogawa, K., & Kanzaki, J. (2001). Quality of life of vestibular schwannoma patients afte surgery. *Acta Otolaryngology, 12*(1), 59-66.

Ishikawa, K., Wang, Y., Wong, W., Shibata, Y., & Itasaka, Y. (2004). Gait instability in patients with acoustic neuroma. *Acta oto-laryngologica, 124*(4), 486-489.

Keller, H. (2005). Helen Keller quotes. http://womenshistory.about.com/od/disabilities/a/qu_helen_keller.htm.

Kurata, C. (2006). Medical check-up findings characteristic of smokers: Aimed at improving smoking cessation interventions by physicians. *Internal Medicine, 45*(18), 1027-1032.

Ladd, P. (2005). Deafness: A concept stressing possibilities, not deficits. *Scandinavian Journal of Public Health Supplement, 66*, 12-17.

Lamoureux, E., Hassell, J., & Keeffe, J. (2004). The impact of diabetic retinopathy on participation in daily living. *Archives of Ophthalmology, 122*, 84-88.

Lautenbacher, S., Kunz, M., Strate, P., Nielsen, J., & Arendt-Nielsen, L. (2005). Age effects on pain thresholds, temporal summation and spatial summation of heat and pressure pain. *Pain, 115*(3), 410-418.

Martha's Direct. (2005). http://www.marthasdirect.com/deafness/community.html.

Meador, H., & Zazove, P. (2005). Health care interactions with deaf culture. *The Journal of the American Board of Family Practice, 18*(3), 218-222.

Meldrum, M. (2005). The ladder and the clock: Cancer pain and public policy at the end of the twentieth century. *Journal of Pain and Symptom Management, 29*(1), 41-54.

Melzack, R. (2001). Pain and the neuromatrix in the brain. *Journal of Dental Education, 65*(12), 1378-1382.

Merck. (2000). Ophthalmologic disorders. In *The Merck manual of diagnosis and therapy*. Whitehouse Station, NJ: Author.

Mosby's dictionary of medicine, nursing, & health professions (7th ed.). (2006). St. Louis, MO: Elsevier.

Murphy, C., Schubert, C., Cruickshanks, K., Klein, B., Klein, R., & Nondahi, D. (2002). Prevalence of olfactory impairment in older adults. *Journal of the American Medical Association, 288*(18), 2307-2312.

Pasero, C., & McCaffery, M. (2005). No self report means no pain-intensity rating. *American Journal of Nursing, 105*(10), 50-53.

Pasquet, P., Monneuse, M., Simmen, B., Marez, A., & Hladik, C. (2006). Relationships between taste thresholds and hunger under debate. *Appetite, 46*(1), 63-66.

Pizzarello, L., Abiose, A., Ffytche, T., Duerksen, R., Thulasiraj, R., Taylor, H., et al. (2004). VISION 2020: The right to sight: A global initiative to eliminate avoidable blindness. *Archives of Ophthalmology, 122*, 615-620.

Scharff, L., Langan, N., Rotter, N., Scott-Sutherland, J., Schenck, C., Tayor, N., et al. (2005). Psychological, behavioral, and family characteristics of pediatric patients with chronic pain: A 1-year retrospective study and cluster analysis. *Clinical Journal of Pain, 21*(5), 432-438.

Stork, W., Kreiner, C., & Rentsch, F. (2002). Bifocal ultra thin intraocular lens—optical properties and clinical results. *Biomedical Technology (Berlin), 47*(Suppl. 1 Pt. 1), 184-185.

Uchida, Y., Nakashimat, T., Ando, F., Niino, N., & Shimokata, H. (2003). Is there a relevant effect of noise and smoking on hearing? A population-based aging study. *International Journal of Audiology, 44*(2), 86-91.

University of Washington, Department of Neurological Surgery. (2000). *Treatment of acoustic neuroma*. Seattle, WA: Author.

U.S. Department of Health and Human Services. (2000). *Healthy People 2010: Understanding and improving health*. Washington, DC: Author.

Wehberg, K., Kendrick, D., & Leventhal, J. (2004). Recognizing and rewarding: A review of OpenBook and Kurzweil 1000. *AccessWorld, 5*(5). Available from http://www.afb.org/afbpress/pub.asp?Doc ID=aw050504.

Work Loss Data Institute. (2004). *Pain*. Corpus Christi, TX: Author.

Wright, W. (2005). *Physical assessment and health history for the adult examination* (4th ed.). North Andover, MA: Fitzgerald Health Education Associates, Inc.

Yancey, P. (1977). *Where is God when it hurts?* Grand Rapids, MI: The Zondervan Corp.

Yueh, B., Shapiro, N., MacLean, C., & Shekelle, P. (2003). Screening and management of adult hearing loss in primary care. *Journal of the American Medical Association, 289*, 1976-1985.

24

Communication: Language and Pragmatics

Barbara J. Boss, PhD, RN, CFNP, CANP
Robin Wilkerson, PhD, RN

Communication is more than talk. Communication is a rich and complex social activity involving linguistic, cognitive, and pragmatic competence. Linguistic competence is the ability to form and use symbols. Language is the symbolic signal system used by a person to communicate with others and is composed of expressive (production) and receptive (comprehension) speech. Problems can occur in either or both of these areas. Effective language involves many processes: development of thoughts to be communicated; selection, formulation, and ordering of words; application of rules of grammar; and initiation of muscle movements to produce speech or written output. Speech output also requires control of respiration to produce the required sounds and verbalization. Individuals listen to or look at their language output, evaluate the output, and correct the language when necessary. Language, speech, and writing provide individuals with a well-ordered, rule-bound system of communication. But communication is more than language. Pragmatic competence is the ability to use language appropriately in situational and social contexts and involves all nonlanguage aspects of communication. Cognitive competence is required for communication to be relevant, to be accurate, and to evidence clear thinking. All aspects of communication are active processes, initially learned within the family and deeply influenced by culture.

A working knowledge of the types of communication deficits helps rehabilitation nurses recognize and assess communication deficits experienced by their patients. This knowledge is invaluable in planning appropriate therapeutic interventions to assist with communication and helps the nurse appreciate the prognosis for recovery, which is fundamental to facilitating the patient and family in their adaptation and coping.

LANGUAGE DEVELOPMENT

Language development requires the substitution of a series of sounds or marks for objects, persons, and concepts and is similar across racial, cultural, and socioeconomic groups. The first stage of language development is the infantile languageless phase, in which there is inability to comprehend or produce language and only phonological aspects are present. In the second stage of language development, semantic aspects appear where there is auditory comprehension of language, but oral communication is fragmentary, ineffective, and contextually meaningless. The toddler begins to use words intentionally and demonstrates behavior that indicates developing understanding of words in context. Between 18 and 24 months the child says single words with meaning, evidencing the beginning of the third stage of language development: the use of substantive words, called *semantics*. The final and highest stage of language development is the ability to apply rules of grammar to language, called syntax. Table 24-1 details language development by age.

Linguistic competence does not appear to decline with normal aging. Linguistic disintegration is evidence of a presence of a pathological process.

Three levels of language production/availability (levels of intention) also are described:
1. Automatic language: the basic level of language output consisting of habitual responses such as prayers, social responses, curses, and songs
2. Imitation (language heard before): a higher level of language output that requires the person to hear what is said, process the messages, produce the appropriate response, and evaluate the context of the transmission (e.g., "Repeat after me, 'no ifs, ands, or buts'")
3. Symbolic language: the highest level of language produced without the benefit of a model and expression of one's own choice (language or original intention); it involves the use of words with the correct meaning, application of rules for ordering sounds and words, and use of appropriate tense and plurality (e.g., "I want to describe for you how my reading difficulty is affecting my life; this has been very hard to deal with")

TABLE 24-1 Language Development in Children

Stage/Age	Language Development
Stage 1. Languageless Stage	
Newborn	Reflexly vocalizes by crying to indicate discomfort, vegetative sounds only (groan, scream)
2-4 months	Cooing. laughing, experimenting with various sounds, vowel sounds emerge
3-4 months	Consonants *b, g, k, n,* and *p* appear
4 months	Gurgling, babbling, repeating alternating consonant and vowel sounds such as dadada
6-9 months	Recitation of heard sounds or lalling
8 months	Consonants *d, t,* and *w* appear
1 year	Intonations approximate adult speech
Stage 2. Beginning Semantic Stage	
8-12 months	Understands 3 to 50 words
	First words used are names of familiar people and objects
	Words are applied to communicative games and routines
	Talk is about appearance, disappearance, and recurrence
12-18 months	25% of speech is intelligible
	Average expressive vocabulary is 50 to 100 words
	One-word speech exists (one-word sentences), about agents, action, object, location, possession, rejection, disappearance, nonexistence, and denial
	Words are understood outside of routine games
Stage 3. Semantic Language Stage (Use of Substantive Words)	
18-24 months	Understands single words for objects out of sight
	Utterances are "telegraphic" with few grammatical markers
	Words consist primarily of the smallest form of sound that possesses meaning (e.g., "go, bye, me, eat")
24 months	50% of speech is intelligible
	70% of consonants are correct
	Two-syllable words emerge
	Average expressive vocabulary is 200-300 words, predominantly nouns and verbs
	Two-word relationships are understood
	Two-and three-word combinations are used to express needs or ideas (e.g., "me go bye bye")
	Phonologically uses 9-10 initial consonants and 5-6 final consonants
24-30 months	Understands and uses questions about objects (what?), people (who?), basic events (what [x] doing?, where [x] going?)
	Phonologically aware of rhyme
	Syntactically uses *no, not, can't, don't*
	Forms questions with rising intonation; forms sentences with semiauxiliaries *gonna, wanna, gotta, hafta*
30-36 months	Uses and understands "why" questions
	Understands and uses basic spatial terms—*in, on, under*
	Phonologically all vowels are mastered
	Ability to produce rhymes emerges
	75% of speech is intelligible
	Syntactically child talks in sentences
	Overgeneralized past-tense forms appear
Stage 4. Syntax Stage (Ability to Apply Rules of Grammar to Language)	
36-42 months	Vocabulary rapidly expanding, increasing use of pronouns, adverbs, and adjectives
	Understands and uses basic color words, kinship terms, semantic relations between adjacent and conjoined sentences
	Consonant mastery continues with *m* and *h* mastered early, but *w* may be substituted for *l* and *r* (e.g. "wice" for "rice," "wook" for "look")
	Syntactically complex sentences appear, use of articles *(a, the)* and possessive *('s)* is acquired
4-5 years	Phonologically speech is fully intelligible, *f* and *v* are mastered, but *r, l, s, z, sh, ch, yt,* and *th* may still be distorted
6 years	*R, l,* and *th* are mastered
7 or 8 years	*S, z, sh, ch,* and *j* are mastered

NEUROANATOMY AND NEUROPHYSIOLOGY RELATED TO LINGUISTICS

The left hemisphere's mediation of language function in nearly all persons regardless of handedness is well accepted. The primary neuroanatomical structures involved with language competence are Wernicke's area, the angular gyrus, and Broca's area (Figure 24-1). The angular gyrus at the temporoparietal occipital junction is thought to link the visual impression of an object carried via the primary visual cortex and visual association areas of the occipital and posterior temporal lobes to the spoken word carried via the primary auditory cortex and auditory association areas. After the initial linkage is made, when the name is registered by the auditory areas, it is transmitted to Wernicke's area for recognition of the sound patterns of the word. This stimulates the angular gyrus, evoking a visual memory of the seen object.

Brain imaging studies consistently remind researchers and clinicians that this is an oversimplification. The language network is complex and involves many regions of the brain, including subcortical structures such as the basal ganglia and thalamus (Figure 24-2). For example, in the past several years, the cerebellum, in particular, the neodentate of the dentate nucleus, has been linked to word-selection tasks. Not only the left Broca's area, Wernicke's area, and the angular gyrus, but also the superior temporal lobes bilaterally and the left frontal cortex, increase activity on reading sentences in English. In addition, individual variation was found among subjects. In learning a second language, adults and children use the same Wernicke's area, but adults who learn a second language use a different region in Broca's area for each language, whereas children use the same region for both languages. The secondary region of the auditory cortex is activated when persons with hearing impairment interpret sign language, which argues for the brain's ability to recruit one area for use by another sensory modality.

LINGUISTIC DEFICITS

A language disorder can be defined as an impairment in comprehension and/or use of spoken, written, and/or other symbol system. It may involve (1) the form of language (phonological, morphological, and syntactic systems), (2) the content of language (semantic system), and/or (3) the function of language in common (pragmatic system). Aphasia is defined as the loss or impairment of a previously established capacity for comprehension and/or formulation of language caused by injury to the brain. There is a phonetic, semantic, and/or syntactic disintegration at the production and/or comprehension level of communication. The language dysfunction is manifested by incorrect word sounds, incorrect choice of words, or incorrect grammar. For infants and young children the term applied to this problem is controversial and argued. The debated terms include *language delay*, *developmental language disorder*, and *developmental aphasia*. These terms are contrasted to specific language impairment, which is more associated with a localized brain lesion. The former terms do not appear associated with localized brain lesions per se but are associated with structural anomalies that may not permit the optimal function for left hemisphere dominance. The process underlying linguistic deficits in either adults or children is not known, however.

The history of modern aphasiology dates back to Broca, who correlated the clinical picture of individuals with the location of the anatomical lesion. Despite critics who argued that there was only one type of aphasia—a general disturbance of language produced by injury—this localization approach dominated the field until after World War I, when a holistic

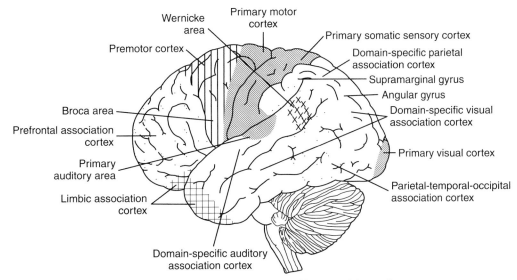

Figure 24-1 Cortical areas of the left (dominant) hemisphere.

view gained predominance. Since the mid-1960s, with improved imaging techniques, most researchers and clinicians have returned to a modified localization viewpoint. Therefore one of the useful classification systems for the aphasias, based on the neuroanatomical localization of the lesions, names the aphasias using anatomical terms (Table 24-2).

Broca's Aphasia

Broca's aphasia reflects a loss of syntax (agrammatism) due to damage in and around Broca's area. The person has impoverished syntax, short utterances, and a tendency to delete inflections or other grammatical forms. Contradictory research data related to linguistic deficits have led some aphasiologists to suggest agrammatism represents several different deficits. Some persons with Broca's aphasia appear to have a disorder of omission of structural form and simplification of the grammatical structure of speech production but retain the ability to understand syntactic relations and to use this understanding to analyze intended sentences. Other persons appear to have a central disorder affecting appreciation of syntactic relations in all modalities. Still other persons appear to have intact syntactic comprehension; written production is intact, and only verbal output is affected. In addition to the communication deficit, right-sided hemiplegia/paresis is present, with little use of the right arm and limited use of the right leg. Usually an anterior ideomotor apraxia of the face and left arm to verbal commands also is present.

Wernicke's Aphasia

In contrast, Wernicke's aphasia represents a semantic problem due to damage to Wernicke's area. The person is unable to understand verbal language. Interestingly, often understanding of axial (truncal, whole body) commands such as "stand up" or "turn around" is intact. However, extremity commands such as "point to the door" are not understood. Reading comprehension and writing are seriously impaired, although one may be more impaired than the other. Related to language production, the output is fluent, that is, a normal or above normal number of words per minute. There is ease of language production and normal phrase length. Articulation is normal, as are melody and inflection qualities. Syntax (grammar) is normal, but semantics are abnormal. Words lack specific meaning, and little information is communicated. Nonspecific words such as *it, thing,* and *us* are used. There is a tendency to use both verbal and semantic paraphasia—that is, substitution of one word for another (e.g., "The car would spit sweetly down the road" instead of "The car sped swiftly down the road")—and to a lesser extent, phonetic or literal paraphasia—that is, a phonetic substitution (e.g., "mesatence is instans" instead of "persistence is essential"), as well as nonsense or nonexistent words, called *neologisms* (e.g., "logper" for "plant") (Boss, 1984a). Repetition and naming are impaired. To communicate with this person, one must depend on facial expressions, gestures, pantomime, and tone of voice. In addition to the communication deficit, sensory loss may be present. If a visual field cut is present, it is usually of the upper quarter of the visual field caused by involvement of the pathway in the temporal lobe. The person may show a lack of concern, especially early after sustaining the injury. Paranoid behavior more commonly is seen later, after injury.

Conduction Aphasia

Conductive aphasia, currently recognized as more common than previously thought, involves a striking repetition problem. The language output is fluent. Literal paraphasia is more common than verbal paraphasia or neologism. Naming is impaired mostly due to the literal paraphasia problem. Reading aloud also is impaired. Writing may be less impaired but contains spelling errors, omitted words, and altered letter and word sequencing. Verbal comprehension is relatively intact. The pathological process producing conduction aphasia is in the supramarginal gyrus (see Figure 24-1) and/or in the area adjacent to the arcuate fasciculus. With conduction aphasia, paresis or a visual field cut also may be present. A cortical sensory loss involving position sense and stereognosis—that is, the ability to recognize forms of objects by touch—is common.

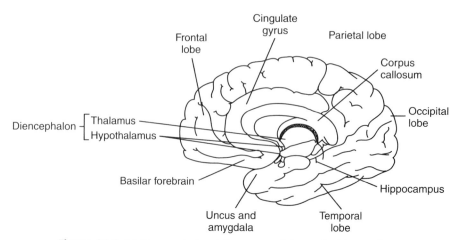

Figure 24-2 Midline cortical and deep areas of the cerebral hemisphere.

TABLE 24-2 Clinical Features of Aphasias

Aphasias	Spontaneous Speech	Auditory Comprehension	Repetition	Naming	Reading	Writing
Broca's	Nonfluent	Preserved	Impaired	Often impaired	Impaired	Impaired
Wernicke's	Fluent, paraphasic	Impaired	Impaired	Impaired	Impaired	Impaired
Conduction	Fluent, paraphasic	Preserved	Impaired	Often impaired	Preserved	Impaired
Global	Nonfluent	Impaired	Impaired	Preserved	Impaired	Impaired
Aphemia (apraxia)	Nonfluent	Preserved	Impaired	Impaired	Preserved	Preserved
Pure word deafness	Fluent	Impaired	Impaired	Preserved	Preserved	Preserved
Transcortical motor	Nonfluent	Preserved	Preserved	Impaired	Preserved	Impaired
Transcortical sensory	Fluent, paraphasic	Impaired	Preserved	Impaired	Impaired	Impaired
Mixed transcortical	Nonfluent	Impaired	Preserved	Impaired	Impaired	Impaired
Anomic	Fluent	Preserved	Preserved	Impaired	Occasional impairment	Often impaired

Modified from Mesulam, M-M. (Ed.). (1985). *Principles of behavioral neurology*. Philadelphia: F. A. Davis. Copyright by F. A. Davis. Modified by permission.

Global Aphasia

Global (total) aphasia involves a striking inability to understand verbal and written language and to write. Naming and repetition are seriously impaired, and the person is nonfluent. Global aphasia often is accompanied by right-sided hemiplegia, visual field loss, and sensory abnormalities. Persistent global aphasia involves damage to a large area of the frontal and parietotemporal language areas.

Transcortical Aphasias

If repetition is intact despite other language comprehension and/or production deficit, transcortical aphasia is present. There are three types of transcortical aphasias: motor, sensory, and mixed.

When aphasia resembles Broca's aphasia but repetition is intact, transcortical motor aphasia is present. Transcortical motor aphasia often is accompanied by hemiplegia. Apraxia is common, and a eye deviation may be seen occasionally. The area of damage may be anterior or superior to Broca's area or to the supplementary motor area (SMA) and its pathways, causing a disconnection of the SMA from Broca's area.

When aphasia resembles Wernicke's aphasia but repetition is intact, transcortical sensory aphasia is present. The syndrome often is accompanied by agitation. The area of damage is the border zone of the parietotemporal junction, which is at the end of the arterial supply. Often the middle and lower temporal gyri are damaged also.

When aphasia resembles global aphasia but repetition is intact, the disorder is called *mixed transcortical aphasia* or *isolated speech area*. In this rarely occurring aphasia, the person does not speak unless spoken to and then echoes (repeats) what the other person says. The language areas are preserved, but there is extensive damage to the surrounding cortical areas. The right hemisphere may also be involved. The syndrome may follow head injury and acute carotid occlusion but most often follows hypoxia.

Anomic Aphasia

Anomic aphasia, a phonological problem involving a word-finding failure, is the most common type of aphasia. The person has an inability to find the correct word in spontaneous speech and writing and when asked to name objects. Many other aphasias resolve into persistent anomic aphasia. Some persons with predominant anomic aphasia also lack comprehension of verbal and written language to some degree and display impaired writing, especially when fatigued. Severe anomic aphasia of acute onset typically involves damage in the left temporoparietal junction area. The site of injury of mild anomic aphasia may be the left frontal, parietal, or temporal area; a subcortical area; or even a right-sided cortical injury. Anomic aphasia is associated with head injury, Alzheimer's dementia, and space-occupying lesions, as well as metabolic or toxic encephalopathies, although in the last case, writing usually is more dramatically affected.

Pure Word Deafness

Pure word deafness is now recognized not as an aphasia but as a prelanguage syndrome. It manifests as an inability to comprehend verbal language. Repetition also is seriously impaired. Earlier after injury, there may be some degree of paraphasia in the person's language production, but the output is fluent. Reading and writing are intact, and ability to name is adequate. A superior quadrantanopia—that is, loss of vision in one fourth of the visual field—may be present. Pathologically there is a single lesion deep in the superior temporal region affecting the primary auditory cortex or the pathways to it from the medial geniculate nucleus isolating it from receiving auditory input, or there is a bilateral pathological condition involving the midportion of both superior temporal gyri (Swanberg, Nasreddine, Mendez, & Cummings, 2003).

LANGUAGE DISORDERS IN CHILDREN

Language disorders are considered a major developmental disability in children and may include an inability to assign meaning to words (vocabulary); an inability to organize words into sentences; or an inability to alter the form to tense, possession, or plurality (Paul, 2001). Language and speech (discussed later in the chapter) disorders characteristically are more common in males. A family history of language and learning difficulties often exists. Although there is no single definite cause, an association with chromosomal abnormalities is present. Global language problems, repetitive problems, expressive problems, articulation problems, and phonological problems may be found. Warning signs that a child is having difficulty assigning meaning to words include not speaking first words before 2 years of age, having a vocabulary size that is reduced for age or is not steadily increasing, having difficulty describing characteristics of objects even though able to name them, infrequently using adjectives and adverbs, and using excessive jargon past 18 months of age (Hockenberry, Wilson, Winklestein, & Kline, 2003). Clinical signs that the child may have an inability to organize words into sentences include not uttering first sentences before 3 years of age; using short and incomplete sentences; omitting words like articles and prepositions; misusing the verb forms for *be, do,* and *can;* having difficulty understanding and producing questions; using easy speech patterns; and reaching plateaus early in language development (Hockenberry et al., 2003). Cues that the child is not able to alter word forms include omitting endings for plurals and tenses, inappropriately using plurals and tense endings, and inaccurately using possession words (Hockenberry et al., 2003).

Concerns about language delay usually emerge around 2 years of age. Global mental retardation is the most common cause of delayed language development. In the past mental retardation was considered the diagnosis. Now with more sophisticated genetic testing most cases of mental retardation can be diagnosed specifically. Syndromes associated with both mental retardation and speech disorder can range from delayed speech (such as Down syndrome) to essentially total lack of verbal speech (Angelman's syndrome). Hearing impairment and specific development language disorders, called *developmental aphasia,* may present as language delays. Affected children have normal cognition and often develop elaborate gestural communication systems to convey their needs and thoughts. Children with infantile autism, in contrast, show a global lack of communication and use neither language nor nonlanguage communication systems. Children with hearing impairment and language disorders may have difficult behavioral problems, in part due to their frustration over their inability to communicate. In fact, until proven otherwise, all behaviors exhibited by those with communication disorders should be considered attempts at communication (including negative/interruptive behaviors). Development and disability in children are discussed further in Chapter 31.

Dyslexia

Brain imaging studies used to study dyslexia have isolated multiple areas of disruption of brain activity. Persons with dyslexia have a difficult time applying appropriate sounds to the letters that make up written words. On brain imaging studies this network dysfunction includes Wernicke's area, parts of the visual

cortex, and a section of the association cortex that integrates sight of printed letters with their corresponding sound. The primary auditory cortex yields only weak, disorganized responses in persons with dyslexia. The angular gyrus may be dysfunctional. Readers who have dyslexia have also been found to have greater activity in the inferior frontal gyrus and Broca's area.

PRAGMATICS

"Pragmatics is that component of communication that transcends language in terms of its isolated words and grammatical structure" (Milton, Prutting, & Binder, 1984). "Pragmatics refers to a system or rules that clarify the use of language in terms of situational or social context" (Sohlberg & Mateer, 1989). Pragmatics is heavily culturally laden. Pragmatics may be viewed as a distinct component of language, or it may be viewed as an umbrella function overlying all other aspects of language. The richness and complexity of a person's communication exists because of the contributions of both the right and left cerebral hemispheres. The right hemisphere is now known to play a major role in the prosody, attitude, emotions, and gestural behaviors involved in language and communicative behaviors. The right hemisphere is dominant for organizing the affective-prosodic component of language and gestural behavior, and the cerebellum may coordinate physical cues through which nonverbal communication occurs.

Pragmatics is a young area of speech and language pathology. Tracking of its development in childhood has not yet been extensively reported. It is known that before children begin to talk they use prosodic features (detailed in the following material) to express themselves. They learn from family and other caretakers how to alter pitch, loudness, tone, inflection, and duration to achieve a desired effect. Thus the quality of the child's cry may be different to indicate different needs. Around 6 months of age, the infant begins to experiment with inflections heard in other voices. By listening to prosodic features in the language of others, the child learns their meaning. Children imitate rhythm and pacing of vocalization, which results in different dialects. Pragmatics has not been specifically examined in elderly persons as yet, but retrieval of visual-spatial memories is known to decrease more than retrieval of language-related memories after age 70 years.

Prosodia

Prosodia, referring to the melody, pause, intonation, stresses, and accents applied to the articulatory line, is the most studied aspect of pragmatics to date. Prosodia imparts affective tone, introduces subtle grades of meaning, and varies emphasis in spoken language. Prosodia is primarily responsible for both the richness and the complexity of communication with its many familial and cultural nuances. Crystal, Lewis, and Monrad-Krohn believe that prosodia, not linguistics, forms the fundamental building blocks for language.

Prosodia was studied first by Monrad-Krohn (1947), who theorized that prosodia has four components: intrinsic, intellectual, emotional, and inarticulate prosodia. "Intrinsic prosodia serves specific linguistic purposes and gives rise to dialectical and idiosyncratic differences in speech quality" (Ross, 1985). Examples of intrinsic prosody are as follows:

1. Stress differences on segments of word to clarify whether it is a noun or a verb (e.g., the noun *combine* [com′ bin] or the verb *combine* [com bin′])

2. Differences in pause structure of a sentence to clarify potentially ambiguous or unclear statements: "the boy and girl with the dog" (said with no pauses and meaning that the dog was with both children) versus "the boy" (pause) "and the girl with the dog" (the four words said together and meaning that the dog was with the girl only)

3. Changing pitch of voice to indicate a question rather than a declarative statement: "Not true?" (high-pitched ending) versus "Not true" (low-pitched ending)

Intellectual prosody conveys the speaker's attitude about the information being communicated (e.g., "He is smart" with *is* stressed reflects the speaker's acknowledgment that the person possesses the characteristic). Stress placed on *smart* may convey that although the person is smart, the use of the quality may not meet the speaker's approval.

Emotional prosody contributes emotion to speech and has a large cultural component. Inarticulate prosody is the use of paralinguistic elements such as sighs, grunts, and groans.

The right brain has a role in the emotional aspects of communication. The left ear (right hemisphere) is better at understanding the intonational aspects of speech. The right ear (left hemisphere) is better at linguistic aspects of speech. Right hemisphere brain injury very seriously impairs affective components of prosody and gestures. Persons with right hemisphere damage are unable to insert affective and attitudinal variation into speech and gestural behavior. Affected persons cannot put any emotion into their voices and actions and are aware of this. They speak in monotone and do not use gestures. Right hemisphere damage also disrupts comprehension of the affective components of language. The listener cannot tell the difference between a flat command statement (e.g., "Get the door") and a pleasant request (e.g., "Get the door?"). They cannot insert intonation on request or by imitation.

The linguistic (i.e., intrinsic) component of prosody can be impaired by either right hemisphere brain injury or left hemisphere brain injury. The basal ganglia most frequently is involved in aprosodia followed by anterior temporal lobe and insular involvement. A transient flatness of emotions occurs with cerebellar injury.

Kinesics (Gestures)

Kinesics is the study of limb, body, and facial movements associated with nonverbal communication. When kinesic activity has a semantic purpose—that is, conveys a specific meaning—it often is referred to as *pantomime*. Pantomime conveys specific semantic information. When movements convey an emotional and attitudinal component, they often are referred to as *gestures*. Gestures are movements used to color, emphasize, and embellish speech and are highly reflective of the speaker's cultural background.

Both the right and left hemispheres appear to contribute to kinesic comprehension and production, but the specific neuroanatomy/neurophysiology involved is not yet well understood. Disturbances in performance and comprehension of pantomime are found in persons with left hemisphere injury along with aphasia. Pantomime comprehension deficit is attributed to an inability to comprehend symbols. The deficit, in execution of pantomime, is associated with the presence of ideomotor apraxia. Persons with Broca's aphasia use more pantomime, whereas persons with Wernicke's aphasia use more gestures. Loss of kinesic activity also occurs with right-sided brain injury. Injury to the right frontal inferior area results in complete loss of spontaneous gestural activity without the presence of apraxia.

The development of kinesic comprehension and production has not yet been explicated. It is known that at 9 months of age an infant gives attention to gestures. Infants have the ability to gesture and use sign before they have the ability to speak. The expressions of meaning through body movement, or kinesics, are learned through observation initially within the confines of the family and other caretakers. Children learn meanings associated with certain body movements or gestures and how to use movement to accompany language or to substitute for language. One of the earliest gestures learned is that of the hand wave to indicate good-bye and, later, hello. The child also learns that a shoulder shrug can indicate "I don't know." It has also been demonstrated that hearing infants actually babble with their hands (Petitto, Holowka, Sergio, Levy, & Ostry, 2004). The effects of aging in kinesics have not been specifically studied.

Facial Recognition and Facial Expression

Facial recognition impairment (prosopagnosia), a right-sided temporal function, is an inability to recognize previously known faces, including one's own, or to learn new ones. Actually the deficit is not limited to faces but extends to individuals in groups. Minor distinguishing features cannot be recognized.

Facial expressions convey mood and emotional state. They set the stage for the dynamics of communication. The right hemisphere is held to be crucially concerned in the appreciation and production of emotional messages via facial expression. Recognition of fear in others' faces activates the left amygdala (review Figure 24-2).

The development of facial recognition begins in the first months of life within the family and progresses as the temporal, parietal, and occipital lobes develop in childhood. The development of facial expression, comprehension, and production has not been specifically examined. Facial recognition declines after 70 years of age.

Pragmatic Deficits

Monrad-Krohn (1947) defined dysprosody as a change in voice quality giving a different accent because of inability to properly stress segments and words. This definition limits dysprosody to a disorder of intrinsic prosody. Aprosodia for Monrad-Krohn referred to a general lack of prosodia such as found in a person with parkinsonism because of akinesia and masked facies. Mesulam (1990) defined aprosodias as encoding and decoding disorders of affective behavior. Hyperprosodia is the excessive use of prosodia such as often found in persons with mania or persons with Broca's aphasia, who may be able to use few words effectively to communicate.

Ross, Holzapfel, and Freemen (1983) described an anatomical/functional classification model for the aprosodias that mirrors the organization for language presented earlier (Figure 24-3). Table 24-3 summarizes the characteristics of these aprosodias.

Motor Aprosodia. A motor aprosodia is characterized by flat, monotone speech with loss of spontaneous gesturing. Repetition of affective prosodia (e.g., repeating "I am having company for dinner" in a happy voice) is severely compromised. However, comprehension of affective prosodia and visual comprehension of emotional gesturing are intact. Motor aprosodia is associated with right frontal and anteroinferior parietal damage and occasionally with subcortical right-sided basal ganglia and internal capsule damage. Accompanying clinical findings include moderate to severe left-sided hemiplegia, variable left-sided sensory loss, and transient dysarthria and anosognosia (e.g., inability to recognize the neurological deficits being experienced). Under extreme emotional conditions, persons with motor aprosodia often are able to laugh or cry in a fleeting all-or-none fashion, resembling the pathological affect found in pseudobulbar palsy.

Sensory Aprosodia. In sensory aprosodia there is severely impaired auditory comprehension of affective prosody, visual comprehension of emotional gesturing, and repetition of affective prosodia. Affective prosodias in speech and active gesturing, however, are intact. In fact, the person may appear somewhat euphoric and overly happy even when talking about serious topics. Sensory aprosodias is associated with right-sided posterotemporal and posteroinferior parietal injury. Sensory aprosodias may be accompanied by moderate deficits in left-sided vibration sense, position sense, and stereognosis, as well as a dense left-sided hemianopia.

Global Aprosodia. The person with global aprosodia has severely compromised comprehension and repetition of affective prosodia, severely compromised visual comprehension of emotional gesturing, and an inability to display affect through prosodia and gestures. The person exhibits a very flattened affect. Global aprosodia is associated with a large right-sided injury involving the inferior frontal and parietal lobes and the superior temporal lobe and occasionally with deep right-sided intracerebral hemorrhage. Global aprosodia is accompanied typically by severe left-sided hemiplegia, left-sided hemisensory loss, and left-sided hemianopia.

Transcortical Aprosodias. Descriptions of transcortical motor aprosodia, transcortical sensory aprosodia, and mixed transcortical aprosodia are based on limited data and so must be discussed with caution. Transcortical motor aprosodia appears to manifest as aprosodic-gestural speech with preserved repetition and comprehension of affective prosodia

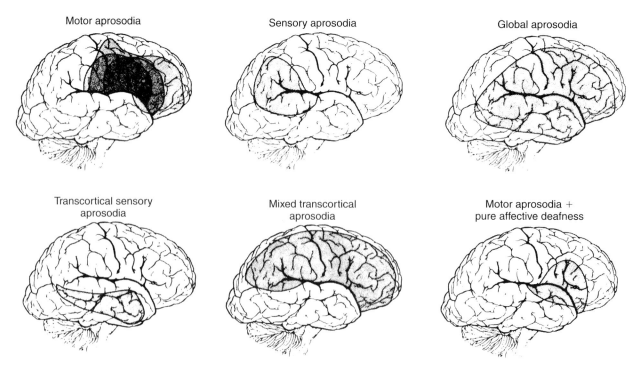

Motor aprosodia   Sensory aprosodia   Global aprosodia

Transcortical sensory   Mixed transcortical   Motor aprosodia +
aprosodia   aprosodia   pure affective deafness

Figure 24-3 Right lateral brain templates showing the distribution of infarctions seen on computed tomography scans of 8 of 10 patients with various aprosodias. (From Mesulam, M-M. [1985]. *Principles of behavioral neurology.* Philadelphia: F. A. Davis.)

TABLE 24-3 The Aprosodias

Aprosodias	Spontaneous Affective Prosody and Gesturing	Affective Prosodic Repetition	Affective Prosodic Comprehension	Comprehension of Emotional Gesturing
Motor	Poor	Poor	Good	Good
Sensory	Good	Poor	Poor	Poor
Global	Poor	Poor	Poor	Poor
Conduction	Good	Poor	Good	Good
Transcortical motor	Poor	Good	Poor	Good
Transcortical sensory	Good	Good	Poor	Poor
Mixed transcortical	Poor	Good	Poor	Poor
Anomic	Good	Good	Good	Poor

From Mesulam, M-M. (Ed.). (1985). *Principles of behavioral neurology.* Philadelphia: F. A. Davis. Copyright by F. A. Davis. Reprinted by permission.

and emotional gesturing. Left-sided hemiparesis without sensory loss may be present. A right-sided basal ganglion injury is thought to produce such an aprosodia. Transcortical sensory aprosodia appears to manifest as a severely impaired comprehension of affective prosody, whereas emotional gesturing, spontaneous affective prosody, and its repetition are intact. A right-sided anteroinferior temporal lobe injury is believed to account for this aprosodia. Mixed transcortical aprosodia is believed to manifest as absent gesturing and spontaneous affective prosody, impaired but present repetition of affective prosody, and poor comprehension of affective prosody and emotional gesturing. The lesion is thought to be in the right inferior frontal and parietal regions and a small portion of the posteroinferior temporal lobe. Severe left-sided hemiplegia and hemisensory loss also are present.

Pure Affective Deafness. Pure affective deafness plus motor aprosodia is thought to be characterized by a flattened voice devoid of affective variation, blunted gesturing, poor comprehension and repetition of affective prosody but intact comprehension of emotional gesturing (i.e., visual comprehension is intact). This aprosodia is accompanied by severe left-sided hemiplegia without sensory loss or aphasia. The right-sided inferior frontal, anterior insular, and anteroinferior temporal areas are believed to be the locations of the injury.

Developmental Affective-Prosodic Deficits

Developmental affective-prosodic deficits may occur in children with congenital or very early right hemisphere injury. Acquired motor type of aprosodias after acute right-sided focal brain injury have been documented in school-age children.

Other pragmatic deficits in the literature are inappropriate reactions to humor and misinterpretation of metaphors. These deficits may arise with right hemisphere injury.

HIGH-LEVEL LANGUAGE SKILLS

Language is a cognitive network, and at the same time many cognitive functions mediated by the left hemisphere are language dependent. Human beings use language when performing cognitive activities. For example, the left hemisphere transfers memory and permanently stores memory in a language format. Persons form language concepts using symbolic representations and move from literal interpretations to abstract principles and meanings. Human beings think in symbols, that is, in words referred to as internal speech. Dysfunction in any of the cognitive networks may seriously influence communication.

According to Groher (1977), confused language may result from disorientation in time and space, faulty short-term memory, poor thinking, mistaken reasoning, poor understanding of the environment, and inappropriate behavior. Aphasia may resolve into a more confused language profile. Development of cognitive functions and dysfunctions in cognitive networks are discussed in Chapter 25.

Attention Networks

Dysfunction in attention networks, either arousal or selective attention, produces altered communication patterns. Without arousal—that is, without wakefulness or consciousness mediated by the ascending reticular activating system of the brainstem—communication is tremendously restricted. There is no language and only inarticulate prosody (the most primitive nonverbal output). Reception of communication is limited and at a primary sensory level at best.

The selective attention network facilitates orienting to specific information of interest. Selective orienting of attention may be either overt (movement of the head, eyes, and body to the point of interest) or covert (mental shifting of attention to the source of interest). Evidence supports that the thalami mediate the engage component of selective attention (Figure 24-4). The right-sided parietal area also has been demonstrated to mediate the disengage component of selective attention. With a weak orienting network, a unilateral neglect syndrome develops. When this syndrome is present, the person cannot orient to any sensory stimuli coming from the contralateral left side. This dysfunction will influence any communication embedded in spatial, tactile, auditory, or visual information on which the person cannot focus.

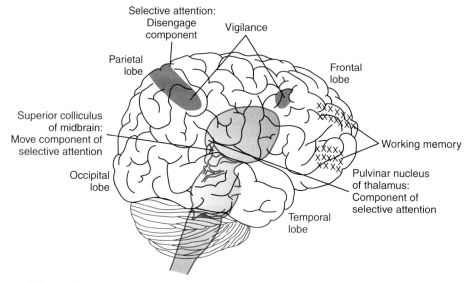

Figure 24-4 Right cortical, subcortical, and brainstem areas of the brain mediating cognitive functions.

Pragmatics is impaired. Cerebellar damage in human beings has been linked to an impaired ability to shift attention quickly from one task to another.

Lack of visual selective attention after 6 weeks of age raises the question of the presence of a visual impairment. Likewise, a dissociation between visual stimuli and motor behavior during the first 6 months of life may suggest a visual impairment. Failure to "listen" or to pay attention to auditory stimulation in the environment is seen in children with autism. In any of these situations communication is affected at the time as well as in the future.

Declarative Memory Network

Memory is the recording, retention, and retrieval of information. The declarative memory system involves learning and remembrance of episodic memories, that is personal history, events and experiences, and semantic memories, that is facts and information. Declarative memory is mediated by domain-specific cortical areas of the association areas of the temporal, parietal, and occipital lobes, where long-term memories are thought to be stored, and by domain-independent areas of the medial temporal lobe, the diencephalon, and the basal forebrain, where it is thought that distinct domain-specific features of an experience are related or bound (Gabrieli, Preston, Brewer, & Vaidya, 2003) (see Figure 24-1).

Related to domain-independent memory (formerly called recent memory or short term memory), the left hippocampus and related temporal areas encode and consolidate language-related memories. The right hippocampus and related temporal areas encode and consolidate nonlanguage auditory and visual-spatial memory stores. The amygdalae (see Figure 24-2) are believed to participate in emotional modulation of memories transferring the affective component of the experience into a permanent memory store. Domain-independent memory appears to be functional shortly after birth. The hippocampi

develop quite early and have reached 40% of maturation by birth, 50% by 1 month, and 100% by 15 months of age. The person with a domain-independent memory deficit cannot learn any new information and is disoriented to all new persons, all new places, time, and the current situation. Affected individuals do not remember what they have been told, what they have read, or what they have experienced. The individual's communication appears confused and not very meaningful, although syntax and semantics may be intact. The person appears forgetful.

Domain-independent memory decreases with aging but not sufficiently to impair cognitive functioning. This may be related to hippocampal changes.

With regard to domain-specific memory (formerly called remote or long term memory), relevant aspects of incoming information are thought to be processed by domain-specific memory networks. Domain-specific memory involves pattern recognition and stores long-term memories. These memories are believed to be stored within the association areas of the parietal, temporal, and occipital lobes appropriately reflecting the content of the memories. The left hemisphere association areas store memories related to language, mathematics, and abstractions in language format. The right hemisphere association areas store nonlanguage sounds such as music, spatial relationships, and visual experiences. During the time that the parietal, occipital, and temporal lobes undergo marked development between ages 1 and 7.5 years, children perfect their ability to form images, use words, and place things in serial order. By about age 10 years, children begin to perform simple operational functions such as weight determination and logical mathematical reasoning. Parietal occipital development is enhanced from 11 to 13 years of age. The temporal lobes mature further between 13 and 17 years of age. Dysfunction in domain-specific memory of the left hemisphere association areas may produce a loss of comprehension of verbal and/or written language, that is, an aphasia. Some of the deficits that may be produced by dysfunction in domain-specific memory of the right hemisphere association areas are aprosody, loss of facial recognition, loss of facial expression, and loss of comprehension of gestures and pantomime. Visual-spatial memory retrieval is more impaired in normal aging than language-related memory retrieval.

Executive Attention Networks

Dysfunction in the executive attention networks—vigilance, detection, and working memory—alters communication patterns. The vigilance network enables a person to maintain a sustained state of alertness for searching and scanning activities. Related to communication, the vigilance network, for example, would help a person scan the environment when there is a competing sound that is not part of the ongoing conversation. Right frontal areas (see Figure 24-4) and the locus ceruleus of the brainstem contribute to the vigilance network. The detection network provides target selection among competing complex contingencies, referred to as *object identification*, and realization that the object fills a desire. The anterior cingulate cortex (see Figure 24-2), basal ganglia, and other frontal lobe areas participate in the network. Motivation, self-monitoring, and use of feedback (self-correction) are mediated by this network. One of the striking communication deficits in persons with diffuse traumatic brain injury (TBI) is their loss of motivation to initiate communication. The apathy blocks their ability to communicate and hinders, if not totally discourages, other persons who may be trying to communicate with them. Akinetic mutism exemplifies a severe detection deficit. Persons with detection network dysfunctions, because of their impaired ability to self-monitor, cannot recognize their communication deficits and cannot understand what is wrong with the other person. Feedback from others cannot be used, nor can this individual use self-feedback. This detection network dysfunction makes rehabilitation extremely difficult and places most of the change on the other persons in the communication rather than on the affected person.

The working memory network mediated by the anterior cingulate (see Figure 24-2) and more lateral areas of the frontal lobes (see Figure 24-4) provides the person with temporary storage areas for information, such as instructions needed to process incoming sensory information and guide behavioral responses to that sensory information. Courtney, Petit, Maisog, Ungerleider, and Haxby (1998) have evidence to support that there are at least two distinct types of working memory located in different areas of the prefrontal cortex—one for objects and another for spatial relationships, which is located near eye movement control. The function mediated by working memory has been called *sustained attention* or *concentration over time*. A more complex form is called *tracking*, the ability to maintain focus despite the presence of competing stimuli or the need to engage in alternating tasks. This network enables a person to choose or set goals; to make plans and "think things through"; and to initiate, maintain, and discontinue

activities and behaviors. This ability to temporarily hold and interrelate several pieces of information allows for understanding of language and pragmatic communication. Holding newly acquired communication temporarily is essential to interrelating it with previous knowledge to generate a more permanent memory storage. With an inability to goal form or goal select, the person is unable to communicate goals because they do not exist; therefore the person appears indecisive. Communication is one way, with the other person forming goals and making decisions. The person's communication evidences little if any planning and more often reflects ill-conceived needs, wants, and desires that cannot be realized. Often the person acts without any preliminary communication of intentions. The person with a working memory dysfunction is inattentive or distractible. Concentration on the communication, in all of its fullness and complexity, is not possible. The person does not retrieve and register the communication. These persons do not hear, see, or feel the communication. The inattentive behavior is difficult for other persons to deal with and communicate around. There is evidence that in schizophrenia there is an inability to clear working memory of irrelevant information and preserve useful visual material no longer in view. These findings help account for the confused language often present in persons with schizophrenia.

The detection and working memory networks develop in early childhood until 6 years of age. At about 7.5 years of age, these frontal areas undergo accelerated development for a few years. These areas continue their maturation between the ages of 17 and 21 years.

Concept Formation

Concept formation (image processing, semantic processing) involves the ability to (1) categorize, sort, and analyze relationships between objects and their properties; (2) perform deductive and inductive reasoning; and (3) abstract. Concept formation and storage are accomplished by the memory networks. The same neural areas used for sensory-specific computations are used for higher-level thoughts. The differences is these areas are activated from the detection and working memory networks rather than from sensory areas by specific sensory stimuli (Boss and Wilkerson, 2006). Related to incidents in one's life, the left prefrontal cortex participates in the acquisition of novel information (learning) while the right prefrontal cortex consistently aids in remembering that material later on (recall). These areas receive information from specific parts of the brain that deal with content, location, or time of various events. The left hemisphere mediates formation of language concepts. The right hemisphere mediates formation of visual-spatial concepts. Concept formation is fundamental to language development. The ability to form concepts develops throughout childhood, as was previously described in the declarative memory network section. Even before 6 years of age, children begin to develop tactics for problem solving. The continuing development of the visual and auditory regions of the cortex permits children from 10 to 13 years of age to perform formal operations such as calculations and to perceive new meaning in familiar objects. The continued development of the visual-auditory, visual-spatial, and somatic systems in the early teenage years permits the adolescent to review formal operations, find flaws with them, and create new operations.

Because of their developmental level, young children cannot draw relationships; therefore their communication uses concrete, literal interpretations. No richness and fullness to the communication is present. The communication of an individual unable to form and use concepts resembles the communication of a young child and requires persons trying to communicate with the individual to use concrete, literal language as well.

Older persons appear to form language concepts and to use abstract concepts as readily as younger persons. However, older persons form visual-spatial concepts and abstract less readily.

SPEECH

Speech is a highly coordinated, sequential pattern of muscular contractions of the respiratory, larynx, pharynx, palate, tongue, and lip musculature. This results in verbal output. Speech development is considered part of language development and was discussed in the Language Development section. Speech does not decline with normal aging. Speech disorders are classified as dysphonia, dysarthria, or speech-related disorders.

Dysphonia

Dysphonia is the inability or reduced ability to vocalize due to disorder of the larynx or its innervations. Laryngeal hypophonia (decreased voice sounds) is due to damage to the superior laryngeal nerve, nodules or polyps of the larynx or vocal cords, carcinoma involving the larynx, muscle paralysis or fatigability. Spasmodic dysphonia is dystonic spasms of the laryngeal muscles. Adductor spasms produce a voice that is strained, high pitched, and commonly punctuated with repetitive brief interruptions of speech. Abductor spasms produce a voice with a whispering, breathy quality.

Dysarthria

Dysarthria has been defined as a defect in articulation. *Anarthria* has been defined as the complete loss of articulation. However, speech problems that arise in dysarthrias are not exclusively articulatory but include respiratory deficits, phonation problems, and resonation difficulties. Loss of control of the vocal tract muscles produces phonation deficits that distort consonant and vowel sound production, which distorts the language.

Dysarthrias are caused by central or peripheral nervous system motor disorders that produce weakness or paralysis, incoordination, or alteration in the muscle tone of the speech musculature. Different forms of dysarthria have specific characteristics.

Flaccid Dysarthria. Flaccid dysarthria, the most common type of dysarthria, is caused by paresis or paralysis of the muscles used for articulation. The neurological damage is located in the motor nuclei of the lower brainstem or in cranial nerves VII (the facial nerve), IX (the glossopharyngeal nerve), X (the vagus nerve), and XII (the hypoglossal nerve). With this dysarthria, there is a marked hypernasality (nasal speech) due to palatal immobility. Speech sounds are thick and slurred but feeble. Indistinctness of speech results from paresis or paralysis of the tongue musculature. Consonant production is imprecise, especially with vibratory consonants such as r. With severe paresis or complete paralysis of all three cranial nerves, no lingual or labial consonants can be pronounced. Inspiration is audible. The voice is breathy. Persons with myasthenia gravis have flaccid dysarthria.

Hypokinetic Dysarthria. With hypokinetic dysarthria there is a slowness of articulatory movements. The range, direction, and force of muscle contraction are limited, making speech muffled and indistinct. Speech is monopitch and monoloud. Clusters of prosodic insufficiencies are present. Persons with extrapyramidal system disorders (e.g., parkinsonism or Wilson's disease) may have this dysarthria.

Hyperkinetic Dysarthria. Hyperkinetic dysarthria is also caused by extrapyramidal system dysfunction. Hyperkinetic dysarthria is characterized by movements that are irregular, random, unpatterned, and rapid. Patterns of articulation are highly varied. Sudden variations in loudness are present. Rhythmic hypernasality is present. Speech is described by Adams, Victor, and Ropper (1997) as "hiccup speech," a speech pattern with abrupt breaks in flow due to the superimposed abnormal movements of the muscles used to speak. Persons with Huntington's chorea have this type of dysarthria.

Spastic Dysarthria. Spastic dysarthria is caused by the loss of inhibitory cortical influxes on the brainstem reflexes due to damage within the corticobulbar system. This is called a *spastic bulbar palsy* or *pseudobulbar palsy*. In spastic dysarthria diffuse reduction, weakening, or loss of motor speech movement activity is present. Speech usually is slow with short utterances. Articulation is imprecise, and pitch is low. The voice is harsh. An acute brainstem trauma or stroke producing bilateral injury may initially produce complete flaccid anarthria. If there is some improvement with time, the person may exhibit the slow, thick, and indistinct speech of spastic dysarthria.

Ataxic Dysarthria. Ataxic dysarthria results from a cerebellar dysfunction. Ataxic dysarthria is characterized by errors in timing, speed, range, and force of vocal tract muscles. These errors result in dysrhythmia of speech manifested by explosive and intermittent speech. Some words and syllables are spoken with too great a force, and other words and syllables are not audible because the person's breath is gone. Syllable repetition may be present. Phoneme and interval prolongation produce an unnatural separation of the syllables of words called *scanning speech*. Imprecision in enunciation is present, speech is monotonous, and the rate of speech is slow. Respiratory and speech patterns are not coordinated. Persons with multiple sclerosis may have ataxic dysarthria, as may an intoxicated person.

Mixed Dysarthria. In mixed dysarthria, two or more of the previously described types of dysarthria are present in the same person. Two or more different neurological systems have sustained injury. Persons with amyotrophic lateral sclerosis (ALS) may have combined flaccid and spastic mixed dysarthria.

Speech-Related Disorders

Speech-related disorders include phonetic tics and vocalizations, reiterative speech, echolalia (that is echoing another's words/speech), and stuttering. Only stuttering is discussed here. Stuttering is a tendency to repeatedly iterate an uttered sound and is especially common among boys. The most common stuttering is developmental stuttering characterized by involuntary repetition of first syllables of a word. Initiation of the word is followed by either machinelike repetition (stutter) or the presentation of the syllable followed by a prolonged silence. Acquired stuttering involves repetition and prolongations that are not restricted to the initial syllable.

As with dyslexia, in stuttering multiple areas of disruption are found. Stuttering has been demonstrated to produce widespread activity in motor areas throughout the brain, particularly the right hemisphere. The cerebellum has also been shown to be particularly active during stuttering On the other hand, stuttering is correlated with a nearly complete absence of neural activity in parts of the cortex that regulate conscious monitoring of one's own speech and in areas that are thought to provide the ability to string words together fluently. More specifically, stuttering may be caused by a strong left cerebral dominance and abnormal levels of the neurotransmitters dopamine and serotonin in regions of the brain controlling coordination of language processing and motor activity of the voice (Friedlander, Noffsinger, Mendez, & Yagiela, 2004). No focal site or sites are associated with acquired stuttering.

Dysfluency in Children

In children, speech impairment may be classified as a dysfluency (rhythm disorders), an articulation deficiency, or a voice disorder. Dysfluencies are usually characterized by repetition of sound, words, or phrases. The disturbance in the normal fluency and time pattern of speech is inappropriate for the child's age. Frequent occurrences of sound and syllable repetitions, sound prolongations, interjections, broken words, audible or silent blocking, circumlocutions, words produced with excess physical tension, and monosyllabic whole-word repetitions are present (Hockenberry et al., 2003). Stuttering is the most common dysfluency. Articulation errors are sounds that the child makes incorrectly or inappropriately. Clinical signs of an articulation problem include unintelligible conversational speech after age 3 years, omission of consonants at beginnings of words after age 3 years and at the end of words after age 4 years, persisting articulation errors after age 7 years, omission of a sound where one should be, distortion of a sound, and substitution of an incorrect sound for a correct one (Hockenberry et al., 2003).

Voice disorders involve deviations in pitch (too high or too low, especially for age and sex), monotone speech, deviations in loudness, and deviations in quality (hypernasal or hyponasal speech) (Hockenberry et al., 2003).

PATTERNS OF RECOVERY AND FACTORS INFLUENCING RECOVERY

Brain imaging technology is now allowing researchers to examine the brain as it recovers from an aphasia. Using imaging, training-induced improvement in verbal comprehension is correlated with activity in the posterior part of the right superior temporal gyrus and the precuneus (Musso et al., 1999). Left hemisphere activation on imaging has also been found in persons recovering from aphasia. Often this activity is localized around the injured areas (Samsom et al., 1999).

A strong tendency for some degree of spontaneous recovery from aphasia exists. At times, recovery is early, rapid, and extensive. Early recovery (i.e., in 1 to 2 weeks) is due to improvement in anoxia, edema, cellular infiltration, and intracranial pressure. The most dramatic language recovery is seen in the first 2 or 3 weeks after a cerebrovascular accident, less so with anoxia or TBI. Striking language recovery may still be found in the first 3 months, but there is a considerable decrease in language recovery after 6 months. Spontaneous recovery follows the path of a return of old knowledge and in no way resembles relearning of a child. Comprehension recovers more quickly and more completely than expression. Oral language improves more than written language. Language training centered on oral remediation also improves written language.

Related to pragmatics, cognitive systems, and speech, empiric evidence of the factors influencing recovery is lacking.

NURSING PROCESS

Assessment of Communication

Nurses and other health-related professionals, as well as families and significant others, ignore or dismiss language and speech errors. It would be rude to focus on the deficit. Nurses mistakenly may view this deficit as solely within the arena of the speech-language pathologist and beyond the assessment skills of the nurse. Unfortunately such attitudes may mean that the deficit is never carefully and thoroughly evaluated, and appropriate therapeutic interventions are not instituted. The informality possible with the nurse and the continuous intimate contact with the nurse make nursing contribution to the assessment valuable. The best assessment takes place by observing patients in natural communication situations conversing with a partner, who may be the nurse.

A comprehensive nursing assessment concerning communication includes information on health history, developmental level of the patient, previous cognitive and communication abilities, and present communication abilities. A comprehensive evaluation of communication function would include assessment of language, cognition, pragmatics, and speech. An aphasia battery in particular is not sufficient for the diagnosis and description of language impairments associated with diffuse brain injury such as in closed head injury because it does not address cognitive factors and pragmatic skills. This comprehensive nursing assessment also is used to identify areas of competence that may help the person cope with the communication deficits.

Before the assessment is begun, its purpose needs to be explained to the patient. Describe what is to be done and why. Acknowledge the difficulty for the patient. During the assessment, observe for fatigue, pain, and undue frustration. Stagger the assessment as needed.

Aphasia Assessment. An aphasia assessment includes evaluation of spontaneous speech, comprehension of verbal language, comprehension of written language, ability to name, ability to repeat, and ability to write. The nurse observes the following:

Spontaneous speech
- Is the patient fluent or nonfluent?
- Is the speech hesitant and slow?
- Are there misused words, grammatical errors, word substitutions, or neologisms?
- What is the patient's response to his or her own speech?

Comprehension of the spoken word
- Ask the patient to follow simple midline (truncal) commands (e.g., "Stand up" or "Sit down").
- Ask the patient to follow simple extremity commands (e.g., "Point to the floor" or "Point to the door").
- Increase the complexity of the commands by joining two or more requests together (e.g., "Stand up and walk to the bed"). Be careful not to give nonverbal cues.

Comprehension of written language
- Ask the patient to read aloud.
- Ask the patient to follow a written command (e.g., write out "Point to the chair").
- If reading is impaired, determine the patient's ability to recognize letters and words.

Ability to name objects
- Ask the patient to name objects in the room.

Ability to repeat
- Ask the patient to repeat what is said (e.g., "It is a cloudy day").

Ability to write
- Ask the patient to write a spontaneous thought in a sentence (e.g., "Write in a sentence what you are thinking"). If this does not work, be more structured (e.g., "Write a sentence about your breakfast this morning").
- Ask the patient to write what is dictated (e.g., "It is a sunny, warm day") (Boss, 1984b).

Language Disorders in Children. Related to assessing for language disorders in a child, ask the parents the following questions:
- How old was your child when he or she began to speak his or her first words?
- How old was your child when he or she began to put words into sentences?
- Does your child have difficulty learning new vocabulary words?
- Does your child omit words from sentences or use short or incomplete sentences?
- Does your child have trouble with grammar, such as the verbs "is," "am," "are," "was," and "were"?
- Can your child follow two or three directions given at once?
- Do you have to repeat directions or questions?
- Does your child respond appropriately to questions?
- Does your child ask questions beginning with "who," "what," "where," and "why"?
- Does it seem that your child has made little or no progress in speech and language in the last 6 to 12 months? (Hockenberry et al., 2003, p. 1012)

Pragmatic Assessment. Pragmatic assessment is not well established. A screening assessment includes evaluation of prosody, gestures, pantomime, facial recognition, and facial expression. The nurse observes the following:

Spontaneous use of affective prosody and gesturing during conversation
- Is there affective prosodia in the patient's voice, especially to emotionally loaded questions (e.g., "How do you feel?")?
- Does the patient convey emotional or attitudinal information appropriate to the situation?

Ability to repeat through imitation or linguistically neutral sentences with affective prosodia
- Select a declarative sentence with no emotional words (e.g., "It is cloudy").
- Ask the patient to repeat the sentence with same affective tone used by the examiner: happy, sad, tearful, angry, surprised, or disinterested voice.

Ability to auditorily comprehend affective prosodia
- Select a declarative sentence with no emotional words in it (e.g., "It is cold").
- Standing behind the patient so he or she cannot see gestures and facial expression, ask the patient to identify the affect voiced by the examiner in saying the sentence.

Ability to visually comprehend gestures
- The examiner conveys an affected state by using gestures of face and limbs (e.g., "It is hot") said neutrally but with facial expression indicating happiness, sadness, or anger.
- Ask the patient to identify emotion or describe emotion.

In addition, the nurse asks about the patient's internal emotional state (e.g., "How does this news make you feel?" or "Tell me how you feel inside"). It is important to remember that patients with motor aprosodia will not display depression but remain able to experience depression.

Cognitive Assessment. Cognitive networks assessment that must accompany language, pragmatic, and speech assessment includes evaluation of arousal, selective attention, declarative memory, concept formation, and executive attention networks. The nurse observes the following:

Arousal
- Is the patient awake?

Selective attention
- Is the patient able to focus his or her attention?
- Does the patient focus on external stimuli? If so, to what does the patient respond?
- What overt orienting behaviors are evidenced?

Domain-independent declarative memory (recent memory or short-term memory)
- Is the patient oriented? If not, to what is the patient disoriented: self, person, place, time, situation? Is the patient confused? What confuses the patient?
- Is the patient able to learn new information? Language-related memory? Non–language-related memory? If so, to what degree? Is emotional memory affected?

Domain-specific declarative memory (pattern recognition, long-term memory)
- Is the patient able to recall (retrieve) previously learned information? Language-related memory? Non–language-related memory? If so, to what degree?

Concept formation (semantic processing)
- Does the patient misinterpret information (illusion)?
- Is the patient able to categorize? Sort? Identify similarities and differences?
- Is the patient able to interpret the current situation? Does the patient exhibit concrete thinking?
- Can the patient abstract?

Vigilance
- Does the patient search his or her environment?
- Does the patient scan his or her environment?

Detection
- Does the patient lack motivation? Initiative? Does the patient initiate communication?
- Does the patient exhibit a flat affect? Appear emotionless?
- Is the patient able to self-monitor communication? Is the patient able to appreciate his or her communication deficits? Does the patient recognize communication omissions and errors in communication? Does the patient recognize mistakes in speech?
- Does the patient exhibit careless speech?
- Does the patient overestimate his or her communication ability?
- Does the patient lack social graces in conversation?
- Is the patient able to use communication cues?

Working memory
- Is the patient distractible or inattentive?
- Is the patient's communication impulsive?
- Is the patient able to attend to and respond to questions?
- Does the patient require redirection?
- Can the patient maintain attention with the presence of competing stimuli?

- Is the patient able to form or set communication goals?
- Is the patient able to make decisions about communication?
- Does the patient think through his or her communications?
- Is the patient able to initiate, maintain, and/or terminate communication activities? Does the patient know where to begin? Is the patient able to carry out a communication sequence?
- Is the patient slow to shift or alter his or her communication responses?
- Is speech perseveration present?

High-level language tests reflecting sensitivity to abstract language such as thematic pictures, synonyms, antonyms, metaphors, verbal power, and speed (e.g., word fluency) exist. The neuropsychologist is the resource person to consult for further information on such tests. However, clinical utility in rehabilitation populations of most neuropsychological measures has not been demonstrated.

Dysarthria Assessment. A dysarthria assessment includes evaluation of articulation, respiration, phonation, resonation, and prosody. Listen to the patient during normal conversation or while the patient reads aloud, and note the speech pattern. With a dysarthria the same speech sounds are equally affected consistently; self-correction is minimal, and articulation errors are consistent throughout repeated testing. Ask the patient to repeat test phrases or to rapidly repeat lingual (la-la-la-la), labial (me-me-me-me), or guttural (k-k-k-k) sounds. Assess movement of the pharynx, tongue, face, and lips. The motor function of the facial, vagus and hypoglossal nerves is tested. Note muscle tone of the facial, palatal, and tongue muscles. Are there signs of spasticity, rigidity, or flaccidity? Identify any other factors that may contribute to a speech problem (e.g., drooling, ill-fitting dentures) (Boss, 1984b).

To assess for speech impairment in a child, ask the parents the following questions:
- Does your child ever stammer or repeat sound or whole words?
- Does your child seem anxious or frustrated when trying to express an idea?
- When your child stammers, have you noticed certain behaviors, such as blinking the eyes, jerking the head, or attempting to rephrase thoughts with different words? What do you do when any of the above occurs?
- Does your child omit sounds from the words?
- Does it seem as though your child uses *t*, *d*, *k*, or *g* in place of most other consonants when speaking?
- Does your child omit sounds for words or substitute the correct consonant with another one (such as "wabbit" for "rabbit")?
- Do you have any difficulty in understanding your child's speech? How much of it is intelligible?
- Has anyone else remarked about having difficulty in understanding your child?
- Have there been any recent changes in the sound of your child's voice? (Hockenberry et al., 2003, p. 1012)

When a speech disorder is present, the rehabilitation nurse also assesses the patient for other health problems often associated with a speech problem, including eating difficulties (see Chapter 16), inability to cough (see Chapter 17), and skin integrity problems (see Chapter 15).

The nurse documents the findings of these assessments in the patient record. Serial assessments are performed to evaluate and document changes over time so that the treatment plan may be modified appropriately.

Magazines and books are excellent resources for pictures that can be used in assessing language, speech, pragmatics, and cognition. Standardized tests for aphasias, pragmatics deficits, and dysarthria are available.

Nursing Diagnosis

The accepted diagnostic category is impaired verbal communication (NANDA International, 2007). Other relevant nursing diagnoses are impaired written, emotional, and/or gestural communication; anxiety; and impaired social interaction (Table 24-4).

Therapeutic Goals

Comprehensive assessment provides a method for translating information gleaned through observation into treatment goals and establishing objectives such as assist the patient in achieving optimum communication, establish a functional means of communication, establish an environment conducive to communication, prevent injury, preserve the patient's self-esteem,

promote social interaction, assist the patient in returning to social roles, provide communication opportunities, educate the patient and family regarding the communication deficit or deficits, and assist the patient and family in establishing effective support systems.

Specific therapeutic goals for dysarthria are (1) to improve articulation and (2) to improve respiration, phonation, and resonance, which will make speech more intelligible. These goals and related nursing interventions are appropriate to inpatient, outpatient, and home health care situations. They are applicable to acute, subacute, long-term care, and rehabilitation settings.

Likewise these goals fall under the broad goals of *Healthy People 2010* to increase the span of healthy life for Americans, to reduce health disparities among Americans, to harness technology, and to heighten demands for quality in health care services. The more specific *Healthy People 2010* indicators are survival disability free and health system access.

Interventions

Rehabilitation nursing interventions for the patient with a communication deficit depend on the patient's unique needs. The members of the rehabilitation team, in addition to the nurse, who most commonly work with the patient with a communication deficit are the speech-language pathologist, physical therapist, occupational therapist, audiologist, dentist,

---

TABLE 24-4 Nursing Diagnoses, Interventions, and Outcomes Applicable to Communication Deficits   `NIC/NOC`

Nursing Diagnosis	Nursing Interventions	Nursing Outcomes
Impaired verbal communication	Communication enhancement: speech deficit Environment management Presence Energy management Support system enhancement	Communication Communication: expressive Communication: receptive
Impaired written, emotional and/or gestural communication	Support system enhancement Energy management Presence Environment management	Communication: expressive Communication: receptive
Impaired social interaction	Socialization enhancement Support group Support system enhancement	Social interaction skills Social involvement Role performance
Anxiety	Anxiety reduction Coping enhancement Presence Anticipatory guidance	Anxiety level Coping Rest
Deficient knowledge	Teaching: disease process Teaching procedure/treatment Teaching: prescribed activity/exercise Teaching: individual Anxiety reduction	Knowledge: disease process Knowledge: treatment regimen Family participation in professional care

Data from Moorhead, S., Johnson, M., & Maas, M. (Eds.). (2004). *Nursing outcomes classification (NOC)* (3rd ed.). St. Louis, MO: Mosby; Dochterman, J. M., & Bulechek, G. M. (2004). *Nursing interventions classification (NIC)* (4th ed.). St. Louis, MO: Mosby; and NANDA International. (2007). *NANDA-I nursing diagnoses: Definitions & classification 2007-2008.* Philadelphia: Author.

social worker, psychologist, nutritionist, clergy member, and primary physician or psychiatrist. A primary nursing role in this team is communicating to all members of the team information about the whole patient so that they all know the patient's underlying diseases, the patient's physical/cognitive/psychological/social communicative limitations, the patient's coping and adaptation styles, and any current changes in the patient. Nursing interventions are designed to provide a therapeutic, supportive environment for the patient to facilitate actual communication and to educate the patient and family. The Nursing Interventions Classification (NIC) is communication enhancement: speech deficit. Other nursing interventions are given in Table 24-4.

Therapeutic Environment. The rehabilitation nurse plays a primary role in creating an environment that makes attempts at communication easier and less stressful. Specific interventions to promote the existence of a therapeutic environment are given in Box 24-1.

In the acute rehabilitation setting, when a room is shared, the patient with a problem in communication output (e.g., Broca's aphasia, motor aprosody, or dysarthria) benefits most from having a roommate who can understand the patient's communication problem. The environment most supportive of the patient with a comprehension problem is one that does not cause excessive auditory or visual stimulation. The roommate of a patient with Wernicke's aphasia who is talkative should not be troubled by frequent spontaneous, meaningless verbalizations.

Impaired communication may seriously compromise the patient's safety. Careful assessment of each patient with a communication deficit for any needed safety precautions is appropriate. Ways to call for help either in the acute rehabilitation setting or at home need to be established, and the patient should be taught how to use them. The patient needs to be informed about environmental hazards despite the communication deficit by pictures, pantomime, or whatever means necessary.

Supportive Behaviors. All rehabilitation team members who interact with the patient need to monitor themselves for postures, behaviors, tone of voice, and facial expressions. All of these types of communications need to be positive and supportive. Team members need to behave as if communications are understood when in the presence of the patient and need to assume that misunderstanding because of the communication deficit may readily occur. Misunderstanding is assessed continuously, and corrective actions are taken immediately.

Embarrassment about the inability to communicate in a meaningful way can discourage the patient from interacting with others and participating in treatment. The nurse, other rehabilitation team members, and family can help reduce

---

BOX 24-1 Creating a Therapeutic Environment

With Any Communication Deficit
- Maintain a calm, relaxed, and unhurried environment.
- Maintain an uncluttered environment with equipment placed in least distracting areas.
- Maintain a routine in the schedule of activities.
- Avoid isolation.
- Recognize anxiety-provoking stimuli, and eliminate stressors.
- Institute anxiety-reducing measures as appropriate.
- Recognize that negative or interruptive behaviors may be attempts at communication.

When Output of Communication Is Impaired While Comprehension Is Relatively Preserved
- Help patient to communicate; create an environment where communicating is a pleasant experience, and praise patient for trying to communicate even when the results are far from perfect.
- Stimulate communication during routine nursing care activities.
- Provide patient with frequent opportunities to experience communication: hear speech; practice listening to family and social conversation; read; and practice interpretation of emotion, gestures, and pantomime as appropriate; radio and television may be used to some degree.
- Encourage patient to participate in group activities for social value and communication stimulation.
- Offer and encourage multimodal communication (speech, sign, gestures, augmentative communication devices).

When a Comprehension Deficit Is Present
- Avoid continuous noise and interaction.
- Avoid fatigue.
- Set limits on amount of praise given.
- Limit frequency and length of time that communication is stimulated.
- Limit frequency and length of group activities.
- If activity or interaction is confusing or stressful, discontinue the activity or interaction (Boss, 1984b).

embarrassment by demonstrating acceptance and interest. Supportive behaviors are listed in Box 24-2.

As the patient physically recovers from the nervous system injury that produced the communication deficit, social interactions are encouraged. Initially interactions involve rehabilitation team members with whom the patient regularly interacts, family, and close friends. Interaction involving one or two persons usually is best because this makes it easier for the patient to focus. Visitors or other patients need to be instructed regarding appropriate communication techniques. The nurse monitors visits to ensure that the encounters are pleasant and not too long.

When a patient returns home, resumption of a "normal" social life often is difficult. Frustration and embarrassment about communication may result in a loss of interest in socializing: the stress itself is fatiguing.

Old friends often feel uncomfortable in initiating interactions because the interests once shared can no longer be pursued. Friends also may be frustrated by their inability to communicate effectively or to help the patient communicate more effectively. They may be frightened by the changes seen in their friend. The nurse and the family can teach the patient's friends ways to communicate. Friends, like family, need to be encouraged to visit and should receive recognition for the support offered. They also need a chance to verbalize their fears and frustrations.

Self-help organizations such as the American Heart Association stroke clubs, the National Head Injury Association chapters, and the National Alzheimer's and Related Disorders Association chapters help fulfill social, support, and education needs. These organizations are helpful not only to the patient experiencing the communication deficit but also to spouses and family members. These organizations may be particularly valuable when the patient and/or family have few support systems. These organizations can serve as a source of new friends who understand, share good ideas regarding mutual problems, and are seeking new friends themselves.

BOX 24-2 Supportive Behaviors

- Show genuine concern for patient.
- Recognize frustration and difficulty patient is experiencing; be patient and accepting of his or her anger and depression.
- Recognize that negative behaviors may be attempts at communication.
- Treat patient as an adult even during times when his or her behavior may regress; involve patient in decision making regarding his or her care and activities.
- Attempt to anticipate patient's needs and validate specific needs with patient; be observant and sensitive.
- Encourage patient in all of his or her communication efforts.
- Praise even the smallest gain.
- Help patient develop constructive and positive outlook: emphasize things that patient can do, build his or her confidence, reassure patient that everyone has difficulty at times with self-expression.
- Do not be overly helpful; allow patient to take pride in being able to provide self-care as much as possible.
- Encourage patient to be as independent as he or she wishes regardless of the communication deficit.
- Be honest with patient regarding prognosis and difficulties in regaining communication abilities.
- Limit communication goals to those that can be accomplished; emphasize short-term goals.
- Avoid placing unreasonable demands on patient.
- Do not force patient to communicate or to see persons when he or she does not wish.
- Do not remind patient that once the patient communicated well.
- If patient laughs or cries uncontrollably, attempt to change subject or activity; if crying or laughing continues, remove patient from situation.
- Begin speech-language therapy when patient is interested and psychologically ready.
- Offer and encourage the use of multimodal communication (any combination of speech, sign, gestures, augmentative communication devices).

When Comprehension and Cognition Are Intact
- Do not behave or permit other persons to behave as if patient does not understand or has lost some of his or her cognitive abilities.

When Comprehension Is Impaired
- Do not discuss patient in the patient's presence without direct attempts to communicate information to patient as well.
- Accept paraphasia, "jargon speech," cursing, and other such output nonjudgmentally, but attempt to inform patient that you do not understand his or her communication.
- Use touch, tone of voice, and other nonverbal behaviors to communicate calmness, reassurance, and trustworthiness when language comprehension is impaired; when prosodic comprehension is impaired, put all emotions and gestural intentions into verbal language and say what you mean.
- Carry out all activities in an unhurried manner (Boss, 1984b).

Facilitation Techniques to Improve Communication.

All members of the rehabilitation team need to be knowledgeable about communication processes and facilitation techniques used to promote effective communication in patients with communication deficits. Often experimentation with various techniques is necessary to determine what works best for a particular patient. Offer and encourage the use of multimodal communication strategies with any combination of verbal speech, signs, gestures, and augmentative communication devices. Behaviors the rehabilitation nurse can use to facilitate communication are shown in Box 24-3.

Therapeutic efforts generally are tailored on an individual basis. Generally therapies concentrate on improving spoken language. Impaired auditory language comprehension often is directly approached by exercises in listening to words and sentences. In severe cases lipreading or reliance on writing may be used. Alexia and agraphia commonly are treated with traditional classroom work and then homework assignments. Children usually are taught language by traditional educational methods. The communication problems most resistant to direct therapeutic approaches and substitute skills models are profound anomia, severe agrammatism, severe alexia, profound impairment of word retrieval and language comprehension via both speech and writing, and severe impairment initiating or formulating an utterance (e.g., transcortical motor aphasia).

General Therapeutic Considerations.

Some general principles that may help guide rehabilitation nurses as they attempt to facilitate the patient's communication include the following:

1. It is common to distinguish between comprehension of communication and production of communication and reeducate each separately.
2. Because comprehension is believed to be easier than production, target it first.
3. Language in context is easier to deal with than words or phrases isolated from immediate experience. Nurses have ample opportunity to provide language exchange in context.
4. Improvement brought about by retraining in one modality may be accompanied by corresponding improvement in untrained skills.
5. With sufficient repeated practice, it is possible either to restore functional efficiency to a defective capacity or to bring an alternative route to a level of voluntary and eventual automatic skill. Interact with the patient while giving care and during activities as well as in practice sessions. Use facilitation techniques given in Box 24-3.

Pragmatic Treatment Protocols.

With regard to pragmatics, treatment protocols are in the very early stages of development. There are some trial remediation programs mostly for patients with head injuries. Some therapists have used a group approach. Solhberg and Mateer (1989) use a modular format to address four behaviors: nonverbal communication, communication in context, message repair, and cohesiveness of the narrative. The module is introduced by describing and demonstrating target behaviors to be learned. Then role-play is videotaped, followed by review by the group. Participants are helped to look at specific behaviors that increase success or failure and identify ways to modify the communication behavior. Other therapists use an individual approach targeting particular communication behaviors that are deficient in individual patients. The therapist attempts to address the communication behaviors in a broad range of naturalistic communication environments. Family members receive descriptions of communication goals and suggestions for providing appropriate feedback. Opportunity is provided to practice appropriate behaviors and to modify existing problem areas as well as to establish new, effective modes of communication.

Dysarthria Therapy.

With regard to dysarthria, rehabilitation nurses need to understand the specific treatments prescribed and the methods for applying the treatments during nurse-patient interactions. Dysarthria therapy may be directed at phonation using prosthetic and/or behavioral management; resonance using surgical, prosthetic, and/or behavioral management; articulation using surgical, prosthetic, and/or behavioral management; or a combination (Duffy, 2005). Another way to conceptualize approach to dysarthria treatment is as follows:

1. Medical care of the underlying neurological disorder to prevent further deterioration
2. Phonation-medical treatment via laryngeal surgery, collagen and Teflon injections, Botox injection, prosthetic management, pharmacological agents
3. Speaker-oriented treatments that are directed to a specific type of dysarthria and may include increasing respiratory support, prosthetic assistance, and behavioral compensation techniques such as breathing techniques and instrumental biofeedback implemented usually by a speech pathologist
4. Communication-oriented treatments that are independent of any specific type of dysarthria and may include speaker strategies, listener strategies, and interaction strategies (Duffy, 2005).

Speech therapy is basically symptomatic and supportive or compensatory. To improve articulation, the speech pathologist determines the reason for the articulatory errors and designs and implements a hierarchy of exercises starting with sounds that sometimes are correct and ending with those sounds impaired most seriously. To improve resonance, which will reduce hypernasality, the palatal muscles (palatine vault) are strengthened using exercises such as sucking and blowing and by producing oral and nasal sounds alternately (e.g., "pa, ma, pa, ma"). To improve phonation, laryngeal valve exercises may be used (e.g., production of "i-i-i" or rapid pitch changes). To strengthen the respiratory muscles, patients may use incentive spirometry, count aloud during expiration, and increase loudness rapidly and dramatically. Exercises to help prevent air waste may be prescribed (e.g., "pa-pa-pa" to improve bilabial air control and "ta-ta-ta" for linguoalveolar air control).

BOX 24-3 Behaviors to Facilitate Communication

- Use spontaneous communication topics that are of interest to patient or of immediate importance to him or her.
- Recognize that frequent but short communications are more beneficial.
- Postpone communication if patient is fatigued or upset.
- Encourage use of gestures and other forms of communication when patient's verbalizations are misunderstood.
- Wait a long enough period of time to allow opportunity for patient to communicate.

When Communication Output Is Disturbed But Comprehension Is Intact

- Allow patient to communicate for himself or herself; provide opportunity for patient to speak first, and provide the necessary time to communicate.
- Encourage all attempts to verbalize by acknowledging attempts and efforts; encourage automatic speech or imitation (e.g., prayers, social responses such as hello); encourage singing if patient enjoys singing.
- Use self-talk (i.e., speaking about the activity as nurse performs it).
- Use parallel talk (i.e., describing aloud the activity patient is carrying out with nurse).
- Use expansion, which adds substance to the statement (e.g., adding to statement "drink of water," "You want a drink of water").
- Attend very carefully to communications.
- With dysarthria, encourage patient to say one word at a time with all sounds in each word produced and consonants emphasized; encourage patient to increase volume of voice.
- React with physical actions or verbalizations to convey your understanding of verbalizations.
- Assume some responsibility for misunderstanding communications.
- Do not interrupt while patient is trying to communicate unless patient becomes frustrated; only then interpret to supply words.
- Encourage use of shorter phrases, single words, or slower verbalization if patient is distressed or fatigued or if verbalizations are misunderstood.
- Allow mistakes; only occasionally correct patient, if clearly appropriate; do not insist that each word be pronounced perfectly.
- If patient is having trouble with a word, use cueing (i.e., pronouncing the initial syllable of word), have patient repeat the word after you, give an open-ended sentence to fill in the blank, or try writing down word for patient to read.
- Request statements be repeated or rephrased if not understood.
- Serve as a good communication model to imitate when patient is having difficulty.

When Even a Slight Comprehension Deficit Is Present (as With Any Aphasia or Aprosodia)

- Provide a quiet environment for communication on a one-to-one basis at least initially.
- Turn off televisions and radios; remove unnecessary items and equipment from patient's visual field.
- Gain patient's attention first, get patient to look at communication partner, and redirect patient to communication partner if patient becomes distracted.
- Speak slowly and distinctly, using natural pauses; use short, simple instructions and/or explanations, and use gestures and pantomime along with verbalizations.
- Use simple, direct questions that are answerable with one word or short phrases; use gestures and pantomime with verbal questions.
- Reinforce appropriate responses.
- Tell patient when you do not understand him or her; ask simple questions, and systematically point and gesture until the point is uncovered.
- Do not raise your voice if patient fails to understand or misunderstands; signal patient that there was a miscommunication, and reword the communication; try to use strong gestures and facial expressions; do not become annoyed (Boss, 1984b).

When Helping a Child Learn Language

- Select a small group of words connected to a specific activity (e.g., say "close" each time a door is closed); repeat the word with the activity several times, and then repeat the word but wait for the child to initiate the activity.
- Choose vocabulary that is useful, easy to pronounce, and understandable to the child.
- Encourage vocabulary development by having the child say the word rather than gesture the word before fulfilling a request.
- Speak at a level slightly above the child's level.
- Expand the statement, preserving the child's intent.
  Expand the statement using the same noun.
     Child: Dog runs.
     Adult: The dog is running into the house.
  Replace the noun with a pronoun.
     Child: Dog runs.
     Adult: He is running.
  Expand the statement, adding new information.
     Child: Dog runs.
     Adult: The cat is running, too.
- Respond by indicating the meaning of the child's utterance, rather than its linguistic accuracy (or inaccuracy).
- Substitute questions with statements about an observed activity (Hockenberry et al., 2003, p. 1013).

The nurse needs knowledge about the use of prosthetic devices and alternate forms of communication used by the patient. Some common strategies used when interacting with the person who has dysarthria are given in Box 24-3.

Patients with aphasia, pragmatic deficits, and cognitive impairments need time to process incoming information. If the nurse has trouble eliciting a response from the patent, the nurse's own communication needs to be examined.

Augmentative and Alternative Communication.
Some persons with only speech problems, such as dysarthria involving only speech, can communicate in writing. Other persons, because of speech and fine motor problems, cannot put out verbal or written language but can use augmentative and alternate communication (AAC), defined as any mode or channel of communication that replaces or supports speech and/or writing systems and include gestures, sign language, picture or word boards, alphabet boards, and systems of synthesized or digitalized speech. When aphasia is present, the communication boards, notebooks, or cards must use pictures of objects, persons, needs, actions, faces expressing moods, and so on.

AAC can be categorized as (1) written signs (2) graphic representation of meaning other than written words, generally pictorial (e.g., universal warning symbols), (3) a symbol set that is a vocabulary or lexicon of symbols that tend to be pictographic, (4) a symbol system that represents language and has its own phonology and grammar (e.g., sign language), and (5) communication aids, which can be high-technology systems like electronic communication devices, speech synthesizers, or digitalized voice, or low-technology systems using paper systems such as word or picture books, picture or word cards/boards and charts, or alphabet boards (Kersner & Wright, 2001). All patients with speech problems may benefit from the use of alternative and augmentative communication. Many sophisticated computerized augmentative communication devices are now available for patients with any type of communication disorder. These devices range from a simple one-hit device to very sophisticated computerized devices using their own iconic language system.

Patient and Family Education

Both the patient and family need to understand the cause of the communication deficit, understand the purpose of speech-language therapy, and have a realistic view of the potential for recovery. All rehabilitation team members need to have knowledge of what the patient and family have been told and by whom. Information on prognosis for recovery initially may be presented by the primary physician, physiatrist, or speech-language pathologist. Realistic hope for recovery of communication ability by the patient and family is supported, but the patient and family are informed that full recovery is not common.

The family is taught the importance of creating an environment that is physically and emotionally supportive and how to create that environment. Facilitation techniques found to promote more effective communication are taught to all persons who interact with the patient. A team approach for education of patients, family, and friends begins with their learning about the communication deficit. Patients learn self-help techniques, including ways to assist others with using supportive behaviors that enhance communication. In turn, family and friends can use supportive behaviors to facilitate communication. They need reassurance about the patient's behavioral changes resulting from language and prosodia comprehension deficits, and they need to understand why these changes occur. Patients also learn how to participate in daily home activities and to manage their environment. Family and friends learn ways to help patients, such as offering them encouragement to participate in appropriate activities and including them in making mutually satisfying decisions, without allowing insignificant daily hassles to be burdensome or becoming overly protective (Boss, 1984a).

Referrals

The nurse assumes a key role in the referral of patients to various health disciplines within rehabilitation institutions and the community. Close and often long-term interactions with the patient provide the opportunity for identifying obvious and subtle problems. The nurse's findings need to be carefully and completely documented in the patient's record.

Nurses can assume a major role in seeing that information regarding communication techniques used with the patient is communicated to other health care professionals. Nurses need to ensure that techniques health care providers have found useful are noted and shared both in the acute care facility and in the community setting.

Growing numbers of patients are receiving speech-language therapy on an outpatient basis in clinics and private practice settings. Likewise, more and more community health agencies and home health care organizations are beginning to offer speech-language therapy services. Because of prohibitive costs for continued therapy, some speech-language pathologists have designed programs that the family can use with the patient. They see the patient only for reevaluation and adjustment of the therapy program. The nurse may need to be involved in finding such resources for patients and encouraging the development of such programs.

Evaluation

Evaluation is an essential component of the nursing process to document quality of care and cost-effectiveness. Both process and outcome evaluations are appropriate when providing health care to a person with a communication deficit.

Process evaluation provides a means to judge and document the caregiving process and behaviors carried out for a person who has a communication deficit. The Association of Rehabilitation Nurses' (ARN's) standards of care provide one means to conduct a process evaluation and document nurses' as well as other health providers' actions.

BOX 24-4 Outcome Criteria for Communication Deficits

- Patient participates in all activities planned to improve communication:
  - Participates in speech therapy sessions and periodic evaluation
  - Interacts and communicates with health team members, family, and friends
  - Explains, demonstrates, or recognizes speech therapy methods and communication techniques designed to improve communication
  - Explains and appropriately uses alternate forms of communication
- Patient is in control of anxiety and frustration, permitting patient to:
  - Participate in speech therapies
  - Effectively express anxieties and frustrations via verbalizations or gestures
  - Communicate needs to others
- Patient functions safely and independently, including searching for and accepting assistance of others as needed
- Patient establishes a defined method of communication
- Patient demonstrates ways to maximize communication
- Patient demonstrates attitude of self-worth as evidenced by:
  - Spontaneous communication to others
  - Awareness and interest in other persons and environment
  - Expression of interest in appearance
- Patient enjoys social interactions as evidenced by:
  - Identification of opportunities for social interaction
  - Participation in chosen activities
- Family provides effective support for patient by:
  - Identifying safety needs of patient
  - Explaining cause of communication deficit
  - Explaining expected prognosis for recovery of communication
  - Providing realistic and honest support for patient
  - Identifying importance of psychological support for themselves as well as patient
  - Explaining and using facilitation techniques, methods for maximizing communication, and augmentative and alternative communication
  - Explaining importance of promoting maximum independence
  - Identifying methods for promoting maximum recovery

Outcome evaluation provides a means to judge and document the effects of the care provided at the patient level. Although outcome criteria for the patient experiencing a communication deficit are determined individually based on the patient and situation, three nursing-sensitive patient outcomes with specific indicators and measurement scales have been developed in the Iowa Outcomes Project (see Table 24-4). Other potential outcome criteria are presented in Box 24-4. The nursing-sensitive outcomes can be used for initially documenting the patient's performance, for monitoring changes over time, and for documenting outcomes at specific points in time (e.g., at inpatient discharge, at outpatient discharge, or on home visits). Outcome criteria shown in Box 24-4 can also be used at specific points, such as discharge to home or discharge from outpatient therapy.

IMPLICATIONS

New technologies have opened the way to study communication networks in healthy children and adults and in adults and children who have sustained neurological insult. With these studies comes a better understanding of how complex and overlapped the networks involved in communication really are.

These networks involve many different specialized areas and require remarkable coordination and synchronization. In addition, genes are increasingly being linked to language and speech as well as to cognition (Fisher, 2005; Haines & Camarata, 2004). These advances also open the way to examine the effectiveness of language, speech, and pragmatic therapies in both children and adults. Genetic interventions may become feasible in the future for some communication deficits.

Rehabilitation nurses traditionally remain on the sidelines in the area of communication rehabilitation, but the ever-increasing demand for cost containment, cross-trained rehabilitation specialists, early return to the community, and home-based health care services mandate that nurses play a larger role in communication interventions. Evidence-based nursing practices with established efficiency and effectiveness grow out of process and outcome evaluations related to communication enhancement. Payers and more recently the public are increasingly demanding these data-based interventions from all health providers, including nurses.

Resource allocation and distribution of services remain issues for patients, families, nurses, and other health care providers.

Case Study

Terri Ross, a 29-year-old woman, experienced an ischemic stroke involving the left superior trunk of the middle cerebral artery 2 weeks after oral anticoagulation therapy was discontinued. She had been receiving anticoagulation drugs for 6 months because of deep venous thrombosis (DVT). She initially presented with a right hemiparesis (arm>face>leg) and a Broca's (motor, expressive) aphasia.

Her relevant medical history related to this cerebrovascular accident included the following: (1) a history of DVT immediately after resection of a right ovarian cyst at the age of 24 years and (2) an iliofemoral DVT (confirmed by echo Doppler imaging and phlebography) at the age of 28 years that developed in her right leg a few days after hospital admission for a fractured left tibia that required casting. At this time her coagulation screening tests were abnormal, affirming her hypercoagulable state. For 6 months after anticoagulation with heparin, warfarin therapy was initiated. When Ms. Ross had completely recovered from the DVT, the warfarin was discontinued. She had no history of nicotine use, hyperlipidemia, vascular abnormalities, or vasculitis.

Relevant family history obtained during hospitalization was that two of her female cousins had had episodes of DVT while taking oral contraceptives.

Relevant physical examination findings included vital signs within normal limits, regular rate and rhythm of heart without murmurs or extra sounds, absence of carotid and abdominal bruit, good peripheral pulses, and awake and alert neurologically but with an apprehensive and frustrated mood. Memory networks and executive attention networks appeared to be intact. On cranial nerve testing, Ms. Ross was weak, related to the motor component of cranial nerves V, VII, IX, X, XI, and XII. The sensory components of V, VII, and IX were intact. Cranial nerves II, III, IV, and VIII were intact. Motor testing demonstrated movement against gravity in the right face and arm, but mild weakness was present with hypotonia in the lower right extremity. Sensation was intact. Deep tendon reflexes on the right side were diminished. Specifically related to communication, Ms. Ross attempted little spontaneous speech (nonfluent). Ms. Ross' comprehension of both verbal and written language was generally intact; comprehension of pragmatics was intact. Language output both verbally and in writing was minimal with slow speech and much hesitation. Mostly the output was one or two words. Repeating was more fluent, and she could swear and sing. Use of pictures, drawing, and gestures was intact. Ms. Ross could not name objects but understood their purpose and use. There was a fairly dense Broca's (nonfluent) aphasia.

Diagnostic Testing

Computed tomography (CT) initially showed no mass lesion or bleeding. Transcranial Doppler imaging suggested an occlusion of the left middle cerebral artery. Carotid Doppler study results were normal. Transthoracic echocardiogram findings were normal. A transesophageal echocardiogram showed no embolic source and no patent foramen ovale or shunt. There was no reoccurrence of DVT by compression ultrasound. The second CT a few days later showed a large hypodense area consistent with ischemia in the left inferior-posterior frontal area. Clotting studies confirmed an abnormal tendency to clot. Her lipid profile was within normal limits, and there was no laboratory evidence of an autoimmune process.

Medical Diagnosis

The medical diagnosis included left inferior-posterior frontal cerebrovascular accident (CVA) with hemiparesis, Broca's aphasia, dysarthria (presence or absence of an apraxia was not able to be determined in view of the weakness), and a primary hypercoagulable state.

Nursing Diagnosis

The nursing diagnosis included impaired verbal communication (written language was also impaired).

The remainder of this case study addresses only communication issues. The therapeutic goals listed on p. 513 are all appropriate for Ms. Ross.

Ms. Ross began receiving heparin therapy and was discharged to the rehabilitation center on 7500 units of subcutaneous heparin twice daily for 1 month. At that time warfarin therapy in conjunction with a lower dose of subcutaneous heparin was planned, and intermittent international normalized ratios (INRs) were to be maintained after discharge to home.

During the acute care hospitalization Ms. Ross was provided with a calm, relaxed, and unhurried environment and as routine a schedule of activities as possible in light of the numerous diagnostic studies undertaken in a short period of time. Staff demonstrated concern, patience, acceptance, and recognition of her frustration. She was treated as a capable adult and was encouraged to carry out as much self-care as feasible with the right hemiparesis. She was encouraged to socialize with staff, her family, and other patients. Generally, effective communication was achieved by her using gestures, pictures, and drawings. Education of the patient and family focused on the nature of the communication problem, its cause, and ways to enhance communication using environmental manipulation, supportive behaviors, and facilitation techniques. The speech therapy department was consulted and worked predominantly to provide alternate means of communication and help the family communicate effectively with the patient.

On completion of the stroke workup and confirmation of the hypercoagulable state, Ms. Ross was transferred to an inpatient rehabilitation center. Speech therapy addressing both the aphasia and dysarthria was started along with other physical and occupational therapies. Rehabilitation staff continued to provide a therapeutic environment, to exhibit supportive behaviors, and to facilitate verbal language output. Family support and education continued as well. The patient was discharged to home with ongoing outpatient therapy in 2 weeks. The hemiparesis and Broca's aphasia persisted to a large degree, but Ms. Ross learned compensatory techniques readily and showed little disability at the end of her rehabilitation period. Her anticoagulation regimen continues.

The outcome criteria listed in Box 24-4 can be used to document the progression and effectiveness of communication enhancement across inpatient acute care, inpatient rehabilitation, and outpatient rehabilitation. Likewise the nursing-sensitive patient outcome titled "communication: expressive" is an appropriate tool to document progression and effectiveness of language rehabilitation over time for Ms. Ross.

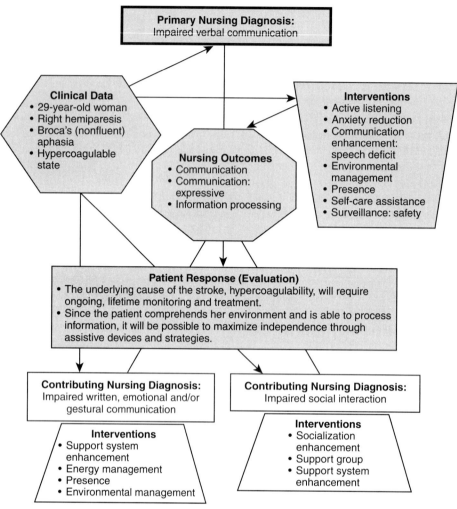

Concept Map. Terri's problems with communication are significant, but she is quickly learning to manage her environment within the hospital setting. The rehabilitation nurse will focus on coordinating interventions to achieve the support as Terri transitions from hospital to home.

CRITICAL THINKING

1. Who in Ms. Ross' family needs to be tested for a hypercoagulability syndrome? How does the rehabilitation nurse facilitate their referral and diagnostic workup?

2. Several years later Ms. Ross experienced another thrombotic CVA involving the left inferior branch of the middle cerebral artery. She was left with a dense Wernicke's aphasia. She had no additional motor or primary sensory deficits. Ms. Ross will be returning to live alone at home. During the course of her stroke workup, she was diagnosed with diabetes mellitus. She has been prescribed an 1800-calorie American Dietetic Association diet, a walking regimen, and 70/30 insulin daily with frequent glucose level checks while her diabetes is regulated. She understands no verbal or written language. Develop a teaching plan so that she can learn about the disease, its signs and symptoms, complications, her diet, glucose testing, insulin injection, foot care, and other related information.

REFERENCES

Adams, R., Victor, M., & Ropper, A. H. (1997). *Principles of neurology* (5th ed.). New York: McGraw-Hill.

Boss, B. J. (1984a). Dysphasia, dyspraxia, and dysarthria: Distinguishing features, part 1. *Journal of Neurosurgical Nursing, 16,* 151-160.

Boss, B. J. (1984b). Dysphasia, dyspraxia, and dysarthria: Distinguishing features, part 2. *Journal of Neurosurgical Nursing, 16,* 211-216.

Boss, B. J., & Wilkerson, R. (2006). Concepts of neurologic dysfunction. In S. E. K. L. McCance & S. E. Huether (Eds.), *Pathophysiology: The biologic basis for disease in adults and children* (pp. 491-546). St. Louis, MO: Mosby.

Courtney, S. M., Petit, L., Maisog, J. M., Ungerleider, L. G., & Haxby, J. V. (1998). An area specialized for spatial working memory in human frontal cortex. *Science, 179*(5355), 1347-1351.

Duffy, J. R. (2005). *Motor speech disorders: Substrates, differential diagnosis and management* (2nd ed.). St. Louis, MO: Mosby.

Fisher, S. (2005). On genes, speech, and language. *New England Journal of Medicine, 353,* 1655-1657.

Friedlander, A., Noffsinger, D., Mendez, M., & Yagiela, J. (2004). Developmental stuttering: Manifestations, treatment, and dental implications. *Special Care in Dentistry, 24*(1), 7-12.

Gabrieli, J. D., Preston, A. R., Brewer, J. B., & Vaidya, C. J. (2003). Memory. In C. G. Goetz, *Textbook of clinical neurology* (pp. 61-75). Philadelphia: Saunders.

Groher, M. (1977). Language and memory disorders following closed head trauma. *Journal of Speech and Hearing Research, 20,* 212-223.

Haines, J., & Camarata, S. (2004). Examination of candidate genes in language disorder: A model of genetic association for treatment studies. *Mental Retardation and Developmental Disabilities Research Reviews, 10*, 208-217.

Hockenberry, M. R., Wilson, D., Winklestein, M. L., & Kline, N. E. (2003). *Wong's nursing care of infants and children* (7th ed.). St. Louis, MO: Mosby.

Kersner, M., & Wright, J. A. (2001). *Speech and language therapy: The decision-making process when working with children.* London: David Fulton.

Mesulam, M-M. (1990). Large-scale neurocognitive networks and distributed processing for attention, language, and memory. *Annals of Neurology, 28,* 597-613.

Milton, S. B., Prutting, C. A., & Binder, G. (1984). Appraisal of communicative competence in head injured adults. In R. H. Brookshire (Ed.), *Proceedings from the clinical aphasiology conference.* Minneapolis, MN: BRK Publishers.

Monrad-Krohn, G. H. (1947). Altered melody of language ("dysprosody") as an element of aphasia. *Acta Psychiatrica Neurologica, 46*(Suppl.), 204-212.

Musso, M., Weiller, C., Kiebel, S., Muller, S. P., Bulau, O., & Rijntjes, M. (1999). Training-induced brain plasticity in aphasia. *Brain, 122,* 1781-1790.

NANDA International. (2007). *NANDA-I nursing diagnoses: Definitions & classification 2007-2008.* Philadelphia: Author.

Paul, R. (2001). *Language disorders from infancy through adolescence: Assessment and treatment.* St. Louis, MO: Mosby.

Petitto, L., Holowka, S., Sergio, L., Levy, B., & Ostry, D. (2004). Baby hands that move to the rhythm of language: Hearing babies acquiring sign languages babble silently on the hands. *Cognition, 93,* 43-73.

Ross, E. D. (1985). Modulation of affect and nonverbal communication by right hemisphere. In M-M. Mesulam (Ed.), *Principles of behavioral neurology* (pp. 239-257). Philadelphia: F. A. Davis.

Ross, E. D., Holzapfel, D., & Freemen, R. (1983). Assessment of affective behavior in brain damaged patients using quantitative acoustical, phonetic and gestural measurements. *Neurology, 33*(Suppl. 12), 219-220.

Samson, Y., Belin, P., Zilbovicius, M., Remy, P., Van Eeckhout, O., & Rancurel, G. (1999). Mechanisms of aphasia recovery and brain imaging. *Revue Neurologique, 155*(9), 725-730.

Sohlberg, M. M., & Mateer, C. A. (1989). *Introduction to cognitive rehabilitation: Theory and practice.* New York: Guilford Press.

Swanberg, M. M., Nasreddine, Z. S., Mendez, M. F., & Cummings, J. L. (2003). Speech and language. In C. G. Goetz, *Textbook of clinical neurology* (pp. 77-97). Philadelphia: Saunders.

RESOURCE

National Aphasia Association. *The aphasia handbook: A guide for stroke and brain injury survivors and their families,* www.naa.org, 800-922-4622.

25

Cognition and Behavior

Cindy Gatens, MN, RN, CRRN-A
Maureen Musto, RN, BSN, CRRN

Rehabilitation nurses provide care for patients who have experienced cognitive and behavioral alterations due to illness or injury across the continuum of rehabilitation care and throughout the life span. Cognition plays a major role in the determination of a person's rehabilitation potential—including the ability to (1) remember and learn new information, (2) relearn self-care, (3) return to an appropriate lifestyle, and (4) maintain independence despite specific deficits in cognitive function.

Cognition is the ability to process and act upon information with awareness and judgment. Intact cognitive function reflects the highly integrated functions of many parts of the cerebral hemispheres. The functional components of cognition include attention, memory, orientation, judgment/reasoning, problem solving, and executive function. Causes of cognitive impairment vary with the patient's age, severity of injury, geographical location, and even season of the year. The location and nature of the insult or disease bear a direct relationship to the cognitive impairment incurred.

BRAIN FUNCTION

The nervous system is most central to our functioning as human beings. The body receives information, and the brain integrates the information to determine a response from the body. The brain is the command center for the nervous system. The brain controls or influences most organs and cell functions, either directly though nerves or indirectly though hormones.

Reticular Activating System

The brain is divided into various parts. The reticular formation of the brain lies within the central core of the brainstem. It is a system of neurons and their axons, which extend from the brainstem and thalamus to the cerebral cortex. Fibers project diffusely from the reticular core to all areas of the cerebral cortex. This reticular core plus the projections are known as the reticular activating system (RAS) (Figure 25-1). The RAS is responsible for arousal, alertness, sleep, wakefulness, and basic orientation, and alerts the cerebral hemispheres to incoming stimuli. If injury occurs to this area, loss of arousal or coma may occur. Cerebral thrombosis, traumatic brain injury, intracerebral lesions, intracerebral hemorrhage, hydrocephalus, and a variety of metabolic disorders can affect consciousness, leading to confusion and decreased attention when information received from the reticular core is disrupted.

Brainstem

The RAS works in harmony with the brainstem reflexes, which are responsible for controlling circulation and breathing. The midbrain area plus the pons and medulla oblongata constitute the portion of the brain called the brainstem, which serves as conduction pathways and modulating centers between the spinal cord and other parts of the brain. The brainstem houses cell bodies for most cranial nerves and areas responsible for specific reflex centers. Nuclei in the midbrain control various visual, auditory, and postural reflexes. The pons area houses reflex centers that control respiratory rhythm. Because the critical reflex centers for cardiac, respiratory, and vasomotor functions are located in the medulla, any injury to the brainstem may result in death.

Cerebellum

The cerebellum is located behind the brainstem. The purpose of the cerebellum is to coordinate voluntary movement, maintain trunk stability, and maintain equilibrium. Cerebellar function is essential for normal execution of movement (see Chapter 20 for additional discussion). It is also recognized as playing an important role in regulating such processes as language, visual spatial organization, memory, planning, sequencing, emotional response, and personality (Powell & Voeller, 2004). Numerous studies have demonstrated that cognitive deficits following damage to the cerebellum bear a strong resemblance to the pattern of deficits following lesions to the prefrontal cortex.

Cerebrum

The cerebrum, the largest part of the brain, is composed of two hemispheres separated by a longitudinal fissure.

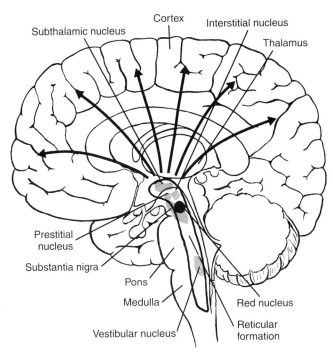

Subthalamic nucleus
Cortex
Interstitial nucleus
Thalamus
Prestitial nucleus
Substantia nigra
Pons
Medulla
Red nucleus
Vestibular nucleus
Reticular formation

Figure 25-1 Reticular activating system. (From Thompson, J. M., McFarland, G. K., Hirsch, J. E., & Tucker, S. M.: *Mosby's clinical nursing* [5th ed.]. [2002]. St. Louis, MO: Mosby.)

The corpus callosum, a band of nerve fibers, connects the two cerebral hemispheres and allows sharing of information between them. The cerebral hemispheres mediate motor, sensory, and cognitive functions in specialized areas of the hemispheres. The hemispheres participate differently in various kinds of cognitive activity. The left hemisphere appears to be more active in cognitive activities that involve sequences of events, understanding the order of events, communication skills, mathematic sequences, and analytic skills. In contrast, the right hemisphere appears to specialize in situations in which the whole is evaluated, rather than its parts. Spatial and pattern perception and artistic forms of intelligence such as painting, music, and three-dimensional objects also appear to be predominantly right hemisphere functions. From birth, one hemisphere (usually the left) develops more highly than the other and becomes dominant.

Each hemisphere contains four major lobes named for the skull bones that lie over them: frontal, parietal, temporal, and occipital (see Figures 24-2 and 24-4). The frontal lobes appear to be particularly important components related to judgment, attention span, abstraction, sequencing thoughts, transference of knowledge from one situation to another, social inhibition, intellectual function, storage of sensory information, and motor activity. The frontal lobe and the limbic system interact to produce an individual's affective behavior and distinctive personality. The limbic system also has projections into the RAS and the cortex and is located anterior to the brainstem. The limbic system controls emotions (rage, fear, pleasure, sorrow), and some automatic functions. Damage to or malfunction of a person's limbic system may affect a person's

sexual behavior, emotional responses, motivation, and biological rhythms.

NEUROBEHAVIORAL PROCESSES AND DEFICITS

Neurobehavioral Processes

No one area of the brain is the primary section for cognition. Cognitive function is made of many components. The most crucial processes involved in carrying out daily living activities include orientation, memory, attention, judgment/reasoning, problem solving, intellectual function, organization, initiation, sequencing, and motivation. Refer to Chapter 24 for discussion of these processes. A fully functioning person has intact cognition. Being independent requires consciousness, mentation, and the ability to integrate cognitive and motor functioning.

Behaviors Associated With Cognitive Deficits

The brain functions as a whole with lesions of specific areas of the hemispheres producing characteristic dysfunctions of confusion, impaired judgment, disinhibition, lability, depression, perseveration, aggression, agitation, and apathy (Box 25-1). The effects of altered cognition can range from minor annoyances to profound disruption of every aspect of living.

Most patients with cognition impairments from any source may exhibit a broad range of behaviors. These behaviors are apt to be most evident in situations in which the brain is being asked to process multiple stimuli or to respond to new situations. The source or cause of the behavior may be different depending on the type of insult, injury, or disease that the individual has experienced, but the techniques of management often are similar. The following are behaviors that often accompany altered cognition:

- *Disorientation/confusion* can be a result of attention problems, fluctuating states of alertness, and memory problems. An individual often appears incoherent. As a result of the loss in sense of direction, getting lost may be a real problem. The disoriented or confused individual most often does not know where he or she is, what time it is, or have the ability to recall minute-to-minute, hour-to-hour, or day-to-day events. As a result the individual is unable to understand his or her current situation in light of what has happened or will occur.
- *Apathy* presents as bland affect, general lethargy, and low motivation. This individual may not have interest in participating in rehabilitation.
- *Lack of initiation* is the inability to start actions independently, continue the actions, and carry them through to completion.
- *Impulsivity* is the tendency to act without thought of consequences. Impulsive individuals may appear to act quickly, making continuous and unrelenting demands.
- *Depression* is sadness that may be evident in social withdrawal, crying, self-degrading comments, anxiety, and irritability.

BOX 25-1 Cognitive Functions Affected by Brain Injury

Area of Brain	Function	Results of Injury
Reticular activating system	Arousal, alertness, orienting of attention (selective attention)	Loss of arousal, coma, confusion, decreased selective attention
Frontal lobe	Working memory (concentration over time, sustained attention) and tracking necessary for sequencing thoughts, judgment and problem solving, and inhibition of impulsive behavior	Poor thinking, poor judgment, mistaken reasoning, inability to problem solve, poor understanding of the environment, loss of social graces, inappropriate social and sexual behaviors, impulsiveness
Domain-specific cortical association areas of temporal, parietal, and occipital lobes	Declarative (explicit) episodic and semantic memory	Impaired long-term memory and recall for personal history, events and experiences, facts and information
Left hemisphere	Long-term memory for language (spoken language, reading, written language), mathematics, and abstractions in language format, analysis skills	Aphasias (see Chapter 24), loss of calculation and mathematical skills, disorientation to time, loss of analytical ability
Right hemisphere	Long-term memory for nonlanguage sounds such as music, spatial relationships, facial recognition and visual experiences	Aprosodias (see Chapter 24), loss of facial recognition, loss of comprehension of gestures and pantomime, change in music and artistic ability and appreciation, spatial disorientation
Limbic system	Motivation, part of detection network	Lack of motivation, failure to self-monitor and use feedback (self-correct)
Left hippocampus	Domain-independent memory that encodes and consolidates language-related memories	Temporary loss of ability to learn new information, disorientation (memory loss), lack of contralateral orientation, distractibility, hyperactivity, attention deficits, perseveration
Right hippocampus	Domain-independent memory that encodes and consolidates nonlanguage-related auditory and visual-spatial memories	Temporary loss of ability and visual-spatial information, lack of contralateral orientation
Amygdala	Participates in emotional modulation of memories	Unexplained emotional states and responses

- *Perseveration* is reflexive repetition of certain behaviors, either verbalizations or actions. There often is a consistent theme to perseverance, such as "I want to go home" or washing one extremity repeatedly during a bath.
- *Confabulation* is inventing details to compensate for memory loss and other deficits, not done purposefully. The patient is unable to find other explanations for what is occurring. It may serve a purpose, such as to reduce anxiety.
- *Emotional lability* is the inability to control emotions and is generally evidenced in easily triggered bouts of crying or laughing even though the individual is not sad or happy. An exaggerated emotion may occur suddenly and then disappear suddenly.
- *Lack of inhibition, or disinhibition*, is the inability to control verbalizations or behaviors in a socially appropriate way. For individuals to function within the social and cultural norms of society, they must be aware of behavioral norms and the feelings and needs of others.
- *Impaired judgment* is the inability to determine what the consequences of a given action may be and the inability to act in a safe and appropriate manner.

- *Impaired problem solving* is the inability to define and analyze a problem, choose and execute a problem-solving strategy, and evaluate the results.
- *Agitation* can be generally defined as excesses of behavior, often characterized by restlessness, inability to focus or maintain attention, and irritability that may escalate to combativeness.
- *Lack of insight* results in denial. Individuals may lack motivation for rehabilitation because they do not have internal feedback about their capabilities. They may blame others for their frustrations.

The cumulative effects of these behavioral changes often cause problems with personal and social relationships that can lead to increasing isolation for individuals and their families. Because the primary goal of rehabilitation is a return to family and community, simple containment or toleration of inappropriate behaviors within rehabilitation is not enough. The community does not tolerate such behavior. The plan for management includes elimination of socially unacceptable behaviors and restoration of self-regulated and socially acceptable responses to environmental demands. The basic premise is to acknowledge an individual's limitation, but provide structure and guidance to enable the person to gain control over behavior. It is essential that rehabilitation nurses teach family members about an individual's cognitive impairment and resulting behavior changes so they can deal with the behaviors appropriately.

DISORDERS CAUSING COGNITIVE DEFICITS

Traumatic Brain Injury

The Brain Injury Association of America (BIAA) (1997) defines traumatic brain injury (TBI) as "an insult to the brain, not of a degenerative or congenital nature but caused by an external force, that may produce a diminished or altered state of consciousness, which results in an impairment of cognitive abilities or physical functioning. It can also result in disturbance of behavioral or emotional functioning. These impairments may be either temporary or permanent and cause partial or total functional disability or psychosocial maladjustment." According to the Centers for Disease Control and Prevention (CDC) (2003a), an estimated 5.3 million Americans live with disability resulting from TBI, and 1.4 million people sustain a TBI annually. Persons at highest risk are young males 15 to 30 years of age. Fifty percent of the injuries are caused by motor vehicle accidents, 21% by falls, 10% by sports, and 12% by violence (McCance and Huether, 2006). TBI previously accounted for 14% to 20% of surviving combat casualties; this number is increasing (Defense and Veterans Brain Injury Center [DVBIC], 2004).

Causative Factors. Motor vehicle accidents are the primary cause of TBI in the United States. Seat belts and air bags prevent or decrease severity of brain injury and are 57% effective in preventing traumatic and fatal brain injuries (BIAA, 2001c). Motorcycle accidents are a significant cause of TBI with 80% resulting in death or injury. The National Highway Transportation Safety Administration (NHTSA) reports that motorcycle helmets may be up to 67% effective in preventing brain injury.

Falls are the leading cause of TBI among the elderly and children under 4 years of age (National Association of State Head Injury Administrators [NASHIA], 2002). Approximately 30% of people older than 65 years of age fall each year (Gillespie, Gillespie, Robertson, Cumming, & Rowe, 2005). See Chapter 32 on geriatric rehabilitation for more detail.

Sports and recreational activities are another source of TBI. There is a paucity of information in the literature evaluating sports activities and the incidence of TBI. Concussion is the most common brain injury associated with sports. For high school team sports, ice hockey has the highest incidence of concussion (Koh, Cassidy, & Watkinson, 2003). In addition, American football, rugby, and soccer are other team sports that have increased risk of concussion. Boxing has the highest concussion rate for individual sports. Repeated concussions from sports injuries have been shown to cause cumulative cognitive dysfunction affecting memory and processing speed (Iverson, Gaetz, Lovell, & Collins, 2004).

A rare but potentially lethal complication of concussion is second impact syndrome. This syndrome results from acute brain swelling that occurs when a second concussion is sustained before complete recovery from a previous concussion.

Brain injuries do not always happen on the sports field. Each year 130,000 children sustain a brain injury due to bicycle accidents (BIAA, 2001a). Helmets have been shown to reduce the risk of severe brain injury (American Academy of Pediatrics, 2001). Helmets absorb energy and dissipate the energy peak of a blow over a larger area for a slightly longer time. Other sports and recreational activities that would potentially benefit from implementing helmets into the practice include riding scooters, rollerblade skating, ice skating, and snowboarding.

Violence is a large contributing causative factor to brain injury. Firearms cause about 10% of all TBI but are attributed to 44% of TBI-related deaths (CDC, 2003b). Shaken baby syndrome (SBS) is another type of violent TBI. SBS is a serious acquired brain injury caused when someone "shakes" a young child. The shaking causes the brain to bounce back and forth within the skull, causing damage to brain tissue (BIAA, 2001b). In addition, blood vessels may be torn, leading to hemorrhages and intracranial pressure. Clinical presentation of SBS may be subtle or profound (Fulton, 2000). In less severe cases the baby may show failure to thrive, vomiting, lethargy/ increased sleepiness, hypothermia, or failure to show expressions/ vocalize. In severe cases the signs may be more pronounced and include decreased level of consciousness, seizures, coma, bulging fontanel, periods of apnea, and bradycardia. The long-term consequences of SBS are varied depending on the seriousness and complications of injury. Long-term outcomes range from no deficits to multiple cognitive and physical disabilities to death.

There has been increased awareness of combat-related brain injury in recent years. The Defense and Veterans Brain Injury Center (DVBIC) suggests that blast injuries are a major factor in the increased incidence of brain injury (DVBIC, 2005). Soldiers are exposed to attacks by rocket-propelled grenades, improvised explosive devices, and land mines. It has been suggested that 50% of injuries in combat are associated with blasts. Primary brain injury may occur from the resulting complex pressure waves generated by an explosion. Secondary causes of blast brain injury include impact from blast-energized debris, as well as the individual's being physically thrown, burned, and/or experiencing inhalation of gases.

Substance abuse is a significant problem associated with TBI. Almost two thirds of adolescents and adults admitted for rehabilitation have histories of alcohol or other drug abuse (Corrigan, Bogner, & Lamb-Hart, 1999). Kolakowsky-Hayner et al. (2002) found that many patients continue to use alcohol after injury, and those persons who drink are unlikely to be "light" or social drinkers. Factors associated with higher risk of postinjury abuse are preinjury history of alcohol or drug abuse, intoxication at time of injury, history of legal problems related to substance abuse, substance abuse problems among family and/or friends, denial or lack of knowledge about the dangers associated with substance abuse, age less than 25 years, and good physical health with income and transportation access

(Taylor, Kreutzer, Demm, & Meade, 2003). Numerous negative outcomes have been documented regarding alcohol abuse and brain injury, including higher mortality rates, increased risk of reinjury, local brain atrophy, longer hospital stays, and poorer discharge status.

Types of Brain Injury. TBI may be focal, diffuse, or mixed in nature. Each individual injury is different due to the various mechanisms and extent of injury. Primary injury occurs from open head injury, including those injuries caused by fractures and projectiles, and closed head injury, including such injuries as concussion, diffuse axonal injury, contusions (either coup or contrecoup in nature), and hematomas. Open head injury occurs when the brain matter is exposed to the environment. A closed head injury involves either the head striking a hard surface or a rapidly moving object striking the head. The meninges remain intact, and brain tissue is not exposed to the environment. Concussions are mild temporary disturbances of synaptic connections that may or may not produce a brief loss of consciousness, whereas diffuse axonal injury occurs when there is more widespread and often permanent damage to the brain's delicate synapses by tearing and stretching. Contusions are bruising of the brain tissue caused when the brain tissue strikes the skull across from the impact (contrecoup injury) and then rebounds to strike the skull near the impact area (coup injury). Hematomas are collections of blood often caused by a strong blow to the head leading to heavy bleeding (hemorrhage) or slow leakage of blood from the vessels. Hematomas are further subcategorized depending on location primarily between the meningeal layers (epidural, subdural, subarachnoid, and intracerebral) (Figure 25-2).

Secondary traumatic damage to the brain confounds primary damage occurring after injury. These may be intracranial or systemic events and can occur during initial injury or within the first few days after injury. Secondary injury can occur from cerebral edema, seizures, increased intracranial pressure, brain herniation, hematoma development, elevated temperature, hypoxia, and ischemia.

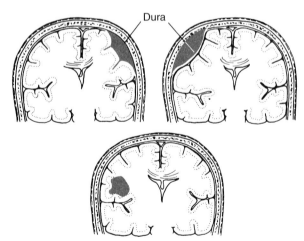

Figure 25-2 Meninges of brain. (From Thompson, J. M., McFarland, G. K., Hirsch, J. E., & Tucker, S. M. [2002]. *Mosby's clinical nursing* [5th ed.]. St. Louis, MO: Mosby.)

Hydrocephalus is a late secondary complication resulting from obstruction of cerebrospinal fluid circulation or absorption. Other late complications include abscesses and seizures.

Anywhere from 4% to 53% of patients experiencing TBI develop a seizure disorder after brain injury (Frey, 2003). This variance is due to the time period after injury, population age range, and the spectrum of severity of injury. Katz and Black (1999) classify seizure events as immediate, early, or late. Immediate seizures (within minutes after injury) are frequent among children but do not necessarily mean that the child will have posttraumatic epilepsy. Early seizures (within the first week after injury) have an incidence of approximately 5% and present a 20% to 30% risk of late seizures. For those with late seizures (after the first week following injury), the risk of late posttraumatic epilepsy may be as high as 70%. More than half of patients with posttraumatic seizures experience onset within the first year, and 75% to 80% by the second year. At 5 years the risk is most likely back to preinjury levels, but seizures can still occur (Katz & Black, 1999). Posttraumatic seizures may be generalized onset (grand mal), absence (petit mal) petit mal, focal, or complex partial.

Tools Used to Evaluate Brain Injury. The Glasgow Coma Scale (GCS) is a simple tool used in acute care to describe severity of brain injury with classifications of mild, moderate, and severe (Box 25-2). A mild TBI is indicated by a

BOX 25-2 Glasgow Coma Scale	
Response	**Points**
Eye Opening	**E**
Spontaneous	4
To speech	3
To pain	2
None	1
Best Motor Response	**M**
Obeys commands	6
Localizes pain stimuli	5
Withdraws from pain stimuli	4
Abnormal flexion	3
Extension response	2
None	1
Verbal Response	**V**
Oriented	5
Confused conversation	4
Inappropriate words	3
Incomprehensible sounds	2
None	1
Coma score (E + M + V): 3 to 15 points.	

Teasdale, G. & Jennett, B. (1974). Assessment of coma and impaired consciousness: A practical scale. *The Lancet 13(2)*, 81-84.

BOX 25-3 Levels of Cognitive Function Scale

Level	Description
I—No response	No response to pain, touch, sound, or sight
II—Generalized reflex response	Generalized response, responses are inconsistent and not specific to stimuli
III—Localized response	Blinks to strong light, turns toward or away from sound, responds to physical discomfort, gives inconsistent response to commands
IV—Confused-agitated	Alert, very active, aggressive, or bizarre behaviors; performs motor activities but behavior is nonpurposeful; extremely short attention span
V—Confused-nonagitated	Gross attention to environment, highly distractible, requires continual redirection, difficulty learning new tasks, agitated by too much stimulation
VI—Confused-appropriate	Inconsistent orientation to time and place, retention span/recent memory impaired, begins to recall past, consistently follows simple directions, goal-directed behavior with assistance
VII—Automatic-appropriate	Performs daily routine in highly familiar environment in nonconfused but automatic (robotlike) manner, skills noticeably deteriorate in unfamiliar surroundings, lack of realistic planning for own future
VIII—Purposeful-appropriate	

Modified from Downey, C.A. (1979). *Levels of cognitive function scale.* Rancho Los Amigos Medical Center, Adult Brain Injury Service. Copyright 1979 by Rancho Los Amigos Medical Center. Reprinted with permission.

GCS score of 13 or greater, moderate TBI with a GCS score between 9 and 12, and severe TBI with a GCS score of 8 or less. There is a pediatric version of this scale. Patients who sustain a moderate or severe TBI are likely to require acute rehabilitation services and have long-lasting cognitive deficits. However, those who sustain a mild TBI also often have long-lasting cognitive deficits. The GCS is often used to measure serial changes but is not a determinant of prognosis or length of recovery. Many variables may affect the score, such as substance abuse, induced comas, and other complications of injury.

The Galveston Orientation and Amnesia Test (GOAT) is a simple, 10-item, reliable tool used in rehabilitation to assess cognition and orientation after brain injury (Levin, O'Donnell, & Grossman, 1979). Points are tallied for areas of orientation; however, error points are subtracted for incorrect responses. A score of 75 or higher indicates that the patient has cleared posttraumatic amnesia (PTA). PTA is the period of time after injury when patients have impaired consciousness that manifests in a variety of neurobehavioral impairments (Nakase-Thompson, Sherer, Yablon, Nick, & Trzepacz, 2004). Although the patient may be clear of PTA, judgment and safety awareness may continue to be impaired.

The Rancho Los Amigos Levels of Cognitive Function Scale is primarily used to differentiate levels of cognitive functioning (Box 25-3). The scale starts at a coma or vegetative state and ends with higher-functioning cognitive skills. The scale has been revised to 10 levels, but levels 1 to 7 are still the most commonly used in practice. The higher levels (8 to 10) differentiate deficits of higher function. Higher-functioning cognitive skills may return years after recovery.

Patients progress through the scale while recovering. Patients may plateau or demonstrate only partial improvement at the next level. It is important to assess the Rancho level because a sudden decline to another level may indicate a complication such as an infection, hemorrhage, or an adverse medication reaction.

There are other tools used in brain injury assessment. The Agitated Behavior Scale (ABS) is helpful in behavioral management (Box 25-4). It measures behavioral excesses associated with agitation that interfere with daily functioning and present a significant barrier to treatment (Bogner, Corrigan, Bode, & Heinemann, 2000). The total score of this scale can be further divided into three subsets of behavior: aggression, disinhibition, and lability (Corrigan & Bogner, 1995). This scale can be administered at different times of the day to identify time variances of behavior. The ABS allows for objective measurement of identified behavior with serial assessment of improvement.

TBI Management. Comprehensive TBI management requires utilization of the interdisciplinary team, including physical therapy, occupational therapy, speech therapy, pharmacy, physicians, psychology, nutrition, and nursing. The team needs to be astute in identifying subtle and blatant deficits. Each brain injury is unique because different parts of the brain are affected and often various other comorbidities coincide with the brain injury. Medications such as anticonvulsants and anticoagulants are used to prevent or treat secondary complications.

Medication selection is based on four components: targeting symptoms, route of administration, onset of action, and side effect profile (O'Shanick, 2001). Targeting symptoms could include problems such as headache, neurogenic bowel and bladder, depression, initiation, and seizure prophylaxis. The underlying neurochemical problem can be addressed if the region of the involved area is known or there is a known neurochemical deficiency. Route of administration, dosage, and onset of action are considered in recognizing when a medication is efficacious. Health care providers also monitor for adverse

---

BOX 25-4 Agitated Behavior Scale

Patient_____   Period of Observation
Obser. Environ._____   From:_____   a.m./p.m. ____ / ____ / ____
Rater/Disc. _____   To: _____   a.m./p.m. ____ / ____ / ____

At the end of the observation period indicate whether the behavior described in each item was present and, if so, to what degree: slight, moderate or extreme.

Use the following numerical values and criteria for your ratings.

1 = **absent:** The behavior is not present.

2 = **present to a slight degree:** The behavior is present but does not prevent the conduct of other, contextually appropriate behavior. (The individual may redirect spontaneously, or the continuation of the agitated behavior does not disrupt appropriate behavior.)

3 = **present to a moderate degree:** The individual needs to be redirected from an agitated to an appropriate behavior, but benefits from such cueing.

4 = **present to an extreme degree:** The individual is not able to engage in appropriate behavior due to the interference of the agitated behavior, even when external cueing or redirection is provided.

DO NOT LEAVE BLANKS.

____ 1. Short attention span, easy distractibility, inability to concentrate
____ 2. Impulsiveness, impatient, low tolerance for pain or frustration
____ 3. Uncooperative, resistant to care, demanding
____ 4. Violent and/or threatening violence toward people or property
____ 5. Explosive and/or unpredictable anger
____ 6. Rocking, rubbing, moaning or other self-stimulating
____ 7. Pulling at tubes, restraints, etc
____ 8. Wandering from treatment areas
____ 9. Restlessness, pacing, excessive movement
____ 10. Repetitive behaviors, motor and/or verbal
____ 11. Rapid loud or excessive talking
____ 12. Sudden changes of mood
____ 13. Easily initiated or excessive crying and/or laughter
____ 14. Self-abusiveness, physical and/or verbal
____ **Total score**

Courtesy Corrigan, J. D., & Bogner, J. A. (2000). *Agitation Behavior Scale*. Copyright 2000 by The Ohio State University Medical Center. Reprinted with permission.

---

reactions and toxicity. Both may be dose dependent, and route of administration may be a factor. All medications have side effects, and benefits are weighed against risk. Many medications affect cognition and have sedating effects. Care is taken to use medications that have less adverse effects on cognition and arousal. The goal is to use the lowest possible effective dose.

Every rehabilitation program serving people with brain injuries screens for risk of substance abuse, provides patient and family education related to alcohol and drugs, and provides appropriate referrals for those identified at risk. The Ohio Valley Center for Brain Injury Prevention and Rehabilitation (1997) also developed a guide for professionals to intervene with those patients who have substance abuse problems.

Prevention fact sheets are available from the Violence and Brain Injury Institute. The set of nine fact sheets contains information about the prevention of violence, accidents, and brain injury. Topics include bicycle safety, SBS, motorcycle safety, motor vehicle safety, playground safety, school bus safety, firearm safety, sports and concussions, and pedestrian safety (Violence and Brain Injury Institute, 2000).

The Division of Research Sciences of the National Institute on Disability and Rehabilitation Research (NIDRR) awards grants for TBI model systems. These grants are competitively awarded to rehabilitation hospitals, centers, and universities to carry out research, demonstrate and evaluate a comprehensive, multidisciplinary service delivery system to improve the care, rehabilitation, and community reintegration of individuals who have experienced TBI. The network of these centers has established a national database (BIAA, 2004).

Anoxia

Anoxic brain injury (ABI) is caused by a decrease in blood flow to the brain, thereby causing inadequate perfusion of oxygen (Goldberg & Ellis, 1997). Causes of ABI include trauma, lightning injuries, choking on food, near drowning, drug overdose, and perioperative complications (Long, 1989). Frequently ABI occurs secondary to cardiac arrest. Fertli, Vass, Sterz, Gabriel, & Auff (2000) found that 30% to 50% of surviving patients with out-of-hospital cardiac arrest sustained some degree of anoxic brain injury. This finding may be consistent with the increased availability of portable defibrillators.

Although cardiopulmonary resuscitation restores some circulation, it is difficult to estimate the duration and severity of compromise of oxygen supply to the brain. When the oxygen supply to the brain is interrupted for a period of time, brain cells die and serious ABI can occur.

Depending on the severity of the ABI, certain "generic" symptoms may be characteristic (Box 25-5). Other signs secondary to anoxia/hypoxia are aphasia, apraxia (difficulty performing requested tasks despite adequate comprehension, strength, and coordination), and visual agnosia (inability to recognize something despite seeing it adequately). Individuals with ABI may experience damage to the hippocampus, junctional areas of the parietal-occipital-temporal cortices called the watershed areas, neocortex, prefrontal lobe, cerebellum, and basal ganglia (Goldberg & Ellis, 1997). Signs specific to brain regions/lobes occur depending on the severity of the anoxia. If the oxygen deprivation is prolonged and severe, numerous brain cells are damaged and the effects can be severe. Improvement is often slow, and independence is rarely achieved with severe anoxic injury (Fertli et al., 2000). Despite current critical care practices, the outcomes from these injuries are often lifelong neurological deficits (Biagas, 1999).

Patients with anoxia have difficulty in cognition that manifests as problems with attention, concentration, and memory that can severely limit a person's safety and ability to function independently in society (Long, 1989). More specifically, research indicates that memory processes are impaired after hypoxic brain injury. Implicit memory (cognitive skill learning that occurs without awareness) appears to be spared after ischemic hypoxic encephalopathy, whereas explicit memory is impaired (Mecklinger, Von Cramon, & Matthes-Von Cramon, 1998).

Cerebrovascular Accident/Stroke

Cerebrovascular accident (CVA) is the leading cause of disability in older adults and the third leading cause of death in the United States. The risk of CVA increases with advancing age. In the over-75 age-group, approximately 10% will experience a CVA. The factors precipitating CVA seem to be age-related progressive changes in blood vessels, whereas the factors associated with those younger than 75 years old appear to be related to lifestyle choices. More than half a million people experience a new or recurrent CVA each year; about 500,000 of these are new CVAs and 100,000 are recurrent CVAs. About 150,000 people die each year from a CVA. CVAs account for half of all patients hospitalized for acute neurological disease. Twenty-eight percent of those who have CVAs are younger than age 65.

Generally, men are at greater risk of CVA than women; however, women have a higher mortality from CVA. African American women have a higher mortality rate than white women. Women are reported to survive longer than men. These differences are directly related to their risk factor of hypertension. Hypertension occurs more frequently in certain African and Hispanic cultures. Hypertension is a major risk factor for CVA. One in every five Americans has hypertension, putting them at risk for a CVA.

CVA is closely associated with certain risk factors divided into three categories: nonreversible, partially reversible, and reversible. The nonreversible risk factors are sex, age, race, and heredity. The partially reversible risk factors are hypertension, diabetes mellitus, cardiac impairments, and blood lipid abnormalities. Any of these diseases significantly increases a person's risk for CVA. The reversible risk factors are smoking, obesity, sodium intake, cholesterol level, sedentary lifestyle, and the use of some oral contraceptives. Smoking increases risk in both men and women, and the risk increases directly with the number of cigarettes smoked. Increased total serum cholesterol and low-density lipoprotein levels, as well as low levels of high-density lipoprotein, correlate with increased production of plaques in the arteries causing a narrowing of the lumen of blood vessels.

CVAs result from impaired blood flow to a particular area of the brain. The carotid and vertebrobasilar arteries are the main arterial blood systems to the brain. The vertebral arteries enter the brain to form the basilar artery. The Circle of Willis is a ring of arteries formed by the major arteries and shunts the blood to the right and left hemispheres of the cerebrum. Factors that affect cerebral blood flow can be divided into extracranial and intracranial factors. Extracranial factors are related to the circulatory diseases such as hypertension. Intracranial factors are related to diseases causing an increase in intracranial pressure such as hemorrhage and tumors.

BOX 25-5 Characteristics of Anoxic Brain Injury

Mild Anoxic Brain Injury
- Decreased attention/concentration
- Memory impairment (amnesia)
- Decreased balance
- Agitation/restlessness

Severe Anoxic Brain Injury
- Decreased attention/concentration
- Memory impairment (amnesia)
- Agitation (may be persistent)
- Soft, mumbled speech
- Dysphasia
- Balance/coordination difficulty
- Seizures
- Spasticity (may be monoclonus—sudden muscle jerking caused by movement)

Most Severe Anoxic Brain Injury
- Inability to communicate consistently
- Not fully comatose
- Able to open eyes
- Inconsistent response to the environment

ssifications of CVA. Thrombosis, the most common
f stroke, is the formation of a blood clot that results in
wing of the lumen of a blood vessel with eventual occlusion.
Atherosclerosis also contributes to the narrowing of the
lumen. Gradual occlusion of an artery allows time for development of collateral circulation, and thus a less serious
neurological deficit may result. Collateral circulation can
develop via the Circle of Willis and other cerebral blood
vessels thus preventing ischemia if a relatively large vessel is
occluded by a clot or complete occlusion resulting from
atherosclerosis. Because thrombotic CVA follows a pattern of
a gradual narrowing of a blood vessel, sometimes with rupture
of the plaque, which then becomes a clot-generating site, a
person may exhibit signs referred to as transient ischemic
attack (TIA) warning signs. This occurs when a person experiences a neurological deficit lasting no more than 24 hours and
is usually caused by a platelet clot released from an ulcerated
atherosclerotic plaque impeding constant blood flow through
the vessel or spasm of blood vessels for a short period of time
before breaking up.

Embolic CVA is the second most common type of CVA
and is usually the result of cardiovascular disease. People with
atrial fibrillation are most likely to experience this CVA.
Blood clots formed in the quivering left atrium are released
into the general circulation and may traverse the cerebral
circulation to lodge in a cranial vessel. The clot (embolus)
lodges at the point where an artery becomes too narrow for it
to pass, causing ischemic infarction. Rapid occlusion, as
with an embolus, does not allow for collateral circulation
development. Neurological deficits are more sudden and
often more severe.

Regardless of whether the stroke is thrombotic or embolic,
edema forms in the area of the infarction and contributes to
the neuronal dysfunction. Edema can cause compression of
brain structures or herniation of the brain. Brain edema develops within a few minutes of artery occlusion and peaks 3 to
4 days after the stroke. The location, extent of infarction, and
severity of edema determine the neurological manifestations.

Hemorrhagic stroke occurs when a blood vessel in the
brain leaks or bursts. The blood extravasates into the brain or
subarachnoid space. Blood compresses and displaces the brain
tissue. In a large hemorrhage, herniation of the brain tissue
may occur. The signs and symptoms are drastic and sudden
when a large vessel is involved. Death may be immediate.

Signs and Symptoms. Signs and symptoms of a TIA or
CVA include speech difficulties, numbness or tingling,
blurred vision, dizziness, loss of consciousness, loss of balance,
lack of comprehension, amnesia, loss of muscle control, or
sensory disturbances. The problem with CVA identification is
that many of these symptoms are vague and similar to other
problems, especially if they resolve in less than 24 hours, so
persons ignore them. However, when a person experiences an
abrupt and severe onset of a neurological deficit, he or she is
more apt to seek medical attention urgently. But irreversible
damage may still have already taken place.

The neurological manifestations of CVA depend on brain
site, rate of onset, size of lesion, presence of collateral circulation,
and timeliness of seeking medical treatment. Neuromuscular
deficits are the obvious manifestations of CVA. The left hemisphere is language mediating (dominant) for 93% of the
population, the majority of whom are also right-handed. When
a CVA, regardless of type, occurs in the dominant hemisphere,
the person may experience an aphasia because the language centers are located in the left hemisphere (see Chapter 24).

Other manifestations associated with left hemisphere
damage are paralysis or paresis on the right side, cautious
behavioral manner, and cognitive deficits. Manifestations of a
right hemisphere CVA include paralysis or paresis on the left
side, spatial-perceptual deficits, impulsive behavior, and cognitive deficits. Regardless of location or type of CVA, many
people experience some form of cognitive impairment and
behavior change.

CVA Management. Medical treatment is aimed at reducing
neurological deficits and complications associated with the stroke
and improving functional outcome. The initial concern with a
CVA is assessing the damage, cause, and onset. This requires thorough assessment and computed tomography (CT) or magnetic
resonance imaging (MRI) studies to determine the location and
cause of the stroke. After the type of CVA is identified (ischemic
versus hemorrhagic), treatment is determined.

Several drugs are used to prevent thrombotic stroke by
reducing blood coagulability, including aspirin, warfarin, and
clopidogrel bisulfate. People with acute nonhemorrhagic
strokes are given a drug such as tissue plasminogen activator
(TPA), which must be given within 3 hours of onset of symptoms. The problem occurs when a patient waits to seek
medical attention, hoping signs and symptoms will resolve. If
a person seeks care after 3 hours from onset of symptoms,
drugs like TPA are not given due to risk of bleeding.
Treatment at this point usually consists of heparin or warfarin,
which have not proven to be as effective in halting the stroke,
but do prevent additional clots. Steroids and osmotic diuretics
are commonly used to reduce increased intracranial pressure.
Carotid endarterectomy is the treatment of choice in 70% to
90% of patients with carotid stenosis. However, CVA is a
possible complication to this procedure.

When designing a rehabilitation plan for a person with a
CVA, attention needs to be on physical, functional, emotional,
and cognitive changes. Cognitive deficits can affect a person's
rehabilitation outcome. Galshi, Bruno, Zorowitz, and Walker
(1993) found that cognitive deficits from the CVA directly predict functional status. People who experienced a CVA with
cognitive changes in the areas of abstract thinking, judgment,
declarative memory (explicit memory), comprehension, and
orientation performed poorly in self-care activities at discharge
from rehabilitation.

Incorporating cognitive rehabilitation into the traditional
physical/language rehabilitation makes a person's recovery
following CVA more meaningful. Sisson (1998) found that
stroke survivors with changes in mood, judgment, memory,

and personality during rehabilitation continued with problems such as depression, memory loss, nervousness, irritability, frustration, lack of energy, and decreased initiative 6 months after rehabilitation. Pound, Gompertz, and Ebrahim (1998) found that CVA survivors reported that in addition to the common physical limitations (in mobility and self-care), confusion and deteriorating memory were also issues.

Recovery and Rehabilitation After CVA. Recovery after a CVA has predominantly been focused on independent mobility and self-care activities. However, learning to perform old skills or new skills requires the ability to think and process information. Studies are beginning to identify neuropsychological consequences of stroke and their role in a person's recovery after a CVA. Hochstenbach and Mulder (1999) found the most relevant cognitive dysfunctions after a CVA include "disorders in attention, memory, executive functions, perception, selection, and evaluation, communication, emotion, and behaviors." Patients with problems in attention had a decline in their flexibility, difficulties in concentrating on a task for a longer time, difficulties performing tasks in a stimulating, noisy environment, and difficulty performing more than one task at a time. Many patients experiencing CVA have problems with processing information, causing a delay in thinking and response.

Problems in executive function lead to problems in planning and carrying out activities, thus forcing the person to be dependent on others. Neglect is another common deficit that impedes cognitive performance. Neglect occurs when a person has difficulty in reporting or responding to stimuli on the contralateral side of the stroke. Neglect is commonly referred to as a perceptual dysfunction. It significantly impedes a person's understanding of self and environment, thus hindering his or her cognitive rehabilitation.

In addition to cognitive deficits following a stroke, many people experience emotional and behavioral problems. Compulsive laughing or crying, often referred to as emotional lability, is a classic behavior. The person's reaction or emotion is not appropriate. Depression is also another common manifestation appearing after the CVA and should be addressed because it can impede recovery. Other behavioral problems identified following a stroke are impulsivity, impatience, or being overly cautious. All of these neuropsychological factors need to be assessed carefully so that a plan of treatment can be activated to minimize the consequences (Hochstenbach & Mulder, 1999).

It is well known that rehabilitation after a CVA provides most CVA survivors with functional improvement. A comprehensive rehabilitation program tailored to a patient's physical and cognitive impairments can better facilitate a patient's return to a worthwhile life.

Alzheimer's Disease

Alzheimer's disease (AD) is the leading cause of dementia, a group of conditions that gradually destroy brain cells and lead to progressive decline in cognitive function. Vascular dementia, another common form of dementia, results from reduced blood flow to the brain nerve cells. In some cases, AD and vascular dementia can occur together in "mixed dementia" (Alzheimer's Association, 2005c).

AD is an insidious, progressive disorder that alters memory, executive function, language, visual spatial orientation, and other cognitive abilities. In addition to cognitive deficits, behavioral disturbances occur such as agitation, hallucinations, delusions, and a decline in self-care function. An estimated 4.5 million Americans have AD. The number of Americans with AD continues to grow; by 2050 the number of individuals with AD could range from 11.3 million to 16 million (Herbert, Scherr, Bienias, Bennett, & Evans, 2003).

Risk Factors. Increasing age is the greatest risk factor for AD. One in 10 individuals over 65 and nearly half over 85 are affected. Having a close family member with AD increases the chances of developing AD. People with a first-degree relative, such as a parent or sibling, with AD have a 10% to 30% chance of developing the disease. The risk is probably higher if the person developed AD at a younger age and lower if the person did not develop AD until later in life. A person with AD lives an average of 8 years and up to as many as 20 years from the onset of symptoms as estimated by relatives. From the time of diagnosis, people with AD survive about half as long as those of similar age without dementia (Larson & Shadlen, 2004).

Etiology. The etiology of AD is unclear. Pathological changes associated with the disease include neurofibrillary tangles and beta-amyloid (neuritic) plaques in the cerebral cortex and hippocampus. The neuritic plaque is a cluster of degenerating axonal and dendritic nerve terminals that contain an abnormal protein, beta-amyloid. Neurofibrillary tangles are bundles of abnormal proteins within the cytoplasm. There is also an excessive loss of cholinergic neurons, particularly in the regions essential for memory and cognition. Gross atrophy occurs as neurons die. Loss of neurons occurs primarily in the neocortex and hippocampus, essential structures for cognition. Loss of cholinergic innervation is one of the major biochemical changes that occur in AD. It is generally agreed that a diagnosis of probable AD can be made on typical findings during life and confirmed by studying brain tissue at death. The definitive diagnosis of AD can be made only at autopsy when the presence of plaques and neurofibrillary tangles is observed.

Signs and Symptoms. Although AD symptoms can vary widely, the first problem that many people notice is forgetfulness at a level that affects performance at home, work, or in favorite activities. The memory decline is often more obvious to family members and close friends than to the individual. Other common symptoms include confusion, getting lost in familiar places, and difficulty with language. Normal daily tasks such as naming objects and people, preparing meals, eating, and personal care become difficult. Agitation, restlessness, wandering, and inappropriate behavior develop as the disease progresses.

The patient's speech eventually becomes difficult to understand, and swallowing problems develop. The individual usually requires total care during advanced stages of the disease.

Progressive impairment of memory and other cognitive skills have been outlined in three stages (Box 25-6). These stages are only a guide to function and capacity and help to monitor or anticipate the progression of the disease. Symptoms and behaviors often overlap stages. Many factors beyond the disease can contribute to cognitive changes or loss of functional capacity, such as illness, changes in the environment, medications, sensory changes, excess alcohol, and nutritional imbalances. When a deficit occurs, attention is toward identifying the potential cause.

Tools for Evaluating AD. A medical history, physical examination, and standard laboratory tests including blood, urine, thyroid, and liver function may help eliminate other possible conditions. A CT or MRI scan may be done to rule out brain tumor or ischemic stroke as the cause of the symptoms. A clinical history based upon information gathered from the patient and family, neuropsychological testing, and serial observations provide essential data to diagnosis AD.

The most widely used screening test of cognitive function for patients with suspected dementia is the Mini-Mental State Examination (MMSE) (Folstein, Folstein, & McHugh, 1975) (see Chapter 32). It takes a clinician a few minutes to complete and evaluate a range of mental functions from knowing the day, month, and year to being able to remember a short list of words or write a full sentence spontaneously. There are similar tests utilized by trained clinicians to more precisely evaluate

---

BOX 25-6 Outline of Progressive Impairment of Memory and Other Cognitive Skills

Stage I (1 to 3 Years)
- Mild memory impairment
- Some naming errors
- Indifference, occasional irritability

Stage II (2 to 10 Years)
- Moderate memory impairment
- Spatial disorientation
- Fluent aphasia
- Ideomotor apraxia (difficulty dressing and difficulty using utensils of daily living)
- Indifference or irritability
- Delusions in some
- Restlessness, pacing

Stage III (11 Years and Longer)
- Severely impaired cognitive function
- Limb rigidity, flexion posture
- Urinary and fecal incontinence

From Luckman, J. (1997). *Manual of nursing care* (p. 714). Philadelphia: W. B. Saunders.

---

patients with more advanced AD. The Severe Impairment Battery (SIB) more easily detects changes in moderate to severe AD. Emphasis is on language/social interaction more than orientation/memory. Testing directions are often simple commands or requests with gestural cues (Panisset, Roudier, Saxton, & Boller, 1994).

AD Management (Pharmacological). Progress has been made in medication management for memory and cognitive impairment as well as behavioral problems. Ongoing research also shows promise for developing treatments to modify (delay or prevent) the disease course. Four commonly used drugs are currently approved in the United States for treatment of the cognitive symptoms of AD. The cholinesterase inhibitors are galantamine, rivastigmine tartrate, and donepezil. Each acts in a different way to delay the breakdown of acetylcholine, a brain chemical that facilitates synapse among nerve cells and is important for memory. AD is associated with inadequate levels of this transmitter. The fourth is memantine, which acts by a different mechanism. It shields brain cells from overexposure to the neurotransmitter glutamate. Excess levels of glutamate contribute to the death of brain cells in those with AD. Memantine helps to regulate the activity of glutamate, which plays a role in learning and memory. In a 2003 study, 252 patients with moderate to severe AD participated in a double-blind study to receive a placebo or 20 mg of memantine daily for 28 weeks. Patients receiving memantine had better outcomes on cognition, behavior, and activities of daily living. Caregivers of this group also reported significantly fewer hours of care assistance (Reisberg et al., 2003).

Cholinesterase inhibitors are more effective when treatment is started in the early AD stages. All AD medications modestly slow the progression of cognitive dysfunction and reduce problematic behaviors in some people. At least half of patients treated with these medications do not respond (Alzheimer's Association, 2005a).

Medical treatments have also been studied that alter the course of dementia and treat the symptoms. Vitamin E (alpha-tocopherol) and selegiline may slow AD progression.

Vitamin E, selegiline, and a combination of the two were equally effective—but no advantage was seen in the group who received both (Sano, Ernesto, & Thomas, 1997). Currently physicians are recommending that patients with AD take Vitamin E, which has fewer adverse reactions than selegiline.

Early studies suggested that estrogen might help prevent the onset of AD. But the data from the Women's Health Initiative Memory Study (WHIMS) did not support this and suggested that estrogen may increase the risk of dementia (Espeland, Rapp, & Shumaker, 2004; Shumaker, Legault, & Thal, 2003).

AD Management (Nonpharmacological). Frequently it is the behavioral symptoms of AD that have a negative affect on patients, their families, and caregivers. Some of the widely used interventions include auditory and tactile stimulation and exercise/movement therapy. Music therapy has been shown to decrease agitation. Touch can significantly reduce behavioral symptoms. Aromatherapy and massage in combination have been shown to reduce behavioral symptoms. Exercise and movement can also decrease agitated behavior. Nurses can take an important role in helping family and caregivers learn of these potential strategies to lessen these negative behaviors of AD over time (Souder & Beck, 2004).

Researchers are investigating how AD develops and progresses over time, the potential for statins to prevent dementia, and how to prevent or remove beta-amyloid plaques. As the pace of research accelerates, scientists funded by the Alzheimer's Association, pharmaceutical industry, universities, and federal government have gained understanding of the basic disease process at work in the Alzheimer's brain. These processes may offer promising targets for new treatments to prevent, slow, or even reverse damage to nerve cells. The Alzheimer's Association and National Institute on Aging estimate the current direct and indirect costs of caring for the 4.5 million Americans with AD are at least $100 billion annually (Alzheimer's Association, 2005b). By 2030, when the entire baby boom generation is over 65, the number of Americans with AD will reach such high levels that costs will be prohibitive.

Mild Cognitive Impairment

Mild cognitive impairment (MCI) is a general term describing subtle but measurable memory deficits. A person with MCI experiences memory problems greater than normally expected with aging but experiences no other symptoms of dementia, such as impaired judgment or reasoning. It is a relatively new syndrome that is currently thought of as a transition phase between healthy cognitive aging and dementia. In 2001 the American Academy of Neurology published practice guidelines for the early detection of memory problems. The following criteria for an MCI diagnosis were identified (Petersen et al., 2001).

- An individual's report of his or her own memory problems, preferably confirmed by another person
- Measurable, greater than normal memory impairment detected with standard assessment tests
- Normal overall thinking and reasoning skills
- Ability to perform normal daily activities

Researchers continue to investigate MCI, and there are varying differences of opinion about the precise definition and classification of MCI. There are also questions about whether MCI could be a transition phase to AD. Because of the inconsistencies, there is no widely accepted professional guideline for a standard approach to MCI treatment (DeCarli, 2003). If a person is diagnosed with MCI, the individual will most likely be monitored over time for changes in memory and thinking skills that indicate a worsening of symptoms or development of a disease such as AD.

Multiple Sclerosis (also see Chapter 21 for further discussion of MS)

It is estimated that between 40% and 70% of people with multiple sclerosis (MS) develop some degree of cognitive dysfunction.

Cognitive deficits are relative to both the extent and location of demyelinative lesions. Cognitive impairment in MS often goes undetected or is misattributed to other problems (Lincoln et al., 2002). Research has shown that memory, learning, conceptual reasoning, speed of information processing and reaction time, attention, concentration, and executive function are affected (MS Exchange, 2005). The cognitive symptoms can be subtle and gradual. During stressful times and exacerbations, cognitive function can be significantly impaired, while improving during periods of remission.

In managing MS the focus is on altering the course of the disease and improving quality of life. Studies indicate that early treatment delays disability, concurrently decreasing the injury to the nervous system, which may delay deficits in cognition. Cognitive impairment can be related to other factors such as medication, depression, stress, or fatigue. Patients should be evaluated for other causes before attributing these deficits to MS. No medication has been Food and Drug Administration (FDA) approved for the treatment of cognitive dysfunction in patients with MS. There is promising preliminary data suggesting that donepezil (an acetylcholinesterase inhibitor) may be effective in improving memory (Krupp et al., 2004).

MS-related cognitive decline might improve with cognitive rehabilitation—which has been a part of treatment for patients with cardiovascular accidents or brain trauma for years. It has recently been applied to MS. Cognitive rehabilitation includes two approaches: the use of compensatory strategies and cognitive retraining. They may be combined, but compensatory strategies tend to be used for mild or moderate cognition problems, whereas cognitive retraining is used for more severe deficits. In using compensatory strategies, patients find ways to capitalize on strengths and circumvent weaknesses. For example, if a patient with MS has an auditory processing problem, utilize written instructions in e-mail, tape lectures, or hire a note taker. If there is difficulty concentrating, the patient should focus on tasks in a quiet place with minimal distractions. The patient can compensate for memory problems by list making, appointment books, calendars, electronic organizers, and limiting clutter.

Solari, Motta, and Mendozzi (2004) studied cognitive retraining in an MS population. In a double-blind, controlled trial, 82 patients with MS were randomized into two groups. One group received a computer-assisted retraining interaction focused on memory and attention; the control group received a visuoconstructional and visuomotor coordination intervention. Improvement was seen in neuropsychological testing with both groups.

Other ways to address MS-related cognitive dysfunction include the use of workbooks, puzzles, and board games that involve cognitive strategies. Health care professionals can also set up tasks that utilize multiple cognitive skills such as planning a community outing or organizing a meal.

Evaluations of specific interactions for cognitive problems have been shown to be beneficial with inpatient groups such as CVA and TBI. But to date little research has been undertaken to assess the benefits of cognitive rehabilitation in individuals with MS.

AGE-RELATED COGNITIVE INJURY

Children and Adolescents

Brain injury at different developmental stages produces different challenges for the child as well as family and rehabilitation professionals. Because children are "in development," brain injury not only has the potential to take away knowledge and skills already learned and create obstacles to success at the current developmental stage, but also can jeopardize the child's ability to master new skills, acquire new knowledge, and successfully negotiate progressively more difficult developmental challenges over the years after injury (Ylvisaker, Chorazy, Feeney, & Russell, 1999).

Piaget emphasized the importance of early physical experience and motor activity in cognitive and intellectual development. Refer to Piaget's stages of intellectual development in Chapter 31. A child in elementary school may perform adequately without obvious problems during the first few years of life after a mild brain injury because the developmental stage is the same after injury as before the injury. When this same child transitions from elementary to middle school and thus moves from a highly structured setting to a more flexible setting requiring organization and independent functioning in a number of classes, this adolescent may begin to have difficulty (Christensen, 1997). After children with cognitive deficits reach adolescence there is a tendency for development of personality and behavior problems secondary to the cognitive deficits and difficulty adjusting to the residual disabilities.

A student must meet the Individuals With Disabilities Education Act (IDEA) definition of TBI to receive special education services. "A TBI is an acquired injury to the brain caused by an external physical force, resulting in total or partial functional disability or psychological impairment, or both, that adversely affects a child's educational performance" (NASHIA, 2002). Once the student is identified as eligible, the student's team develops an Individualized Education Plan (IEP). The IEP describes the student's specific strengths and weaknesses and includes goals that specifically focus on strengthening weak areas while reinforcing the student's strengths. The IEP team meets as needed to accommodate the rapid changes that can occur among students with TBI.

Rehabilitation goals for the child with altered cognition promote age-appropriate growth and maturation. A child's altered cognition affects the entire family (Gill & Wells, 2000; Rocchio, 2000). Rocchio (2000) supports the need for increased and more productive dialogue between service providers and parents and better access to community support systems over the life span of individuals with brain injuries. Gill and Wells (2000) examined the experiences of siblings living with a brother or sister who had experienced a TBI and found one overwhelming theme: the well sibling's life was forever different. There were four primary supporting themes: change in the sibling with a brain injury (the reason for the difference in the well sibling's life), mixed emotions change in the sibling with a brain injury (the reason for the difference in the well sibling's life), mixed emotions (well sibling's reactions to the experience), different life rhythm (changes in the way the well sibling went about day-to-day life), and change in self (ways that the well sibling became a different person). Education and appropriate support services are essential in empowering and enabling family members to become advocates—not only for their child with a brain injury, but for the entire family.

Aging

Older adults may experience alterations or impairments in cognition as a result of falls, motor vehicle accidents, and cerebrovascular accidents, or secondary to illness or drugs. Falls are a serious often preventable problem for older adults. The leading causes of TBI in those 65 years and older are falls and motor vehicle accidents (Coronado, Thomas, Sattin, & Johnson, 2005). Older adults experience worse outcomes than younger persons even when they experience minor brain injuries or other general trauma (Susman, Di Russo, & Sullivan, 2002). Falls occur more frequently in people with cognitive impairment than in normal-functioning older adults. The estimated annual incidence of falls for people with dementia ranges from 70% to 85%, nearly double the fall risk of cognitively normal older adults (Tinetti, Speechley, & Ginter, 1988).

Motor vehicle traffic accidents are the second leading cause of TBI hospitalization. Even though elder adults wear seat belts more often than those in other age-groups except for infants and preschoolers and are less likely to drink and drive than other adults, drivers 65 or older have higher crash death rates per mile driven than all groups except teenage drivers (Coronado et al., 2005; Insurance Institute for Highway Safety, 2001). Their percentage of alcohol-related crashes increased slightly from 1999 to 2001 (NHTSA, 2001). The NHTSA in 2002 found that fatalities among alcohol-intoxicated drivers and pedestrians age 70 or older accounted for 5% and 8% of driver- and pedestrian-related fatalities in this age-group in the United States (Coronado et al., 2005). Interventions such as better vehicle design (seat and pedal adjustment), roadway design (better visibility/signs), and improved prevention education for elders may decrease these numbers.

Once an older adult enters rehabilitation, the intensities of the daily therapies must be tailored to meet the individual's tolerance. Reconditioning presents greater risk for older adults. Ability to learn is preserved, but elders often learn at a slower rate. Overall, the more complex the mental task, the greater the effects of aging. Long-term outcomes for the elderly with altered cognition are related to cognitive status, behavioral status, and social situation. Because much of rehabilitation requires learning, there are major implications for rehabilitation professionals.

NURSING PROCESS

Assessment

Because cognition has a major impact on a patient's rehabilitation potential, nursing has a major role in determining baseline cognition, participating with the interdisciplinary team in formulating a plan of care to treat the deficits, monitoring for changes in cognition, carrying out the treatment plan, and evaluating outcomes. To begin the assessment, the nurse needs to talk with family members and significant others to determine the patient's preinjury cognitive abilities. This assists in defining the baseline normal cognitive strengths and weaknesses. The neuropsychologist's assessment provides a description of the patient's mental status, covering both cognitive processes and affective status. Among the major cognitive processes that are assessed are attention, executive function, perception, memory, motor performance, language, and intelligence. It is equally important that the presence of depression, agitation, and emotional lability be evaluated because these affective disturbances are prime determinants of a patient's ability to participate in rehabilitation.

Preinjury Nursing Assessment. It is imperative to acquire knowledge about baseline function. Obtain data before disease, injury, or alteration in thought processes, including medical history in regard to thought processes and cognitive and behavioral functioning. Ask family and friends to describe an individual's preinjury behaviors and intellectual functioning. Also ask about the individual's preinjury recreation, socialization, and occupation. Assess a pediatric patient's preinjury level of development by talking with parents and the pediatrician. Obtain history of medications, alcohol, or substance abuse. Obtain history of activities of daily living, functional ability, and sleep-wake patterns.

Postinjury Nursing Assessment. Obtain data immediately after injury or onset of disease or alteration in thought process. Assess level of consciousness, cognition, or behavior with the Glasgow Coma Scale (see Box 25-2) or the Children's Coma Scale (modified from the Glasgow Coma Scale). Assess short-term memory, attention span, and concentration (refer to Chapter 24). Monitor judgment, intellectual functioning, and thought content. Assess cognitive function with Rancho Los Amigos Levels of Cognitive Function Scale (see Box 25-3). Obtain sequence of recovery from coma and tracking of behaviors.

Assess body systems. Identify onset of symptoms, gradual onset versus sudden onset, and the etiology of impairment. Apply tactile stimulation to skin, and monitor response. Assess level of responsiveness. Assess visual-spatial alterations. Monitor for seizures and signs of increased intracranial pressure. Observe physical status and motor functioning. Assess language and nonlanguage communication. Assess sensory and perceptual function. Review medications, and identify those that could alter thought processes.

Assessment Concurrent With Rehabilitation. Assessment data is collected throughout the rehabilitation process by nurses and members of the rehabilitation team including general orientation to person, place, time, and situation. The GOAT can be used to assess progression through posttraumatic amnesia. Refer to Chapter 24 for further discussion of memory.

Monitor for phobias, perseveration of thought, or delusions. Assess for changes in behavior. The Agitated Behavior Scale may be used to denote excesses in behaviors (see Box 25-4). Note any changes in medications, and observe patterns of seizures. Monitor vital signs and test values.

Observe progression of physical status and motor control. Note patterns of communication/language skills. Monitor changes in sensory and perceptual functioning. Assess the patient's ability to perform activities of daily living. Observe motivation and cooperation with the rehabilitation program. Note sleep-wake cycles. Assess available community and social support systems available to the patient.

Cognitive impairments can affect how well an individual functions in rehabilitation and in society. Neuropsychological assessment tests have been developed to quantitate the severity of cognitive deficits by identifying brain-behavior relationships. For many the deficits are transient; for some the cognitive deficits are permanent. In either situation a neuropsychological assessment test is used to clarify the nature and type of cognitive deficits. Vast numbers of neuropsychological tests are available. They derive from many scientific and clinical traditions. A neuropsychologist is an essential member of the rehabilitation team who identifies the most appropriate tests. As a result of the diversity in tests, a single index or measure cannot capture the pattern of cognitive strengths and weaknesses. Comprehensive neuropsychological assessment is done with overlapping tests to survey cognitive functions. Comprehensive sampling permits the analysis of patterns of cognitive performance within an individual patient. After specific deficits are identified and quantified, a plan of individual care can be established and implemented.

Commonly used neuropsychological tests in rehabilitation include the Halstead Reitan Battery, Wechsler Memory Scale III, and Luria-Nebraska Neuropsychological Battery. Halstead Reitan Battery measures problem solving, attention, vigilance, abstraction, motor speed, and incidental memory (Putnam & Fichtenberg, 1999). The Wechsler Memory Scale III measures verbal and nonverbal memory functioning. It measures the level of cognitive functioning and allows a quantitative discrimination between verbal and performance abilities (Fisher, Ledbetter, Cohen, Marmor, & Tulsky, 2000). The Luria-Nebraska Neuropsychological Battery measures simple and complex abilities in each sensory area under varying conditions (Bondy, 1994).

Nursing Diagnoses

Experiencing cognitive deficits is a frightening experience for the patient as well as for his or her family. Patients respond differently to problems with cognition depending on many factors including etiology, age, prior health status, education about and understanding of injury or disease, support systems, and available treatments. When a rehabilitation nurse identifies that a person is having cognitive problems, an essential management strategy is consistency. A number of nursing diagnoses can be formulated for the person with impairment in cognition (Table 25-1).

TABLE 25-1 Nursing Diagnoses: Defining Characteristics

Nursing Diagnosis	Functional Health Pattern*	Definition	Defining Characteristics	Common Medical Diagnoses/Concerns
Disturbed thought processes	Cognitive-perceptual pattern	Disruption in cognitive operations or activities relative to chronological age expectation	Cognitive dissonance Memory deficit/loss Impaired perception/judgment/decision making Distractibility Inappropriate behavior Impaired attention span	Dementia Alzheimer's disease Neurological diseases, such as brain tumors, seizures, stroke, multiple sclerosis Head injuries Anoxia/hypoxia injuries Mental disorders Drug and alcohol abuse Fluid and/or electrolyte imbalance Infections (older adults)
Chronic confusion	Cognitive-perceptual pattern	Irreversible long-standing or progressive deterioration of intellect and personality, characterized by decreased ability to interpret environmental stimuli and decreased capacity for intellectual thought processes, and manifested by disturbances of memory, orientation, and behavior	Disoriented to person, place, or time Clinical evidence of organic impairment Altered interpretation or response to stimuli Progressive or long-standing cognitive impairment No change in level of consciousness Impaired memory Altered personality Impaired socialization	Alzheimer's disease Multiinfarct dementia Stroke Head injury Anoxia/hypoxia injuries Multiple sclerosis
Impaired memory	Cognitive-perceptual pattern	Inability to remember or recall bits of information or behavioral skills	Memory problems only Forgetfulness Difficulty learning new skills or information Inability to perform a previously learned skill Inability to recall recent or past events Forgetting to perform a behavior at a scheduled time	Hypoxia/anoxia injuries Anemia Congestive heart failure Neurological disturbances, such as multiple sclerosis, mild-moderate Alzheimer's disease, brain injury, dementia, stroke Fluid and electrolyte imbalance Excessive environmental disturbances Stress/fatigue
Impaired environmental interpretation syndrome	Cognitive-perceptual pattern	Consistent lack of orientation to person, place, time, or circumstances over more than 3-6 months that necessitates a protective environment	Consistent disorientation in known and unknown environments for more than 3-6 months Chronic confusional states Loss of occupation or social functioning from memory decline Inability to follow simple directions Inability to reason Inability to concentrate Slow in responding to questions	Alzheimer's disease AIDS dementia Parkinson's disease Huntington's disease Depression Alcoholism Head injury

*Functional health pattern data from Gordon, M. (2005). *Manual of nursing diagnosis* (9th ed.). St. Louis, MO: Mosby.
AIDS, Acquired immunodeficiency syndrome.
Other potential nursing diagnoses are Impaired memory, Risk for cognitive impairment, Acute confusion, and Deficient knowledge.

Implications for the Family

Rocchio (2000) describes the emotions that families experience from the moment of injury to various levels of patient recovery. No family is ever prepared to comprehend the full magnitude of the life changes that brain injury or chronic disease affecting cognition creates. Most manage from day to day—learning as they go and drawing on resources to get through what they hope is a short-term situation that comes to a satisfactory conclusion. Family and friends share relief at the first signs of awakening after a brain injury, get excited at the first attempts to communicate and walk, and feel confident that rehabilitation can restore functional abilities. But the physical recovery may be misleading, and families are often not prepared for the cognitive and behavioral changes that may persist.

Because of the consequences of TBI, young adults often lose recently attained independence and regress to a stage of dependency on family members. Many move back to their parents' home. Typically family members rely on themselves to care for an adult member with a severe disability. This forced self-reliance creates over time a burden, more stresses than family members can handle, and generally decreases life satisfaction (see Chapter 22 for patient and family coping).

For those whose family members sustain severe brain damage to the frontal and temporal lobes of the brain from trauma or disease, life may never be the same. The public seems to accept physical limitations, but few understand and/or tolerate cognitive deficits and the accompanying behaviors. The manner in which the family deals with the residual deficits in cognition determines the quality of life for the person with the injury, as well as for the remaining family. The more time that health care professionals spend gathering data and planning interventions to help the family deal with these issues, the more positive results can be expected.

It does not take long for the individual with brain injury to realize that life is not the same. Friends stop visiting, driving privileges are gone, and life can become mundane. This may begin a vicious cycle of behavioral deterioration. The goal of treatment is to circumvent this cycle by advance planning.

Benn and McColl (2004) interviewed parents of children with acquired brain injury to investigate coping, social support, and family environment. Their findings note the importance of recognizing parents' individual coping styles, enhancing the development of positive strategies for coping, and emphasizing the importance of social support and a positive family environment. All the above facilitate the potential of parents' coping positively with their child's brain injury.

Not only parents but siblings are affected by their brother's or sister's disability as well. Opperman and Alant (2003) conducted open-ended structural interviews with adolescents who had a sibling with severe disabilities. Their subjects reported limited family interactions and limited information and guidance regarding their sibling's disability. There were also reticent to express their feelings about their disabled sibling and felt guilty about their sibling. Their need for professional support and strong support networks to facilitate adolescent coping was emphasized.

The review by Verhaeghe, Defuor, and Grypdonck (2005) of the literature on stress and coping among families of patients with TBI revealed that professional intervention for family coping is appropriate even 10 to 15 years following injury. Attempts should be made to develop models of long-term support and care that can alleviate sources of burden on relatives. Findings included that good communication, positive coping, professional support, strong support networks, and development of models for long-term support are also essential for other diseases or injuries that alter cognition.

In AD, because of the older age of the individual affected, primary caregivers often are the children or spouses who are elderly. Because the cognitive deficits associated with AD progress over time, the needs of the individuals with AD and caregivers are somewhat different. Common needs may include clear communications between caregiver, patient, and health professionals, especially related to disease progression and prognosis. Flexible services provide continuity and reliability in support of the patient and caregiver (i.e., respite care). Provide information about entitlements from federal, state, and local programs. Survivor support services should be provided after patient's death.

Rehabilitation nurses who provide care at all points along the continuum are in an essential position to educate, support, and advocate for patients and caregivers for those with cognitive deficits.

Goals

Many goals are appropriate for people with cognitive deficits. Goals are formulated based on the etiology of the problem. Goals need to target interventions that focus on assisting the person in using effective communication, improving memory, increasing sensory awareness, and promoting safety.

Identifying the numerous settings in which rehabilitation nurses practice while caring for people with cognitive deficits serves as a guide in planning quality care. If the etiology of a cognitive deficit is abrupt and sudden, such as a stroke or brain injury, the person usually enters into the health care system through the emergency department. Depending on the seriousness of the injury, a person may enter a critical care life supportive environment, where the goal is survival. For a person with cognitive deficits or behavioral problems, other primary goals are safety and effective communication. The cognitive problem may be temporary or permanent. Once stabilized, the person is most likely admitted to an acute care unit.

After entering the acute care unit, the goals for the patient are prevention of complications and return to medical stability. Many times patients are admitted to acute care medical units because of acute confusional states, change in level of consciousness, altered personality, new onset of dementia, or behavioral disturbances. Through examination, testing, and assessments the etiology of cognitive dysfunctions is identified—such as MS, AD, MCI, CVA, or TBI. If the person needs therapy to regain strength, to practice activities of daily living, for speech enrichment, or for memory strategies, it may be initiated in acute care. Because of shortened length of stay in acute care, there is not much time for improvement. If acute care treatment does not promote the person's ability to return to his or her premorbid living situation, other options may be needed.

Rehabilitation Nursing Levels of Care

Each level of care has a unique purpose and criterion for admission. The major options of rehabilitation care include acute rehabilitation, subacute rehabilitation, outpatient rehabilitation therapies, day rehabilitation care centers, home health care services, transitional living homes, memory special care homes, and long-term convalescent homes. People may enter and leave many levels of care. The goals of each level of care usually involve a team effort between nurses,

physicians, physical therapists, occupational therapists, speech therapists, recreation therapists, social workers, dietitians, psychologists, vocational counselors, and the patient and family. Reimbursement can range from 100% coverage by health insurance providers to 100% private pay. Because of the cost of various care levels and the nonreimbursement issues, many patients do not enter into the appropriate level of care.

Acute Rehabilitation Units. Acute rehabilitation units are inpatient short-term units in which the patient receives intense therapy that may include physical therapy, occupational therapy, speech therapy, social services, nursing care, psychology, and ancillary services to promote his or her return to home or the next level of care. Table 25-2 delineates

TABLE 25-2 Rehabilitation Nursing Outcomes and Interventions for Cognitive Deficits in an Acute Rehabilitation Unit

Potential Rehabilitation Nursing Outcomes	Potential Rehabilitation Nursing Interventions
Cognitive ability intact as evidenced by ability to execute complex mental processes	Promote cognitive function: • Identify/assess current cognitive status via Mini-Mental State Examination/Ranchos Los Amigos Scale • Facilitate reality orientation • Label items in environment to promote recognition • Provide access to current news events • Encourage participation in decision making • Encourage use of aids (e.g., eyeglasses, hearing aids, and dentures) • Dress patient in personal clothing • Speak in concrete terms, avoid abstract terms
Decision making intact as evidenced by the ability to choose between two or more alternatives	Promote appropriate decision making: • Identify potential choices such as allowing the patient to pick daily clothing • Allow the patient to make choices in daily care • Help patient identify the advantages and disadvantages of each alternative • Encourage the patient to make decisions about self and care • Provide positive reinforcement when appropriate choices are made • Provide simple problems that can be controlled (e.g., card games, meal selection) • Gradually increase complexity of tasks (e.g., computer games, planning daily activities) • Develop a problem-solving training program that allows patient to practice responses to common problem situations • Gradually introduce common problems the patient may face in the community • Encourage patient to participate in community outings to test decision-making skills • Use computer programs to practice decision making
Thought control as evidenced by appropriate perception, thought processes, and thought content	Promote appropriate control of thoughts: • Monitor patient's statements of self • Provide experiences that increase patient's autonomy • Assist patient with identifying positive responses from others (discourage negative criticizing and teasing) • Identify patient's inappropriate behavior when it occurs: provide feedback in behavior; if patient cannot identify inappropriate behavior, nurse identifies it for patient and provides counsel (videotape patient when acting inappropriately and show to patient for educational purposes), role-playing • Establish consistent interdisciplinary plan to deal with inappropriate behaviors • Establish a behavior modification plan • Provide positive reinforcement for appropriate behavior

TABLE 25-2 Rehabilitation Nursing Outcomes and Interventions for Cognitive Deficits in an Acute Rehabilitation Unit—cont'd

Potential Rehabilitation Nursing Outcomes	Potential Rehabilitation Nursing Interventions
Information processing is consistently demonstrated as evidenced by acquiring, organizing, and using information	Promote accurate information processing: • Assess level of comprehension • Encourage the patient to ask for clarification • Assess for nonverbal and verbal behaviors that would indicate the degree of understanding • Converse with patient in one-on-one conversation • Provide discussion about events, current news, items found in print (reading is the highest level of comprehensive skills)
Memory intact as evidenced by ability to retrieve and report previously stored information	Promote memory function: • Assess memory problems • Stimulate memory by repeating patient's last expressed thought • Implement appropriate memory techniques (i.e., memory cues, making lists, memory games, mnemonic devices, computers, rehearsing information) • Assist in associated learning tasks (such as practical learning and recalling information) • Provide for orientation training (e.g., patient rehearsing personal information and dates) • Provide opportunities to use memory for recent events (e.g., questioning patient about recent event) • Encourage patient to participate in group memory training program • Provide repetition of information and make verbal or visual association that promotes remembering • Teach patients to organize information in a logical way (e.g., when dressing teach person to plan events in sequence of bathing, hygiene, underclothes, and clothes) • Model calm and friendly behavior to reduce fear and anxiety
Safety behavior as evidenced by fall prevention	Promote safety: • Assess patient for potential for injury/risk for fall • Educate patient and family about potential hazards in current environment and home • Assess environment for potential or actual risks, and eliminate problem area • Use less-restrictive devices to prevent falls from bed, wheelchair, commode, etc., such as a bed alarm, chair alarm, and constant supervision; restraint options include locking bed belt, side rails, and wheelchair belt • Identify risk factors, and design plan of care to lessen the risk (i.e., call light within reach, toileting program, frequent observation checks, consistent caregivers and routine, adhering to schedule, visual cues in environment, anticipating patient's needs, wearing shoes or nonskid slippers) • Use wheelchair tippers to prevent wheelchair from tipping over • Consult physical therapist for wheelchair and ambulation safety • Use safety ambulation device (e.g., merry walker), if needed • Use specialty beds that are low or set up on the floor if frequent falls out of bed • Limit access to windows that can be opened by patient • Avoid stairways, but if stairs are used make sure handrail is available • Manipulate lighting for therapeutic viewing of environment
Aggression control as evidenced by self-restraint of assaultive, combative, destructive, or agitation behaviors	Promote control of aggression: • Assess level of cognition in relation to potential for agitation and behavior control • Identify situations that precipitate aggression or agitation • Set up behavior management plan: communicate expectations to patient and family about the need to maintain control; set limits; refrain from arguing; establish routines; employ consistent caregivers; use soft, low speaking voice; redirect agitation away from source; ignore inappropriate behavior; praise efforts at self-control; provide consistent consequences for desired and undesired behaviors; break multiple-step instructions into simple steps; provide aids that increase environmental structure, concentration, and task (i.e., watches, calendars, signs, step-by-step instructions, schedules); monitor and regulate level of activity and stimulation in environment; limit choices as necessary; use external controls as needed to control patient (i.e., time-out, physical restraint, chemical restraint); limit caffeinated foods and fluids; and teach/reinforce appropriate social skills • Teach behavior management plan to family and significant others • Facilitate family coping through support groups, respite care, and family counseling as needed

rehabilitation nursing interventions and outcomes for cognitive disturbances in acute rehabilitation.

Subacute Rehabilitation Units. Subacute care units are considered to be less acute than a medical unit, yet they provide interdisciplinary therapies, as does a traditional inpatient rehabilitation unit, but on a smaller scale. Table 25-3 presents rehabilitation nursing interventions and outcomes for cognitive disturbances in a subacute rehabilitation.

TABLE 25-3 Rehabilitation Nursing Outcomes/Interventions for Cognitive Deficits in a Subacute Rehabilitation Unit

Potential Rehabilitation Nursing Outcomes	Potential Rehabilitation Nursing Interventions
Cognitive orientation intact as evidence by identifying person, place, and time	Promote comfort, safety, and reality orientation by the following activities: • Maintain safe environment • Provide appropriate level of supervision • Decrease environmental stimuli • Maintain daily, consistent routine • Assign consistent caregiver • Educate family and significant others about orientation strategies • Post calendars, clocks for visual aids • Encourage patients to participate in orientation, reality groups (if available) • Maintain daily log • Keep schedule with patient at all times
Concentration intact as evidenced by the ability to focus on a specific task or stimulus appropriately	Promote attention span and the ability to focus, which allows the patient to participate in an activity: • Minimize environmental stimuli • Keep distractions to a minimum • Promote adequate rest and sleep • Individualize schedule of activities and therapies • Gradually increase complexity of schedule as ability to focus improves
Neurological status: consciousness as evidenced by the individual's ability to arouse, orient, and attend to the environment	Promote recovery of consciousness by coma-stimulation activities such as: • Familiar strong odors (coffee, chocolate) • Familiar sounds (family member's voice, music) • Tactile stimulation with different fabric textures • Visual pictures or large colored codes
Activity tolerance increased to the point where the patient can participate in daily activities	Promote frequency and duration of individual's activity: • Establish baseline activity tolerance, and gradually increase • Assist with choosing appropriate activities consistent with cognitive capabilities (focus on what can be and not deficits) • Provide activities to increase attention span and concentration in therapies • Provide positive reinforcement for engaging in activities • Assist the patient and family with monitoring own progress toward goal achievement
Family participates in professional care as evidenced by their involvement in making decisions, delivering care, and evaluating care provided by health care professionals	Promote family participation: • Educate family about disease, situation, and their role responsibilities • Facilitate coping and problem-solving skills • Assist family with maintaining positive relationships • Facilitate open communication between health care workers and family • Encourage families to participate in support groups • Encourage family participation in care as appropriate • Schedule and facilitate family conferences to discuss and evaluate care
Family has the knowledge to understand the illness or injury causing deficits in cognition	Promote family understanding for reasons of deficits in cognition: • Assess family's education level (learning style and ability to learn new information) • Use resources from appropriate agencies such as American Heart Association, Multiple Sclerosis Society, Brain Injury Association of America, or Alzheimer's Association • Encourage interdisciplinary team strategies to provide information about deficits • Provide education one-on-one or in small groups as appropriate • Facilitate family participation in managing the cognitive deficits
Patient and family participate in health care decisions regarding next level of care	Promote appropriate decision making by patient and family regarding next of level of care: • Keep family informed • Encourage participation in rehabilitation program • Use discharge planning resources (i.e., case manager, social worker, patient advocates) • Provide them with information about options and resources based on situation and benefits

Outpatient Rehabilitation. Outpatient rehabilitation consists of day rehabilitation care centers or home health care services provided while the patient resides at home but receives support and therapy. Table 25-4 provides a list of rehabilitation nursing interventions and outcomes for cognitive disturbances in outpatient rehabilitation.

Other Residential Facilities. Other residential facilities of care include transitional living centers, special memory care homes, assisted living homes, and long-term convalescent homes. These are considered a patient's home in which he or she receives specialized care services. Table 25-5 lists rehabilitation nursing interventions and outcomes for cognitive disturbances in these facilities.

TABLE 25-4 **Rehabilitation Nursing Expected Outcomes and Interventions for Cognitive Deficits in Outpatient Rehabilitation**

Possible Rehabilitation Nursing Outcomes	Potential Rehabilitation Nursing Interventions
Home physical environment: safety as evidenced by no physical harm or injury in the home	Promote home safety: • Assess home by interdisciplinary team to assess for potential hazards • Provide good lighting • Place handrails, ramps, and grab bars • Arrange furniture to reduce risk • Notify community safety personnel about cognitively impaired patient at home in community (e.g., local police, neighborhood watch patrol) • Place telephone or communication device in an accessible location with phone numbers posted nearby • Ensure smoke detectors are in working condition in the home • Remove environmental hazards (e.g., rugs, cords, sharp objects) • Provide adaptive equipment for cooking (e.g., mirrors over stove so patient can see, large knobs, key and lock use) • Secure rooms to keep patient in to avoid elopement
Caregiver home health care readiness as evidenced by being prepared to assume responsibility for the health care of family member with cognitive deficit	Promote caregiver readiness: • Assess caregiver potential to assume the role/responsibilities (emotional readiness, knowledge, stress/coping) • Participate in home health care decisions • Return demonstration and information about home health care management/care plan: treatments, activity plan, schedule, emergency care, follow-up care/appointments, when to seek medical attention, identification of plans for home health care backup, management of equipment/supplies • Establish a respite plan if needed
Caregiver performance, direct care, and indirect care given as evidenced by provision and oversight of appropriate care by family member or significant other	Promote caregiver performance, direct and indirect care: • Implement a care plan identified in acute or rehabilitation level of care • Monitor behavior of care recipient and anticipation of care recipient needs • Demonstrate confidence in monitoring caregiver skills • Demonstrate positive regard for care of recipient, confidence in performing needed tasks, and confidence in problem solving • Recognize changes in behavior and health status of recipient and care • Obtain and oversee needed services for care recipient
Caregiver physical and emotional health as evidenced by physical and emotional well-being of family care provider while caring for family member or significant other over extended period	Promote caregiver's physical and emotional health by continually assessing energy level, sleep pattern, physical function, perceived general health, mobility level, resistance to infection, medication use, use of health care providers, and physical comfort Promote wellness behaviors: • Encourage social support system • Identify stressors • Identify limitations in caregiving • Identify role performance • Use health care services • Encourage involvement in activities • Identify satisfaction/dissatisfaction with caregiver's role • Identify other potential needs for caregiver support

Continued

TABLE 25-4 Rehabilitation Nursing Expected Outcomes and Interventions for Cognitive Deficits in Outpatient Rehabilitation—cont'd

Possible Rehabilitation Nursing Outcomes	Potential Rehabilitation Nursing Interventions
	• Identify potential support groups • Monitor factors promoting endurance • Observe satisfaction of care recipient/caregiver relationship • Master indirect/direct care activities • Identify services/social support needs for caregiver • Provide health care system support, resources, and respite for caregiver
Family normalization as evidenced by the ability of the family to develop and maintain routines and management strategies that contribute to optimal functioning when a member has a cognitive impairment	Promote family normalization and integrity: • Assess family roles and structure preinjury/disease and current status • Identify family's ability to maintain usual routines • Monitor family's ability to accommodate the needs/care of recipient • Identify potential resources to support family integrity (counseling, psychology, social work, support groups) • Facilitate participation in the role changes required by cognition deficit of care recipient (e.g., breadwinner, parent, spouse no longer able to fulfill previous role responsibilities) • Promote communication between family members • Encourage problem solving and conflict resolution • Encourage participation in family events (e.g., meals, leisure activities, family traditions, rituals) • Identify potential support/resources in times of crisis
Health-seeking and health-promoting behaviors as evidenced by actions promoting and sustaining optimal wellness, recovery, and rehabilitation	Promote health-seeking and health-promoting behaviors: • Assess family and patient's ability to implement healthy behaviors: asking questions appropriately, completing health-related tasks, performing daily activities with energy tolerance • Describe strategies to eliminate unhealthy behaviors • Describe strategies to maximize health • Encourage health-promoting behaviors • Monitor personal behaviors for risk • Seek balance among exercise, work, leisure, rest, and nutrition • Use effective stress reduction behaviors • Maintain satisfactory social relationships • Use financial, physical, and social support resources to promote health • Facilitate the reentry into school and work by monitoring current and ongoing cognition needs and potential services to improve cognitive recovery • Facilitate work site assessment, and visit to determine appropriateness and potential resources for return • Promote work-simulated opportunities • Monitor performance, and make changes based upon individual patient's needs • Identify the child's or adolescent's ability to participate in formal schooling • Provide cognitive appropriate resources or sites for ongoing education • Promote long-term monitoring for changes in educational support based on changes in cognition/problems that may occur with developmental levels • Provide educational support based on developmental needs
Social interaction skills/involvement as evidenced by a patient's ability and frequency of social interactions	Promote social interaction skills and involvement: • Encourage involvement within already established relationships • Encourage relationships with people who have common interests/goals • Encourage honesty in presenting oneself to others • Encourage respect for the rights of others • Refer patient to a program that teaches appropriate social skills • Help patient increase awareness of strengths and limitations in communicating with others • Use role-playing to practice communication and social skills • Confront patient about impaired judgment when appropriate • Give positive feedback when patient reaches out to others • Encourage patient to participate in leisure activities

TABLE 25-5 Rehabilitation Nursing Expected Outcomes and Interventions for Cognitive De[...] in Other Potential Rehabilitation Facilities

Potential Rehabilitation Nursing Outcomes	Potential Rehabilitation Nursing Interventions
Safety behavior as evidenced by caregiver's ability to control patient's behaviors that might injury	Promote personal safety: • Assess patient's risk for injury/falls assessment tool • Create a safe environment for the patient • Remove potentially harmful objects from the environment • Provide low-height beds or floor mats as appropriate • Provide adaptive devices (e.g., handrails) • Place frequently used objects within reach (e.g., urinal) • Monitor environmental stimuli (e.g., noise, lighting, contact stimulation) • Individualize daily routine • Maintain consistency of staff assignment • Provide frequent or ongoing monitoring • Ensure patient has access to nursing call light at all times (mark it with bright color such as orange) • Educate patient and family about safety plan • Monitor patient for inappropriate behaviors, attempt to identify trigger stimuli • Redirect patient's attention away from agitation source • Ignore inappropriate behavior • Praise efforts at self-control • Use chemical restraints as a last option • Use restraints or immobilization devices, if appropriate and according to facility's policy (may no longer allow them)
Aggression control as evidenced by self-restraint of assaultive, combative, or destructive behavior toward others	Promote control of aggressive behavior: • When aggressive outbursts occur, assess situation for patterns such as time of day, circumstances before event, environmental factors (lighting, noise, overstimulation or understimulation), caregiver's approach, food/drinks (e.g., caffeinated products, high-sugar foods) eaten before episode, and visitors/people surrounding patient before or during event • Refrain from arguing with patient • Ensure patient does not strike out at staff or other patients by removing them from scene • Secure environment so patient does not have access to sharp objects • When patient's anger escalates, assist patient in identifying behavior (e.g., voice gets louder, makes threatening comments, strikes out), and provide patient with alternative solution (e.g., throw pillow, hug stuffed animal, ambulate [if able to safely] or propel self in wheelchair, push in wheelchair [motion can have a calming effect], try rocking chair, put on calming music, dim lights, remove people [avoid gathering staff; this feels like an attack], or avoid conversation) • After outburst, discuss the situation to educate patient on aggressive behaviors • Educate family about aggression and plan of care
Caregiver adaptation to patient institutionalization as evidenced by family caregiver's adaptation role when the care recipient is transferred outside the home	Promote caregiver's adaptation to patient's institutionalization: • Assess caregiver's understanding/belief of institutional care • Promote a trusting relationship between family and staff • Encourage family to be involved in decision-making regarding care • Offer to let family participate in care • Establish a means of communication • Encourage family and patient to express feelings about change or being in institution • When conflicts arise, promote family's being part of resolution • Allow patient to be as independent as possible • Encourage family to bring in patient's personal items/clothes to make the environment feel more familiar
Quality of life as evidenced by an individual's or family's expressed satisfaction with current life circumstances	Promote quality of life: • Assess patient's code status and living will status • Promote patient's productivity or usefulness by having patient participate in self-care activities and mobility, as appropriate • Encourage patient to express thoughts about past, present, and future • Assist patient in recognizing strengths • Encourage patient to engage in social support system, leisure activities, and daily routine • Seek psychological support, if appropriate • Administer medications, if appropriate • Promote comfort and prevention of complications • Provide a balance between rest and activity • If not a group activity person, provide one-on-one activities

Continued

...ehabilitation Nursing Expected Outcomes and Interventions for Cognitive Deficits
...n Other Potential Rehabilitation Facilities—cont'd

...itation ...mes	Potential Rehabilitation Nursing Interventions
	• Maintain consistency in schedule; dress patient in street clothes during the day and pajamas for bedtime
	• Provide meals at a table/dining room experience
	• Promote toileting in a bathroom environment
	• Provide hygiene and baths appropriately
	• Use pastoral and social services when indicated

Case Study

History of Present Illness

Brutus Gray is a 68-year-old man who experienced a subdural hematoma after a fall on the ice. Recovery was complicated with respiratory failure and encephalopathy. Glasgow Coma Scale score upon arrival at the emergency department was 9. He spent 7 days in critical care before being admitted to acute rehabilitation. At the time of admission to rehabilitation, he was a Rancho level V with a disturbance in his sleep-wake cycle.

Past Medical History

Past medical history includes hypertension and mild TBI secondary to motor vehicle accident 30 years ago.

Social History

Mr. Gray is a retired high school math teacher. He is married with three children, who live within 50 miles of his home. His wife is also retired and does volunteer work at the local hospital. He and his wife live in a ranch style home with a one-step entrance. There is no history of alcohol, drug, or tobacco use. Mr. Gray's immediate family history includes a father with myocardial infarction and a grandmother with Alzheimer's disease.

Physical Examination

Vital signs are within normal limits, and he is oriented to name only. Mini-Mental State Examination score is a 9. He needs maximum assistance with activities of daily living and transfers. He requires cues for bowel and bladder management with frequent episodes of incontinence. He is confused and impulsive.

Nursing Diagnosis

Disturbed thought processes: Rancho level V related to TBI

Nursing Outcome

Caregiver performance: Direct care as evidenced by family able to provide appropriate care for patient in their home; patient will not leave home without supervision

Nursing Goal

Nursing goals include actions that promote the family's providing appropriate care for Mr. Gray.

Nursing interventions include the following:
- *His wife's understanding of her husband's cognitive status and potential safety concerns was assessed. After assessment, it was discovered that his wife did not have an understanding of the need for continuous supervision for safety.*
- *In mutual decision making, it was decided that Mr. Gray needed a planned routine and structure. Mr. Gray would attend a rehabilitation day care center from 8:00 AM to 4:30 PM, where he would receive therapy, social activities, leisure activities, and home management activities.*
- *His wife participated in the plan. After day care she would pick him up and bring him home.*
- *A planned schedule was established weekly.*
- *His wife agreed that supervision would include close monitoring at all times.*
- *Bells were added to all doors to alert the family when doors were opened.*
- *Bright red STOP signs would be placed on the inside of all doors to remind Mr. Gray not to leave.*
- *Mr. Gray agreed to wear an alert bracelet stating "Memory Problems" with a home phone number until his memory improved.*
- *Local community emergency medical services (police, fire department) were notified of Mr. Gray's condition and risk for elopement.*
- *Mr. Gray and his wife were encouraged to participate in a local TBI support group.*
- *Return appointment was made with outpatient rehabilitation services to evaluate the plan of care and formulate necessary changes.*

Other expected outcomes that may be a part of Mr. Gray's recovery once living at home include the following:
- *Home physical environment safety*
- *Caregiver home readiness*
- *Caregiver physical and emotional health*
- *Family normalization*
- *Social interaction skills and involvement*

Specific nursing interventions for each of these outcomes are detailed in Table 25-4.

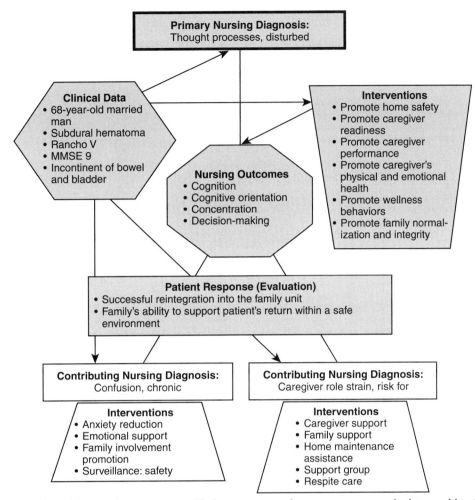

Concept Map. Mr. Gray's problem with cognition and behavior present long-term concerns for him and his family. The concept map depicts initial concerns, including disturbed thought processes, chronic confusion, and risk for caregiver stress. The rehabilitation nurse will focus on coordinating interventions to achieve the outcomes of reintegration of Mr. Gray into the family, while ensuring his safety and family support.

Evaluation

To evaluate the effectiveness of nursing interventions, compare actual patient and family behaviors with the expected patient and family outcomes.

CRITICAL THINKING

The discharge plan is for Mr. Gray to return home to live with his wife. His cognitive status in acute rehabilitation is severely impaired. The goal at discharge is that Mr. Gray needs 24-hour supervision for his cognitive deficits. He is physically independent in mobility and self-care. His specific cognitive impairments include confusion, impulsiveness, impaired judgment, and poor safety awareness.

1. Identify potential nursing diagnoses and interventions specific to Mr. Gray's cognitive deficits.
2. What questions do you ask in evaluating the potential for his wife to take him home?
3. Identify potential strategies and resources that will facilitate Mr. Gray's success at home.

REFERENCES

Alzheimer's Association. (2005a). *Materials and treatment plans for dementia*: NCGNP Mental Health Kit. Available from http://www.alz.org.

Alzheimer's Association. (2005b). *Statistics about Alzheimer's disease*. Available from http://www.alz.org/AboutAD/statistics.asp.

Alzheimer's Association. (2005c). *What is Alzheimer's disease?* Available from http:www.alz.org/AboutAD/WhatIsAD.asp.

American Academy of Pediatrics. (2001). Bicycle helmets. *Pediatrics, 108*(4),1030-1032.

American Stroke Association. (2006). *Impact of stroke*. Available from http://www.strokeassociation.org/presenter.jhtml?identifier=1033.

Benn, K. M., & McColl, M. A. (2004). Parental coping following childhood acquired brain injury. *Brain Injury, 18*(3), 239-255.

Biagas, K. (1999). Hypoxic-ischemia brain injury: Advancements in the understanding of mechanisms and potential avenues for therapy. *Current Opinions in Pediatrics, 1*, 223- 228.

Bogner, J. A., Corrigan, J. D., Bode, R. K., & Heinemann, A.W. (2000). Rating scale analysis of the agitated behavior scale. *Journal of Head Trauma Rehabilitation, 15*(1), 656-669.

Bondy, K. N. (1994). Assessing cognitive function: A guide to neuropsychological testing. *Rehabilitation Nursing, 19*, 24-30.

Brain Injury Association of America. (1997). *Causes of brain injury*. Available from http://www.biausa.org/Pages/causes_of_brain_injury.html.

Brain Injury Association of America. (2001a). *Bicycle safety*. Available from http://www.biausa.org/word.files.to.pdf/good.pdfs/2002.Fact.Sheet.bike.safety.pdf.

Brain Injury Association of America. (2001b). *Shaken baby syndrome.* Available from http://www.biausa.org/pdf/baby.pdf.

Brain Injury Association of America. (2001c). *Transportation safety.* Available from http://www.biausa.org/word.files.to.pdf/good.pdfs/2002. Fact. Sheet. transportation.pdf.

Brain Injury Association of America. (2004). *TBI model systems.* Available from http://www.biausa.org/Pages/modelsystems/tbi_model_systems.html.

Centers for Disease Control and Prevention. (2003a). *Traumatic brain injury facts–NCIPC.* Available from http://www.cdc.gov/ncipc/factsheets/tbi.htm.

Centers for Disease Control and Prevention. (2003b). *Traumatic brain injury in the United States: A report to Congress.* Available from http://www.cdc.gov/doc.do/id/0900f3ec8001012b/.

Christensen, J. R. (1997). Pediatric traumatic brain injury rehabilitation: Challenges in care delivery. *Neuro Rehabilitation, 9,* 105-112.

Coronado, V. G., Thomas, K. E., Sattin, R. W., & Johnson, R. L. (2005). The CDC traumatic brain injury surveillance system: Characteristics of persons aged 65 years and older hospitalized with a TBI. *Journal of Head Trauma Rehabilitation, 3,* 215-228.

Corrigan, J. D., & Bogner, J. A. (1994). Factor structure of the Agitated Behavior Scale. *Journal of Clinical and Experimental Neuropsychology, 16,* 386-392.

Corrigan, J. D., & Bogner, J. A. (1995). Assessment of agitation following brain injury. *Neurorehabilitation, 5,* 205-210.

Corrigan, J. D., Bogner, J. A., Lamb-Hart, G. C. (1999). Substance abuse and brain injury. In M. Rosenthal, E. R. Griffith, J. S. Kreutzer, & B. Pentland (Eds.), *Rehabilitation of the adult and child with traumatic brain injury* (3rd ed., pp. 556-571). Philadelphia: F. A. Davis.

DeCarli, C. (2003). Mild cognitive impairment: Prevalence, prognosis, etiology, and treatment. *Lancet Neurology, 2*(1), 15-21.

Defense and Veterans Brain Injury Center. (2004). *What's new?* Available from http://www.dvbic.org/whatsnew_bd.html.

Defense and Veterans Brain Injury Center. (2005). *Blast injury.* Available from http://www.dvbic.org/blastinjury.html.

Espeland, M. A., Rapp, S. R., & Shumaker, S. A. (2004). Conjugated equine estrogens and global cognitive function in postmenopausal women: Women's Health Initiative Memory Study. *JAMA, 291,* 2959.

Fertli, E., Vass, K., Sterz, F., Gabriel, H., & Auff, E. (2000). Neurological rehabilitation of severely disabled cardiac arrest survivors. Part 1. Course of post-acute inpatient treatment. *Resuscitation, 47*(3), 231-239.

Fisher, D. C., Ledbetter, M. F., Cohen, N. J., Marmor, D., & Tulsky, D. S. (2000). WAIS-III and WMS-III profiles of mildly to severely brain-injured patients. *Applied Neuropsychology, 7*(3), 126-132.

Folstein, M., Folstein, S., & McHugh, P. (1975). *Mini Mental State Exam.* Lutz, FL: Psychological Assessment Resources, Inc.

Frey, L. C. (2003). Epidemiology of posttraumatic epilepsy: A critical review. *Epilepsia, 44*(Suppl. 10), 11-17.

Fulton, D. (2000). Shaken baby syndrome. *Critical Care Nursing Quarterly, 23*(2), 43-50.

Galshi, T., Bruno, R. L., Zorowitz, R., & Walker, J. (1993). Predicting length of stay, functional outcome and after care in the rehabilitation of stroke patients. *Stroke, 24,* 1794-1800.

Gill, D. J., & Wells, D. L. (2000). Forever different: Experiences of living with a sibling who has a traumatic brain injury. *Rehabilitation Nursing, 25,* 48-53.

Gillespie, L., Gillespie, W., Robertson, M., Cumming, R., & Rowe, B. (2005). Interventions for preventing falls in elderly people. *The Cochrane Database of Systemic Reviews,* (2).

Goldberg, K.B., & Ellis, D.W. (1997). Anoxic encephalopathy: A neurobehavioral study in rehabilitation. *Brain Injury, 11*(10), 743-750.

Herbert, L. E., Scherr, P. A., Bienias, J. L., Bennett, D. A., & Evans, D. A. (2003). Alzheimer's disease in the U.S. population: Prevalence estimates using the 2000 census. *Archives of Neurology, 60*(8), 1119-1122.

Hochstenbach, J., & Mulder, T. (1999). Neuropsychology and the relearning of motor skills following stroke. *International Journal of Rehabilitation Research, 22,* 11-19.

Insurance Institute for Highway Safety. (2001). Older drivers up close: They aren't dangerous except maybe to themselves. *Insurance Highway Safety Status Report, 36*(8), 1-8.

Iverson, G., Gaetz, M., Lovell, M., & Collins, M. (2004). Cumulative effects of concussion in amateur athletics. *Brain Injury, 18*(5), 433-443.

Katz, D., & Black, S. E. (1999). Neurological and neuroradiological evaluation. In M. Rosenthal, E. R. Griffith, J. S. Kreutzer, & B. Pentland (Eds.), *Rehabilitation of the adult and child with traumatic brain injury* (3rd ed., pp. 89-116). Philadelphia: F. A. Davis.

Koh, J. O., Cassidy, D., & Watkinson, E. J. (2003). Incidence of concussion in contact sports: A systematic review of the evidence. *Brain Injury, 17*(10), 901-917.

Kolakowsky-Hayner, S. A., Gourley, E. V., III, Kreutzer, J. S., Marwitz, J. H., Meade, M. A., & Cifu, D. X. (2002). Post-injury substance abuse among persons with brain injury and persons with spinal cord injury. *Brain Injury, 16*(7), 583-592.

Krupp, L. B., Christodoulou, C., Melville, P., Scherl, W. F., McAllister, W. S., & Elkins, L. E. (2004). Donepezil improved memory in multiple sclerosis in randomized clinical trial. *Neurology, 63,* 1579-1585.

Larson, E. B., & Shadlen, M. F. (2004). Survival after initial diagnosis of Alzheimer's disease. *Annals of Internal Medicine, 140*(7), 501-509.

Levin, H. S., O'Donnell, V. M., & Grossman, R. G. (1979). The Galveston Orientation and Amnesia Test. *Journal of Nervous and Mental Disease, 167,* 675-684.

Lincoln, N. B., Dent, A., Harding, A., Weyman, N., Nicholl, C., & Blumhardt, L. D. (2002). Evaluation of cognitive assessment and cognitive intervention for people with multiple sclerosis. *Journal of Neurology, Neurosurgery, and Psychiatry, 72*(1), 93-98.

Long, D. F. (1989). *What is anoxic brain injury?* Washington, D.C.: National Head Injury Foundation.

McCance, K. L., & Huether, S. E. (2006). *Pathophysiology: The biologic basis for disease in adults and children* (5th ed.). St. Louis, MO: Mosby.

Mecklinger, A., Von Cramon, Y., & Matthes-Von Cramon, G. (1998). Event-related potential evidence for a specific cognition memory deficit in adult survivors of cerebral hypoxia. *Brain, 121,* 1917-1935.

MS Exchange. (2005). Treatment of cognitive dysfunction in MS. *Consortium of MS Centers Newsletter, 9*(2), 4, 9.

Nakase-Thompson, R. N., Sherer, M., Yablon, S. A., Nick, T. G., & Trzepacz, P. T. (2004). Acute confusion following traumatic brain injury. *Brain Injury, 18*(2), 131-142.

National Association of State Head Injury Administrators. (2002). *Traumatic brain injury facts: Children and youth.* Available from http://www.nashia.org/pdocfiles/children.pdf.

Ohio Valley Center for BI Prevention and Rehabilitation. (1997). *Substance use and abuse BI: A programmer's guide.* Columbus, OH: Author.

Opperman, S., & Alant, E. (2003). The coping responses of the adolescent siblings of children with severe disabilities. *Disability Rehabilitation, 25*(9), 441-454.

O'Shanick, G. (2001). *The road to rehabilitation. Part 6. Mapping the way: Drug therapy & brain injury.* Available from http://www.biausa.org/Pages/road_to_rehab.html.

Panisset, M., Roudier, N., Saxton, J., & Boller, F. (1994). The Severe Impairment Battery: A neuropsychological test for severely demented patients. *Neurology, 51*(1), 41-45.

Petersen, R. C., Stevens, J. C., Ganguli, M., Tangalos, E. G., Cummings, J. L., & DeKosky, S. T. (2001). Practice parameter: Early detection of dementia—Mild cognitive impairment (an evidenced based review). Report of the Quality Standards Subcommittee of the American Academy of Neurology. *Neurology, 56,* 1133-1142.

Pound, P., Gompertz, P., & Ebrahim, S. (1998). A patient-centered study of the consequences of stroke. *Clinical Rehabilitation, 12,* 338-347.

Powell, K., & Voeller, K. (2004). Prefrontal executive function syndromes in children. *Journal of Child Neurology, 19*(10), 785-797.

Putnam, S. H., & Fichtenberg, N. L. (1999). Neuropsychological examination of the patient with traumatic brain injury. In M. Rosenthal, E. R. Griffith, J. S. Kreutzer, & B. Pentland (Eds.), *Rehabilitation of the adult and child with traumatic brain injury* (3rd ed., pp. 147-166). Philadelphia: F. A. Davis.

Reisberg, B., Doody, R., Stottler, A., Schmitt, F., Ferris, S., & Mobius, H. (2003). Memantine in moderate-to-severe Alzheimer's disease. *New England Journal of Medicine, 348*(14), 1333-1341.

Rocchio, C. (2000). *Family news and views–impaired cognition and behavior problems: Double trouble!* Available from http://www.biusa.org/famviewnws/impairedcog_behaveprob.htm.

Sano, M., Ernesto, C., & Thomas, R. G. (1998). A controlled trial of selegiline, alpha-tocopherol, or both as treatment for Alzheimer's disease. The Alzheimer's Disease Cooperative Study. *New England Journal of Medicine, 336,* 1216.

Shumaker, S. A., Legault, C., & Thal, L. (2003). Estrogen plus progestin and the incidence of dementia and mild cognitive impairment in postmenopausal women: The Women's Health Initiative Memory Study—A randomized controlled trial. *JAMA, 289,* 2651.

Sisson, R. (1998). Life after stroke: Coping with change. *Rehabilitation Nursing, 23,* 198-203.

Solari, A., Motta, A., & Mendozzi, L. (2004). Computerized retraining of memory and attention in people with MS: A randomized double blind controlled trial. *Journal of Neurology & Science, 222,* 94-104.

Souder, E., & Beck. C. (2004). Overview of Alzheimer's disease. *Nursing Clinics of North America, 39*, 545-559.

Susman, M., Di Russo, S. M., & Sullivan, T. (2002). Traumatic brain injury in the elderly: Increased mortality and worse functional outcome at discharge despite lower injury severity. *Journal of Trauma, 53*(2), 219-224.

Taylor, L. A., Kreutzer, J. S., Demm, S. R., & Meade, M. A. (2003). Traumatic brain injury and substance abuse: A review and analysis of the literature. *Neuropsychological Rehabilitation, 13*(1/2), 165-188.

Tinetti, M. E., Speechley, M., & Ginter, S. F. (1988). Risk factors for falls among elderly persons living in the community. *New England Journal of Medicine, 319*, 1701-1707.

Verhaeghe, S., Defuor, T., & Grypdonck, M. (2005). Stress and coping among families of patients with traumatic brain injury. *Journal of Clinical Nursing, 14*(8), 1004-1012.

Violence and Brain Injury Institute. (2000). *Violence and brain injury.* Available through electronic mail from biausa.org.

Ylvisaker, M., Chorazy, A. J. L., Feeney, T. J., & Russell, M. L. (1999). Children and adolescents: Assessment and rehabilitation. In M. Rosenthal, E. R. Griffith, J. S. Kreutzer, & B. Pentland (Eds.), *Rehabilitation of the adult and child with traumatic brain injury* (3rd ed., pp. 353-392). Philadelphia: F. A Davis.

26

Sleep

Pamela M. Duchene, DNSc, RN, CRRN

According to Shakespeare, sleep is "nature's soft nurse." In the United States, however, most adults sleep less than the recommended 7 to 9 hours a night (National Sleep Foundation, 2005). The National Sleep Foundation, in their omnibus, annual "Sleep in America Poll" conducted a telephone poll of 1006 adults living within the continental United States. They questioned sleep habits, problems, and disorders and found that most Americans sleep an average of 6.8 hours during work nights, and an average of 7.4 hours on weekends. Results of the poll indicate that during the past year only 49% of American adults report having a good night's sleep most nights. Unfortunately, Americans consider sleep a waste of time, robbing the sleep hours for daytime activities. During the past century, average sleep time decreased by 20%, whereas work and commute times increased by a month. In a national poll conducted through the American Academy of Family Physicians (2002), 40% of respondents attributed lack of sleep to too little time for sleep, and 13% attributed lack of sleep to stress. Although culture has changed, the physiology of the body and the need for sleep have not, resulting in the problems indicated in Box 26-1.

OVERVIEW OF SLEEP

Purpose of Sleep

Sleep is necessary for restoring energy and other anabolic processes. The actual homeostatic contribution of sleep is unknown (National Center on Sleep Disorders Research, 2003). Although sleep serves the purpose of providing rest and maximizing wakefulness, the functions of sleep are not well understood. Studying the effects of sleep loss, or deprivation, provides clues to the purpose of sleep. Sleep deprivation leads to problems with simple, short activities. An absence of sleep causes irritability, fatigue, decreased motivation, a shortened attention span, and reduced problem-solving capacity. Sleeplessness is a predictor of absenteeism and is estimated to be linked to more than 270,000 motor vehicle accidents annually (Czeisler & Fryer, 2006). Drowsiness increases the risk of a traffic accident fourfold according to the National Highway Traffic Safety Administration (2006). Such information

indicates that sleep plays a major role in physical and emotional health and promotes healing from illness and injury.

Sleep requirements vary throughout the life span according to the National Sleep Foundation (2005). Although new parents may disagree with the following statement, infants 2 months of age or younger require as much as 18.5 hours of sleep during a 24-hour period. The requirement for sleep decreases to 15 hours from 2 to 12 months of age. Toddlers require around 15 hours of sleep per day. The requirement continues to decrease as children age. Adolescents require 8.5 to 9.5 hours of sleep. Adults of all ages require 7 to 9 hours of sleep.

Process of Sleep

Through polysomnography, a process involving electroencephalogram, electrooculogram, and electromyogram studies, sleep may be classified into two major categories: slow eye movement or non–rapid eye movement (NREM) sleep, and rapid eye movement (REM) sleep. Slow eye movement sleep can be subdivided into four stages, with REM composing a fifth stage (Table 26-1).

In REM sleep there are rapid oscillations of the eyes, with muscle atonia (linked with deep sleep), whereas with wakefulness the electroencephalographic activity is low volume and high frequency (Russo, 2005). Bursts of electroencephalographic activity in conjunction with decreased muscle activity occur during REM sleep.

During sleep a person shifts through stages, initially proceeding through stages 1, 2, 3, and 4, and then reversing through stages 3 and 2, followed by an REM episode every 90 to 120 minutes. A sleeping individual will pass through the stages several times during the night, with five or six cycles during the night. Age, medication, and other differences will have an impact on sleep cycles, as discussed later in this chapter.

Physiology of Sleep

The midline raphe system, located in the midbrain, is considered a center for sleep activity. Serotoninergic mechanisms originating in the midline raphe affect the noradrenergic and cholinergic systems. During NREM sleep there is increased secretion of growth hormone (70% of secretion occurs during sleep), luteinizing hormone, and prolactin and decreased secretion of adrenocorticotropic and thyroid-stimulating hormones. During deep sleep (stages 3 and 4), blood pressure and respiratory function decrease, whereas vagal tone in the cardiovascular system increases.

The systems work in a balance to prevent an immediate change from a wakeful state to REM sleep. One hypothesis on the cause of narcolepsy is an imbalance in the systems, with immediate change to REM sleep becoming possible. In such a situation (REM intrusion), an individual would be wide awake one minute and in a state of atonia with active hallucinations, or visual dreams, the next.

Circadian rhythm is linked with sleep-wake cycles. Stemming from the 24-hour Earth rotation, the term *circadian* means "around a day." During a 24-hour period many changes occur within physiological parameters, including changes in temperature, respiratory rate, heart rate, and wakefulness. Minimum body temperature and maximum sleepiness coincide

in time during the nighttime hours. A second point of low temperature and sleepiness typically occurs at 3 P.M., a common time for naps and siestas. The suprachiasmatic hypothalamic nucleus is an important anatomical structure in the wakefulness-sleep cycle. The retina provides stimulation to the suprachiasmatic hypothalamic nucleus, cueing the body to the light-dark cycle and influencing wakefulness/sleep. Lesions of this area result in an impairment of circadian rhythm.

FACTORS AFFECTING SLEEP

Healthy Sleep Habits

Obtaining a good night's sleep is an elusive goal to many individuals. To ensure the optimal chances of getting enough sleep and of obtaining enough rest through sleep, the following strategies may be of assistance:

- Go to bed at a regular time every night.
- Establish a consistent waking time, and do not vary the time during weekends and holidays.
- Develop and maintain bedtime rituals, such as a warm bath or relaxation exercise, reading a book, or having a snack such as cookies and milk (Barrett, 2006).
- Exercise during the daytime, and avoid strenuous activity immediately before sleeping.
- Reduce fluid intake close to bedtime.
- Avoid eating a heavy meal right before going to bed.
- Avoid alcohol, caffeine, and nicotine.
- Use the bed only for sleeping and sex.
- If unable to fall asleep within 15 minutes, get out of bed.

The most common thieves of sleep are listed in Table 26-2.

Shift Work

Shift work is well known to nurses, and the impact and disruption of typical sleep-wake cycles is personally an issue for many nurses. Shift work results in alteration of core body temperature, immune functioning, hormonal levels, and

---

BOX 26-1 Qualities of Sleep in America

Results of the 2005 Omnibus Sleep in America Poll indicate the following about U.S. adults with sleep problems:

- 32% receive less than the 6 hours of sleep during weeknights
- 91% report one or more symptoms of insomnia
- 24% are at risk for restless legs syndrome
- 39% report less sleep than needed to perform well
- 67% report a "good night's sleep" less than a few nights each month
- 54% perceive themselves as "evening" people
- 46% require more than 30 minutes to fall asleep
- 61% report daytime sleepiness
- 49% have missed one or more days of work or made mistakes at work in the last 3 months

Modified from National Sleep Foundation. (2005). *National Sleep Foundation's 2005 "Sleep in America Poll."* Available from http://www.sleepfoundation.org/.

TABLE 26-1 Stages of Sleep

Stage 1	The onset of sleep, identified by muscle relaxation, slow side-to-side eye movements, and reduction in eye blinking. Slow eye movement (non–rapid eye movement [NREM]). Normally this stage lasts 5% of the night. EEG shows theta waves (3-7 Hz); EOG shows slow rolling eye movements (SREMs); EMG shows slightly elevated waves.
Stage 2	Slightly deeper sleep with muscle relaxation and little eye movement. Slow eye movement (NREM). Normally this stage lasts 50% of sleep. EEG shows K-complexes and sleep spindles.
Stage 3	Deep sleep, with slow waves noted on electroencephalography, and some side-to-side eye rolling. Slow eye movement (NREM).
Stage 4	Deep sleep, similar to stage 3, with high-voltage and slow-frequency electroencephalographic activity. Slow eye movement (NREM). Stage 3 and 4 are 20-25% of sleep time. EEG shows delta or slow wave sleep.
Stage 5	Rapid eye movement (REM) sleep, characterized by dreams with vivid visual content. Normally this stage is 20-25% of sleep. EEG shows sawtooth or theta waves (3-7 Hz), alpha waves 1-2 Hz slower than in wake cycle. EOG may show rapid eye movements. Phasic REM shows rapid eye movement. Tonic REM shows no eye movement. EMG is significantly reduced compared with NREM sleep.

Data from Jackson, W. J. (1999). Brain function: Sleep. In T. Nosek (Ed.), *Essentials of human physiology.* Atlanta: Gold Standard Multimedia Inc. and Medical College of Georgia.

EEG, Electroencephalogram; *EOG,* electrooculogram; *EMG,* electromyogram.

activity-rest cycles. Because there is no potential possibility of eliminating shift work for nurses and for many other 24/7 occupations, methods of reducing the negative impact are critical for health, personal well-being, and safety. Keys to reducing the impact of shift work include ensuring the optimal rotation pattern, 12 or more hours off between shifts, and elimination of overtime for shifts over 8 hours (Berger & Hobbs, 2006).

Specific tips for nurses working night shifts include the following (Martin, 2006):
- Promote great daytime sleeping:
  - Take a warm bath when you get home
  - Avoid caffeine and nicotine for several hours before sleeping
  - Avoid spicy foods and heavy meals before sleeping
  - Do a generalized relaxation exercise to reduce the time to fall asleep
  - Use blackout shades for windows
  - Keep the room on the cool side
  - Use an air cleaner or fan to reduce daytime sounds
  - Don a sleep mask and earplugs
  - Plan on 8 hours of sleep, even if divided into morning sleep and evening sleep times
- Avoid wake-time sleepiness:
  - Exercise or take a walk
  - Take a 20- to 30-minute nap
  - Stay safe on the drive home by pulling over for a short nap if wakefulness is compromised

Alcohol Use

Alcohol acts as a central nervous system depressant, inducing sleep; however, alcohol is linked with delay and disruption of REM sleep. Short-term intake of alcohol may have no effect on sleeping. Moderate intake (blood alcohol level of 0.1%) before bedtime will act as a hypnotic, with a suppression of REM density. As the alcohol is metabolized, a rebound may occur with REM sleep late in the sleep cycle, resulting in increased light sleep (Feige et al., 2006).

Medications

Many medications have an impact on sleeping cycles—in particular, those known to influence mood (Table 26-3). Monoamine oxidase–inhibiting drugs suppress REM sleep more than any other drug class.

Natural Sleep Factors and Dietary Supplements to Induce Sleep

With the trend to look to natural and herbal remedies for relief of common problems, there is research on natural sleep factors. In the 2002 National Health Interview Survey (Pearson, Johnson, & Nahin, 2006), 17% of the 31,000 adults interviewed indicated a problem during the past 12 months with insomnia. Complementary or alternative medications were used by 4.5% of those reporting insomnia.

Naturally occurring substances such as tryptophan (found in turkey and milk), melatonin, and valerian root may induce sleep. A bedtime snack of milk or potatoes will provide sufficient tryptophan to induce sleep. A long-held myth is that the postprandial sleepiness that individuals experience after a large Thanksgiving dinner is due to tryptophan in the turkey. However, although tryptophan, an amino acid essential to nutrition, is present in turkey, an empty stomach and a low protein intake are necessary to produce the sleep-inducing effect of tryptophan. L-tryptophan, a synthetic form of tryptophan, was produced originally in 1989, and the use was linked with an outbreak of eosinophilia-myalgia syndrome. Around 1,500 cases were identified, and 37 deaths occurred linked with the use of L-tryptophan, 95% of which were associated with distribution from Japan. The Food and Drug Administration (FDA) reviewed the possible link between eosinophilia-myalgia syndrome and ingestion of L-tryptophan and concluded that safety risks exist. As a result, the FDA issued a special alert limiting the importation of L-tryptophan into the United States (U.S. Food and Drug Administration, 2001). As a result of such alerts, synthetic tryptophan should be used with caution, if at all.

TABLE 26-2 Sleep Stealers

Psychological factors	The most common cause of sleep problems is stress, pressure, illness, or marital problems.
Shift work	Around 20% of workers in the United States are shift workers. For shift workers, sleep must occur while others are awake, resulting in a need to compete with usual biological rhythms developed over decades of life. Shift workers are as much as five times more likely to fall asleep at work as non–shift work employees.
Environmental interferences	Issues such as the room temperature, noise level, or lighting will influence the ability to sleep soundly. Likewise, the size of the bed, comfort of the mattress, and habits of the individual's sleep partner will influence sleep.
Physical factors	Pain, hormonal shifts, breathing issues, and pregnancy are just a few of the physical factors that can interfere with sleep.
Jet lag	Biological rhythms can be disturbed by traveling across time zones.
Lifestyle stressors	Intake of alcohol or caffeinated beverages before sleeping can interfere with sound sleep or the ability to fall asleep. Exercise or heavy mental activity completed immediately before sleep may interfere with the ability to sleep.
Medications	Steroids, antihypertensives, and antidepressants may interfere with sleeping.

National Sleep Foundation. (1999). *ABC's of ZZZ's*. Available from http://www.sleepfoundation.org/.

TABLE 26-3 Impact of Medications on Sleep

MEDICATION		EFFECT ON SLEEP		
Generic Name	Classification	Heavy Sedation	Moderate Sedation	Low Sedation
Amitriptyline	Tricyclic antidepressant	X		
Amoxapine	Tricyclic antidepressant	X		
Bupropion	Dopamine uptake inhibitor		X	
Desipramine	Tricyclic antidepressant			X
Doxepin	Tricyclic antidepressant	X		
Fluoxetine	Selective serotonin reuptake inhibitor			X
Fluvoxamine	Selective serotonin reuptake inhibitor	X		
Imipramine	Tricyclic antidepressant		X	
Mirtazapine	α_2-adrenergic blocker antidepressant	X		
Nefazodone	Postsynaptic serotonin 5-HT$_{2A}$ antagonist and presynaptic serotonin reuptake inhibitor	X		
Nortriptyline	Tricyclic antidepressant	X		
Paroxetine	Selective serotonin reuptake inhibitor	X		
Phenelzine	Monoamine oxidase inhibitor		X	
Sertraline	Selective serotonin reuptake inhibitor		X	
Venlafaxine	Serotonin and norepinephrine reuptake inhibitor			X

Data from Burnham, T. (Ed.). (2000). *Drug facts and comparisons*. St. Louis, MO: Facts and Comparisons.

Melatonin is a neurohormone produced through tryptophan in the pineal gland of the brain. Associated with the circadian rhythm and light and dark, melatonin is referred to in research as the "hand of the clock" (Arendt, 2005). Levels of melatonin in the body are highest at bedtime. As melatonin levels rise, the level of alertness declines and body temperature drops. Light suppresses the secretion of melatonin, and ingestion of synthetic melatonin is linked with sleep induction (Arendt, 2006). Melatonin has demonstrated efficacy with sleep inducement for individuals doing shift work and for individuals who are blind. Concerns with melatonin include disruption of the sleep-wake cycle and lack of standardization of production, because melatonin is an herbal supplement. Long-term studies on the use of melatonin are needed.

Valerian root is effective in improving deep sleep. It has a very safe profile but requires consistent use over 2 to 3 weeks for efficacy (Wheatley, 2005). Synthetic valerian root is available; however, the extract (400 to 450 mg) is most effective. As with melatonin, long-term safety has not been documented. Other herbs and natural agents that may induce sleep include chamomile, catnip, hops, kava, lavender, and St. John's wort (Wheatley, 2005) (Table 26-4). Because of the accessibility of such natural agents and their purported claims, many individuals with sleep disturbances are using them. In one study of 937 individuals with arthritis, 32.8% reported sleep disturbances. The most common reason for use of complementary relief strategies cited was sleep disturbance (Jordan et al., 2000). Alternative and complementary interventions are discussed in Chapter 6.

Relaxation and Music

Although relaxation and sleep are not synonymous, they are related states. Without relaxation, one will find it difficult to sleep. Without sufficient sleep, a person may find it difficult to relax without sleeping. Relaxation exercises will aid in assisting a person with falling asleep. One manner of achieving a state of relaxation is through the use of music. In a study of 60 older adults, the use of 45 minutes of music at bedtime was found to decrease sleep latency, increase the depth of sleep, and decrease daytime sleepiness. The effects were found to be cumulative and continued to improve for the 3-week study period (Lai & Good, 2005). Johannes Brahms is best known for his lullabies, which many find sleep inducing. There is some evidence to show that Brahms himself may have suffered from sleep apnea (Margolis, 2000). Brahms had difficulty with heavy snoring, an obese neck, irritability, and was frequently seen sleeping at unusual times and places (most often in Viennese cafes). Each of these symptoms is associated with sleeping issues. Whether such problems with sleep led Brahms to compose beautiful lullabies is unknown; however, his music continues to lull people to sleep today.

Stimulants

The use of caffeine, nicotine, and other stimulants may significantly affect sleep. Coffee, tea, chocolate, and colas taken within 6 hours of bedtime may interfere with sleep. For some individuals, even a small amount of caffeine taken as much as 10 to 12 hours before sleep may prove problematic.

Psychological Stressors

Of the most common factors that interfere with sleep is psychological stress, including depression and anxiety. In a study of 25,580 subjects the Stanford Sleep Epidemiology Research Center (2005) found that correlates of nonrestorative sleep included stressful life, anxiety, and physical disease among other factors.

TABLE 26-4 Dietary Supplements Used to Impact Quality and Quantity of Sleep

Herb/Dietary Supplement	Description	Comments
Chamaemelum nobile [L] (chamomile)	• Antispasmodic • Diaphoretic • Sedative and sleep inducement • Folk remedies have used the plant for asthma, fevers, colic, inflammation, and cancer	• Herbal plant, creeping perennial • Native to western Europe and North Africa
Garcinia mangostana L.	• Used to treat diarrhea, dysentery, cystitis • Acts as a central nervous system depressant • May cause elevation of blood pressure	• Derived from the fruit, mangosteen • Grown in Malaysia, Thailand, and Burma
Humulus lupulus L. (hops)	• Sedative • Primary use is as a flavor for beer	• Perennial vine • Native to Europe
Hypericum perforatum L. (St. John's wort)	• Relieve or reduce depression • Antibacterial • Spasmolytic • Antiseptic • Increases latency to rapid eye movement sleep • Increases amount of deep sleep in total sleeping period	• Native to Russia • Wild, flowering plant • Used in teas • Most popular drug (herbal or otherwise) in Germany for treatment of depression
Lavandula sp. (lavender)	• Used to induce sleep • Used to reduce depression • Gives sense of happiness and relaxation • Antispasmodic • Diuretic • Tonic • Used for treatment of colic and headaches	• Aromatic shrub • Native to Europe • Fragrant blue and purple flowers
Melissa officinalis L. (balm or lemon balm)	• Sedative, central nervous system depressant • Used for fever, flatulence, diaphoretic • Used to treat influenza, headaches, and toothaches	• Perennial herb • Native to southern Europe and North America
Nepeta cataria L. (catnip)	• Used as an antispasmodic, diaphoretic, stimulant • Mild sedative • Used to treat diarrhea, colic, colds, and cancer	• Perennial herb • Native to Eurasia • Grown in North America • Smoking catnip causes euphoria and hallucinations
Papever somniferum L. (opium poppy)	• Habit-forming narcotic used for manufacture of morphine, papaverine, codeine, and heroin • Used as a hypnotic, sedative, antitussive, and analgesic • Seeds contain no opium and are a source of energy	• Annual or biennial herb • Native to Mediterranean areas east of Iran
Tagetes minuta (Asteraceae)	• Remedy for colds • Diarrhea • Stomach upset • Liver ailments • Oil of the plant has tranquilizing properties, and may promote hypotension, bronchodilation, anti-inflammation	• Erect annual herb • Native to South America • Has a slightly sweet taste and is similar to the taste of licorice
Valerian officinalis (valerian)	• Used to shorten sleep latency and to increase length of sleep • Used as a flavor for tobacco • Antispasmodic, calmative • Used for fever, fatigue, headaches • Used to relieve stress and hysteria	• Tall, perennial herb • Native to western Asia and Europe • Linked with liver disease
Ziziphus sp. (jujube)	• Used for memory enhancement • Anti-inflammatory • Analgesic • Sedative, used for insomnia • Antispastic	• Native to China • Medium-sized tree with deciduous foliage • Fruit is similar to figs • Used in candies and cooking

From Tyler, V.E. (1999). Herbs affecting the central nervous system. In J. Janick (Ed.), *Perspectives on new crops and new uses* (pp. 442-449). Alexandria, VA: ASHS Press.

Health Care Issues

Pain. Many of the issues that coincide with health care problems affect sleep. Health care problems associated with pain will interrupt sleep. Although analgesics may be necessary to decrease pain levels to allow sleep, the medications themselves will affect the architecture of sleep. Narcotics will facilitate relaxation and pain relief; however, they interfere with both deep and REM sleep. An individual using narcotics for pain relief may experience daytime sleepiness and nighttime restlessness, with reduced dreaming and deep sleep. In a study of the correlation of sleep impairment with painful diabetic peripheral neuropathy, patients reported sleeping the same number of hours as the diabetic control group. Sleep adequacy, however, for those with pain was markedly less effective (p <0.0001). The researchers recommend including sleep assessment and treatment of sleep disturbance as a component of care for individuals with pain (Zelman, Brandenburg, & Gore, 2006).

Cardiopulmonary Problems. Individuals with cardiopulmonary problems may experience shortness of breath and orthopnea. These issues often result in sleep hypoxemia, which causes alterations in pulmonary, cardiac, and hematological functions. Obstructive sleep apnea is linked with hypertension and may in fact, be a causative factor (Phillips & Cistulli, 2006). Researchers have found that correcting obstructive sleep apnea may result in lowering blood pressure and may decrease the resistance to antihypertensive agents.

A significant clue to cardiopulmonary problems is the question of sleep efficacy and pillow use. Persons with orthopnea frequently sleep with multiple pillows to ease the breathing difficulty they experience. With cardiopulmonary compromise, patients with orthopnea experience difficulty breathing within 1 minute of assuming a flat supine position. Clinicians should inquire about multiple pillow use by patients because it may be a key indicator of cardiac failure or significant obstructive pulmonary disease. The elevated position is helpful for lung fluid clearance but is problematic for sleep, resulting in daytime drowsiness.

Urinary Problems. Urinary problems, including frequency and urgency, whether the result of diuretic use, urinary tract infection, or benign prostatic hypertrophy, may result in sleep disruption. Individuals waking multiple times during the night may have difficulty falling back asleep and will not cycle through deep and REM sleep in the manner necessary. Individuals with incontinence will, likewise, experience sleep disturbance, whether because of becoming wet or because of the disruption of nursing and hygiene care.

Sleep Apnea. Sleep apnea occurs as a result of relaxation and collapse of the upper airway during sleep, resulting in snoring and lowered oxygen saturation. As the individual continues to sleep, relaxation increases and oxygen saturation decreases until the point at which the individual wakes, gasps for breath, and falls back asleep. The individual's sleeping partner may be aware of this cycle, but often the affected person is oblivious to the problem. The indicators of this problem may be daytime sleepiness and excessive fatigue. A self-administered questionnaire may be a good first effort at problem identification. The Berlin questionnaire (Hiestand, Britz, Goldman, & Phillips, 2006) is a low-cost, valid tool for early identification of individuals suspected of having sleep apnea. It includes questions about weight, snoring, witnessed apneic periods, and daytime drowsiness.

The utility of the apnea index (AHI) has been subjected to considerable controversy. The recommended intervention for sleep apnea is based on clinical symptoms as discussed in this chapter and a response to airway pressure (CPAP). Treatment should be initiated based on the clinical indicators of sleep apnea.

Musculoskeletal Problems. Spasticity and limited mobility may affect sleep architecture. Individuals with spasticity may find the spontaneous movement of limbs and muscles awakens them. Although with neurological diseases such as Parkinson's, tremors may cease during sleep, they may reoccur during times of body movement and sleep arousal. In able-bodied individuals, position changes occur about every half hour during sleep. For those with weakness or impaired mobility, it may be difficult or impossible to obtain positions of comfort. Requesting and waiting for the assistance of others in order to move to a comfortable position may be difficult and result in an additional loss of sleep.

Cognitive Changes. Disorders that affect cognition, including Alzheimer's disease, may lead to impairment of normal circadian control of sleep and alertness, which may result in sundowning (increased confusion and behavioral changes during the late afternoon and early evening), nighttime insomnia, and wandering.

Aging

Although individuals of all ages sleep, the amount of time spent in stages of sleep varies with age. The amount of REM sleep is highest in neonates and decreases steadily until 20 years of age. REM sleep continues to decrease after 20 years of age but at a slower rate of reduction. Older persons spend little time in REM, stage 3, and stage 4 sleep and awaken during the night. As a result of these changes, as an individual ages, it may take longer to gain the needed amount of sleep in REM and stage 4.

SLEEP ASSESSMENT

Subjective

Few individuals will seek health care for sleep issues, although many people are affected. Because problems with sleep do not trigger a visit to a health care practitioner, sleep may be overlooked in the assessment process. A critical question to ask any patient is, "Do you have difficulty getting enough sleep, and do you have problems staying awake during the day?"

One of the most common tools for sleep assessment is the Epworth Sleepiness Scale (Parish & Lyng, 2003), which is available on the Internet (http://www.sleepquest.com/). Individuals completing the questionnaire by Internet send the results to the SleepQuest site, where the results are interpreted and correspondence is returned to the individual. The website is managed through Stanford University and is linked with Dr. William Dement, a founder of the study of sleep.

The following questions should be included in an assessment of sleep hygiene and quality:

- Do you have difficulty sleeping?
- Do you feel rested upon rising?
- Do you keep a regular sleep schedule (go to bed and rise at consistent times)?
- Do you have any difficulty falling asleep?
- Do you use any routines to assist you in falling asleep?
- Do you use any medications to assist you in falling asleep?
- Do you drink alcohol? How often? Do you use alcohol to assist with sleep?
- Do you drink coffee, tea, or colas? Do you drink caffeinated beverages before bedtime?
- Do you smoke?
- Do you awake chocking and gasping?
- Do you experience drowsiness during the daytime?
- Do you nap during the daytime? If so, for how long and how often?
- Do you rise during sleep time for any reason, for example, to urinate?
- Approximately how many times during an episode of sleep do you rise?
- Are you able to return to sleep after an interruption?

Objective

Observation of sleep patterns should include an hour-by-hour assessment of the time the patient spends sleeping, the number of times the patient is awakened because of pain, voiding, incontinence, and interruptions. According to one study (Hoekert, der Lek, Swaab, Kaufer, & Van Someren, 2006), nurses' observations of sleep patterns overestimated patient sleep by an average of 96 minutes, usually underestimating the delay in falling asleep (sleep latency). In addition to assessing the pattern of sleep, nurses should review the environment, including lighting, noise level, and temperature. If lighting and noise levels are elevated, the individual attempting to sleep may be unable to achieve a deep sleep or REM sleep. Temperature is significant in that individuals who are too cold or too warm may not be able to achieve a sense of comfort and may not be able to sleep uninterrupted. Foot bathing to promote warmth may decrease sleep latency and improve sleep (Liao, Landis, Lentz, & Chiu, 2005). Another factor that should be assessed is the perceived comfort of the bed, pillows, and linens. The need for comfort during sleep is critical in attaining deep and REM sleep.

NURSING DIAGNOSIS: INSOMNIA (SPECIFY TYPE)

Disturbance of sleep patterns may occur because of a variety of factors. Nursing assessment information appropriate to the nursing diagnosis of insomnia is included in this section. Nursing diagnosis, outcomes, and interventions are included in Table 26-5.

Sleep pattern disturbances may present in different ways, including parasomnias, dyssomnias (insomnia and hypersomnia),

and medical/psychiatric sleep disorders (discussed in the Health Care Issues section). Each pattern will be discussed in the following section.

Parasomnias

Disorders that disrupt sleep events and processes are known as parasomnias. Arousal disorders and sleep-wake transition disorders are also considered parasomnias. Abnormal arousal disorders include sleepwalking (somnambulism), confusional arousals, and sleep terrors. In these disorders, individuals are sufficiently awake to act, but not aware of their actions. Somnambulism results in walking during sleep and most often starts before puberty. Complex behaviors are initiated during slow-wave sleep, usually during the first third of sleeping time. Individuals are difficult to arouse during such episodes and do not recall the event on waking. Intervention revolves around making the environment safe and preventing injury to the affected person. Benzodiazepines (diazepam and alprazolam) may be of assistance in preventing somnambulism activity. Relaxation before sleeping and prevention of overexertion may also be of help.

Nightmares. Frightening dreams occurring during REM sleep are nightmares. Alcohol, excess fatigue, and fever may lead to the occurrence of a nightmare. Night terrors are nightmares with screaming and flailing. As with nightmares, the development of night terrors in adults is linked with alcohol use and psychological stress.

Nocturnal Leg Cramps. Muscle cramps of the lower calf or foot may occur in middle-age and older individuals who are otherwise healthy. The cramps are severe and make cause an individual to awaken suddenly. Relief may be obtained through stretching the muscles after the spasm has subsided.

Restless Legs Syndrome. Uncomfortable sensations such as a crawling sensation, paresthesia, and dysesthesia occurring in the legs associated with motor restlessness may be restless legs syndrome. The problem may affect the arms also and is typically worse during times of rest. This problem may result in sleep loss and distress because the legs may move every 20 seconds with bursts of movement. Individuals are unable to find a position of comfort because of the sensations, thereby delaying sleep. The individual affected with restless legs syndrome suffers sleeplessness, as does his or her sleeping partner. The problem is associated with peripheral neuropathy, uremia, anemia, and rheumatoid arthritis (National Center on Sleep Disorders Research, 2000).

Dyssomnias (Insomnia and Hypersomnia)

Interruption of sleep may be linked with alcohol use, psychological stress, or pain. Initial insomnia may be caused by pain, emotional stress, respiratory problems, and problems with sleep hygiene. Early morning awakening is common with aging and with individuals experiencing depression. Sleep rhythm reversals are associated with disturbance of circadian rhythms and tend to affect night shift workers and those with brain injury or damage to the hypothalamus. Lesions of the

TABLE 26-5 Nursing Diagnoses, Interventions, and Outcomes Applicable to Sleep

NIC/NOC

Nursing Diagnosis	Nursing Interventions	Nursing Outcomes
Insomnia: sleep disruption	Dementia management Environmental management Environmental management: comfort Medication administration Medication management Medication prescribing Security enhancement Simple relaxation therapy Touch Anxiety reduction Autogenic training Bathing Calming technique Coping enhancement Energy management Exercise promotion Exercise therapy: ambulation Meditation facilitation Music therapy Nutrition management Pain management Positioning Progressive muscle relaxation Self-care assistance: toileting Simple massage Urinary incontinence care: enuresis	Anxiety control Rest Sleep Well-being Comfort level Leisure participation Medication response Mood equilibrium Pain level Psychosocial adjustment: life change Respiratory status: ventilation
Sleep deprivation	Anxiety reduction Coping enhancement Dementia management Energy management Environmental management: comfort Medication management Meditation facilitation Pain management Progressive muscle relaxation Simple guided imagery Surveillance safety Music therapy Simple massage	Sleep Anxiety control Cognitive ability Concentration Distorted thought control Endurance Energy conservation Information processing Memory Mood equilibrium Pain control Rest

Data from Moorhead, S., Johnson, M., & Maas, M. (Eds.). (2004). *Nursing outcomes classification (NOC)* (3rd ed.). St. Louis, MO: Mosby; Dochterman, J. M., & Bulechek, G. M. (2004). *Nursing interventions classification (NIC)* (4th ed.). St. Louis, MO: Mosby; and NANDA International. (2007). *NANDA-I nursing diagnoses: Definitions & classification 2007-2008*. Philadelphia: Author.

hypothalamus may cause hypersomnia, as may encephalitis, depression, and increased intercranial pressure. In addition, hypersomnia may be seen with hyperglycemia, hypoglycemia, hypothyroidism, uremia, anemia, hypercalcemia, liver failure, hypercapnia, multiple sclerosis, and epilepsy. Narcolepsy is an infrequent form of hypersomnia in which there is a sudden change from wakefulness to deep sleep with cataplexy (momentary paralysis with no loss of consciousness), hypnagogic phenomena (vivid visual and auditory hallucinations), and sleep paralysis (loss of voluntary movement as falling asleep or awakening). The majority of individuals with narcolepsy do not experience all of the symptoms of narcolepsy.

Although longevity is not affected, there are clinical accounts of individuals who have experienced an episode of narcolepsy while driving, resulting in a collision or fatality.

SUMMARY

Sleep is essential for life satisfaction, yet it tends to be overlooked as "nonessential" or not critical to an individual's outcome. Rehabilitation nurses must recognize the key element that sleep plays in recovery and rehabilitation from illness and disability. Through attention to sleep, individuals are able to make the gains necessary at the rate possible in therapy.

Case Study

Mr. Kessler had recently survived a triple coronary artery bypass, a new diagnosis of type 1 diabetes mellitus, and 6 weeks in intensive care, 2 weeks on an acute telemetry and surgical unit, and a left below-the-knee amputation. After his prolonged and arduous recovery, he found himself on the physical rehabilitation unit. During the first week of therapy, he was unable to tolerate the required 3 hours of therapy a day. He was so tired, he felt all he could or should do was sleep. He and the therapists were disappointed with his progress, and there was discussion of transferring him to a less acute level of rehabilitation care. The evening nurse, Charlene, commented to the physiatrist that no matter what she did, Mr. Kessler did not seem to sleep at night. The physiatrist prescribed 400 mg of Skelaxin as needed at bedtime. Charlene administered the medication.

When she entered Mr. Kessler's room at 11 P.M., he was sitting up in bed, watching television, and requested a cup of hot tea. Although Mr. Kessler was adamant about his desires, Charlene questioned the wisdom of his choices. She made him a cup of hot herbal tea and requested his permission to talk with him about his sleeping habits. After completing a sleeping history, she learned that ever since his time in the intensive care unit (ICU), whenever he drifted to sleep, he experienced severe nightmares. His attempt to stay up was an effort to avoid them.

Charlene learned that Mr. Kessler enjoyed classical music and that a prior bedtime routine was a warm bath just before bed. She offered him a back rub with lavender lotion, located and played a classical radio station on the radio, and ensured he was in a position of comfort for the initial part of the night. She explained that she would have Elaine, the night shift nurse, not waken him for vital signs or assessment, unless he requested that she do so or a change was noted in his status.

Charlene repeated the process each night she was working. She updated his care plan to ensure continuity of care. Mr. Kessler began to sleep soundly at night. He no longer needed the bedtime medication, and he began to make progress in therapy.

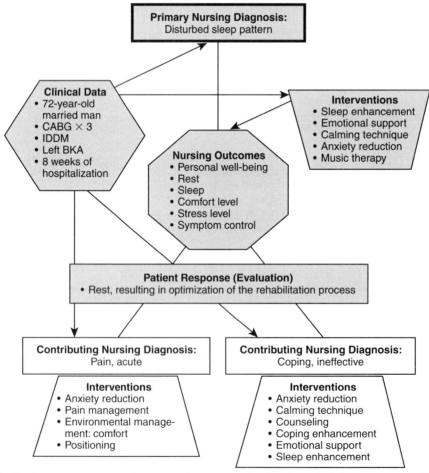

Concept Map. Mr. Kessler has many nursing diagnoses that are involved in his rehabilitation care. Unless the issue of sleep is addressed, however, Mr. Kessler will have difficulty attaining any gains. The concept map therefore focuses on sleep, pain, and coping, which will maximize Mr. Kessler's ability to make functional gains.

CRITICAL THINKING

1. A colleague approaches you and tells you that she is calling the physician for an order for a sleeper for Mr. Kessler. She states that she does not have time for the music and tea routine. Do you intervene? If so, how?

2. You are working the evening shift, and a nurse on the night shift calls in sick for the night. The supervisor asks you to stay, and you agree, although you have been up all day and will not be able to sleep the next day until nighttime. You are also scheduled to work the following evening shift. Will this compromise your ability to practice safety? What are other options?

REFERENCES

American Academy of Family Physicians. (2002). Why don't I get enough sleep? *American Academy of Family Physcians/2002 Wirthlin Worldwide poll*. Available from http://www.aafp.org/online/en/home/press/newskits/acfpresskit/pollfindings/sleep.html.

Arendt, J. (2005). Melatonin: Characteristics, concerns and prospects. *Journal of Biological Rhythms, 20*(4), 291-303.

Arendt, J. (2006). Melatonin and human rhythms. *Chronobiology International, 23*(1-2), 21-37.

Berger, A., & Hobbs, B. (2006). Impact of shift work on the health and safety of nurses and patients. *Clinical Journal of Oncology Nursing, 10*(4), 465-471.

Barrett, R. (2006). Personal communication.

Czeisler, C., & Fryer, B. (2006). Sleep deficit: The performance killer. *Harvard Business Review*, 53-56.

Feige, B., Gann, H., Brueck, R., Hornyak, M., Litsch, S., Hohagen, F., et al. (2006). Effects of alcohol on polysomnographically recorded sleep in healthy subjects. *Alcoholism: Clinical and Experimental Research, 30*(9), 1527-1537.

Hiestand, D., Britz, P., Goldman, M., Phillips, B. (2006). Prevalence of symptoms and risk of sleep apnea in the US population: Results from the national sleep foundation sleep in America 2005 poll. *Chest, 130*(3), 780-786.

Hoekert, M., der Lek, R., Swaab, D., Kaufer, D., & Van Someren, E. (2006). Comparison between informant-observed and actigraphic assessments of sleep-wake rhythm disturbances in demented residents of homes for the elderly. *American Journal of Geriatric Psychiatry, 14*(2), 104-111.

Jackson, W. J. (1999). Brain function: Sleep. In T. Nosek (Ed.), *Essentials of human physiology*. Atlanta: Gold Standard Multimedia Inc. and Medical College of Georgia.

Jordan, J., Bernard, S., Callahan, L., Kincade, J., Konrad, T., & DeFriese, G. (2000). Self-reported arthritis-related disruptions in sleep and daily life and the use of medical, complementary, and self-care strategies for arthritis. *Archives of Family Medicine, 9*, 143-149.

Lai, H., & Good, M. (2005). Music improves sleep quality in older adults. *Journal of Advanced Nursing, 49*(3), 234-244.

Liao, W., Landis, C., Lentz, M., & Chiu, M. (2005). Effect of foot bathing on distal-proximal skin temperature gradient in elders. *International Journal of Nursing Studies, 42*(7), 717-722.

Margolis, M. (2000). Brahms' lullaby revisited: Did the composer have obstructive sleep apnea? *Chest, 118*, 210-213.

Martin, L. (2006). Good night, sleep tight. *Modrn, 2*(6), 22-25.

National Center on Sleep Disorders Research. (2000). *Restless legs syndrome: Detection and management in primary care* (NIH Publication No. 00-3788). Washington, DC: National Institutes of Health: National Heart, Lung and Blood Institute.

National Center on Sleep Disorders Research. (2003). *2003 National Sleep Disorders Research Plan* (NIH Publication No. 03-5209). Washington, DC: National Institutes of Health: National Heart, Lung and Blood Institute.

National Highway Traffic Safety Administration. (2006). *NHTSA, Virginia Tech Transportation Institute release findings of breakthrough research on real-world driver behavior, distraction and crash factors*. Available from http://www-nrd.nhtsa.dot.gov/departments/nrd-13/newDriverDistraction.html.

National Sleep Foundation (1999). *ABC's of ZZZ's*. Available from http://www.sleepfoundation.org/ publications/ZZZs.html.

National Sleep Foundation. (2005). *The National Sleep Foundation's 2005 "Sleep in America Poll."* Available from http://www.sleepfoundation.org/.

Parish, J., & Lyng, P. (2003). Quality of life in bed partners of patients with obstructive sleep apnea or hypopnea after treatment with continuous positive airway pressure. *Chest, 124*(3), 942-947.

Pearson, N., Johnson, L., & Nahin, R. (2006). Insomnia, trouble sleeping, and complementary and alternative medicine: Analysis of the 2002 National Health Interview Survey data. *Archives of Internal Medicine, 166*, 1775-1782.

Phillips, C., & Cistulli, P. (2006). Obstructive sleep apnea and hypertension: Epidemiology, mechanisms and treatment effects. *Minerva Medica, 97*(4), 299-312.

Russo, M. (2005). Normal sleep, sleep physiology, and sleep deprivation: General principles. *eMedicine*. Available from http://www.emedicine.com/neuro/topic444.htm.

SleepQuest. (2006). *The Epworth Sleepiness Scale*. Available from http://sleepquest.com/s_sleepquestionnaire2.html.

Stanford Sleep Epidemiology Research Center. (2005). Prevalence and correlates of nonrestorative sleep complaints. *Archives of Internal Medicine, 165*(1), 35-41.

Tyler, V. E. (1999). Herbs affecting the central nervous system. In J. Janick (Ed.), *Perspectives on new crops and new uses* (pp. 442-449). Alexandria, VA: ASHS Press.

U.S. Food and Drug Administration. (2001). Information paper on L-tryptophan and 5-hydroxy-L-tryptophan: Background on L-tryptophan and 5-hydroxy-L-tryptophan and the eosinophilia myalgia syndrome. Retrieved October 16, 2006, from http://www.cfsan.fda.gov/~dms/ds-tryp1.html.

Wheatley, D. (2005). Medicinal plants for insomnia: A review of their pharmacology, efficacy and tolerability. *Journal of Psychopharmacology, 19*(4), 414-421.

Zelman, D., Brandenburg, N., & Gore, M. (2006). Sleep impairment in patients with painful diabetic peripheral neuropathy. *Clinical Journal of Pain, 22*(8), 681-685.

27

Sexuality Education and Counseling

Pamela M. Duchene, DNSc, RN, CRRN

One of the most contemplated, and least discussed areas of rehabilitation—sexual activity, is a topic of concern to rehabilitation nurses. Given the inherent aspects of physical care and intimacy involved in nursing practice, rehabilitation nurses often receive questions from patients and partners about sexual function. Reviewed in this chapter are commonly held myths of sexuality and disability, sexuality and sexual function, physiology of sexual response, and assessment and interventions for sexual dysfunction applicable to the rehabilitation setting.

MYTHS OF SEXUALITY AND DISABILITY

Although sexual images are ubiquitous in society, there is a paucity of factual, valid information on sexuality and disability. As a result, the rehabilitation nurse needs to understand and anticipate that laypersons, including patients, may believe the following commonly held myths.

Myth #1: Individuals with disabilities and chronic illnesses are not sexual. Obviously this is untrue. Disability does not preclude sexuality. Although the circumstances of an illness or injury may complicate the sexual act, human beings are sexual by nature. Social psychological theories of disability (Tomes, 2005) hold that able-bodied individuals believe that those with disability are in a perpetual state of grieving. However, a disability, regardless of the physical or intellectual nature, does not change the fact that the basic nature of humans is a sexual one (Blackburn, 2002).

Myth #2: Chronic illness and disability render individuals undesirable. The common association of sex is with young, attractive adults—not with individuals who are elderly, sick, or disabled. However, just as sex is more than a physical act, the concepts of sexuality and physical attraction transcend physical attributes (Peck, 2006).

Consider the example of Christopher Reeve. The addition of a wheelchair and the loss of ambulatory status did not make Christopher Reeve less attractive.

Myth #3: "Real" sex is not possible for individuals with disability and chronic illness. Of course, this is not accurate. Although sex may require more planning and preparation, in addition to flexibility for the partners, the act of sex is as "real" as for individuals who are able bodied (Kaufman, Silverberg, & Odette, 2003). According to the *American Heritage Dictionary of the English Language* (2000), sex is defined as the behavior manifested with a sexual urge or instinct. Using this definition, the act of sex includes kissing, foreplay, and orgasm in addition to the traditional concept of intercourse. Sex acts are possible for individuals with disabilities, and like those without a disability, through experimentation and opportunity, sex may be as pleasurable for couples with disabilities as for those who are able-bodied.

SEXUALITY AND SEXUAL FUNCTION

A holistic view of sexuality embraces biology, psychology, sociology, relationships, and spirituality. Biological factors dictate sexual development from conception to birth, reproductive ability after puberty, and certain sex differences in behavior; they also elicit physical responses, such as with sex organs or pulse rate. Sexual desire, functioning, and satisfaction have physical and psychological components. The psychosocial dimension, the sense of gender identity, is shaped by information and attitudes transmitted by parents, peers, teachers, and society. Because sexual behavior is a product of biological and psychosocial forces, it sheds light on why and how persons act, not only what they do (Blackburn, 2002). Sex is part of the mind, body, and soul connection and involves intimacy. As such, it is dependent on relationships with sexual acts and response dependent on interpersonal dynamics.

Ultimately sexuality is a construct of one's body image and self-concept. The sexual drive is a basic human need that varies with culture, life stage and status, physical and emotional well-being, and available opportunities. In 2002 the World Health Organization (WHO) (2005) formed a Technical Consultation on Sexual Health group. The members of this group provided WHO with the following working definition of sexual health: "a state of physical, emotional, mental and social well-being in relation to sexuality; . . . not merely the absence of disease, dysfunction or infirmity."

Sexual Response

Sexual function is determined by sexuality and the sexual response, which includes a complex interrelationship of neurotransmitters and psychological and physiological factors. There are five stages to sexual response: desire, arousal, plateau, orgasm, and resolution (King, 2005). *Desire* is the strong wanting of a sexual experience. Influenced by an individual's experiences, thoughts, and feelings, it is more of a mental or psychological experience than a physical experience. *Arousal* or excitement is the body's response to desire. For both genders, arousal occurs with an increase in pulse and blood pressure. Vasocongestion occurs in genital areas, and the nipples become erect. Men will develop an erection during this stage. Women will experience lubrication of the vagina. During the *plateau* stage respiratory rate, heart rate, and blood pressure continue to rise, and the individual experiences a sense of impending orgasm. In the *orgasm* stage, the respiratory and heart rate reach their peak, with a loss of muscle control or spasms. Women experience orgasms in short bursts, whereas men experience ejaculation. During the *resolution* stage, there is a refractory period during which there is relaxation and a return to a preexcitement stage.

PHYSIOLOGY OF SEXUAL RESPONSE

Overview

Before an individual initiates or performs sexually, there must be a psychological desire. The sexual response is contingent on a synergistic connection of vascular, hormonal, and neurological systems, which must work in balance in either gender. Male and female sexual physiology is discussed in the following sections.

Male Sexual Physiology

Male erection requires neurological innervation of a competent vascular response in a sequence of events. Male sex organs receive somatic innervation as sympathetic fibers (T11 to L3) synapse on the sympathetic chain ganglia and then onto the pelvic plexus via the hypogastric nerve. This efferent and afferent innervation to the testes, prostate, seminal vesicles, and vas deferens allows seminal emission by causing contraction of the prostate while closing the bladder neck. Parasympathetic innervation, responsible for erections, is via the pelvic nerves that are formed by the preganglionic fibers originating in the intermediolateral nuclei (sacral spinal cord S2 to S4).

The fibers innervate the penis, prostate, seminal vesicles, and vas deferens. The pudendal nerve, a mixed motor and sensory nerve, supplies motor innervation to the pelvic floor (S2 to S4), and the sensory dermatomes are from S2 to S5 (King, 2005). Somatic neural stimulation (S2 to S5) is necessary for sensation and contraction of the bulbocavernous and ischiocavernous skeletal muscles during erection and ejaculation. Distally the pudendal nerve becomes the dorsal nerve of the penis and carries the messages for somatic neural stimulation (Figure 27-1). Other important components are the arteries that bring blood to the penis via the internal pudendal artery to the penile artery and the venous drainage, which comes from variable areas of the penis. Neurotransmitters help norepinephrine act on smooth muscle to cause detumescence via sympathetic nerve fibers; acetylcholine acts on parasympathetic fibers.

Erections in neurologically intact men can begin through both reflexogenic and psychogenic pathways (Figure 27-2). Reflexogenic erections occur when tactile genital stimulation is conveyed to the sacral spinal cord via the pudendal nerve. Activation of the sacral parasympathetic outflow via the pelvic nerve to the cavernosal nerve leads to relaxation of the corporal smooth muscle and erection. Reflex erections are poorly maintained without constant tactile stimulation and require intact S2 to S4 nerve roots. Impairments that interfere with transmission to or from S2 to S4, such as multiple sclerosis or spinal cord injury affecting S2 to S4, often result in an inability to develop or sustain a reflex erection.

Psychogenic erections are activated by stimuli from the brain, mental images, or nontactile sensory stimulation, including thoughts, sights, sounds, tastes, and smells, and travel via the thoracolumbar sympathetics (T10 to L2) to the sex organs (Figure 27-3). The phenomenon of psychogenic erections in paraplegics with complete motor neuron lesions and abolished reflexogenic erections indicates that pathways exist for erection from the sympathetic outflow (McKenna, 2001). Impairments that interfere with transmission to or from T10 to L2, such as multiple sclerosis or spinal cord injury affecting T10 to L2, often result in an inability to achieve a psychogenic erection. With such an injury the individual may be able to have a reflex erection, with a response to tactile stimulation.

Semen arriving at the prostatic urethra is dependent on intact hypogastric sympathetic nerve function, whereas true ejaculation results from pudendal nerve activity and contraction of the pelvic floor muscles. Diseases affecting the peripheral or autonomic nervous system can impair erectile capacity, and almost any pathological process involving the spinal cord may lead to ejaculation dysfunction. True ejaculation is rare in men with spinal cord injuries (SCIs), especially with complete tetraplegia; it is more common with lower motor neuron lesions and more caudal lesions. It is possible to induce ejaculation following spinal cord injury through vibratory stimulation and through abdominal electrical stimulation (Goetz & Stiens, 2005). Sperm, however, may deteriorate after spinal injury (Das, Soni, Sharma, Gazvani, & Lewis-Jones, 2006).

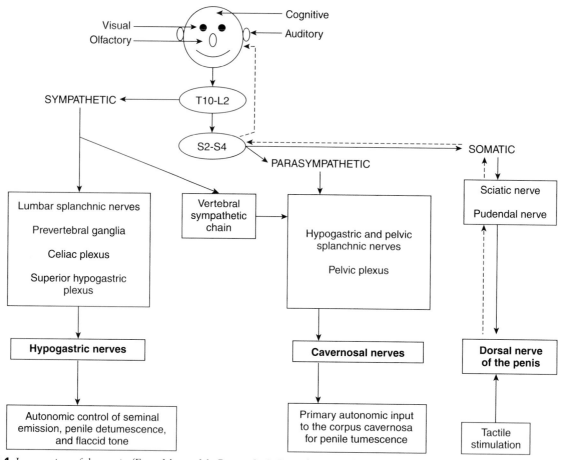

Figure 27-1 Innervation of the penis. (From Monga, M., Bernie, J., & Rajasekaran, M. [1999, October]. Male infertility and erectile dysfunction in spinal cord injury: A review. *Archives of Physical Medicine and Rehabilitation, 80,* 1332.)

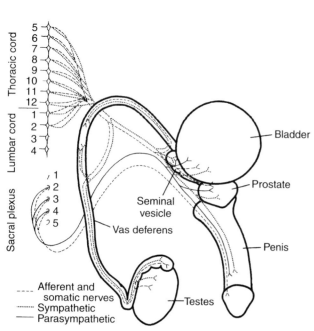

Figure 27-2 Reflexogenic erections and psychogenic pathways in male reproductive organs. (From Woods, N. F. [1984]. *Human sexuality in health and illness* [3rd ed.]. St. Louis, MO: Mosby.)

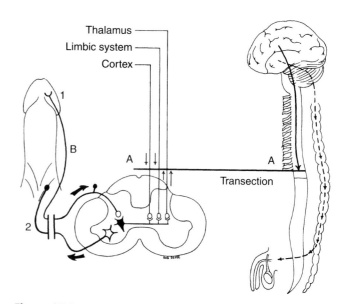

Figure 27-3 *A,* Psychogenic erection: messages from the brain are blocked at the level of the lesion but may bypass the lesion via the autonomic nervous system. *B,* Reflexogenic erection: sensory nerve *(1)* relays message to the spinal cord and synapses with the nerve that carries information to the genitals *(2)* and produces erection. (From Woods, N. F. [1984]. *Human sexuality in health and illness* [3rd ed.]. St. Louis, MO: Mosby.)

Female Sexual Physiology

The sensory pathways from the clitoris and vagina are in the pudendal nerves. The pelvic nerves innervate the vagina, clitoris, and fallopian tubes via the hypogastric and uterine plexus and receive mixed autonomic innervation. Clitoral swelling and reflex vaginal secretions are triggered by parasympathetic activity (S2 to S4). Psychogenic lubrication involves both the thoracolumbar sympathetics and sacral parasympathetics. The ovaries and uterine smooth muscle are innervated by the sympathetic nervous system (T10 to L2) sympathetic pathways. The female sympathetic nerve supply is mixed and carried by the preganglionic splanchnic nerves and the postganglionic fibers to the ovarian plexus. When the somatic pudendal nerves activate, the vaginal wall and pelvic floor musculature contract (Guaderrama et al., 2005) (Figure 27-4). Spinal cord injury or impairment of the T10 to L2 area will impact the woman's ability to feel penetration, and psychogenic lubrication will be impaired. The autonomic nervous system is not as critical to fertility in women with SCI; those fecund before injury may become pregnant.

Brain Structures' Effect on Sexuality

The brainstem maintains arousal and alertness in sexual function; the reticular activating system prepares information processing so that behavior keeps its driving force. Libido and potency may require specific activation within certain limbic and cortical structures, initiated by externally or internally generated stimuli. The brainstem also carries motor and

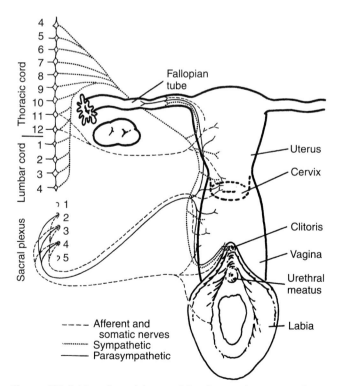

Figure 27-4 Neurological bases of female sexual response. (From Woods, N. F. [1984]. *Human sexuality in health and illness* [3rd ed.]. St. Louis, MO: Mosby.)

sensory messages via the spinal tracts, which allow participation in sexual activity. The hypothalamic-pituitary axis functions in the production of sex-related hormones, including gonadotropin-releasing hormone, follicle-stimulating hormone, luteinizing hormone, and prolactin. Epilepsy and antiepileptic drugs may cause sexual dysfunction due to hormonal alterations. In particular, the hypothalamic-pituitary axis may be disrupted by temporal lobe epileptic discharges (Morris & Vanderkolk, 2005).

Other higher brain centers affect sexual function; damage to the frontal cortex may produce disinhibited, sexually inappropriate verbal behavior, devoid of true sexual arousal, or, more rarely, increased promiscuity with full arousal but difficulty with erection or emission. Injury to the dorsolateral convexities of the frontal lobe produces a more apathetic and akinetic effect. Initiation is impaired, but the patient can be led step by step through erection and copulation. Frontal injury may affect attention and impair the ability to fantasize.

Problems in the left hemisphere can affect sexual function. Language problems, as with aphasias, may impede comprehension of verbal requests or directions for sexual activity. Motor apraxia may impair motor movement. The right hemisphere is more active during orgasm; damage may produce impulsiveness, denial, and occasionally euphoria. Visual-perceptual problems make aligning the body with a partner difficult and hamper interpretation of nonverbal cues or expressing emotional communication (Sapire, 2005).

Hormonal Influence on Sexual Function

Hormones influence sexual activity from conception. Brain injury or stroke can affect structures that regulate hormone balance, such as with secondary hypogonadism or with damage to the pituitary. Present in both men and women, testosterone is the most important biological determinant of the sex drive; deficiencies reduce sexual desire, and excess heightens sexual interest. The ovaries and testes manufacture estrogens. In women estrogen maintains vaginal elasticity, lubrication, and condition of the lining and preserves breast texture. Excessive estrogen in males can reduce libido, affect erection, and enlarge the breasts. No direct or individualized relationship exists between hormone levels and sexual ability or behavior, although deficient testosterone reduces sexual interest in both sexes (Vignozzi et al., 2005).

SEXUALITY THROUGHOUT THE LIFE SPAN

Maturation

From the time of conception throughout the life span, humans are sexual beings. Children are taught societal expectations for gender from the time of birth. The process of puberty toward sexual and reproductive maturity is marked by various highly individualized physical, psychological, and social changes. The process begins before birth and unfolds as hormones effect changes to stimulate physical development and intensified sexual feelings and fantasies in the brain, combining to cause spontaneous erections, increased vaginal lubrication, and tendency for masturbation (King, 2005).

For boys the first changes of puberty, between 9 and 15 years of age, are internal as testicles begin to mature and produce increased amounts of testosterone, in turn causing growth of the prostate gland and other internal organs related to male reproduction. Girls begin to develop sexually at an earlier age, with changes appearing in a different order, beginning some time between 8 and 11 years of age. Internal changes are initiated by hormones, particularly estrogen. Puberty normally is completed by the early 20s.

Aging

Sexual changes occur with aging. Male testosterone declines and may alter libido, with fewer viable sperm. Muscle tone decreases, the testes become more flaccid, and the diameter of the testicular tubules narrows, predisposing benign prostatic hypertrophy. Weakened prostate contractions reduce the volume and viscosity of the seminal fluid and decrease ejaculation force; the postejaculation refractory period increases at 12- to 24-hour intervals. Although erection requires longer, more intense, direct stimulation, it can be maintained longer and may satisfy a partner. The Sexuality Study Group (Araki, 2005) researched sexuality and sexual feelings of middle-age and older adults. They found that the key components of a mature sexual relationship are to build relationships with physical contact such as caressing and to engage in casual conversation. Slow sex and pillow talk with physical contact are more critical to a mature sexual relationship than sex alone. For those in nursing homes, all sexual activity is reduced. In fact, nursing home residents are seen as sexually invisible—despite the known positive physical and emotional impact of continued sexual activity (Hajjar & Kamel, 2003).

The onset of menopause and associated hormone deprivation directly affects women's interest in sex and performance. The lowered estrogen levels during menopause result in gradual atrophy of the uterus and vagina, concurrent with reduced firmness and size of genital tissues. The vaginal mucosa thins, the canal shortens, and lubrication decreases with fewer, less active Bartholin's glands; a friable vagina may make intercourse painful. The excitement level of the sexual response is slowed, the plateau stage lasts longer, and orgasm takes longer. Longer times may enhance a woman's sexual experience both physically and emotionally, but orgasmic capacity is decreased. Estrogen deficiency may cause pain during normal uterine contractions during orgasm. With pelvic relaxation and tissue atrophy, a woman may have urinary stress incontinence, adversely affecting the couple's sexual experience. The negative effects of vaginal atrophy may be partially or fully relieved through topical estrogen creams and regular sexual activity (Society of Obstetricians and Gynecologists of Canada, 2005).

RELATIONSHIP FACTORS THAT MAY AFFECT SEXUALITY

There are many threats to a satisfactory sexual relationship. Factors within a couple's interpersonal relationship affect the quality of sexual relationships and responses. Marginal relationships, however, are stressed by disability, which may lead to separation. Relationships that are solid and healthy are able to overcome many obstacles to a satisfactory sexual relationship. With a healthy relationship before an injury, an impairment may give partners a focus on factors that maintain relationships, such as love, communication, maintaining trust, intimacy, affection, romance, timing, sensory stimulation, fantasy, and self-concept.

"Love is patient, love is kind. It does not envy, it does not boast, it is not proud. It is not rude, it is not self-seeking, it is not easily angered, and it keeps no record of wrongs. Love does not delight in evil but rejoices with the truth. It always protects, always trusts, always hopes, always perseveres. Love never fails" (1 Cor. 13:4-8a; the Bible, New International Version). Effective communication is a cornerstone of interpersonal and sexual intimacy that occurs in a committed, intimate, and caring relationship within a safety net of trust and support. Communication is essential when one partner has impaired or altered functions. With sensory loss, partners must find ways to share feelings of pleasure, lack of sensation, or pain or discuss potential incontinence beforehand. Communication adds stability and satisfaction that may suffer when a person is unable to use or understand language; concepts are difficult to convey without words. Some couples find the sexual relationship conveys their love when language can not.

Trust necessary for intimacy develops over time as partners learn to rely on each other's words, commit to value and honor each other, and mutually solve problems. Love is a choice to build security into a relationship (Smalley & Trent, 2006). Intimacy builds commitment through crises, boredom, and fatigue, not only joy, prosperity, and excitement. Affection may be transmitted when spoken, by touch, or by other direct behavior. Consistent, gentle touching is a powerful message of security, emotional bonding, and romance, superseding sexual activity for some. Without words of affection, caring is questioned. Persons with sexual impairments may find fulfillment in intimacy, communication, meaningful touch, affection, and eye contact with caring partners.

Romance helps set the stage for a positive sexual experience and demonstrates value in togetherness. Taking time for romance affords a chance for preparation, relaxation, and enjoyment, limited only by one's imagination, privacy, and safety. Timing and mood for sexual activities occur day or night, when both partners feel rested and relaxed. Impairments affect timing; function improves with arthritis after morning stiffness subsides, and incontinence is less likely after bowel programs for those with SCI. With cardiac or pulmonary dysfunction, sexual activity should be scheduled before a heavy meal accompanied by alcohol.

The brain is the central coordinating center for sensory stimulation or fantasy. Sexual desire begins in this great sense organ fueled by sights, sounds, tastes, smells, or touches. For some, fantasy is a powerful producer of sexual desire, as well as a means of expression. Sexual fantasies vary widely, but generally fall into one of four categories: exploratory, impersonal sex, intimacy, and dominance (King, 2005).

Stimulating the senses enhances psychological sexual desire, and partners may sense or emit natural body scents or pheromones during arousal.

Arousing touch includes massage with body oils, creams, or lotion; light touch to sensitive areas; kissing; or licking. Hot or cold applications, rubbing, textures, or vibrators enhance sexual arousal and increase sensory input. Sight is a powerful sensory tool. For instance, positioning a person to see what is occurring, lighting the room, and strategically placing mirrors allow the brain to enjoy what the eye can see when the body is impaired. The technique of sensate focus encourages partners to explore each other's bodies without leading to intercourse or orgasm. Concentration on touching all areas and telling the partner what is pleasuring helps restore focus on the other.

ALTERATIONS IN SEXUAL FUNCTION

Physiological Alterations

Patients with chronic disease or disability involving the neurological, musculoskeletal, respiratory, cardiovascular, or digestive systems are at risk for altered sexual function. Fatigue with arthritis or cardiac or pulmonary conditions and positioning for lower extremity spasticity necessitate adjustments for both partners. Many fear that sexual activity may cause harm or adverse effects. Table 27-1 discusses functional complications that may affect sexuality.

Effects of Medication

Analgesic drugs that depress the central nervous system are similar to alcohol in their effect on sexual function. Addictive narcotic drugs produce erectile dysfunction (ED), retarded ejaculation, low libido in men, and low sexual interest and orgasmic dysfunction in women. Many patients with neurological involvement take medication to manage health problems or control neurological symptoms only to find effects on sexual function. Diazepam decreases the hypertonic response of spasticity but also reduces sexual desire, and like baclofen (Lioresal) it can contribute to problems with ejaculation or orgasm (Table 27-2).

Antihypertensives, antidepressants, antipsychotics, antiulcer agents (cimetidine, finasteride), 5-alpha reductase inhibitors,

TABLE 27-1 Relationship of Chronic Diseases to Sexual Dysfunction

Factors Related to Preparation for Sexual Activity	Diseases/Conditions	Effects
Impaired mobility	Neurological conditions: SCI, stroke, Parkinson's disease, multiple sclerosis, cerebral palsy, amyotrophic lateral sclerosis, muscular dystrophy, brain injury, Guillain-Barré syndrome, chronic pain, cancers Musculoskeletal conditions: rheumatic disease, fractures, limited range of motion, amputations	Hypertonia affects most positions for intercourse; hand function deficits affect manual stimulation of partner; transfers to bed, chair, etc.; dressing/undressing; personal hygiene; insertion/application of birth control devices; coordination of motion/apraxia or ataxia; balance/positioning; no pelvic movement
Increased or decreased sensation	Neurological conditions or peripheral nerve damage in musculoskeletal injuries	No/decreased sensation in genital area or other erogenous zones Cervical SCI—most of skin surface may be affected CVA—decrease to affected side of body or painful touch to upper extremity or shoulder Brain injury—may be defensive to areas of altered sensation
Pain/discomfort	Neurological, musculoskeletal, respiratory, cardiovascular, digestive dysfunction, or cancer in any system	Affects libido, limits positions, limits movement, depression
Bowel/bladder incontinence	Effects from neurological/urological deficits/cancer surgeries Incontinence types: stress; urge; overflow; neurogenic bladder, reflexic or hyporeflexic; neurogenic bowel, reflexic or hyporeflexic	Incontinence, increased risk of infection For females the steady stretch from the penis in the vagina can activate bowel reflexes and initiate bowel emptying; fecal odor can decrease libido Urine smell and wetness can damage surfaces such as mattresses Determine who will provide assistance with bowel/bladder management before sexual activity
Fatigue	Brain injury, stroke, rheumatic disease, multiple sclerosis, cancer, respiratory disease, cardiovascular disease, deconditioning	Decreased libido; depression; ADLs take so much energy there is none left for sex; scheduling/pacing issues

Continued

TABLE 27-1 Relationship of Chronic Diseases to Sexual Dysfunction—cont'd

Factors Related to Preparation for Sexual Activity	Diseases/Conditions	Effects
Changes in libido	Hypersexuality (sexual addiction); brain dysfunction, especially in thalamus, limbic system, bitemporal injury, or disinhibition from frontotemporal damage; hyposexuality; brain injury; stroke; depression; stress/anxiety; Parkinson's disease; affective disorders	Partners have difficulty fulfilling the multiple requests for sex or partners miss the sexual sharing in their relationship Disinhibition can lead to problems of STDs, undesired pregnancy, relationship problems, especially if multiple partners In facility settings overt sexual behavior distresses staff Alcohol is physically inhibiting, but in some is psychosocially disinhibiting and lowers testosterone levels
Female genital sexual function: dysfunction, excitement disrupted, insufficient vaginal lubrication, orgasm decreased or absent	Diabetes; alcoholism; drug use; medications like antihistamines can increase dryness; neurological disturbances; hormone deficiencies; postmenopausal and cancer treatments, which result in lack of estrogen; pelvic disorders (i.e., infections, trauma, scarring from surgery)	Dyspareunia (painful intercourse), decreased satisfaction with the sexual experience, altered spontaneity due to need to apply lubricants Vaginal atrophy and friability can result from lack of estrogen
Male genital sexual function: erectile dysfunction (impotence), premature ejaculation, delayed or absent ejaculation, orgasm	Diabetes, alcoholism, neurological dysfunction (particularly spinal cord injury and multiple sclerosis), prostrate surgery, infection or injury to sex organs, hormone deficiencies, circulatory problems	Impotence/inability to maintain an erection firm enough for coitus at least 25% of the time; may affect 1 of 10 men in the United States; may have physiological and/or psychological component; SCI, once spinal shock subsides, reflex erections occur if injury at T11 or above; paraplegics with no S2-S4 reflex connection have psychogenic erections via the sympathetic pathway, T10-L2; ejaculation is rare in men with SCI (reports of from 10% to 32%), but orgasm has been shown to be present in approximately 50% of sexually active men and women
Female fertility	SCI during initial onset when menses ceases Damage to endocrine system Brain injury or disease that affects ovarian endocrine dysfunction Polycystic ovaries, hypogonadism Alcohol detrimental to unborn child Some medications contribute to birth defects	All women should know that generally fertility is unchanged once menses resumes, unless there is damage to the endocrine system or ovarian function Birth control options can be affected by the disease/injury (i.e., with an increased risk of deep venous thrombosis in persons with SCI who smoke, the birth control pill may not be the best option)
Male fertility	SCI Endocrine dysfunction—decreased serum testosterone levels Alcoholism	Semen has lowered volume and sperm counts overall and progressively slower sperm motility, impaired sperm membrane integrity, and poor oocyte-penetrating capabilities of the sperm Retrograde ejaculation can occur, altering fertility; retrograde ejaculation contributes to infertility Decreased libido Erectile dysfunction Altered secondary sex characteristics

ADLs, Activities of daily living; *CVA*, cerebrovascular accident; *SCI*, spinal cord injury; *STDs*, sexually transmitted diseases.

TABLE 27-2 Sexual Problems Resulting From Medication

Sexual Problem	Medication
Reduced desire and sexual function	Tranquilizers, SSRIs; most drugs listed below can reduce desire for sex in men and women
Erectile dysfunction	Diuretics, exogenous hormones, H_2 blockers, tricyclic antidepressants, antihypertensives, street drugs
Ejaculation problems	Diazepam (Valium), methyldopa (Aldomet), ranitidine (Zantac), phenytoin, baclofen (Lioresal), cimetidine (Tagamet), carbamazepine
Priapism	Hydralazine (Apresoline), prazosin (Minipress), labetalol (Trandate)
Gynecomastia	Methyldopa (Aldomet), hydrochlorothiazide and spironolactone (Aldactazide), raudixin, Rauzide, reserpine (Serpasil), spironolactone
Menstrual changes	Hydrochlorothiazide and spironolactone (Aldactazide), spironolactone
Drowsiness, decreased vaginal lubrication	Antihistamines
Impaired arousal/anorgasmia	Alprazolam (Xanax), amitriptyline (Elavil), amphetamines, fluoxetine (Prozac), haloperidol (Haldol), molindone (Moban), nortriptyline (Pamelor), thiothixene (Navane), doxepin, paroxetine (Paxil), sertraline (Zoloft), and similar drugs of the same class

SSRIs, Selective serotonin reuptake inhibitors.

and cholesterol-lowering agents may contribute to impotence (Brosman & Leslie, 2004). Antidepressants and antipsychotics may reduce sexual desire and may cause difficulty with ejaculation and orgasm. Antiepileptic medications used by patients who have posttraumatic seizure disorder after a head injury can affect ejaculation. Diuretics may cause reduced sexual desire and erection problems in men and painful intercourse from vaginal dryness in women.

Psychosocial Alterations

Psychosocial alterations, social isolation, role changes, and issues with partnership or self-esteem, along with physical problems of chronic, disabling conditions, may affect sexuality. Decrease in sexual activity is frequent following a stroke (Giaquinto, Buzzelli, DiFrancesco, & Nolfe, 2003). There is no correlation between hemisphere affected, gender of the stroke patient, or length/strength of the marriage and sexual decline. Psychological factors account for the sexual difficulties, rather than physical or medical issues. Counseling may provide the most effective intervention.

Self-concept includes all the beliefs concerning the ideal self, the value of self or self-esteem, and internal feelings about body parts and body image. Cosmetics, clothes, and jewelry, as well as input from the environment or genetics, are external factors. Knowledge of self related to positive or negative views or gender identity develops early in life as individuals interact with others; in adolescents and adults homosexuality is a function of self-concept. Adjustment to changes with chronic or disabling conditions varies but always challenges body image and self-concept (King, 2005). Having a positive body image before impairment tends to allow more effective coping with body changes than a negative image. Independence in self-care and social roles eliminates barriers and promotes a positive self-concept. Education from rehabilitation nurses, counselors, and support groups may help individuals with disability overcome self-esteem and relationship issues.

Partnership issues arise when a spouse becomes disabled, especially when cognition is impaired, and the partner and

usually the entire family sense the lost contribution to the relationships. When one partner serves dual caregiver and provider roles, such as after SCI, the burdens can lead to burnout and imbalance in the relationship. Too often a partner becomes preoccupied with tasks or financially unable to continue participating in activities that brings zest to life. Communication and problem-solving skills to bridge the strains of financial, health, and physical needs are vital issues for couples dealing with disability.

Cognitive and Behavioral Alterations

Attention, memory, executive function, communication, mood, social perceptiveness, and behaviors affect sexual function and sexuality. Although cognition and behavior are significant components of sexuality, deficits do not preclude sexual activity but may impact the satisfaction of the partner. Cognitive impairments or alterations occur with brain injury, stroke, multiple sclerosis, Parkinson's disease, and other neurological diseases. Dementia of the Alzheimer type and other types of dementia may be linked with hypersexual behavior, or aberrant sexual behavior and verbal comments (Alagiakrishnan et al., 2005). The impact of impairment is presented in this section. For each of the deficits discussed, anticipation, planning, and preparation for the potential issues by the partner may be of benefit. With cognitive and behavioral alterations, partner education is critical to achieving a healthy sexual relationship.

Deficits in attention affect the ability to attend to a task for a required time. A doorbell or telephone ringing can break attention to or concentration on sexual activity, but persistent partners can help refocus attention. When inattention disrupts concentration, the partner may fantasize or use sexual play or psychogenic means to maintain erection. When one partner is egocentric, focusing on self needs, it detracts; equal contributions by persons focused on the other create balance in a sexual relationship.

Executive function impairments affect the quality of reasoning, planning, organization, and judgment. Sexual function is a high-level social skill that requires planning, preparation, and anticipation. In a sexual scenario this translates to understanding nonverbal and verbal signals, knowing what is expected of each partner, anticipating what comes next, and selecting the best approach, all of which are difficult for those with impaired executive function. Similarly, when a partner lacks social perceptiveness skills to express personal feelings or show love through actions, words, and nonverbal communication, the entire intimate relationship, not only sexual activity, is threatened. Truly understanding and comprehending how one is perceived may be altered by brain injury, causing other relationship problems.

Effective communication sharing hopes, dreams, values, and critical needs maintains and enhances intimacy but requires high-level communication skills. With altered communication, such as after stroke or brain injury, couples may have a signal to initiate sexual intimacy when they cannot communicate verbally.

Mood disturbances, often depression after chronic or disabling conditions, can adversely affect libido and sexual performance. Depression may decrease libido or, alternatively with euphoria, increase libido. The cycle in which depression leads to decreased sexual activity and, in turn, to depression alters sexual function. Irritability occurs more frequently in persons with brain injury, stroke, or neurological diseases. An irritable person does not make the best partner because incorrect perception of a behavior may elicit an irritable response, disrupting the sexual encounter.

Disinhibition differs greatly from depression but can change the nature of the sexual encounter for some spouses. Sexual function has social and cultural rules that vary greatly in practice among couples. For instance, a verbal interaction may carry over into sexual relations, becoming a turnoff for some partners. Children need to learn the social rules to overcome their inherent disinhibition, by learning to differentiate public from private behavior. For some who are without a partner, sexual disinhibition can cause problems in the community; the person relearns that sexual activity is only performed in private and among consenting adults.

ASSESSMENT OF SEXUAL FUNCTION

A holistic assessment for sexual function considers impaired or altered sexual function and sexuality in relation to the relationship, as well as work, home maintenance, and recreation. Sexuality and sexual response may not be a priority early in a patient's rehabilitation process; later sexual function may be a major concern. At various stages in the process, rehabilitation nurses are responsible for addressing the topic and assessing, educating, and counseling patients; assessment of sexual function is an interdisciplinary process. Rehabilitation nurses integrate data from assessment with information from other team members to provide sexual education or counseling as a therapeutic intervention.

The sexual assessment obtains a sexual history, identifies physical and psychosocial strengths and limitations, determines the patient's sexual values, and assists with performing diagnostic tests. The rehabilitation nurse prepares for the assessment, after establishing trust and rapport with the patient, by assuring privacy and confidentiality. Sexual health is conveyed as an integral part of personal health. The rehabilitation nurse should inquire about cultural or ethnic needs and evaluate language and understanding, in addition to the patient's general level of sexual knowledge. Teaching and counseling should be individualized and proceed logically with information, allowing time for questions and reassessment through feedback from the patient.

Patients are informed that they can refuse to answer any questions. Sociocultural factors, such as considering sex a taboo topic, may be barriers that dissuade patients from answering questions. Respect for moral and ethical views is a core element of successful assessment. A referral to someone from the same religious or cultural background may be in order. Questions proceed from less to more sensitive areas. A life cycle chronology provides a logical unfolding of events, as well as a progression from less to more threatening topics. The impact of any questions can be softened by making a general statement and then proceeding with the question. For instance, the nurse can make a general statement about sexual activity as a normal form of sexual release and then ask the patient's opinion about this practice. Or ask about the ideal rather than the real to facilitate communication such as, "Statistically, persons near your age have intercourse from three times a week to once a month. How often do you have intercourse?"

Sexual History

The purpose of the sexual history is to identify problems and misconceptions, as well as areas requiring education and counseling regarding sexual issues (Box 27-1).

Sexual Physical Examination

Findings from the physical examination guide content of sexual education and counseling. External genitalia are inspected in both male and female patients. It is prudent to have another nurse or assistant present during the physical examination of the genitalia. Women may have a pelvic examination and complete breast inspection. Assess both for sexually transmitted diseases (STDs) using urine cultures or wet pap smears. A neurological examination of the genital area is useful to determine rectal sphincter tone; normal sphincter tone indicates both the lumbar and sacral segments of the spinal cord are intact, allowing strong reflex erections in the male. Ask the patient to contract the rectal sphincter voluntarily; ability to do this implies preservation of efferent motor fibers in the pyramidal tract system essential for ejaculation.

Pain and temperature presence in the saddle area (S2 to S4) mean sensory awareness of orgasm. Sensation from the testes enters the spinal cord at the T9 level, so if squeezing the testicle elicits a pain response, psychogenic erections are likely because their pathway is through the T11 to T12 spinal nerves via the sympathetic nervous system (see Figure 27-2).

Assess the bulbocavernosus reflex manually by compressing the penis while palpating the perineum or anus for a reflex

---

BOX 27-1 Sexual History Form

Name _____ Age_____ Occupation _____ Highest education _____
Marital/partnership status (includes quality, duration)_____
Religion _____ Interests/hobbies _____

Medical History
☐ Psychological/psychiatric problems ☐ Behavioral/emotional problems ☐ Diabetes
☐ Cognitive dysfunction ☐ Renal insufficiency ☐ Hypertension ☐ Hereditary disorders ☐ Neurological conditions ☐ Endocrine disorders
☐ Sexually transmitted diseases

Current Medications
☐ Antihypertensives ☐ Antipsychotics ☐ Antihistamines ☐ Alcohol ☐ Analgesics ☐ Narcotics ☐ Recreational drugs

Premorbid Sexual Function
Preferred sexual activities (description): _____ Sexual activity frequency: _____ Initiating partner: _____
Sexual preferences: _____ Sexual importance in relationship: _____

Physical Issues That Affect Sexual Function
☐ Transfers ☐ Ability to dress/undress ☐ Monoplegia/hemiplegia/hemiparesis
☐ Paraplegia/quadriplegia ☐ Limited range of motion ☐ Hypertonicity ☐ Hypotonicity ☐ Endurance ☐ Balance ☐ Decreased sensation
☐ Hypersensation ☐ Incontinence
☐ Pain (describe presence/location): _____
☐ Genitourinary/gastrointestinal collection devices (position): _____
☐ Vision, hearing, oral motor control, memory, communication limitations: _____
☐ General and genital hygiene and cleanliness limitations (describe): _____

Sexual Response Issues

Female	**Male**
Menstrual history _____	Sexual interest _____
Sexual interest _____	Morning erections: ☐ present ☐ absent
Sexual frequency _____	Erections with manual stimulation:
Vaginal lubrication: ☐ present ☐ impaired	☐ present ☐ absent
Sensation: ☐ present ☐ impaired	Process for ejaculation: _____
Orgasms: ☐ present ☐ impaired	Sensation: ☐ present ☐ impaired
Fertility/birth control: _____	Type of ejaculation/volume: _____
Pregnancy/childbirth _____	Fertility/birth control: _____

---

contraction, present in approximately 70% of neurologically intact males. In female patients press on the clitoris to contract the rectal sphincter. In both, contraction of the anal sphincter is a positive response that indicates an intact reflex arc, allowing reflex erections in males.

Diagnostic Tests

Because the urinary tract and genital organs share much innervation, tests of bladder function (urodynamics) help estimate the neurological integrity of the genital system. Urodynamic testing identifies a person's reflexic versus areflexic neurological status and sphincter dyssynergia. If reflexes are present, reflex erections are possible; if not, psychogenic erections may be tried. Efferent neurological pathways can be assessed by nocturnal penile tumescence testing, a measure of penile erection during sleep conducted in a sleep laboratory or at home. The test provides a reliable report of all nighttime penile activity for frequency, quality, duration, and amplitude of any nighttime erections. If erections occur during sleep, or

if the patient wakes with an erection, the clinician has some information about the motor and autonomic efferents involved in penile erection.

Another method to evaluate erection potential is intracavernosal injection of pharmacological agents. When all physical components of erection are present, vasodilators such as papaverine, phentolamine, or prostaglandin E_1 are injected into the corpus cavernosum of the penis, leading to erection. Failure of the injection to produce erection suggests the vascular system to the penis is not intact and functioning, leading to impotence. Other tests of erection and ejaculation potential include nocturnal penile tumescence and sensitivity of the penis to vibration. In nocturnal penile tumescence, a band is placed around the penis before the patient falls asleep. Changes in penis size are measured during two to three nights. If erection does not occur, the problem is likely organic rather than psychogenic (Brosman & Leslie, 2004). Penile biothesiometry is done through placing an electromagnetic probe to the right and left of the penis. The vibration

TABLE 27-3 Nursing Diagnoses, Interventions, and Outcomes Applicable to Sexual Function

NIC/NOC

Nursing Diagnosis	Nursing Interventions	Nursing Outcomes
Sexual dysfunction or ineffective sexuality pattern	Sexual counseling, anticipatory behavior guidance, sexual management, anxiety reduction, body image enhancement, role enhancement, self-esteem enhancement, coping enhancement Teaching: sexuality, safe sex, fertility (preservation, reproduction technology enhancement, birth control)	Sexual functioning, child development for children and adolescents, sexual identity acceptance, self-esteem, body image, psychosocial adjustment to life change, social interaction skills, role performance Risk control: unintended pregnancy, sexually transmitted diseases Abuse recovery
Activity intolerance	Exercise promotion Strength training Energy management Body mechanics promotion Pain management Therapy	Activity tolerance Endurance Energy conservation Cardiac pump effectiveness Respiratory status: gas exchange Meets physiological mobility level
Disturbed body image, chronic low self-esteem	Counseling, body image enhancement, coping enhancement, emotional support, pain management, self-esteem enhancement, socialization enhancement, support system enhancement Teaching: urinary, bowel incontinence care related to preparation for sex	Body image, psychosocial adjustment to life change, self-esteem, acceptance of health status, social involvement, social interaction skills, development commensurate with age, bowel/bladder managed during sexual activity
Altered sexual role performance, social isolation leisure	Role enhancement, caregiver support, complex relationship building, normalization promotion, socialization enhancement, self-awareness enhancement, self-esteem enhancement, mutual goal setting, values clarification, socialization enhancement	Adjustment to life change, social interaction skills, social involvement, social support, well-being, participation
Deficient knowledge: sexual health	Teaching: sexuality, safe sex Sexual counseling, health education, health system guidance, preconception counseling	Knowledge: sexual functioning Information processing: memory Communication: receptive ability Cognitive ability

Data from Moorhead, S., Johnson, M., & Maas, M. (Eds.). (2004). *Nursing outcomes classification (NOC)* (3rd ed.). St. Louis, MO: Mosby; Dochterman, J. M., & Bulechek, G. M. (2004). *Nursing interventions classification (NIC)* (4th ed.). St. Louis, MO: Mosby; and NANDA International. (2007). *NANDA-I nursing diagnoses: Definitions & classification 2007-2008*. Philadelphia: Author.

level is increased while questioning the patient. Impaired response indicates a sensory deficit.

INTERVENTIONS

Education for Patient and Partner

Rehabilitation nursing roles in sexual counseling are education and counseling. Refer to Table 27-3 for nursing diagnoses, interventions, and outcomes related to sexual function. Sexual education offers suggestions about interventions and provides information to a patient and partner (or to a patient through the course of daily interactions) about sexual options, positions for sexual activities, management or relief of pain, management of bowel and bladder function, psychosocial aspects of human sexuality, effects of medications on sexual function, prevention of STDs, and birth control methods. A session on human sexuality included in education programs reaches groups who experience altered sexual function, similar to community support groups for men experiencing impotence. Composed of patients at similar

adjustment stages or with diagnoses that risk similar sexual problems, groups may mix patients and partners or segregate by gender. Either way, groups focus on education and management strategies.

Even if not leading a group or class on sexual health, rehabilitation nurses provide sexual information during daily contact. Essential knowledge about sexuality and function is only effective when nurses also are comfortable with their own sexuality, with discussing sexual topics with patients, with a patient's "need to know" apart from sexual preferences and practices, and with not discussing sexuality when a patient so chooses. Preparation for sexual counseling begins with self-education and knowledge about the following topics:

- Human sexual response, variety and prevalence of sexual behaviors, and anatomy and physiology of sexual function
- Types of sexual dysfunction and other deficits that affect sexual function (e.g., paralysis, especially potential experiences for patients counseled)

- Relationship of age, life events, pathological conditions, behavior problems, or pharmaceuticals with sexual function
- Signs of fertility in females and appropriate effective contraception methods
- Benefits of abstinence and assertive communication skills to resist peer pressure and social pressure of sexual activity
- Professional responsibility for holistic care

Compensation Strategies for Sexual Dysfunction or Altered Sexuality Pattern

Alternative Techniques. Patients may learn to compensate for sexual dysfunction in all areas of deficit, but when intercourse is not an option, strategies for satisfying sexual activities are especially important. Physical impairment usually does not reduce interest in sex or capacity for sexual functioning, except when intercourse is too difficult or impossible. Many patients report difficulty in finding sexual partners and thus masturbate to orgasm. Patients with partners may find masturbation helpful. In particular, if a patient with intact sensation has difficulty achieving an orgasm, masturbation may allow the patient an opportunity to find pleasure points in privacy (Kaufman et al., 2003).

Options with a partner are diverse, including manual sexual stimulation, and orogenital stimulation (cunnilingus and fellatio). Concerning cunnilingus, educate patients never to blow air forcibly into the vagina, because fatal air embolism may result for the woman and/or fetus if the woman is pregnant. Patients with sensory loss may find fulfillment from pleasing a partner by performing manual or orogenital sexual stimulation. Touch, slow sex, and gentle caressing will heighten pleasure during sex.

The use of aroma therapy, lotions, and lubricants may be of assistance. Because many medications decrease natural lubrication, lubricants may decrease pain associated with penetration. When providing advice on lubricants, consider the type, water-based, oil-based or silicone-based. Lubricants containing spermicide should be avoided by patients who are prone to urinary tract infections (Car, 2006).

Strategies to compensate for ED involve the partner. When a man has ED, his female partner positions the soft penis into her vagina and contracts vaginal (pubococcygeal) muscles; this action holds the penis in the vagina ("stuffing technique") (Kaufman, Silverberg, & Odette, 2003). With the man on top and the woman's legs drawn upward, the woman moves her hips. Even though the penis is soft, a vacuum is created within the vagina, and an erection can develop. Clitoral stimulation also occurs, resulting in pleasure, even if ejaculation does not occur. Another variation of stuffing involves the use of a harness with a dildo strapped around the male. The genitals remain exposed and can be stimulated. The dildo should be lubricated before insertion.

Vacuum entrapment systems or pumps are external devices that can produce or maintain erection (Figure 27-5). The man lubricates the flaccid penis and places it into a clear acrylic tube that is held tightly against the body. Then he uses the pump device to produce a vacuum in the acrylic tube, which

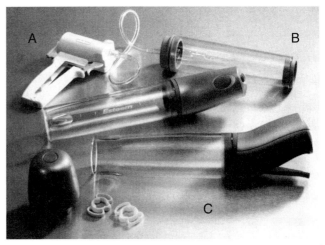

Figure 27-5 A, Classic Erect Aid. B, Esteem battery-operated system. C, Manual system. (Courtesy Timm Medical Technology, Eden Prairie, MN.)

encourages blood flow into the penis. Once the penis is engorged, a ring is placed around the base of the penis to hold the erection. The ring should be removed no later than 30 minutes after placement. There are many varieties of pumps available, ranging in price from $30 to $300 (Kaufman et al., 2003). It is best to start with a low-cost pump because there is often some disappointment with them, because the advertisements often overstate the advantages of use. The pump is **not** recommended for patients with coagulation disorders, diabetes, hypertension, or peripheral vascular disease. When using a pump, a ring may be used to maintain the erection. Pumps and rings are available through the Internet or medical supply stores. If purchased as a medical device, the expense is significantly higher, and a prescription is required. Potential problems are damage to the penile shaft, damage to internal penile tissue, and infection of or irritation to the urinary tract (Kaufman et al., 2003).

Penile vibrators such as the FertiCare Personal Vibrator are safe and effective alternatives for individuals with spinal cord injury who have difficulty obtaining and sustaining an erection. The FertiCare Personal Vibrator is linked with successful ejaculation following spinal cord injury (Laessoe, Nielsen, Biering-Sorensen, & Sonksen, 2004). The device requires a prescription and is available for $695 (http://www.medicalvibrator.com).

Pharmacological Agents. One of the most remarkable developments in recent decades is the discovery of the molecule UK-92-480, later named sildenafil citrate. Originally tested for antianginal effects, the use of sildenafil citrate resulted in an adverse erectogenic effect. Clinical trials of sildenafil citrate for erectile dysfunction were so effective that subjects protested when the trials ended and the medication was withdrawn. Open trials were added to provide humanitarian relief for couples who had experienced relief from erectile dysfunction during clinical trials. As a result, more than 4,500 men were involved in testing sildenafil citrate, a much higher number than usually included in clinical trials. Before the Food and Drug Administration (FDA) approval of sildenafil citrate, around 4% of men with erectile dysfunction sought medical attention for it, and sales of $4 million annually were expected. Within 2 years of release of sildenafil citrate, the drug had captured 98% of the market with 20% of those with erectile dysfunction using the drug. Because sildenafil citrate has few side effects, is easy to use, and requires only 20 minutes for onset of action, it dramatically displaced less-convenient methods and radically changed the lives of men affected by erectile dysfunction (McCullough, 2002).

According to the National Guideline Clearinghouse (Erectile Dysfunction Guideline Update Panel, 2005), the first-line therapy option for erectile dysfunction is an oral phosphodiesterase-5 (PDE-5) inhibitor such as sildenafil citrate, vardenafil, or tadalafil. Oral PDE-5 inhibitors are contraindicated in patients taking organic nitrates because profound and fatal hypotension may result from the drug-drug interaction (Cheitlin et al., 1999). The drug is used with caution in persons with retinal damage, such as retinitis pigmentosa. Sildenafil citrate is taken 20 to 60 minutes before intercourse but can be used only once in 24 hours; the dose is not to be exceeded. Vardenafil is effective within 20 minutes of ingestion. Tadalafil is taken 1 to 2 hours ahead of time and is effective for 36 hours.

Patients for whom one of the PDE-5 inhibitors is not effective should be offered a different PDE-5 inhibitor. Second-line therapy options include alprostadil intraurethral suppositories and intracavernous drug injection. Each of these options will be discussed briefly.

Alprostadil (Caverject, Edex, or Muse) intraurethral suppositories relax the arterial smooth muscle and allow the penile sinusoids to fill with blood (Kava, 2005). The initial dose of an alprostadil intraurethral suppository should be done under medical supervision, because syncope may result. The syncopal side effect is of particular concern for patients with spinal cord injury. A venous constrictor band can be placed at the base of the penis before inserting the alprostadil to prevent systemic absorption of the prostaglandin. Once the alprostadil is inserted, the penis must be rubbed for 10 seconds to help with absorption of the medication, and the penis must be held upright to keep the medication from falling out.

Intracavernosal vasoactive drug injection therapy with alprostadil, papaverine (Pavabid), and phentolamine should be initiated under health care provider supervision. Medications that relax smooth muscle and allow for an increase in penile blood flow can be prescribed for penile intracavernosal injection. Cavernosal fibrosis is a concern with long-term use in a small percentage of men; fibrosis may adversely alter erectile ability. The injections effect erection only and do not increase ability to ejaculate or experience orgasm. Priapism occurs in 3% to 10% of men, and a plan should be developed before the use of an intracavernosal vasoactive drug injection.

Penile Implants. Penile implants are options for some men impotent as a result of SCI, diabetes, arterial ischemia, extensive pelvic surgery, or long-term use of drugs, such as antihypertensives. Implantation may diminish the ability to achieve partial erection, but presurgical sperm count and sensations during intercourse will remain as before surgery. Penile implants or prostheses can be hydraulic inflatable, noninflatable semirigid, or malleable. Inflatable prostheses are three-piece devices with two cylinders implanted in the corporal bodies of the penis, a pump placed in the scrotum, and a fluid reservoir located behind the abdominal wall (Figure 27-6). The 5-year failure rate is between 6% and 16% (Coughlin, 2006).

Patients who cannot tolerate or do not want penile implant surgery may decide to use an artificial penis, a device strapped onto the groin that simulates natural erection. Some use a vibrator to intensify stimulation in the genital area to facilitate erection or ejaculation. Because rough handling damages genital tissues and structures, a vibrator is used gently with a water-soluble lubricant and is halted immediately on discomfort or irritation. Vibrator stimulation may enhance sexual function for some; however, those who become dependent on intense stimulation may find it difficult to achieve orgasm from less-stimulating touch. Electrovibration is used to collect sperm for fertility treatments because it increases the possibility of antegrade ejaculation.

Compensation for Motor Dysfunction. Persons with central nervous system injury, including SCI above T12 or L1, multiple sclerosis, stroke, cerebral palsy, spina bifida, or brain injury experience hypertonicity. Not only do they have difficulty attaining and remaining in a position, but involuntary movements may be embarrassing, inconvenient, or even a safety hazard during sexual activity. Medications to relieve or reduce the spasticity also reduce libido. Steady stretching of a hypertonic muscle and avoiding jerking movements may relieve an isolated spasm, but it also may interfere with sexual activity. For persons with hemiplegia, positioning the affected side downward helps by allowing the unaffected side to move freely. Those with hypotonicity find careful positioning can defend against subluxation at involved joints. Pillows or other supports prevent further stretching of ligaments, and joints are supported in proper alignment at all times.

A patient's inability to move the lower body places the responsibility for motor movement on the partner. Waterbeds allow one partner to initiate movement of the water as though the other person were moving also. Waterbeds have hazards for those with limited head control while lying prone or for transfers (in or out) with paralysis. A person with apraxia, motor planning dysfunction, may not be able to initiate the thrusting motor movement but can participate in the movement once initiated by the partner. The partner must be willing to assume the dominant role in motor movement, which may be difficult for some women. Patients with ataxia, uncoordinated muscle movement, need guidance to find a position sufficiently stable for them to perform the motor components of coitus. With motor perseveration that

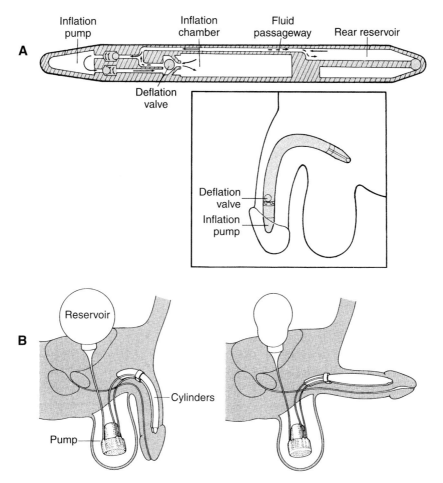

Figure 27-6 *A,* One-piece inflatable penile prosthesis. *B,* Scott inflatable penile prosthesis. (From Thompson, J. M., McFarland, G. K., Hirsch, J. E., & Tucker, S. M. [1998]. *Mosby's clinical nursing* [4th ed.]. St. Louis, MO: Mosby.)

interferes with a patient moving from one activity to another, the partner can redirect the activity verbally or physically.

In the individual with SCI, especially complete injury at the T6 level or above, sexual activity may elicit autonomic dysreflexia or hyperreflexia, notably in certain positions that provide greater stimuli below the level of injury. Should symptoms of dysreflexia occur, the couple is taught to cease sexual activity so that symptoms subside or to seek help as indicated. In general, the patient sits upright, monitors blood pressure, and takes prescribed medications. Mecamylamine hydrochloride (Inversine) may prevent dysreflexia symptoms but may reduce desire and lead to erection problems. Refer to Chapter 18 for complete information about autonomic dysreflexia.

Compensation for Sensory Dysfunction. Persons who have lost sensation to the genital area include those who have experienced SCI (complete or that affects sensation), those with diabetes or multiple sclerosis, and a few with heightened or diminished sensation on the affected side after stroke or brain injury. Persons with SCI report a wide variety of sexual sensations ranging from anesthesia to orgasm, and some report

heightened pleasurable sensation similar to sexual orgasm in other areas of the body, especially intact areas generally considered erogenous zones, such as the breasts, ears, eyes, neck, lower abdomen, groin, inner thighs, and back above the level of the spinal cord lesion (Woods, 1984). Literature about SCI has information concerning true versus pseudoorgasm, with true orgasm being experienced by those with a neurologically intact nervous system and pseudoorgasm being related to emotional components. In the last few years research studies have demonstrated orgasm in a number of women with complete and incomplete SCIs. Self-report and laboratory studies of orgasm indicate that almost half of all persons with SCI experience orgasm unrelated to the level or completeness of injury. Most report that a relationship with a trusted sexual partner was the pathway to achieving pleasure and orgasm and also added emotional and spiritual aspects to the experience (Tepper, 1999). Sensory amplification involves thinking intensely about a physical stimulus and mentally amplifying that sensation; in some instances this technique facilitates orgasm.

Sensory stimulation may enhance sexual enjoyment; especially for men, viewing the activity may compensate for

BOX 27-2 Pain Control for Sexual Activity for Persons With Rheumatic Disease

- Practice muscle relaxation techniques and mental imagery to promote comfort and tranquility.
- Practice range-of-motion exercises without resistance to promote comfortable movement.
- Apply moist heat to painful joints 10 to 15 minutes before sexual activity to reduce swelling and promote increased range of motion.
- Rest after completing bathing and grooming activities.
- Position pillows under affected painful limbs for support; always remove the pillows after sexual activity to prevent contractures.
- Schedule pain medications and arrange for sexual activities around the period of maximum drug effectiveness and when less fatigued, when possible.
- Explore massage, vibration, or self-hypnosis to relieve pain, and use effective techniques before sexual activity.
- Explore alternative styles of sexual expression to convey caring, concern, and love.
- Use a warm waterbed, an electric blanket over the patient, or a bed warmer under the sheets to ease pain or stiffness; use a moist heating pad for a particularly painful joint.
- Precede sex by a warm bath or massage and mild exercise.
- Try cold rather than hot applications, especially for inflamed joints; some may have better relief from these.
- Understand that frequent sexual activity may reduce pain of arthritis by stimulating adrenal glands to increase production of the body's own natural antiinflammatory and pain-reducing corticosteroids.
- Be aware that joint injections of corticosteroid for pain relief at joints impacted by sexual activity may help.

decreased genital sensation. Light the room, place mirrors, and position for visualization; use the senses to promote fantasy through pleasant sounds, music, or the noises and words uttered during sexual activity to increase sexual desire or release. Touching intact areas of sensation; rubbing or caressing with various textured items or lotions; or smelling pleasant odors in the environment, on the person, and from sexual activity can be powerful precursors to sexual pleasure. The taste of the partner is unique, and the special taste during sexual excitement brings sexual pleasure to some.

Pain Control. Persons with chronic pain, with rheumatic diseases, or after joint replacement surgery may experience pain that inhibits sexual activity. Rehabilitation team members can suggest techniques to control pain during sexual activity. Hill (2004) suggests that although fatigue and pain may negatively impact sexual function, most partners are sympathetic. Avoiding fatigue, engaging in anticipatory planning, and managing activity will reduce pain with sexual function. These suggestions also apply to patients with other conditions involving painful muscles and joints (Box 27-2).

Couples develop techniques to alert a partner that a particular activity or position is painful. The "hand riding" technique signals distress when one person places a hand on the partner's hand. Women experiencing painful intercourse should have a gynecological referral to rule out or identify organic causes and suggest corrections.

Women, particularly those who are postmenopausal or those with neurological or vascular compromise, may experience discomfort during intercourse because of vaginal dryness. Vaginal lubrication is very helpful. Water-soluble lubricants are recommended, such as KY Jelly (reapply frequently); longer-lasting lubricants, including KY Long Lasting and Replens, provide a consistent vaginal moisture and are applied periodically during the week. Estrogen creams have the best restorative value to vaginal and external orifices but cannot be used by all women, especially those with estrogen-dependent cancers. Oil-based lubricants (Vaseline, baby oil) are not recommended because they increase risk of infection and interfere with the effectiveness of latex condoms, diaphragms, and cervical caps.

Continence Management. Because the autonomic nervous system regulates sexual function and influences bowel and bladder control, activation of one set of neurons can activate the others. A partner is advised when potential for incontinence exists to prevent embarrassment and allow for preparation. Use protection for bed covers, rinse items in white vinegar while washing to eliminate any urine odor, and use incense or cologne to mask odor if no one is sensitive or allergic. Sexual activity should be scheduled to prevent conflict with an established bowel program. Prepare by emptying the bladder and limiting liquid intake.

Indwelling catheters require special precautions. An indwelling catheter may be removed before sexual activity and replaced following it. The catheter should not be disconnected from the drainage tubing. Suprapubic or ileoloop appliances need not be removed but are taped to the abdomen. Urinary flow to any catheter cannot be obstructed for long periods without increasing the risk for urinary tract infection. The newer continent internal urinary storage pouches require no special preparation; catheterizing before sexual activity will ensure the pouch is empty.

Medication Management. Medications and other ingested substances can affect sexual performance. Antihypertensive agents, antidepressants, antiandrogens, alcohol abuse, and smoking are just a few of the substances that may affect sexual functioning (Lue, 2000). Patients should be advised of the side effects of medications, including sexual dysfunction. If such develops, a different dosage or alternative drug may be discussed with the physician or nurse practitioner.

Reproduction Issues. Fertility and infertility are major issues during childbearing years. *Healthy People 2010* objectives concerning family planning apply to all, regardless of disability. Guidelines include reducing unintended pregnancies, postponing sexual activity among adolescents, increasing education and counseling, and reducing the prevalence of infertility (U.S. Department of Health and Human Services, 2000). Birth control information should be shared with all fertile patients and partners. The commonly held myth that disability may cause infertility should be corrected. Likewise, the rehabilitation nurse should provide patients with infertility information and resources available for childbearing or adoption when desired.

Fertility instruction includes information on sexual anatomy, the physiology of contraception, and birth control devices or methods. A contraceptive method is chosen based on accurate information about failure rates, reversibility, safety, and personal health status. The nurse obtains feedback from the couple about premorbid birth control practices, as well as their preparation to meet future birth control needs. Referral to a gynecologist or urologist may be required for the birth control method of the couple's choice. Birth control pills do not protect from sexually transmitted diseases and may reduce antibiotic and anticonvulsant efficacy. Table 27-4 and related material provide a brief discussion of birth control methods, including effectiveness, availability, and advantages and disadvantages for certain disability groups.

Pregnancy and Disability. Women with chronic illnesses or traumatic injuries generally maintain fertility and childbearing options and usually can carry and delivery health full-term infants. Labor and delivery present specific risks for women with chronic illness or injury, and the obstetrical team should include physicians knowledgeable about the disability. Mothers with disability or chronic illness should be considered high risk for complications during labor and delivery. As an example, labor and delivery may trigger an exacerbation of multiple sclerosis. Women with high-level spinal cord injury may experience autonomic dysreflexia during labor.

Spinal Cord Injury and Pregnancy. Most patients with spinal cord injury are able to delivery vaginally at full term. The most significant complication during intrapartum care is autonomic dysreflexia. Epidural anesthesia is noted to reduce the risk of autonomic dysreflexia (Pereira, 2003). Skin integrity must be assessed and preserved, especially during labor and delivery. Should a pressure area develop, the resulting nutritional catabolic state or anemia is treated aggressively to avoid inhibiting fetal growth. Attention to decreased gastrointestinal motility with pregnancy may prevent constipation and maintain bowel programs.

Autonomic dysreflexia may occur during labor and delivery. Box 27-3 lists interventions; refer to Chapter 18 for full description and management information. Breast-feeding is not contraindicated in women with SCI, but with lesions at T6 they may have decreased milk supply after 6 weeks because of the lack of sensory input when breast-feeding. Women with lesions at T6 or above should be taught to carefully monitor their nipples, because they will not be aware of soreness or infection, which could lead to mastitis.

Infertility. Many conditions contribute to infertility: erectile or ejaculation dysfunction, decreased sperm quality and quantity, altered thermoregulation to the testicles from autonomic nervous system dysfunction in men, and genitourinary infection or hormonal irregularities in both sexes. Infertility treatment has grown in many rehabilitation centers as results have improved. Specific programs offer education for couples with disabilities who are infertile but wish to bear children. Couples who have had successful unprotected intercourse for 1 full year during the woman's most fertile time in each cycle without pregnancy benefit from fertility evaluation. Refer to an accessible clinic with expertise on infertility management for couples with disabilities; many conduct research on each aspect of the cause for infertility. One example of research concerns sperm retrieval and quality and applications of findings for families with disabilities. Sperm collection uses electrovibratory stimulation applied directly to the penis or electroejaculation techniques. The semen is washed and used for artificial insemination or in vitro fertilization. Vibroejaculation used at home requires little sperm preparation of the semen. In research, approaches to improve sperm quality for men with SCI include bladder management, early treatment of urinary tract infection, and reduced scrotal temperatures.

Interventions for Activity Intolerance

The plan of care for activity intolerance involves the patient and partner in active therapy; they identify deficits in activity level and receive instruction in how to perform the desired activity, make adaptations, and modify the environment to accommodate it. Rehabilitation activities that build strength and endurance for activities of daily living and community living can include those to enable sexual activity once the patient returns home (McCloskey & Bulechek, 2000).

Positions for Sexual Activity. A nurse may encourage patients to experiment with positions that are comfortable and appropriate for them, that is, those that enhance comfort and facilitate sexual activity. Couples often welcome information about alternate positions, as well as encouragement to experiment. Assistive devices or adapted equipment, such as side rails, bed loops, or an overhead trapeze, may ease changing positions and be safe for those with difficulty in bed mobility. Loss of range of motion in the joints, particularly the hips, limits movements during sexual activity and restricts favorite positions. Pillows are for positioning; those shaped like an armchair back can position the person with high SCI to see what is transpiring. Some persons are more comfortable in a recliner or other chairs than in a bed. Helping couples select positions that place the least stress on involved body parts manages pain, reduces potential for injury or complications, and allows the most sexual pleasure.

Specific disabilities preclude certain positions. For example, patients who have cardiac problems should avoid positions that place undue stress on the arms for sustained periods. The supine position is less stressful physically, as long as breathing is not restricted. The side-by-side position and face-to-face position create less worry about compromising

TABLE 27-4 Birth Control Methods and Disability

Method	Effects	Advantages	Contraindications
Oral contraceptives	Alter hormone patterns to suppress ovulation; cervical mucosa and endometrium resist sperm	2%-3% failure rate due to irregular use	Those with a history of blood clots, such as after SCI, multiple trauma, stroke, or coronary artery disease; those with hypertension, diabetes, gallbladder disease, or irregular menses
Norplant	Levonorgestrel released steadily into the bloodstream through small implanted tubes; drug inhibits ovulation, thickens mucosa to inhibit sperm motility	No estrogen; 1% failure rate in 5 years	No research regarding persons with disabilities; not used with breast cancer, liver disease, uterine bleeding problems, breast-feeding, or pregnancy
Depo-Provera (medroxyprogesterone acetate)	Hormone that regulates the menstrual cycle; one injection intramuscularly prevents pregnancy for 12 weeks by keeping the ovaries from releasing eggs and thickening cervical mucosa to keep sperm from joining with eggs	Failure rate is 3 per 1000 in 1 year; can be used while breast-feeding	Not used if planning to become pregnant within 18 months; not used with unexplained vaginal bleeding, with serious liver disease, after a heart attack, stroke, breast cancer, or with severe high blood pressure, long-standing or complicated diabetes
Intrauterine device (IUD)	Appears to act by preventing implantation of ovum; monthly check required for string placement	5% failure rate with ParaGard; 2% fail with Progestasert; reversible	Some women with disabilities are unable to check the string; those with decreased sensation in saddle area may not notice pain or bleeding
Male condom	Only latex protects from HIV and hepatitis B; use new condom for each encounter and discard after use; may use spermicide in addition to condom	10% failure due to improper use or product failure; 2%-3% failure with proper use; high failure rate with nonlatex condoms	Allergies to latex may develop; oil-based lubricants destroy latex; partner may have to apply condom for male patient
Diaphragm	Barrier to sperm; placed over female cervix; may be used with various spermicides; must be used each time	As low as 2% failure when correctly sized, placed, and used; 10%-19% failure in some studies	Use during menstruation may lead to toxic shock; allergies to latex or spermicide may develop; with limited saddle sensation, patient may not notice dislodgment; partner may have to insert, remove, or apply
Spermicidal foams, jellies, creams, dissolving tablets, suppositories NOTE: Mountain Dew and Coke are not spermicides	Chemical attacks sperm, while base forms mechanical barrier; renew application with each encounter	Protects against many STDs when ingredients include nonoxynol-9 or octoxynol; 18%-21% failure rate when used alone; increased effectiveness when used with condom or diaphragm	Douche may wash away spermicide prematurely; partner may need to apply; difficult for those with impaired hand function, balance, or flexibility
Sponge	Soft, round polyurethane sponge fits over cervix; sponge contains spermicide that is activated when moistened with water before insertion; for a second encounter, reapply spermicide	10%-20% failure rate	Do not use during menses or 3-4 weeks postpartum to avoid toxic shock syndrome; partner may need to insert and remove
Withdrawal (coitus interruptus)	Removal of penis from vagina before ejaculation; man determines timing unless woman controls movement	23% failure rate; cooperation, communication, and timing are essential	Enjoyment may be decreased or partner may miscalculate
Natural methods: rhythm, fertility awareness techniques, calendar, basal body temperature, cervical mucus test	Abstinence during at-risk times as determined by different methods; abstinence during fertile times and ovulation is required (approximately 10 days/month)	Inexpensive, reversible, no chemicals or hormones; 2%-10% failure rate for those with regular cycles and proper use; 24% failure rate overall; 40% failure rate with cervical mucus test alone; promotes awareness of bodily functions in women	Persons not cognitively able to calculate and those who do not adhere to schedules are not candidates

TABLE 27-4 Birth Control Methods and Disability—cont'd

Method	Effects	Advantages	Contraindications
Permanent sterilization: vasectomy or tubal ligation	Vasectomy: vas deferens is cut to block sperm ejaculation Tubal ligation: fallopian tubes are blocked or cut to prevent ova from reaching the uterus or from fertilization in the tubes	Vasectomy is effective and popular; failure rate is 160 per 100,000 Tubal ligation is effective and popular; failure rate is 276-326 per 100,000	Permanent; very difficult to reverse Ethical issues may arise when used with vulnerable populations Both are surgical techniques and require some recovery time

SCI, Spinal cord injury; *STDs,* sexually transmitted diseases; *HIV,* human immunodeficiency virus.

BOX 27-3 Autonomic Dysreflexia: Interventions During Labor and Delivery

- Differentiate from toxemia of pregnancy (i.e., blood pressure rises associated with uterine contractions)
- Monitor blood pressure frequently
- Avoid external restraints
- Use anesthetic ointments during insertion of an indwelling catheter and during vaginal examinations, enemas, and the like
- Position upright to decrease symptoms and shorten labor
- Use an epidural anesthetic
- Use medications as prescribed for blood pressure control
- Know that when dysreflexia is uncontrolled by medications and anesthesia; prompt delivery by cesarean section may be the most expedient method of management

Data from Pope, C., Markenson, G., Bayer-Zwirello, L., & Maissel, G. (2001). Pregnancy complicated by chronic spinal cord injury and history of autonomic hyperreflexia. *Obstetrics & Gynecology, 97,* 802-803.

BOX 27-4 Guidelines for Sexual Intercourse After Myocardial Infarction

The patient and partner should:
- Wait after eating for 1 to 3 hours to allow digestion.
- Choose an interruption-free setting that is familiar, comfortable, and peaceful.
- Prepare by ensuring rest and relaxation before sexual activity.
- Consult with the physician to determine if medications are needed before sexual activity.
- Person on the bottom position causes less stress because person on the bottom is not supporting the body.
- Orogenital sex and masturbation cause no undue strain, so they may be used for sexual expression.
- Notify physician if a rapid heart rate persists longer than 15 minutes after intercourse.
- Sex with a new partner may increase stress to the heart.

Data from American Heart Association. (2006). *Sexual activity and heart disease or stroke: AHA recommendation.* Retrieved September 30, 2006, from http://www.americanheart.org/presenter.jhtml?identifier=4714.

---

cardiac function. Sexual activity for the patient with cardiac problems is resumed based on the cardiologist's recommendations; generally as soon as the patient feels ready for it (American Heart Association, 2006). Energy requirements range between 3 and 6 METs (metabolic equivalent units), that is, from light to moderately heavy activity. Chapter 32 discusses more about specific activity levels following myocardial infarction. Refer to Box 27-4 for guidelines for sexual intercourse following myocardial infarction.

Common Positions and Precautions. Persons with disabilities may use variations of the four basic positions; all provide access for genital-to-genital contact, cunnilingus, and fellatio.
- Face-to-face, man above (or missionary position)
- Face-to-face, woman above
- Side-lying, with one leg of the woman over the man's hips (provides for freedom of movement for both partners)
- Rear entry, which is possible from a side-lying or sitting position or when the woman is kneeling or lying prone; hand stimulation is possible for both partners, and penetration into the vagina may be regulated.

Some precautions are sensible in sexual positioning for patients who have been immobile for long periods or who cannot bear weight on their lower extremities. Weight of a partner on a patient's osteoporotic bones may be sufficient to cause fractures; others with recent orthopedic injuries and concomitant neurological injuries may require bracing for bone stabilization. Until the physiatrist or orthopedist determines a brace can be removed safely during sexual activity, the person wears it, even if the brace is removed in bed otherwise. A brace also can dictate positions because undue pressure is not applied to any area of the body that is braced. Persons with heterotropic ossification may have limited joint motion and painful joint areas; they benefit from positioning that allows them maximum functional mobility without pain.

Avoiding complications and providing comfortable sexual activity are goals when experimenting with positions. Persons with rheumatic disease, for example, select positions that place the least stress on the involved joints. Although patients with restricted joint motion must limit movements during sexual activity, experimenting with several positions may yield one that permits both comfort and flexibility. Many persons with arthritic hip joint problems (70%) report sexual difficulties. Women whose arthritis affects the hip joint find the spoon position, side-lying with the man behind the woman, more comfortable. Recommended for men with hip joint problems is a position with the couple lying facing and side by side; the woman wraps her upper leg around the man's upper hip or both legs around his hips. Alternatively the man lies supine while the woman sits astride his hips with her knees, lower legs, and feet on either side of his body. Her knees provide support, and she can put her hands on the bed to control her weight on his pelvis. Pillows all around help support the weight and cushion painful joints.

Those with multiple sclerosis who experience fatigue and spasticity consider scheduling and positioning that is the most comfortable and least tiring. Persons with SCI may need encouragement to experiment with various positions. Often the person with SCI takes the bottom position because of the motor dysfunction and lack of movement. Pillows placed under a woman's hips make this a comfortable position, but the couple may experiment with prone or side-lying positions. Couples are educated to manage autonomic dysreflexia, should it occur.

Psychosocial Interventions

Disturbed Body Image and Chronic Low Self-Esteem.
Body image and self-esteem may be affected adversely by altered sexual abilities. Nurses assess the patient's body image expectations based on developmental stage and provide anticipatory guidance about predictable changes, such as with a congenital condition, injury, disease, or surgery. Children or adolescents may draw pictures that reflect their body image perceptions. They need to learn how their impairment affects sexuality and effective strategies to accept their appearance. Sexuality is more than sexual activities, and the groundwork is laid in early developmental stages.

Nurses can find ways to enhance a patient's life satisfaction through rehabilitation interventions because success with bowel and bladder retraining, success with transfers, and independence in activities of daily living improve self-concept. Self-esteem thrives in a therapeutic environment with trusting relationships between nurses who communicate acceptance and include patients as worthwhile and unique apart from the impairment. The sooner a patient returns to meaningful work and resumes roles in the family and community, the greater the self-esteem and role balance. All factors that build self-concept contribute positively to the sexual relationship. On the other hand, a decrease in sexual abilities and performance has a negative impact. Men anxious about sexual problems may voice concern about their ability to satisfy their partners. When role changes become necessary for sexual activities, rehabilitation nurses can support and encourage individuals and couples, including educating them about compensation strategies, fertility clinics, and other options, as appropriate.

Interventions for Ineffective Role Performance/Social Isolation

Social Isolation. A patient whose self-concept is threatened may avoid contact with others and become socially isolated. Involving the patient in social interaction as early as possible, complimenting efforts to appear attractive, discussing individual sexual concerns, and accepting concerns as a matter of course may help maintain or restore self-concept. As children grow, they need the same interventions as adults to develop a social network. Planning involves assessing whether altered body image contributes to increased social isolation. Reducing the impact of physical changes with accessories, such as scarves, manageable clothing, wigs, or cosmetics as appropriate may help some to feel more comfortable in public and avoid social isolation. Peer counseling with someone who has similar alterations in body image helps some to find support (McCloskey & Bulechek, 2000).

Social isolation also restricts opportunities to meet that special someone and build a strong interpersonal or sexual relationship. Tips concerning fostering relationships include the following:
- Do not believe that no one will love you because you have a disability.
- Do not build your life in search of romance; use activities to meet others.
- Be a friend first.
- Keep up on current events.
- Be patient in your search for connection with others.
- Be open about your disability.
- Know that regardless of your disability, lovemaking is possible.

Building and Maintaining Relationships. Information concerning building and maintaining relationships is an essential component of education programs for patients and their partners. High levels of subjective quality of life and life satisfaction are possible for couples with disability. Emphasizing sexual rehabilitation, encouraging positive communication patterns, and encouraging mutually enjoyable activities are keys to ensuring an optimal sexual relationship (Box 27-5).

Couples can not assume that talk about sex is something to do once and then put aside. Like all forms of intimate communication, this topic benefits from the ongoing dialogue that permits a couple to learn about each other and resolve confusion or uncertainties over time. One area where men and women differ is communication. In general, men process and remember in conversation mainly through the left side of the brain, and focusing on the literal words and factual data, they miss the underlying emotions. Women, however, store nonverbal and emotional communication, perceiving the tone of voice as well as the emotional or pictorial messages. One technique to reconcile the differences is using word pictures or analogies that bridge both sides of the brain, enabling a couple to be open to intimacy (Smalley & Trent, 2006).

BOX 27-5 Communicating About Sex

- Talk with your partner about how and when it would be most comfortable to discuss sex. This will let your partner know you are interested in feedback about your sexual interaction.
- Consider the possibility of using books or other media sources to initiate discussions. One disadvantage is that books do not always suit the personal style of the couple, so choose one that is not offensive.
- Use "I" language as much as possible when talking about sex together, and try to avoid putting blame on your partner for your own patterns of response (or lack thereof).
- Remember that if your partner rejects a type of sexual activity that you think you might enjoy, he or she is not rejecting you as a person.
- Be aware that sexual feelings and preferences change from time to time.
- Do not neglect the nonverbal side of sexual communication because these messages often speak louder than words.
- Do not expect perfection.

Relationships are nurtured by the daily sharing of our feelings, needs, hopes, and dreams and by active listening when a partner shares. Effective social interaction skills incorporate elements of disclosure, receptiveness, cooperation, sensitivity, assertiveness, confrontation, consideration, genuineness, warmth, poise, relaxation, engagement, trust, and compromise (Johnson, Maas, & Moorhead, 2000). Building trust and honor is a choice for a lifelong commitment, to understand each other's needs, to develop the skills to meet those needs, and for a desire to resolve conflicts and promote harmony. After an illness or injury partners who commit to each other choose to accept each other as unique, complete persons who are loved and to look for ways to comfort and nurture.

Affection and Romance. Privacy for a hug or kiss and to express affection with meaningful touch are encouraging during hospitalization and rehabilitation. Most persons retain some areas of intact sensation, making meaningful touch effective. Eight to 10 meaningful touches a day keep fires of a relationship burning. Verbal communication, verbal communication with signals such as gestures or facial movements, and sign language are all means of communicating feelings. Romance is a shared emotional experience of special times in which couples focus on how valuable each is to the other, but couples may require careful planning and conversation to rediscover romance and to build it into their lives. They are encouraged to schedule intimate times together despite the pressures of life with a chronic condition or disability (Smalley & Trent, 2006).

Sexual role performance can be enhanced by sexual education and by introducing role models who have overcome a similar problem. Roles are discussed with the

partner, and compensation strategies for role performance are included in the education program (McCloskey & Bulechek, 2000).

Interventions for Deficient Knowledge

The Rehabilitation Nurse's Role as Counselor.

Counselors become aware of their personal value systems, including biases and beliefs about appropriate and inappropriate sexual behavior; all rehabilitation team members ideally understand their own sexuality. Nurses are never to negate their own beliefs, but while acknowledging their validity should be aware of what they can or cannot acceptably teach. Should conflicts interfere with counseling or education, the nurse refers patients to other health professionals. All persons providing counseling or education have limitations and at times refer to others qualified in specific areas or able to provide the counsel or education the patient wants or needs.

A therapeutic relationship based on trust and respect enhances counseling; patients are more open when assured of privacy and confidentiality. The individual is of primary importance; certainly group classes are useful in rehabilitation and for sharing basic information; however, each patient's needs are worth private discussion. Timing is important when opening the door for sexuality discussions. Patients and partners learn that sexuality is an important part of life that is affected by their current physical condition or functional ability. Holistic care means the rehabilitation nurse is poised to provide information and support at the time sexual function problems are discovered, observed, or expressed. Communication is on the patient's level, using language the patient understands and discussing sexuality with ease and confidence. Communication skills include active listening, techniques to elicit feelings, strategies for showing acceptance, goal setting, and problem solving. Compassion, a sense of humor, patience, perceptiveness, ingenuity, and flexibility are strengths in counseling relationships. It is helpful to preface questions with a statement that tells patients they are not alone in experiencing sexual difficulties (e.g., "Some persons with SCI experience problems with ejaculation; is that something you have had a problem with since your injury?"). Moving from a less sensitive to a more sensitive topic keeps the information flow from disruption.

Effective counseling begins with a willing, available listener who spends quality time listening to a patient express needs as a sexual being. Empathetic and active listening is a foundational technique for counseling, guiding a patient through problem solving toward being comfortable in discussing sexuality and eliciting specific needs relative to self and family members. Counseling is an opportunity for patients to express grief and anger about altered body image and function and for their partners to learn to accept the changes. Guilt expressed during counseling may relate to the cause, or beliefs about the cause, of the illness or accident (McCloskey & Bulechek, 2000).

Counseling the Sexual Partner. Partners need counsel about how to react to changes in body image, in preparation for what can happen during sexual intercourse, and to understand effects of medications and certain disabilities on sexual function. This counsel can help alleviate a partner's anxiety about engaging in sexual acts. Both the patient and partner may need to dispel myths and correct misconceptions about sexual options. The nurse can confirm that a particular sexual practice is acceptable and not harmful, but responses must be appropriate to patients' lifestyles, beliefs, and needs. The couple makes final decisions and sets the guidelines for their comfort. Successful coping strategies used in the past will help place events in proper perspective and assist with identifying strengths and previous successes. When couples can reframe a situation knowing that things have changed but are not necessarily worse than before, they may adjust to altered sexual ability more readily.

All too often in Western culture, sexual acts are taken seriously, without humor. In a trusting relationship, humor can serve as a form of tension release and a means of dealing with problematic or potentially embarrassing situations. Counselors anticipate a patient's reactions to surgeries, procedures, or impairments and supply information before events occur, strategies that may alleviate threats to self-esteem or perceived loss of control. A nurse counselor builds expertise with counseling patients who have similar disabilities, as well as gaining knowledge for comprehensive health assessment and improving competency in intervening with persons of various developmental levels and cultural or religious values.

The PLISSIT Model. The PLISSIT model developed by Annon (1976) helps nurses evaluate their role and level of comfort in sexual counseling. The acronym PLISSIT defines possible levels of involvement for nurses: permission, limited information, specific suggestions, and intensive therapy. With increased comfort and experience, a nurse may use more complex levels while choosing to refer at any time. The nurse gives the patient permission to discuss concerns and problems related to sexuality—permission to be a sexual being. For instance, when a patient is queried concerning sexuality during an admission assessment, the door is open for any questions or discussion by the patient. The nurse may give permission by reassuring that sexual practices of the patient are appropriate and healthy and that worrying about sexual function is common, or the nurse may give permission to experiment with new forms of sexual expression.

Patients should not leave the rehabilitation setting without limited information concerning how their illness or accident has or has not affected their sexual function. Part of the basic education for patients, information must answer their questions about sexual function.

The nurse can offer specific suggestions to address specific concerns. For example, patients with total hip replacements need specific suggestions about positions for sexual function that are not contraindicated. Specific suggestions include

strategies for direct problem solving or referrals for medical interventions. Suggestions may help patients to rethink a problem and make changes to alleviate the concern. Patients can practice the suggestions and evaluate progress and problems.

Intensive therapy uses the referral process to meet the needs of a patient whose problems cannot be solved using the first three levels. This level of intervention is required by some patients and especially appropriate for those with significant psychosocial sexual dysfunction (Annon, 1976). Rehabilitation nurses who are uncomfortable with any of these levels refer patients to team members who are skillful and knowledgeable in specific areas for counseling and education. Other team members who may be skilled in sexual counseling include the clinical nurse specialist, nurse practitioner, psychologist, social worker, rehabilitation counselor, therapy staff, gynecologist, physiatrist, urologist, and sex therapist. The team approach offers opportunity for individual or group counseling and the resources of a number of health care professionals. Couples who require a higher level of expertise can contact professional organizations such as the Society for Sex Therapy and Research (New York) and the American Association of Sex Educators, Counselors, and Therapists (Washington, D.C.). They publish national directories of qualified sex therapists. Local medical societies, psychological associations, certified psychiatric or mental health nurses, mental health associations, and other nurses working in rehabilitation centers or as members of a sexual management team may be helpful in identifying qualified sex therapists in an area.

Many rehabilitation facilities have initiated sexual education programs after educating members of the team for sexual counseling. Information is gathered from professionals with expertise, literature reviews, conferences and seminars, and other resources. Planned, structured opportunities allow health care providers to become desensitized to hearing sexual terms and concepts, to evaluate their values and cultural practices through role-playing and small-group discussion, and to consider personal feelings and beliefs about sexual behavior for themselves and others. Such opportunities help prepare rehabilitation nurses to provide support and encouragement to patients and partners who face impairment of sexual function.

Counseling for Children. Although sexual counseling is primarily directed toward adults and older persons, sexual counseling is not an adults-only activity. When children and adolescents require sexuality information and counseling, parents are involved in setting up any individualized or group sexual education programs. Understandably parents may be anxious concerning sexual education for their children. More often they allow sexual education that does not teach simply "how to do it," but rather, material emphasizing sex roles, understanding of the body, and socialization skills. Programs on sexual abstinence, especially in younger teens, have been well received by parents and teens.

Research findings indicate that students who understand their sexuality and the responsibilities that go with it are less likely to encounter sexual troubles than students who are uninformed. Parents have legal and ethical rights to retain primary responsibility for transmitting values and building morality in their children. When teaching sexual information in the rehabilitation setting or any setting, it is imperative to receive permission from parents before providing information to teenagers or children.

Rehabilitation nurses and case managers who work with pediatric and adolescent patients may become the providers of sexual education when parents are unable or unwilling to do so. In group homes, where young persons with chronic, disabling, or developmental delays live, staff members may impart sexual information through daily contacts and as part of the fabric of daily life, as well as in formal classes.

Sexual education programs for youth and adolescents include content on responsible sexual behavior such as social skills, how to avoid being sexually exploited, appropriate body exposure, privacy of sexual behavior, responsibility of sexual behavior including abstinence, and how to prevent pregnancy. Children with disabilities will mature sexually. They need to be prepared for the changes that will occur in their bodies. Social skills concerning sexuality are very important for children with disabilities. Children in some settings, where personal assistance with bowel/bladder management and assistance with dressing are provided, are more vulnerable to sexual exploitation. Children and adults with cognitive dysfunction should be taught appropriate social behavior concerning sexuality, including what constitutes proper touching.

The following information might be shared with parents of children with disabilities to enhance sexual education:
- Parents should demonstrate acceptance of the child's body.
- Parents and siblings will provide the first experience with love and socialization.
- Social relationships with siblings and friends should be encouraged.
- Children need to understand the difference between private and public behavior.
- Sexuality information is presented related to a child's age (Box 27-6).

Prevention of Sexually Transmitted Diseases. STDs are at near-epidemic levels in the United States. Uncomfortable or painful, inconvenient, embarrassing, anxiety producing, and sometimes fatal, many STDs persist or leave residual damage, as with chlamydia and gonorrhea. Any symptoms of genital infection need immediate diagnosis and treatment for protection of all involved parties. Sexually active persons, especially those not in monogamous relationships or who change partners, need to recognize symptoms and have annual tests. Early diagnosis and treatment may prevent some long-term complications. Prevention involves education, counseling, increased abstention, and partner notification.

Teenagers are noted for their risky sexual behavior, exemplified in teen pregnancies. Feelings of invincibility and denial influence risk-taking behaviors, such as unprotected sexual activity. However, with the spread of STDs, including human immunodeficiency virus (HIV) and acquired

---

BOX 27-6 Age-Related Sexual Information for Children and Adolescents

Ages 5 to 7 Years	Ages 8 to 11 Years	Ages 12 to 18 Years
Correct name of body parts and their functions	Girls learn about menses; boys learn about nocturnal emissions	Health maintenance (regular examination of breasts or testicles by self-examination and primary care provider)
Differences and similarities between boys and girls	Signs and variations of puberty	Sexuality as part of the total self, to include communication, love, dating, and intimacy
Elements of reproduction and pregnancy	Sexuality as part of the total self	Masturbation becomes a private practice
Qualities of good relationships (love, friendship, communication, and respect)	Information on reproduction and pregnancy	Importance of values in guiding one's behavior
Decision-making skills; all decisions have consequences	Importance of values in decision making	How alcohol and/or drugs influence decision making
Beginning social responsibility, values, and morals	Communication within family unit about sexuality	Intercourse and other ways to express sexuality
Masturbation may be found pleasurable	Masturbation	Birth control and the responsibilities of childbearing, reproduction, and pregnancy
Ways to avoid and report sexual exploitation	Abstinence from sexual intercourse	Pros and cons of condoms in disease prevention
	Avoidance and reporting of sexual abuse	
	Sexually transmitted diseases, including HIV/AIDS	

From National Information Center for Children and Youth With Disabilities. (1992). *Sexuality education for children and youth with disabilities. Fostering relationships: Suggestions for young adults. News digest.* Washington, DC: Author.
HIV, Human immunodeficiency virus; *AIDS,* acquired immunodeficiency syndrome.

immunodeficiency syndrome (AIDS), the consequences have escalated from unwanted pregnancy to long-term illness and even death. Cervical cancer is linked with exposure to the sexually transmitted human papillomavirus (HPV). Although a vaccination exists for prevention of HPV, there is concern that screening for cervical cancer may take lower priority than vaccination (Collins et al., 2006). Recommendations for providing the most effective sex education programs for teenagers include the following:

- Deliver a clear message: Delay sex until you are older, of if you have sex, use a latex condom.
- Focus on setting peer norms: Not everyone is doing it, and you do not have to either.
- Teach resistance skills through role-playing and group discussion on how to say no without hurting someone's feelings and how to avoid situations in which you might have to say no. Repetition of the practice builds learning.
- Include special training for teachers. The SHARE program is one abstinence program that can be used in schools for education (refer to Resources). Safer sex guidelines were developed for all persons, although they originated in response to the AIDS epidemic (Box 27-7). The goals are to reduce risks of STDs, as well as unplanned pregnancy, when used properly and every time. Guidelines for safe sex include abstinence until marriage, monogamous sex, and marriage for life.

EVALUATION

Evaluation of nursing interventions for education or counseling follow the nursing process. Evaluation methods are patient demonstrations of learned skills and verbal repetition of the information. Because sexual activity is a private matter, the socially acceptable evaluation is questioning and evaluating the verbal responses. A nurse might ask about achievement of individualized goals, and the patient and partner decide how or if they wish to reply. When teaching psychomotor domain skills, such as using devices to promote erections (injections or a vacuum device) or applying birth control devices, patients can perform return demonstrations. Performance criteria, such as correct placement and use of the device or adaptations for impairments, ensure quality. The effectiveness of birth control methods is evaluated readily by the absence of pregnancy and side effects.

Sexual function outcomes for patients include expressing sexual interest; attaining sexual arousal; sustaining penile/clitoral erection through orgasm; using assistive devices safely; adapting sexual techniques as needed; and being able to perform sexually, despite physical impairments (Johnson et al., 2000). Activity intolerance outcomes are evaluated by physiological signs of tolerance to activity. Outcomes include compensated heart rate, respiratory rate, blood pressure, skin color, and ability to speak while sexually active as signs of increased activity tolerance. Those related to sexual activity are best assessed by the couple in private.

BOX 27-7　Safer Sex Guidelines

- Delay engaging in sexual intercourse as long as possible. Abstinence is the only completely safe behavior for preventing sexually transmitted diseases (STDs) and pregnancy.
- Learn proper use of effective birth control methods and regard abstinence as a best practice for birth control.
- Restrict the number of sexual partners; the fewer sexual partners in a lifetime, the less chance of exposure to any STD.
- A mutually exclusive sexual relationship (sex with only one partner) lowers the risk for STDs. Avoiding body penetration or exchange of body fluids decreases risk of some STDs.
- Be selective when choosing sexual partners; learn as much as possible about them, including their sexual history. Never assume that a woman is automatically in a low-risk group for STDs or that a male partner has never had sex with other men; bisexual behavior occurs among some groups.
- Avoid high-risk sexual behavior until you know with certainty that your partner is not infected with an STD. The most risky behaviors are unprotected anal intercourse and unprotected vaginal intercourse.
- Any activity that exposes a person to blood, semen, vaginal secretions, menstrual blood, urine, feces, or saliva is high-risk behavior, unless partners are in a mutually exclusive sexual relationship and neither is infected. A condom for oral, anal, and/or vaginal sex, with a spermicide containing nonoxynol-9 or octoxynol added for vaginal or anal intercourse, can help to prevent STDs. If engaging in cunnilingus, a barrier in the mouth, such as a dental dam, may add some protection where it covers oral parts.
- Condoms do not provide protection when an infectious area is not covered. For example, a herpes sore on the scrotum would not be covered. Condoms do fail on occasion, creating risk. Natural skin condoms do not protect from the AIDS virus, and oil-based products weaken latex condoms, encouraging breakage.
- Good hygiene, lubrication, and voiding after intercourse decrease some susceptibility to infections.
- Vibrators, dildos, or other items used for sexual stimulation are not shared with others until thoroughly washed with soap and water. Plenty of lubricant and gentle use prevent skin irritation or breakdown of vaginal or rectal tissues.
- Those at risk for STDs need to have regular examinations, including testing, by their health care provider (McCloskey & Bulechek, 2000).

AIDS, Acquired immunodeficiency syndrome.

Outcomes for self-esteem and disturbed body image might include the following: expresses self-esteem, challenges negative images of sexual self, expresses willingness to be sexual, and expresses comfort with body and satisfaction with body appearance.

Relationship factors are evaluated by observing interactions between the patient and partner. Outcomes for sexual functioning that involve relationship factors include the following: expresses ability to be intimate, reports access to consenting partner, expresses respect/acceptance of partner, and expresses knowledge of partner's sexual capabilities (Johnson et al., 2000).

Knowledge outcomes concerning sexual function include identification of body part and understanding physical/emotional changes of puberty and reproduction for younger patients, understanding of physical/emotional changes with aging for older patients, and knowledge of safer sexual practices and cultural influence on sexual behavior. Key outcomes are all related to evaluation of knowledge. Some research exists on physiological function with observations of actual sexual activity, but most knowledge and data have been gathered through communication techniques (Johnson et al., 2000).

IMPLICATIONS FOR PRACTICE

Rehabilitation nursing assessment and interventions during hospitalization are instrumental in identifying sexual problems requiring early intervention, discharge planning, and follow-up, especially because a great deal of adjustment to disability will occur in the community. Problems resolved during the hospitalization with team collaboration lay groundwork for decision making and problem solving at home.

Ideally, rehabilitation facilities, nursing homes, and other residences provide privacy for patients and spouses or partners to experiment with techniques. Facilities, personnel, and patients need to know what is provided and allowable. Visiting for sexual purposes may be possible only in certain areas and where more privacy can be afforded. Weekend passes from the facility or hospital provide patients and partners opportunities to explore sexual options in the privacy of their own home. Time set aside to discuss the weekend experiences and offer additional information is often overlooked but can be a planned method for intervention and evaluation. Staff and visitors tend to disregard common courtesies for persons in hospitals or other residences, taking liberties with privacy and personal effects that would be unacceptable by any standards elsewhere. The patient's right to privacy dictates that all staff members knock on a patient's closed door and wait for permission to enter.

Rehabilitation nurses also need to know community resources and nurses working in various community-based programs including home health care, case management, and specialized programs. Arranging appropriate referrals for patients who require continuing services is part of the team plan. Basic sexuality education and counseling are available from nurses in the community.

Ideally, sexual assessment is part of assessment in all health care settings, and providers are educated to provide information related to sexual health. The relationship-building component must not be neglected when counseling on sexual health. Behavior, self-determination, and self-concept are essential for improving outcomes and topics for research. Information on sexual function incorporated into the basic curricula for health care providers can address interventions and specific suggestions related to sexual function. More research is needed in all areas of sexual function for enhancement, as well as prevention and treatment of STDs.

Education content needs to include evidence from research because information about sexuality has changed over time. For example, the sexual function of persons with SCIs was believed to be related to category of spinal injury (i.e., complete versus incomplete injury) or level of function. Although physiologically true for many activities and abilities, research demonstrates that the ability to experience orgasm is based on the physiology as well as behavioral and relationship issues; a higher percentage of persons experience orgasm than originally believed (Tepper, 1999). What an encouragement to persons with SCIs and a mandate to health professionals to share this information.

Sexual issues are worldwide and affect all persons, including the disabled. Those with impairments are exposed to the negative impact of violence, abusive behavior, STDs, rape, incest, and substance abuse and may be more vulnerable in some situations because of economic, social, or cognitive/behavioral issues. Preventing these negative events is a goal for all persons and a major challenge for the health professional, as well as for societies.

SUMMARY

The ability to function as a sexual being is a basic need of all persons. This need coexists with chronic illness or disability, where sexual concerns may become a major focus. Because sexual concerns are tremendously complex, no simple behavioral or medical approach will suffice to assess or treat individual sexual problems. Ideally a team approach—with members who are comfortable with their own sexuality, knowledgeable about sexuality, and willing to commit a considerable amount of time—is required to plan and implement with the individual experiencing sexual problems.

Rehabilitation nurses frequently deal with patients' sexual problems at their level of comfort, refer to other team members when unable to address the problems expressed, and participate as members of the sexuality management team. It is the responsibility of every rehabilitation nurse to give the patient permission to discuss sexual concerns and then to deal with any expressed difficulties appropriately. Patients should leave rehabilitation settings knowledgeable concerning their sexual function, with their questions answered, and prepared to manage their sexual function independently or direct their partner in the process.

Case Study

Mike was 18 at the time of his spinal cord injury (SCI). He fell from a tree into a swimming pond and fractured his neck at the C5-6 level, resulting in tetraplegia. His rehabilitation program progressed uneventfully, and he was discharged to home, with his parents serving in the caregiver capacity. With much effort, he was able to complete college and accepted a position as a chaplain in the local hospital. Although he had a steady girlfriend throughout high school, their relationship did not withstand the trial of Mike's injury. He did not date in college,

choosing to focus specifically on his college work. Shortly after accepting the position at the hospital, Mike met a nurse. After several dates, Mike brought her home to meet his parents, who were thrilled that he had found a wonderful woman. Mike desired a long-term relationship with her; he wanted to marry her but was concerned about the sexual aspect of their relationship. He had no actual sexual experience. Mike discussed his concerns with his primary care physician, who referred him to a rehabilitation clinical specialist at the hospital.

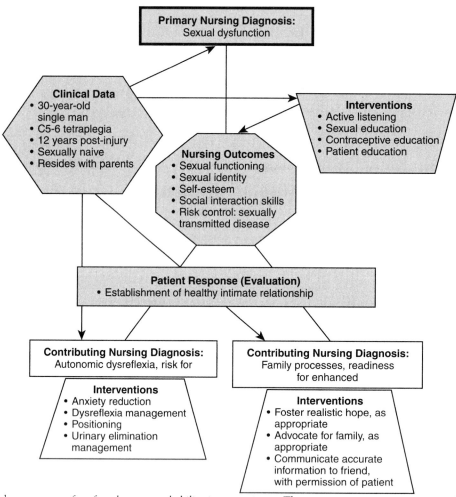

Concept Map. Mike's case occurs far after the acute rehabilitation experience. The concept map portrays nursing diagnoses that revolve around one key issue for Mike, that of establishing initimacy with another individual. The rehabilitation nurse will assist him through working with Mike and his girlfriend in answering questions and assisting them as concerns regarding intimacy develop.

CRITICAL THINKING

1. You are providing a patient with nursing care when the patient reaches out and touches you inappropriately. If the patient is cognitively intact, how would you respond? How would you respond if the patient cognitively could not distinguish cause and effect, and what should your interventions be?

2. The husband of a married couple is no longer cognitively intact due to stroke. What would you assess, and how would you advise the wife on their sexual relationship?

3. Sexual relationships are often linked with morality. If a rehabilitation nurse has a strong belief that a patient's premorbid sexual activities were morally wrong, how should he or she proceed with counseling?

RESOURCES

General

Abstinence education: The SHARE program, provides sexual health and relationship education; http://www.share-program.com/default.htm; 425-284-2945.

AIDS and STD Hotline: Program of the Centers for Disease Control, open 24 hours per day, with multilingual translators to answer questions; 800-342-2437.

American Association for Marriage and Family Therapy: http://www.aamft.org/index_nm.asp.

American Association of Sex Educators, Counselors, and Therapists (AASECT): http://www.aasect.org/ (a list of therapists is available through a searchable map).

American Fertility Society: http://www.theafa.org/.

National Abstinence Clearinghouse: http://www.abstinence.net.

Paralyzed Veterans of America: http://www.pva.org.

RESOLVE, The National Infertility Association: http://www.resolve.org/ (sponsors a help line, publications, and support groups for members).

SIECUS—Sex Information and Education Council of the United States: http://www.siecus.org/.

REFERENCES

Alagiakrishnan, K., Lim, D., Brahim, A., Wong, A., Wood, A, Senthilselvan, A., et al. (2005). Sexually inappropriate behavior in demented elderly people. *Postgraduate Medical Journal, 81*(957), 463-466.

American Heart Association. (2006). *Sexual activity and heart disease or stroke: AHA recommendation.* Retrieved September 30, 2006, from http://www.americanheart.org/presenter.jhtml?identifier=4714.

The American Heritage Dictionary of the English Language (4th ed.). (2000). Houghton Mifflin Company. Available from http://www.eref-trade.hmco.com/.

Annon, J. S. (1976). The PLISSIT model: A proposed conceptual scheme for behavioral treatment of sexual problems. *Journal of Sex Education Therapy, 2,* 1-15.

Araki, C. (2005). Sexuality of aging couples—From women's point of view. *Hinyokika Kiyo, 51*(9), 591-594.

Blackburn, M. (2002). *Sexuality and disability.* Boston: Butterworth and Heinemann.

Brosman, S., & Leslie, S. (2004). Erectile dysfunction. *eMedicine.* Available from http://www.emedicine.com/med/ topic3023.htm.

Burnette, A. L. (1999). Oral pharmacology for erectile dysfunction: Current perspectives. *Urology, 54,* 392-399.

Car, J. (2006). Urinary tract infections in women: Diagnosis and management in primary care. *British Medical Journal, 332*(7533), 94-97.

Cheitlin, M., Hutter, A., Brindis, R., Ganz, P., Kaul, S., Russell, R., et al. (1999). ACC/AHA expert consensus document on use of sildenafil (Viagra) in patients with cardiovascular disease. *Journal of the American College of Cardiology, 33*(1), 273-82

Collins, Y., Einstein, M., Gostout, B., Herzog, T1., Massad, L., Rader, J., et al. (2006). Cervical cancer prevention in the era of prophylactic vaccines: A preview for gynecologic oncologists. *Gynecologic Oncology, 102*(3), 552-562.

Committee on Psychosocial Aspects of Child and Family Health and Committee on Adolescence. (2001). Sexuality education for children and adolescents. *Pediatrics, 108*(2), 498-502.

Coughlin, L. (2006). Practice guidelines: AUA updates guidelines on management of erectile dysfunction. *American Family Physician, 73*(2), 340.

Das, S., Soni, B., Sharma, S., Gazvani, R., & Lewis-Jones, D. (2006). A case of rapid deterioration in sperm quality following spinal cord injury. *Spinal Cord, 44*(1), 56-58.

Dobson, J. (2000, February). Solid answers. *Focus on the Family, 5.*

Doerfler, E. (1999). Male erectile dysfunction: A guide for clinical management. *Journal of the American Academy of Nurse Practitioners, 11*(3), 117-123.

Erectile Dysfunction Guideline Update Panel. (2005). *The management of erectile dysfunction: An update.* Rockville, MD: National Guideline Clearinghouse. Retrieved September 30, 2006, from www.guideline.gov.

Giaquinto, S., Buzzelli, S., DiFrancesco, L, & Nolfe, G. G. (2003). Evaluation of sexual changes after stroke. *Journal of Clinical Psychiatry, 64*(3), 302-307.

Goetz, L., & Stiens, S. (2005). Abdominal electrical stimulation facilitates penile vibratory stimulation for ejaculation after spinal cord injury: A single-subject trial. *Archives of Physical Medicine and Rehabilitation, 86*(9), 1879-1883.

Goodwin, A. J., & Agronin, M. E. (1997). *A woman's guide to overcoming sexual fear and pain.* Oakland, CA: New Harbinger Publications.

Guaderrama, N., Liu, J., Nager, C., Pretorius, D., Sheean, G., Kassab, G., et al. (2005). Evidence for innervation of the pelvic floor muscles by the pudendal nerve. *Obstetrics and Gynecology, 106*(4), 774-781.

Hajjar, R., & Kamel, H. (2003). Sex and the nursing home. *Clinics in Geriatric Medicine, 19*(3), 575-586.

Hill, J. (2004). The impact of rheumatoid arthritis on patients' sex lives. *Nursing Times, 100*(20), 34-35.

Kaufman, M., Silverberg, C., & Odette, F. (2003). *The ultimate guide to sex and disability.* San Francisco: Cleis Press.

Kava, B. (2005). Advances in the management of post-radical prostatectomy erectile dysfunction: Treatment strategies when PDE-5 inhibitors don't work. *Reviews in Urology, 7*(Suppl. 2), S39-S50.

King, B. (2005). *Human sexuality today* (5th ed.). Upper Saddle River, NJ: Pearson Education, Inc.

Korpelainen, J. T., Nieminen, P., & Myllyla, V. V. (1999). Sexual functioning among stroke patients and their spouses. *Stroke, 30,* 715-719.

Kuric, J. (1999). How do I find what I want on the Internet? *SCI Nursing, 16*(4), 137.

Laessoe, L., Nielsen, J., Biering-Sorensen, F., & Sonksen, J. (2004). Antispastic effect of penile vibration in men with spinal cord lesion. *Archives of Physical Medicine and Rehabilitation, 85*(6), 919-1024.

Lue, T. (2000). Erectile dysfunction. *New England Journal of Medicine, 342*(24), 1802-1813.

McCloskey, J. C., & Bulechek, G. M. (Eds.). (2004). *Nursing interventions classification* (4th ed.). St. Louis, MO: Mosby.

McCullough, A. (2002). Four-year review of sildenafil citrate. *Reviews in Urology, 4*(Suppl. 3), S26-S38.

McKenna, K. (2001). Neural circuitry involved in sexual function. *Journal of Spinal Cord Medicine, 24*(3), 148-154.

Moorhead, S., Johnson, M., & Maas, M. (Eds.). (2004). *Nursing outcomes classification* (3rd ed.). St. Louis, MO: Mosby.

Morris, G., & Vanderkolk, C. (2005). Human sexuality, sex hormones and epilepsy. *Epilepsy Behavior, 7*(Suppl. 2), 22-28.

National Information Center for Children and Youth With Disabilities. (1992). *Sexuality education for children and youth with disabilities. Fostering relationships: Suggestions for young adults.* News digest. Washington, DC: Author.

Peck, L. (2006). Sexuality and disability fact sheet. *MossRehab ResourceNet.* Philadelphia: Albert Einstein Healthcare Network.

Pereira, L. (2003). Obstetric management of the patient with spinal cord injury. *Obstetrical & gynecological survey, 58*(10), 678-687.

Pope, C., Markenson, G., Bayer-Zwirello, L., & Maissel, G. (2001). Pregnancy complicated by chronic spinal cord injury and history of autonomic hyperreflexia. *Obstetrics & Gynecology, 97,* 802-803

Sapire, K. (2005). Sex after stroke. *Cardiovascular Journal of South Africa, 16*(Suppl. 2), 21.

Smalley, G., & Trent, J. (2006). *The language of love.* Carol Stream, IL: Tyndale House Publishing.

Society of Obstetricians and Gynaecologists of Canada. (2005). The detection and management of vaginal atrophy. *International Journal of Gynaecology and Obstetrics, 88*(2), 222-228.

Tepper, M. S. (1999). *Attitudes, beliefs, and cognitive processes that impede or facilitate sexual pleasure in people with spinal cord injury.* Unpublished doctoral dissertation. University of Pennsylvania, Philadelphia.

Tomes, H. (2005). Civil rights for people with disabilities. *Monitor on Psychology, 36*(6), 34-62. Available from http://www.apa.org/monitor/jun05/itpi.html.

U.S. Department of Health and Human Services. (2000). *Healthy people 2010.* Washington, DC: Author.

Vignozzi, L, Corona, A., Petrone, L., Filippi, S., Morelli, A., Forti, G., et al. (2005). Testosterone and sexual activity. *Journal of Endocrinological Investigation, 28*(Suppl. 3), 39-44.

Woods, N. F. (1984). *Human sexuality in health and illness* (3rd ed.). St. Louis, MO: Mosby.

Woods, N. F. (1988). Human sexuality: An overview. In P. H. Mitchell, L. C. Hodges, M. Muwases, & C. A. Wallick (Eds.), *Neuroscience nursing* (pp. 459-469). Norwalk, CT: Appleton & Lange.

World Health Organization. (2005). Sexual health—A new focus for WHO. *Progress in Reproductive Health Research, Issue 67,* 2-4.

28

Lifestyle and Recreation

Pamela M. Duchene, DNSc, RN, CRRN

RECREATIONAL, LIFESTYLE, AND DIVERSIONAL ACTIVITY

It is 2 weeks before you are scheduled to take a much-needed vacation to visit California. You have worked at least 56 hours a week each week for the past 2 months. When you are not working, you are attending graduate school classes in an effort to complete the course work for a nurse practitioner certificate. At home the situation is grim. The laundry has accumulated, and although a source of embarrassment, you have resorted to purchasing additional pairs of underwear in an effort to stay the need to do laundry a few more days. It has been at least 2 weeks since you made a trip to the grocery store. The milk in the refrigerator soured about 3 days ago, and you have been using ice cream for your morning and evening coffee.

The day for the start of vacation finally arrives. You finish last-minute packing, slip in a few articles to read during the flight, and board the plane for California. You spend the first 2 days of vacation worrying about work, graduate school, mounting laundry, and other tasks left undone. By day 3, you are able to sleep without setting an alarm clock, and you are able to leave the unfinished articles for review in your carry-on bag for the return trip home. It has taken 3 full days for you to remember how to rest and enjoy leisure time and activities.

Is vacation linked with physical and psychological well-being and health? According to the results of a study of 109 white-collar men and women, vacation can provide recuperation from stress, exhaustion, and sleep deficit (Strauss-Blasche, Reithofer, Schobersberger, Ekmekcioglu, & Marktl, 2005). The researchers noted that a well-planned vacation involving warmer climates tends to result in better recuperation.

The above illustration is one to which many can relate. It is crucial that rehabilitation understand that, as important as lifestyle and recreation are to able-bodied individuals, they are equally important concepts for individuals with disabilities. Chronic illness and disability create changes in abilities for many activities of daily living, including recreational activities. Although acute rehabilitation frequently focuses on regaining function, medical stability, and activities of daily living, successful rehabilitation outcomes are enhanced with an emphasis on a balanced lifestyle, inclusive of recreational and diversional activity.

Consider the example of Sheila Burnham (60 years) of Madison, Mississippi. On a warm January day, with the leaves gone, the sun tucked behind cloud cover, and the landscape a subtle study in taupes and grays, the thrill of the hunt is in Sheila's quick eyes and head-to-toe camouflage. In a wheelchair since a 1992 accident, Sheila took to the sport after her injury. "It's a de-stressor, sitting out in the woods—it is my God time," she said. Her brother and father hunted, and through the years she listened to their adventures. Sheila was a natural and quickly excelled in the sport. She was invited to hunts in Mississippi and Alabama and as far away as North Dakota, Wyoming, and Minnesota.

Sheila, a former English teacher and retired insurance adjuster, has worked with outdoor and hunter education programs in Mississippi and Alabama. An advocate for hunters with disabilities, she emphasizes safety, promotes awareness, and addresses accessibility issues. Always teaching, motivating, encouraging, and continuing to learn, Sheila has helped pave the way and opened up the great outdoors for hunters with disability in the state of Mississippi—available funding for hunts, adaptable equipment, knowledgeable personnel, accessible hunting sites, and the satisfaction of hunting once again.

In 2005 Sheila was the first-ever female recipient of Safari Club International's Pathfinder Award, which honors physically challenged hunters. The award came with a 10-day hunt in South Africa in September 2005. She always has a positive attitude and commonly says, "I take pause at anyone labeled 'disabled.' I don't know of anyone who is completely disabled. I like to use the term 'differently able,'" (G. Boydston, personal communication, 2006). This chapter will provide a discussion of recreational, lifestyle, and diversional activity and the significance to rehabilitation of individuals with disability.

OVERVIEW OF RECREATIONAL, LIFESTYLE, AND DIVERSIONAL ACTIVITY

In order to gain an understanding of the need for recreational and diversional activity, it is helpful to look at situations in which such activities are notably absent. The question of a link between the "joyless striving" of the type A personality and cardiac disease has existed since the mid-nineteenth century (Januzzi, Stern, Pasternak, & DeSanctis, 2000). In 1910 Sir William Osler noted that the individual with angina pectoris is frequently a worrier and "a man whose engine is always set full speed ahead" (Larkins, 2000). The type A personality is characterized by hostility, aggressiveness, and a perpetual sense of urgency and is linked with an increased risk of cardiovascular disease (Trigo, Silva, & Rocha, 2005). Studies to reduce cardiovascular risks through stress reduction indicate that including stress reduction programs may positively affect morbidity and mortality (Saner, 2005).

Stress reduction and physical activity are linked with positive health and well-being. Benefits of physical activity are correlated with positive health impact; however, the effect may be influenced by the type of physical activity. In one study involving patients with chronic back pain, routine back exercises were linked with increased pain, whereas recreational exercise resulted in physical improvement (Hurwitz, Morgenstern, & Chiao, 2005). For those unable to participate in recreational physical exercise, alternative methods of simulating the exercise experience have been noted to positively affect risk factors.

In addition to the research findings identified above, recreational activities have a significant impact on the well-being of individuals with physical impairment and disability. Therapeutic recreational activities are linked with the outcomes indicated in Box 28-1. Through therapeutic interventions including recreational, leisure, and diversional activities, the physical, emotional, cognitive, and social functioning of individuals may be enhanced. Such therapeutic interventions include the environment and support systems of individuals and focus on maximizing physical and psychosocial well-being. Activities are structured around specific goals targeting improved independence, function, and symptom reduction.

Participation in recreational physical activities result in enhanced cardiovascular and respiratory function, in addition to improved coordination, strength, and endurance (Duncan et al., 2005). These improvements affect those who are able bodied, as well as those with physical disabilities and chronic illness (Karason, Lindroos, Stenlöf, & Sjöström, 2000). Related to the improvements in cardiopulmonary status, secondary medical complications that are associated with spinal cord injury and chronic illnesses are reduced through recreational physical activities (Wannamethee, Shaper, & Alberti, 2000). Specifically, complications such as pressure ulcers and urinary tract infections are less common in those participating in recreational physical activities. Health risk factors, including cholesterol and blood sugar levels, are improved through recreational physical activities. In a study comparing the use of omega-3 supplementation with regular exercise, researchers found that the combination of omega-3 with exercise resulted in lowering of low-density lipoprotein (LDL) level and raising of high-density lipoprotein (HDL) level, combined with a 5% loss of body fat (Hill et al., 2005). Memory, attention, organizational skills, and perception may be enhanced through participation in recreational activities. In addition, depression may be decreased and body image enhanced through recreational exercise and lifestyle activity.

Leisure is, of course, more than just exercise and physical activity. The pursuit of leisure activities counteracts boredom. Whether reading, playing a video game, watching a great movie, or playing a game of cards, leisure activities keep the mind active while promoting stimulation, interaction, and problem solving. Because leisure activities and the balance between recreation and work impact an individual's well-being and outcome, nurses need to be cognizant of premorbid and postmorbid activities and abilities.

THE ROLE OF NURSES IN RECREATIONAL, LIFESTYLE, AND DIVERSIONAL ACTIVITY

Regardless of the setting in which the rehabilitation nurse practices, nursing care tends to revolve around implementation of the plan of care and often is focused on physical needs and treatments. Rehabilitation nurses have a clear and necessary role in therapeutic recreation activities. Such activities are often designed and coordinated by therapeutic recreation specialists. A specific role within the rehabilitation team, therapeutic recreation specialists use activities in creative ways to foster physical, cognitive, social, and emotional independence. In many facilities, therapeutic recreation specialists design outings, such as theater attendance or visits to ballparks, and work with the other members of the team to meet therapeutic goals. Through encountering architectural barriers during a therapeutic outing, patients have an opportunity to learn independence while remaining in the rehabilitation program. Often the nursing role in outings focuses on the need for safety.

BOX 28-1 Outcomes of Recreational Therapy

- Improvement in physical, social, cognitive, and emotional function
- Enhanced functional independence and improved quality of life
- Prevention of physical, cognitive, and psychosocial functional declines
- Reduction of secondary disability and prevention of increased health care costs

Modified from Coyle, C., Kinney, W., Riley, B., & Shank, J. (Eds.). (1998). *Benefits of therapeutic recreation: A consensus view.* Ravensdale, WA: Idyll Arbor, Inc.

For example, during a therapeutic outing, nurses may accompany the patients to ensure their physical needs are met and to provide assistance should a medical complication develop.

Rehabilitation nurses can be involved in promoting access and encouraging participation in recreational activity, in addition to ensuring safety. Nurses are in a unique place to foster participation and involvement. As an example, in one rehabilitation center the therapeutic recreation specialist for the spinal injury program continually ran into difficulty with evening activities because of competition from scheduled bowel programs. The timing of the programs was done for staffing convenience, rather than patient request of need. Collaboration with the nurses resulted in a modification of the program to allow those interested in evening activities to move their programs to later in the evening or night. Because it is unlikely that young individuals with spinal cord injury will opt for a bowel program over a trip to a baseball game or the movies, this change was perceived positively by all involved.

Whether in a hospital, long-term care, or home health care setting, nurses have a key role in promoting participation in activities. Social activities and recreational events facilitate interaction and counteract boredom. Nurses are in positions where they may be first to identify signs and symptoms of boredom and depression. Individuals with devastating diseases, threatening prognoses, and altered lifestyles are faced with overwhelming reasons for discouragement. Nurses have the privilege of caring for patients during their most intimate and vulnerable times. Adding the tools of recreation to the existing nursing interventions may make a difference in the ultimate patient outcome. To intervene in boredom and provide an opportunity for diversional activity, in one rehabilitation unit the unit advisory committee (a shared governance committee composed of nurses, assistants, and therapists) designs celebrations throughout each month. Some of the celebrations have included school days, where the therapists, nurses, assistants, and physicians brought in old school photos. Patients, visitors, and staff members were encouraged to identify the staff member in the photo. The staff had a celebration and party to disclose the identities of the individuals in the photos. Patients were involved in designing the party and of course participated in the event.

The inclusion of recreation and diversion as components of nursing care can be simple and easy to initiate. For example, in an oncology rehabilitation unit the evening charge nurse purchased margarita glasses for evening medications. With the traditional evening medications, she passed out margarita glasses filled with sparkling cranberry juice or diet ginger ale. Patients looked forward to the evening medication pass, simply because they never knew what crazy stunt she would plan next. With one of the patients who had particular issues with constipation, she blew up balloons and broke open the sparkling cider when the bowel program worked successfully. Photos of the party were taken and posted at the nursing station. When asked about the cause of the party, the nurse responded, "John's program worked—and we needed to celebrate!"

Too often, recreation and diversion are viewed as the responsibility of the therapeutic recreation specialist. Incorporating activities into the nursing plan actually saves nursing time. As an example, on a small rehabilitation unit the nursing assistants organized evening activities, which included a different event each evening. The activities are simple to design—movies, bingo, and games. Two nursing assistants run the activity program each evening following the dinner meal. Family members are encouraged to attend the activity program. Call light usage during the activity time is virtually absent. Evening medications are passed during the activity, requiring less walking time for each nurse because the patients are located in one central area. Patients not involved in the activity are offered a book or video in their rooms to encourage some diversional activity time and promote rest for the next full day of therapy.

There are activities for all interests. BlazeSports is a national program designed to ensure all children and adults with disabilities have access to sports of their liking (http://www.blazesports.com). With core sports in basketball, rugby, swimming, track and field, and tennis, BlazeSports offers many options and provides links to other sports such as hiking, fishing, and golf. Another resource for individuals with disabilities is the Society for Accessible Travel & Hospitality (SATH). SATH (http://www.SATH.org) provides links to travel agents that will guide individuals through the maze of preparing for trips while avoiding environmental barriers. In addition to providing a list of all major airlines and a review of accessibility, SATH provides tips for travelers when planning a trip by air, ship, or train. For those with interests such as hunting, the Buckmasters American Deer Foundation (www.badf.org) provides support and resources to individuals with disabilities who have interest in hunting. Refer to Box 28-2 for a listing of web resources for travel, leisure, and diversional activities.

FACTORS AFFECTING RECREATIONAL, LIFESTYLE, AND DIVERSIONAL ACTIVITY

Although aspects of physical disability and chronic illness may impact *how* one participates in recreational and leisure activities, *whether or not* one participates is the result of inclusion and accessibility more than a restriction imposed by physical limitations. For example, a man who enjoyed golfing before a stroke should be able to participate in the sport after the illness. If, however, his friends perceive him as disabled and unable to participate or believe that he will be embarrassed by the limitations imposed by the stroke, they may opt to not include him in outings.

Inclusion

The philosophy of inclusion holds that individuals with and without physical disabilities and chronic illnesses should

---

BOX 28-2 Web Resources for Leisure, Travel, and Recreation

http://www.badf.org/	Buckmasters American Deer Foundation: Provides tips on accessible hunting, an overview of national and local regulations on hunting with disability, and resources for hunters with disabilities.
http://fhnbinc.org/	Fishing Has No Boundaries, Inc.: Provides information on adaptive equipment for individuals with disabilities who have an interest in fishing. Sponsor events for anglers with disabilities.
http://www.activeamp.org/	Provides information on adaptive equipment, resources, and tips for individuals with amputation who are interested in archery.
http://www.ableproject.org/	Information on mobility, adaptive and assistive products for individuals with disabilities.
http://www.aquaticaccess.com/	Aquatic Access Inc.: information on pool lifts and adaptive equipment for inground and above-ground pools.
http://www.sitski.com/	Features extreme adaptive sports with inspirational video clips of athletes.
http://www.abilityplus.org/	Sponsors accessible events, including ski trips, day camps, bike trips, and golfing for New England.
http://www.windsurf.org/	AccesSportAmerica provides access to water sports including windsurfing.
http://www.mankatoleep.org/	Leisure Education for Exceptional People: According to LEEP, recreation has no limits. Offers recreational events for individuals with disabilities in Minnesota.
http://www.usolympicteam.com/paralympics/	Official site for the U.S. Paralympics.
http://www.nps.gov/	Website for the National Park System. From this website, links are available to all national parks, each of which describes accessibility within the parks.
http://www.blazesports.com	National program to ensure individuals with disabilities have access to sports.
http://www.SATH.org	Provides links to travel agents to guide individuals in preparing for trips.

participate in activities together. The perception of limitation should not interfere with an invitation to participate in an event. Rehabilitation professionals must understand that it is better to make the error of assuming an individual will want to participate in an event than to fail to invite the individual. Many individuals have painful memories of being the last individual selected for a team. The failure to include an individual in an event is far worse than simply being selected late.

According to the National Center on Accessibility (2005), there are three levels of inclusion. A person's right to access is considered *physical integration*. The Americans With Disabilities Act ensures that all buildings receiving federal funding are accessible. Individuals with disabilities must by law be able to enter such facilities. This is only the first step in inclusion. The implementation of a ramp or elevator provides physical integration for some facilities. The second step is *functional inclusion*, which describes the ability of individuals to enjoy a recreational event equally regardless of a disability. The National Park Service provides information on the accessibility of areas within the parks and ensures that the trails and hiking paths indicate levels of accessibility available. Although not all areas may be accessible, many of the parks provide a ranger service to ensure that individuals with disabilities are able to fully enjoy the park experience. The third step in inclusion is perhaps the most salient and most difficult to achieve (Figure 28-1). *Social inclusion* describes the individual's ability to gain social acceptance during recreational activities. Although physical integration and functional inclusion are mandated through the Americans With Disabilities Act, it is not possible to legislate social inclusion. For example, public

schools struggle with the philosophy of inclusion for children with physical and intellectual disabilities. Although classrooms may be modified, it is difficult to alter attitudes and perceptions of teachers and other students (Swain & Cook, 2001). Although the child with a disability is a member of the classroom (physical integration), and all activities are developed to enable the child's participation (functional inclusion), the child may not be invited to birthday parties or other out-of-school events (social inclusion). Awareness of the need for inclusion is the key to correcting the problem. Students' response in one church outing shows a positive example of inclusion. One of the adolescent girls is a dwarf with Ellis-Van Creveld syndrome, or chondroectodermal dysplasia. She participated in a recent trip to a theme park and was excluded from many of the rides because of height restrictions. The other adolescents tried to assist her by stuffing her shoes to increase her height. The small increases were not sufficient, and the adolescents banded together and uniformly boycotted the rides. The attempts, although unsuccessful in gaining her access to the rides, were highly successful in promoting her inclusion within the group (social inclusion).

Accessibility

According to the Centers for Disease Control and Prevention (CDC), there are an estimated 54 million individuals in the United States who report a disabling condition (CDC, 2000). Given such a high prevalence, it is common to see individuals with disabilities in all settings. In fact, if individuals with disabilities are not evident in a public area, it is likely due to problems with access rather than interest. For example, the

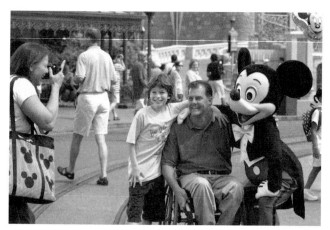

Figure 28-1 Many recreational facilities have made considerable efforts to accommodate guests with disabilities. (Photo courtesy © Disney Enterprises, Inc.)

absence of accessible trails limits the ability of individuals with disabilities to visit parks and conservation areas. When problems of accessibility are corrected, it is evident that individuals with disabilities have the same interests in recreational and diversional activities as able-bodied individuals (Figure 28-2).

Therapeutic recreation specialists work to design "ways around physical limitations" to enable individuals with physical disabilities and chronic illness to participate in recreational and leisure activities. In Jackson, Mississippi, one therapeutic recreation specialist, Ginny Boydston (personal communication, December, 30, 2005), has devoted her career to creating opportunities for individuals with significant physical disabilities to participate in sports activities. She offers a scuba program for individuals with quadriplegia. After participants have passed an initial training program at the local pool, she takes them to the Gulf of Mexico for actual diving experiences. Ginny has developed a program known as "Victory Sports" for racing, basketball, and other team types of activities for individuals with spinal cord injury. She coaches the team, Jackson Jags, a rugby team similar to the team featured in the film *Murderball* (Rubin & Shapiro, 2005), which was the winner of Best Documentary at the 2005 Sundance Film Festival. In addition, she offers sports clinics throughout the state of Mississippi for individuals with significant physical limitations. The clinics include water skiing and bowling. Ginny's efforts provide proof that the extent of physical limitation need not interfere with participation in recreational and leisure activities (Figure 28-3). She has noted patients have increased self-esteem, body image, and social interaction as results of the unique sports clinics.

NURSING DIAGNOSIS: DEFICIENT DIVERSIONAL ACTIVITY

Deficits in diversional activities may occur as a result of variety of factors. Nursing assessment should include a review of the individual's likes and dislikes with respect to activities and lifestyle interests. An individual who routinely refuses to join the afternoon bingo game may simply not enjoy bingo. Not all individuals enjoy arts, crafts, or movies. In the rehabilitation setting the more diverse the activities and leisure opportunities, the more likely that some activity will appeal to most individuals. Arts, crafts, and cooking are popular activities because they convey a sense of accomplishment, and many individuals find the activities relaxing with easy opportunities for socialization, fine motor exercise, and hobby development (Dixon, 2005).

In addition to assessing likes and dislikes, the nurse designing a therapeutic recreation program should assess energy and endurance levels. Individuals who are tired from a full day of therapy may not have an interest in an evening movie or game. Assessing the individual's exercise tolerance and the impact on cardiopulmonary function will be helpful. The therapeutic recreation program should be designed to accommodate changes in exercise tolerance, muscular fitness, and range-of-motion limitations (Petajan & White, 2000).

Assessment

Assessment of individual strengths and limitations in leisure, play, and recreation are part of a comprehensive rehabilitation nursing assessment. The rehabilitation nurse considers cultural and age-related information in completing the assessment. In addition to assessing the patient's occupational interests and concerns, the nurse assesses how the patient spends leisure and recreational time. Understanding the patient's interests enables the nurse to connect with the patient and to ensure that the plan of care developed meets the patient's individual needs.

Past behaviors are often the best indicators of future actions. Because this adage applies to recreation and leisure as it does to other aspects of life, the rehabilitation nurse collaborates with the therapeutic recreation specialist to identify possible options for recreational, diversional, and leisure activities. Factors that are included in the assessment include attention span, motor and sensory skills, social and comprehension skills, and coping skills. Does the patient's attention span exclude some activities or events? If so, what techniques are effective in motivation and redirection? Does the patient have limitations of fine or gross motor skills that will impact recreation or leisure? Is the patient able to communicate? What is the patient's level of comfort in social situations? If the patient was shy before the injury or illness, it is unlikely he will be comfortable in social interactions. Such information should be used to plan optimal recreational and leisure activities for patients (City of Eden Prairie, 2006).

Plan/Intervention

Rehabilitation nurses collaborate with therapeutic recreation specialists and other therapists in designing a plan for recreation and leisure time that meets the patient's needs. After they review the patient's likes and dislikes, past activities, and any needed modifications, recreational activities are incorporated into the plan of care.

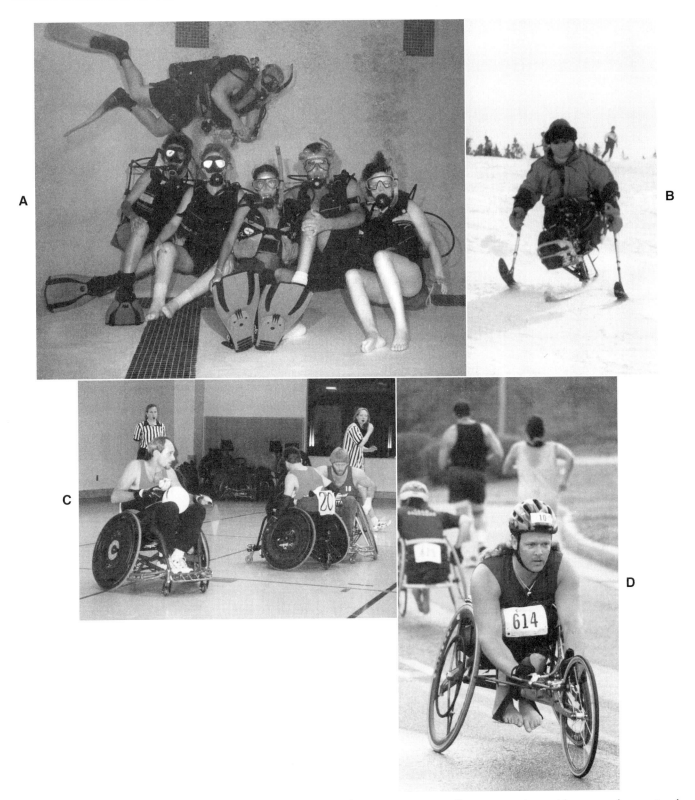

Figure 28-2 A to D, Patients with chronic illnesses and physical impairments can still participate in a wide range of recreational activities. (**A,** Reproduced with permission of Ginny Boydston, Jackson, MS. **D,** © Greg Campbell Photography, Jackson, MS.)

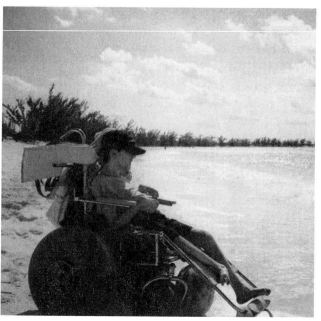

Figure 28-3 A. J. Swanson enjoys the beach, thanks to a beach wheelchair. Many recreational facilities have made considerable efforts to accomodate guests with disabilities. (Photo used with permission.)

Rehabilitation nurses use creativity to implement optimal recreational and leisure plans. For example, the patient who was an avid reader before a stroke can listen to books on tape, if the stroke has resulted in acquired dyslexia. The patient who enjoyed gardening before an injury can continue to work with plants in an area on the unit.

Evaluation

Evaluation of the plan for recreation and leisure is done with patients in determining if the plan meets their needs and if they are able to tolerate and enjoy the activity. Does the activity fit within the patient's lifestyle? Does the patient enjoy the activity? Refer to Box 28-1 for a list of therapeutic recreation outcomes. These can be incorporated into the evaluation of a plan for therapeutic recreation.

Is the patient improving in physical, social, cognitive, or emotional function through participation in the activity or plan? Is there improvement in functional independence or quality of life? Does the activity or plan show promise for preventing physical, cognitive, or psychosocial functional declines?

SUMMARY

Lifestyle and recreation are activities essential for life satisfaction, yet both tend to be overlooked by nurses as "nonessential" or extracurricular in nature and therefore not critical to an individual's functional outcome. Rehabilitation nurses must recognize the key element that lifestyle and recreation play in recovery and rehabilitation from illness and disability. Input and involvement from the patient are key to development of an optimal therapeutic recreation plan. Through attention to recreational and lifestyle activities, individuals may have the drive to regain function and to return to lives filled with adventure, excitement, and fun.

Case Study

Joe, 42, was diagnosed with amyotrophic lateral sclerosis in 1997. He is able to reside at home through home health care nursing, personal attendants, and a dedicated, caring, and supportive extended family. Joe's physical limitations have progressed to the point that he has a tracheostomy and respiratory assistance and uses a power chair for mobility. His voluntary muscle control is limited to flexion and extension of the index finger of his right hand. Joe's quality of life is linked with his involvement with his family and with his ability to remain current in news events and reading.

Through extensive modification of the living environment and the installation of an environmental control unit, Joe is able to use the limited range of his index finger to control the world around him.

Of most significance to him, however, through the use of his single digit, Joe is able to access a control switch to run the computer system for leisure and recreation. Although the computer system does not provide Joe with physical exercise, it facilitates recreation and allows his mind to continue to stretch and grow. This is critical to Joe's position as professor of information technology at the University of Massachusetts. Computers have long been his life, and continued access is essential for leisure and for his vocation.

With the progression of his illness, Joe's goals shifted to the use of technology for recreation and leisure and to continue to participate in his children's lives as long as possible.

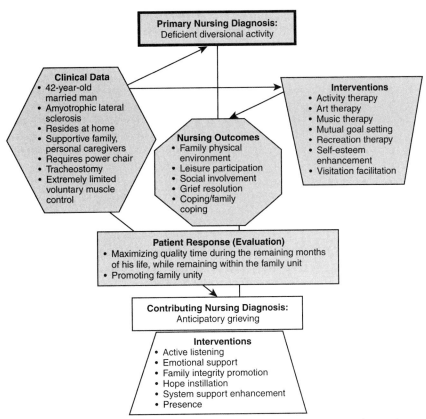

Concept Map. The trajectory of Joe's illness is such that the rehabilitation nurse must focus on quality in the present, with an awareness of the future needs of the family. Focusing on diversional activity is logical, because many family memories of strong family times can be developed through such activities. Focusing on both diversional activity and anticipatory grieving should allow the rehabilitation nurse to maximize Joe's remaining months of life.

CRITICAL THINKING

1. What are three ways of facilitating recreation in a home health care environment?

2. Identify two programs to encourage social interaction within an inpatient rehabilitation program.

3. Recreational activities are not generally considered reimbursable; however, if combined with therapeutic activities and individualized goals, the activity may be considered a therapy session. Identify therapeutic goals that might be met through a trip to a local restaurant.

REFERENCES

Centers for Disease Control and Prevention. (2000). State specific prevalence of disability among adults—11 states and the District of Columbia. *MMWR, 49*(31), 711-714.

City of Eden Prairie. (2006). *Therapeutic recreation.* Eden Prairie, MN: Author. Retrieved September 4, 2006, from http://www.edenprairie.org/.

Coyle, C., Kinney, W., Riley, B., & Shank, J. (Eds.). (1998). *Benefits of therapeutic recreation: A consensus view.* Ravensdale, WA: Idyll Arbor, Inc.

Dixon, C. (2005). *Therapeutic recreation activities and treatment ideas: Arts and crafts.* Available from http://www.recreationtherapy.com.

Duncan, G., Anton, S., Sydeman, S., Newton, R., Corsica, J., Durning, P., et al. (2005). Prescribing exercise at varied levels of intensity and frequency: A randomized trial. *Archives of Internal Medicine, 165*(20), 2362-2369.

Hill, A., Buckley, J., Murphy, K., Saint, D., Morris, A., & Howe, P. (2005). Combined effects of omega-3 supplementation and regular exercise on body composition and cardiovascular risk factors. *Asia Pacific Journal of Clinical Nutrition, 14*(Suppl.), S57.

Hurwitz, E., Morgenstern, H., & Chiao, C. (2005). Effects of recreational physical activity and back exercises on low back pain and psychological distress: Findings from the UCLA low back pain study. *American Journal of Public Health, 95*(10), 1817-1824.

Januzzi, J., Stern, T., Pasternak, R., & DeSanctis, R. (2000). The influence of anxiety and depression on outcomes of patients with coronary artery disease. *Archives of Internal Medicine, 160*, 1913-1921.

Karason, K., Lindroos, A., Stenlöf, K., & Sjöström, L. (2000). Relief of cardiorespiratory symptoms and increased physical activity after surgically induced weight loss. *Archives of Internal Medicine, 160*, 1979-1802.

Larkins, R. (2000). A great life in medicine. *Lancet, 9206*, 852-856.

National Center on Accessibility. (2005). Best practice of inclusive services: The value of inclusion. *Access Today, 19.* Bloomington, IN: Author. Retrieved September 4, 2006, from http://www.ncaonline.org/monographs/19inclusion.shtml.

Petajan, J., & White, A. (2000). Tailored physical activity programmes beneficial for patients with multiple sclerosis. *Drug and Therapeutic Perspectives, 15*, 7-9.

Rubin, H., & Shapiro, D. (Directors). (2005). *Murderball* [Motion picture]. United States: ThinkFilm Company.

Saner, H. (2005). Stress as a cardiovascular factor. *Therapeutische Umschau. Revue thérapeutique, 62*(9), 597-602.

Strauss-Blasche, G., Reithofer, B., Schobersberger, W., Ekmekcioglu, C., & Marktl, W. (2005). Effect of vacation on health: Moderating factors of vacation outcome. *Journal of Travel Medicine, 12*(2), 94-101.

Swain, J., & Cook, T. (2001). In the name of inclusion: 'We all, at the end of the day, have the needs of the children at heart.' *Critical Social Policy, 21*(2), 185-207.

Trigo, M., Silva, D., & Rocha, E. (2005). Psychosocial risk factors in coronary heart disease: Beyond type A behavior. *Revista Portuguesa de Cardiologia, 24*(2), 261-281.

Wannamethee, S., Shaper, A., & Alberti, K. (2000). Physical activity, metabolic factors, and the incidence of coronary heart disease and type 2 diabetes. *Archives of Internal Medicine, 160*, 2108-2116.

29

Spirituality

Darlene N. Finocchiaro, MSN, RN, CRRN, PN

Nurses have an ethical responsibility to consider a patient's value system and religious beliefs when establishing a plan of care (American Nurses Association, 2001). A comprehensive plan includes helping patients recognize and manage their spiritual needs. Nurses may be uncertain of their roles with spirituality and pay more attention to immediate realities of physical care than on reflection. When assessing religious preferences and practices, they may ignore spirituality. Experts cannot agree upon a definition of "spiritual," much less differentiating between spirit and soul. Rehabilitation nurses practice holistically and may affect a patient's spiritual quality of life.

HOLISM AND PARADIGM SHIFTS

Florence Nightingale originated the scientific, professional perspective in nursing as a practical art (Macrae, 1995). Her spiritual beliefs that all creativity, insight, and sense of purpose were evidence of divine intelligence and a potent resource for healing shaped her programs. "Nurses were to be handmaidens of God and to emulate Jesus Christ in their work" (Grypma, 2005). A nurse's white "cap," worn until the 1980s, was a modification of the veil favored by women in religious orders; it symbolized service, humility, and love (Donohue, 1985).

Conventional medicine, based on empirical science, ignored spirituality in the health paradigm until recently. Now medicine and nursing have revisited the mind/body/spirit interaction and its role in health. The result is a broader perspective and a new paradigm shift (Barnum, 2003). Holistic theory originated in physics (von Bertalanffy's general system theory in 1955), with parallel developments in the biological, behavioral, and social sciences, opening a previously mechanistic world to sets of integrated systems. In 1926, Jan Christian Smuts coined the word *holism* to refer to a concept of "wholeness."

Laszlo (1972) identified humans as self-contained living systems, challenging Descartes' notion of the body as a machine,

isolated from the mind/soul. Holism is *not* "New Age" or mechanistic reductionism and not the same as alternative/complementary approaches. Holism is to understand the whole person in the context of his or her total environment and to consider the impact of multiple sources of causality (Vash, 1994). By definition, "nursing is not medicine" (Rosenberg, 1998). Nurses embrace conventional medicine and incorporate physical, psychological, social, and environmental factors to enhance health, emphasize prevention, and encourage patients to participate in decision making and self-care. They can encourage patients to interact with their environments and a higher being for well-being and health, realizing the system has intimately interconnected parts. Figure 29-1 illustrates the model.

Longway's "Circuit of Wholeness" (1970) was the first theory based on spirituality and God as a power source. Nursing theorists advanced disparate views of holism and incorporated the concept of soul into theory. Newman (1986) viewed disease as opportunity for expanding consciousness, her notion of spirituality, and with the shock of illness or injury a patient must repattern for health. Watson (1988) focused on a mental-spiritual-nursing role, with the body as access; disease is, or gives, disharmony. Dossey & Guzzetta (2000) defined the bio-psycho-social-spiritual person as an integrated, interconnected system. Disease is a blockade to life stage progression, and the mind is a tool for healing. They combined the *"doing/being"* therapies with the mechanisms of conventional medicine.

SPIRITUAL CARE CONCEPTS

Soul, Spirit, and Spirituality

The *soul* is the depth and inner-self helper interpreting life's relationships, pleasures, pains, emotions. Although rational or intellective, it lacks composition. The three powers of the soul are memory, understanding, and will. Karasu (1999) differentiated the soul from the spirit. It is the inner-man (conscience),

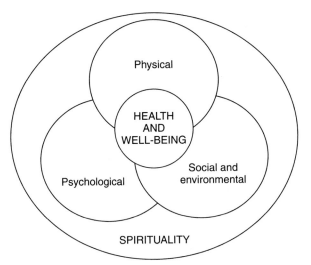

Figure 29-1 A model for incorporating spirituality into holistic biopsychosocial health.

the place of connection with God from within, a symbol with religious tones, and the point of contact with intuitive, even miraculous experiences (Hillman, 1972). Secular language speaks to an intensity of something called soul; "living or singing with all their soul." Christians believe God creates each soul and it endures after death (Stravinskas, 1991). Watson, the only nursing theorist to conceptualize the soul, defined the spirit, inner-self, and soul interchangeably. The mind and emotions are windows to the soul, not confined by the physical universe. The body, mind, and soul are interconnected into the whole person (Tomey & Alligood, 1998).

Spirit is essence of being and is to the soul what blood is to the body (Karasu, 1999). Spirit breathes, pervading and integrating the system, and is a repository of morality, energy, force, and life-giving power. It is inseparable from the body, intangible; its presence is obvious even though it cannot be observed (Buchholz & Schwartz, 2004).

Spirituality is an individual paradigm, dynamic and constant, with an activating force, which can be (the person's) God (Delaney, 2005). It may or may not be associated with religion, which is an organized set of holy traditions, rituals, beliefs, values, and practices from a doctrine of faith. Relationships with transcendence or God, with other persons (spouse), with nature, and life events (helping, career, sports), and the context in which a person views his or her place in the universe reflects how a person views self, God, and others. It is a connectedness within oneself, a relationship with a higher being, God or universe (Reed, 1992). Stoll (1989) stated "spirituality is my being, my inner person ... it is me expressed through my body, my thinking, my being, my judgments, my creativity ... I respond to and appreciate God, other people, a sunset." Spirituality is a quality that invokes a need to transcend the self in a way that is empowering, not devaluing to the individual (Sherwood, 2000). The greater the degree of spirituality, the more it influences life and health. Impaired spirituality ("dis-spiriting") is manifested by physical or

psychosocial disquietude. Figure 29-1 shows spirituality may be affected by multiple factors.

Spiritual Crisis

A spiritual crisis occurs when a person of faith no longer feels God is present; the connection is broken. "God, the rock of a person's life is suddenly gone" (Penson et al., 2001), and problems extend beyond their capacity to cope. Patients and families need to make sense of their circumstances and to find meaning in daily events, relationships, and life. Mild concerns or anxiety, discouragement, or anticipatory grief can escalate to distress manifested by crying, silence, expressed guilt, sleep pattern disturbances, anger, and increasing anxiety. Without intervention, the situation may lead to despair and a patient might exhibit psychotic behavior or depression. Enhanced, inclusive spiritual support is a patient's right; care that considers the patient's personal dignity and respects the patient's values as he or she works toward spiritual well-being (Sumner, 1998). Also consult Chapter 22.

FACTORS INFLUENCING SPIRITUAL CARE

Religions, Cultures, and Care

Whether consciously, or unconsciously, many persons only acknowledge their spiritual relationship with or dependency on God when faced with illness or incapacity. Surveys and in-depth studies report greater impact and intensity of spiritual experience when a person is under stress related to illness or trauma; a major trauma may draw a patient closer to God. Or it may lead to alienation, where the patient feels abandoned, "Where is God when I need Him most?" (O'Brien, 2003), or believes the injury is God's punishment. Gathering data about a patient's religious affiliation is *insufficient* to understand how beliefs, practices, and attitudes may influence responses to illness or disability, but it is a starting place.

Many patients are without spiritual services or are unable to access them and cannot participate fully within their faith communities. Too often religious organizations have inadequate knowledge about persons with disabilities, hold conflicting worldviews about illness and disability, or show dissonance between their ideals and practices. People of many faiths consider suffering a product of wrongdoing or failure to perform some action. Patients from differing cultures will have their own explanations for suffering, loss, or disability. Recognizing patterns of behavior without relying on stereotypes increases a nurse's cultural competences. The nursing literature references many guides that detail specific cultural and religious beliefs; refer to Chapter 6 for more information about culture and health systems.

Patients may respond more openly to a nurse who offers opportunities for discussions about beliefs and practices and who asks perceptive questions indicating an awareness and respect. A patient's education, economic status, length of time in the dominant culture, and personal goals are factors in care.

Nurses may have regularly planned events or contacts with religious leaders who serve as professional resources when a patient goes home. A spiritual leader can lend insight to rehabilitation team members and help them form therapeutic liaisons within the religious community. Spiritual interventions will vary according to cultures of both patient and nurse. At no time are professionals required to abdicate their own beliefs, and likewise they cannot impose their beliefs on patients, which would raise ethical questions.

Health Services and Parish Nursing

Parish nursing is a concept of working with faith communities to deliver holistic health care nursing. Religious communities and organizations can help change attitudes and often provide care to members. Parish nursing is embraced by some cultural groups who associate spirituality with healing through prayer and rituals. Nurses may work with one or a group of parishes, or collaborate with various community health agencies. In addition to self-care programs and preventive care, parish nurses use many rehabilitation principles. Some rehabilitation facilities offer ecumenical prayer groups for patients who already share goals and therapies in rehabilitation. A goal is to foster self-esteem, mutual support, and prayer.

The Health Ministries Association developed standards for parish nursing as an advanced practice professional role. Parish nurses serve by advocating, outreaching, teaching (patients and volunteers), listening, counseling, referring, empathizing, and praying. They can spearhead services, such as home visitation and respite and peer counseling programs. They do not provide home health care services or perform invasive nursing procedures but work collegially with agencies. Not every function is spiritual; they collaborate with clergy to establish programs for health promotion, education about chronic health problems, and information about impairment and healing from a more spiritual viewpoint (Easton & Andrews, 2000).

Perceptions of Pain and Suffering

Pain is physical, and suffering is mental; both are part of human life and caring. Pain signals that the body is in danger, whereas suffering is the state of severe distress associated with events that threaten the intactness of a person: the strain of trying to endure, the alienation of forced exclusion from everyday life, the shock of institutionalization, and the uncertainty of anticipating the ramifications of disability (Hinds, 1993). Foley (1988) reviewed the various meanings for suffering found in our society and categorized them into 11 "interpretations of suffering" (Box 29-1). Suffering and its meaning are personally owned. As suffering intensifies, the person begins to feel anguish that becomes so deep that it affects the mind and body; envisioning a normal life seems impossible.

"Why do good people suffer?" Only a spiritual answer satisfies because a secular response is random chance and the question can never really be answered. Christians view suffering as part of this earthly life but may use it to God's glory. Response to suffering is compassion and keeping faith; once a

---

BOX 29-1   Interpretations of Suffering

- Punishment (such as for sins)
- Testing (such as loyalty to God)
- Bad luck (negative odds)
- Submission to the laws of nature (nature taking its course)
- Resignation to the will of God (accepting what happened without knowing why)
- Acceptance of the human condition (including suffering and pain)
- Personal growth (becoming a better person as a result of suffering)
- Defensiveness and denial (not thinking about it)
- Minimalization (downplaying the severity or significance of suffering)
- Divine perspective (transcending personal perspective)
- Redemption (finding joy in suffering)

Data from Foley, D. P. (1988). 11 interpretations of personal suffering. *Journal of Religion & Health, 27,* 321-328.

---

person understands the spiritual significance of suffering, a life of hope and joy is possible (Wong, 2005). In both Jewish and Christian views, how one responds to suffering is more important than trying to answer the question of *why.* Muslim patients may not seek a miracle or cure but endure believing that Allah heals through medicine and that illness (or disability) may be for a purpose, even a test, for the person to become more faithful (Hoeman & Haddad, 1999).

Frankl's concentration camp experiences (1984) produced logotherapy, a model for overpowering suffering by finding meaning in it. Logos, from the ancient Greek word translated as thought or logic, is the controlling principle in the universe. Frankl's version of modern existentialism proposes that each life has meaning under all circumstances, even the most miserable, and that a person has a will to meaning (i.e., their main motivation for living). People have freedom to find meaning in what they do, what they experience, or at least in the stand they take in the face of a situation of unchangeable suffering. The object and challenge of logotherapy is to weave the slender threads of a broken life into a firm pattern of meaning and responsibility, focusing on the future.

SPIRITUAL LOSS AND CHANGE

Any deficit or impairment is a loss that forces confrontation with limitations in life, a recognition of events, and reevaluation of goals and hopes. Early on, patients must be allowed to grieve for what they had, and now lack, and what "might have been." Mourning affirms life, but the pace and pathways differ. Patients need time to become accustomed to an altered body image and to regain a sense of purpose, reestablish priorities and goals, make moral choices, and develop a new philosophy of life and spiritual orientation. They must learn to take self-responsibility without fostering self-blame; otherwise they may engage in demands and faultfinding, withdrawal, and inability to control frustration. Whatever people value is what gives them meaning and purpose and inherently influences their response and adjustment to the event, even a traumatic one. An independent person, with a positive and stable sense of self, can come to accept personal limitations and accept the person he or she has become. Spiritual health encourages reevaluation of the meaning of pain and suffering in our lives so as to give purpose to the experience. Ideally, patients will be uplifted spiritually to regard whatever occurs, including their struggle against frustration, as opportunity for spiritual growth.

Spirituality and Chronicity

A chronic condition requires letting go in a myriad of small stages, with the person often being healthy between times. This "health in illness" is understood as coping in the best way possible with inevitable physical and psychological changes. Researchers investigating spirituality and chronic illness identified spirituality, with faith and prayer, as a powerful tool for coping with chronic illness (Narayanasamy, 2002). Other studies found that patients with a chronic illness or disability had a greater sense of life satisfaction when they also had a high level of spirituality (Brillhart, 2005; Riley et al., 1998). Kim (2002) found faith was important in the lives of patients with disabilities (n = 28). They increased their faith practices following onset of their disability, and 89% described both spiritual crisis and spiritual awakening.

Rehabilitation Nursing Roles

The spiritual roles for rehabilitation nurses are comforter, counselor, and challenger; necessary skills include self-awareness and the ability to communicate, build trust, and encourage hope (Narayanasamy, 1996). Nurses can target interventions that improve a patient's comfort, strength, well-being, and attitude by establishing a spiritual presence. However, a patient whose condition is potentially threatening or terminal may need time to express feelings and deal with sadness before becoming receptive to a spiritual intervention, even prayer.

A patient who has a chronic illness or disability tends to set goals that are general rather than specific, open-ended rather than finite, and focused on adapting to altered functional status, reflecting expectations and avoiding disappointment. Rehabilitation nurses help patients set goals that are mutually agreed upon, feasible, realistic, and appropriate that help to integrate hope into the patient's existence. Nurses can refer a patient for *Spiritual care* upon request or when uncomfortable with spiritual care and can collaborate with the chaplain or spiritual leader to support or assist the patient (O'Brien, 2003).

SPIRITUALITY AND DEVELOPMENTAL STAGES

Child and Adolescent Spirituality

Barnum asks, "Is there a spiritual phase in development?" Maslow (1971) discussed potential for transcendence for the self-actualized person. Erikson (1963) posited that psychological development must resolve conflicts at successive, cumulative stages beginning with the first year of life (trust versus mistrust). Resolution impacted a child's spiritual growth and determined the response to God in later stages. Both Fowler (1974) and Aden (1976) state that developing trust is basic to a relationship with God. Bradford (1995) suggests that hopes and fears are aspects of spirituality, and that positive experiences can be fostered in a child through love and affection, security, and a stimulating environment. During the "autonomy versus shame and doubt" stage, children interpret meaning literally, such as looking up to the sky toward heaven and wanting to see God (Smith & McSherry, 2004). Aden (1976) describes development of faith for the 4- or 5-year-old child as obedience, such as to rules given by parents and teachers, because "God sees everything." A school-age child views God as communicated through family and community and wants to learn about God and the child's faith tradition. According to Fowler (1974), a child will attempt to control or manipulate God through prayer requests. At this level the child learns to serve others so as to please God, believing there is punishment for wrongdoing and reward for good deeds (Carson, 1989). The child may believe in a universal power or only in the capabilities of others to provide (Carson, 1989). School-age children develop a personal image of God that is often framed on whether (or not) they believe prayers have been answered (Fowler, 1974).

Children in rehabilitation may be slow to enter into a relationship with nurses who are responsible for painful procedures and the invasion of their privacy; however, they do value the times when a nurse is willing to listen when they question pain and suffering. Although it is difficult to have no answers to questions about why and to whom accidents and illness happen, nurses should understand that children recognize honesty and need a nurse who will honor them with truth. Children have a fine-tuned relationship with God, taking each day as it comes. A trusted nurse can reassure that God looks beyond their imperfections and sees them as special, not punishing them with disability. With this knowledge they can gain strength to survive, come to terms with their condition, or move forward with the power of prayer and relationships. A visit from the family's spiritual leader early on may open communication and lay groundwork for future support.

Preschoolers enjoy picture books or puzzles with religious themes and small meaningful items. Their vivid imaginations respond to games and techniques for relaxation, imaging, and centering. Therapeutic play with puppets, equipment models, storytelling, and drawing materials allow children to work through feelings and gain a different perspective on the situation. Some cultures do not use religious objects, pictures, or other materials, so ask before introducing the items. Families will have their own ways of making contact with key people, relating the stories and performing the ceremonies important to their children. Faith rituals appropriate to family culture and beliefs are important and comforting at all ages. Rituals, such as bedtime prayers, are ways for children to know that they are remembered by their families and that their God will always be with them (Sommer, 1989).

Hopefulness contributes to the psychosocial development of adolescents. They are inclined to look to God as they move toward independence from authority, questioning family values and ideals. Given to emotion and introspection, they need support while sorting out conflicts; peer influence is highly valued and may create conflict with values gained during formative years. Adolescents may reject formal services and then worship in the privacy of their rooms or reveal deep spiritual concerns and then act silly and deny the feelings. Responses of hospitalized adolescents (ages 11 to 19 years) to a questionnaire indicated that importance of spirituality and religious experiences was related directly to the severity of their condition, a finding usually attributed to the elderly (Silber & Reilly, 1985). Westerhoff (1976) studied how adolescents experience affiliated faith derived from group interactions and activities. They were more likely to engage in religious worship and socialization when peers shared their values and beliefs. Youth groups in a faith community may affirm the adolescent's identity, provide comfort and support, and encourage commitment to religion. Adolescents are searching for values and may welcome discussion about interventions such as meditation, visualization, and relaxation. Refer to Chapter 31 for specific developmental stage information.

NURSING PROCESS

A rehabilitation nurse builds patients' spiritual resources, needs, or distress into an individualized plan of care. Observations, such as religious books or objects, facial expressions and gestures, or references to God or religion must be validated to eliminate false assumptions. Religious items or practices from some cultures may not be recognized, especially when a patient and nurse have different cultures or faiths. "An individual's lifestyle, value system and religious beliefs should be considered in planning health care with and for each patient" (American Nurses Association, 2001; International Council of Nurses, 2000). Not all patients seek spiritual care, but they might need the presence of the nurse or a loved one. Nurses are not to postulate their own religion to patients; some nurses are uncomfortable providing spiritual care and may need training to assess the spiritual needs of their patients (McSherry & Ross, 2002).

Though spiritual care may improve outcomes, there are dilemmas. Various definitions of spirituality and religion and beliefs about cultural practices have led to confusion, ambiguity, and subjectivity. Rehabilitation nurses need accurate information and insight into a variety of faith communities and familiarity with beliefs and practices. Having a faith leader forms a dilemma; it begs the question, who is qualified and acceptable to provide spiritual care? Chaplains complain they are not invited to participate in care conferences (McSherry & Ross, 2002); the patient's faith leader should be a member of the rehabilitation team.

Spiritual Assessment

The initial spiritual assessment best occurs later in the admission history, when there has been opportunity to assess psychosocial factors and gain trust and rapport with the patient. Patients need reassurance that they can or someone will attend to basic religious needs, such as dietary requirements, receiving sacraments, access to water for washing, or the means to perform other rituals. A number of multidimensional tools measure religious parameters based on patients' responses in an attempt to identify and define true needs over vague or elusive concepts. Using a meaningful and effective assessment tool is imperative (Delaney, 2005).

However, data alone do not offer insight into spiritual recesses. Patients may not discuss their spiritual needs or coping strategies because the information collected was limited to religion. When a nurse remains open and respectful of privacy, a patient may be relieved to share spirituality; conversely, a patient may express offense, feel threatened, or appear to be puzzled by spiritual assessment. The way a patient responds and the content, not the degree of expressed concern or absence of it, may be meaningful for care. A patient has a right to object and not to answer questions; others may manifest spiritual needs, recall spiritual events, spontaneously acknowledge problems, and confide in the nurse. Spiritual needs may emerge as conversation during daily care, providing opportunity for intervention.

Questions in the spiritual history must be validated as relevant, sensitive, and reflective of the fundamental values of respect, understanding, caring, and fairness—both for patient and nurse. Nurses may benefit from a continuing education program about how to anticipate patient needs and ways to learn specific information about common beliefs and practices held by patients in the community. Stoll's spiritual history guide (1979) (Box 29-2) is a screening tool that can be incorporated readily into any general nursing history. The questions may be asked in any order.

Spiritual Assessment Measurements

The Spiritual Well-Being Scale (SWBS) is a 20-item Likert scale that measures the individual's relationship with God and satisfaction with life (Ellison, 1982). Used for two decades, the SWBS has been criticized for limitations: it may not address several key components of spirituality, has a potentially narrow focus within the Judeo-Christian religious perspective, and focuses on assessing spiritual beliefs rather than actions. Still, the SWBS is the most widely used tool in studies of spirituality (Delaney, 2005).

The Spiritual Assessment Scale (SAS) is a standardized instrument that measures the construct of spiritual well-being using a 21-item Likert scale to evaluate personal faith, religious practices, and spiritual contentment (O'Brien, 2003). The Spiritual Scale (SS) (Delaney, 2005) is a holistic assessment instrument of beliefs, institutions, lifestyle choices, practices, and rituals that goes beyond religious beliefs to represent the spiritual dimension. It is an ideal tool for determining possible interventions.

Maddox (2001) recommended a short spiritual assessment tool with open-ended questions to investigate a patient's faith as part of life, the influence of faith on health care needs,

BOX 29-2 Spiritual History Guide

Sources of Hope and Strength (Support System)
Who is the most important person to you?
To whom do you turn when you need help? Are they available?
In what ways do they help?
What is your source of strength and hope?
What helps you most when you feel afraid or need special help?

Concept of God/Deity
Is religion or God significant to you? If yes, can you describe how?
Is prayer helpful to you? What happens when you pray?
Does God/deity function in your personal life? If yes, can you describe how?
How would you describe your God or what you worship?

Relation Between Spiritual Beliefs and Health
What has bothered you most about being sick (or in what is happening to you)?
What do you think is going to happen to you?
Has being sick (or what has happened to you) made any difference in your feelings about God or the practice of your faith?
Is there anything that is especially frightening or meaningful to you now?

Religious Practices
Do you feel your faith (or religion) is helpful to you? If yes, would you tell me how?
Are there any religious practices that are important to you?
Has being sick made any difference in your practice of praying? Your religious practices?
What religious books or symbols are helpful to you?
To this might be added:
Is there anything I can do to help you in your practice of faith?

involvement in a religious community, and permission to discuss spiritual needs. Assessment models may use acronyms, such as for the popular hospital model, SPIRIT (Spiritual belief system, Personal spirituality, Integration/involvement in a spiritual community, Ritualized practices and restrictions, Implications for care, and Terminal events planning) (Maugans, 1996).

The Spiritual Involvement and Beliefs Scale (SIBS) (Hatch, Burg, Naberhaus, & Hellmich, 1998) (Box 29-3) has a broader scope, uses terms without cultural bias, and assesses both beliefs and actions. The Jarel Spiritual Well-Being Scale is a brief, reliable, and valid scale to assess spiritual well-being in older adults (Hungleman, Kendel-Rossi, Klassen, & Stollenwerk, 1989), and the Correlates of Spiritual Well-Being Scale measures spiritual well-being, loneliness, health hardiness, social support, functional status, and pain (Pace & Stables, 1997). The Index of Core Spiritual Experience is a sample of an instrument that measures intrinsic spirituality (McBride, Arthur, Brooks, & Pilkington, 1998). The Spirituality Index of Well-Being (SIWB) instrument has strong validity and reliability. It was developed to examine relationships between patient spirituality and quality of life or well-being for persons with illness or disability (Daaleman & Frey, 2004).

Nursing Diagnoses: Spiritual Needs

Spirituality fits within the value-belief pattern that is used to identify patients' actual or at-risk health problems or wellness regarding their spiritual well-being (Gordon, 2006). Patients may have clinical manifestations of loneliness, despair or discouragement, expressing no reason to live. They may become alienated and withdraw from friends or their usual religious practices. They may express resentment and anger; fear or anxiety; grief with hopelessness, powerlessness, or ineffective coping; all are verbal and nonverbal indicators of spiritual distress. Spiritual distress is "the state in which an individual or a group experiences, or is at risk of experiencing a disturbance in the belief or value system that provides strength, hope and meaning in life" (Carpenito-Moyet, 2004). Nursing diagnoses, interventions, and outcomes applicable to spirituality are presented in Table 29-1.

Nursing Interventions

It can be difficult for the nurse to distinguish spiritual needs from distress or religious needs (Cavendish, 2003). Patients will have spiritual or religious questions and need interventions, as discussed below, and appropriate referrals.

Spiritual Listening or Presencing. "I was afraid and the procedure was going to be quite uncomfortable. The nurse leaned over to help me into position, but also gave me an extended hug; I couldn't see her after that, but I could feel her hand on my shoulder and I knew she was there with me. It still was painful, but I knew I wasn't alone amidst all the medical technology; I am not sure I learned her name, but I knew her presence" (Hoeman, 2000). Presence is defined as being with another, both physically and psychologically, during times of need, acting as an advocate for patients of other faiths (Cavendish et al., 2003).

In an age when communication tends to be swift, short, and superficial, many patients affirm "presencing" or "accompanying." They simply want someone to be present to listen, acknowledge, touch, empathize, show concern, quietly reassure, patiently explain, allow their crying or crying out, or exercise nonjudgmental understanding. Nurses often provide the greatest amount of spiritual care to patients simply by being there (Mauk, Russell, & Schmidt, 2004). Risks are feeling awkward or uncomfortable, possibly fear, pain, or vulnerability in silence. The voice of the spirit in silence is intuition; listening develops wisdom and is "skilled companionship" through which a nurse honors the spirituality of others (Keating, 1996). Presencing is a primary spiritual nursing intervention and may be the most effective. Once established in a relationship, presencing does not require time.

The Relaxation Response. The relaxation response decreases anxiety and fatigue and helps patients rest and dissociate from pain. A patient may be trained through autogenic means (self-hypnosis), deep-breathing exercises, progressive muscle relaxation, prayer repetition, techniques such as the

BOX 29-3 Spiritual Involvement and Beliefs Scale

Respondents are asked to rate how strongly they agree or disagree with each statement. The seven response categories are: (7) Strongly Agree, (6) Agree, (5) Mildly Agree, (4) Neutral, (3) Mildly Disagree, (2) Disagree, and (1) Strongly Disagree.

To score the results, add the corresponding numbers except for negatively worded items (3, 6, 9, 15, 16, 21, 28, 29, 37)—for these results reverse the scoring (Strongly Agree will be 1).

How strongly do you agree with the following statements?
1. I set aside time for meditation and/or self-reflection.
2. I can find meaning in times of hardship.
3. A person can be fulfilled without pursuing an active spiritual life.
4. I find serenity by accepting things as they are.
5. Some experiences can be understood only through one's spiritual beliefs.
6. I do not believe in the afterlife.
7. A spiritual force influences the events in my life.
8. I have a relationship with someone I can turn to for spiritual guidance.
9. Prayer does not really change what happens.
10. Participating in spiritual activities helps me forgive other people.
11. I find inner peace when I am in harmony with nature.
12. Everything happens for a greater purpose.
13. I use contemplation to get in touch with my true self.
14. My spiritual life fulfills me in ways that material possessions do not.
15. I rarely feel connected to something greater than myself.
16. In times of despair, I can find little reason to hope.
17. When I am sick, I would like others to pray for me.
18. I have a personal relationship with a power greater than myself.
19. I have had a spiritual experience that greatly changed my life.
20. When I help others, I expect nothing in return.
21. I don't take time to appreciate nature.
22. I depend on a higher power.
23. I have joy in my life because of my spirituality.
24. My relationship with a higher power helps me love others more completely.
25. Spiritual writings enrich my life.
26. I have experienced healing after prayer.
27. My spiritual understanding continues to grow.
28. I am right more often than most people.
29. Many spiritual approaches have little value.
30. Spiritual health contributes to physical health.
31. I regularly interact with others for spiritual purposes.
32. I focus on what needs to be changed in me, not on what need to be changed in others.
33. In difficult times I am still grateful.
34. I have been through a time of great suffering that led to spiritual growth.

Please indicate how often you do the following:
(The scale is (7) Always, (6) Almost Always, (5) Usually, (4) Sometimes, (3) Not Usually, (2) Almost Never, (1) Never.)
35. When I wrong someone, I make an effort to apologize.
36. I accept others as they are.
37. I solve my problems without using spiritual resources.
38. I examine my actions to see if they reflect my values.
39. How spiritual a person do you consider yourself? (With "7" being the most spiritual.)

From Hatch, R. L., Burg, M. A., Naberhous, D. S., & Hellmich, L. K. (1998). The spiritual involvement and beliefs scale: Development and testing of a new instrument. *Journal of Family Practice, 46,* 485-486.

exercises in Box 29-4, or guided sessions via audiotapes. Biofeedback may be a complementary intervention when a patient is weaning from a ventilator.

Meditation. Meditation is an age-old means of relaxation used in many cultures. Meditation is finding the quiet within. It is listening long and deeply with calmness and concentration for the subtleties and sensibilities of the spirit that evoke intuition, nurturing one's spiritual voice with open-mindedness and without judgment. Meditation techniques include yoga, Zen, transcendental meditation, and hypnosis. Regular meditation improves overall well-being and mental alertness.

TABLE 29-1 Nursing Diagnoses, Interventions, and Outcomes Applicable to Spirituality

Nursing Diagnosis	Nursing Intervention	Nursing Outcomes

Decisional conflict	Decision making support, Mutual goal setting
	  Meditation facilitation
	  Music therapy
	  Simple guided imagery
	  Simple relaxation
		Decision making, Information processing,
		Values clarification

Grieving; dysfunctional	Grief work facilitation, Guilt work facilitation	Grief resolution, Acceptance

Hopelessness	Hope instillation, Mood management
	  Coping enhancement
	  Emotional support
	  Energy management
		Hope, Mood equilibrium, Effective coping

Spiritual distress; At risk for	Spiritual support
	  Dying care
	  Forgiveness facilitation
	  Grief work facilitation
	  Hope installation
	  Music therapy
	  Touch
		Acceptance: health status
		Personal actions to maintain control during
		  approaching end of life

Spiritual well-being; Readiness for enhanced	Spiritual growth facilitation, Hope instillation
	  Coping enhancement
	  Emotional support
	  Religious ritual enhancement
	  Self-esteem enhancement
		Personal well-being, Spiritual health
		Purpose in life; connectedness with others and/or
		  a higher power

Classic meditation requires a comfortable position and passive attitude within a quiet environment (the spirit loves silence), while dwelling on some object, mantra, or thought. At any time the patient can engage in thoughts or in conversation with God, returning to the simple breathing formula. Practicing breathing techniques, with eyes averted and mentally repeating the chosen words, ensures a patient inner contact with a spiritual presence. Some patients focus on an image of their higher power. This breath of spirit flows out with whatever the patient chooses for holy words, verses, mantra, or other. When thoughts intrude during meditation, they are acknowledged, not engaged, and then deliberately set aside for later consideration. Thus, someone who meditated after breakfast and continued it during therapy could make the work of therapy a prayer offering. Nurses may help patients plan time and find seclusion for meditation.

Centering, performed by nurses who practice the principles of therapeutic touch (TT), has been likened to the sensations attained through meditation. Although TT is not associated directly with meditation techniques or mental effort, it depends on the universal healing power being channeled through the nurse as a conduit to provide comfort or healing.

Visualization and Imagery. Nurses can guide patients to visualize their lives and purpose by asking questions such as, "How does life look?," "How do I feel inside?," "What am I doing?," "How do I interact, and with whom?," and "What is a typical day?" Journal writing is a complementary method to track life goals and guide discussions of visualizations to help in making decisions or taking actions toward the goals.

Imagery, related closely to visualization, is an internal experience of memories, dreams, and fantasies. It requires focused concentration because it uses imagination and all the senses in attempts to dismiss anxiety and reach inner spiritual resources. Imagery techniques may reduce stressors and speed recovery, as well as help change perceptions about disability or treatment. Art therapy and scripted audiotapes are complementary interventions; they may reveal areas where patients retain negative images. Nurses who plan to use imagery first become familiar with the types, methods, and resources before using it as an intervention.

Prayer. Prayer is communication between a patient and his or her God. More than talking or making requests, prayer means active listening. A response may come from another person or read in sacred literature. For Mother Teresa (1998), "real prayer is union with God. Prayer is the very life of oneness, of being one with Christ." Prayer has been shown to affect persons who pray for themselves, as well as those prayed for by others (Deachter, 2002). Prayer and the relaxation process use the same biochemical pathways, and prayer may activate a location in the brain. It is not necessary to understand how prayer works to use it. Although intercessory prayer does not always yield the precise desired benefit from the human point of view, the results over time may be welcomed, and faith need not be validated by science. Meditative prayer may be part of the relaxation response intervention; thus, prayer may be an attribute of being spiritual or characterized as an outcome of spirituality. A patient in spiritual distress feels apart from God's presence and unable to pray; then prayer becomes an outcome rather than an intervention.

BOX 29-4   Relaxation Exercises

Exercise 1

Slow, rhythmic breathing for relaxation requires a comfortable position and the ability to put aside distractions. Instruct patients to breathe in and out slowly and deeply. Guide them to concentrate on releasing tension, relaxing, and breathing regularly; try abdominal breathing. On inspiration they silently count 1-2-3 and, maintaining a slow rhythm, count 1-2-3 while exhaling, or they concentrate on a word or thought. Perform relaxed breathing for 5 to 10 minutes initially, working up to 15 to 20 minutes. Patients end the exercise with a slow, deep breath, saying, "I feel alert and relaxed."

Exercise 2

The examples of simple touch, massage, or warmth for relaxation can be integrated with other nursing interventions and activities of daily living. Touch is useful contact for infants and older persons. Massage can be whole body or a 3- to 10-minute massage of the back, hands, and feet. Use a warm lubricant, and as patients prefer and are permitted, vary massage techniques or add aromatics. Place the person in an appropriate position, and use rhythmic stokes (60 per minute) with continuous hand contact during a back rub. Begin at the crown of the head, and move to the lower back, avoiding the spine.

Exercise 3

Drawing on memories of peaceful past experiences helps some persons to gain present calm and comfort. However, avoid this technique for persons who may draw on sad or uncomfortable memories. Patients may recall special times with family or events or religious experiences and try to regain those happy feelings. Music, poetry, daydreams, photographs, or memorabilia may help patients. Patients may choose to write or tape record their memories and review them later.

Exercise 4

For patients who are able, active listening to recorded books, old radio or comedy programs, music, or religious messages is a popular and inexpensive form of relaxation. Materials are available from a variety of public and private sources. A comfortable position, appropriate volume, and pleasurable content aid relaxation. Patients may choose their level of participation, such as keeping time with a musical selection or focusing steadily, to bypass discomfort.

The best prayer petition is open-ended and not specific. O'Brien (2003) found a patient to benefit most from prayer petitions after writing concerns, needs, and thoughts on paper and placing it in a "prayer box" or "God box." Similar to journaling or hanging prayers on a Buddhist wheel, he felt free; all his worries were leaving his body and mind and going to God, and God would take over the situation.

Prayer has cultural roots but remains highly personal. Thus a Jewish patient might believe that sympathetic prayer by others is a value in itself and part of a larger sympathetic act. Native Americans may pray for dreams, spirited insight, or wisdom. Some of Hispanic heritage might ask for penance or divine intervention from patron saints; Islamic patients may invoke Allah's blessing for their fate; or those communing with nature may invoke channels.

Not offering an opportunity to pray is tantamount to withholding medication. If patients indicate any interest in prayer, a nurse first tells them to pray, then offers presence during prayers, and finally may choose to offer to pray with them. Prayer is the sense of being aligned with something higher; prayers are not sent into the universe, but directed inward to the spirit. Overt demonstration does not indicate quality or level of prayer, but a faith or spiritual leader may assist patients with meditation or by performing prayer rituals or ceremonies. In a prayerful state, patients have had "a sense in which a 'cure' can occur—the realization that physical problems, no matter how painful or severe, are of secondary importance in the total scheme of existence. One's authentic higher self is completely impervious to the ravages of any ailment whatsoever—utterly beyond the ravages of disease and death" (Dossey, 1993, p. 36).

Generating Hope. In rehabilitation, recent developments have given patients optimism and generated hope. Progress in understanding disease etiology, improved treatment methods, validated research findings, and interdisciplinary teamwork have created more choices for interventions and stimulated social services and programs for patients and their families—more reasons for hope. Hope is defined as "optimism that is personally satisfying and life supporting" (Moorhead, Johnson, & Maas, 2004). Hope is conceptualized as vertical and horizontal and usually is experienced simultaneously.

When oriented towards earthly goals, actions, and relationships, it is horizontal. Vertical hope depends on eternal goals, actions, and relationships with a divine being (Carson, 1989). Hope is future oriented and may change across the illness trajectory. When earthly hope fades or does not materialize, eternal hope carries the person through the earthly disappointment, allowing a healthy perspective and individual peace and joy (Roberts, 1982). Essential to achieving goals and strong interpersonal relationships, it is a force binding patients to their perception of God.

When a patient achieves a goal that dissipates a stressful experience, the success creates an immediate sense of peace and well-being. A generalized hope emerges for future success. Hope is a powerful, positive, and active phenomenon that promotes effective coping, it is not passive. Post-White (2003) found it sustains life and is necessary for healing; without hope, patients find no reason or confidence to get up in the morning. The process and meaning of hope across cultures requires further investigation.

Pain and suffering, depleted energy, and impaired cognition impede hope. Hopelessness is often accompanied by helplessness that is preceded by loss of control of one's own life and independence. Ironically, the same life situation can be an occasion for hope or hopelessness or both. Patients who feel hopeless are not demanding or noisy; rather, they appear passive and depressed, wreaking further adversity on their quality of life. Acknowledging that a patient seems hopeless or in grief and despair, then offering to discuss problems or assist may initiate a relationship from which to foster hope rather than focusing on a premature goal. Assessment for potential self-injury may be appropriate. Helping patients realize that hope develops as an evolving process allows them to identify outcomes and resources that have little meaning now, but may be meaningful when pursued later.

Hope and effective coping are especially difficult for the patient with spinal cord injury, even after a year after injury. Patients were found to move between experiences of suffering that entailed feelings of loneliness, impatience, disappointment, bitterness, waiting, and dependency. Hope was finding a way out of the vicious circle (Lohne & Severinsson, 2005). Strategies that built hope were teaching effective coping, setting mutual goals, reframing health problems as opportunities for adaptation and physical growth, and fostering improved self-esteem and social supports. Although hope is directive and willful, spiritual hope is most likely to emerge when a patient lets go of will and opens self to trust in God.

Humor. Humor has physiological and psychological effects to ease tension in situations, act as a great distraction, and play up the eustress (positive, motivating energy) in situations, and it can be shared. Laughter may play a role in increasing blood flow to the heart with resulting cardiovascular benefits (Miller, Mangano, Park, et al., 2006). It is thought to be one way to help distract patients from or to dull pain. As a spiritual intervention, humor helps patients to think creatively; it may give a feeling of belonging and social cohesion, facilitate coping, and counteract feelings of alienation and give a sense of control or improved quality in life (Provine, 2000). The benefits of comedy have been likened to the functions of religion: to raise self-awareness and one's spirits; to accept reality and its contradictions; to reveal harmony by increasing connections to each other and to life.

Laughter provides a perspective for suffering, acknowledging it while momentarily relieving the tension and grief suffered from illness or injury (Miller, 1998). As with any intervention, it is wise to assess the patient's sense and use of humor to learn if and what type of humor is appropriate. Some facilities have collections of small toys, games, comedy tapes, and joke books; a recreation department can host a humor cart. Nurses' continuing education venues often include humorists who impart wise humor skills for patients and also attend to teaching stressed-out nurses how to laugh and replenish their own cheer.

Utilizing the Arts for Therapy. Typically *the arts* refers to the creative and interpretive works that express perceptions, feelings, and intuitions. The symbolism inherent in dance, painting, poetry, music, quilting, gardening, and other arts communicates a powerful language of the soul (Vash, 1994). A patient's preferred music can enhance the relaxation response and imagery states. For example, an elderly woman was comforted by a piano music box that played waltz tunes because she recalled pleasant memories that made her feel as though she were in a different place and time. Ecumenical chants of Taize are a popular choice that brings all cultures and religions together to share the healing, prayer, and reconciliation (O'Brien, 2003).

Music has demonstrated positive effects on patients experiencing conditions such as Alzheimer's disease or coma. A student nurse cared for a comatose patient for a long period of time and was instructed to communicate to the patient; eventually she began to sing hymns, spirituals, and pop songs. Years later, now a registered nurse, she was walking down the hall of a rehabilitation hospital when a man asked, "Aren't you the nurse who sang to me?" She recognized him as he recalled her care; it was the songs he remembered most (Smith & Wiebe, 1998).

Bibliotherapy. In bibliotherapy, medical librarians join the rehabilitation team by identifying appropriate readings in the literature that can guide patients to cost-effective, low-technology, and high-quality tools. Patients can learn about their disabilities or conditions, as well as about the spiritual and emotional aspects. At first they may prefer "escape" literature and progress to material that aids nurse-patient discussions. Patients may identify with others having similar problems through uplifting narratives or biographies. *When God Weeps* is a true story of a woman's relationship with Christ following her spinal cord injury (Tada & Estes, 1997). Librarians are aware of resources such as book reading groups or spiritual and poetry readings, multilingual volunteer readers, videotapes and audiotapes, and specialized materials online (Tada, 1999). They help nurses locate organizations, education programs, support groups, and treatments relevant to any particular illness or disability (Solimine, 1995).

Reminiscence Therapy. Reminiscence therapy is characterized by bringing conscious and progressive positive experiences from the past into current memory. A type of bibliotherapy, it involves listening, being present, and caring for the distinct purpose of encouraging a patient to recall memories. Evocative questions help recall successful victories over challenges in life. Other memories are retrieved only upon request, and then only if patients desire to explore what actually happened to cause them distress. The goal is to achieve closure; rehashing failures or renewing old wounds is counter to the therapy.

Photographs and memorabilia can enhance memory and create an atmosphere for family storytelling. Recalling stories, patients can make sense of life, connect with listeners, and even make recordings as a legacy. When patients share images etched in their imagination or their life story, they are sharing part of their soul they carry within, and this should be honored (Hillman, 1972). Other strategies are to create a time line, a collage, or a journal for reflection. Writing about stressful experiences to reduce symptoms may be helpful (Smyth, Stone, Hurewitz, & Kaell, 1999).

Spiritual Growth Facilitation. Cavendish et al. (2003) found spiritual growth facilitation and spiritual support to be the two main spiritual interventions performed by nurses. Spiritual growth facilitation is the "facilitation of growth in patient's capacity to identify, connect, and call on the source of meaning, purpose, comfort, strength, and hope." Activities include spending time with the patient, encouraging talk about spiritual concerns and help to sort them out, offering individual and group support prayer, encouraging participation in devotions and study groups and use of rituals or celebrations, and referring for pastoral care, if desired. Spiritual support is "assisting the patient to full balance and connection with a greater power" Activities include taking the patient to services or hospital chapel, encouraging use of spiritual literature and resources, offering inspirational care for agnostics, making religious or sacred articles available, and ensuring patients receive a sacrament, diet, other specific spiritual requirements (Cavendish et al., 2003; Dochterman & Bulechek, 2004).

Outcomes

Forgiveness. One of the most powerful things a person can accomplish is to decide to make peace with oneself and others, letting go of grudges and the pain of hurtful relationships—forgiving oneself and others—and say yes to life. It is the necessary first step in the passage to spiritual quality of life. It entails a struggle with feelings of denial, anger, bargaining, and depression, much as the dying patient makes.

Although anger is an appropriate initial response to hurt, patients may become victims of their own mistaken judgment. The error of the self as right and powerful prevails, and patients damage themselves, for anger weakens rather than empowers (Borysenko, 1987). When a person cannot find it in his or her heart to forgive, the other party may or may not experience grief, but the person will continue to anguish and mourn and cannot be a loving, peace-filled person. It restrains and limits spiritual growth. Mickley and Cowles (2001) recount how a patient was able to recognize the actions necessary for her to move forward and heal after she shared her story with an objective professional listener.

When a nurse listens in a nonjudgmental manner as patients speak about past hurts, helping them express the hurts may lead to their forgiving the offender. Forgiveness gives peace and a sense of freedom and of becoming unburdened. It takes grace to forgive and ask God's forgiveness; forgiving others follows. The process of forgiving is a dynamic energy force—an act of will consciously undertaken to heal self and memories, to restore self-determination and strengthen spirituality.

Asking for another's forgiveness for any conscious or unconscious sorrow one has inflicted means learning about responsibility, sensitivity, empathy, and kindness—and internalizing them. When a person forgives self, loses any attachment to the deed, and considers the consequences of not forgiving, then a person can celebrate becoming a new being. However, telling someone he or she has been forgiven may not be necessary or even wise; forgiveness is an internalized process. An amputee, Andre Dubus (1991) says: "After the physical pain of grief has become, with time, a permanent wound in the soul, . . . then comes the transcendent and common bond of suffering, and with that comes forgiveness, and with forgiveness comes love. . . ."

Serenity. Trauma, major illness, and aging stimulate a search for inner peace, or serenity, to be sustained regardless of life events. Serenity, an awakened state, "gives one a healthy mastery of emotions, decreases stress, and leads to improved relationships with others, and especially with God, through prayer, zest for living, acceptance of one's self as worthy, increased compassion and self-possession during trying times, and trust in a higher power" (Dossey, 1993). A serene person is caring, active, involved, and responsible, not passive or detached. Serenity is not always being happy, rather it is being able to have a quiet inner-directed action and calm despite negative circumstances. Conversely, anxiety, anger, lack of faith, impatience, and unhealthy lifestyle behaviors are samples of emotion and behaviors found in the nonserene.

Nurses themselves benefit from acquiring serenity to reach their own inner haven where they find detachment, belonging, giving, trust in a higher power, acceptance, problem solving, presentness, forgiveness, and a view of the future. One who is able to achieve serenity has a strategy for coping with chronic illness, other comorbid conditions, or addictive behaviors that may accompany disabilities. Patients may suffer a spiritual emergency that leads to a crisis of their spirituality, and potentially they experience a spiritual transformation. One addicted to food, gambling, drugs, alcohol, nicotine, and the like may be longing for wholeness. Consider references to "drinking spirits" and "using drugs to get high." Alcoholics Anonymous (AA) and similar programs ground their recovery in a relationship to a higher power. Many have gained insights after breaking through addiction and having a spiritual focus instead of an addiction. The AA prayer is, "God grant me the serenity to accept the things I cannot change, courage to change the things I can, and wisdom to know the difference" (Niebuhr, 1943).

Healing. Disability and chronic illness interrupt the fabric of life; patients adjust by weaving their lives together in whatever ways make sense to them. This is a healing, but it does not cure the physical problem. Authentic healing is an expression of spiritual maturity that leads to integrity and wholeness, and psychospiritual growth may be nearly equivalent to healing. Self-healing can bring patients to meaningfulness in life through separation from daily routine, transition to the inner self, and finally a return with an inner peace.

"Healing is an active and internal process that includes investigating one's attitude, memories and beliefs with the desire to release all negative patterns that prevent one's full emotional and spiritual recovery" (Myss, 1996). Healing must be distinguished from curing and cannot be measured in the same manner. "It is one thing to evaluate whether the signs and symptoms of disease are still present. It is quite another to determine if there has been a shift at any level of this person's body-mind-spirit" (Quinn, 2000). The process of *curing* is passive; the patient authorizes physicians and healers to apply treatments that do not necessarily alleviate the accompanying psychological and emotional stressors; indeed the stressors may trigger return of illness. Healing means emotional, psychological, physical, and spiritual recovery.

Healer is a nursing role that involves presencing, respecting, and caring apart from a patient's culture or personal qualities, listening actively, being nonjudgmental, and viewing time with patients as times of sharing and serving. The nurse and patient are mutually involved as healers, and healing may mean the patient finds a purpose in life, regardless of impairment. The nurse guides patients toward discovery of possible health behaviors and new insights and helps them make choices for coping effectively. In a facilitator role a nurse acts to "evoke the patient's process of inner healing" (Dossey & Guzzetta, 2000).

SPIRITUALITY FOR THE REHABILITATION NURSE

Rehabilitation nurses can and should provide spiritual care for patients, but what about the plight of the overworked, underspiritualized nurses? Basic nursing education traditionally included lists and reviews of major religions and their tenets, with no attempts to infuse spiritual purpose or belief. Many nurses have no idea of a role with spirituality, and there are different levels of religious maturity. Nurses are only able to provide care within their own limitations and talents (Barnum, 2003). Although nurses are trained to care, ethically their first care should be themselves so they are able to care and minister to others. Nurses who choose to be spiritual resources must replenish and revitalize their body, mind, and spirit. Are you caring for your whole self as conscientiously as you do for others? Take responsibility for your own spiritual health by focusing creatively on your needs and ways to achieve better balance. Use a list of things you do for your physical, emotional, intellectual, social, and spiritual growth. Identify categories that need enhancement, where you need more "re-creation."

To strengthen wellness and self-esteem, use the same list and state what characteristic you like best about yourself in each category. Add what others say they like about you and for what you would like to be remembered. If you are critical of yourself, target this to cultivate something positive. A personal wellness prescription is to focus on your positive aspects, set realistic goals and reward yourself for progress, be gentle, practice centering, learn to ask for what you need, learn to say no, and think and say positive things to yourself. Develop intuitive skills, take time for fun and laughter, walk a labyrinth, and learn to take mental health breaks and mini-vacations. Identify your stressors and develop effective coping mechanisms, and mentally inventory the good things that happen to you daily and give thanks. We are all eligible for small pleasures (Uustal, 1992).

In practice, trust your intuition; trust in change from day to day. Walk the path of humility, let go of control outcomes, hold your highest healing intention in your thoughts and actions, and be open (Towey, 1997). To all of these add praying for guidance and seeking counsel when needed. Sharing and demonstrating the benefits of personal renewal with a patient may result in mutual reinforcement.

Barriers to Spirituality in Practice

Nurses may agree spirituality is important but respond negatively to its use in their practice. At times a nurse's own beliefs/culture may differ from that of the patient to the point of contradicting the patient's perspective or demanding self-expression. Box 29-5 identifies beliefs that may arise from patient or nurse or both and form barriers to spiritual care in practice.

However, patients choose nurses second to clergy as those with whom they wish to discuss spiritual matters. This is not surprising because nurses educate patients about their condition and rehabilitation interventions they may find strange or frightening, address most physical needs without a physician, and intervene with many psychosocial or emotional responses without relying on a psychologist. A nurse is an advocate who understands when a referral is needed and selects an appropriate professional. When a patient believes illness or impairment is punishment for wrongdoing (especially perceived sexual transgressions), the nurse includes a clerical or

---

BOX 29-5 Beliefs That Form Barriers to Spiritual Care

- Patients are uncomfortable discussing spiritual matters with a nurse (social restraint).
- Spirituality matters do not concern nurses, but rather psychologists or pastoral caregivers.
- Nurses lack time to devote to what is perceived as an arduous or uncomfortable task.
- Nurses are technologically oriented and not comfortable with spirituality.
- A nurse lacks maturity or education necessary to have anything to do with spiritual issues (own shortcomings).
- A nurse's own spiritual wellspring is depleted and not equal to the task (vulnerability; emotional risk).
- A nurse may not prepared to deal with the issues (counseling skills) when a patient's spiritual fears surface.
- Nurses fear they are meddling in a patient's spiritual life.

spiritual leader. When serious adjustment problems of conscience persist, patients are referred for psychological help. Recall that religious belief is formed during the same developmental stage as the ability to trust. Thus fostering an atmosphere of trust, confidentiality, and respect may allow a patient to confide needs and promote spiritual healing.

Research Directions

Research in the field of spirituality remains sparse. Although conceptual frameworks and definitions are challenging, a definition of spirituality that will accommodate the uniqueness of all patients and nurses is a need. Few reliable tools measure the effects of interventions used with disabled patients and control groups or validate changes. Questions for investigation include nurses' perceptions of spirituality, techniques that facilitate spiritual healing, and patients' responses and values. Other spiritual factors that influence outcomes with disability or chronic illness, complications from spiritual interventions, and the roles of lay and religious communities in rehabilitation need to be investigated. Further research is needed to find out why nurses sometimes find it difficult to provide spiritual care and what spiritual interventions by nurses would be more effective with rehabilitation patients, which interventions would provide more positive outcomes.

Interdisciplinary Focus

Spiritual care is an inseparable part of patient care and has an intrinsic value and importance, beginning with basic professional education. Increasingly, schools of nursing and other health professions are incorporating spiritual care into their curricula. The diagnosis of religious or spiritual problems was added to the *Diagnostic and Statistical Manual of Mental Disorders*. The diagnosis includes the loss or questioning of faith or spiritual values and is considered a problem, not a mental disorder (American Psychiatric Association, 1994).

Spirituality is a sought-after topic in professional conferences, continuing education, publications, media, and websites. Often spiritual and ethical issues are discussed alongside alternative or complementary therapies. However, a great deal of confusion and disagreement exists about whether spiritual interventions are to be performed, by whom, and under what circumstances. Hospitals offer continuing education for staff that includes ways to work closely with the chaplain or other faith leaders. Lesser known journals may publish more spiritual articles, such as *The Journal of Religion in Disability and Rehabilitation*, the *Journal of Christian Healing*, the *Journal for the Scientific Study of Religion*, and the *International Journal for the Psychology of Religion*.

SUMMARY

The rehabilitation nurse has the opportunity to guide patients through their journey of suffering, confusion, and then a new life. The rehabilitation nurse has the opportunity to help the patient find peace, hope, and God during this trial. Pope John Paul II (1999) stated, "It is Christ to whom you minister in the suffering of your brothers and sisters." The challenge is for nurses to determine the most effective means of facilitating spirituality and life satisfaction through this suffering for their patients and families. Nurses who use the nursing process according to standards for spirituality are ensuring "care" and make a difference in outcomes for their patients in rehabilitation.

Case Study

Dinh is a 39-year-old Vietnamese man who suffered a gunshot wound to his spine while eating at a restaurant. This resulted in the medical diagnosis of C-6 tetraplegia, changing his life forever. Before his spinal cord injury Dinh was a machinist, a job he could not do following his injury. He decided to attend school and now. He is near completion of his master's degree in social work. He states, "I want to use my personal experience of dealing with a life-changing injury to help other people cope and move on in life." Dinh has a strong family support system and lives at home with his mother.

Dinh grew up following the Buddhist philosophy and rituals, such as meditation. Nine years ago Dinh converted to Catholicism and was fully initiated into the church. Following his injury, Dinh lived in a long-term care facility where members of the Catholic faith, including a priest and a nun, visited him, comforted him, and shared scripture with him. Their example led to Dinh's decision to become a Catholic.

Assessment

The spiritual history scale was part of the assessment tool used with Dinh, providing open-ended questions in an interview process.

Dinh was interviewed using the Spiritual Involvement and Beliefs Scale (SIBS) and Stoll's spiritual history guide assessment tools in a private room at a rehabilitation facility. Dinh was receiving treatment for a stage three pressure ulcer to the sacral area, ultimately requiring surgery. Dinh was asked, "How strongly do you agree with the following statements?" from the SIBS (see Box 29-3). Dinh scored 100% on SIBS. The direct interview questions from the spiritual history guide were presented to Dinh. Dinh stated the following: "Religion and God are significant to me; absolutely I can see God in myself during the many blessings I have received during my difficult times. Prayer is helpful to me; I feel inner-peace, relief of stress. . . . God functions in my daily life. When in time of need, some people come into my life and help me. It is a blessing from above, especially during desperate times. He is always present. . . . I describe my God as love. . . . Even though my SCI isn't painful; sometimes I cannot do all the things I need to do."

When asked "What do you think is going to happen to you?" Dinh replied, "Whatever happens, I have to accept it. If it is good, thanks be to God. If it isn't good, I need to just accept it."

Case Study—cont'd

In response to other interview questions, Dinh stated: "The SCI brought me closer to God. . . . My strength comes from God, because God is my strength. . . . the most meaningful things to me in life now are spiritual,. . . . I feel my faith is guiding me down the right pathway leading me to a more meaningful way of life, to go to school and to do volunteer work at a hospital, helping others. I enjoy it because I get good feedback from the people I help."

Regarding religious practices, Dinh stated: "I practice the Catholic doctrines of faith, go to mass and receive communion. . . . Having an SCI, made a difference in my praying because I didn't pray before I got injured, I didn't know God before. I love reading the Bible and learning more about it. . . . spiritual practices most helpful to me are the Bible, prayer, communion, presence, or another person, meditation, and group faith sharing and support."

Nursing Diagnosis

The wellness diagnosis of readiness for enhanced spiritual well-being was selected for Dinh because there was no evidence of his being in spiritual distress. Also, he expressed hope for the future, having purpose in life, and being connected to his God.

Nursing Outcomes

Dinh's outcome was that he would continue to experience spiritual health. Spiritual health is defined as "connectedness with self, others, higher power, all life, nature, and the universe that transcends and empowers the self" (Moorhead, Johnson, & Maas, 2004). Dinh ranked a 5 in all the indicators listed except in ability to worship (3), expression through art (2), and expression through writing (2). Sometimes Dinh has difficulty getting his family members to drive him to church. Because of his tetraplegia, Dinh has limited use of his hands to draw or write.

Nursing Interventions Used With Dinh
Nursing Diagnosis: Readiness for Enhanced Spiritual Well-Being

Nursing Interventions Classification (NIC)	Nurse Activity
Spiritual support	• Provide privacy and quiet times for spiritual activities • Encourage participation in support group of SCI Christian individuals
Simple guided imagery	• Teach/review methods of relaxation, meditation, guided imagery • Pray with the individual • Communicate to staff necessity to keep Dinh's Bible available
Religious ritual enhancement	• Make arrangements for Dinh to receive communion daily while in hospital • Discuss with family Dinh's need to go to mass weekly, and consider transportation options available

Rationale

Support Groups. In a study of battered women the women participated in spiritual discussions weekly (Humphreys, 2000). The findings showed that among these women, spirituality may be linked with greater internal resources that lighten anxious feelings and give peace to the mind and spirit.

Relaxation. A survey of parish nurses showed they used guided imagery as an intervention for spirituality with patients (Tuck, Wallace, & Pullen, 2001).

Keep Religious Materials Available. In a survey of battered women, church attendance and reading the Bible were rated highly in promoting spiritual well-being (Humphreys, 2000).

Communion. Findings from a survey of parish nurses showed religious rites and rituals, such as offering communion and anointing, supported patient's spiritually (Tuck et al., 2001).

Evaluation

Dinh still experiences hope, serenity, and wholeness. He has effective coping skills and has no current issues with forgiveness. He feels forgiveness and extends forgiveness to anyone who has hurt him. Regarding Nursing Outcomes Classification (NOC) indicators, Dinh's score on ability to worship went from a 3 to a 5. His family has been making more efforts to get him to mass on Sundays. Indicators of expression through art and writing remained a 2. Arrangements were made for Dinh to receive communion 3 times a week while in the hospital, and this gave Dinh great joy. NIC interventions were effective, and no modification of plan was necessary.

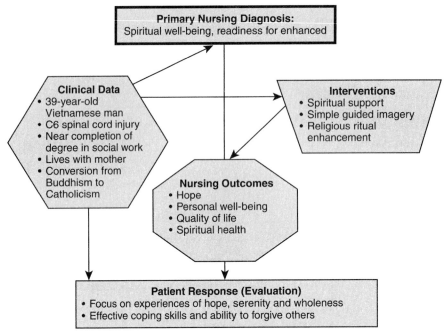

Concept Map. Dinh's nursing diagnosis focuses on wellness, rather than a specific problem. The rehabilitation nurse will focus on coordinating interventions to achieve the outcomes of hope, personal well-being, quality of life, and spiritual health.

CRITICAL THINKING

At the time of assessment Dinh was in a state of spiritual well-being. However, since an individual's spirituality can change, it is possible that Dinh may experience spiritual distress in the future. The following questions explore the meaning and consequences of spiritual distress and the role that the rehabilitation nurse plays in restoring spiritual well-being:

1. What subjective and objective data might Dinh exhibit indicating spiritual distress?
2. What response should the rehabilitation nurse give when Dinh states, "God has abandoned me."
3. What interventions might the rehabilitation nurse implement to help Dinh recover his spiritual well-being? What interventions could the nurse use if Dinh were not practicing a religious faith?
4. How might the nurse evaluate Dinh's spiritual progress?

REFERENCES

Aden, L. (1976). Faith and the developmental cycle. *Pastoral Psychology, 24*(2), 215-230.

American Nurses Association. (2001). *Code of ethics for nurses with interpretive statements.* Silver Spring, MD: Author.

American Psychiatric Association. (1994). *Diagnostic and statistical manual of mental disorders* (4th ed.). Washington, DC: Author.

Barnum, B. S. (2003). Spirituality in nursing, (2nd ed.).

Borysenko, J. (1987). *Minding the body, mending the mind.* Reading, MA: Addison-Wesley.

Bradford, J. (1995). *Caring for the whole child: A holistic approach.* London: The Children's Society.

Brillhart, B. (2005). A study of spirituality and life satisfaction among person with spinal cord injury. *Rehabilitation Nursing, 30*(1), 31-34.

Buchholz, S. W., & Schwartz, K. (2004). The nurse's spiritual health. In K. L. Mauk & N. K. Schmidt (Eds.), *Spiritual care in nursing practice* (pp. 327-357). Philadelphia: Lippincott Williams, & Wilkins.

Burkhart, L. (2005). A click away: Documenting spiritual care. *Journal of Christian Nursing, 22*(1), 6-13.

Carpenito-Moyet, L. J. (2004). *Handbook of nursing diagnosis* (10th ed.). Philadelphia: Lippincott Williams & Wilkins.

Carson, V. B. (1989). *Spiritual dimensions of nursing practice.* Philadelphia: W. B. Saunders.

Cavendish, R., Konecny, L., Mitzeliotis, C., Russo, D., Luise, B. K., Lanza, M., et al. (2003). Spiritual care activities of nurses using nursing interventions classification (NIC) labels. *International Journal of Nursing Terminologies and Classifications, 14*(4), 113-124.

Daaleman, T., & Frey, B. (2004). The Spirituality Index of Well-Being: A new instrument for health-related quality-of-life research, *Annals of Family Medicine, 2,* 499-503.

Deachter, J. (2002). Use of prayer in diabetes self-management. *The Diabetes Educator, 28*(3), 390-394.

Delaney, C. (2005). The spirituality scale: Development and psychometric testing of a holistic instrument to assess the human spiritual dimension. *Journal of Holistic Nursing, 23*(2), 145-167.

Dochterman, J. M., & Bulechek, G. M. (2004). *Nursing interventions classification (NIC)* (4th ed.). St. Louis, MO: Mosby.

Donahue, M. P. (1985). Nursing: The finest art, an illustrated history. St. Louis, MO: Mosby.

Dossey, B. M., & Guzzetta, C. E. (2000). Holistic nursing practice. In B. M. Dossey, L. Keegan, & C. Guzzetta (Eds.), *Holistic nursing: A handbook for practice* (3rd ed.). Gaithersburg, MD: Aspen.

Dossey, L. (1993). Healing words: The power of prayer and the practice of medicine. San Francisco: Harper & Row.

Dubus, A. (1991). *Broken vessels.* Boston: D.R. Godine.

Easton, K. L., & Andrews, J. C. (2000). The roles of the pastor in the interdisciplinary rehabilitation team. *Rehabilitation Nursing, 25,* 10-12.

Ellison, C. W. (1982). Spiritual well-being: Conceptualization and measurement. *Journal of Psychology and Theology, 11,* 330-340.

Erikson, E. H. (1963). *Childhood and society* (2nd ed.). New York: W. W. Norton & Co.

Foley, D. P. (1988). 11 interpretations of personal suffering. *Journal of Religion & Health, 27,* 321-328.

Fowler, J. W. (1974). Toward a developmental perspective on faith. *Religious Education, 69*(2), 207-219.

Frankl, V. (1984). Man's search for meaning: An introduction to logotherapy (Reprint). New York: Simon & Schuster.

Gordon, M. (2006). *Manual of nursing diagnosis* (11th ed.). Boston: Jones and Bartlett.

Grypma, S. (2005). Florence Nightingale's changing image? Part 2. From saint to fiend to modern mystic. *Journal of Christian Nursing, 22*(4), 6-15.

Haddad, L. G., & Hoeman, S. P. (2000). Home healthcare and the Arab-American client. *Home Healthcare Nurse, 18*(3), 189-197.

Hatch, R. L., Burg, M. A., Naberhaus, D. S., & Hellmich, L. K. (1998). The spiritual involvement and beliefs scale: Development and testing of a new instrument. *Journal of Family Practice, 46,* 476-486.

Hillman, J. (1972). *The myth of analysis.* New York: Harper & Row.

Hinds, C. (1993). Suffering: A relatively unexplored phenomenon among family caregivers of non-institutionalized patients with cancer. *Journal of Advanced Nursing, 17,* 718-725.

Hoeman, S. P. (2000). Patient interview.

Humphreys, J. (2000). Spirituality and distress in sheltered battered women. *Image: Journal of Nursing Scholarship, 32,* 273.

Hungleman, J., Kendel-Rossi, E. Klassen, L., & Stollenwerk, R. (1996). Focus on spiritual well-being: Harmonious interconnectedness of mind-body-spirit—including the use of the Jarel Spiritual Well-Being Scale. *Geriatric Nursing, 17,* 262-266.

International Council of Nurses. (2000). Code of ethics. Geneva: Author. Available from http://www.icn.ch/icncode.pdf.

John Paul II, Pope. (1999, October 1). *Letter of His Holiness Pope John Paul II to the elderly.* Vatican City: Author.

Moorhead, S., Johnson, M., & Maas, M. (Eds.). (2004). *Nursing outcomes classification (NOC)* (3rd ed.). St. Louis, MO: Mosby.

Karasu, T. B. (1999). Spiritual psychotherapy. *American Journal of Psychotherapy, 53,* 143-145.

Keating, T. (1996). *Intimacy with God.* New York: Crossroads.

Kim, J. J. (2002). *Spirituality and the disability experience: Faith, subjective well-being, and meaning and purpose in the lives of persons with disabilities.* Doctoral dissertation, Northwestern University, UMINo.AA13050545. Retrieved from Ebsco Host Database, http:80-search-epnet.com.mimas. calstatela.edu/login.aspx?direct=true&db=c8h&an2004115152.

Laszlo, E. (1972). The systems view of the world: The natural philosophy of the new developments in the sciences. New York: George Braziller.

Lohne, V., & Severinsson, E. (2005). Patient's experiences of hope and suffering during the first year following acute spinal cord injury. *Journal of Clinical Nursing 14,* 285-293.

Longway, I. (1970). Toward a philosophy of nursing. *Journal of Adventist Education, 32,* 20-23, 27.

Macrae, J. (1995). Nightingale's spiritual philosophy and its significance for modern nursing. *Image—The Journal of Nursing Scholarship, 27,* 8-10.

Maddox, M. (2001). Teaching spirituality to nurse practitioner students. The importance of the interconnectiveness of mind, body, and spirit. *Journal of the Academy of Nurse Practitioners, 13,* 134-139.

Maslow, A. H. (1971). *The farther reaches of human nature* (2nd ed.). New York: Viking.

Maugans, T. (1996). The spiritual history. *Archives of Family Medicine, 5*(1), 11-16.

Mauk, K. L., Russell, C. A., & Schmidt, N. A. (2004). Planning, implementing and evaluating spiritual care. In K. L. Mauk & N. K. Schmidt (Eds.), *Spiritual care in nursing practice* (pp. 243- 275). Philadelphia, PA: Lippincott Williams & Wilkins.

McBride, J. L., Arthur, G., Brooks, R. E., & Pilkington, L. (1998). The relationship between a patient's spirituality and health experience. *Family Medicine, 30,* 122-126.

McSherry, W., & Ross, L. (2002). Dilemmas of spiritual assessment: Considerations for nursing practice. *Journal of Advanced Nursing, 38*(5), 479-488.

Mickley, J. R., & Cowles, K. (2001). Ameliorating the tension: Use of forgiveness for healing. *Oncology Nursing Forum, 28*(1), 31-37.

Miller, J. (1988). Jokes and joking: A serious laughing matter. In Durant, J., & Miller, J. (Eds.). *Laughing matters: A serious look at humor* (pp. 5-16). Essex, England: Longman Scientific and Technical.

Miller, M., Mangano, C., Park, Y., Goel, R., Plotnick, G. D., & Vogel, R. A. (2006). Impact of cinematic viewing on endothelial function. [Scientific letter.]. *Heart, 92,* 261-262.

Moorhead, S., Johnson, M., & Maas, M. (Eds.). (2004). *Nursing outcomes classification (NOC)* (3rd ed.). St. Louis, MO: Mosby.

Myss, C. (1996). *Anatomy of the spirit: Seven stages of power and healing.* New York: Harmony.

Narayanasamy, A. (1996). Spiritual care of chronically ill patients. *British Journal of Nursing, 5,* 41-46.

Narayanasamy, A. (2002). Spiritual coping mechanisms in chronically ill patients. *British Journal of Nursing, 11*(22), 1461-1470.

Newman, M. (1986). *Health as expanding consciousness.* St. Louis, MO: Mosby.

Niebuhr, R. (1943). *Serenity prayer.* Heath, MA: Written for service in the Congregational Church.

O'Brien, M. E. (2003). *Spirituality in nursing: Standing on holy ground* (2nd ed.). Sudbury, MA: Jones & Bartlett.

Pace, J. C., & Stables, J. L. (1997). Correlation of spiritual well-being in terminally ill patients with AIDS and terminally ill patients with cancer. *Journal of the Association of Nurses in AIDS Care, 8,* 31-42.

Penson, R. T., Yusuf, R. Z., Chabner, B. A., LaFrancesca, J. P., McElhinny, M., Axelrad, A.S., et. al. (2001). Losing God. *The Oncologist, 6,* 286-297.

Post-White, J. (2003). How hope affects healing. *Creative Nursing, 1,* 10-11.

Provine, R. R. (2000). *Laughter: A scientific investigation.* New York: Viking.

Quinn, J. F. (2000). Transpersonal human caring and healing. In B.M. Dossey, L. Keegan, L.G. Kolkmeier, & C. E. Guzzetta (Eds.), *Holistic health promotion: A guide for practice* (3rd ed., pp. 37-48). Gaithersburg, MD: Aspen.

Reed, F. C. (2003). *Suffering and illness: Insights for caregivers.* Philadelphia: F. A. Davies Co.

Reed, P. (1992). An emerging paradigm for the investigation of spirituality in nursing. *Research in Nursing and Health, 15,* 349-357.

Riley, B. B., Perna, R., Tate, D. G., Forchheimer, M., Anderson, C., & Luera, G. (1998). Types of spiritual well-being among persons with chronic illness: Their relation to various forms of quality of life. *Archives of Physical Medicine and Rehabilitation, 79,* 258-264.

Roberts, R. C. (1982). *Spirituality and human emotion.* Grand Rapids, MI: Wm. B. Erdmans.

Robinson, V. (1946). *White caps: The story of nursing.* Philadelphia: J. B. Lippincott.

Rosenberg, C. E. (1998). Holism in 20th century medicine. In G. Lawrence & G. Weisz (Eds.), *Greater than the parts: Holism in biomedicine, 1920-1950* (pp. 335-355). New York: Oxford Press.

Sherwood, G. D. (2000). The power of nurse patient encounters. *Journal of Holistic Nursing, 18*(2), 159-175.

Silber, T. J., & Reilly, M. (1985). Spiritual and religious concerns of the hospitalized adolescent. *Adolescence, 20,* 217-223.

Smith, J., & McSherry, W. (2004). Spirituality and child development: A concept analysis. *Journal of Advanced Nursing, 45*(3), 307-315.

Smith, S. M., & Wiebe, S. (1998). *Meeting patient's spiritual needs.* In P. A. Chin, D. Finocchiaro, & A. Rosebrough (Eds.). *Rehabilitation nursing practice* (pp. 196-220). New York: McGraw-Hill.

Smyth, J. M., Stone, A. A., Hurewitz, A., & Kaell, A. (1999). Effects of writing about stressful experiences on symptom reduction in patients with asthma or rheumatoid arthritis: A randomized trial. *Journal of the American Medical Association, 281,* 1304-1309.

Solimine, M. A. E. (1993). Seek and you will find: The librarian and the team. *Holistic Nursing Practice, 7,* 82-90.

Sommer, D. R. (1989). The spiritual needs of dying children. *Issues in Comprehensive Pediatric Nursing, 12,* 225-233.

Smuts, J. (1970). *Holism and evolution.* New York: MacMillan.

Stravinskas, P. M. (1991). *Our Sunday visitor's: Catholic encyclopedia.* Huntington, N: Visitor Publishing.

Stoll, R. (1979). Guidelines for spiritual assessment. *American Journal of Nursing, 1,* 1572-1577.

Stoll, R. (1989). *The essence of spirituality.* In V. B. Carson (Ed.), *Spiritual dimensions in nursing practice* (pp. 4-23). Philadelphia: W. B. Saunders.

Sumner, C. H. (1998). Recognizing and responding to spiritual distress. *American Journal of Nursing, 98,* 26-30.

Tada, J. E. (1999). How to minister to the disabled: Q and A with Joni Eareckson Tada. Available from http://www.rts.edu/quarterly/spring99/ qa.html.

Tada, J. E., & Estes, S. (1997). When God weeps: Why our sufferings matter to the almighty. Grand Rapids, MI: Zondervan.

Teresa, Mother. (1998). *On prayer.* In D. Salwak (Ed.), *The power of prayer* (pp. 3-11). New York: MJF Books.

Tomey, A. M., & Alligood, M. R. (1998). Nursing theorists and their work (4th ed.). St. Louis, MO: Mosby.

Towey, S. (1997). Spiritual self-care: The healer's journey. *Creative Nursing, 3,* 12.

Tuck, I., Wallace, D., & Pullen, L. (2001). Spirituality and spiritual care provided by parish nurses. *Western Journal of Nursing Research, 23,* 144

Uustal, D. B. (1992). Rx: Holistic caring in the caregiver. In B. M. Dossey, C. E. Guzzetta, & C. V. Kenner (Eds.), *Critical care nursing: Body-mind-spirit* (3rd ed., pp. 41-50). Philadelphia: J. B. Lippincott.

Vash, C. L. (1994). *Personality and adversity: Psychospiritual aspects of rehabilitation.* New York: Springer.

von Bertalanffy, L. (1955). *General system theory: Foundations, developments, applications.* New York: George Braziller.

Watson, J. (1988). *Theory of nursing: Human science and human care.* New York: National League for Nurses.

Westerhoff, J. (1976). *Will our children have faith.* New York: Seabury Press.

Wong, P. T. P. (2005). *Pope John Paul II on the meaning of life and dignity of suffering.* Retrieved August 4, 2005, from http://www.meaning.ca/articles05/wong-pope.htm.

30

Rehabilitation Nursing Care of People With Intellectual/Developmental Disabilities

Dalice L. Hertzberg, RN, MSN, APRN, BC

OVERVIEW

"*Intellectual and developmental disability* refers to a wide variety of mental and/or physical conditions that interfere with the ability of an individual to function effectively at an expected developmental level" (American Nurses Association & the Nursing Division of the American Association on Mental Retardation, 2004). However, universal agreement on terminology is lacking. The term *developmental disability* is defined by the U.S. Developmental Disabilities Assistance and Bill of Rights Act of 2000 and is used primarily in state and federal policy documents to refer to those individuals who qualify for specific public services and civil rights. Many health care professionals use the term *mental retardation*, which is a specific medical and psychiatric diagnosis referring solely to cognitive deficit and is listed in the American Psychiatric Association's (APA's) *Diagnostic and Statistical Manual of Mental Disorders* (4th ed., text revision) *(DSM-IV-TR)* as such (APA, 2000). Advocates, families, and *self-advocates* (individuals who themselves have a developmental disability) believe the terms *mental retardation* and *developmental disability* have negative connotations, that the terms focus more on the deficits of a person than on the person's strengths, and that the terms create stigma for the individual and family. The term *intellectual disability* has arisen more recently to avoid the growing stigma of *developmental disability* or *mental retardation* to individuals who carry that label. The American Association on Mental Retardation has changed its name, as of January 1, 2007, to the American Association on Developmental/Intellectual Disability.

The term *intellectual disability* is used internationally and is promoted by the International Association for the Scientific Study of Intellectual Disability (IASSID). In addition, in Great Britain the term *learning disability* is used to refer to developmental disability.

There is also a historical perspective to terminology. The term *mental retardation* was primarily used in the 1960s, when federal legislation supported by the Kennedy family was initially passed. John F. Kennedy's sister, Rosemary, had mental retardation, and his personal perspective on this disability was the basis for legislation providing services and rights for this population. Later administrations continued to support similar legislation but changed the term to *developmental disability*, which it remains to this day (Minnesota Governor's Council on Developmental Disabilities, 1996).

Developmental Disability

The Developmental Disabilities Assistance and Bill of Rights Act of 2000 (DD Act) defines a developmental disability as

a severe, chronic disability of an individual that—(i) is attributable to a mental or physical impairment or combination of mental and physical impairments; (ii) is manifested before the individual attains age 22; (iii) is likely to continue indefinitely; (iv) results in substantial functional limitations in 3 or more of the following areas of major life activity:

(I) Self-care.
(II) Receptive and expressive language.
(III) Learning.
(IV) Mobility.

(V) Self-direction.

(VI) Capacity for independent living.

(VII) Economic self-sufficiency; and

(V) (above) reflects the individual's need for a combination and sequence of special, interdisciplinary, or generic services, individualized supports, or other forms of assistance that are of lifelong or extended duration and are individually planned and coordinated (Developmental Disabilities Assistance and Bill of Rights Act, 2000).

The DD Act puts forth this definition for the purpose of identifying recipients of specifically stated services, rights, and responsibilities. This definition is purposefully broad, including the presence of physical disabilities, such as cerebral palsy and other conditions originating in childhood. The services specified in the Act include health care, the practice of inclusion, respite care, rehabilitation and assistive technology, personal assistance services, parent training and counseling, support for families headed by aging caregivers, appropriate modifications of homes and vehicles, and assistance for families with unexpected expenses associated with the needs of individuals with developmental disabilities. The law outlines specific terminology to describe mandated services, such as the term *individualized supports*. The term *individualized supports* means services, tailored to the needs of the individual, that enable an individual with a developmental disability to be as independent, productive, and integrated into all facets of community life as possible. *Natural supports* consist of assistance given to a child, adult, or family by neighbors, friends, fellow members of a religious group—in short, nonpaid, nonprofessional caregivers. For example, a toddler play group organized by neighbors might be a natural support, as opposed to a formal early intervention program. Important to the concept of individualized supports is the concept of self-determination, which means that the individual be allowed choice and the ability to determine the course of his or her life, instead of having his or her life directed by others. Although this concept may seem self-explanatory, the history of services for people with intellectual/developmental disability (I/DD) has been primarily that of little or no choice and of professionals determining all facets of a person's life, based on the idea that this population is incapable of making choices for themselves.

Inclusion is the term used for community integration, that is, children or adults with a developmental disability are able to participate with their nondisabled peers in activities that are typical for their age and ethnic group. *Typical or natural environments* are those that would be the usual setting of activities for nondisabled peers of the same age and ethnic group. For more information on natural environments, see Table 30-1.

State Definitions. Although states operate under the federal definition of developmental disabilities, many states offer their own definitions of developmental disabilities in order to limit eligibility for service. For example, although the federal definition is quite general and might include a larger number of individuals, many state definitions are less inclusive and may define a developmental disability solely on the basis of intellectual function, using intelligence quotient (IQ) of 70 or less as the criteria for service eligibility.

Mental Retardation

Although the term *mental retardation* (MR) is defined differently by different organizations, all the definitions have in common the characteristic of limitations in intellectual functioning originating in childhood. Health, social, educational, and vocational service systems use these definitions to define populations and to qualify individual children or adults for services, as well as to determine the intensity and degree of services needed. The major organizations defining mental retardation are the American Psychological Association, the American Psychiatric Association (APA) and the American Association on Mental Retardation (Poindexter & Nehring, 2005).

The *DSM-IV-TR* (APA, 2000) offers perhaps the most medically oriented of the definitions:

Significantly sub average intellectual functioning: an IQ score of approximately 70 or below on an individually administered IQ test. (b) Concurrent deficits or impairments in present adaptive functioning in at least two of the following areas: communication, self-care, home living, social/interpersonal skills, use of community resources, self-direction, functional academic skills, work, leisure, health and safety. (c) The onset is before age 18 years.

TABLE 30-1 Typical or Natural Environments

Typical Community Setting	Example
Home	Personal apartment, group home, host (foster) home, family home
Neighborhood/community	Friend's home, neighbor's home, park, community common area
Places of worship	Church, synagogue, temple, mosque, prayer group
Workplace	Private business, public agency, sheltered workshop
School	Child care, family child care home, preschool, public or private school, community college, vocational school, university
Social setting	Meeting in public place (e.g., coffee shop or cafe), organized group activities, support group activities
Recreation	Gym, organized sports, park, informal recreational get-togethers, organized walk/run, roll

There are five degrees of severity of intellectual impairment, which are accompanied by a specific ICD-9 code (International Classification of Diseases and Related Health Problems). These are mild (IQ 50 to 70); moderate (IQ 35 to 55); severe (IQ 20 to 35); profound (IQ below 20 to 25); and severity unspecified (untestable or uncooperative) (APA, 2000).

The American Psychological Association defines mental retardation as "(a) significant limitations in general intellectual functioning; (b) significant limitations in adaptive function, which exist concurrently; and (c) onset of intellectual and adaptive limitations before the age of 22 years" (Editorial Board, 1996). Four categories of severity are used, roughly equivalent to the first four categories of the American Psychiatric Association. In addition, in the mild and moderate categories, adaptive behaviors are limited in two or more domains, whereas in the severe and profound categories, there are limitations in adaptive behavior in all domains. Adaptive behavior is essentially the ability to solve problems in various conceptual, social, and practical situations and change behavior accordingly. The APA states that socioeconomic status, language and communication, ethnicity, and environment must also be considered in determining the diagnosis of mental retardation.

According to the American Association on Mental Retardation (AAMR), mental retardation is not a diagnosis but a disability "characterized by significant limitations both in intellectual functioning and in adaptive behavior ... disability originates before age 18" (Luckasson et al., 2002). Assessment also includes consideration of cultural and linguistic diversity. Other domains of function, including motor, communication, behavior, and sensory, are assessed as well. Instead of identifying deficits, as did earlier published definitions, the 2002 definition focuses on the determination of strengths, as well as the limitations or needs, to determine the required level of supportive services to promote optimal development and quality of life. Therefore, according to AAMR, an individual's function is classified not by IQ, but by the intensity of support needed at a certain time (Table 30-2). Support intensity may change based on changing circumstances in the environment and/or changes in adaptive skills. The definition is based on the person's level of functioning at the time of assessment and is not a long-term prognosis. In addition, the level of functioning is assessed based upon the context of the environment that is typical for the person's age and ethnicity, not in an isolated clinical setting, but in a setting where people of similar age spend their time (Luckasson et al., 2002).

For the purpose of this chapter, the term *intellectual/developmental disability* (I/DD) will be primarily used. Because research articles and other professional publications often use specific terminology, such as *mental retardation*, the term will

TABLE 30-2 Classification of Mental Retardation by IQ, Support Needs, and Developmental Characteristics

Level of MR	IQ Score	Characteristics
APA: Mild mental retardation AAMR: Intermittent or "as needed" supports	55-70	Minimal impairment, develop social and communication skills, able to acquire academic skills up to about the sixth grade. Able to meet physical developmental milestones. Usually able to provide self-support but may need guidance particularly when under unusual stress. Likely to be integrated into general society.
APA: Mental retardation AAMR: Limited supports; time-limited, more than	40-55	Develop communication skills, difficulty with social skills. Often have physical developmental delays, particularly in fine motor areas; also communication delays. Able to provide personal self-care with guidance. Achieve academically to about the second-grade level. Can perform unskilled or semiskilled work under supervision. Intermittent, involve fewer staff members and limited cost.
APA: Severe mental retardation AAMR: Extensive supports characterized by daily, long-term supervision.	25-40	Few or no communication or social skills, may learn only basic self-care skills and limited academic skills. Obvious developmental delays in all areas. May be able to perform simple tasks with close supervision. Require supervised living situation.
APA: Profound mental retardation AAMR: Pervasive, high-intensity supports continually, which are usually life-sustaining in nature	Less than 25	Significant impairment in sensorimotor function usually due to congenital or neurological condition causing the MR.
APA: Mental retardation, severity unspecified AAMR: Included in above level	IQ untestable by standard tests, lack of cooperation, or in the case of an infant	Substantial delays in all developmental areas, usually noted at birth. Require extensive or total assistance with personal care, may be able to develop rudimentary communication.

Modified from American Psychiatric Association. (2000). *Diagnostic and statistical manual of mental disorders* (4th ed., text revision). Washington, DC: Author.
AAMR, American Association on Mental Retardation; *APA,* American Psychiatric Association; *MR,* mental retardation.

be used in accordance with the *DSM-IV-TR* definition as a diagnosis rather than a descriptive term.

HISTORY OF DEVELOPMENTAL/ INTELLECTUAL DISABILITIES NURSING

In the past, individuals with I/DD were seen as inferior, less than human, and objects of ridicule, and they were segregated and excluded from society (Minnesota Governor's Council on Developmental Disabilities, 1996). The nineteenth century brought about the rise of institutions or large congregate living facilities that segregated individuals. "Training schools," which also segregated children and adults with I/DD, continued as the predominate type of services until the 1960s and 1970s. In 1972 an expose of the Willowbrook State School in New York by journalist Geraldo Rivera publicized the appalling conditions within the institution and greatly contributed to the deinstitutionalization movement. The concept of *normalization*, which was first introduced in 1969, focused on assisting individuals with I/DD or MR to experience a typical schedule, life cycle, and living experiences and also contributed to deinstitutionalization (Nirje, 1973). More recently the self-advocacy movement has allowed and supported individuals with I/DD and MR to speak for themselves in obtaining needed services and life opportunities (Minnesota Governor's Council on Developmental Disabilities, 1996).

By the turn of the nineteenth century nurses were specifically identified as having a role in caring for people in institutions as assistants to the physician. In the 1930s, nursing care for individuals with MR was differentiated from nursing care for people with mental illness. The care provided was custodial. Although most nursing care in the first half of the twentieth century occurred in institutions, public health nurses were involved with children with MR and their families in homes and communities, often recommending institutionalization to parents. Early public health nurses who cared for "the sick poor" in their homes often provided the only habilitative or rehabilitative care individuals with disabilities, such as "crippled" children, living in the tenements received (Buhler- Wilkerson, 2006). By the 1960s and 1970s, public health and pediatric nurses were involved in case finding in the community and teaching families about development and child welfare, as well as caring for children and adults with I/DD and MR in hospitals and institutions, providing both custodial and habilitative care. During the 1960s the role of the nurse in caring for children with MR was proposed, and nurses were actively involved in remedial training programs or habilitation for children and adults with I/DD, such as sensory-motor training. The 1970s brought about the "modern era" of nursing care, which included the following habilitative/rehabilitative roles and functions: prevention, counseling, developmental screening, behavior modification, counseling, interdisciplinary care, and sex education. I/DD nursing was not recognized as a specialty until 1997, largely because the majority of the population was institutionalized until the 1960s and 1970s (Nehring 1999).

IMPLICATIONS FOR REHABILITATION NURSES

Nurses specializing in the care of children and adults with I/DD practice across all levels and settings of care. Rehabilitation nurses working with patients with I/DD who wish to consult with nurses specializing in this population can look to a number of sources, including the membership of the Nursing Division, American Association on Mental Retardation; the Developmental Disabilities Nurses Association (DDNA), and the University Centers of Excellence in Training, Research and Service in Developmental Disabilities (UCEDD). Also, Healthsoft Incorporated has produced an online and CD educational resource on caring for individuals with I/DD. The *International Journal of Nursing in Intellectual and Developmental Disabilities* is also an easily accessible source of information, and is accessible on the DDNA website (http://journal.hsmc.org). For websites where these organizations may be contacted, see Box 30-1.

Providing rehabilitation nursing care for individuals with I/DD across the continuum of care requires knowledge based on the principles of rehabilitation nursing. However, information specific to the condition and issues that are common to people with I/DD is necessary. One of the primary areas of difference in caring for patients with I/DD is in the very important role of advocacy for these very vulnerable individuals, who may or may not have legal guardians or decision makers and who have significant communication deficits. Also, although there are some similarities among all adults with cognitive disabilities (e.g., people with traumatic brain injury), the differing experiences of growing up with an intellectual disability uniquely influence behaviors, self-concept, coping skills, and other adaptive skills. Adults with I/DD who have experienced the effects of stigma and prejudice all their lives may respond differently to standardized interventions than those with acquired disability who have not had those experiences.

BOX 30-1 Resources for Nurses Specializing in the Care of People With I/DD

Association of University Centers on Disability (AUCD): www.AUCD.org; links to websites of University Centers of Excellence in Developmental Disabilities Education, Research and Service (UCEDD) in each state, with e-mail addresses of the interdisciplinary faculty members at each center

American Association on Mental Retardation (AAMR): www.AAMR.org; go to the links for Divisions/Special Interest Groups (SIGs), and click on Nursing

Developmental Disabilities Nurses Association: http://www.ddna.org/

HealthSoft Inc. Developmental Disabilities Courses: http://www.nursingresourcecenter.com/hsi/index.asp

---

I/DD, Intellectual/developmental disability.

Nursing interventions for children and adults with I/DD are most effective when based on the person's developmental or functional level, rather than on chronological age. However, if a person is clearly a physiological adult with a chronological age of 38 years and a developmental or functional age of 6 months, that person should still be treated with the respect of an adult while teaching and other nursing interventions are targeted at the functional age. Table 30-3 provides an outline of aspects of the nursing knowledge base that are helpful in the care of children and adults with I/DD.

REHABILITATION AND HABILITATION

Whereas rehabilitation seeks to aid people in relearning skills, habilitation focuses on the initial learning of life skills for an individual with a developmental or intellectual disability. Examples of life skills include activities of daily living (ADLs), play skills, social skills, recreation, communication, and mobility. Habilitation is "the provision of medical, psychological, educational and family services to people with (developmental) disabilities in order to maximize their vocational, mental, physical and social abilities and to facilitate functioning as independently as possible" (Accardo & Whitman, 2003).

Most people with developmental/intellectual disabilities have fewer deficits in gross motor skills and more deficits in fine motor, communication, sequencing, social skills, and academic skills. However, individuals with I/DD may also have physical disabilities, such as cerebral palsy or spina bifida, which may require rehabilitation throughout the life span (Klingbeil, Baer, & Wilson, 2004). Those individuals whose disability is primarily cognitive, such as those with autism, Down syndrome, fragile X, and mental retardation, are susceptible to the same effects of aging as anyone else, such as arthritis and sensory loss (Fisher & Kettl, 2005). Individuals with I/DD may be candidates for rehabilitation if they lose skills already learned due to disease or trauma.

Injury Risk in People With I/DD and Potential for Rehabilitation

Children with developmental disabilities are more likely to become injured when the demands of a task exceed the individual's ability to complete the task safely. One study found that children in special education have a disproportionate

TABLE 30-3 Nursing Knowledge Base for Caring for People With I/DD

Domain	Topics
Physiologic	Causes of I/DD Genetic conditions and syndromes Secondary conditions of specific diagnoses Common medications used and effects/side effects Influence of I/DD on common chronic diseases (e.g., type 2 diabetes, cardiac disease)
Psychosocial	Co-occurring mental health diagnoses Challenging behavior, and the importance of environment on behavior Communication disorders (e.g., nonverbal, speechprocessing problems) Social communication disorders (e.g., autism spectrum disorders) Poor social skills Developmental effects of growing up with an I/DD Importance of self-advocacy
Family	Family-centered care and collaboration Family adaptation Response to stigma Effects on the family of initial diagnosis of child and how diagnosis was given to family Understanding that parents experience joy from their child with I/DD as well as chronic sorrow Lifetime economic and health effects on caregivers
Community Service System	Early Intervention service system and the Individualized Family Service Plan (IFSP) Educational system and the Individualized Education Plan (IEP), and transition planning Individualized Plan (IP) or Individualized Habilitation Plan (IHP) Health disparities and quality of health and preventative care Where people with I/DD commonly live (e.g., large institutionalized population vs. group homes or other settings) Issues of consent and guardianship DD service system in state of practice Advocacy and support for self-advocacy of people with I/DD Funding issues Policy issues

Modified from American Nurses Association & the Nursing Division of the American Association on Mental Retardation. (2004). *Intellectual and developmental disabilities nursing: Scope and standards of practice* (p. 1). Silver Spring, MD: American Nurses Association.
DD, developmental disability; *I/DD,* intellectual/developmental disability.

number of injuries compared with children who were in regular education (Ramirez, Peek-Asa, & Kraus, 2004). Individuals with I/DD may be at a higher risk than the general population due to decreased coping skills, lack of the ability to "read" a situation and determine what comes next (e.g., an injury), impulsivity, and hyperactivity. Attention-deficit/hyperactivity disorder (ADHD), for example, occurs at an increased prevalence in people with fragile X syndrome and may also co-occur with other types of I/DD (Hastings, Beck, Daley, & Hill 2005).

Some children and adults with autism tend to act impulsively and are often not aware of safety factors; in addition, they are very physically active and rarely have any activity limitations. Co-occurring sensory deficits, such as vision or hearing, may compromise the ability of an individual with MR to hear a warning siren or see a missing step (Petridou et al., 2003). Children with sensorimotor deficits such as poor coordination or lack of sensitivity to temperature are at greater risk for severe burns and bear higher morbidity and mortality risks (Ramirez, Behrends, Blakeney, & Herndon 1998). For children with developmental problems living in poverty with their families, there is a greater risk for accidental injury as well as for abuse (Aber & Bennett, 1997). Among young adults with I/DD in Australia, Sherrard, Tonge, and Ozanne-Smith (2002) found that individuals with disruptive behavior patterns, anxiety, difficulty with social skills, and difficulties with communication had a higher rate of unintentional injury requiring medical care.

In noninstitutionalized adults with I/DD and activity limitations, falls cause an increased prevalence of injury (Xiang, Leff, & Stallones, 2005). Comorbid medical conditions, such as epilepsy and osteoporosis, increased the risk of disabling injury from fractures in adults residing in a developmental center (Lohiya, Crinella, Tan-Figueroa, Caires, & Lohiya, 1999).

People with Down syndrome are more prone to developing heart disease as adults, due to congenital conditions, and some may also develop dementia earlier than it is known to occur in the general population. In addition, undiagnosed atlantoaxial instability can potentially result in trauma to the spinal cord (Down Syndrome Medical Interest Group, 1999).

Aging in Persons With I/DD and Rehabilitation

As people with cerebral palsy age, they may experience central nervous system degeneration and joint problems that interfere with ADLs and can seriously affect functioning. In addition, swallowing disorders and bowel and bladder function may deteriorate (Klingbeil et al., 2004). As individuals with all types of I/DD age, there are declines in ambulatory status as well as in ADLs. In all of these cases, rehabilitation services may be needed, and the success of rehabilitation interventions may be compromised by the underlying developmental disability.

EPIDEMIOLOGY OF DEVELOPMENTAL DISABILITY

Prevalence

Due to the varying definitions of developmental/intellectual disability and MR, as well as different methodologies for determining the condition, there is a great deal of variation in published prevalence rates. In addition, these definitions may change over time due to changes in philosophy and technical advances (Leonard & Wen, 2002). Differences in measures of intelligence, difficulty in testing the intelligence of children and adults who are nonverbal, and differences among age-groups, gender, and socioeconomic status all contribute to this variation in prevalence (Leonard & Wen, 2002). For example, there is a greater prevalence of mental retardation in school-age children than in infants and toddlers, because school-age children are easier to test using standardized intelligence testing. There are lower prevalence rates in adults partly due to the lack of intellectual testing in this age-group, improved adaptive skills in adults, and early death. Rates of mental retardation are higher in males, individuals from lower socioeconomic settings, and in African American children (Bhasin, Brocksen, Avchen, & Van Naarden Braun, 2006). Mental retardation is present in about 2% to 3% of the population; of these, about 75% to 90% have mild MR. Severe mental retardation occurs in about 3 to 4 per 1000 children or adults, with moderate levels of MR at about 10% to 25% of all cases of MR. It is estimated that in 30% to 50% of school-age children with MR the cause cannot be identified (Croen, Grether, & Selvin, 2001).

According to the Centers for Disease Control and Prevention (CDC) (1996), rates of mental retardation can be estimated for states using data about individuals who receive specialized services through entitlement programs (such as special education programs for children age 6 to 17 years) and the Social Security Administration (for adults age 18 to 64 years receiving disability services due to MR). Using this data from the year 1993, the CDC estimated that 1.5 million persons age 6 to 64 years in the United States were identified as having MR, and the overall rate of MR for the United States was 7.6 cases per 1000 population (CDC, 1996). Interestingly, rates per state varied widely, with the lowest rates of MR found in the Pacific and Mountain states. For children the rate of MR was 11.4 per 1000, and for adults it was 6.6 per 1000. It is important to note that the prevalence rates for mild mental retardation are higher than for moderate or severe MR and are estimated at approximately 75% to 90% of all people with MR (Daily, Ardinger, & Holmes, 2000).

Etiology of I/DD

The causes of I/DD are many and include genetic conditions and heavy metal poisoning; prenatal and perinatal insults; multifactorial causes such as neural tube defects; postnatal trauma and environmental causes; and idiopathic, or unknown causes. Children who are born with birth defects are more likely to be diagnosed with MR by age 7 years (Jelliffe-Pawlowski, Shaw, Nelson, & Harris 2003). The majority of causes of mental retardation lie in the prenatal period, with relatively few etiologies in the postnatal period.

Prenatal Causes of I/DD

Genetic causes account for the majority of identified causes of mental retardation. There are at least 500 different genetic disorders that are identified as causes of I/DD, including chromosomal abnormalities, single-gene disorders, and multifactorial conditions. Monogenic (single-gene disorders) are often causes of metabolic disorders, which are a significant cause of MR (Aicardi, 1998). Chromosomal disorders constitute from 4% to 28% of the total causes of MR (Curry et al., 1997). Down syndrome is one of the most common birth defects that is caused by a chromosomal abnormality. The most common inherited cause of I/DD is fragile X syndrome (March of Dimes, 2006). For an overview of genetic causes of I/DD, see Table 30-4.

Other prenatal causes include congenital infection, teratogens, maternal disease (e.g., seizure disorder, diabetes), as well as maternal medications and use of drugs of abuse (alcohol, cocaine, heroin, marijuana, methamphetamine). The issue of maternal drug use is difficult to sort out, because multiple substances are often used and drug use often is accompanied by poverty, malnutrition, and poor prenatal care. Alcohol abuse by the mother of the child is thought to be the most common single, nongenetic prenatal cause of mental retardation. Prenatal alcohol exposure may result in fetal alcohol syndrome (FAS), which is the most common prenatal cause of mild to moderate mental retardation. For a list of prenatal causes of I/DD other than genetic causes, see Box 30-2.

Perinatal Causes of I/DD

Perinatal causes of I/DD account for about 10% of all known causes. Anoxia to the brain, resulting from birth trauma, is associated with physical disability, such as cerebral palsy, and often seizures. Premature infants are more likely to experience intraventricular hemorrhage resulting in damage to the brain. Infections, such as bacterial meningitis, due to premature rupture of membranes may also result in I/DD (Futagi, Toribe, Ogawa, & Suzuki, 2006).

Postnatal Causes of I/DD

Trauma and disease are the primary postnatal causes of I/DD. About 3% to 15 % of all causes of I/DD are postnatal causes. Bacterial meningitis and nonaccidental trauma account for the majority of cases. Individuals who have acquired I/DD postnatally tend to have greater disability and more comorbidities. Other postnatal causes of I/DD include near-drowning, stroke, and motor vehicle accidents. Additional causes include noninfectious disease conditions such as brain tumor or other cancers and negative sequelae from surgery such as cardiac surgery or transplants. However, these noninfectious disease conditions account for a very small number of individuals with I/DD (CDC, 1996).

Environmental factors are also potential causes of I/DD. Exposure to toxins such as lead and mercury are known causes of cognitive sequelae. Children who lack exposure to an

TABLE 30-4 Common Genetic Disorders Causing I/DD

Types of Genetic Malformation	Condition Associated With I/DD

Chromosomal disorders causing I/DD	Down syndrome (trisomy 21)
	 Edwards syndrome (trisomy 18)
	 Patau's syndrome (trisomy 13)
	 Disorders of the X chromosome
	   Klinefelter's syndrome (XXY)
	   Turner's syndrome (XO)
	 Microdeletion disorders on chromosomes
	   Prader-Willi syndrome*
	   Angelman's syndrome*
	   Williams syndrome

Single-gene (Mendelian) disorders	*X-linked recessive*
	   Fragile X syndrome
	   Lesch-Nyhan syndrome
	 Autosomal recessive
	   Phenylketonuria
	   Congenital hypothyroidism
	   Galactosemia
	   Maple syrup urine disease
	   Tay-Sachs
	   Metachromatic leukodystrophy
	 Autosomal dominant
	   Neurofibromatosis
	   Tuberous sclerosis

Multifactorial	Spina bifida (myelomeningocele) Mild mental retardation

Modified from Curry, C. J., Stevenson, R. E., Aughton, D., Byrne, J., Carey, J. C., Cassidy, S., et al. (1997). Evaluation of mental retardation: Recommendations of a Consensus Conference: American College of Medical Genetics. *American Journal of Medical Genetics*, 72(4), 468-477.
I/DD, Intellectual/developmental disability.
*These two conditions are due to the same deletion on chromosome 15. If the deletion is transmitted paternally, Prader-Willi results; if the deletion is transmitted maternally, Angelman's results.

BOX 30-2 Common Nongenetic Prenatal Causes of I/DD

Common Prenatal Infections Causing I/DD
- Cytomegalovirus (most common infectious prenatal cause)
- Toxoplasmosis
- Rubella
- Syphilis
- Herpes

Maternal Disease

Untreated Hypothyroidism

Untreated or Inadequately Treated Phenylketonuria

Maternal Medications Causing I/DD
- Phenytoin (Dilantin)

Maternal Substance Abuse
- Alcohol
- Cocaine
- Heroin
- Marijuana
- Methamphetamine

I/DD, Intellectual/developmental disability.

BOX 30-3 Common Perinatal and Postnatal Causes of I/DD

Perinatal Causes	Postnatal Causes
Prematurity (hypoxia)	Meningitis/encephalitis
	Accidental trauma (e.g., falls, motor vehicle accidents)
Sepsis meningitis	Nonaccidental trauma (child abuse, shaken baby syndrome)
Perinatal trauma	Malnutrition
	Environmental pollutants (e.g., lead, mercury)

I/DD, Intellectual/developmental disability.

BOX 30-4 Outline of Diagnostic Process for Mental Retardation

- Extensive medical and developmental history, including gestational history, prenatal exposure to disease or toxins, and birth history; prior pregnancy history for any fetal loss; family history, particularly looking for consanguinity, any family members with developmental problems or school problems
- Thorough physical examination, particularly for any dysmorphic or unusual physical features
- Developmental testing using a standardized, norm-referenced test such as the Bayley Scales of Infant Development
- Laboratory investigations such as metabolic testing; neuroimaging and electrophysiology (in selected situations); and chromosomal testing

Modified from Curry, C. J., Stevenson, R. E., Aughton, D., Byrne, J., Carey, J. C., Cassidy, S., et al. (1997). Evaluation of mental retardation: Recommendations of a Consensus Conference: American College of Medical Genetics. *American Journal of Medical Genetics, 72*(4), 468-477.

---

enriched environment may also be diagnosed with mental retardation; whether due to poverty or other family factors such as malnutrition (Valent et al., 2004). For a summary of perinatal and postnatal causes, see Box 30-3.

DIAGNOSIS

Diagnosis of mental retardation is usually performed by a multidisciplinary team in a hospital, a clinic, or the school. Intelligence testing is generally conducted by a psychologist. The etiology of the mental retardation is determined by a physician, usually a developmental pediatrician or a pediatric neurologist. If dysmorphic features are recognized, genetic testing is required to determine the cause, and geneticists or genetic counselors may be involved in the diagnosis.

Both cognitive testing and developmental testing are involved in the diagnosis of mental retardation. Unless they are severely affected, children with MR are first identified by delays in development, usually speech and communication delays, in the preschool and early school-age period. Cognitive, or IQ, testing can only be performed once a child has sufficient language to communicate with the tester. Before this period, children may be diagnosed with developmental delay, instead of mental retardation. Using developmental tests such as the Bayley Scales of Infant Development, infants and toddlers who have little or no language may be evaluated, and delays in specific domains may be quantified. Although it is not completely necessary to providing treatment, determining the cause of the mental retardation can offer information about the natural history of the condition, identify conditions that may be treatable (e.g., phenylketonuria, a metabolic disease causing MR), provide genetic information for family members, and aid in planning services (Curry et al., 1997). For an outline of the diagnostic process, see Box 30-4.

Once the diagnosis is made, a treatment plan is developed to minimize developmental delays and improve the child's functioning. A diagnosis of mental retardation is sufficient to qualify a child age 6 to 21 years for special education and related services. At the time of diagnosis, the family is faced with both learning about the diagnosis and providing the additional care and instruction the child with MR needs.

CONDITIONS ASSOCIATED WITH MENTAL RETARDATION AND INTELLECTUAL/DEVELOPMENTAL DISABILITIES

Associated conditions (conditions that occur as part of the condition or syndrome) or comorbidities that may occur in people with MR and I/DD include seizures, speech and language disorders, and sensory disorders such as hearing deficit or visual deficit. Neurodevelopmental disorders, such as those listed above, are the most common. Some genetic conditions predispose a child or adult to specific problems; for example cardiac defects are common in individuals with Down syndrome and are thought to be genetic in origin (Roper & Reeves, 2006). Some syndromes, such as Lennox-Gastaut syndrome, a seizure disorder resulting in deteriorating cognitive abilities, often include mental retardation as a comorbidity (Trevathan, Murphy, & Yeargin-Allsopp, 1997). Swallowing disorders occur primarily in individuals with cerebral palsy and other neuromuscular disorders that may co-occur with mental retardation and are addressed in Chapter 16.

Associated or Comorbid Conditions

Seizure disorders occur more frequently in individuals with I/DD, at a rate of about 20% in children with MR. As people with I/DD age, seizure disorders increase in frequency (McDermott et al., 2005). Individuals with I/DD who also have seizure disorders tend to have more difficulty managing seizures and have a greater risk of death. Other conditions involving MR, such as autism spectrum disorders and Down syndrome (in association with Alzheimer's dementia), all have an increased risk of seizure disorders associated with the conditions (Menendez, 2005).

Communication disorders are common in individuals with I/DD. Children are often identified first with a language delay as the initial sign of an I/DD. People with cerebral palsy may have spasticity, which affects the muscles of speech. Autism spectrum disorders are defined as social communication disorders, and difficulties with communication are a hallmark of these conditions. Individuals with developmental disorders such as Williams syndrome and Down syndrome have unique speech and language disorders that most likely derive from their genetic origins (Ypsilanti, Grouios, Alevriadou, & Tsapkini, 2005).

Other communication problems arise from sensory disorders, such as hearing impairment, as well as from the cognitive disability itself, and can result in behavioral problems. Communication problems in people with I/DD are associated with both receptive and expressive language disorders. Difficulty communicating with others results in social isolation and difficulty making and keeping friends. Inability to communicate feeling ill or other physical symptoms may complicate health care. Audiologists and speech and language pathologists are involved in both assessment of and treatment of communication disorders in I/DD.

Sleep problems may affect children and adults with MR and I/DD, particularly in response to stressors. Co-occurring health problems, such as obstructive sleep apnea, ADHD, or anxiety may complicate sleep disorders. Medications used to treat ADHD or mental health disorders may also cause insomnia. In many cases the interventions are behavioral or may involve adjustment of medications (Luiselli, Magee, Sperry, & Parker, 2005).

Sensory disorders such as vision and hearing deficits are more common in individuals with I/DD than in the general population (Owens, Kerker, Zigler, & Horwitz, 2006). Sensory disorders require ongoing assessment and treatment through the life span and can worsen as people with I/DD age.

Sensory processing, or sensory integration (SI) disorders also occur more frequently in people with I/DD, particularly those with autism spectrum disorders and fragile X syndrome. Impairments in sensory processing may result in tactile sensitivity of the skin and/or the mouth, abnormalities of proprioception, and unusual sensitivity to odors, sounds, or tastes and textures. This unusual sensitivity can result in avoidance of crowds or certain activities because of the overwhelming sensory input, as well as avoidance of physical contact, such as hugs or holding hands. Some people may experience a lack of sensory input and seek more sensory input, such as rocking, vocalization, and/or seemingly purposeless movement. Individuals with SI disorders may have related fine and gross motor disorders, as well as academic problems. Treatment of SI disorders consists of desensitization, the use of stimulating activities directed toward the nervous system, and directed play activities (Baranek, Foster, & Berkson, 1997; Baranek, et al., 2002).

Secondary Conditions

Secondary conditions are those that may arise from the underlying condition, such as contractures in cerebral palsy, or as a result of familial or lifestyle factors such as cardiac disease or obesity. Secondary conditions are largely preventable by good health care and health promotion interventions, to which many individuals with I/DD lack access.

Frey, Szalda-Petree, Traci, and Seekins (2000) reviewed the literature for the most commonly identified secondary conditions in adults with developmental disabilities. They found communication problems, injuries due to self-inflicted abuse, dental hygiene problems, difficulties with memory, difficulties with persistence, and mobility deficits. As more people with I/DD live in the community, substance abuse can become a problem, although rates are lower than in the general population. Cigarette smoking and other tobacco abuse, alcohol abuse, and illicit drug use can increase health risks and result in need for additional health and psychological services. In the interest of brevity, the most common and/or limiting secondary conditions will be discussed here.

Obesity is a significant problem in individuals with I/DD. Some genetic conditions, such as Down syndrome, predispose to obesity. Prader-Willi syndrome, a genetic disorder with the characteristics of short stature, hypogonadism, and hyperphagia, frequently results in obesity (Butler et al., 2002). In part due to low literacy and cognitive disability, people with I/DD are less likely to be able to access healthy lifestyle information, which promotes weight control and exercise. Health disparities often interfere with the receipt of quality health care in this population, and people with I/DD may not receive interventions that are routinely offered to people without disabilities, such as weight loss programs (Havercamp, Scandlin, & Roth, 2004). In some cases food may take the place of satisfying social interactions. The best intervention for obesity is prevention by promoting regular exercise and a healthy diet, but weight loss programs can be effective for this population as well. Living situations, that is institutionalization versus living in the community in a group home or apartment with assistance or living with their family of origin, may influence health promotion activities. The concept that the more choices people with I/DD have, the less likely they are to engage in health-promoting activities has been supported by several studies (Frey, Buchanan, & Rosser Sandt, 2005). However, provision of positive role models, accessible health information, and accessible exercise opportunities can counter this trend (Frey et al., 2005).

Lack of adequate dental care is another health disparity that contributes to poor dental hygiene, tooth decay, infections and pain and can impact nutritional status of the individual with I/DD. Physical and cognitive disabilities, as well as tactile defensiveness, can interfere with dental hygiene. Seizure medication, such as Dilantin, can cause gingival hyperplasia. This common secondary condition is preventable with regular dental care and cleaning and dental hygiene (Havercamp et al., 2004).

Common functional deficits in this population include poor social skills and lack of or limited self-care skills. Mobility deficits occur primarily in people with I/DD who also have physical disabilities, such as people with cerebral palsy or other motor disorders, and/or those with very severe MR.

Individuals with MR and I/DD are prone to difficulties with social skills, which can result in difficulty making and keeping friends and developing romantic relationships and can lead to social isolation. Although some of these difficulties may be related to lack of language skills, the majority are related to the cognitive deficit and resulting difficulties with learning or perception. Even individuals with very mild or borderline MR may have difficulty making friends. Although social skills training and interventions may ameliorate this problem to some degree, the practice of inclusion of people with I/DD at an early age can facilitate greater acceptance of disability diversity among the general population.

DUAL DIAGNOSIS: MENTAL RETARDATION AND MENTAL ILLNESS AND BEHAVIORAL DISORDERS

In the I/DD field, dual diagnosis is defined as the co-occurrence of mental retardation and mental illness. Although published statistics vary, psychiatric disorders are thought to occur more frequently in people with MR than in the typically developing population, with some conditions more frequent than others. Although the cause is unknown, a number of risk factors may predispose children and adults with I/DD to mental illness, including the presence of injury to the brain, adverse life events such as repeated losses or abuse, communication difficulties and sensory impairments, limited coping abilities, untreated or inadequately treated medical problems, and genetic factors. Although developmental/intellectual disability does not cause mental illness, it may cause disorders to manifest differently and complicates diagnosis and treatment. ADHD, for example, is more common in people with I/DD than in the general population (Rush & Frances, 2000).

Behavioral disorders are also common in children and adults with I/DD. Particularly in persons who are nonverbal or have limited language and communication skills, challenging behavior may be functional for the individual. Behaviors may serve to gain attention for the person, avoid unpleasant demands being made upon them, obtain desired actions or objects (e.g., toys or food), reduce arousal and anxiety, and offer a sense of control over the environment. Also, some behaviors, such as hand flapping, head banging, or even masturbation, may serve only for purposes of self-stimulation. However, these behaviors may be annoying for others, dangerous to the individual, or even illegal, such as masturbation in public, and may need to be addressed. Individuals with I/DD often have very little control over their lives and tend to rely on external structure and routine in order to cope. Even well-meaning changes in the environment by caregivers may result in increased anxiety and challenging behaviors in order to exert some control or to express dissatisfaction with the environment or stimuli.

Diagnosis is generally accomplished by a psychiatrist or psychologist with special training in the area. Depending on the level of mental retardation present and the individual's age, adaptive skills, and communication skills, many children and adults can be assessed for behavioral and mental health disorders using standardized instruments used in the general population. Assessment methods may include a family or caregiver interview, direct observation of behavior, medical examination, and a psychiatric diagnostic interview. In addition, there are screening tools that have been specifically developed for people with I/DD. There are several rating scales that have been found to be helpful in diagnosing behavioral and psychiatric disorders in the general population that can be helpful for people with I/DD, such as the Conners Parent and Teacher Rating Scales for ADHD, the Child Behavior Checklist, and the Vineland Adaptive Behavior Scales. Specific rating scales exist for children and adults with I/DD, such as the Psychopathology Inventory for Mentally Retarded Adults and the Reiss Scale for Children's Dual Diagnosis. However, these tools are useful only for individuals with mild to moderate intellectual disability, because diagnosis is much more difficult in people with severe I/DD (Rush & Frances, 2000).

Diagnosis of psychiatric disorders in individuals with I/DD is challenging, as is differentiating the symptoms of a specific DSM-IV-TR psychiatric disorder from the symptoms of challenging behavior due to nonpsychiatric causes. Children and adults with I/DD may experience any of the more common psychiatric disorders, including but not limited to schizophrenia and psychotic disorders, mood disorders including depression and bipolar disorder, anxiety disorders and obsessive-compulsive disorder, posttraumatic stress disorder, ADHD, and others. Perhaps the most challenging aspect of diagnosing psychiatric disorders among people with I/DD, particularly those with significant communication problems, is distinguishing a true mental illness from the behavioral manifestations of physical illness. In order to rule out physical illness as a cause of symptoms, a complete physical examination and laboratory tests are necessary, such as thyroid testing, toxicology screens, and blood levels of medications. Behavioral outbursts or uncharacteristic aggressive behaviors, withdrawal, poor appetite and weight loss or gain, or delirium may result from physical disorders ranging from an ingrown toenail or abscessed tooth to elevated blood levels of medication or electrolyte disorders (Rush & Frances, 2000).

Treatment of psychiatric and behavioral disorders initially focuses on alteration of the environment or behavioral modification. In some cases, cognitive behavioral therapy can be useful, particularly with anxiety disorders in children and adults with mild intellectual disability. For more severe behavioral disorders or specific psychiatric disorders, psychotropic medication is frequently used. Hyperactivity and ADHD are treated in a similar manner as is seen in the nondisabled population. Polypharmacy may be a significant problem with this population, and side effects must be monitored with vigilance to avoid medical problems as well as exacerbating behavioral issues (Rush & Frances, 2000). For an overview of commonly used medications, their indications in individuals with I/DD, and possible side effects, see Table 30-5.

TABLE 30-5 Medications Commonly Used to Treat Psychiatric Disorders in Adults With I/DD

Psychiatric Disorder	Recommended Medication	Side Effects/Implications
Psychosis	First-generation antipsychotic medications: Haldol (haloperidol). Atypical antipsychotic medications: Clozaril (clozapine), Risperdal (risperidone), Zyprexa (olanzapine), Seroquel (quetiapine)	Weight gain, hyperglycemia, extrapyramidal symptoms (tardive dyskinesia)
Depression, posttraumatic stress disorder, anxiety disorders	Selective serotonin reuptake inhibitors (SSRIs): Prozac (fluoxetine), Zoloft (sertraline), Celexa (citalopram), Luvox (fluvoxamine). Other antidepressants: Serzone (nefazodone), Effexor (venlafaxine), Wellbutrin (bupropion). Antianxiety medications: BuSpar (buspirone)	Irritability, digestive problems
Bipolar disorder	Mood stabilizer: Lithium Anticonvulsants: Depakote (divalproex), Tegretol (carbamazepine).	Narrow therapeutic window, interaction with NSAIDs and thiazide diuretics for lithium
Self-injurious behaviors, aggression	Atypical antipsychotic medications (see above), SSRIs	

Data from Rush, J. A., & Frances, A. (Eds.). (2000). Expert Consensus Guideline Series: Treatment of psychiatric and behavioral problems in mental retardation. *American Journal of Mental Retardation, 105*(3), 159-228.
I/DD, Intellectual/developmental disability; *NSAIDs*, nonsteroidal antiinflammatory drugs.

COMMON DEVELOPMENTAL DISABILITIES

Autism Spectrum Disorders

A number of distinct conditions with specific diagnostic criteria are associated with I/DD. Autism spectrum disorders (ASDs) are a group of neurodevelopmental conditions characterized by impairments in interpersonal communication and reciprocal social interactions. This group of conditions is also referred to as *pervasive developmental disorders* (APA, 2000).

The prevalence rate for autism has been increasing in the past 10 to 15 years and is estimated at about 11 to 17 children per 10,000. It is unclear whether this represents a true increase in prevalence or improved recognition and diagnosis. Autism is more common in males than females, with a ratio of about 6 to 8 males to 1 female (Fombonne, 2005).

Current theories about the etiology of ASDs implicate an abnormality of brain development and function, most likely due to a combination of genetic factors and other etiologies (Beversdorf et al., 2005). There are associated medical conditions in many individuals on the spectrum, which include tuberous sclerosis, fragile X syndrome, Down syndrome, cerebral palsy, phenylketonuria, neurofibromatosis, congenital rubella, hearing and visual disorders, and seizure disorders (Fombonne, 2005). There is recent evidence that familial factors contribute to ASDs. One study identified risks for ASDs in California, finding a greater risk in males, in multiple births, in children with African American mothers, and in children with mothers who are older and well educated (Croen, Grether, & Selvin, 2002).

Individuals with an ASD exhibit a range of communication disorders and deficits, difficulties with social interaction, and stereotypic interests, activities, and behaviors. A large proportion of individuals with ASD have mental retardation, but not all. Behavioral disorders, such as angry outbursts or self-injurious behavior are common, as are co-occurring mental illnesses such as anxiety disorders or attentional disorders. Sensory integration disorders also occur frequently. There have been anecdotal reports of gastrointestinal problems such as celiac disease and "leaky gut" in a small population of children with autism, but this has not been substantiated in the literature.

The ASDs occur on a continuum with variable severity and presentation of symptoms. All of the ASDs have onset before 36 months of age but may not be diagnosed until the child is older. ASD includes the following diagnoses: autistic disorder, Asperger's disorder or syndrome, atypical autism or pervasive developmental disorder not otherwise specified (PDDNOS), Rett syndrome, and childhood disintegrative disorder (APA, 2000). For more information on ASDs, see Table 30-6.

Symptoms of the characteristic impairments in communication and play may include speech delay without any other form of communication, such as gestural, or in people who do have speech, inability or difficulty in initiating and sustaining a conversation. People with ASD often use a very stereotypical language, often referring to objects or people in their own way. Children with ASD show rigid, stereotypical play, often having more interest in repetitive activities than in creative, reciprocal play. Older children or adults with ASD may have interests that are very narrow, very intense, or unusual and may show a great deal of inflexibility when it comes to routines. They may have repetitive motor mannerisms such as hand flapping or finger flicking and may show a persistent preoccupation with parts of objects, instead of the entire object.

TABLE 30-6 Overview of Autism Spectrum Disorders

Disorder	Prevalence	Level of MR	Characteristics
Autistic disorder, infantile autism, childhood autism, Kanner's autism	5-20 cases per 10,000	Mild to profound	Behavioral symptoms (e.g., hyperactivity, impulsiveness, aggressiveness, self-injury) Marked impairment in social interaction particularly in the use of nonverbal behaviors (e.g., eye contact, facial expression, posture, and gestures). Communication impairment including delay or lack of speech, inability to sustain a conversation, stereotypical or repetitive language; lack of imitation or make-believe play Restricted and stereotypic patterns of behavior, interests, and activities
Asperger's disorder, or Asperger's syndrome	2.6 per 10,000	None	Impairment in social interaction, particularly nonverbal behaviors. Lack of developmentally appropriate peer relationships. Lack of social or emotional reciprocity. Restricted repetitive and stereotypical patterns of behavior, interests, and activities. No significant language delay, or delay in cognitive development, or age-appropriate self-care skills or adaptive skills
Rett's disorder, also Rett syndrome	1 per every 10,000 to 15,000, only in females	Moderate to severe	Normal prenatal and perinatal development, normal head circumference at birth. Normal psychomotor development up to 5 months of age only Deceleration of head growth between 5 and 48 months of age. Loss of hand skills with development of stereotypical hand movements (wringing or "washing" of hands); poor motor coordination in general. Severe impairment of expressive and language development Loss of the ability for social engagement, with severe psychomotor retardation
Childhood disintegrative disorder	Rare, may be slightly more common in males; 1-2 per 100,000	Severe	Marked regression in function after normal development for first 2 years of life. Regression occurs between 2 and 10 years of age, with loss of skills that were previously acquired in expressive or receptive language, social skills/adaptive behavior, bowel or bladder function, play and/or motor skills Frequent association with EEG abnormalities and seizure disorder. May be associated with other neurological conditions

Modified from American Psychiatric Association. (2000). *Diagnostic and statistical manual of mental disorders* (4th ed., text revision). Washington, DC: Author.; and Fombonne, E. (2005). Epidemiology of autistic disorder and other pervasive developmental disorders. *Journal of Clinical Psychiatry, 66*(Suppl. 10), 3-8.

MR, Mental retardation; *EEG,* electroencephalogram.

For example, an adult with ASD may seem obsessed with a certain topic, such as the history of a certain country, and talk about it all the time. Young children may be preoccupied with lining up shoes instead of playing with age-appropriate toys (APA, 2000).

Symptoms of impairment of social interaction include difficulty initiating and maintaining friendships or even social exchange, avoidance of eye contact, the inability to perceive or understand social rules, and inability to use or understand nonverbal behaviors on the part of others. The concept "Theory of Mind" is used to describe the lack of ability of persons with ASD to perceive or understand the motivations, perspective, or feelings of others (Fischer & Happe, 2005). Despite these considerable difficulties, people with ASD are capable of affection and long-term attachments and experience sadness and grief with loss. They are also able to learn and are

capable of behavior change with consistent intervention and therapy (Cashin, 2005; Sperry & Mesibov, 2005).

ASDs are usually diagnosed in early childhood, and most children are diagnosed by school age. The presence of communication disorders, behavioral problems, and social concerns are the usual triggers for developmental evaluation, particularly with regard to delayed or regressed language. A few individuals with Asperger's syndrome, a high-functioning form of autism, may not be diagnosed with the condition until adolescence or adulthood.

Treatment of children and adults with ASDs includes long-term behavioral interventions at home and at school and the use of speech-language and psychological therapy to develop communication and interpersonal skills. Children with autism generally receive special education (Hutchins & Prelock, 2006). Individuals with co-occurring mental illness

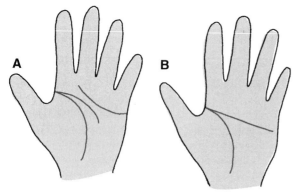

Figure 30-1 Examples of flexion creases on palm. **A,** Normal. **B,** Transpalmar crease. (From Hockenberry, M. R., Wilson, D., Winklestein, M. L., & Kline, N. E. [2003]. *Wong's nursing care of infants and children* [7th ed.]. St. Louis, MO: Mosby.)

require treatment, both behavioral and pharmacological, for those diagnoses. Individuals with persistent behavioral issues, even in the absence of diagnosed mental illness, may also require treatment with psychopharmaceuticals (Rush & Frances, 2000). Provision of social and educational services such as school-to-work transition, vocational rehabilitation, and job support are critical. Because of the often profound communication deficits and significant behavioral disorders, family members of children and adults with autism experience a great deal of stress and often require respite services (Lecavalier, Leone, & Wiltz, 2006).

Down Syndrome

Down syndrome (DS) is the most common genetic condition resulting in mental retardation. Trisomy 21 (extra chromosome number 21), resulting in 47 chromosomes instead of the usual 46, is the most common genetic malformation causing Down syndrome and may occur through nondisjunction or mosaicism (NICHD, 2005). Although maternal age is a risk factor for Down syndrome, older mothers (age 35 years and older) have fewer children, so a greater number of children with this disorder are born to younger women. About 75% of children born with Down syndrome are born to younger mothers. The genetic error that results in Down syndrome may be familial or may be a spontaneous mutation, the cause of which is unknown. The prevalence rate for Down syndrome is about 1 in 650 to 1000 births (NICHD, 2005).

Usually diagnosed at birth, infants with Down syndrome have characteristic flattened facial features, epicanthal folds and slanted eyes, and a small mouth with large, protruding tongue. Other characteristic features include a flattened occiput and short neck and small hands with very short fifth fingers, which are curved inward. Approximately 50% of the time the infant has a transverse crease in the palm of the hand (American Academy of Pediatrics (AAP), 2001) (Figure 30-1).

Comorbid conditions at birth may include congenital heart defects such as endocardial cushion defects and septal defects, gastrointestinal malformations such as esophageal

atresia, and hypotonia causing motor delays and joint dislocations, most commonly dislocated hips and a poor suck, causing difficulty with breast-feeding. Presence or absence of the above-mentioned congenital defects appears to be genetically determined, because the comorbidities do not occur across the board in all individuals with DS. Some children with DS may have a seizure disorder, and others may develop seizures in adulthood in combination with early Alzheimer's dementia (Roper & Reeves, 2006). Although all children with DS have some level of mental retardation, the degree ranges from mild to severe, with the majority in the moderate range. Children with DS are at increased risk for a number of secondary conditions such as feeding disorders, vision and hearing abnormalities, constipation, thyroid and other endocrine problems, obesity, and skin conditions. Altered immune function combined with a short ear canal contributes to an increased risk of respiratory disease and frequent ear infections, which may lead to hearing loss. Periodontal disease and other infections also occur more frequently than in the general population. In addition, growth retardation results in short stature and can contribute to obesity. Other conditions that occur more frequently in children with DS are leukemia and celiac disease. Atlantoaxial instability is found in about 14% of children with DS on radiological evaluation; however, actual cord compression occurs in less than 1% of the population (Down Syndrome Medical Interest Group, 1999).

As with other people with I/DD, behavioral problems may arise as a result of communication deficits or environmental influences. Some authors suggest that individuals with DS have fewer behavioral problems than people with mental retardation from other causes. Autistic behavior is more common in individuals with DS than in the general population, with symptoms of stereotypic mannerisms, compulsive behaviors, and self-injurious behaviors (Chapman & Hesketh, 2000).

Adults with DS are more likely to develop Alzheimer's disease and at an earlier age than the general population (Aisen et al., 2005). Males with DS tend to be infertile, and females have a reduced level of fertility, although without extensive testing, contraception is the safest course. In addition, women with DS experience earlier menopause (Down Syndrome Medical Interest Group, 1999). For adults with DS the median age of death is 49, but many survive into the sixth decade (Yang, Rassmussen, & Friedman, 2002).

Treatment for DS includes surgical repair of congenital defects, such as heart and gastrointestinal problems, and medical diagnosis and treatment of associated conditions. Developmental therapies include early intervention, special education, speech and language therapy, and physical and occupational therapies. Participation in Special Olympics provides a source of self-esteem, as well as exercise and camaraderie. Life expectancy for people with DS is reduced due to the many associated disorders, premature aging, and Alzheimer's disease. Despite these challenges, people with DS are capable of living productive and happy lives (Down Syndrome Medical Interest Group, 1999).

Fragile X Syndrome

Fragile X syndrome is a complex sex-linked genetic condition causing mental retardation and a range of communication and behavioral disorders. Fragile X syndrome is the most common inherited cause of mental retardation, with a prevalence rate of about 1 per 4000 to 6000 in the general population and a slightly higher prevalence in African American boys (Crawford et al., 2002).

Although the syndrome occurs primarily in males, females are carriers and can also show clinical affects. There is a fragile site, or break, in the X chromosome, caused by a mutation in the fragile X mental retardation gene 1 (FMR1). The mutation can be partial or full and can worsen in the expression of symptomatology as it is passed on down to the next generation through a male or female carrier. Males who are carriers may pass that state on to their daughters, who then become carriers. Despite the prevalence of this condition, the majority of individuals with MR caused by fragile X syndrome go undiagnosed (Hagerman, 2004).

Many young children with fragile X syndrome have such severe attention, communication, and behavioral disorders that they are unable to remain in a preschool and/or may have been expelled numerous times. Most males with fragile X syndrome have poor eye contact and perseveration in speech, and many have unusual hand movements such as hand flapping or hand biting and severe learning disabilities or mental retardation. In addition to the developmental symptoms, the physical features associated with fragile X syndrome in about 80% of males include a long narrow face; large, prominent ears (Figure 30-2); and macroorchidism, or enlarged testicles (Hagerman, 2004). However, the physical characteristics are usually most evident in older children, adolescents, and adults, particularly the macroorchidism, which develops with puberty. Other physical characteristics that may be seen in males and females include hyperextensible finger joints and pes planus. A high arched palate may interfere with feeding as a child. Mitral valve prolapse may lead to cardiac problems as an adult (Hagerman, 2004).

Females who show clinical effects tend to be more mildly affected than males, with anxiety, depression, attention problems, language delays, and mild cognitive effects particularly in executive functioning and in mathematics skills. There is a significant comorbidity of autism in fragile X, which compounds the socialization skill deficits in people with fragile X syndrome (Hagerman, 2004). A neurodegenerative syndrome involving ataxia, tremor, and cognitive disability has recently been identified in older adult male carriers of fragile X (Hagerman, Greco, & Hagerman, 2003).

Fragile X syndrome is diagnosed by DNA genetic testing. Individuals with fragile X syndrome may be diagnosed at any age, but the condition is most commonly recognized during childhood. Delayed language skills, hyperactivity and attention problems, and developmental delay are initially what brings the child to the attention of diagnostic professionals. Many clinicians are unaware of this syndrome, which complicates

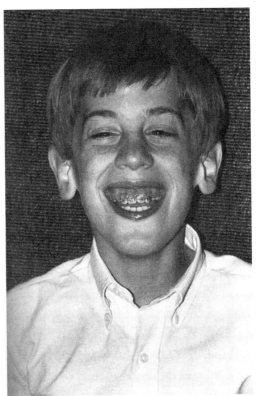

Figure 30-2 Prepubertal fragile X male. (From Jackson, P. L., & Vessey, J. A. [Eds.]. [2000]. *Primary care of the child with a chronic condition* [3rd ed.]. St. Louis, MO: Mosby.)

diagnosis and treatment. In addition, the heritable characteristics of this condition have significant implications for childbearing family members. If one family member is diagnosed with fragile X syndrome, all members of the extended family must be considered in genetic counseling.

Treatment for individuals with this condition includes early intervention, special education, and speech therapy. Depending on the level of mental retardation and behavior disorder, a number of people with fragile X syndrome may be capable of self-care, but most males with the full mutation will need some level of custodial care throughout their lifetimes. Behavioral treatment is often necessary, with some children and adults benefiting from psychopharmacological interventions to reduce anxiety and improve attention and social interactions. Adolescents and adults need vocational training, and some are capable of supported employment. Families of individuals with fragile X syndrome experience a great deal of stress and family disorganization due to both the severity and complexity of the disorder, the wide-reaching genetic risk, and the asymptomatic carrier status of parents and other family members.

COMMUNITY SERVICE SYSTEMS

Legislation and Key Government Actions

Knowledge of federal regulations that influence the lives of people with I/DD and their families provides the rehabilitation

TABLE 30-7 Disability Agencies

Agency	Website
U.S. Administration on Developmental Disabilities, Health Resources and Services Administration (U.S. Government)	ADD home page: http://www.acf.dhhs.gov/programs/add/index.html
University Centers of Excellence in Developmental Disabilities (UCEDDs)	Association of University Centers on Disability (national association): www.AUCD.org
Protection and Advocacy agencies for individuals with disabilities (P&As)	State Protection and Advocacy agencies from ADD: http://www.acf.dhhs.gov/programs/add/states/pas.html National Disability Rights Network (national association for P&As): http://www.ndrn.org
State Councils on Developmental Disabilities	Information on State Councils on Developmental Disabilities from ADD: http://www.acf.dhhs.gov/programs/add/states/ddcs.html National Association of State Councils on DD: http://www.nacdd.org

ADD, U.S. Administration on Developmental Disabilities; *DD*, developmental disabilities.

nurse with the information to better advocate for this population. The U.S. Administration on Developmental Disabilities (ADD), a department of the U.S. Department of Health and Human Services, administers the DD Act, which provides federal regulations that guide service delivery. In addition, ADD regulates funding for state agencies dedicated to research and training (University Centers of Excellence in Developmental Disabilities [UCEDD]); the protection of rights for people with I/DD, other disabilities, and elders (Protection and Advocacy agencies); and advocacy, policy, and systems change (State Councils on Developmental Disabilities). These agencies are represented in each state. For information about how to contact the agencies in individual states, see Table 30-7.

In 2001 the U.S. Supreme Court entered a decision, called the Olmstead decision, which required federal and state governments to provide documentation of plans to move people with developmental and psychiatric disabilities from institutions into less-restrictive community settings. The Olmstead decision has had a tremendous impact on deinstitutionalization and led to greater development of community-based services for people with I/DD. The decision put a great deal of pressure on state and community agencies, which often lack the capacity to provide support, health, and social services for this population. Although spending by states and the federal government has dramatically increased over the last 20 years, many states still lack resources to adequately meet the needs of their populations of people with I/DD. This has led to an increase in numbers of people on waiting lists for developmental disabilities services—people with I/DD who qualify for services, but for whom services are not available (Rizzolo, Hemp, Braddock, & Pomeranz-Essley, 2004; Hemp, Braddock, Parish, & Smith, 2001).

DEVELOPMENTAL DISABILITIES SERVICE SYSTEM

Unlike services funded to support other disabilities, a comprehensive, dedicated, federally funded system of services,

administered through the states, provides funds to support children and adults with developmental disabilities. The service system is administered on a federal level by the Administration on Developmental Disabilities and is guided by the DD Act. Although some services are available for children and youth with I/DD, the majority of state and local funds are spent on adult residential services. Children and youth primarily receive services through the early intervention systems, the school systems, and occasionally through the child welfare system in the state. States have various funding mechanisms to assist families with service coordination and family support funds during this period and with respite care. The great majority of children with I/DD live with their parents or in foster homes and do not reside in institutions. States receive federal funding to provide services, as well as some state, municipal, and often private funding.

In the last 20 years, public spending on developmental disabilities services has dramatically increased, particularly for community-based services and family support. Funding for institutionalization of individuals with developmental/intellectual disability has greatly decreased, mostly due to changing philosophies in service provision and recent legal actions, such as the Olmstead decision (Braddock et al., 2005).

Residential living options for adults with I/DD range from group homes or host homes (adult foster care) to supported living in the individual's own apartment, with or without a roommate. For group homes, supervision is provided 24 hours a day. Host homes provide a family-like living situation for adults with I/DD whose own families either are not capable of caring for them, have passed away, or who have relinquished care. People with I/DD who are capable of independence may live on their own with intermittent supervision as needed. Supported living services have been found to be less expensive than institutions and are more likely to involve residents in the community and to contribute to an improved quality of life. Some individuals own their own homes and can live independently. In some states, families have the option to set up their adult child in their own home or in an apartment, so that the family functions as an agency, providing care and oversight according to state laws. These arrangements provide an opportunity for families to hire and fire caregivers and to control state funds to benefit their family member with I/DD (Caldwell & Heller, 2003). Individuals with significant medical and physical care needs may reside in nursing facilities.

Most state I/DD service agencies provide employment services for patients whom they serve. Employment services may range from coordination with state and county vocational rehabilitation, to personal job coaches, to sheltered workshops. The concept of supported employment has enabled more people with I/DD to work in community settings instead of sheltered or segregated programs. People with I/DD in the mild or moderate range are usually able to work in low to moderately skilled positions such as cleaning or grocery stocking and bagging or in hospitals. Some people are able to perform more complex skills, such as clerical and filing or retail checkout, or jobs with more responsibility. In many cases it is not the presence of MR per se that influences employment options, but the individual's social skills, that is, the ability to get along with co-workers, to get to work on time and complete the assigned task, and to dress and act appropriately to the job requirements. With job adaptations, people with more physical disability and less cognitive deficits have fewer limitations in employment options. Once they have mastered the skills, most people with I/DD make loyal and reliable employees.

Adults with I/DD who qualify for supported living, usually called *comprehensive community-based services*, generally have the most significant supervision, health, or mental health needs. Each individual has a yearly Individualized Plan (IP), similar to the Individualized Education Plan that children in special education receive. The IP specifies the type of services the adult will receive for the next year, where he or she will live, the health care or health promotion plan, and even the type of diet the person will receive. Traditionally the IP is put together at a meeting of agency professionals and caregivers, who then determine the plan. Although the person with I/DD may be present, he or she often is not a real participant. Past program models were governed with a philosophy that individuals with mental retardation were incapable of expressing choices or aspirations for the future and were then not able to carry out responsibilities.

However, a growing advocacy movement for the rights of people with I/DD has developed a planning process called "person-centered planning," which includes the individual with I/DD in the planning process and even puts him or her in the center, much as a traditional rehabilitation team includes the patient or person with a disability in the team. Secondary to the provider agency, the person-centered planning model puts the needs of the individual with I/DD first and enlists natural supports from the community, instead of relying solely on paid caregivers.

HEALTH CARE SERVICES

Individuals with I/DD experience significant health disparities (U.S. Public Health Service, 2001). Negative attitudes, lack of training in working with the population, and reluctance on the part of providers to take on patients insured by Medicaid all contribute to these disparities. Also, challenging behaviors and learning difficulties may take more time than busy health care providers can afford. For example, women with I/DD lack adequate screening for breast and cervical cancers, and adults in general are less likely to receive recommended preventive screenings for age (Davies & Duff, 2001; Fisher, 2005). As a result, many children and adults with I/DD lack access to basic health services, as well as to needed specialty services, often resulting in more severe or complex medical problems or late diagnosis of conditions such as cancer (Havercamp, Scandlin, & Roth, 2004).

Health promotion and prevention are important nursing interventions and have a significant role in both habilitation and rehabilitation in all settings and for all persons with I/DD. Health education is most effective when tailored to meet the intellectual level of the individual, and frequent reinforcement is helpful. Rehabilitation nurses can encourage group home staff and caregivers to initiate walking programs or schedule time at the gym to increase exercise. Obesity is a significant problem for people with I/DD, and both good nutrition and increased exercise can ameliorate this (Marks & Heller, 2003). Promoting good nutrition is also very important, and nutritionists who have experience with the population can aid rehabilitation nurses in preventing obesity and teaching individuals with I/DD about healthy food choices.

Special Olympics was started in 1962 by Eunice Kennedy Shriver as a day camp for children with I/DD at her home (Special Olympics, 2005a). The program provides physical fitness for people with I/DD, as well as socialization and the opportunity to compete with others and to excel at something, which is an important factor in the development and maintenance of self-esteem. Recent research has suggested improvements in social skills and social interactions as well (Special Olympics, 2005a). More recently, Special Olympics has been in the forefront of promoting quality health care, including dental care, for participants and others with I/DD (Special Olympics 2005b).

Issues of Consent and Guardianship

Adults with I/DD may often serve as their own guardians in most matters of daily living, unless they have severe intellectual or social communication impairments. However, if during the course of health or rehabilitative services certain issues arise, then court appointment of a legal guardian or medical decision maker may be necessary, if not previously established. These issues include the following situations: interventions that carry significant risk; situations in which there is disagreement among family members, or a family member and physician, or the patient and physician; situations in which there are significant ethical issues (e.g., in the case of major organ transplant in a person who may not be able to comply with follow up treatment); the establishment of an advanced directive; and treatments that may infringe on the individual's rights, such as sterilization. In any situation the ability of the patient with I/DD to legally consent to treatment should be assessed, and a formal evaluation by a psychologist may be required. Legally an adult with MR is assumed to be competent, unless proven otherwise. In reality, most individuals may have the capacity to make many day-to-day decisions, or at least some daily decisions, but may require assistance to make more complex decisions significantly affecting health or life (Lyden, 2006).

In order to consent to a health care treatment, the patient should understand the treatment itself; the treatment options, the risks and benefits of the proposed treatment, and other options; and the risk and benefits of doing nothing. At the core of assisting a person with I/DD with making a decision is clear, developmentally appropriate teaching that takes into consideration any sensory or communication difficulties and the determining of the person's understanding of the instruction. The decision should be voluntary and not coerced, and the patient with I/DD should understand that the patient can change his or her mind at any time regarding the treatment (Lyden, 2006).

PREVENTION OF PHYSICAL AND SEXUAL ABUSE

Individuals with I/DD are at increased risk for both physical and sexual abuse throughout their lives, and some intellectual disabilities may be caused by abuse during early childhood. In one study almost 80% of those interviewed reported 1 sexual assault, and of those, 20% reported more than 10 incidents of sexual assault. Frequently abusers are known to the individual and family and are often paid caregivers or health care providers. People with I/DD who have communication difficulties or who are unable to physically resist aggression are the most likely to experience abuse. Often people with I/DD are not believed when they give a history of abuse, or the symptoms of abuse go unnoticed. Community agencies that provide services experience a great deal of turnover of caregiving staff and often fail to properly screen applicants (Ayelott, 1999).

Prevention of sexual abuse is best accomplished by educating people with disabilities how to avoid sexual exploitation and dangerous situations. Physical and sexual abuse can be prevented on the part of agencies by careful screening of caregivers, by assigning caregivers of the same gender to perform personal care, by training all caregiving staff in empathy, and in apprising all providers of the responsibility to report suspected abuse, physical or sexual, to the appropriate authorities (Ayelot, 1999). For more information on the symptoms of physical or sexual abuse in individuals with I/DD, see Box 30-5.

TRANSITION TO ADULTHOOD

As adolescents with I/DD mature and prepare to exit the educational system, comprehensive transition services are necessary to enable the youth to gain the necessary skills to

---

BOX 30-5 Signs of Physical or Sexual Abuse

- Unusual bruising or injuries without a reasonable explanation
- Behavioral changes without other clear cause, particularly agitation, fearful behavior, or reluctance to go to a certain place (e.g., a day program) or to be around a certain person or people
- Increase in self-inflicted injury
- Aggressiveness around a certain individual
- Emotional outbursts when around a certain person
- Withdrawal from usual activities
- Injury to the genital or anal area
- Unusual bleeding
- Presence of sexually transmitted infection in a person who is not known to engage in consensual sex

All allegations of injury should be investigated.

Modified from Krajicek, M. J., Thomas, D., & Hertzberg, D. (2005). Sexuality. In W. Nehring (Ed.), *Core curriculum for specializing in intellectual and developmental disability, a resource for nurses and other health care professionals* (pp. 183-206). Sudbury, MA: Jones & Bartlett.

---

emancipate and live independently. The adult service systems that youth with I/DD must transition to are often difficult to navigate and can be very confusing for youth and families. Historically people with I/DD are less likely to be employed than those with physical disabilities (Olney & Kennedy, 2001). Although transition services are necessary for all youth with disabilities, the presence of intellectual disability, as well as potential communication problems, makes both health and vocational transition somewhat more challenging. In addition, these same needs make placement in a community living setting more difficult to achieve. Simply stated, the greater the level of supervision and assistance most people with I/DD need in their daily lives, the more challenging the transition. Depending on the needs of an adolescent with I/DD, the ability of the family to care for them, and the availability of residential placements, the youth can be placed on a waiting list for adult services.

Transition begins in the educational system at about 16 years of age. A transition plan is formulated as part of the Individualized Education Plan (IEP), and the youth, the family, and school staff begin to plan the remainder of the youth's education for a future vocational and independence goal. As part of the Individuals with Disaabilities Education Act (IDEA) (2004), a youth with I/DD or other disability may remain in school until age 21 years if a plan is included in the IEP and transition plan. This would allow for further instruction in vocational skills, social skills, and self-care skills. Often the state vocational rehabilitation office is included in the transition planning process. However, because this process is initiated and led by the educational system, health transition is not included. Health transition can be very challenging for youth and families, because many adult health care providers do not take Medicaid, which is the main health insurance for most adults with developmental and other disabilities, and they lack education in working with this population. If the youth has complex health needs in addition, specialty care is even more difficult to arrange and may not even be available in some rural areas (Betz, 2003).

AGING AND DEVELOPMENTAL DISABILITIES

As more and more people with I/DD are living longer, issues of declining health and end-of-life care are arising. Aging parents who have put off obtaining community services from an agency may die and leave their adult offspring with I/DD without care.

Aging adults with I/DD experience many of the same health problems as the general population, with the addition of conditions specific to their disability, such as obesity the earlier onset of dementia in persons with Down syndrome (Down Syndrome Medical Interest Group, 1999). Research suggests that adults with I/DD without Down syndrome have no greater risk of dementia than the general population. Indeed, adults with Down syndrome experience more health problems and disruptive life events as they age than aging adults with nongenetic forms of MR (Patti, Amble, & Flory, 2005). Studies differ on the rate of health impairments as a result of aging; however, existing health conditions and functional impairments are likely to worsen with age. The impairments most commonly identified were sensory impairments such as visual and hearing deficits, mobility impairments, and increasing self-care deficits with age (Fisher, 2004). There is an increased risk for osteoporosis in people with I/DD in part due to the wide use of antipsychotic and antiseizure medication in this population, as well as mobility impairments in persons with CP and other comorbid physical disabilities. Risk is particularly high in women and individuals with Down syndrome. Screening for all of these conditions and impairments early in adulthood is indicated in this population.

Most state developmental disabilities service systems are ill prepared to face the needs of their aging individuals with I/DD. The majority of senior programs and senior living centers are designed for typical seniors, and although they may be accessible to people with mobility impairments, they are less accessible to people with intellectual impairments or who need closer supervision. Also, government funding guidelines for senior programs often unintentionally exclude individuals with I/DD on the basis of health insurance (e.g., Medicaid versus Medicare) or living situation (group homes). Currently state and national organizations are focusing more on the needs of aging adults with I/DD in hopes of expanding care and eliminating barriers to improve services (Parish & Lutwick, 2005). Palliative care needs will also increase in this population, and there is currently little research in end-of-life care for people with I/DD, as well as a lack of experience in this area on the part of health care and human service providers (Service & Hahn, 2003).

Aging adults with I/DD present opportunities to rehabilitation nurses with knowledge of geriatric care principles and the aging process in adults with and without disabilities. Rehabilitation nurses have the ability to perform functional assessments; to evaluate living situations and the need for assistive devices; to provide interventions for sensory impairments, mobility impairments, and bowel and bladder dysfunction; and to help families and other caregivers (Service & Hahn, 2003).

Family Issues

Families face a number of issues beginning with the initial diagnosis of an I/DD whether during infancy, childhood, or adolescence. The manner in which families hear the news can influence their view of the child's potential and their view of health care providers. In cases of prenatal diagnosis, prospective parents often receive inaccurate information or recommendations to discontinue the pregnancy (Skotko, 2005).

Family-centered care is the philosophy and model of care that recognizes the enormous importance of the family to the child's development and well-being and respects the family's culture, ethnicity, goals, and hopes for the child when designing interventions. Families are the "ultimate decision makers for their children, with children gradually taking on more and more of the decision-making themselves" as they mature (U.S. Department of Health and Human Services, 2006). In family-centered care, families and professionals work together to share information and make decisions on behalf of the child and to support and strengthen the family.

Families are faced with the need to maintain equilibrium while providing for the special needs of their child. They must master a treatment regimen for their child in addition to maintaining relationships with spouses and other children. Often family members may experience "chronic sorrow," when the initial grief and loss of the diagnosis is revisited at critical periods of development, for example, when the child fails to walk at age 1 year or to emancipate at 18 or 20 years of age. Additional stressors on the family may result in marital problems. Children or adults with comorbid MR and mental illness or who have severe behavioral problems present additional lifelong challenges to family coping (Kim, Greenberg, Seltzer, & Krauss, 2003). However, most parents express satisfaction with their marriages and derive a great deal of satisfaction from their child with I/DD (Stoneman & Gavidia-Payne, 2006).

Families of different cultural and ethnic backgrounds may view intellectual disability somewhat differently, and this will influence whether they seek assistance with their child or how they respond to treatment recommendations or make decisions (Bailey et al., 1999). As the child grows and develops, parents must navigate different service systems from early intervention to schools and health care. In addition to coping with the changes in lifestyle and relationships necessitated by the child's diagnosis, families must also develop skills in service coordination or learn where they can obtain services for their child. Some parents are overwhelmed by their child's physical and educational needs and have difficulty managing daily care, whereas other families become experts at maneuvering among the systems of care and establish programs to aid other parents and health care providers, such as Family Voices (Family Voices, 2006).

Social support is crucial to the success of families in adapting to the needs of their child with I/DD, and families who lack this critical component often remain isolated. Although fathers certainly participate in the care of the child with I/DD, mothers remain the primary caregivers, particularly when adult children remain in the home. Social support can contribute to the well-being of the caregiver and aid coping (Magaña, 1999). Siblings of children with I/DD may also be involved in the care or supervision of their brother or sister and may feel stigmatized or resentful. Sibling support groups have grown in the past few years and can be a valuable asset to families.

Particularly for families with a child or adult who has challenging behavior or significant physical needs, respite care can provide a needed break. Respite care programs are often offered through developmental disabilities agencies as part of their family support program and may also be available through advocacy groups, such as The Arc.

As adult children with I/DD age, families are faced with planning for the future, when parents may be gone. Some families set up trusts to fund additional services or housing for their child with I/DD or may designate a sibling to carry on as guardian. Although many adults with I/DD can take care of themselves day-to-day, they need assistance to make complex decisions, such as decisions about medical care. In these situations an individual may be his or her own guardian but may have a designated medical decision maker to assist the individual when the possibility of surgery or some other complex medical treatment looms. However, most parents do not plan at all for the eventuality of their demise, and their aging adult children with I/DD are left needing crisis placement services.

SUMMARY: IMPLICATIONS FOR REHABILITATION NURSING CARE

Individuals with I/DD are truly patients with special needs in the rehabilitation setting. Because of their unique matrix of skills in restorative and rehabilitative care, rehabilitation nurses are particularly well suited to provide care to this population across health care settings: inpatient rehabilitation, outpatient services, and home health care. In order to provide quality rehabilitation services, nurses must be aware of the lifelong nature of disability in this population. Growing up with I/DD influences the individual's behavior and interaction with the environment as much as the intellectual disability itself. The frequent presence of significant social communication disorders, such as autism, complicates the nurse's task in enlisting the patient's cooperation and collaboration in the rehabilitation process. The process of restoring the patient's prior level of function is complicated by the intellectual disability and its impact on learning. In some cases the prior level of function may not be clear, depending on the circumstances of the injury or disease. Factors such as premature aging and occurrence of dementia in people with Down syndrome and comorbidities such as congenital heart defects, mental illness, and epilepsy may compromise the rehabilitation process. Finally, obtaining consent for treatment can be difficult if the patient with I/DD is his or her own guardian, yet has difficulty understanding the impact of the decisions to be made. Although working with this population in the rehabilitation setting can be frustrating, it can also be rewarding, and many rehabilitation nurses will be ready to take on the challenge of providing quality, comprehensive rehabilitation nursing care to meet the complex needs of these unique patients.

Case Study

Deana is a cheerful, well-nourished, friendly young woman with Down syndrome. She participates in Special Olympics in track and skiing and has won a gold medal in skiing. She has friends from school and from Special Olympics. Her dream is to work with animals, and she would like to have a boyfriend and get married someday.

Deana is 21 years old and living with her parents. She just completed high school and is now looking for a job. She would like to have her own apartment, but her family and her case manager are concerned that she is not "safe" enough to live by herself. Several times she has left soup on the burner and forgotten it until it has burned and set off the smoke alarm. She loves surfing the Internet but is so trusting she gives out personal information in chat rooms, putting herself at risk for exploitation. Deana takes the bus from her home to the mall and to the county workforce center where she looks for employment. She is able to negotiate buses, change routes, and ask for help if she needs it.

Deana has a case manager from the developmental disabilities service agency in her state. The agency provides recreational opportunities

for Deana and some family support funds for her family for respite care and recreation. Although Deana qualifies for Comprehensive Community Services through the agency, including employment support, residential placement, and personal care and training, the agency is underfunded and she is on a waiting list for these services. In the meantime, she lives at home with her parents, who both work and who worry about needing to leave her home by herself during the day. Because she is diagnosed with a developmental disability, she qualifies for state Medicaid services for health care.

Last year she broke her right leg skiing when practicing for Special Olympics. Deana had a severe, compound fracture, and she required rehabilitation following surgery. She was hospitalized on the rehabilitation unit for 2 weeks and then received outpatient therapy and follow-up in the rehabilitation clinic, with the clinical nurse specialist (CNS). The CNS worked with the physical therapist, the physiatrist, Deana, and Deana's family to help her return to her preinjury level of function, so she could participate in skiing again.

CRITICAL THINKING

1. Based on the case study, formulate a nursing care plan for Deana, the young woman with Down syndrome who sustained a lower extremity fracture. Be sure to account for her desire to return to skiing in the Special Olympics, her wish to live independently, and her unique educational needs.

2. Discuss similarities and differences between rehabilitation nursing care of the individual with a traumatic brain injury and an individual with an intellectual/developmental disability.

3. Identify at least three resources in your local community and/or your state of residence for information on nursing care of individuals with intellectual/developmental disability.

REFERENCES

Aber, J. L., & Bennett, N. G. (1997). The effects of poverty on child health and development. *Annual Review of Public Health, 18*, 463-483.

Accardo, P. J., & Whitman, B. Y. (2003). *Developmental disabilities dictionary online* (2nd ed.). Paul H. Brookes. Available from http://www.brookespublishing.com/cgi-bin/dictionary.pl.

Aicare, J. (1998). The etiology of development delay. *Seminars in Pediatric Neurology, 5*(1), 15-20.

Airaksinen, E. M., Matalainen, R., Mononen, T., Mustonen, K. Partanen, J., & Jokela, V. (2000). A population based study on epilepsy in mentally retarded children. *Epilepsia, 41*, 1214-1220.

Aisen, P. S., Dalton, A. J., Sano, M., Lott, I. T., Andrews, H. F., Tsai, W.-Y., et al. (2005). Design and implementation of a multicenter trial of vitamin E in aging individuals with Down syndrome. *Journal of Policy and Practice in Intellectual Disabilities, 2*(2), 86-93.

American Academy of Pediatrics. (2001). Health supervision for the child with Down syndrome. *Pediatrics, 107*(2), 442-449.

American Nurses Association & the Nursing Division of the American Association on Mental Retardation. (2004). *Intellectual and developmental disabilities nursing: Scope and standards of practice* (p. 1). Silver Spring, MD: American Nurses Association.

American Psychiatric Association. (2000). *Diagnostic and statistical manual of mental disorders* (4th ed., text revision). Washington, DC: Author.

Ayelott, J. (1999). Preventing rape and sexual assault of people with learning disabilities. *British Journal of Nursing, 8*(13), 871-875.

Bailey, D. B. Jr., Skinner, D., Correa, V., Arcia, E., Reyes-Blanes, M. E., Rodriguez, P., et al. (1999). Needs and supports reported by Latin families of young children with developmental disabilities. *American Journal of Mental Retardation, 104*(5), 437-451.

Baranek, G. T., Foster, L. G., & Berkson, G. (1997). Tactile defensiveness and stereotypical behaviors. *American Journal of Occupational Therapy, 51*(2), 91-95.

Baranek, G. T., Chin, Y. H., Hess, L. M., Yankee, J. G., Hatton, D. D., & Hooper, S. R. (2002). Sensory processing correlates of occupational performance in children with fragile X syndrome: Preliminary findings. *American Journal of Occupational Therapy, 56*(5), 538-546.

Baxley, D. L. (2006). Thinking and planning for end of life: Some ideas for parents of a child with a developmental disability. *Exceptional Parent, 36*(4), 10-11.

Betz, C. (2003). Nurse's role in promoting health transitions for adolescents and young adults with developmental disabilities. *Nursing Clinics of North America, 38*(2), 271-289.

Beversdorf, D. Q., Manning, S. E., Hillier, A., Anderson, S. L., Nordgren, R. E., Walters, S. E., et al. (2005). Timing of prenatal stressors and autism. *Journal of Autism & Developmental Disorders, 35*(4), 471-478.

Bhasin, T. K., Brocksen, S., Avchen, R. N., & Van Naarden Braun, K. (2006, January 27). Prevalence of four developmental disabilities among children aged 8 years—Metropolitan Atlanta Developmental Disabilities

Surveillance Program, 1996 and 2000. *Morbidity and Mortality Weekly Report. Surveillance Summaries, 55*(1), 1-9.

Braddock, D., Hemp, R., Rizzolo, M. C., Coulter, D., Haffer, L., & Thomson, M. (2005). *The state of the states in developmental disabilities, 2005: Preliminary report.* Boulder, CO: The University of Colorado, Department of Psychiatry and the Coleman Institute for Cognitive Disabilities.

Brezeniak, J. (1998). The effects of aging on the ambulation activities of a developmentally disabled population. *Topics in Geriatric Rehabilitation, 12*(4), 22-29.

Buhler-Wilkerson, K. Our history. The call to the nurse: Our history from 1893 to 1943. Visiting Nurse Service of New York. Available from http://www.vsny.org/a_history_more.html 4-5-06.

Butler, J. V., Whittington, J. E., Holland, A. J., Boer, H., Clarke, D., & Webb, T. (2002). Prevalence of, and risk factors for, physical ill-health in people with Prader-Willi syndrome: A population-based study. *Developmental Medicine & Child Neurology, 44*(4), 248-255.

Caldwell, J., & Heller, T. (2003, May-June). Management of respite and personal assistance services in a consumer-directed family support programme. *Journal of Intellectual Disability Research, 47*(Pt. 4-5), 352-366.

Cashin, A. J. (2005). Autism: Understanding conceptual processing deficits. *Journal of Psychosocial Nursing and Mental Health Services, 43*(4), 22-30.

Centers for Disease Control and Prevention. (1996, February 16). *MMWR. Morbidity and Mortality Weekly Report, 45*(6), 10-14.

Chapman, R. S., & Hesketh, L. J. (2000). Behavioral phenotype of individuals with Down syndrome. *Mental Retardation & Developmental Disabilities Research Reviews, 6*(2), 84-95.

Crawford, D. C., Meadows, K. L., Newman, J. L., Taft, L. F., Scott, E., Leslie, M., et al. (2002). Prevalence of the fragile X syndrome in African-Americans. *American Journal of Medical Genetics, 110*(3), 226-233.

Croen, L. A., Grether, J. K., & Selvin, S. (2001). The epidemiology of mental retardation of unknown cause. *Pediatrics, 107*(6), E86.

Croen, L. A., Grether, J. K., & Selvin, S. (2002). Descriptive epidemiology of autism in a California population: Who is at risk? *Journal of Autism & Developmental Disorders, 32*(3), 217-224.

Curry, C. J., Stevenson, R. E., Aughton, D., Byrne, J., Carey, J. C., Cassidy, S., et al. (1997). Evaluation of mental retardation: Recommendations of a Consensus Conference: American College of Medical Genetics. *American Journal of Medical Genetics, 72*(4), 468-477.

Daily, D. K., Ardinger, H. H., & Holmes, G. E. (2000). Identification and evaluation of mental retardation. *American Family Physician, 61*(4), 1059-1067, 1070.

Davies, N., & Duff, M. (2001, June). Breast cancer screening for older women with intellectual disability living in community group homes. *Journal of Intellectual Disability Research, 45*(Pt. 3), 253-257.

The Developmental Disabilities Assistance and Bill of Rights Act, 42 U.S.C. 15002 §102 (2000).

Dochterman, J. M., & Bulechek, G. M. (2004). *Nursing interventions classification (NIC)* (4th ed.). St. Louis, MO: Mosby.

Down Syndrome Medical Interest Group. (1999). Health care guidelines for individuals with Down syndrome: 1999 revisions. *Down Syndrome Quarterly, 4*(3). Retrieved August 24, 2006, from http://www.denison.edu/collaborations/dsq/health99.html.

Editorial Board. (1996). Definition of mental retardation. In Jacobson, J. W., & Mulick, J. A. (Eds.), *Manual of diagnosis and professional practice in mental retardation* (pp. 13-41). Washington, DC: American Psychological Association.

Family Voices. (2006). *About Family Voices—mission, principles, our children and families.* Retrieved September 2, 2006, from http://www.familyvoices.org/about.htm.

Fisher, N., & Happe, F. (2005). A training study of theory of mind and executive function in children with autistic spectrum disorders. *Journal of Autism and Developmental Disorders, 35*(6), 757-771.

Fisher, K. (2004). Nursing care of special populations: Issues on caring for elderly people with mental retardation. *Nursing Forum, 39*(1), 28-31.

Fisher, K. (2005). Health disparities and mental retardation. *Journal of Nursing Scholarship, 36*(1), 48-53.

Fisher, K., & Kettle, P. (2005). Aging with mental retardation: Increasing population of older adults with MR require health interventions and prevention strategies. *Geriatrics, 60*(4), 26-29.

Fombonne, E. (2005). Epidemiology of autistic disorder and other pervasive developmental disorders. *Journal of Clinical Psychiatry, 66*(Suppl. 10), 3-8.

Freedman, R. I., Krauss, M. W., & Seltzer, M. M. (1997). Aging parents' residential plans for adult children with mental retardation. *Mental Retardation, 35*(2), 114-123.

Frey, G. C., Buchanan, A. M., & Rosser Sandt, D. D. (2005). "I'd rather watch TV": An examination of physical activity in adults with mental retardation. *Mental Retardation, 43*(4), 241-254.

Frey, L., Szalda-Petree, A., Traci, M. A., & Seekins, T. (2001). Prevention of secondary health conditions in people with developmental disabilities: A review of the literature. *Disability and Rehabilitation, 23*(9), 361-369.

Futagi, Y., Toribe, Y., Ogawa, K., & Suzuki, Y. (2006). Neurodevelopmental outcome in children with intraventricular hemorrhage. *Pediatric Neurology, 34*(3), 219-224.

Hagerman, P. J., Greco, C. M., & Hagerman, R. J. (2003). A cerebellar tremor/ataxia syndrome among fragile X premutation carriers. *Cytogenetic & Genome Research, 100*(1-4), 206-212.

Hagerman, R. (2004). Fragile X syndrome. In P. Allen & J. Vessey (Eds.), *Primary care of the child with a chronic condition* (4th ed.). St. Louis, MO: Mosby.

Hastings, R. P., Beck, A., Daley, D., & Hill, C. (2005). Symptoms of ADHD and their correlates in children with intellectual disabilities. *Research in Developmental Disabilities, 26*(5), 456-468.

Havercamp, S. M., Scandlin, D., & Roth, M. (2004). Health disparities among adults with developmental disabilities, adults with other disabilities, and adults not reporting disability in North Carolina. *Public Health Reports, 119*(4), 418-426.

Hemp, R., Braddock, D., Parish, S., & Smith, G. (2001). Leveraging federal funding in the states to address Olmstead and growing waiting lists. *Mental Retardation, 39*(3):241-243.

Hutchins, T. L., & Prelock, P. A. (2006). Using social stories and comic strip conversations to promote socially valid outcomes for children with autism. *Seminars in Speech & Language, 27*(1), 47-59.

Janicki, M. P., Davidson, P. W., Henderson, C. M., McCallion, P., Taets, J. D., Force, L. T., et al. (2002, May). Health characteristics and health services utilization in older adults with intellectual disability living in community residences. *Journal of Intellectual Disability Research, 46*(Pt. 4), 287-298.

Jelliffe-Pawlowski, L. L., Shaw, G. M., Nelson, V., & Harris, J. A. (2003). Risk of mental retardation among children born with birth defects. *Archives of Pediatrics & Adolescent Medicine, 157*(6), 545-550.

Johnston, C., Hessl, D., Blasey, C., Eliez, S., Erba, H., Dyer-Friedman, J., et al. (2003). Factors associated with parenting stress in mothers of children with fragile X syndrome. *Journal of Developmental & Behavioral Pediatrics, 24*(4), 267-275.

Kim, H. W., Greenberg, J. S., Seltzer, M. M., & Krauss, M. W. (2003, May-June). The role of coping in maintaining the psychological well-being of mothers of adults with intellectual disability and mental illness. *Journal of Intellectual Disability Research, 47*(Pt. 4-5), 313-327.

Klingbeil, H., Baer, H., & Wilson, P. E. (2004). Aging with a disability. *Archives of Physical Medicine & Rehabilitation, 85*(7 Suppl. 3), S68-S73, quiz S74-S75.

Krajicek, M. J., Thomas, D., & Hertzberg, D. (2005). Sexuality. In W. Nehring (Ed.), *Core curriculum for specializing in intellectual and developmental disability, a resource for nurses and other health care professionals* (pp. 183-206). Sudbury, MA: Jones & Bartlett.

Lacavlier, L., Leone S., & Wiltz, J. (2006). The impact of behavior problems on caregiver stress in young people with autism spectrum disorders. *Journal of Intellectual Disability Research, 50*(Pt 3): 172-183.

Leonard, H., & Wen, X. (2002). The epidemiology of mental retardation: Challenges and opportunities in the new millennium. *Mental Retardation & Developmental Disabilities Research Reviews, 8*(3), 117-134.

Lohiya, G. S., Crinella, F. M., Tan Figueroa, L., Caires, S, & Lohiya, S. (1999). Fracture epidemiology and control in a developmental center. *Western Journal of Medicine, 170*(4), 203-209.

Luckasson, R., Borthwick-Duffy, S., Buntinx, W. H. E., Coulter, D. L., Craig, E. M., Reeve, A., et al. (2002). *Mental retardation: Definition, classification, and systems of support.* Washington, DC: American Association on Mental Retardation.

Luiselli, J. K., Magee, C., Sperry, J. M., & Parker, S. (2005). Descriptive assessment of sleep patterns among community-living adults with mental retardation. *Mental Retardation, 43*(6), 416-420.

Lyden, M. (2006). Capacity issues related to the health care proxy. *Mental Retardation, 44*(4), 272-282.

Magaña, S. M. (1999). Puerto Rican families caring for an adult with mental retardation: The role of familism. *American Journal of Mental Retardation, 104*(5), 466-482.

March of Dimes. (2006). *Quick reference fact sheets.* Retrieved August 21, 2006, from http://www.marchofdimes.com/professionals/14332.asp.

Marks, B., & Heller, T. (2003). Bridging the equity gap: Health promotion for adults with intellectual and developmental disabilities. *Nursing Clinics of North America, 38*(2), 205-228.

McDermott, S., Moran, R., Platt, T., Wood, H., Isaac, T., & Dasari, S. (2005). Prevalence of epilepsy in adults with mental retardation and related disabilities in primary care. *American Journal of Mental Retardation, 110*(1), 48-56.

Menendez, M. (2005). Down syndrome, Alzheimer's disease and seizures. *Brain & Development, 27*(4), 246-252.

Minnesota Governor's Council on Development Disability. (1996). *Parallels in time.* Available at http://www.mnddc.org/parallels/menu.html.

National Institute for Child Health and Human Development (NICHD). Facts about Down syndrome. Available at http://www.nichd.gov/publication/pubs/downsyndrome/down.htm.

National Survey of Children with Special Healthcare Needs. U.S. Department of Health and Human Services. Available at http://mchb.hrsa.gov./chscn/pages/family.htm.

Nehring, W. M. (1999). *A history of nursing in the field of mental retardation and developmental disabilities.*Washington, D.C.: American Association on Mental Retardation.

Nirje, B. (1973). The normalization principle—implications and comments. In H. C. Gunzberg (Ed.), *Advances in the care of the mentally handicapped.* Baltimore: Williams & Wilkins.

Olney, M. F., & Kennedy, J. (2001). National estimates of vocational service utilization and job placement rates for adults with mental retardation. *Mental Retardation, 39*(1), 32-39.

Owens, P. L., Kerker, D. D., Zigler, E., & Horwitz, S. M. (2006). Vision and oral health needs of individuals with ID. *Mental Retardation and Developmental Disabilities Research Reviews, 12*(1), 28-40.

Parish, S. L., & Lutwick, Z. E. (2005). A critical analysis of the emerging crisis in long-term care for people with developmental disabilities. *Social Work, 50*(4), 345-354.

Patti, P. J., Amble, K. B., & Flory, M. J. (2005). Life events in older adults with intellectual disabilities: Differences between adults with and without Down syndrome. *Journal of Policy and Practice in Intellectual Disabilities, 2*(2), 149-155.

Petridou, E., Kedikoglou, S., Andrie, E., Farmakakis, T., Tsiga, A., Angelopoulos, M., et al. (2003). Injuries among disabled children. *Injury Prevention, 9*(3), 226-230.

Ramirez, M., Peek-Asa, C., & Kraus, J. F. (2004). Disability and risk of school related injury. *Injury Prevention, 10*(1), 21-26.

Ramirez, R. J., Behrends, L. G., Blakeney, P., & Herndon, D. H. (1998). Children with sensorimotor deficits: A special risk group. *Journal of Burn Care & Rehabilitation, 19*(2), 124-127.

Rizzolo, M. C., Hemp, R., Braddock, D., & Pomeranz-Essley, A. (2004). *The state of the states in developmental disabilities: 2004.* Boulder: University of Colorado, Coleman Institute for Cognitive Disabilities and Department of Psychiatry.

Robertson, J., Emerson, E., Gregory, N., Hatton, C., Turner, S., Kessissoglou, S., & Hallam, A. (2000). Lifestyle related risk factors for poor health in residential settings for people with intellectual disabilities. *Research in Developmental Disabilities, 21*(6), 469-486.

Roper, R. J., & Reeves, R. H. (2006). Understanding the basis for Down syndrome phenotypes. *PLoS Genetics, 2*(3), e50.

Rush, J. A., & Frances, A. (Eds.). (2000). Expert Consensus Guideline Series: Treatment of psychiatric and behavioral problems in mental retardation. *American Journal of Mental Retardation, 105*(3), 159-228.

Service, K. P., & Hahn, J. E. (2003). Issues in aging. The role of the nurse in the care of older people with intellectual and developmental disabilities. *Nursing Clinics of North America, 38*(2), 291-312.

Sherrard, J., Tonge, B., & Ozanne-Smith, J. (2002, January). Injury risk in young people with intellectual disability. *Journal of Intellectual Disability Research, 46*(Pt.1), 6-16.

Skotko, B. G. (2005). Prenatal diagnosis of Down syndrome: Mothers who continued their pregnancy evaluate their health care providers. *American Journal of Obstetrics & Gynecology, 192*(3), 670-677.

Special Olympics. (2005a). *Changing attitudes, changing the world. Changing lives through sport—a report card on the impact of Special Olympics.* Available from http://www.specialolympics.org/NR/rdonlyres/eatyprlxrjepub5h6ja56gs7 bplo3fouqn4mx7l1326rpevzf6ee2nd5vo3dw46vrgudz7a2qfyan2h5ls7hup4 byx4f/CACW_Sports.pdf.

Special Olympics. (2005b). *Changing attitudes, changing the world. The health and health care of people with intellectual disabilities.* Available from http://www.specialolympics.org/NR/rdonlyres/e75okatixbkneht- tnruutheossutueniq7hsd6ev6bg3astpgwfmbbzfwy5ph2tbjojz3gnjuzum6hh bjgljh6nl36d/CACW_Health.pdf.

Sperry, L. A., & Mesibov, G. B. (2005). Perceptions of social challenges of adults with autism spectrum disorder. *Autism, 9*(4), 362-376.

Stoneman, Z., & Gavidia-Payne, S. (2006). Marital adjustment in families of young children with disabilities. *American Journal on Mental Retardation, 111*(1), 1-14.

Trevathan, E., Murphy, C. C., & Yeargin-Allsopp, M. (1997). Prevalence and descriptive epidemiology of Lennox-Gastaut syndrome among Atlanta children. *Epilepsia, 38*(12), 1283-1288.

Trumble, S. (1999). Down syndrome. In N. Lennox & J. Diggens (Eds.), *Management guidelines, people with developmental and intellectual disabilities* (1st ed.). Melbourne, Australia: Therapeutic Guidelines Limited.

U.S. Department of Health and Human Services, Health Resources and Services Administration, Maternal and Child Health Bureau. (2004). *The National Survey of Children With Special Health Care Needs chartbook 2001.* Rockville, MD: U.S. Department of Health and Human Services.

U.S. Public Health Service. (2001). *Closing the gap: A national blueprint for improving the health of individuals with mental retardation. Report of the Surgeon General's Conference on Health Disparities and Mental Retardation.* Rockville, MD: U.S. Department of Health and Human Services.

Valent, T., Little, D., Bertollini, R., Nemer, L. E., Barbone, F., & Tambrulini G. (2004). Burden of disease attributes to selected environment factors and injury among children and adolescents in Europe. *Lancet, 363*(9426), 2032-3039.

Xiang, H., Leff, M., & Stallones, L. (2005). Non-fatal injuries among adults with activity limitations and participation restrictions. *Injury Prevention, 11*(3), 157-162.

Yang, Q., Rasmussen, S. A., & Friedman, J. M. (2002). Mortality associated with Down's syndrome in the USA from 1983 to 1997: A population-based study. *Lancet, 359*(9311), 1019-1025.

Ypsilanti, A., Grouios, G., Alevriadou, A., & Tsapkini, K. (2005). Expressive and receptive vocabulary in children with Williams and Down syndrome. *Journal of Intellectual Disability Research, 49*(Pt. 5), 353-364.

31

Pediatric Rehabilitation Nursing

Deirdre F. Jackson, MSN, APRN, CRRN

Pediatric rehabilitation nursing is a specialty practice area that continues to grow within the field of rehabilitation. This chapter traces the evolution and the expanding scope of this specialty. The unique role of the pediatric rehabilitation nurse is described. A developmental framework is suggested as a conceptual model for practice and applied to discussion of the impact of disabilities across pediatric age-groups. Medical and societal trends that affect the field are examined. Public laws protecting the educational rights of children with disabilities are identified. Strategies for assessment are presented along with interventions and outcomes based on nursing diagnoses commonly associated with selected chronic illnesses and disabilities. The chapter concludes with a case history that highlights the complexity of care needs—a common finding in children receiving pediatric rehabilitation services.

EVOLUTION OF PEDIATRIC REHABILITATION

The field of pediatric rehabilitation has experienced marked development over the past century. In the late nineteenth century, "homes" and training schools were established for individuals with specific problems such as blindness and disabling conditions (Edwards, 1992). Near the turn of the twentieth century the concept of a multidisciplinary approach emerged as restorative and reconstructive procedures were incorporated into the care of people with disabilities. During the 1940s many new rehabilitation facilities were established, some of which specialized in the care of children (Allan, 1958). Congenital neurological and orthopedic problems commonly were seen.

Through the end of the twentieth century the scope of the field has continued to broaden. Many pediatric rehabilitation facilities now provide care for children with chronic conditions or, acquired disabilities, and developmental disabilities,

as discussed in Chapter 30. Some of these children are also dependent on technology for their survival.

UNIQUENESS OF THE PEDIATRIC REHABILITATION NURSE

Although rehabilitation services have been provided for children for quite some time, the field of pediatric rehabilitation nursing is relatively new (Selekman, 1991). In the mid-1980s the Pediatric Special-Interest Group was formed within the Association of Rehabilitation Nurses. The membership described the role of the pediatric rehabilitation nurse in the publication *Pediatric Rehabilitation Nursing–Role Description* (Pediatric Special Interest Group, 1992). Pediatric rehabilitation nurses are both specialists and generalists: specialists by virtue of the age of their patients and generalists as a result of the broad diagnostic categories they serve.

Inherent in the specialized approach is the nurse's acceptance of a child with disability as a valued member of society who is first and foremost a child and secondly a child with special needs. This approach requires the nurse to be able to accept and celebrate small accomplishments and establish outcomes that focus on optimal levels of performance for that child.

Pediatric rehabilitation nurses can assume a wide variety of roles across the health care continuum, including expert clinician, care coordinator, early intervention nurse, school nurse, educator, consultant, researcher, or political activist. Advanced practice pediatric rehabilitation nurses can also function as primary care providers, administrators, or managers (Neal, 1997). Regardless of the role assumed or the practice setting, pediatric rehabilitation nurses must have in-depth knowledge of the theories, issues, and legislation affecting the pediatric rehabilitation population. They must also have a strong knowledge of patient management strategies, such as life care planning and self-care management, across pediatric rehabilitation settings and be able to effect positive outcomes through teams of professionals and in collaboration with patients and families (Jackson & Wallingford, 1997).

PEDIATRIC REHABILITATION POPULATION

Approximately 13% of children in the United States have a special health care need (Child and Adolescent Health Measurement Initiative, 2005). The Maternal Child Health Bureau defines children with special health care needs as

> Those who have or are at increased risk for, a chronic physical, developmental, behavioral, or emotional condition and who also require health and related services of a type or amount beyond that required by children generally (McPherson et al., 1998).

Children with special health care needs may have congenital or acquired disorders. Many of these disorders are also rare. The increased numbers of survivors of childhood illness, prematurity, and serious injuries contribute to this population. This variety in disorders is a defining characteristic of pediatric rehabilitation (Box 31-1). Two groups of children that are relatively new to pediatric rehabilitation settings are discussed below.

Childhood Cancer Survivors

As more children survive childhood cancers, the sequelae of hematology/oncology problems are being seen more frequently in rehabilitation settings. Psychological support, rehabilitation, and increased physical activity can have positive effects on functional outcome and quality of life after treatment for childhood cancer (Parsch, Mikut, & Abel, 2003; Philip, Ayyanger, Vanderbilt, & Gaebler-Spira, 1994; Poggi et al., 2005; Robertson & Johnson, 2002). Goals in the rehabilitation setting are generally focused on managing complications from surgeries, radiation, and chemotherapy; increasing exercise tolerance; and reintegrating the child into the community. Complications include cardiomyopathies, pulmonary fibrosis, orthopedic problems, and neurological deficits.

Technology-Dependent Children

Another population that is increasing is that of children who are dependent on or assisted by technology for survival (e.g., total parenteral nutrition, oxygen, or ventilators). Dependence on technology can result from a variety of conditions such as spinal cord injury, brain injury, or prematurity. These children may be cared for in intensive care units, long-term care facilities, or pediatric rehabilitation centers. Each setting has its own unique limitations. Intensive care units are extremely costly. These units are generally not able to meet the long-term developmental needs of these children and their families. There are a very limited number of long-term care facilities that accept children on ventilators. Often the staffing ratios of a long-term care facility do not provide for developmental interventions, intensity of care, or the vigilance that some children on ventilators require. In each of these hospital-based settings the child has limited exposure to the real world (e.g., sunshine, breezes, rain, and snow) and too much exposure to hospital routines

---

BOX 31-1 Common Pediatric Rehabilitation Conditions

Acquired Disabilities
- Burns
- Traumatic brain injury
- Spinal cord injury
- Anoxic brain injury
- Stroke

Problems of Prematurity and Low Birth Weight
- Bronchopulmonary dysplasia
- Short gut
- Feeding disorders

Developmental Disabilities
- Cerebral palsy
- Muscular dystrophy
- Autism
- Sensory integration disorders
- Learning disabilities

Congenital Conditions
- Congenital heart disease
- Spina bifida
- Limb deficiencies
- Down syndrome
- Miscellaneous syndromes

Chronic Illnesses
- Juvenile diabetes
- Juvenile rheumatoid arthritis
- Seizure disorders
- Renal failure
- Cancer
- Hematologic disorders
- Chronic pain

Miscellaneous Disorders
- Neuromuscular diseases
- No diagnosis
- Orthopedic conditions
- Obesity

---

and infections. In most cases, pediatric rehabilitation centers are better able to meet the ongoing developmental needs of patients and prepare them for transition to the community.

The home setting provides another care alternative. Discharge to the home setting requires an extensive and comprehensive multidisciplinary plan. Community resources such as a primary care pediatrician, a case manager, home nursing services, and durable medical equipment must be available. School systems must be able to accommodate and provide a safe environment for the child who is dependent on technology. Common stressors for families in the home setting are fear of technological failure, exhaustion from constant care needs, inadequate respite, loss of personal freedom and employment opportunities, lack of full-time nurses, transportation challenges, and financial issues. Although home health care presents a more cost-effective alternative to long hospital stays, there are many "hidden" expenses that are not covered by insurance—such as utility bills, electrical renovations, and lost income (Capen & Dedlow, 1998; Hewitt-Taylor, 2005). Despite these stressors most families find a higher quality of life at home than in the hospital (Heaton, Noyes, Sloper, & Shah, 2005; Lumeng, Warschausky, Nelson, & Augenstein, 2001).

DEVELOPMENTAL FRAMEWORK

Developmental theory is fundamental to pediatric rehabilitation nursing because children are continuing to grow and mature throughout the rehabilitation process. The pediatric rehabilitation nurse must continuously revise goals and tailor interventions to the child's currently expected level of development. For example, goals set for a child who enters the care setting at 9 months of age would need adjustment when the child reaches 12 months of age and maybe sooner. Age-specific communication skills, knowledge of developmentally appropriate play, and creative problem solving are necessary skills for promoting developmental milestones (Selekman, 1991). In addition, emphasis should always be placed on the child's abilities rather than limitations. Clearly, special skills are needed to optimally care for children with disabilities, because "children are not small adults" (Figure 31-1).

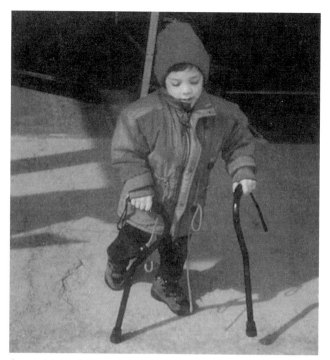

Figure 31-1 Children are not miniature adults. They require care and equipment designed especially for their growth, development, and disabling disorders. (From Wong, D. L., Hockenberry-Eaton, M., Wilson, D., Winkelstein, M. L., & Schwartz, P. [2003]. *Wong's essentials of pediatric nursing* [7th ed.]. St. Louis, MO: Mosby.)

Children grow and develop in several realms: physical, cognitive, social, and emotional. Growth and development proceed in a predictable, sequential fashion for all children. It is the individual rate and level of achievement that vary.

Physical Growth and Gross Motor and Fine Motor Skills

In the physical realm, growth occurs in a cephalocaudal manner. Height, weight, and head circumference are important indicators of health and disease. These growth parameters should be tracked serially and plotted on standardized charts. Children must also acquire mobility to negotiate their environment and fine motor skills to eat, dress, toilet, and groom themselves.

Cognitive, Social, and Emotional Development

Cognitive development progresses from concrete to abstract thinking, which ultimately provides for learning and problem solving (Piaget, 1952). In the social realm children develop a trusting relationship first with their parents or primary caregivers, then their siblings, and ultimately with strangers (Erickson, 1963). They also learn socially appropriate behavior and culturally acceptable norms. A positive body image and self-esteem are essential building blocks of healthy emotional development.

Play, Sports, and Recreation

Play is the life work of children, occupying the majority of the day. It is the child's vehicle for exploration and learning. Play also helps children to master anxiety-provoking situations—for instance, catheterizing a doll during medical play. Involvement in sports and recreation provides fun and exercise, while allowing for development of peer relationships and self-esteem. There are a wide range of adapted equipment, adapted toys, and organized programs available to enable children with special health care needs to participate in sports and recreational activities. Refer to Box 31-2 for a list of some of the many organizations involved in providing sports and recreation for children with special health care needs.

Camps provide another recreational outlet for children with disabilities and chronic illnesses. Camps may be organized around a particular disability or chronic illness, or they may provide the opportunity for children to be mainstreamed into programs for children without disabilities. Some camping programs operate year-round to provide recreation during school vacations or ongoing respite for families.

BOX 31-2 Sports and Recreation Organizations

- Disabled Sports USA
- National Center on Accessibility
- National Disability Sports Alliance
- National Sports Center for the Disabled
- Special Olympics International
- VSA Arts
- Wheelchair Sports, USA

IMPACT OF DISABILITY

The meaning and impact of chronic illness and disability varies for each child. However, the effects of disability are similar in that they create "differentness" in performance or achievement, services required, participation in life events or sequences, and connectedness. Physical growth and development may be below expected age or qualitatively unusual. Special services or assistive technology and devices may be necessary for success and participation in school and recreation. Relationships with family, peers, and significant others may be altered (Crocker, 1996). These psychosocial factors may be greater determinants of overall success in life than the severity of the child's disability (Easton, Rens, & Alexander, 1999). The following sections discuss the impact of disability across pediatric age-specific populations. Developmental tasks, effects of disability, and intervention strategies are summarized in Table 31-1.

Infancy (Birth to 1 Year of Age)

When a child is born with or acquires a chronic or disabling condition during infancy, the implications are far reaching.

TABLE 31-1 Summary of Developmental Tasks, Effects of Disability, Coping Skills, and Intervention Strategies

Stage	Developmental Profile	Effects of Disability	Coping Skills	Intervention Strategies
Infancy	Trust versus mistrust Sitting, crawling, walking Sensorimotor exploration and discrimination Visual tracking Pincer grasp Recognizes bottle Eats solid foods Differentiate self from environment Cause and effect Separation anxiety Object permanence (beginning)	Unpredictable caregivers Delays in having needs met Pain Limited exploration of environment Inappropriate sensory stimulation	Crying Motor activity (e.g., kicking legs, thumb sucking, pacifier sucking)	Give parents information about child's condition and trajectory of condition Provide consistent nurturing and caregiving Support breast-feeding, if desired Respond to infant's needs in a timely fashion Give appropriate sensory stimulation Permit freedom to move and explore Provide verbal and vestibular soothing Provide toys and activities adapted to disability (e.g., switch-activated)
Toddlerhood	Autonomy versus shame and doubt Walks alone Climbing Hand dominance (beginning) Drinks from cup Language acquisition and development Says "no" Begins toilet training Object permanence (established) Asserts independence Separation from parents Imitation, fantasy, and play Concrete thinking Egocentricity (limited ability to see another viewpoint)	Separation difficulties Limited mobility and exploration Forced dependence Overprotection No limit setting Lack of ability to control elimination functions	Crying Protest Temper tantrums Demanding attention Repetitive activity Play and fantasy Behavioral regression	Allow parents and siblings to be involved in care Provide independent mobility Promote independence in activities of daily living (ADLs) Provide safe outlets for tension reduction Set limits Break instructions down into small parts Teach basic sign language to communicate needs Teach parents caregiving and limit-setting skills Use time-outs for discipline
Early childhood (preschool)	Initiative versus guilt Exploration and mastery of environment Running Rides tricycle	Lack of stamina Difficulty establishing body image Overprotection No limit setting	Routines and ritualized activities Imaginative play Physical or verbal aggression	Use pictures to help communication Integrate play and fantasy into therapies and treatments

Continued

TABLE 31-1　Summary of Developmental Tasks, Effects of Disability, Coping Skills, and Intervention Strategies—cont'd

Stage	Developmental Profile	Effects of Disability	Coping Skills	Intervention Strategies
	Toilet trained Independence in self-care activities Fantasy and magical thinking Fears (e.g., dark, body mutilation) Asks why, when, how Identifies self as boy or girl	Limited mobility Impaired communication Lack of normal routine Lack of choice		Support established routines Allow parents to be present to decrease anxiety Provide independent mobility Offer realistic choices Encourage and assist with independence in ADLs Teach parents caregiving and limit-setting skills
Middle childhood (school-age)	Industry versus inferiority Rides bicycle Roller skates Increased independence Starts school Competition and cooperation Starts to read Same-sex peer relationships Consideration of other points of view Logical thought Develops academic skills of conservation, reversibility, and time	Lack of stamina Inability to participate in social/recreational activities Inaccessible schools Missed school Feelings of inferiority Forced dependence Incontinence (when should be continent)	Humor Withdrawal Verbal aggression Physical aggression Depression Hides disability or chronic illness from peers and others	Allow participation in or direction of self-care and procedures Use models and diagrams to teach self-care Correct disability-related misconceptions Maintain peer and sibling relationships when hospitalized Assign household responsibilities and chores Set up situations where child can be successful Educate school personnel and classmates about child's disability Obtain assistive devices and adaptations to make schools and playgrounds accessible Foster friendships with sleepovers and outings Enhance opportunities to relate to others with similar difficulties Facilitate participation in organized sports and recreation expectations
Adolescence	Identity versus role confusion Rapid growth Puberty Establishes sexuality identity Increased emotional independence Need for privacy Conflicts with parents Peer relationships with larger groups Dating Driving Sets future career and personal goals Abstract thinking Transition to adult roles	Altered body image Separation from peers Missed school Forced dependence Delayed puberty Limited behavioral and style experimentation (hair color, tattoos, piercings) Limited risk taking Vocational and social limitation	Denial Intellectualization Despair Resentment Conformity Withdrawal Noncompliance Risk-taking behavior	Give independence in self-care and decision making as much as possible Allow to fail Respect need for privacy Listen to perceptions of illness and clarify misconceptions Give honest, accurate sexuality information Dress in developmentally appropriate clothing Assist in giving attention to overall appearance and cleanliness

TABLE 31-1 Summary of Developmental Tasks, Effects of Disability, Coping Skills, and Intervention Strategies—cont'd

Stage	Developmental Profile	Effects of Disability	Coping Skills	Intervention Strategies
				Teach how to deal with unwanted sexual advances and emergency situations Provide electric wheelchairs for independent mobility Facilitate peer interactions through clubs, dances, and sports and recreation

Data from Jackson, D., & Wallingford, P. (1997). Nursing care across the age continuum: Children and adolescents. In K. M. M. Johnson (Ed.), *Advanced practice nursing in rehabilitation: A core curriculum* (pp. 87-108). Glenview, IL: Association of Rehabilitation Nurses.

Parent-infant bonding may be interrupted or impaired because of the physical or behavioral characteristics of the infant. Infants with disabilities are often difficult to calm, and they may have impaired ability to communicate their basic needs (Easton et al., 1999). Separation anxiety may be exacerbated by multiple hospitalizations.

Toddlerhood (1 to 4 Years of Age)

The toddler is a concrete thinker who affords life and function to all objects. Reasoning is transductive; therefore illness may be viewed by the child as a consequence of "bad" behavior (Pontious, 1982). Disability and hospitalization may separate parents and children for extended periods of time. Equipment and physical environments may limit mobility. Toddlers are often forced to be dependent (e.g., spica cast prevents getting to toilet independently or safety dictates that child sleep in crib). At times parents may be reluctant to set appropriate limits for children with special health care needs; however, failure to do so may interfere with development of impulse control (Perrin & Gerrity, 1984).

Early Childhood/Preschool (4 to 6 Years of Age)

The preoperational phase of cognitive development (Piaget, 1952) provides the preschool child with a basic understanding of rules of social behavior and a basic sense of right and wrong (Kohlberg, 1969). Disability and chronic illness can limit mobility and disrupt established routines. Body invasion and mutilation are key fears; thus treatments including burn dressings, bladder catheterization, and injections may be perceived as punishment for bad behavior. Time constraints and overprotection may prevent parents from allowing children to perform activities of daily living (ADLs) independently.

Middle Childhood/School Age (6 to 12 Years of Age)

The school-age child has a greater understanding of the body, causation of illness, and treatment processes than does the younger child. There is a shift in emphasis from home to peers and school. School-age children with special health care needs may need help with personal care and often take more time to move through the environment. Learning disabilities may also become evident during early elementary school years. In addition to academic learning, the structure of the classroom and interactions with classmates provide an opportunity for learning social skills and making friends. But having the "opportunity" does not guarantee these children will be accepted. School-age children with disabilities need to develop the social skills to overcome the fears and prejudice they may face (Easton et al., 1999). Isolation, withdrawal, depression, and social dysfunction can result if the child is not well integrated into family, school, and community life. Whenever possible, therapies and other health-related activities should be scheduled so that they do not interfere with critical academic subjects and peer relationships.

Adolescence (12 to 18 Years of Age)

Adolescence is a period marked by rapid growth, profound physiological changes, development of higher-order reasoning abilities, an emerging personal identity, and a budding interest in the opposite sex (Molnar, 1988). The peer group is highly influential, and there is a strong need to be a part of the crowd. It is a tumultuous time for adolescents as they strive to attain independence from their parents.

Whether the disability is congenital, as with limb deficiency, or acquired, such as traumatic amputation, the impact on psychosocial functioning can be great. The adolescent may have to adapt to separation from school and peers, changes in body image, discomfort, limitations in mobility, and involvement with the health care system.

During adolescence there is a preoccupation with physical characteristics, and "different" automatically implies "imperfect" (Perrin & Gerrity, 1984). A person whose physical appearance is altered or who may require assistive devices for mobility may be perceived as less attractive to members of the opposite sex (Thompson, 1990). Because body image is so important and control over one's body increases self-esteem and confidence, every attempt should be made to promote continence through bowel and bladder programs, intermittent catheterization programs, or external devices (not diapers).

Socialization can be another problem area for adolescents with special health care needs. They may find themselves with limited friends and minimal opportunities for social interactions. Getting to social functions may be logistically difficult. Limited ability to perform the "3Ds"—dating, driving, and dressing—may create social isolation (Thompson, 1990).

Sexuality is a concept that should be addressed throughout the life span of an individual. However, specific issues may surface at this stage related to sexual functioning and fertility. Teenagers who are capable of communicating should be allowed time alone with the physician or nurse to ask questions and voice their concerns. Their goals and issues may be very different from those of their parents. However, it is not uncommon for adolescents to be hesitant about sharing thoughts and feelings, particularly with adults. Therefore clinicians must be alert to cues that may indicate a desire to talk and be willing to listen. The nurse and other members of the rehabilitation team are highly influential in the development and adjustment of children with chronic illness and disability as they mature into productive adults.

TRANSITION TO ADULTHOOD

Barriers to Success

The transition from childhood through adolescence to adulthood is challenging for all children, but often it is more difficult for the child with a special health care need. These adolescents are often not well prepared for the transition to adulthood. People without disabilities often feel the need to protect and make decisions for them; thus an adolescent may not have had the opportunity to develop decision-making skills. Parents often continue to speak for their adolescents (e.g., during visits with nurse practitioners or physicians), further limiting opportunities for the adolescent to express feelings and concerns. The adolescent with a special health care need may have been protected from family responsibilities and therefore may be lacking in basic skills such as performing household chores.

For the first time in history a generation of children born with a chronic illness or disability will survive into adulthood. Unfortunately, unemployment, economic dependence, depression, social isolation, and lack of access to health services and medical care are realities for many adults with disabilities (U.S. Department of Health and Human Services, 2000). In response to these identified issues, the Healthy and Ready to Work National Center works to diminish the disparities and improve the quality of life for children and young adults with disabilities. The mission of the Center is to create changes in policy, programs, and practices that will help children and young adults with special health care needs transition to adult health care, thereby improving employment opportunities

and future independence (Healthy and Ready to Work National Center, n.d.-a). Preparations for a fully functioning adult lifestyle must begin at the person's point of entry into the rehabilitation system.

Health Transition

The passage into adulthood brings with it some unique concerns related to health maintenance. One issue is that of transitioning from the pediatric to the adult rehabilitation team. Ideally the stage is set for this transition in the mid-to-late teenage years. Both adolescents and parents must be prepared to leave the team of health professionals with whom they have a long-standing relationship. Many adolescents and young adults continue to be followed by their pediatrician, but this typically occurs because of difficulty finding an adult general physician willing and capable of providing care rather than unwillingness to transition on the part of the family. The need to coordinate complex care needs among multiple health care providers further complicates the health transition for many of these children. Physicians who are interested in providing care may not have the time or the resources to provide the necessary care management (Healthy and Ready to Work National Center, n.d.-b). It may also be difficult to impossible for young adults to obtain insurance coverage if they are no longer considered a dependent (Healthy and Ready to Work National Center, n.d.-d).

Vocational Transition

At this point in life, most young adults without disabilities have solidified their self-identity and career plans and have established or are working toward personal and financial independence. Transition plans are the tools used to assist adolescents with disabilities in moving toward the same level of independence. Under the Individuals With Disabilities Education Act of 1997, a statement of transition service needs is required at age 14 and then at age 16 a more comprehensive transition plan is developed. Rehabilitation professionals, educators, parents, and the student conduct an assessment of the student's abilities and skills. The plan that is developed includes details of the services and supports needed for successful postsecondary education, job training, employment, and community living (National Dissemination Center for Children with Disabilities [NICHCY], 2002).

Community Mobility

Community mobility is important for employment, as well as participation in social and recreational activities. Driver's evaluation and training programs are available through some vocational rehabilitation centers or departments. Assessments can be made of the cognitive and physical abilities required for safe driving skills. If driving is not feasible, educating the adolescent or young adult in how to use public transportation of all types can increase locus of control. Feeling in control of one's life is essential in establishing the independence and self-determination needed to function as an adult in society.

Improving Transition

The pediatric rehabilitation nurse can play a key role in supporting adolescents through the transition process. Health professionals can assist families in accessing appropriate health care services, encourage parents to allow teens to make informed decisions about their health care, and educate adolescents about their rights. Teaching self-care management strategies, connecting teens with peer or adult mentors with similar disabilities, and assisting in development of personalized criteria for selecting and hiring peer caregivers are other ways that nurses can support transition.

The Maternal and Child Health Bureau's Division of Services for Children With Special Health Care Needs is working to improve transition through the funding and development of model state-funded programs for health transition of children with special health care needs. In 2001 President Bush announced a national effort to remove barriers to community living for people with disabilities called the New Freedom Initiative. It has the following goals:

- Increase access to assistive and universally designed technologies
- Expand educational opportunities
- Promote homeownership
- Integrate Americans with disabilities into the workforce
- Expand transportation options
- Promote full access to community life

Another effort to support effective and smooth transition is the creation of www.disabilityinfo.gov, a website that provides comprehensive information and resources for people with disabilities (Healthy and Ready to Work National Center, n.d.-c).

SUPPORTING FAMILIES

Coping and Adjustment

Disability and chronic illness have a far-reaching impact on the entire family system. A variety of events that may be directly or indirectly related to the child's illness produce "caregiver burden" (Power & Dell Orto, 2004). Travel to distant trauma or rehabilitation centers, high care needs, financial concerns, lost time from work, problems with school systems, fatigue, trouble finding babysitters, and lost leisure time are just a few of the challenges families face (Sterling, Jones, Johnson, & Bowen, 1996). And these are in addition to major and daily life stresses we all experience. Families vary widely in their reaction to having a child with a disability or chronic illness. Typically emotional responses are dynamic and may subside then recur throughout the course of the child's life (Power & Dell Orto, 2004). Having appropriate resources can help families cope with stress and manage care effectively. Important family supports include the following (Cernoch & Newhouse, 1996; Crocker, 1996; Montagnino & Mauricio, 2004; Sterling et al., 1996):

- Nurses and other health professionals
- Support from spouses, extended families, and friends
- Formal parent networks
- Training on the child's health needs
- Adequate transportation
- Education on rights and entitlements
- Available financial resources and insurance coverage
- Religious beliefs and prayer
- Legal services
- Respite care
- Appropriate child care

Siblings' reactions to children with special health care needs can range from positive to negative (Box 31-3). Involvement in sibling support groups, time alone with parents, the ability to continue their own activities, and participation in family decision making can support sibling adjustment (Crocker, 1996). Coping and spirituality related to childhood are discussed further in Chapters 22 and 29.

Respite Care. All parents need an occasional break from parenting, and this is also true for parents of children with special health care needs. In addition to providing direct relief, respite has added benefits for families (Box 31-4).

Federal legislation authorizes funding to states for respite care, but access and affordability are still issues in many communities.

BOX 31-3 Sibling Reactions to Children With Special Health Care Needs

Positive Reactions
- Maturity
- Responsibility
- Altruism
- Tolerance
- Humanitarian concerns and careers
- Sense of closeness
- Self-confidence
- Independence
- Resilience

Negative Reactions
- Feelings of parental neglect
- Feelings of resentment
- Perceived parental demands and expectations for achievement
- Embarrassment
- Guilt about own health
- Extra responsibilities in the home
- Restrictions in social activities
- Sense of distance in the family
- Isolation
- Concerns for child's future

Data from Cate, I. M. P., & Loots, G. M. P. (2000). Experiences of siblings of children with physical disabilities: An empirical investigation. *Disability and Rehabilitation, 22,* 400.

Connecting with groups and professionals in the community that work with children of similar ages to the child with the disability can assist in locating these critical services (National Information Center for Children and Youth With Disabilities, 1996). Assisting parents in locating respite services, either within the extended family network or community, can be an extremely valuable role for nurses and social services.

Child Care. Many children with special health care needs younger than 6 years of age have mothers who could be in the workforce if they could identify safe and appropriate child care. Despite the increasing number of laws and incentives, parents of young children with disability or chronic illness face multiple challenges in locating affordable and appropriate child care. The needs for flexibility to integrate medical and therapy appointments, special accommodations, and the desire for partnerships are just some of the challenges families face (DeVore & Bowers, 2006).

Most mainstream child care centers lack staff that are adequately trained or experienced in the management of children with disabilities. Space, support services, and staffing ratios are also barriers; therefore they are reluctant to undertake this responsibility.

By providing child care personnel with the appropriate resources and training, there is hope that a greater comfort level will be achieved in caring for this population, thus increasing enrollment. Increased enrollment provides opportunities for nurses to become involved in health education of child care providers and in legislative activities, to serve as liaisons to the community, and to advocate with parents for increased services.

BOX 31-4 Benefits of Respite Care

Relaxation. Respite gives families peace of mind, helps them relax, and renews their humor and energy.

Enjoyment. Respite allows families to enjoy favorite pastimes and pursue new activities.

Stability. Respite improves the family's ability to cope with daily responsibilities and maintain stability during crisis.

Preservation. Respite helps preserve the family unit and lessens the pressures that might lead to institutionalization, divorce, neglect, and child abuse.

Involvement. Respite allows families to become involved in community activities and to feel less isolated.

Time off. Respite allows families to take that needed vacation, spend time together and time alone.

Enrichment. Respite makes it possible for family members to establish individual identities and enrich their own growth and development.

Data from National Information Center for Children and Youth With Disabilities. (1996). Respite care: A gift of time. *NICHCY News Digest* (No. ND12). Retrieved February 1, 2006, from http://www.nichcy.org/pubs/outprint/nd12.pdf.

Family-Centered Care

Disability and chronic illness bring families and health care workers together over the continuum of pediatric rehabilitation settings. The family is responsible for advocating for the child's rights to the best care, education, and resources available. Role conflicts, differing opinions, and limiting hospital policies were part of the driving force behind a major philosophical change in care delivery. Many organizations, including the American Academy of Pediatrics, Society for Pediatric Nurses, and Commission on Accreditation of Rehabilitation Facilities (CARF) endorse pediatric family-centered care. This philosophy involves the patient and family at all phases of care with full partnership with the interdisciplinary team. Within family-centered care the child must be viewed as an integral part of a family system, with the family and home as the central focus of the child's world. Key elements of family-centered care include the following:

1. Respecting each child and his or her family
2. Honoring racial, ethnic, cultural, and socioeconomic diversity
3. Recognizing and building on the strengths of each child and family, even in difficult and challenging situations
4. Supporting and facilitating choice for the child and family about approaches to care and support
5. Ensuring flexibility in organizational policies, procedures, and provider practices so services can be tailored to the needs, beliefs, and cultural values of each child and family
6. Sharing honest and unbiased information with families on an ongoing basis and in ways they find useful and affirming
7. Providing and/or ensuring formal and information support (e.g., family-to-family support) for the child and parent(s) and/or guardian(s) during pregnancy, childbirth, infancy, childhood, adolescence, and young adulthood
8. Collaborating with families at all levels of health care in the care of the individual child and in professional education, policy making, and program development
9. Empowering each child and family to discover their own strengths, build confidence, and make choices and decisions about their health

Rehabilitation nurses and other personnel who have contact with children with special health care needs share an important role and responsibility with the families in shaping each child's future.

CARE SETTINGS

Infants, children, and adolescents with special health care needs are major users of health care services in a wide variety of settings.

Acute Inpatient Rehabilitation

Pediatric rehabilitation services were traditionally provided on acute inpatient pediatric rehabilitation units. These units may be part of a larger acute care hospital, a larger rehabilitation facility, or a freestanding pediatric rehabilitation center.

Like many other types of hospitals, changes in reimbursement have had a profound effect on pediatric rehabilitation service delivery during the past decade. Some facilities that have been freestanding for more than 100 years have merged, affiliated, reduced the number of inpatient beds, or closed altogether. Inpatient stays, once long and intensive, have been streamlined significantly. For example, hospitalizations for spinal cord injury, which once spanned 6 to 12 months, have now been reduced to 60 days in some cases.

Day Hospital and Medical Day Care

Today the trend is clearly toward outpatient and community-based services. Children can attend comprehensive outpatient day hospital or medical day care programs during the day Monday through Friday. Nursing care, cognitive retraining, therapies, and educational services are provided by the multidisciplinary team. The children return home each evening. This trend supports the philosophy of keeping children in their most natural environment: family and community. In addition, it provides a more cost-effective alternative to the inpatient approach to rehabilitative care. Unfortunately, these types of programs are not available in all communities and may not be covered by all insurance carriers.

Home Health Care

Home health care is a rapidly growing segment of the health care continuum. This growth has been driven by consumer desire, technological improvements such as portable ventilators, and health care financing issues. To meet the needs of the varied pediatric rehabilitation population, home health care agencies must be able to provide or access a full range of services, including skilled nursing care, home health care aides, professional therapies, infusion services, and durable medical equipment services (Madigan, 1997). They must also have staff with the same level of expertise as hospital- and clinic-based pediatric rehabilitation nurses with the added skill of dealing with situations that happen only in the community environment.

Reimbursement for home health care services varies widely among insurers. State Medicaid programs are the major payment source for the majority of pediatric cases (Clemens, Davis, Novak, & Connell, 1997). Federal Medicaid waiver programs provide coverage for many technology-dependent children cared for in the home setting. Waiver programs allow families to bypass the usual income requirements for Medicaid eligibility. Other sources of payment include funds from state and community organizations for children with special health care needs (Madigan, 1997).

The role of the pediatric rehabilitation nurse in a home health care setting is to teach the family about the chronic illness or disability so that they can provide care, administer medication, identify problems, and intervene appropriately (Madigan, 1997). Insurers may discharge children home with 16 hours of nursing care reimbursed, only to decrease that reimbursement to 8 hours within weeks. As reimbursement from insurers continues to change, parental training and identification of alternate care providers is critical for the health and safety of the child in the home health care setting.

Outpatient Services

Outpatient services include clinics and therapy services. The increased demand for outpatient pediatric rehabilitation services has given rise to private, for-profit outpatient therapy practices. These practices often are appealing because of more convenient locations, flexible service hours, and minimal waiting lists.

School

Pediatric rehabilitation services may also be provided in school settings as an adjunct to facility-based services. Public laws mandating these services in early intervention, preschool, and school settings will be discussed later in this chapter.

ACCESS TO CARE

Access to health care includes having insurance to pay for care and having identified providers for regular and specialty care. In 2004, 11.2% of all children less than 18 years of age in the United States had no health insurance coverage. Moreover, 18.9% of all poor children were uninsured. Of those children with coverage, 26.9% were covered by Medicaid (DeNavas-Walt, Proctor, & Lee, 2005).

In an effort to control health care costs, state Medicaid and other insurance providers have changed from traditional fee-for-service to managed care plans. Most managed care plans require a primary care pediatrician who serves as the gatekeeper to the health system. These plans could benefit children with special health care needs by improving access to primary health care and case management services.

On the other hand, managed care plans can increase the difficulty in accessing rehabilitation services. Families may be "forced" to receive care from physicians who have no interest or time to coordinate and provide care for children with special health care needs. Most pediatricians have little experience and have received limited training in skills needed to manage these children effectively (Sneed, May, & Stencel, 2000). Access to pediatric specialists and other rehabilitation services may also be affected if these providers are not part of the managed care plan (Committee on Children With Special Needs, 1998). As more children with chronic illness and disability survive and return to the community, these issues become more critical. Continued work is needed to educate primary care providers and develop community-based networks to meet the complex needs of these patient populations (American Academy of Pediatrics [AAP], 2005).

Care Coordination

Increased numbers of children with complex care needs and managed care are two factors that have contributed to increased need for care coordination services. Care coordination includes implementation of care plans by a variety of service providers and programs in an organized fashion (AAP, 2005).

Implicit in this definition is the requirement of helping families meet both current and future goals in a timely and cost-effective manner. Children with special health care needs have high care-coordination needs when they are discharged from the hospital, enter school or the special education setting, transition to adulthood, or when their health status changes.

Parents, an agency, a health professional, or a combination of these people may assume the role of care coordinator. Qualifications for a care coordinators include knowledge of the issues of infants, children, and adolescents with special health care needs; knowledge of the requirements of relevant disability legislation; knowledge of the nature and scope of services available in the child's community; and knowledge of insurance benefits and other available funding. Care coordinators must also have expert documentation skills and the ability to effectively communicate information to the rehabilitation team and family. Identifying alternate placement options when families are unable or unwilling to provide care at home is an ongoing challenge in most inpatient pediatric rehabilitation facilities. Pediatric rehabilitation nurses have traditionally cared for children and families from a holistic perspective, thereby uniquely qualifying them to function in the role of care coordinator. With greater numbers of children and families requiring these services, it is likely that pediatric rehabilitation nurses will increasingly assume these responsibilities.

FACTORS ASSOCIATED WITH PEDIATRIC REHABILITATION

Poverty

Poverty is a societal problem that influences chronic illness and disability in children and adolescents. In 2004, 17.8% of children under 18 lived below the poverty level. The typical profile of a child living in poverty is a child younger than the age of 6 years, living in a household led by a single woman, who is African American or Hispanic (DeNavas-Walt et al., 2005). Children who are living below the poverty level or who are homeless are more likely to have no usual source of health care. Health problems among these children include poor general health, underimmunization, malnutrition, high infant morbidity and mortality rates, lead poisoning, illicit drug use, and child abuse.

Foster Care

Many children in foster care come from homes where parents have human immunodeficiency virus (HIV) or acquired immunodeficiency syndrome (AIDS) or problems with drugs and alcohol abuse. Some have suffered child abuse as well. Young children with chronic illness and disability are the fastest growing population of children in foster care. Although there are some families willing to assume the added responsibility of caring for children with complex medical and behavioral problems, more families are needed. Foster parents need adequate financial support, education, and training

regarding the child's care, and support and respect from health care professionals for their knowledge and love of these special children (Barton, 1999).

Unintentional and Intentional Injury

Unintentional injury is the leading cause of death and disability in children ages 14 and under. Motor vehicle–related events (which include children injured as automobile occupants or pedestrians or riding on bicycles, motorcycles, or other recreational vehicles) are the leading cause of injuries in children. Injury profiles are determined by the child's developmental level; the child's gender, race, and socioeconomic level; the prevalence of the threat in the child's community; and prevention strategies in use. For example, burn injuries in young children are generally caused by scalds from hot liquid spills or hot tap water, whereas burns in older children are often the result of playing with fire (e.g., matches, fireworks). Urban African American children have higher overall injury rates from violence than do other children in the United States (National Center for Injury Prevention and Control, 2005). Near-drownings are more prevalent in areas where there are outdoor swimming pools. Children with attention-deficit/hyperactivity disorder are at greater risk for severe injury from motor vehicle–pedestrian and bicycle accidents (DiScala, Lescohier, Barthel, & Li, 1998).

Violence. In 2002 more than 877,700 young people ages 10 to 24 were injured from violent acts, and homicide is the second leading cause of death among young people in this age bracket (National Center for Injury Prevention and Control, 2005). Youth are increasingly involved both as perpetrators and victims. In addition to the deaths, significant numbers of adolescents and children sustain long-term disability as a result of violence. Immediate access to handguns is a major contributing factor. Public awareness, parental involvement in schools, mentoring, education in conflict management skills, primary prevention programs, offering alternative school- and community-based activities, and increasing efforts of mental health and substance abuse programs are among the intervention strategies necessary to reduce violence-related deaths and injuries among our youth (Thornton, Craft, Dahlberg, Lynch, & Baer, 2002).

Child Abuse. Child abuse is another significant contributor to childhood injury, disability, and mortality. In 2002 approximately 1 million children under the age of 18 were reported to be victims of child abuse or neglect. Neglect represents the most commonly reported type of abuse, followed by physical abuse, emotional abuse, and sexual abuse. Children who are victims of abuse are usually very young, and many have a disability (U.S. Department of Health and Human Services, Administration on Children, Youth and Families, 2005). Burns, head injuries, and other injuries that result from child abuse are all too often witnessed in the pediatric rehabilitation setting. By increasing public awareness regarding child abuse and neglect, as well as providing such services as hot lines, parenting classes, and mentor programs, health professionals are attempting to decrease the incidence of abused children.

Special Education and the Laws

Education is a critical aspect of all children's lives. Involvement in a regular school setting promotes normalcy, and education is correlated with higher levels of employment and social and financial independence in adulthood. Special education is instruction provided at no cost to the parents that meets the unique needs of children with disabilities. It can be provided in preschool, elementary, and secondary school settings; hospitals; or at home. Current legislation supports education of children with disabilities alongside children without disabilities. Refer to Chapter 3 for further information on federal legislation with implications for special education.

When the Individuals With Disabilities Education Improvement Act (IDEA) was reauthorized in 2004, changes were made in the new revision. Key aspects are listed below (Individuals With Disabilities Education Improvement Act of 2004):

- Free and appropriate public education for children from 3 through 21 years of age in the least restrictive environment and alongside children who are not disabled
- A system to identify children with special education needs (child find), including those who are homeless or in foster care
- Individualized education plans (IEPs)
- Procedural safeguards for parents that give them the right to review records, participate in meetings, submit grievances, and resolve issues through mediation
- Evaluation procedures
- Confidentiality of records and information
- Services for effective transition from early intervention to preschool and then transition from secondary school to adulthood
- Procedures to prevent overidentification or disproportionate representation of minority children as children with disabilities

IDEA 2004 also provides grants for coordination of early intervention services for children from birth to 3 years of age. Each state has the responsibility to set up systems to serve their children; however, the following components are requirements for all early intervention services (Individuals With Disabilities Education Improvement Act of 2004):

- Child find—Identifies infants and toddlers who have or are at risk for developmental delays, including those in foster care or that are homeless
- Diagnostic evaluation—Multidisciplinary assessment of the child to determine if the child qualifies for services; family assessment is also included
- Individualized family service plan (IFSP)—Plan for needed services that is developed jointly between the family and the health care team; the plan builds on family strengths and supports the family as a unit because they are the best support for the young child

- Early intervention service delivery—Full range of services provided by a multidisciplinary team in the child's natural environment whenever possible.

Despite public laws, parents still face many challenges within the educational system. The "appropriate" placement is not always the best placement in the parents' eyes. There is also wide variability in services between states and different communities within those states. School nurses, teachers, and administrators have unmet needs for health information about individual students; education and training about specific disabilities; and effective, timely communication with the multidisciplinary team. School systems need to continue to develop the structure and personnel to support the child with special health care needs in the school setting (Esperat, Moss, Roberts, Kerr, & Green, 1999). Parents, professionals, and children with disabilities need to have a full awareness of the laws related to special education so they can advocate effectively and work toward making full inclusion a reality. A firm knowledge base also helps families cope with the change in family support that often accompanies the transition from home-based early intervention services to school-based special education services.

NURSING PROCESS

Assessment

Strategies for Assessment. Children with chronic illness or disability are assessed at regular intervals and at all points along the health care continuum. Assessment is a critical element in the nursing process. It is the basis from which planning and evaluation of therapeutic interventions emerge.

Holistic assessments encompass the physical, cognitive, social, emotional, cultural, and spiritual aspects of a child's life. The child also is assessed within the context of the family system. An additional consideration for some children with disabilities is the application of chronological versus developmental age. Neurological deficits and limited or abnormal experiences can delay the child's development. This must be considered during the assessment.

Privacy and dignity must be provided for the child or adolescent during the assessment process. Fear and anxiety can be allayed or minimized by providing honest, concise, and age-appropriate information to the child. Toys for younger children and other age-appropriate items such as puppets, anatomically correct dolls, diagrams, and books may also help to calm and elicit information from the child. Although parents or guardians usually are the primary historians, older children and adolescents should never be overlooked or excluded from conversations regarding themselves. The nurse's behavior must convey the fact that the child is the central focus of the interaction and a valuable source of information.

Tools for Developmental Assessment. Nurses can use screening tools to detect delays in development. The Denver II (the revised Denver Developmental Screening Test) is a standardized basic screening tool that can assist the practitioner in evaluating children from birth to 6 years in the following areas: gross motor, fine motor–adaptive, language, and personal-social. The administration of the Denver II is relatively simple, requiring minimal and easily accessible equipment, and can be done in any pediatric rehabilitation setting. Parent-completed screening tools, such as the Denver Prescreening Developmental Questionnaire (PDQ II), are also available (Denver Developmental Materials Inc., n.d.). They require very little professional time and are a cost-effective alternative for basic developmental screening. More focused assessments should be performed by the appropriate interdisciplinary team member if delays are identified during the basic screening. There are numerous tools available for these diagnostic assessments.

Nursing Diagnoses, Interventions, and Outcomes for Common Chronic Conditions and Disabilities in Children and Adolescents

It is beyond the scope of this chapter to provide a comprehensive review of all the diagnoses encountered in the field of pediatric rehabilitation; however, this section addresses four of the more common conditions with respect to nursing diagnoses, outcomes, and interventions.

Cerebral Palsy. Children with cerebral palsy (CP) are the largest population requiring pediatric (re)habilitative services (Matthews & Wilson, 1999). Bax and Molnar (as cited in Matthews & Wilson, 1999) define cerebral palsy as "a disorder of movement and posture that results from a nonprogressive lesion or injury to an immature brain." The injury may occur in utero, near the time of delivery, or during early childhood. Among the multiple causes of CP (e.g., intrauterine infections, toxins, and delivery complications), prematurity is the most significant contributing factor (Matthews & Wilson, 1999). The National Center on Birth Defects and Developmental Disabilities estimates that for 1991-1994, 28 of every 10,000 children 3 through 10 years of age had cerebral palsy. Lifetime costs for a newly diagnosed child (using 2003 dollar values) are estimated at $921,000, and these estimates do not include family out-of-pocket expenses ("Economic Costs Associated With Mental Retardation," 2004).

CP is classified as spastic, athetoid, ataxic, or mixed. These types are further divided according to the number of extremities or parts of the body involved. The majority of children with CP have the spastic form. CP is usually diagnosed in the second half of the first year of life. Suspicious signs are reflex abnormalities, abnormal muscle tone and posture, delayed development, and poor feeding.

The broad span of causes accounts in part for the number of associated problems seen in children with this condition: hearing, vision, and speech impairments; feeding problems and malnutrition; seizures; and mental retardation; in addition to various motor impairments (Matthews & Wilson, 1999). Not all children with CP have cognitive limitations.

Spasticity is a complication that is particularly difficult to manage. Figure 31-2 illustrates two children who have spasticity producing "scissoring." The goal of spasticity management is functional mobility. Daily passive/active range-of-motion

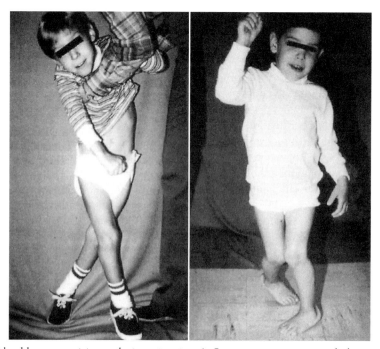

Figure 31-2 Two children with adductor spasticity producing scissoring. **A,** Severe spasticity in nonambulatory child who has adduction deformity and severe scissoring. **B,** Ambulatory child with spastic diplegia whose legs scissor during walking. (From Canale, S. T., & Beaty, J. H. [1991]. *Operative pediatric orthopaedics.* St. Louis, MO: Mosby.)

(ROM) exercises, warm baths, and other relaxation techniques can be used to facilitate movements. Follow-through of physical and occupational therapy exercises in the rehabilitation, home, and school settings is essential. Roughly half of children with CP use assistive devices such as strollers, wheelchairs, walkers, standers, splints and orthotics, or positioning devices. These devices must be evaluated frequently to ensure proper fit as the child grows and develops. Other strategies to manage spasticity and promote mobility include medications, intrathecal baclofen pump, phenol injections, botulin toxin injections, orthopedic surgeries, and rhizotomy. Surgical procedures should be scheduled for summertime or vacation to minimize time lost from school.

The ability to communicate opens doors. Advances in technology in the last 10 to 15 years have greatly advanced long-term well-being for children with CP. Communication skills can be increased with augmentative (enhance existing speech) or alternative (replace written or spoken word) communication devices that are recommended by a speech-language pathologist. If an augmentative or alternative device is recommended, the child, family, school, and health care personnel need education to ensure consistency in use. Children with CP also need adequate time and a supportive environment for communication.

Feeding is a very time-consuming task in caring for many children with CP. Collaboration with the physician and speech-language pathologist is necessary to establish a safe feeding regimen. Swallowing studies may be recommended to rule out aspiration and ensure safe oral feeding. Consistency of food and fluid may need to be adjusted to promote safe consumption. Occupational therapists can provide adaptive feeding utensils and techniques; physical therapists can ensure proper seating and positioning for feeding. Families and school personnel require education regarding feeding regimen and techniques to ensure community follow-through. If adequate nutrition cannot be taken orally in a reasonable time, education in the care and use of an enteral feeding tube may be necessary.

Safe transport is another consideration for children with CP. Convertible car seats approved for the forward-facing semi-reclining position are useful for children with poor head control. Other modifications to maintain appropriate posture and alignment can be made using rolled towels, diapers, or blankets. Parents must be trained in proper techniques so that modifications do not interfere with proper function of safety features of the car seat. Wheelchairs should be secured with proper tie downs with trays and adaptive equipment removed. Community resources to provide specialized restraint systems and training in proper car restraint use should be identified. Transportation should also be incorporated into the individualized education plan at school (Bull et al., 1999).

Constipation in children with CP is related to decreased fluid and bulk intake and decreased mobility. Bowel programs should focus on the least-invasive, most cost-effective measures first (i.e., dietary and fluid measures, regular exercise/increased mobility, and scheduled toileting). Stool softeners and laxatives are added as adjuncts to dietary measures and exercise as necessary. The physical therapist can provide supported seating (commode chair) for relaxation of tone and facilitation of elimination. The child's ability to communicate the need to use the toilet is also a consideration. Support of family and school personnel is necessary for a successful program.

Many children with CP have specialized dental care needs. Consultation with a pediatric dentist who specializes in care of children with special health care needs can provide solutions for problems such as gingival hyperplasia, malocclusion, caries, and periodontal disease (Matthews & Wilson, 1999). Case managers can collaborate with a child's dentist to identify funding for dental care. Routine oral hygiene consisting of toothbrushing and flossing is essential for dental health. Drooling is an additional problem with significant social implications. Medications, oral stimulation, and behavior modification can be effective in reducing this problem. Refer to Table 31-2 for specific nursing diagnoses, outcomes, and interventions for children with CP.

Spina Bifida. Spina bifida is a term used to describe a group of neural tube defects that include spina bifida occulta, meningocele, and myelomeningocele. Neuromuscular function is affected below the level of lesion, resulting in lower extremity paralysis; impaired bowel, bladder, and sexual function; sensory deficits; respiratory problems; and hydrocephalus. Over the past three decades, use of antibiotics and surgical advances have increased survival and life expectancy for children with spina bifida. Spina bifida occurs in about 6 in 10,000 live births in the United States. Although the exact cause of spina bifida is unknown, a contributing factor has been identified—inadequate folic acid intake. The U.S. Public Health Service, Institute of Medicine, and Academy of Pediatrics currently recommend that all women of childbearing age consume 400 micrograms of folic acid daily from fortified foods or supplements before conception and during pregnancy to prevent neural tube defects (U.S. Department of Health and Human Services, 2000).

Controlling incontinence, preventing infections, and preserving kidney function are common rehabilitation goals for the child with spina bifida. Routine urological evaluation by a physician is recommended every 6 to 12 months to monitor these goals. Families are educated regarding urinary tract health maintenance; adequate fluid intake; signs, symptoms, and steps to take for urinary tract infection; prevention of bladder overdistention; and performing clean intermittent catheterization. They must also learn about medications to increase bladder volumes (oxybutynin) and treat infection (nitrofurantoin or trimethoprim). By 4 to 8 years of age, children have the manual dexterity, psychological readiness, and postural balance to learn and perform self-care for clean intermittent catheterization (Edwards, Borzyskowski, Cox, & Badcock, 2004). Appropriate direct care providers should be educated regarding the bladder program so they can provide the support, encouragement, and privacy needed. Families, school

TABLE 31-2 Nursing Diagnoses, Interventions, and Outcomes Applicable to Cerebral Palsy **NIC/NOC**

Nursing Diagnosis	Nursing Interventions	Nursing Outcomes
Impaired swallowing	Aspiration precautions Enteral tube feeding Feeding Nutrition management Medication management Surveillance Positioning Swallowing therapy	Aspiration prevention Swallowing status
Impaired physical mobility	Exercise promotion: stretching Exercise therapy: ambulation Exercise therapy: balance Exercise therapy: joint mobility Exercise therapy: muscle control Splinting Positioning Medication management Positioning: wheelchair Self-care assistance Teaching prescribed activity/exercise	Mobility
Impaired verbal communication	Active listening Communication enhancement: hearing deficit Communication enhancement: speech deficit	Communication
Risk for constipation	Bowel training Constipation/impaction management Bowel management Fluid management Exercise promotion Medication management Self-care assistance: toileting	Bowel elimination
Impaired urinary elimination	Urinary habit training Teaching: toilet training Urinary incontinence care	Urinary continence
Risk for impaired skin integrity	Skin surveillance	Immobility consequences: physiological
Self-care deficit: bathing/hygiene, dressing/grooming, feeding, toileting	Self-care assistance	Self-care: activities of daily living
Impaired dentition	Oral health maintenance	Oral hygiene
Delayed growth and development	Developmental enhancement: child Developmental enhancement: adolescent	Child development: 1 month through adolescence
Social isolation	Socialization enhancement	Social involvement Play participation Leisure participation
Risk for caregiver role strain	Caregiver support Respite care Abuse protection support: child	Family coping Role performance

Data from Moorhead, S., Johnson, M., & Maas, M. (Eds.). (2004). *Nursing outcomes classification (NOC)* (3rd ed.). St. Louis, MO: Mosby; Dochterman, J. M., & Bulechek, G. M. (2004). *Nursing interventions classification (NIC)* (4th ed.). St. Louis, MO: Mosby; and NANDA International. (2007). *NANDA-I nursing diagnoses: Definitions & classification 2007-2008.* Philadelphia: Author.

personnel, and health professionals must encourage the child's progression toward maximal independence with the bladder program because continence gives self-esteem. The need for intermittent catheterization puts the child at personal risk for child sexual abuse. Children should be taught from an early age that they are in charge of their own bodies and that they have the right to say no to anyone who tries to touch them in a private place.

Obesity is another common problem among children with spina bifida that only adds to their musculoskeletal, mobility, and skin problems (van den Berg-Emons, Bussmann, Meyerink, Roebroeck, & Stam, 2003). Children and families need early education regarding healthful nutrition patterns. Even young children can participate in selection and preparation of healthy meals and snacks. Dietitians can assist by calculating appropriate calories for weight control. Regular exercise and involvement in adapted sports and recreational activities should also be encouraged.

Unique safety issues are present for the child with spina bifida. Some children have ventriculoperitoneal (VP) shunts in place to manage hydrocephalus. Parents must be able to identify signs of increased intracranial pressure and shunt failure and perform shunt care. Neurosurgical evaluations are necessary as children grow to ensure they do not outgrow their shunts, which would inhibit function. Families can expect that children will need three or more shunt revisions by age 12 (Hoeman, 1997).

Sensory alterations place these children at risk for pressure ulcers, burns, frostbite, and trauma. Skin checks should be performed at least twice daily to prevent development of impaired skin integrity. A long-handled mirror can increase the child's involvement and promote independence. Special attention should be given to areas under braces and other orthoses. Frequent hygiene care is necessary in children who are incontinent or adolescents who are menstruating.

The child with spina bifida needs adaptive equipment for exploratory play. Adapted seats, carts, standers, and wheelchairs are available to support involvement in play and activities. When children move to the school setting, motorized wheelchairs should be considered so children can keep up with peers. School-age and adolescent children should be able to instruct others in use of their adaptive equipment and wheelchairs. Refer to Table 31-3 for specific nursing diagnoses, outcomes, and interventions for children with spina bifida.

TABLE 31-3 Nursing Diagnoses, Interventions, and Outcomes Applicable to Spina Bifida ▪NIC/NOC▪

Nursing Diagnosis	*Nursing Interventions*	*Nursing Outcomes*
Impaired urinary elimination	Urinary catheterization: intermittent Urinary elimination management	Urinary continence Urinary elimination
Risk for imbalanced nutrition: more than body requirements	Exercise promotion Nutrition management Weight management	Risk control
Risk for latex allergy response	Latex precautions Allergy management	Risk control
Risk for injury	Sports injury prevention: youth Teaching: disease process	Risk control
Bowel incontinence	Bowel training Self-care assistance: toileting Teaching: toilet training	Bowel elimination Bowel continence
Risk for impaired skin integrity	Skin surveillance	Immobility consequences: physiological
Impaired physical mobility	Exercise promotion: strength training Exercise therapy: ambulation Positioning: wheelchair	Ambulation Ambulation: wheelchair
Disturbed body image Risk for situational low self-esteem	Self-esteem enhancement Body image enhancement	Body image Self-esteem
Delayed growth and development	Developmental enhancement: child Developmental enhancement: adolescent	Child development: 1 month through adolescence
Risk for caregiver role strain	Caregiver support Respite care Abuse protection: child	Family coping Role performance

Data from Moorhead, S., Johnson, M., & Maas, M. (Eds.). (2004). *Nursing outcomes classification (NOC)* (3rd ed.). St. Louis, MO: Mosby; Dochterman, J. M., & Bulechek, G. M. (2004). *Nursing interventions classification (NIC)* (4th ed.). St. Louis, MO: Mosby; and NANDA International. (2007). *NANDA-I nursing diagnoses: Definitions & classification 2007-2008.* Philadelphia: Author.

Traumatic Brain Injury. Traumatic brain injury (TBI) is a major and costly cause of disability in children. Among children 0 to 14 years of age TBI results in 2,685 deaths, 37,000 hospitalizations, and 435,000 emergency department visits each year (Langlois, Rutland-Brown, & Thomas, 2004). The highest incidence of traumatic brain injury is in the adolescent and young adult male population (15 to 24 years of age) (Centers for Disease Control and Prevention, 2004). Falls, motor vehicle, pedestrian, and bicycle accidents are responsible for the majority of brain injuries. Sports and recreation, violence, and assault are other major contributors (National Center for Injury Prevention and Control, 2006). Child abuse is the cause of most brain injuries in children under 3 years of age (Reece & Sege, 2000).

A wide spectrum of problems is seen as a result of TBI. The severity and type of disability varies with the amount, type, and location of brain damage. Common motor consequences in children are balance problems, ataxia, hemiparesis, and spasticity. Hearing and vision impairments, dysphagia, and seizures may also be present. But it is the cognitive deficits that have the largest impact on the child and family. Impaired attention, agitation, altered memory and judgment, behavior problems, and emotional lability are all common cognitive consequences of TBI that profoundly affect development (National Institute of Neurological Disorders and Stroke, 2002).

Nursing and rehabilitative intervention to manage these consequences and other associated medical disorders must focus on the child's current level of cognitive functioning. The Rancho Los Amigos Levels Cognitive Functioning is one scale that is used to facilitate use of common language between rehabilitation team members (see Chapter 25). Throughout the rehabilitation process, the three most important strategies are structure, repetition, and consistency.

Stimulation activities are the focus of care before the child is able to follow simple commands (levels I to III). ROM exercises and positioning to prevent pressure ulcers and contractures are also important at this stage. Bowel and bladder programs, tracheostomy care, gastrostomy feedings, and seizure management are common aspects of nursing care during this phase.

When the child is agitated (levels IV to V), safety and limit setting are key. Using simple commands, providing concrete explanations, and providing orientation help the child to cooperate and participate in ADLs. Decreased environmental stimulation (i.e., decrease light, noise, and visitors); relaxation techniques (i.e., warm bath or shower, deep breathing, guided imagery, soft music, comfort items within reach); and scheduling prescribed medical and nursing procedures so that sleep is not disturbed help promote adequate rest during these stages.

By level VI the child is often ready to return to the community and school. Neuropsychological testing should be performed to ensure proper school placement. These tests evaluate higher cortical functioning (e.g., attention span, memory, problem solving, social judgment) as well as sensory motor function. More complex commands can generally be understood and followed. Memory books and daily schedules will help children with TBI gain independence. A low-stimulation environment will increase their ability to attend to tasks. Increased emotional support is often needed as they begin to realize the magnitude of their disabilities. They often lose friends and need to adjust life goals because of their disabilities. Schools are often not prepared to deal with the learning disabilities, attention deficits, poor impulse control, lack of motivation, and impaired social judgment that are common behavioral consequences of TBI. Behavior management programs must be communicated, understood, and implemented consistently by the interdisciplinary team, family, and school personnel.

Families need support during community reentry. Structured counseling sessions and spontaneous interactions through the course of daily activities help family members verbalize feelings related to their situation. Referrals to brain injury support groups and identifying appropriate community resources (i.e., day care programs, respite services, and attendant care) also help families cope with ongoing care needs in the home setting. Refer to Table 31-4 for specific nursing diagnoses, outcomes, and interventions for children with traumatic brain injury.

Bronchopulmonary Dysplasia. Bronchopulmonary dysplasia (BPD) is a chronic lung disease that occurs primarily in premature infants. Excessive intravenous fluid, exposure to high concentrations of oxygen, and mechanical ventilation all contribute to lung injury. Surfactant replacement therapy has improved survival of preterm infants but has not had a conclusive effect on reducing the number of children with BPD (D'Angio & Maniscalco, 2004). Many infants with BPD have additional developmental disadvantages such as extreme prematurity, intraventricular hemorrhage, and prolonged hospitalization.

Early rehabilitation goals for children with BPD are often focused on stabilizing respiratory status. These children may receive supplemental oxygen through nasal cannula, tracheostomy, or mechanical ventilators (Figure 31-3). A common long-term goal is to wean them from respiratory support. Supportive care is needed from both nursing and respiratory staff. Portable oxygen and ventilators enable these children to have mobility despite their need for continuous respiratory support. Activity intolerance is an obstacle to full involvement in the rehabilitation program. Clustering care and paying attention to early signs of distress can help prevent acute deterioration and clinical setbacks.

Oral hypersensitivity, prolonged periods without food or drink, increased caloric demands, and poor feeding skills combine to place many infants at increased nutritional risk. Collaboration with the registered dietitian is important for nutritional planning and growth monitoring. Growth is the key to improving respiratory status. Speech-language pathologists can help enhance these children's oral feeding skills.

Parents of children with BPD require extensive training and support for success in the home environment. Care regimens should be simplified whenever possible to enable parents to get several hours of uninterrupted sleep at night (e.g., eliminate feedings and medications in the middle of the night). Parents should be educated on illness warning signs, respiratory care, feeding, positioning, calming strategies, and cardiopulmonary resuscitation. Health emergency plans must be established before discharge. They should also be encouraged to avoid tobacco smoke exposure and obtain immunizations against respiratory syncytial virus (RSV) infections.

Parents often need training in well child care, because many of these infants have never been home. Positioning devices, age-appropriate toys, and calming strategies promote development in the hospital and at home. Considerations for safe transportation should also be included in the training plan. Strollers can be adapted to accommodate suction equipment, portable oxygen, and ventilators. Infant-only car seats that can be reclined are helpful for children with difficulty breathing in the sitting position. To prevent injury to the neck and face or blockage of the tracheostomy during impact,

premature and small infants and infants and children with tracheostomies should not be placed in car seats with a harness-tray/shield combination or an armrest. According to the American Academy of Pediatrics' Committee on Injury Prevention and Poison Prevention, a rear-facing car safety seat with a three-point harness or a car safety seat with a five-point harness is the best option for children with a tracheostomy. Oxygen tanks and monitors should be secured on the floor of the vehicle (Bull et al., 1999). Refer to Table 31-5 for specific nursing diagnoses, outcomes, and interventions for children with BPD.

EVALUATION

Outcomes

Outcomes have always been important to professionals, patients, and families, but measurement of outcomes has

TABLE 31-4 Nursing Diagnoses, Interventions, and Outcomes Applicable to Traumatic Brain Injury   NIC/NOC

Nursing Diagnosis	*Nursing Interventions*	*Nursing Outcomes*
Disturbed thought processes	Behavior management: overactivity/inattention Cognitive stimulation Elopement precautions Environmental management: safety Medication management Memory training	Cognition Information processing
Disturbed sensory perception (auditory, gustatory, kinesthetic, olfactory, visual)	Communication enhancement: hearing deficit Nutrition management Environmental management	Sensory function: taste and smell Sensory function: proprioception Hearing compensation behavior Vision compensation behavior
Impaired verbal communication	Communication enhancement: speech deficit	Communication
Insomnia	Environmental management Sleep enhancement	Sleep
Risk for injury	Seizure precautions Surveillance: safety Physical restraint	Fall prevention behavior Risk control Seizure control
Impaired physical mobility	Exercise therapy: ambulation Exercise therapy: balance Exercise therapy: joint mobility Positioning: wheelchair	Ambulation Ambulation: wheelchair
Impaired swallowing	Swallowing therapy	Swallowing status
Bowel incontinence	Bowel training Self-care assistance: toileting	Bowel continence
Impaired urinary elimination	Urinary incontinence care Self-care assistance: toileting	Urinary continence
Delayed growth and development	Developmental enhancement: child Developmental enhancement: adolescent	Child development: 1 month through adolescence
Risk for caregiver role strain	Caregiver support Respite care	Family coping Role performance
Impaired parenting	Abuse protection support: child	Abuse protection

Data from Moorhead, S., Johnson, M., & Maas, M. (Eds.). (2004). *Nursing outcomes classification (NOC)* (3rd ed.). St. Louis, MO: Mosby; Dochterman, J. M., & Bulechek, G. M. (2004). *Nursing interventions classification (NIC)* (4th ed.). St. Louis, MO: Mosby; and NANDA International. (2007). *NANDA-I nursing diagnoses: Definitions & classification 2007-2008.* Philadelphia: Author.

become increasingly important in all pediatric rehabilitation settings. In the current health care environment, insurance carriers use outcomes to justify spending of limited health care dollars. Accrediting bodies also integrate outcome data into organizational accreditation processes. Outcomes in pediatric rehabilitation are related to age at initiation of services, severity, extent and location of injury, overall health and nutrition, comorbidities, psychosocial issues, and quality and quantity of interventions. As length of stay decreases, traditional measures of outcomes need to be adjusted to include measures of quality of life and school and community reintegration.

Program Evaluation

Pediatric rehabilitation facilities, like most organizations, use outcome measurement as a method of evaluating the effectiveness of their programs. Outcome measurement tools are used to identify the level at which a patient is functioning on admission and discharge, thus enabling detection of improvement in functional categories or ADLs. These measures are being evaluated for use in home and community settings as well. Some examples of areas that are rated include transferring,

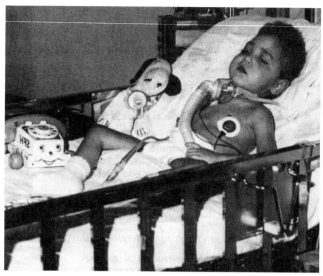

Figure 31-3 Children with BPD often require respiratory support via a tracheostomy. (From Wong, D. L., Hockenberry-Eaton, M., Winkelstein, M. L., Wilson, D, Ahmann, E., & DiVito-Thomas, P. A. [1999]. *Whaley and Wong's nursing care of infants and children* [6th ed.]. St. Louis, MO: Mosby.)

TABLE 31-5 Nursing Diagnoses, Interventions, and Outcomes Applicable to Bronchopulmonary Dysplasia   NIC/NOC

Nursing Diagnosis	Nursing Interventions	Nursing Outcomes
Ineffective airway clearance	Airway management Artificial airway management	Respiratory status: airway patency
Impaired gas exchange	Respiratory monitoring Mechanical ventilation Mechanical ventilation weaning	Respiratory status: gas exchange Respiratory status: ventilation
Activity intolerance	Oxygen therapy	Activity tolerance
Ineffective infant feeding pattern	Enteral tube feeding Nonnutritive sucking Swallowing therapy	Swallowing status
Imbalanced nutrition: less than body requirements	Nutrition management Environmental management: attachment process Nutritional monitoring	Nutritional status: food and fluid intake Nutritional status: body mass
Ineffective protection	Immunization/vaccination management	Immunization behavior
Delayed growth and development and disorganized infant behavior	Developmental care	Child development: 1 month through 3 years
Risk for impaired parent/child attachment	Attachment promotion Parent education: infant	Parent-infant attachment Parenting performance
Risk for caregiver role strain	Caregiver support	Caregiver performance: direct care

Data from Moorhead, S., Johnson, M., & Maas, M. (Eds.). (2004). *Nursing outcomes classification (NOC)* (3rd ed.). St. Louis, MO: Mosby; Dochterman, J. M., & Bulechek, G. M. (2004). *Nursing interventions classification (NIC)* (4th ed.). St. Louis, MO: Mosby; and NANDA International. (2007). *NANDA-I nursing diagnoses: Definitions & classification 2007-2008*. Philadelphia: Author.

toileting, bathing, and cognitive functioning (i.e., communication, problem solving, and memory). Rehabilitation programs use the information to assess their effectiveness and make necessary adjustments to improve patient outcomes.

Individual programs or facilities traditionally developed outcome measurement tools; however, it became apparent that there was a nationwide need for documenting the severity of disability and the outcomes of medical rehabilitation in a uniform language. The Uniform Data System for Medical Rehabilitation (UDSMR) was established to ensure uniformity in definitions and measures of disabilities and outcomes in rehabilitation.

The functional independence measure (FIM) tool was developed to assess 18 items relative to self-care, sphincter management, mobility, locomotion, communication, and social cognition on a seven-level scale. The UDSMR serves as a central repository for patient data and provides reports of comparable data for quality management to subscribing facilities. The process is dependent on reliable data collection and reporting by facilities and quality control of data received by the UDSMR. Raters are credentialed to ensure knowledge of FIM definitions and levels (UDSMR 1991). Chapters 8 and 11 provide additional information on these topics.

A FIM for children (WeeFIM) was developed to reflect functional and criteria differences seen in children as a result of developmental age. The tool is used with children from 6 months to 16 years of age. Although very young children may score with a higher dependency factor at both admission and discharge because of developmental age, scores for older children can reflect gains in any or all areas measured. The WeeFIM can be used in both inpatient and outpatient settings, as well as in schools and community-based agencies. The WeeFIM Instrument: 0-3 Module is a complement to the WeeFIM. It is a family questionnaire that measures precursors to function in children ages 0 to 3 years who have a variety of disabilities (http://www.UDSMR.org).

The pediatric evaluation of disability inventory (PEDI) is another functional evaluation measurement tool (Box 31-5). The PEDI provides a comprehensive clinical assessment of key functional capabilities and performance in children between the ages of 6 months and 7 years. Older children whose functional abilities are not equivalent to chronological norms may also be evaluated. The unique feature of the PEDI is the attempt to include social outcome measures, as well as those for ADLs. The three domains attempt to measure what a child "does do" rather than what cannot be accomplished and the level of caregiver assistance required. A separate scale, the modifications scale, documents environmental modifications or adaptive equipment a child uses to perform ADLs. The PEDI has been standardized on a sample of children without disabilities in the targeted age range (Feldman, Haley, & Coryell, 1990). Rehabilitation professionals administer the PEDI in a clinical setting or by structured interview of parents, requiring approximately 45 minutes. Individual record booklets for maintaining a long-term profile are available. Software for data entry, scoring, and individual profile summaries is also available.

IMPLICATIONS FOR PEDIATRIC REHABILITATION NURSING PRACTICE

Prevention Summary

Prenatal intervention is a major strategy to decrease the incidence of premature and low-birth-weight infants and the associated medical problems. A good prenatal diet with adequate folic acid intake; absence of smoking, alcohol, and recreational drugs; and appropriate medical monitoring increase the chances of having a healthy infant. Teenage pregnancies, which often result in premature deliveries, contribute to the numbers of infants born at risk for special health care needs. Ongoing well-child care, including immunizations, can

---

BOX 31-5 **Functional Skills Content of the Pediatric Evaluation of Disability Inventory**

Self-Care Domain
- Types of food textures
- Use of utensils
- Use of drinking containers
- Toothbrushing
- Hair brushing
- Nose care
- Hand washing
- Washing body and face
- Pullover/front-opening garments
- Fasteners
- Pants
- Shoes/socks
- Toileting tasks
- Control of bladder function
- Control of bowel function

Mobility Domain
- Floor locomotion
- Chair/wheelchair transfers
- Opening and closing doors
- In and out of car
- Bed mobility
- Stand/sit in tub or shower
- Method of indoor locomotion
- Distance/speed indoors
- Pulls/carries objects
- Method of outdoor locomotion
- Distance/speed outdoors
- Locomotion on outdoor surfaces
- Scooting up and down stairs
- Walking up and down stairs

Social Function Domain
- Comprehension of word meanings
- Comprehension of sentence complexity
- Functional use of expressive communication
- Complexity of expressive communication
- Problem resolution
- Social interactive play
- Peer interactions
- Self-information
- Time orientation
- Household chores
- Self-protection
- Community function

From PEDI Research Group, New England Medical Center Hospital, Boston, MA.

potentially prevent disabling illnesses such as measles encephalopathy, influenza, meningitis, and polio.

Unintentional injury is the leading cause of death and acquired disabilities in children older than 1 year of age. Prevention strategies must be multifaceted, focus on the specific type of injury, and be population and culturally relevant. For example, manufacturers' changes in shopping carts have decreased head injuries from falls in young children. Ongoing use of infant and child car seats, car safety belts, and helmets and other protective gear while bicycling or participating in contact sports can continue to decrease disability related to traumatic brain injury and other physical injuries. Offering parenting classes on stress management and expected behavior could reduce the incidence of child abuse. Educating children and adults in all areas of safety and injury prevention is key to decreasing the incidence of injuries. It is clearly less costly from a financial and societal perspective to prevent rather than treat injuries. Combined efforts from many professionals and organizations such as the National Center for Injury Prevention and Control of the Centers for Disease Control and Prevention, *Healthy People 2010*, and the National Safe Kids Campaign are necessary to identify and implement further prevention strategies.

Unmet Needs

The field of pediatric rehabilitation continues to grow and evolve. Federal and state legislation has helped to ensure the rights of children and adults with disabilities. A fully integrated system of health care to meet the needs of children with special health care needs is not yet a reality. This system has been described as the "medical home" by the American Academy of Pediatrics (2005). It includes the following:

1. A plan of care is developed by the physician, practice care coordinator, child, and family in collaboration with other providers, agencies, and organizations involved with the care of the patient.
2. A central record or database containing all pertinent medical information, including hospitalizations and specialty care, is maintained at the practice. The record is accessible, but confidentiality is preserved.

3. The medical home physician shares information among the child, family, and consultant and provides a specific reason for referral to appropriate pediatric medical subspecialists, surgical specialists, and mental health/developmental professionals.
4. Families are linked to family support groups, parent-to-parent groups, and other family resources.
5. When a child is referred for a consultation or additional care, the medical home physician assists the child and family in understanding clinical issues.
6. The medical home physician evaluates and interprets the consultants' recommendations for the child and family and, in consultation with them and subspecialists, implements recommendations that are indicated and appropriate.
7. The plan of care is coordinated with educational and other community organizations to ensure that special health needs of the individual child are addressed.

Nurses at all levels will clearly play an important role in quality, efficiency, and cost-effectiveness in this system. Development of standards for care of special populations in different settings will help in outcome and quality measurements of this system of care.

Other National Resources. State and local disease- or disability-specific associations, such as United Cerebral Palsy and the Spina Bifida Association, are resources for consumers and professional providers. National organizations such as the National Center for Injury Prevention and Control, National Center on Birth Defects and Developmental Disabilities, National Dissemination Center for Children With Disabilities (NICHCY), Maternal and Child Health Library, American Academy of Pediatrics (AAP), and the Academy of Cerebral Palsy and Developmental Medicine are just a few other examples of organizations that provide resources, websites, and information that can assist nurses and families of children with disabilities. Many of these organizations are involved in important research and demonstration models to help advance the available knowledge, train professionals, and develop more effective care models.

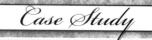

Case Study

Ryan is a 6-year-old child with myelomeningocele who began first grade a few weeks before coming in for an outpatient evaluation. During this evaluation with the rehabilitation team, his mother reported to the nurse that Ryan recently had expressed embarrassment about wearing diapers and had been teased by his classmates. She was concerned that Ryan was becoming more withdrawn and irritable. After completing the assessment, the following short-term goals were identified: establish urinary continence through intermittent catheterization, establish bowel continence through a regulated bowel

program, and promote effective coping for Ryan and his family. Long-term goals included independence in bladder and bowel program and increased self-esteem for Ryan.

In developing an educational plan, it is important to consider both the developmental age and any associated learning disabilities common in children with myelomeningocele. Ryan was encouraged to express his feelings about being different and being teased by peers. His desire to get out of diapers was established, learned how as a goal, and he could participate in the plan. Because school-age children are industrious

Case Study—cont'd

and eager to master skills, Ryan was given clear and concrete information regarding his urinary and gastrointestinal systems. Pictures and anatomically correct dolls were used to facilitate understanding of the body systems and the relationship between dietary measures and elimination.

Both Ryan and his mother were taught how to perform the bladder and bowel programs. Ryan was allowed to practice catheterization skills first on the doll and then on himself. Because he could not yet tell time, the catheterization schedule was linked to familiar events (when he awakened, after lunch and school, and before bedtime). A watch with an alarm helped to remind Ryan of his schedule. The teacher and school nurse were also involved to facilitate success of the

program. Ryan was given the responsibility of recording his catheterization volumes on a chart by coloring in the appropriate amount on a predrawn graduated cup. Ryan's mother was responsible for supervising, coaching, and praising her son's efforts and achievements. She also maintained contact with the teacher, school nurse, and rehabilitation nurse. Both Ryan and his mother were referred to the local Spina Bifida Association for support groups and family activities.

Over time, Ryan gained more control over his body by participating in self-catheterization and bowel regulation. He achieved continence, which increased his self-esteem and allowed him to get out of diapers. Ryan's mother and teacher reported that he seemed happier and more confident and that the teasing had stopped.

Nursing Diagnoses, Interventions, and Outcomes Applicable to Ryan   NIC/NOC

Nursing Diagnosis	Nursing Interventions	Nursing Outcomes
Impaired urinary elimination	Urinary catheterization: intermittent	Self-care: toileting Urinary continence
Bowel incontinence	Bowel training Self-care assistance: toileting	Bowel continence
Situational low self-esteem	Self-esteem enhancement	Adaptation to physical disability Self-esteem
Readiness for enhanced therapeutic regimen management	Self-modification assistance Teaching: procedure/treatment	Family participation in professional care Knowledge: treatment regimen

Data from Moorhead, S., Johnson, M., & Maas, M. (Eds.). (2004). *Nursing outcomes classification (NOC)* (3rd ed.). St. Louis, MO: Mosby; Dochterman, J. M., & Bulechek, G. M. (2004). *Nursing interventions classification (NIC)* (4th ed.). St. Louis, MO: Mosby; and NANDA International. (2007). *NANDA-I nursing diagnoses: Definitions & classification 2007-2008.* Philadelphia: Author.

CRITICAL THINKING

1. What strategies would encourage compliance with the bowel and bladder program?
2. How could you help Ryan plan his medical care needs around his life, rather than his life around his care needs?
3. What nursing interventions would continue to build Ryan's independence in managing his bowel and bladder programs?
4. Could you do in your life the things that the rehabilitation team often ask children and families to do?

REFERENCES

Allan, W. S. (1958). *Rehabilitation: A community challenge.* New York: John Wiley & Sons.

American Academy of Pediatrics. (2005). Care coordination in the medical home: Integrity, health and related systems of care for children with special health care needs. *Pediatrics, 116,* 1238-1244.

Barton, S. J. (1999). Promoting family-centered care with foster families. *Pediatric Nursing, 25,* 57-59.

Biehl, R. F. (1997). Case management and service coordination. In H. M. Wallace, R. F. Biehl, J. C. MacQueen, & J. A. Blackman (Eds.), *Mosby's resource guide to children with disabilities and chronic illness* (pp. 259-267). St. Louis, MO: Mosby.

Bull, M., Agran, P., Laraque, D., Pollack, S. H., Smith, G. A., Spivak, H. R., et al. (1999). American Academy of Pediatrics. Committee on Injury and Poison Prevention. Transporting children with special health care needs. *Pediatrics, 104,* 988-992.

Capen, C. L., & Dedlow, E. R. (1998). Discharging ventilator-dependent children: A continuing challenge. *Journal of Pediatric Nursing, 13,* 175-184.

Centers for Disease Control and Prevention. (2004). *Traumatic brain injury (TBI): Risks and groups at risk.* Retrieved February 6, 2006, from http://www.cdc.gov/node.do/id/0900f3ec8000dbdc/aspectId/AS_C60308.

Cernoch, J. M., & Newhouse, E. E. (1996). Respite care: Support for families in the community. In H. M. Wallace, R. F. Biehl, J. C. MacQueen, & J. A. Blackman (Eds.), *Mosby's resource guide to children with disabilities and chronic illness* (pp. 402-410). St. Louis, MO: Mosby.

Child and Adolescent Health Measurement Initiative. (2005). *National Survey of Children With Special Health Care Needs (NS-CSHCN), 2001.* Retrieved October 26, 2006, from Data Resource Center for Child and Adolescent Health website: http://www.childhealthdata.org/content/Default.aspx.

Clemens, C. J., Davis, R. L., Novak, A. H., & Connell, F. A. (1997). Pediatric home health care in King County, Washington. *Pediatrics, 99,* 581-584.

Committee on Children With Special Needs. (1998). Managed care and children with special health care needs: A subject review. American Academy of Pediatrics. *Pediatrics, 102,* 657-660.

Crocker, A. C. (1996). The impact of disabling conditions. In H. M. Wallace, R. F. Biehl, J. C. MacQueen, & J. A. Blackman (Eds.), *Mosby's resource guide to children with disabilities and chronic illness* (pp. 22-29). St. Louis, MO: Mosby.

D'Angio, C. T., & Maniscalco, W. M. (2004). Bronchopulmonary dysplasia in preterm infants: Pathophysiology and management strategies. *Pediatric Drugs, 6,* 303-330.

DeNavas-Walt, C., Proctor, B. D., & Lee, C. H. (2005). *Income, poverty, and health insurance coverage in the United States: 2004* (U.S. Census Bureau Current Population Reports P60-229). Washington, DC: U.S. Government Printing Office.

Denver Developmental Materials, Inc. (n.d.). The Denver II. Retrieved February 6, 2006, from http://www.denverii.com/home/html.

DeVore, S., & Bowers, B. (2006). Childcare for children with disabilities: Families search for specialized care and cooperative childcare partnerships. *Infants and Young Children, 19,* 203-212.

DiScala, C., Lescohier, I., Barthel, M., & Li, G. (1998). Injuries to children with attention deficit hyperactivity disorder. *Pediatrics, 102,* 1415-1421.

Easton, J. K., Rens, B., & Alexander, M. A. (1999). Psychosocial aspects of childhood disabilities. In G. E. Molnar & M. A. Alexander (Eds.), *Pediatric rehabilitation* (3rd ed., pp. 111-124). Philadelphia: Hanley & Belfus.

Economic costs associated with mental retardation, cerebral palsy, hearing loss, and vision impairment—United States, 2003. (2004). *MMWR. Morbidity and Mortality Weekly Report, 53,* 57-59. Retrieved February 1, 2006, from http://www.cdc.gov/mmwr/preview/mmwrhtml/mm5303a4.htm.

Edwards, M., Borzyskowski, M., Cox, A., & Badcock, J. (2004). Neuropathic bladder and intermittent catheterization: Social and psychological impact on children and adolescents. *Developmental Medicine and Child Neurology, 46,* 168-177.

Edwards, P. (1992). The evolution of rehabilitation facilities for children. *Rehabilitation Nursing, 17,* 191-195.

Erickson, E. H. (1963). *Childhood and society* (2nd ed.). New York: Norton.

Esperat, M. C. R., Moss, P. J., Roberts, K. A., Kerr, L., & Green A. E. (1999). Special needs of children in the public schools. *Issues in Comprehensive Pediatric Nursing, 22,* 167-182.

Feldman, A. B., Haley, S. M., & Coryell, J. (1990). Concurrent and construct validity of the pediatric evaluation of disability inventory. *Physical Therapy, 70,* 602-610.

Healthy and Ready to Work National Center. (n.d.-a). *About us.* Retrieved February 6, 2006, from http://www.hrtw.org/about_us/index.html.

Healthy and Ready to Work National Center. (n.d.-b). *Doctors.* Retrieved February 6, 2006, from http://www.hrtw.org/healthcare/doctors.html.

Healthy and Ready to Work National Center. (n.d.-c). *Federal initiatives.* Retrieved February 6, 2006, from http://www.hrtw.org/systems/federal.html.

Healthy and Ready to Work National Center. (n.d.-d). *Health insurance.* Retrieved February 6, 2006, from http://www.hrtw.org/healthcare/hlth_ins.html.

Heaton, J., Noyes, J., Sloper, P., & Shah, R. (2005). Families' experiences of caring for technology-dependent children: A temporal perspective. *Health and Social Care in the Community, 13,* 441-450.

Hewitt-Taylor, J. (2005). Caring for children with complex and continuing health needs. *Nursing Standard, 19,* 41-47.

Hoeman, S. P. (1997). Primary care for children with spina bifida. *The Nurse Practitioner, 22,* 60-72.

Individuals With Disabilities Education Improvement Act of 2004, Pub. L. No. 108-446, Part C, § 635 (2004).

Jackson, D., & Wallingford, P. (1997). Nursing care across the age continuum: Children and adolescents. In K. M. M. Johnson (Ed.), *Advanced practice nursing in rehabilitation: A core curriculum* (pp. 87-108). Glenview, IL: Association of Rehabilitation Nurses.

Kohlberg, L. (1969). Stage and sequence: The cognitive-developmental approach to socialization. In D. A. Goslin (Ed.), *Handbook of socialization theory and research.* Chicago: Rand McNally.

Langlois, J. A., Rutland-Brown, W., & Thomas, K. E. (2004). Traumatic brain injury in the United States: Emergency department visits, hospitalizations, and deaths. Atlanta, GA: Centers for Disease Control and Prevention, Nation Center for Injury Prevention and Control.

Lumeng, J. C., Warschausky, S. A., Nelson, V. S., & Augenstein, K. (2001). The quality of life for ventilator-assisted children. *Pediatric Rehabilitation, 4,* 21-27.

Madigan, E. A. (1997). An introduction to pediatric home health care. *Journal of the Society of Pediatric Nurses, 2,* 172-178.

Matthews, D. J., & Wilson, P. (1999). Cerebral palsy. In G. E. Molnar & M. A. Alexander (Eds.), *Pediatric rehabilitation* (3rd ed., pp. 193-218). Philadelphia: Hanley & Belfus.

McPherson, M., Arango, P., Fox, H., Lauver, C., McManus, M., Newacheck, P. W., et al. (1998). A new definition of children with special health care needs. *Pediatrics, 102,* 137-140.

Molnar, G. E. (1988). A developmental perspective for the rehabilitation of children with physical disability. *Pediatric Annals, 17,* 766, 768-771, 773-776.

Montagnino, B. A., & Mauricio, R. V. (2004). The child with a tracheostomy and gastrostomy: Parental stress and coping in the home—a pilot study. *Pediatric Nursing, 30,* 373-380.

National Center for Injury Prevention and Control. (2005). *Youth violence: Fact sheet.* Retrieved February 3, 2006, from http://www.cdc.gov/ncipc/factsheets/yvfacts.htm.

National Center for Injury Prevention and Control. (2006). *TBI–Causes: Fact Sheet.* Retrieved November 2, 2006, from http://www.cdc.gov/ncipc/tbi/Causes.htm.

National Dissemination Center for Children With Disabilities. (2002). *Transition planning: A team effort.* Retrieved February 6, 2006, from http://www.nichcy.org/pubs/transum/ts10txt.htm.

National Information Center for Children and Youth With Disabilities. (1996). Respite care: A gift of time. *NICHCY News Digest* (No. ND12). Retrieved February 1, 2006, from http://www.nichcy.org/pubs/outprint/nd12.pdf.

National Institute of Neurological Disorders and Stroke. (2002). *Traumatic brain injury: Hope Through research.* Retrieved November 3, 2006, from http://www.ninds.nih.gov/disorders/tbi/detail_tbi.htm.

Neal, L. J. (1997). Characteristics of the advanced practice nurse in rehabilitation. In K. M. M. Johnson (Ed.), *Advanced practice nursing in rehabilitation: A core curriculum* (pp. 18-22). Glenview, IL: Association of Rehabilitation Nurses.

Parsch, D., Mikut, R., & Abel, R. (2003). Postacute management of patients with spinal cord injury due to metastatic tumour disease: Survival and efficacy of rehabilitation. *Spinal Cord, 41,* 205-210.

Pediatric Special Interest Group. (1992). *Pediatric rehabilitation nursing–role description.* Skokie, IL: Association of Rehabilitation Nurses.

Perrin, E. C., & Gerrity, P. S. (1984). Development of children with a chronic illness. *Pediatric Clinics of North America, 31,* 19-31.

Philip, P., Ayyanger, R., Vanderbilt, J., & Gaebler-Spira, D. (1994). Rehabilitation outcome in children after treatment of primary brain tumor. *Archives of Physical Medicine and Rehabilitation, 75,* 36-39.

Piaget, J. (1952). *The origins of intelligence in children.* New York: International Universities Press.

Poggi, G., Liscio, M., Galbiati, S., Adduci, A., Massimino, M., Gandola, L., et al. (2005). Brain tumors in children and adolescents: Cognitive and psychological disorders at different ages. *Psycho-Oncology, 14,* 386-395.

Pontious, S. (1982). Practical Piaget: Helping children understand. *American Journal of Nursing, 82,* 114-117.

Power, P. W., & Dell Orto, A. E. (2004). *Families living with chronic illness and disability: Interventions, challenges and opportunities.* New York: Springer Publishing.

Reece, R. M., & Sege, R. (2000). Childhood head injuries: Accidental or inflicted? *Archives of Pediatrics and Adolescent Medicine, 154,* 11-15.

Robertson, A. R. R., & Johnson, D. A. (2002). Rehabilitation and development after childhood cancer: Can the need for physical exercise be met? *Pediatric Rehabilitation, 5,* 235-240.

Selekman, J. (1991). Pediatric rehabilitation: From concepts to practice. *Pediatric Nursing, 17,* 11-14, 33.

Sneed, R. C., May, W. L., & Stencel, C. S. (2000). Training of pediatricians in care of physical disabilities in children with special health needs: Results of a two-state survey of practicing pediatricians and national resident training programs. *Pediatrics, 105,* 554-561.

Sterling, Y. M., Jones, L. C., Johnson, D. H., & Bowen, M. R. (1996). Parents' resources and home management of the care of chronically ill infants. *Journal of the Society of Pediatric Nurses, 1,* 103-109.

Thompson, C. E. (1990). Transition of the disabled adolescent to adulthood. *Pediatrician, 17,* 308-313.

Thornton, T. N., Craft, C. A., Dahlberg, L. L., Lynch, B. S., & Baer, K. (2002). *Best practices of youth violence prevention: A sourcebook for community action.* Atlanta: Centers for Disease Control and Prevention, National Center for Injury Prevention and Control.

Uniform Data System for Medical Rehabilitation. (1991). *Uniform data system for medical rehabilitation.* Buffalo: State University of New York at Buffalo. Available at www.udsmr.org.

U.S. Department of Health and Human Services, Administration on Children, Youth and Families. (2005). *Child maltreatment 2003.* Washington, DC: U.S. Government Printing Office. Available from www.acf.hhs.gov/programs/cb/pubs/cm03/index.htm.

U.S. Department of Health and Human Services. (2000). *Healthy people 2010: With understanding and improving health and objectives for improving health* (2 vols.). Washington, DC: U.S. Government Printing Office.

van den Berg-Emons, H. J. G., Bussmann, J. B. J., Meyerink, H. J., Roebroeck, M. E., & Stam, H. J. (2003). Body fat, fitness and level of everyday physical activity in adolescents and young adults with meningomyelocele. *Journal of Rehabilitation Medicine, 35,* 271-275.

32

Gerontological Rehabilitation Nursing

Maria L. Radwanski, RN, MSN, CRRN

Gerontological rehabilitation nursing is a specialty practice within rehabilitation nursing that focuses on the unique requirements of elderly patients 65 years of age and older. Gerontological rehabilitation nurses practice in a variety of settings, and many hold the certified rehabilitation registered nurse (CRRN) credential. Roles include advocating for the rights of older persons and dispelling the myths of aging, providing clinical expertise, educating and promoting activities for healthy aging and prevention of disability, consulting with others who provide geriatric services, and communicating and conducting relevant research (Association of Rehabilitation Nurses, 1995).

The gerontological rehabilitation nurse uses a holistic approach in the assessment and provision of care to help older patients achieve their optimal level of physical, mental, and psychosocial well-being. Normal age-related changes and functional limitations due to illness or injury are considered in developing the plan of care. Chronic disease and disabilities that occur with aging require expert assessment to determine whether a patient's impaired function is related to a preexisting problem or the result of a newly acquired condition or disability. Early, timely intervention and long-term management aimed at health protection ultimately improve outcomes.

THEORIES AND SOCIETAL ATTITUDES OF AGING

A number of theories have been advanced to explain the aging process (Table 32-1). Some theories set forth stereotypes, not only of the elderly, but from a cultural bias against the social, behavioral, and physiological processes of aging. This bias is ageism, that is, prejudice against older adults expressed through beliefs, practices, and attitudes. Society provides many myths and cruel humor about aging that unfortunately mold older adults' beliefs about themselves and their worth, however inaccurate. An older person who has impairments or chronic conditions that prevent independent function bears a double burden. Rehabilitation nurses recognize the role society plays in shaping beliefs and attitudes and assist patients and families with transforming negative beliefs into a more accurate vision of older adults and what they can expect from themselves (see case study). They advocate and support goals of *Healthy People 2010* to reduce disparities in access to health care.

DEMOGRAPHICS

Physiological old age occurs much later in life when compared with half a century ago. Vaccines, antibiotics, surgical advances, and new treatments for cancer, heart disease, and other chronic diseases deserve credit, as well as improvements in the workplace, housing, and sanitation. People are living longer, active lives into their 60s, 70s, and 80s, and their attitudes are more positive. Today's baby boomers anticipate working beyond traditional retirement age for personal and economic reasons.

TABLE 32-1 Theories of Physiological Aging

Aging Theory	Description
Loose cannon theory	Free radicals and glucose slowly disrupt cellular macromolecular elements.
Weak link theory	A specific physiological system has become vulnerable, accelerating the aging process.
Rate of living theory	Free radicals and other metabolic by-products play a role in the aging process.
Error catastrophe theory	Errors in genetic translation lead to genetic errors that promote aging.
Master clock theory	Aging is under direct genetic control.

Modified from Mobbs, C. (2003). Molecular and biologic factors on ageing. In Cassel, C., Liepzig, R., Cohen, H., Larson, E., Meier, D., & Capello, C. (Eds.). *Geriatric medicine* (pp. 15-26). New York: Springer.

The "golden years" have three separate categories: the young old (65 to 74), the old (75 to 84), and the very old, including the frail elderly (85 years and above) (Schrier, 1990). In 2003, the very-old population was 4.7 million. By 2030 it will reach 9.6 million (U.S. Department of Health and Human Services, 2004). Although the young-old adults face fewer health problems than in the past, persons in the very-old group are the frailest, least educated, and have the lowest functional levels. The challenges of aging are compounded by the onset of chronic illnesses and disabling conditions.

Disability status and reported health status are related. In the 2004 U.S Health and Human Services' *Profile of Older Americans*, over half (57.6%) of respondents 80 years and older had one or more severe disabilities, and 34.9% reported they needed assistance as a result of disability. Among those 65 years and older with a severe disability, 68% reported their health as fair or poor. Arthritis was a chief cause of disability, affecting 21% of adults (Centers for Disease Control and Prevention, 2005).

EXPECTED CHANGES WITH THE AGING PROCESS

Many problems previously attributed to aging are now recognized as consequences of chronic disease, illness, or social adversity. Table 32-2 lists normal changes attributed to the aging process. Normal aging-related changes are intensified by

TABLE 32-2 Changes From the Aging Process Versus Chronic Illness or Disease

System	Expected Aging Changes	Changes From Disease or Chronic Illness
Cardiopulmonary	Increased risk for arteriovenous blocks or other arrhythmia Decreased pumping force of heart Reduced work capacity Higher resting systolic blood pressure Decreased vital capacity Increased risk of pulmonary infection Increased significance for risk factors of cardiopulmonary disease Reduced chest wall compliance Reduced cough reflex Reduced ciliary activity	Orthostatic hypotension Reduced reflex tachycardia
Musculoskeletal	Decreased height Decreased mobility Decreased stature and posture Redistribution of bone minerals Redistribution of body mass and fat	Muscle atrophy from disuse Slowed movement to accommodate for decreased range of motion Diminished strength Stiffening of joints
Skin changes	Thinner, paler skin Less vascularity to skin and subcutaneous tissue Fewer sweat and sebaceous glands Drier Less thermoregulatory control Nails more brittle Increased incidence of corns and calluses	Delayed healing time
Neurological	Decreased short-term memory Decreased brain weight Slowed reflexes Increased response time Decreased sensory receptors for temperature, pain, and tactile discrimination	Decreased cerebral blood flow Decreased balance and coordination
Sleep patterns	Longer to fall asleep Less rapid eye movement sleep More nighttime awakenings Quicker transition between sleep cycles	Frequent daytime and early evening "catnaps"
Bowel function	Less saliva Decreased gastric juices Decreased peristalsis Slower absorption	Gastroparesis Dysphagia
Genitourinary function	Vaginal atrophy resulting in urethral changes Prostatic enlargement	Hypertrophy of bladder wall Diverticula formation Decreased size and capacity Elevation of postvoid residual Change in sensation

TABLE 32-2 Changes From the Aging Process Versus Chronic Illness or Disease—cont'd

System	Expected Aging Changes	Changes From Disease or Chronic Illness
Liver function	Decreased size Decreased drug metabolism Decreased protein synthesis	Elevated liver enzyme levels
Renal	Decreased vascularity of nephrons Decreased glomerular filtration rate Decreased creatinine clearance Decreased sodium conservation Slower adjustment to acid-base balance	Increased serum blood urea nitrogen and creatinine levels
Endocrine	Reduced insulin secretion Decreased glucose tolerance Decline, then plateau of estrogen production Gradual decline in testosterone production	Hypoglycemia

Data from Hanson, C. (2005). *Instant nursing assessment: Gerontologic.* Clifton Park, NY: Delmar; and Grundinskas, L., & Nee, M. (2002). Normal aging changes intensify chronic problems in disability. *SCI Nursing, 19*(2), 61-66.

chronic illness. These changes and health problems result in functional decline, which will continue to cause a downward spiral in function if not addressed appropriately (Grundinskas & Nee, 2002).

HEALTH CARE FINANCES

Finances are an issue in the health care of older adults. Social Security benefits and Medicare programs continue to be the sole income and support for many older adults. Nearly all (96%) noninstitutionalized persons 65 years and older were covered by Medicare in 2003; 61% also had some type of private health insurance. Although Medicare covers mostly acute care services, it requires substantial cost sharing, and it is not comprehensive and many services are not covered, including health promotion and disease prevention (U.S. Department of Health and Human Services, 2004). Opportunities for rehabilitation nurses to interact with older adults occur across the health continuum. They can provide information and education to help patients maximize health and wellness, avoid unnecessary health-related expenses, and target services that meet their precise needs.

THE NURSING PROCESS

The nursing process guides care planning with the older adult. Developing rapport with the older adult is crucial to obtaining a thorough assessment. The sections that follow contain assessments that are specific to older adults and are conducted in conjunction with standard nursing assessments. For clarity, each assessment is listed followed by the specific interventions (strategies) for the nursing diagnoses, diagnoses that are of particular importance in the health care of the older adult. Table 32-3 contains the major gerontological nursing diagnoses and outcomes.

Physical Assessment

Physical assessment parameters critical to nursing management of the older adult are outlined in Table 32-4; however, the nurse performs a comprehensive assessment as with any patient. A gerontological assessment enables a rehabilitation nurse to recognize how one factor affecting an older adult's health may exacerbate or aggravate another problem and then identify that it has reappeared to complicate the first problem. To this end, content and concepts are discussed separately, and they are not ranked in order because multiple variables and complex factors interact uniquely in any patient situation. For example, an older adult who is depressed develops urinary incontinence; the incontinence exacerbates the underlying depression, and eventually malaise leads to poor hygiene and skin breakdown.

Medication History

A thorough medication history is conducted with the patient and the family. The goal is to identify beliefs or expectations about the medications and resolve any concerns or problems the patient is experiencing with the medications. Ask specifically about each step of the medication regimen. Assess the older adult's technical skills, including ability to read the labels, open the container, and take the medication properly. Cognitively, assess whether the person understands why the medication is taken, how much and how often it is taken, and any special instructions, such as "take with milk" or "store out of direct sunlight." Patients may not consider over-the-counter preparations, home remedies, herbal products, or folk and cultural treatments to be medications (Kaufman, Kelly, Rosenberg, Anderson, & Mitchell, 2002). Many older adults take vitamins and herbal products in an effort to improve their health (O'Brien King & Pettigrew, 2004).

Medication Management. Reconcile the number of pills in each container with the date of the last refill to obtain a sense of compliance. Inspect all medications and how they are stored. Confusion, diminished eyesight, multiple medications, and other issues make medication assessment crucial to an older person's success with living in the community. Older patients often continue to take medications after they are no longer needed or when the drugs are old or outdated, in

TABLE 32-3 Nursing Diagnoses and Related Outcomes for Gerontological Rehabilitation

Nursing Diagnosis	Suggested Nursing Outcomes	
Risk for injury	Abuse protection Aspiration protection Balance Coordinated movement Fall prevention behavior	Risk control: hearing impairment Risk control: visual impairment Risk detection Safe home environment
Adult failure to thrive	Appetite Cognition Decision making Depression control Endurance Hydration Information processing	Neglect recovery Nutritional status: food and fluid intake Personal health status Psychosocial adjustment: life change Self-care: activities of daily living Social involvement Weight control
Disturbed sleep pattern	Anxiety level Mood equilibrium Personal well-being Rest Sleep Comfort level Leisure participation	Medication response Pain level Respiratory status: ventilation Stress level Urinary incontinence Urinary elimination
Chronic pain	Comfort level Depression self-control Depression level Pain control Pain level Quality of life	Rest Sleep Stress level Symptom control Symptom severity Will to live
Acute confusion	Cognitive orientation Cognition Distorted thought self-control Information processing Memory Neurological status: consciousness Sleep Blood glucose control Concentration	Electrolyte and acid-base balance Fluid balance Infection severity Respiratory status: gas exchange Risk control: alcohol use Risk control: drug use Safe home environment Thermoregulation
Chronic confusion	Cognition Cognitive orientation Concentration Decision making Distorted thought self-control Identity	Information processing Memory Neurological status: consciousness Communication ability Safe home environment Social interaction skills
Ineffective coping	Effective coping Sense of control Decreased stress	Adapts to life changes Seeks information on illness and treatment Increase in psychological comfort

Data from Moorhead, S., Johnson, M., & Maas, M. (Eds.). (2004). *Nursing outcomes classification (NOC)* (3rd ed.). St. Louis, MO: Mosby; and North American Nursing Diagnosis Association (NANDA-I). (2005). *Nursing diagnoses: Definitions and classification 2005-2006.* Philadelphia: NANDA-I.

addition to newly prescribed drugs. They may take them in undesirable food-medication or multiple-medication combinations. Older patients have been known to frugally divide pills and space doses inappropriately, share medications with others, or hoard medications obtained by prescriptions from several providers. Excellent problem-solving and communication skills are needed to determine whether medications are being taken accurately and appropriately.

Assessment of Functional Status

Age-related variables associated with a person's actual age, including cognitive skills, socialization status, physical ability, and presence of depression and comorbid conditions, have potential to influence the outcome of rehabilitation in older adults. However, recent findings indicate that a older adult's functional abilities before admission for rehabilitation are a better predictor of outcomes than are the age-related

TABLE 32-4 Physical Assessment of the Geriatric Rehabilitation Patient

Parameters	Assessment	Comments
General appearance	Height Weight Appropriateness of facial expression Verbal and nonverbal communication Grooming Appropriateness of clothing to the season Grooming of hair, nails Odors	Weight is considered the fifth vital sign of the older adult
Head, eyes, ears, nose, and throat	Extraocular muscle coordination and movement Cranial nerve testing Visual acuity Pupillary reflexes Hearing acuity Patency of ear canals Intactness of tympanic membranes Moisture of tongue Color of lips, tongue, and gingival tissue Condition of teeth/fit of dentures Quality of voice Swallowing ability	
Cardiac	Vital signs Blood pressure and pulse lying, sitting, and standing Carotid pulsations, presence of bruits Jugular venous pressure Hepatojugular reflux Arterial pulses Peripheral edema	Assessment of orthostatic hypotension
Respiratory	Rate and rhythm of breathing Chest expansion Presence of adventitious lung sounds Presence of shortness of breath at rest or with activity	
Abdomen	Presence of bowel sounds in all four quadrants Firmness of abdomen Presence of abdominal pain or tenderness Abdominal circulation Liver tenderness, size	
Rectal and pelvic examination	Rectal sphincter tone Presence of rectal nodules Presence of occult blood Firmness/nodularity of prostate Presence of hemorrhoids Pelvic floor muscle strength Vaginal discharge Presence of rectocele, cystocele	Pelvic floor examination necessary in incontinence evaluation. Older adult should otherwise be counseled to have yearly pelvic examination with primary care physician or gynecologist
Mobility/neurological	Arm and leg strength Range of motion of all joints Gross deformities Atrophy Localized joint or soft tissue inflammation, nodules Joint swelling, tenderness, crepitations Dynamic and static sitting and standing balance; single leg standing balance Quality of gait Speed and coordination of movement Walking posture Range of motion of joints Presence of ataxia	The Timed Up and Go Test is useful as screening of balance and gait function Ataxia can be assessed by finger-to-nose-to-finger testing and the heel-to-shin test

Continued

TABLE 32-4 Physical Assessment of the Geriatric Rehabilitation Patient—cont'd

Parameters	Assessment	Comments
	Romberg test	
	Sensory testing of extremities: position sense, temperature testing, sharp and dull testing	
	Presence of arm drift	
	Rigidity and cogwheeling	
	Position-change induced dizziness and/or vertigo	
	Deep tendon reflexes, including (−, +) presence of Babinski's reflex	
	Presence of kyphosis/scoliosis of spine	
	Deviation of leg lengths	
Skin	Condition of feet and toenails, deformities of toes, feet, and ankles or fingernails	
	Condition of hair	
	Pigmentation	
	Intactness of skin	
	Bruising	
Cognitive	Attention	The Mini-Mental State Examination is useful to use as a screening of cognitive function
	Calculation	The Geriatric Depression Scale is useful as a screen of affect
	Short-term memory	
	Long-term memory	
	Orientation	
	Verbal comprehension	
	Nonverbal comprehension	
	Judgment	
	Insight	
	Affect	

Modified from Hanson, C. (2005). *Instant Nursing Assessment: Gerontologic.* Delmar, NY: Clifton Park, NY.

variables (Yu, Evans, & Sullivan-Marx, 2005; Yu & Richmond, 2005).

Successful discharge or long-term plans take into account the person's lifestyle, health beliefs, and practices. Questions about lifestyle help in understanding the patient's current function and well-being. For example, ask, How do you spend the day? and What leisure, social, or other activities do you participate in outside your home? Do family members, neighbors, or friends assist with any activities of daily living (ADLs)? Instrumental activities of daily living (IADLs), such as grocery shopping, transportation, financial management, laundry, or cleaning are the first activities older adults ask others for assistance with when their function becomes impaired. Chapter 14 lists assessment tools and contains more information about functional abilities and assessment.

If older adults are reluctant to answer assessment questions, ask for details about their premorbid self-care practices, management of health and chronic disease, self-perception of the impairment, and ways altered function affects their health. Assess the home and the environment for safety and well-being of the older adult with disabilities. See Box 14-3 for home assessment guidelines.

Strategies for Health Promotion and Prevention.
Longitudinal studies have demonstrated that older adults lose mobility and function over time. One study examined 21 functional activities for participants for 2 years. At the end of the second year their functional abilities such as sitting, standing, walking distances, and climbing stairs had declined steadily. Early intervention and therapy were variables essential to preventing further decline in function and improvement in specific tasks (Resnick, 2000; U.S. Department of Health and Human Services, 2004). Daily activities need to be adapted to medical conditions, but at the same time, exercise and therapy are necessary to increase muscle mass and maintain balance. Good balance is a prerequisite of mobility and performing ADLs without difficulty, and thus it may enable a physically active life.

Prevention, screening, and wellness programs improve outcomes. Screening for osteoporosis and risk of falls are prevention strategies that rehabilitation nurses can implement within the community for patients and for primary care providers. Tai chi, strength training, and seated "sit and fit" classes have been shown to improve cardiovascular health, as well as physical function including muscle strength, balance, and bone density measures (Zhang, Ishikawa-Takata, Yamazaki, Marita, & Ohta, 2006). Tai chi improves balance through exercise movements consisting of turning, alternate leg weight shifts, bending the legs, and various arm movements. It increases muscle strength and helps prevent physical deterioration (Liu, 1990). Although postural sway increases with age, tai chi

---

BOX 32-1 Strategies for Interventions With Older Adults Who Have Chronic Confusion

- Keep requests and demands relatively simple.
- Keep explanations simple, with one concept or idea stated at a time.
- Avoid complex tasks that might lead to frustration.
- Use distraction rather than confrontation to manage behavior.
- Remain calm, firm, and supportive if the patient becomes upset.
- Allow the patient brief periods of quiet time if he or she becomes upset.
- Identify and move potential dangers in environment.
- Provide a structured routine; be consistent.
- Provide simple explanations and reminders; give one simple direction at a time.
- Provide orientation cues such as clocks, calendars, name outside of room, personal items in surroundings; however, avoid quizzing with orientation questions.
- Recognize decline in function and adjust explanations accordingly.
- Bring sudden changes or decline in function to the physician's attention; evaluate for medical causes of decline.
- Review physical activity limitations, such as no driving, need for supervision at all times, assistance for medication management.

Modified from Dochterman, J. M., & Bulechek, G. M. (2004). *Nursing interventions classification (NIC)* (4th ed.). St. Louis, MO: Mosby.

---

incorporates single-stance postures that aid in balance and thus reduces risks of falling.

Exercise behaviors in older adults are influenced by self-efficacy and outcome expectations (Resnick, 2000). Six factors influence their adherence to an exercise program and need to be addressed with patients: their beliefs about exercise and the benefits of exercise, their goals and personality, experiences with exercise, and unpleasant sensations they associate with exercise (Resnick & Spellbring, 2000).

Self-Care Strategies. The older adult should perform as much self-care as possible. The rehabilitation nurse monitors patients who use adaptive devices to ensure they are able to attend to personal hygiene, grooming, toileting, and eating. Encouragement and a consistent, repetitive routine help most patients to establish patterns so they can perform ADLs and simultaneously incorporate personal health practices. Patients who are confused need additional cues, simple commands, and directions for taking a step at a time. Those who develop receptive aphasia after a stroke or other cognitive impairments may respond to nonverbal gestures. Other strategies to assist the older adult with chronic confusion are described in Box 32-1. A rehabilitation team evaluation with referral to an occupational therapist may be indicated when patients have impairments in ADLs, visual-spatial skills, or perception.

Risk for Falls

After age 75 years 70% of accidental deaths are related to falls (Fuller, 2001). More than 1.8 million older adults were treated in emergency departments for fall-related injuries in 2003; more than 421,000 were hospitalized and placed at risk for further decline in function and mobility (Centers for Disease Control and Prevention, National Center for Injury Prevention and Control, 2005). For patients who sustain hip fractures, 20% become nonambulatory and only 14% to 21% recover their functional ability with ADLs (Agostini, Baker, & Bogardus, 2001). Many elderly live a compromised lifestyle, avoiding any exercise or outings for fear of falling. Less than 5% of community-dwelling adults older than 75 years walk at a gait speed necessary to safely perform common functional activities; pain may impede mobility.

Falls are attributed to a variety of factors, including alcohol and prescription drug use, fear of falling, dizziness, orthostatic hypotension, neuropathy changes, balance problems, urinary urgency, hearing or vision loss, and lack of exercise. Patients may not mention falling episodes when they were not injured. Detecting a patient's history of falls, performing a fall-related assessment, and adding interventions can reduce the probability of falls (American Geriatrics Society, British Geriatrics Society, & American Academy of Orthopedic Surgeons, 2001).

Older adults who fall have characteristics that differentiate them from their healthy age-mates who do not fall. It is generally accepted that falls are caused by multiple factors. Characteristics responsible for falls can be intrinsic or extrinsic in nature. Intrinsic factors include a patient's physical, mental, and cognitive condition, such as age-related physiological changes in balance and gait, cognitive impairments (including awareness and insight, attention, judgment, depression), medical conditions (Table 32-5), visual changes, nutritional status, and the use of certain medications. The chance of falling increases with age when a sedentary lifestyle alters body weight, fat, and muscle distribution and changes the center of gravity. Patient safety is discussed in Chapter 10.

Extrinsic factors are external to the system and relate to a person's physical environment. Identifying extrinsic factors within the environment improves safety for older adults. For example, when mechanical restraints were used for hospitalized patients, their risk for falls increased. Extrinsic factors in the community include living alone and being socially isolated, lack of or inadequate assistive devices, condition of ground surfaces, poor illumination conditions, or wearing poorly designed or ill-fitting footwear (Land et al., 2005).

The Timed Up and Go Test is a quick, sensitive mobility and balance test to identify patients at risk for falls. The patient is asked to perform this sequence: sit in a chair and rise without using arms for support, stand still, walk 10 feet and 9 inches, turn without touching anything, and return to the chair without using arms for support. The test is scored. Difficulty rising or sitting without support or unsteadiness indicates a need for further assessment (Shumway-Cook, Brauer, & Woollacott, 2000). The Berg Balance Scale is a 14-item performance-based scale designed to specifically measure

TABLE 32-5 Chronic Illnesses That Make Older Adults More Susceptible to Falls and Injuries

Type	Illness
Neurological	Transient ischemic attacks, vertigo, syncope, stroke, cerebellar disorders, spinal stenosis, cervical spondylosis, delirium, dementia, myelopathy, normal pressure hydrocephalus, Parkinson's disease, peripheral neuropathy, seizure disorder
Musculoskeletal	Muscle weakness, arthritis, inflammatory joint disorders, myopathy, podiatric problems
Sensory	Vision loss: cataracts, glaucoma, macular degeneration; vestibular disorders: acute labyrinthitis, Meniere's disease, benign positional vertigo, vertebrobasilar disease, drug toxicity
Genitourinary	Incontinence, micturition syncope, nocturia, frequency, urgency leading to unsafe maneuvering to toilet
Cardiovascular	Aortic stenosis, arrhythmia, carotid sinus sensitivity, conduction disorders, myocardial infarction, postural hypotension, syncope, vertebrobasilar insufficiency, volume depletion
Respiratory	Pneumonia, hypoxemia
Environmental/functional	Improper clothing such as long nightclothes or robes, improper use of wheelchairs and walkers, especially on transfers
Psychological	Anxiety, confusion, depression, stress, fear of falling, impaired judgment, impulsiveness, polypharmacy (more than four medications), new medication, increased dosage, type of drug, (alcohol, antihypertensive, barbiturate, diuretics, narcotics, nonmiotic eye medications, phenothiazines, tricyclic antidepressants, oral hypoglycemics, cardiac medications)

balance in detail, a skill important for older adults (Berg, Wood-Dauphinee, Williams, & Maki, 1992).

Fall Prevention Strategies. Preventing falls requires a thorough assessment focusing on identifying and reducing risk factors. Specific interventions include treating underlying medical conditions, removing fall hazards from the home or facility, prescribing exercise programs to improve mobility, and helping patients to minimize their fear of falling (Tideiksaar, 1996). In a classic study by Tideiksaar (1992) multifactorial interventions such as medication adjustments, behavioral changes, and balance-training exercises used in combination were most significant in reducing falls in the community. Strategies aimed at preventing falls among the very old focus on modification of intrinsic factors. Modification of environmental hazards has the greatest potential for prevention among the young old and those living in private homes (Norton, Campbell, Lee-Joe, Robinson, & Butler, 1997). Fall-related consultation services may involve a physical and occupational therapist, physiatrist, and rehabilitation nurse. A home environment assessment can identify and correct potential hazards and prevent further falls (see Chapter 14). Community health and rehabilitation nurses often provide education programs about fall prevention and ways to eliminate risks. Table 32-6 lists nursing interventions to reduce the risk of falls.

Disturbed Sleep Pattern

Although one third of all Americans report sleep-related problems, the elderly are the most deprived. The National Sleep Foundation (2003) reported that 48% of all adults older than 65 years of age and living at home had sleep disturbances. Sleep-related complaints are the second most common reason for elderly visits to physicians. The most common problem

affecting sleep is the need to get up to go to the bathroom, followed by sleep disturbance caused by pain. Other causes include age-related changes such as diminished blood flow, structural changes, and neuron loss that occur as the brain ages. This results in a decline of stages 3 and 4 of the non–rapid eye movement stage of sleep; stage 5 is less prominent. These may be associated with age-related changes in core body temperature, usually occurring between 2:00 and 8:00 A.M. Sleep pathologic conditions, including sleep apnea, neurological diseases affecting the respiratory center and cardiac-respiratory loops, restless legs syndrome in kidney disease, diabetes, and circulatory diseases, account for many sleep disturbances (National Sleep Foundation, 2003). Other conditions contributing to insomnia among the elderly include chronic pain from arthritis and other disorders, esophageal reflux, hiatal hernia, Alzheimer's disease, and Parkinson disease.

Insomnia, the most frequently encountered sleep problem among older adults, is characterized by an inability to fall asleep, fragmented sleep owing to increased arousal, decreased total time asleep, decrease in sleep efficacy, and early awakenings. Insomnia is more prevalent in women and increases with age and lower socioeconomic class. Taking longer than 40 minutes to fall asleep with an average sleep time of less than 6 hours in 24 hours, or feelings of distress, tenseness, or upset resulting from the lack of sleep are diagnostic criteria.

Although there may be a specific reason for insomnia, it is often the result of multiple factors, representing many different underlying causes. Insomnia may begin in response to a crisis situation such as illness or death and progress into a chain of ineffective behaviors. Assessment of all the underlying factors is necessary to resolve the problem of insomnia. One study among caregivers of patients with Alzheimer's disease suggests that sleep hygiene interventions such as

TABLE 32-6 Nursing Interventions to Reduce the Risk of Falls*

Risk Factors	Nursing Interventions
New admission or relocation	Orient thoroughly to environment including use of call bell and bedside items Introduce to staff and roommates Instruct patient to call for assistance with movement Provide agreed-on place to store belongings and personal care items, dentures, prostheses, or assistive devices Place articles within easy reach of the client Encourage family involvement and visits Provide visible clock, calendar, familiar objects, family pictures, favorite pillow Use night-light at bedside at night; keep surroundings well-lit during the day Provide frequent observations by nursing staff, especially at night
History of fall or physical weakness	Assess thoroughly for risk factors and causes Explore associated events (before, during, after falls) Use wheelchair, chair, bed alarm devices Provide antiskid mat at bedside Ensure easy access to bathroom and assure call bell is answered promptly; observe frequently Encourage timed voiding every 2 hours during the daytime, every 4 hours at nighttime Use bedside commode during hours of sleep for patients experiencing severe urgency, frequency, nighttime confusion, dizziness, unsteadiness at night Use comfortable chairs of proper height, with backrests and armrests for easy transfer Use comfortable chairs such as rockers, recliners, instead of wheelchair when client is in bedroom or lounge Encourage mobility and activity Monitor gait, balance, and fatigue level when ambulating Provide close supervision Encourage reconditioning exercises Encourage frequent, short rest intervals Provide nonrestrictive reminders to stay seated Use appropriate assistive devices Remove low-lying furniture that presents a tripping hazard Avoid clutter on floor surface Provide sleeping surface close to floor, as needed
Altered mental status	Provide visual cues to client to remind him to call for help Eliminate unnecessary noise Reduce visual stimulation Assign a room near nurses' station Provide adequate lighting Provide family education and encourage involvement Use companion or closer supervision Implement orientation exercises Consider medication, dehydration, or nutritional or electrolyte imbalances as potential causes
Altered psychosocial or emotional status	Encourage decision making Involve in establishing short-term goals or plan of action Perform psychosocial or psychiatric assessment and treatment as indicated Ask client and family to identify measures to aid in relaxation for inducing sleep (back rub, tea, music) When appropriate, gradually expand psychosocial environment
Visual impairment	Assess vision Ensure eyeglasses are cleaned regularly Assess eyeglasses Encourage use of visual aids Provide adequate lighting Remove unnecessary furniture Avoid highly polished floors that produce glare Have unobstructed and nonskid floor surfaces Use colors to increase visibility (avoid blue-green combinations, use contrasting colors) Instruct patient to wear prescription glasses, as needed, when out of bed

Continued

TABLE 32-6 Nursing Interventions to Reduce the Risk of Falls*—cont'd

Risk Factors	Nursing Interventions
Actual or potential incontinence	Ensure easy access to bathroom and assure call bell is answered promptly
	Assess cause of incontinence
	Encourage time voiding every 2 hours during daytime, every 4 hours during hours of sleep
	Use bedside commode during hours of sleep for patients experiencing severe urgency, frequency, nighttime confusion, dizziness, unsteadiness at night
	Encourage using easily manipulated clothing such as elastic waistbands
Postural hypotension	Perform initial assessment of blood pressure lying, sitting, and standing
	Ensure adequate hydration (1500–2000 ml/24 hours unless restricted)
	Use elastic stockings
	Provide education regarding slow, gradual position changes
Medications	Assess drug actions, interactions, side effects; include self-medication and over-the-counter products
	Assess drug substitutions or elimination
	Consider changing medications that produce adverse side effects or discomfort
	Consider drug holidays with physician's order
Comfort	Use relaxation measures identified as helpful by client and family
	Provide pain medication on a schedule if client is experiencing pain (or when suspected in client who is unable to communicate)

From Strumf, N., Evans, L., & Patterson, J. (1992). *Reducing restraints: Individual approaches to behavior: A teaching guide.* Huntington Valley, PA: Geriatric Research and Training Center. Copyright 1992 by University of Pennsylvania, School of Nursing. Adapted with permission; Dochterman, J. M., & Bulechek, G. M. (2004). *Nursing interventions classification (NIC)* (4th ed.). St. Louis, MO: Mosby.
*This table addresses situations in institutions, including assisted living; the home assessment is in Chapter 14.

changing the sleep schedule, napping habits, and walking routines are very effective (McCurry, Gibbons, Logsdon, Vitiello, & Teri, 2003). Refer to Chapter 26 for additional information concerning sleep.

Behavioral Strategies to Treat Insomnia. Transient and intermittent insomnia of short duration does not require treatment. Longer episodes of insomnia when accompanied by recurrent daytime sleepiness and impaired performance may improve with behavioral interventions, and medications may reverse the insomnia. Sleeping pills remain controversial because of the potential side effects, particularly among the elderly. Even sleep medications considered safe may result in impaired mobility for many older adults. When used, low doses for the shortest duration are recommended. Behavioral techniques to improve sleep include withholding evening fluids to avoid nocturia and eliminating foods and fluids containing caffeine. Caffeine is found in coffee and tea; in carbonated drinks such as Mountain Dew, cola drinks, and Dr. Pepper; and in chocolate.

Relaxation therapy helps reduce or eliminate anxiety and body tension, inducing muscle relaxation and restful sleep. With practice, elders can learn these techniques to achieve effective relaxation. Sleep-deprived older adults spend too much time in bed trying to get to sleep. If sleep does not occur within a half hour after retiring, the person should get up and leave the room for some type of activity and return to bed a half hour later. Other recommendations are to restrict the hours of sleep during the night, gradually reintroducing time until the person is back up to their normal sleep hours.

Another strategy is to recondition elders to associate the bed only with sleep and sexual activity. Activities in bed such as reading or watching television are halted because these activities may stimulate the brain and thus derail sedation and drowsiness in preparation for sleep. Sleep disorders associated with medical problems, such as sleep apnea and depression, require referral for medical evaluation and testing.

Chronic Pain

Pain is not always considered in the care of elders; their perceptions of pain may be devalued or considered inaccurate. Physical signs vary and may be confused with distress or anxiety. Experiences of pain are influenced by culture and social norms and may be altered because of communication and cognitive deficits. Many older adults are reluctant to report pain because they continue to believe that analgesia is addictive and fear they will become dependent on the medication, regardless of past experiences. They are concerned that use of any analgesia will cause confusion.

X-ray examinations and bone density tests of older adults with vertebral fractures reveal that many also have osteoporosis. Pain associated with fractured vertebra leads to lack of sleep, social isolation, and increased dependence; maintaining function prevents debilitation. Active and active-assistive exercises to stretch and exercise to reduce stiffness and pain intensity may be beneficial.

Nurses should take report of pain at the person's word (McCaffery & Pasero, 1999). Older adults with chronic confusion may describe their immediate experience with pain accurately, but when rating their degree of pain, the visual analogue pain scale may be more effective than the numbered scale.

Strategies to Avoid Pain-Related Depression.

Frequent, intense pain may cause depression and affects independence and self-care abilities that are quality-of-life issues (Turner, Ersek, & Kemp, 2005). Assessment of depression is essential. The Geriatric Depression Scale (Table 32-7) has dual use in that it can help evaluate the effects of pain on the person's quality of life as well as depression. Nearly three quarters of community-dwelling older adults acknowledge pain, the greatest prevalence being degenerative joint diseases, rheumatoid arthritis, cancer, and vascular diseases. Impaired or altered sensory function, such as vision or hearing and reduced sensation and perception, alter the pain experience. An older adult may guard movement or positioning, change patterns of walking, pace level of activity, or "work around" painful activities without reporting pain. Those with cognitive or communication impairments may become frustrated, angry, or contentious because they cannot express or explain their pain. Careful interviews are important because older adults may experience chronic transient pain, but describe the experience as discomfort, an ache, or other names that avoid the name or nature of pain (Flahery, 2000). Chapter 23 contains additional information about pain.

Chronic Pain Management Interventions.

Analgesic management of acute, chronic, and neuropathic pain in older adults becomes somewhat cumbersome because of age-related changes in drug metabolism. To offer patients maximum pain relief, it helps to have a menu of at least two prescribed analgesics to administer according to the patient's report of pain severity. For example, a pain report of 8 requires a stronger analgesic than a level 4 report. Acetaminophen and nonsteroidal antiinflammatory drugs (NSAIDS) (Shakoor & Loeser, 2004) are considered the safest analgesic agents for

TABLE 32-7 Geriatric Depression Scale

Question	Score
Are you basically satisfied with your life?	Score 1 if no
Have you dropped many of your activities and interests?	Score 1 if yes
Do you feel that your life is empty?	Score 1 if yes
Do you often get bored?	Score 1 if yes
Are you hopeful about the future?	Score 1 if no
Are you bothered by thoughts that you cannot get out of your head?	Score 1 if yes
Are you in good spirits most of the time?	Score 1 if no
Are you afraid that something bad is going to happen to you?	Score 1 if yes
Do you feel happy most of the time?	Score 1 if no
Do you often feel helpless?	Score 1 if yes
Do you often get restless and fidgety?	Score 1 if yes
Do you prefer to stay at home rather than go out and try new things?	Score 1 if yes
Do you frequently worry about the future?	Score 1 if yes
Do you feel you have more problems with your memory than most?	Score 1 if yes
Do you think it is wonderful to be alive now?	Score 1 if no
Do you often feel downhearted and blue?	Score 1 if yes
Do you feel worthless the way you are right now?	Score 1 if yes
Do you worry a lot about the past?	Score 1 if yes
Do you find life very exciting?	Score 1 if no
Is it hard to get started on new projects?	Score 1 if yes
Do you feel full of energy?	Score 1 if no
Do you feel that your situation is hopeless?	Score 1 if yes
Do you think most people are better off than you are?	Score 1 if yes
Do you frequently get upset over little things?	Score 1 if yes
Do you frequently feel like crying?	Score 1 if yes
Do you have trouble concentrating?	Score 1 if yes
Do you enjoy getting up in the morning?	Score 1 if no
Do you prefer to avoid social gatherings?	Score 1 if yes
Is it easy for you to make a decision?	Score 1 if no
Is your mind as clear as it used to be?	Score 1 if no

From Yesavage, J. A., Brink, T. L., Rose, T. L., Lum, O., Huang, V., Adey, M., et al. (1983). Development and validation of a geriatric depression screening scale: A preliminary report. *Journal of Psychiatric Research, 17,* 37-49. Reprinted with permission.

long-term chronic pain. They may be used concomitantly with neuroleptics or antidepressants depending on the nature and source of the pain. The selective serotonin reuptake inhibitors do not have the anticholinergic, antihistaminic, or α-adrenergic receptor blocking activities of tricyclic antidepressants and thus have low risk for adverse reactions when used for chronic pain in the elderly. Glucosamine and chondroitin have also been shown to improve pain and function and even decrease the progression of osteoarthritis (Shakoor & Loeser, 2004).

Chronic pain also requires a holistic approach, using behavioral strategies along with medications. The impact the pain has on function is one indicator for implementing aggressive pain management strategies and appropriate modalities. Nonpharmacological techniques are helpful before, during, and after painful activities; before pain occurs or increases; and along with other pain relief measures. Alternative methods for pain relief may be effective, especially when used to complement conventional modalities. Older adults who are engaged actively in making decisions about which modalities to use and are willing to participate in planning a program of pain management have a significant impact on the outcome. Examples of alternative methods include biofeedback, hypnosis, music and activity therapies, guided imagery and distraction, applied heat or cold, massage, acupressure, and transcutaneous electrical nerve stimulation (TENS), as well as the relaxation exercises described in Chapter 29.

Access and Driving a Car

The aging process and medical conditions may impair the older adult's ability to operate a car safely. It is essential to identify driving safety hazards resulting from functional impairments that occur from specific medical conditions. Older adults with reduced functional ability and sensory impairments drive with reduced skill, which puts themselves and others at risk for serious injury. Adaptive devices or medical equipment may hinder driving. When older adults stop driving, they must depend on others for trips outside of the home. A few are fortunate to have spouses or family members available to drive them. Reduced access and the resulting decreased participation in leisure activities contributes significantly to social isolation and depression (Azad, Byszewski, Amos, & Molnar, 2002).

Driver Evaluations. Assessment of potential for mobility and functional skills is important before taking the step of revoking an older adult's license to drive because he or she has reduced function and is at risk for injury. Driver evaluation programs, available in most communities, employ occupational and physical therapists to evaluate whether the older adult's function can be enhanced and deficits corrected or adjusted to retain independence. When restricted mobility follows the loss of a driver's license, the rehabilitation nurse must facilitate communication about options with the patient and family. This involves a significant amount of planning to ensure the patient has optimal mobility especially when the older adult does not live in close proximity to shopping

and recreation or does not have appropriate, affordable, or accessible transportation. Rehabilitation nurses have a responsibility for educating patients, families, community agencies, and other providers about access and mobility needs of older adults and the unique needs of individual persons. The nurse can facilitate education and counseling by elder peers and the multidisciplinary team to help people plan ahead to retire from driving, just as they retired from work (Pettersson, Engardt, & Wahlund, 2002).

Adult Failure to Thrive

Four syndromes are prevalent and predictive of adverse outcomes in patients with failure to thrive: impaired physical function, malnutrition, depression, and cognitive impairment (Robertson & Montagnini, 2004). Decreased ability to perform ADLs results in a downward spiral and causes increased frailty, more caregiver services, frequent hospitalizations, and nursing home placements. Using Folstein's Mini-Mental State Examination, researchers found that the domains of cognition most closely associated with ADL dependence were orientation and short-term memory impairments. Furthermore, when older adults lost the ability to manage money or make a telephone call accurately and simultaneously experienced decline in their lower body function, they had higher morbidity rates (Gill, Williams, Richardson, Berkman, & Tinetti, 1997).

Nutritional deficits often contribute to adult failure to thrive. Oral health is a major problem for all ages, but older people often develop difficulty with dentition. Tooth decay and breakage, receding gums that cause dentures to fit poorly, changing food preferences, some brought on by altered glucose tolerance, and chronic diseases such as hypoglycemia and diabetes increase risk. In one study, two thirds of institutionalized or hospitalized older adults had serum albumin levels below normal; only 27% ever received prescriptions for nutritional supplements (Zulkowski & Kindsfater, 2000). Poor nutrition is a known risk for skin breakdown, delayed wound healing, and increased mortality when older adults become ill.

There is often an inaccurate assumption about older adults who are overweight. The obese person appears to be getting adequate protein and nutrients. Foods ingested are often of inferior quality. Alcohol use also affects nutrition. Other factors affecting nutrition include self-care abilities, food preferences, cultural and dietary habits, financial resources, and transportation to obtain food. Weight loss is a significant indicator of health issues for older persons.

Strategies to Improve Nutrition. Remembering to eat is a subtle problem, especially when the older adult has cognitive impairments. When telephoned by family members, older adults with mild to moderate cognitive impairment may confabulate sufficiently to affirm that they have eaten. When queried further to identify what time or what they ate, their answers are vague. Food preparation and shopping may be beyond their abilities.

It is imperative to identify the underlying cause of the nutritional problem and employ nursing interventions. For example, the family of an older adult who experienced chronic confusion believed a microwave would be easier than a gas stove for the person and avoid risk of creating a fire. However, an older adult with chronic confusion is not likely to be capable of new learning; the microwave would most likely be useless. Health promotion interventions for improving nutrition, such as Meals-on-Wheels, or obtaining assistance with instrumental activities of daily living (IADLs) may be indicated.

Acute Confusion

Acute confusion (delirium) is defined as an abrupt onset of global, transient changes and disturbances in attention, cognition, psychomotor activity, level of consciousness, and the sleep-wake cycle. Confusion has become known as a normal part of the aging process. This is inaccurate. As a result, health care providers fail to attend to this significant cause of acute illness. Recent reports demonstrate that acute confusion is prevalent in 22% of older adults in acute care facilities (Pi-Figueras et al., 2004). Acute confusion is present at hospital admission for at least 18% of older adults, increasing to 24% after admission. Those with acute confusion are likely to have chronic cognitive impairment, severe acute illness, multiple comorbid conditions, and functional disability. Acute confusion is characterized by fluctuations in mental function and may be accompanied by hallucinations. Delirium, or acute confusion, is usually caused by sudden changes in environment (sometimes referred to as transfer trauma). Acute confusion may precipitate an acute illness, but more often it develops as a result of iatrogenic factors: infections, polypharmacy use, or other hospital-acquired complications (Insel & Badger, 2002). Acute confusion is treatable but left undiagnosed can continue indefinitely and progress to a chronically confused state and declining health.

Strategies for Eliminating Acute Confusion. A safe and therapeutic environment is essential for the older adult who becomes acutely confused. The cause or source of acute confusion is central to the type of treatment. Assessment includes review of medications, over-the-counter drugs, and any supplements. Review the medical history for possible precursors, including head injury, hypertension, cerebral vascular disease, B_{12} deficiency, and emotional or psychiatric disease. Ask family members about the patient's past and current drug and alcohol use and dietary habits.

The rehabilitation nurse collaborates with the physician to review drugs that may elicit acute confusion in light of the assessment and the individual's history. Avoid medications that aggravate acute confusion in this age-group, namely hypnotics, sedatives, antianxiety agents, tricyclic antidepressants, and others that have anticholinergic side effects (Table 32-8).

TABLE 32-8 Medications That May Cause Delirium/Acute Confusion

Drug Class	Generic Names
Anticholinergic agents	Scopolamine, orphenadrine, atropine, trihexyphenidyl, benztropine, meclizine, homatropine
Tricyclic antidepressants	Amitriptyline, desipramine, doxepin, trazodone, fluoxetine
Antimanic agents	Lithium
Antipsychotics	Thioridazine, chlorpromazine, fluphenazine, prochlorperazine, trifluoperazine, haloperidol
Antiarrhythmics	Quinidine, disopyramide, tocainide
Antifungals	Amphotericin B, ketoconazole
Sedative/hypnotic agents	Diazepam, chlordiazepoxide, lorazepam, oxazepam, flurazepam, triazolam, alprazolam
Barbiturate acid derivative	Phenobarbital, butabarbital, butalbital, pentobarbital
Chloral and carbonate derivatives	Chloral hydrate, meprobamate
Beta-adrenergic antagonists	Propranolol, metoprolol, atenolol, timolol
Alpha-2 antagonists	Methyldopa, clonidine
Alpha-1 antagonists	Prazosin
Calcium channel blockers	Verapamil, nifedipine, diltiazem
Inotropic agents	Digoxin
Corticosteroids	Hydrocortisone, prednisone, methylprednisolone, dexamethasone
Nonsteroidal antiinflammatory agents	Ibuprofen, naproxen, indomethacin, sulindac, diflunisal, choline magnesium trisalicylate, aspirin
Narcotic analgesics	Codeine, hydrocodone, oxycodone, meperidine, propoxyphene
Antibiotics	Metronidazole, ciprofloxacin, norfloxacin, ofloxacin, cefuroxime, cephalexin, cephalothin
Radiocontrast media	Metrizamide, iothalamate, diatrizoate, iohexol
H_2 receptor antagonists	Cimetidine, ranitidine, famotidine, nizatidine
Immunosuppressives agents	Chlorambucil, cytarabine, interleukin-2, spirohydantoin mustard
Anticonvulsants	Phenytoin, valproic acid, carbamazepine
Anti-Parkinson agents	Levodopa, levodopa/carbidopa, bromocriptine, pergolide
Antiemetics	Prochlorperazine, methocarbamol, carisoprodol, baclofen, chlorzoxazone
Antihistamines/decongestants	Diphenhydramine, chlorpheniramine, brompheniramine, pseudoephedrine, phenylpropanolamine

When it is not possible to eliminate an offending drug because it is the only option for treatment of a chronic condition, a short medication holiday may clear the drug from the body. A drug holiday must be supervised. The medication is reintroduced at a lower dose—"start low and go slow." The goal of therapeutic dosing is to optimize function with chronic disease.

Patients experiencing acute confusion have difficulty with abstract concepts. Information is best given in concrete terms. Short-term memory is usually impaired but may cycle as the delirium clears, and many experience delusions and hallucinations. Specific interventions improve outcomes for patients and reduce their anxieties. Recognize and accept the patient's perceptions, stating your perception of the situation in a calm, reassuring, and nonargumentative manner. It is important to respond to the patient's theme or feelings and not focus on the content of hallucinations. Quizzing patients with orientation questions they cannot answer only adds frustration. Anything in the environment that appears to trigger misperceptions should be removed. For example, flower pollen that has fallen onto a tabletop may appear as insects to a person who is acutely confused.

Nursing strategies for interventions with older adults who have chronic confusion are in Box 32-1. These interventions also are appropriate for the patient with acute confusion until the symptoms clear.

Chronic Confusion

Chronic confusion or dementia may be caused by a number of conditions (Table 32-9). Dementia is a progressive decline in several dimensions of cognition that severely interferes with a person's everyday living and ability to perform ADLs, but without a decreased level of consciousness. Dimensions of cognition that may be affected include memory, verbal and nonverbal learning, visual-spatial perception, aphasia, apraxia,

and agnosia. Changes in personality and motor and gait disturbances may occur. Table 32-10 compares characteristics of chronic and acute confusion. Chapter 25 discusses cognition in detail.

Confusion also inhibits functional ability that directly affects the outcome of rehabilitation. For example, complications from failure to thrive may occur in older adults who develop chronic confusion. Their weight loss occurs before cognitive changes are apparent, but this is subtle because the cognitively impaired person is unwilling or unable to eat (Robertson & Montagnini, 2004).

Interventions for Treatment of Chronic Confusion.
Treatment for chronic confusion is targeted to the specific medical or neurological disorder. Some dementia is reversible with treatment. Patients may be able to participate in some decision making, but their degree of insight, reasoning ability, and judgment will vary depending on the diagnosis and the progression of the disease. Use specific examples with families when defining a patient's abilities to participate because it is not unusual for families to seek confirmation with the patient who is chronically confused. They attempt to gain consent from their confused loved one and seek assurance that the family member also understands the new information. By diagnosis, older adults with chronic confusion are not able to remember complex conversation or understand abstract concepts. They need a supportive, structured, and supervised environment. Family education must extend beyond treatments and medications to incorporate their awareness of these more insidious manifestations of chronic confusion.

Rehabilitation is appropriate for older adults with chronic confusion, with some caveats. Chronically confused older adults often experience acute illnesses that alter their function and mobility; however, those with early to middle stages of chronic confusion can perform most ADLs when guided

TABLE 32-9 **Diseases or Conditions and the Relationship of Dementia to the Cause**

Disease or Condition	Relationship of Dementia to Cause
Alzheimer's disease	Degeneration of the cells and neurons of the basal forebrain, cerebral cortex, and other areas of the brain
Multiinfarct dementia	Small and large cerebral infarcts often associated with hypertension
Normal pressure hydrocephalus	Caused by impeded cerebrospinal fluid and absorption
Metabolic disorders	Chronic anoxia, nutritional deficits, hepatic or uremic encephalopathy, hypercalcemia, hypothyroidism, hypoglycemia, B_{12} deficiency
Intracranial mass lesions	Caused by benign as well as malignant masses
Medication toxicity	Benzodiazepines, methyldopa, neuroleptics, cimetidine, anti-Parkinson drugs, and others
Wernicke's dementia	Alcoholism
Dementia pugilistica	Repeated head injuries leading to frontal lobe dementia syndrome
Infections	Tertiary syphilis, human immunodeficiency virus
Other degenerative diseases	Anterior lateral sclerosis, Parkinson's disease, multiple sclerosis, Pick's disease, Huntington's chorea, Wilson's disease, epilepsy

Data from Beers, M., & Berkow, R. (2000). *Merck manual of geriatrics* (3rd ed.). Whitehouse Station, NJ: Merck Research Laboratories.

TABLE 32-10 Characteristics of Confusion States

Acute Confusion (Delirium)	Chronic Confusion (Dementia)
Acute onset, short duration	Long duration
Fluctuation in symptoms	Progressive symptoms
Short attention span	Short attention span
Reduced ability to shift attention	Personality changes and progressive behavioral problems
Impaired orientation (severity fluctuates)	Severe disorientation with confusion and mood fluctuation
Impaired short-term memory	Impaired short- and long-term memory
Distorted thinking	Impaired thinking and judgment
Distorted perception (delusions, hallucinations, or illusions)	Confabulates, no insight into memory deficits; impaired abstract reasoning
Variable psychomotor behavior	Impairments interfere with social and functional abilities
Reversal of sleep-wake cycles	Chronic confused sleep-wake cycles

Modified from Walker, J., Lofton, S., Haynich, L., & Martin, T. (2006). The home health nurse's role in geriatric assessment of three dimensions: Depression, delirium, and dementia. *Home Healthcare Nurse, 24*(9), 572-580.

BOX 32-2 Medications That Can Cause Reactive Depression

Analgesics and antiinflammatory agents
Hormones
Antihypertensives
Anticonvulsants
Antihistamines
Digoxin
Estrogen
Anti-Parkinson drugs
Antibiotics
Cardiac drugs
Chemotherapy agents
Immunosuppressives
Sedatives and tranquilizers

---

by simple verbal and visual cues. The rehabilitation nursing principle of offering guidance to older adults to function within their capabilities applies to family education as well. Emphasize that although it is more time consuming, patients will maintain a higher level of function and general health with fewer complications if they remain engaged and practice self-care as fully as possible.

Reactive Depression

Ten percent of the general population will experience a major depressive episode in their lifetime. Depression can be difficult to distinguish from dementia because some symptoms of depression (disorientation, memory loss, and easy distraction) are similar; it coexists with early to mid dementia in nearly one third of cases. Unrecognized and untreated, depression is life threatening. Biological, social, and psychological changes place older adults at higher risk for developing or having a recurrence of depression. Examples might be central nervous system changes, adjustments in lifestyle, reduced

income, or a decline in physical health that negatively affects the older adult. Medications that may cause depression are listed in Box 32-2.

Symptoms of reactive depression are more difficult to identify in older adults who are less likely to express their feelings when preoccupied with a problem. They may present with masked depression, denying they are depressed and hiding symptoms, such as crying spells, apathy, and diminished appetite. Others who are more anxious and somatic may display vague, nonspecific complaints that cannot be confirmed during physical assessment. The 30-item Geriatric Depression Scale (see Table 32-7) is useful in evaluating depression in older adults. A score of 8 or higher suggests depression and indicates a referral to a psychologist for further evaluation.

Interventions for Treatment of Reactive Depression. Interventions for older adults with depressed mood focus on providing safety, stabilization, recovery, and maintenance. Because older adults are less likely to report feelings associated with depression, the rehabilitation team must weigh the merits of implementing psychotherapy as part of the treatment plan. Psychotherapy has been found to be effective in reducing symptoms of short-term depression in the older adult who is physically ill. Depression is a biochemical illness; antidepressant medications benefit older adults in the same way they do in younger cohorts. Antidepressant drugs may require more time to become effective when patients have chronic conditions.

Many clinicians become frustrated with the high number of side effects reported with antidepressant therapy. However, older adults who have reactive depression exhibit a high level of somatic symptoms that cannot be attributed to medications. It is imperative that patients take their medication as prescribed; they are inclined to discontinue their antidepressant when they begin to feel better. Encourage the patient to continue the antidepressant. As with chronic pain, older adults respond best to selective serotonin reuptake inhibitors for the treatment of depression and experience fewer side effects when compared with more traditional tricyclic antidepressants.

Complementary interventions that are therapeutic to the older adult include regular exercise and involvement in self-care, both of which improve quality of life (Ellingson & Conn, 2000). Social support, loneliness, and conflict affect depression; the most significant factor in avoiding depression is a sense of belonging (Hagerty & Williams, 1999). Increasing socialization may eliminate a cause of depression, particularly in those who have been socially isolated. This intervention is most successful if a companion, perhaps a family member or friend, accompanies the older adult for the initial socialization experience, such as a program at a neighborhood senior center or other community site. A self-report questionnaire (e.g., the Geriatric Depression Scale) is useful for periodic evaluation of outcomes and documenting a need for ongoing follow-up. Ask about any changes in personality.

Alcohol Abuse

Alcohol is a depressant; it affects a patient's judgment, coordination, alertness, and reaction time. Research findings show older adults to be negatively affected by smaller quantities of alcohol than are younger persons. Older adults are also more likely to be taking prescription drugs and over-the-counter medications that potentiate when taken with alcohol (National Institute on Aging, 1999). During assessment the rehabilitation nurse must ask, rather than avoid, questions regarding alcohol use. Several useful screening tools are the Geriatric Michigan Alcohol Screening Test (Hirata, Almeida, Funari, & Klein, 2001), CAGE, and the Alcohol Use Disorders Test (Culberson, 2006). They are not diagnostic.

Misuse of alcohol is often overlooked. It can cause cognitive changes, confusion, depression, elevated blood pressure, weight loss, self-neglect, neuropathy, gait or balance abnormalities, tremors, jaundice, ascites, falls, and other injuries. Zulkowski and Kindsfater's study (2000) of wellness behaviors among independent-living older adults found 71% had at least one alcoholic beverage a day; 15% consume four or more alcoholic beverages daily. The risk for alcohol abuse is greater for older women than for men due to less lean muscle mass and therefore a reduced ability to metabolize alcohol. Older women are more sensitive to over-the-counter medication, and misuse of prescription medications can be a problem. Psychologically women are also at greater risk as they age due to loneliness and depression from outliving their spouses and suffering from other losses (Blow & Barry, 2002). Signs of abuse or misuse include history of falls, self-neglect, confusion, and family problems (Ruth, Sedlak, Doheney, & Martsoff, 2000). It is essential to address the effects of alcohol on existing conditions, interactions with medications, and increased risk for injuries.

Interventions to Manage Alcohol Use. Education and counseling increase awareness of the effects of alcohol. Counseling interventions include socialization for older adults who are isolated. They may be encouraged to join a senior center or social group, such as garden club to meet

---

BOX 32-3 Indications of Possible Elder Abuse

- Poor hygiene
- Unexplained bruises in different stages of healing
- Broken bones
- Malnutrition
- Dehydration
- Depressed mood
- Withdrawn, fearful
- Cowering
- History of treatment in a variety of facilities and by different physicians
- Unattended or untreated health problems
- Person left alone in the home
- Person brought for treatment by someone other than the caregiver
- Elder expresses feelings of hopelessness, helplessness
- Elder expresses ambivalent feelings toward family
- Caregiver refusal to allow visitors to see elder alone
- Unsanitary/unclean living conditions
- Emotionally upset or agitated behavior
- Unusual behavior usually attributed to dementia (e.g., sucking, biting, rocking)

Modified from Easton, K. (1999). *Gerontological rehabilitation nursing.* Philadelphia: W. B. Saunders.

---

people and participate in activities. Many counties, services for the aging, senior centers, or churches offer transportation at no cost or for a small fee. Referral to a drug and alcohol rehabilitation program is indicated for those with severe alcohol dependency. Older adults usually fare well in treatment programs that address the physiological struggles encountered in withdrawal, as well as the psychosocial roots of alcohol dependence, including loneliness.

Abuse of Older Adults

Older adults who are abused most often are women and have dementia. The profiles of their abusers aid in their detection and suggest ways to assist potential victims. Caregivers who have extreme stress, anxiety, lack of knowledge as caregivers, and a maladaptive personality have potential to become abusive (Levine, 2003). The older adult who has been abused may be unable or may not choose to disclose the abuse for fear of retribution. Although many symptoms of abuse may replicate expected changes due to aging, a keen assessment of clusters or specific types of symptoms can detect and differentiate abuse. For example, numerous bruises that are in various stages of healing and in different colors clustered together in the same area on arms, trunk, or legs may indicate repeated squeezes, grabbing, or blows. Verbal abuses are more difficult to detect. Other common indicators are outlined in Box 32-3. Abuse may not only be physical or psychological but can present as physical neglect (failure to provide adequate food, water, clothing, shelter, medicine, safety, or other essentials), financial exploitation (misappropriation of assets) or violation of rights (personal property, privacy, etc.) (Swagerty, Takahashi, & Evans, 1999).

TABLE 32-11 *Healthy People 2010:* Health Promotion and Prevention Topics for the Older Adult

Topic	Key Points
Diet and exercise	Fat, cholesterol, complex carbohydrates, fiber, sodium, calcium Caloric balance Selection of exercise programs
Substance use	Tobacco cessation Alcohol and other drugs: limiting alcohol consumption, driving/other dangerous activities while under the influence, treatment for abuse
Injury prevention	Prevention of falls Medications/abuse practices that increase the risk for falls Safety belts Smoke detectors Smoking near bedding or upholstery Hot water heater temperature Safety helmets Home safety awareness Abuse and neglect awareness Burn prevention
Dental health	Regular dental visits, toothbrushing, flossing
Myths of aging	Dispel myths that urinary incontinence, falls, confusion are normal results of aging
Cardiovascular disease in women	Effects of estrogen as a natural protector, changes after menopause, prevention and treatment
Vaccinations	Flu clinics Pneumonia vaccines
Senior consumer awareness	Scam prevention

Data from U.S. Department of Health and Human Services. (2000). *Healthy people, 2010.* Available from http://web.health.gov/healthypeople/document.

Interventions for Suspected Abuse. All health care providers are mandated by law to report suspected abuse to the state or county division of adult protective services or the state's office of child and family services. Once mistreatment has been reported, a social worker will be assigned to investigate the case. A guardian may be appointed by the state if the older adult is not competent to make decisions (Swagerty et al., 1999).

OUTCOME: COMMUNITY INTEGRATION

Gerontological rehabilitation nurses cannot prevent the aging process; however, they can promote a healthy lifestyle to maximize quality of life and actively engage older adults in the community and in rehabilitation settings. Many older adults maintain a higher level of function and mobility when given the opportunity to interact socially with their peers. Some communities offer wellness-maintenance classes targeted at providing recreational activities, structured but safe standing and modified seated exercises classes, and informal social time as needed. For instance, the local chapter of the Arthritis Foundation rents the heated swimming pool in the acute rehabilitation hospital every day during lunch when it is not used for inpatient and outpatient therapy; in the evening the hospital's community-based wellness program uses the pool for water aerobics classes. The programs are well attended and worth the effort. The rehabilitation team can refer patients and reduce reliance on expensive inpatient and outpatient resources.

Each encounter with an older adult in a rehabilitation setting is an opportunity for rehabilitation nurses to address goals for health promotion and prevention that will affect quality of life positively. A speaker's bureau with lists of topics sent to women's clubs, nonprofit groups, church groups, senior centers, senior clubs, and similar groups offers opportunity for reaching older adults and the family members involved in their care. Suggestions for health promotion and health prevention program topics of interest to older adults are outlined in Table 32-11.

Case Study

Dorothy Walsh is receiving inpatient rehabilitation therapy for an acute stroke with left-sided hemiplegia. The multidisciplinary team reports that she complains of constant tiredness, wants to return to the nursing unit in the middle of therapy sessions to sleep, is irritable, cannot sleep, and has a poor appetite. Dorothy has lost 17 pounds since the stroke, and she is preoccupied by vague somatic complaints. She requests pain medication frequently.

Dorothy reveals to the rehabilitation nurse that she feels hopeless about her condition, thinking that she will never recover from the stroke, despite making gains in function. She is anxious and has poor concentration ability.

Her family views her uncooperative behavior as totally out of character. She denies being depressed, stating she is simply frustrated about being away from home for the past 4 weeks.

Her family reveals that she had an acute myocardial infarction about a year before this stroke. Following the heart attack, she seemed to become reclusive. Before the heart attack she was very outgoing and was constantly on the go with family and friends.

Dorothy's symptoms are suggestive of depression. It is not unusual for an older adult to focus on somatic complaints, deny depression, and experience irritability, loss of appetite, and sleeplessness. Treatment for the depression is required for optimum recovery.

Dorothy is treated with a selective serotonin reuptake inhibitor. The patient and family are instructed by the rehabilitation nurse that it will take at least 4 to 6 weeks for the medication to make a difference. She is encouraged to journal in order to explore her feelings. Dorothy is also encouraged to participate with other senior citizens in an aquatic exercise program upon discharge from outpatient therapy.

Three months after discharge Dorothy attends the stroke follow-up clinic. She and her family report that she is sleeping well. She has gained 10 pounds and reports a good appetite. The family indicates there is no irritability and reports that she is adjusting well.

CRITICAL THINKING

Elderly persons who have experienced chronic illness and functional deficits are at risk for developing other deficits and comorbid conditions. One factor affecting health may exacerbate or aggravate another, then reconfigure and complicate the first situation, and so forth until the seeming "snowball" effect or "cascade" of problems overwhelms patients and their families. Consider this dilemma with patients you encounter in your workplace, clinical site, and community programs for the elderly, or your own circle of family and friends.

1. Identify obstacles to and resources for preventing or ameliorating the "snowball" or "cascade" of problems. What nursing interventions are appropriate at individual, family, and community levels.

2. Identify gaps, barriers, and resources in the health care system, including those occurring at different levels of nursing assessments and interventions, such as primary, acute, or tertiary care, that affect outcomes for elderly persons. Are some nursing processes interfering with rather than improving outcomes?

3. Choose a patient and situation from personal or professional experiences. What are particular changes associated with aging that may contribute to a "snowball" or "cascade" of problems?

REFERENCES

Agostini, J. V., Baker, D. I., & Bogardus, S. T. (2001, July). Prevention of falls in hospitalized and institutionalized older people. In Agency for Healthcare Research and Quality, *Making health care safer: A critical analysis of patient safety practices*. Rockville, MD: U.S. Department of Health and Human Services.

American Geriatrics Society, British Geriatrics Society, & American Academy of Orthopedic Surgeons. (2001). Guideline for the prevention of falls in older persons. *Journal of American Geriatrics Society, 49*(5), 664-672.

Association of Rehabilitation Nurses. (1995). *The gerontological rehabilitation nurse: Role description*. Skokie, IL: Author.

Azad, N., Byszewski, A., Amos, S., & Molnar, F. J., (2002). A survey of the impact of driving cessation on older drivers. *Geriatrics Today: Journal of the Canadian Geriatrics Society, 5*(4), 170-174.

Berg, K., Wood-Dauphinee, S., Williams, J., & Maki, B. (1992). Measuring balance in the elderly: Validation of an instrument. *Canadian Journal of Public Health, 83*(Suppl. 2), S7-S11.

Blow, F. C., & Barry, K. L. (2002). Use and misuse of alcohol among older women. *Alcohol Research & Health, 26*(4), 308-315.

Centers for Disease Control and Prevention. (2005). Racial/ethnic differences in the prevalence and impact of doctor-diagnosed arthritis—United States, 2002. *MMWR Morbidity and Mortality Weekly Report, 54*(5), 119-123.

Centers for Disease Control and Prevention, National Center for Injury Prevention and Control. (2005). *Falls and hip fractures among older adults*. Atlanta, GA: National Center for Injury Prevention and Control.

Culberson, J. W. (2006). Alcohol use in the elderly: Beyond the CAGE: Part 2. Screening instruments and treatment strategies. *Geriatrics, 61*(11), 20-26.

Ellingson, T., & Conn, V. (2000). Exercise and quality of life in elderly individuals. *Journal of Gerontological Nursing, 26*, 17-25.

Flahery, E. (2000). Assessing pain in older adults. *Journal of Gerontological Nursing, 26*(3), 5-6.

Fuller, G. F. (2001). Falls in the elderly. *American Family Physician, 61*, 2159-2168, 2173-2174. Available from http://www.aafp.org/afp/20000401/2159.

Gill, T., Williams, C., Richardson, E., Berkman., L., & Tinetti, M. (1997). A predictive model for ADL dependence in community living older adults based on a reduced set of cognitive status items. *Journal of the American Geriatrics Society, 45*, 441-445.

Grundinskas, L., & Nee, M. (2002). Normal aging changes intensify chronic problems in disability. *SCI Nursing, 19*(2), 61-66.

Hagerty, B., & Williams, R. (1999). The effects of sense of belonging, social support, conflict, and loneliness on depression. *Nursing Research, 48*, 215-219.

Hirata, E., Almeida, O., Funari, R., & Klein, E. (2001). Validity of the Michigan Alcoholism Screening Test (MAST) for the detection of alcohol-related problems among male geriatric outpatients. *American Journal of Geriatric Psychiatry, 9*(1), 30-34.

Insel, K. C., & Badger, T. A. (2002). Deciphering the 4 D's: Cognitive decline, delirium, depression, and dementia—A review. *Journal of Advanced Nursing, 38*(4):360-368.

Kaufman, D. W., Kelly, J. P., Rosenberg, L., Anderson, T. E., & Mitchell, A. A. (2002). Recent patterns of medication use in the ambulatory adult population of the United States: The Slone Survey. *Journal of the American Medical Association, 287*(3), 337-344.

Land, F., Onder, G., Cesari, M., Barillaro, C., Russo, A., & Bernabei, R. (2005). Psychotropic medications and risk for falls among community-dwelling frail older people: An observational study. *Journals of Gerontology Series A Biological and Medical Sciences, 60*(5), 622-626.

Levine, J. M. (2003). Elder neglect and abuse: A primer for primary care physicians. *Geriatrics 58*(10), 37-44.

Liu, D. (1990). *The Tao of health and longevity.* New York: Prager.

McCaffery, M., & Pasero, C. (1999). *Pain clinical manual* (2nd ed.). St. Louis, MO: Mosby.

McCurry, S. M., Gibbons, L. E., Logsdon, R., Vitiello, M., & Teri, L. (2003). Training caregivers to change the sleep hygiene pactices of patients with dementia: The NITE-AD project. *Journal of the American Geriatric Society, 51*(10), 1455-1460.

National Institute on Aging. *Alcohol use and abuse.* (1999). Bethesda, MD: National Institute on Alcohol Abuse and Alcoholism. Available from http://www.nih.gov/nia.

National Sleep Foundation. (2003). *Sleep in America Poll.* Washington, DC: American Academy of Sleep Medicine.

Norton, R., Campbell, J., Lee-Joe, T., Robinson, E., & Butler, M. (1997). Circumstances of falls resulting in hip fractures among older people. *Journal of the American Geriatrics Society, 45,*1108-1112.

O'Brien King, M., & Pettigrew, A. (2004). Complementary and alternative therapy use by older adults in three ethnically diverse populations: A pilot study. *Geriatric Nursing, 25*(1), 30-37.

Pettersson, A. F., Engardt, M., & Wahlund, L. O. (2002). Activity level and balance in subjects with mild Alzheimer's disease, dementia and geriatric cognitive disorders, *Dementia and geriatric cognitive disorders, 13*(4), 213-216.

Pi-Figueras, M., Aguilera, A., Arrellano, M., Miralles, R., Garcia-Caselles, P., Torres, R., et al. (2004). Prevalence of delirium in a geriatric convalescence hospitalization unit: Patient's clinical characteristics and risk precipitating factor analysis. *Archives of Gerontology and Geriatrics Supplement, 9,* 333-337.

Resnick, B., & Spellbring, A. (2000). Understanding what motivates older adults to exercise. *Journal of Gerontological Nursing, 26,* 34-41.

Resnick, P. (2000). Functional performance and exercise of older adults in long term care settings. *Journal of Gerontological Nursing, 26,* 7-16.

Robertson, R. G., & Montagnini, M. (2004). Geriatric failure to thrive. *American Family Physician, 70*(2), 343-350.

Ruth, T., Sedlak, C., Doheney, M., & Martsoff, D. (2000). Alcohol use in elderly women. *Journal of Gerontological Nursing, 26,* 44-49.

Schrier, R. W. (1990). *Geriatric medicine.* Philadelphia: W. B. Saunders.

Shakoor, N., & Loeser, R. F., (2004). Treatment options to provide pain relief and preserve joint function. *Drug Benefit Trends* (Suppl. C) *16,* 18-22.

Shumway-Cook, A., Brauer, S., & Woollacott, M. (2000). Predicting the probability for falls in community-dwelling older adults using the timed up and go test. *Physical Therapy, 80*(9), 896-903.

Swagerty, D. L., Takahashi, P. Y., & Evans, J. M. (1999). Elder mistreatment. *American Family Physician, 59*(10), 2804-2808.

Tideiksaar, R. (1992). Falls among the elderly: A community prevention program. *American Journal of Public Health, 82,* 892-893.

Tideiksaar, R. (1996, February). How to identify risk factors, reduce complications. *Geriatrics, 51,* 43-53.

Turner, J. A., Ersek, M., & Kemp, C. (2005). Self-efficacy for managing pain is associated with disability, depression, and pain coping among retirement community residents with chronic pain. *The Journal of Pain, 6,* 471-479.

U.S. Department of Health and Human Services. (2004). *A profile of older Americans.* Rockville, MD: U.S. Department of Health and Human Services, Administration on Aging.

Yu, F., & Richmond, T. (2005). Factors affecting outpatient rehabilitation outcomes in elders. *Journal of Nursing Scholarship, 37*(3), 229-236.

Yu, F., Evans, L. K., & Sullivan-Marx, E. M. (2005). Functional outcomes for older adults with cognitive impairment in a comprehensive outpatient rehabilitative facility. *Journal of the American Geriatrics Society, 53*(9), 1599-1606.

Zhang, J. G., Ishikawa-Takata, K., Yamazaki, H., Marita, T., & Ohta, T. (2006). The effects of tai chi chuan on physiological function and fear of falling in the less robust elderly: An intervention study for preventing falls. *Archives of Gerontology and Geriatrics, 42*(2), 107-116.

Zulkowski, K., & Kindsfater, D. (2000). Examination of care-planning needs for elderly newly admitted to an acute care setting. *Ostomy Wound Management, 46*(1), 32-36, 38.

33

Cardiac and Cardiovascular Rehabilitation

Linda Brewer, RN, MSN, CFNP, CACNP
Angela L. Boleware, RN, MSN, FNP-C
Barbara J. Boss, PhD, RN, CFNP, CANP

Cardiac rehabilitation nursing is an essential professional nursing area within an interdisciplinary specialty—a specialty that is growing in response to needs of an aging population and an increased awareness of the benefits available from cardiac care programs for persons of all ages. Technological advances, treatment options, early intervention procedures, and medications have rescued many lives.

Cardiac rehabilitation is defined by the World Health Organization as "the sum of activities required to ensure patients the best possible physical, mental and social conditions so that they may resume and maintain as normal a place as possible in the community" (Wenger et al., 1995). The U.S. Public Health Service definition states that cardiac rehabilitation services are comprehensive, long-term programs involving medical evaluation, prescribed exercise, cardiac risk factor modification, education, and counseling (Wenger et al., 1995).

PREVALENCE OF HEART DISEASE

Coronary heart disease (CHD) affects 13 million Americans. Fifty-nine percent of the 1.2 million persons survived their myocardial infarctions (MIs) (45% were younger than age 65 years) in 2002; 6.4 million persons had stable angina; 305,000 persons had coronary artery bypass graft (CABG) surgery (45% younger than age 65 years), and 640,000 had percutaneous transluminal coronary angioplasty (PTCA) (138/100,000 were between 45 and 64 years) in 2002. In addition, 4.9 million persons had congestive heart failure (CHF) (American Heart Association, 2002). The estimated cost of health care services, institutional care, medications, and lost productivity for patients who had cardiovascular disease (CVD) exceeded $142.1 billion in 2005 (American Heart Association, 2005). Cardiovascular diseases and stroke estimated costs exceeded $393.5 billion in 2005 (American Heart Association, 2005). At the same time the pattern of coronary care has changed, as have treatment philosophies, with early hospital discharge being a major force. Supervised programs of exercise, education, and lifestyle changes have improved outcome for patients who have coronary artery disease, MI, and other severe cardiovascular conditions.

CANDIDATES FOR CARDIAC REHABILITATION

The Agency for Healthcare Research and Quality (AHRQ) clinical practice guidelines list candidates for cardiac rehabilitation, which include the survivors of MI, the persons with stable angina, and the persons who undergo CABG surgery and PTCA. In addition, persons with CHF benefit from rehabilitation. However, low utilization rates and unequal access have been repeatedly demonstrated (Bunker & Goble, 2003; Grace et al., 2002). On average only 11% to 20% of eligible patients enroll in cardiac rehabilitation (Blackburn et al., 2000). Patient factors such as age, gender, ethnicity, and social support and clinical characteristics such as comorbidities and CVD risk factors account for low participation rates (Grace, Evindar, Kung, Scholey, & Stewart, 2004; Missik, 2001; Plach, 2002; Stiller & Holt, 2004). Health care systems and provider factors also contribute to underutilization rates (Grace, Evindar, Abramson, & Stewart, 2004; Mitoff, Wesolowski, Abramson, & Grace, 2005).

Some participants in supervised programs would have been rejected as candidates for cardiac rehabilitation programs in the past. Thirty years ago patients were restricted to bed rest with limited activities over several months after an MI. By the early 1970s eligible applicants to participate in hospital-based cardiac rehabilitation programs exceeded the number of programs and trained staff available. By the 1980s community-based cardiac rehabilitation programs and supervised outpatient clinic programs began to serve low-risk patients. Researchers continue to investigate patient risk factors, patient self-help, program methods, and the optimal amount and type of exercise that is safe. Patient characteristics associated with referral to cardiac rehabilitation are under study (Missik, 2001; Stiller & Holt, 2004).

ADHERENCE CHARACTERISTICS

Researchers have examined characteristics of patients who adhere to and benefit from programs. The studies of cardiovascular disease, treatment for cardiovascular disease, and cardiac rehabilitation for many years used predominantly men in the samples. Only recently has this area of research been broadened to study women, minorities, and elders. Eligibility rates compared to referral rates continue to show higher male referral, whereas elders are less frequently admitted to cardiac rehabilitation programs. However, post-CABG surgery elders have increased functional capacity and cardiovascular efficiency with either a low- or high-intensity aerobic exercise program, as well as increased body strength with a combined resistive-aerobic exercise program.

Interestingly, compliance rates have been shown to be higher in men with better physical outcomes. Women's exercise patterns and adherence to recommendations for exercise are well below recommendations. Fewer women complete the early rehabilitation phase. Women tend not to push to peak exercise oxygen consumption maximum with testing. American women have tended to be less athletic in general. This may change now that young women are being encouraged to pursue athletic careers, including professional sports. Women are now being studied in relation to psychosocial factors, social networks, and support as these variables relate to recovery.

PROGRAM SERVICES

A cardiac rehabilitation program may be located in a community health setting, major medical center, local hospital, or self-directed home programs. The scope, size, goals, and variety of services can be expected to vary among programs. Although most patients enter a cardiac rehabilitation program after a cardiac event, secondary prevention is a program cornerstone. Exercise training is a generic ingredient in programs. For patients with severe cardiac disease and who are high risk, programs offering a broad range of services and a full interdisciplinary team is recommended. This chapter provides information that applies to any cardiac rehabilitation program.

Several professional and governmental organizations have developed standard competencies for professionals in cardiac rehabilitation (Box 33-1) that include minimum qualifications as well as additional preferred qualifications. Leading organizations that have set program standards are listed at the end of this chapter.

INTERDISCIPLINARY TEAM APPROACH

The minimum cardiac rehabilitation team is composed of a medical director or supervising physician, a program director

---

> **BOX 33-1 Basic Core Competencies for All Cardiac Rehabilitation Care Professionals**
>
> **Minimum Qualifications**
> - Bachelor's degree in a health field such as exercise science, or licensure in the jurisdiction
> - Experience or specialty training in cardiovascular rehabilitation and secondary prevention
> - Basic knowledge of exercise physiology, nutrition, risk reduction and behavior modification strategies, counseling techniques, and uses of educational programs and technologies as applied to cardiovascular rehabilitation services
> - Successful completion of BLS course
>
> **Preferred Qualifications**
> - Successful completion of ACLS course
> - Certification by a professional organization that documents core competencies

From American Association of Cardiovascular and Pulmonary Rehabilitation. *Guidelines for cardiac rehabilitation and secondary prevention programs* [4th ed., p. 194]. Champaign, IL: Human Kinetics. ACLS, Advanced Cardiac Life Support; BLS, Basic Life Support.

or coordinator, and a registered professional nurse. In some instances the coordinator is an allied health professional rather than a nurse. Although the nurse's role may vary from program to program, the most consistent role functions are (1) program coordination and (2) patient and family education, essential activities in all programs. Nursing is viewed as vital to all phases of cardiac rehabilitation in all settings, largely because of the holistically oriented goals inherent to nursing. Ideally professionals include a cardiologist and a physiatrist with training in cardiac rehabilitation as regular or consulting members, an exercise physiologist, and a specialty trained cardiac rehabilitation nurse. A cardiac rehabilitation team may consist of additional professionals such as registered dietitian, mental health professional, health educator, vocational rehabilitation counselor, physical therapist, occupational therapist, and pharmacist.

Although team members have specialized cardiac knowledge appropriate to their discipline, each professional must understand the role and contribution of the other disciplines. The concept of cross training is valued among members of cardiac rehabilitation teams who regularly share specialty knowledge during team meetings. As a result, the team members participate in developing one another's expertise within the specialty, which subsequently improves outcomes for patients. Regardless of program size, individualized services are one hallmark of quality in a cardiac rehabilitation program, which means the patient and family are always active members of the interdisciplinary team.

The success of a cardiac rehabilitation program has been attributed in part to the professional quality of the team members. Composition of the team reflects the program philosophy, available resources, patient population, demand, and administrative policies of the institution or agency. Taken together, members of a team of cardiac rehabilitation professionals have advanced practice knowledge about (1) cardiovascular disease; (2) current intervention strategies; (3) educational goals, methods, and tools; (4) health psychology; (5) nutrition; (6) exercise physiology; (7) emergency procedures; (8) rehabilitation principles and care for patients with comorbid conditions; (9) prescription medications; and (10) common over-the-counter (OTC) supplements used by patients, especially those with potential risk when used in conjunction with exercise (e.g., ma huang) and with thrombolytics (e.g., ginseng and ginkgo).

An ideally functioning team is characterized by collaborative relationships and collective decision making that includes the patient and family members. The obvious advantage is full integration of professional expertise and an informed and involved patient. However, many teams tend to function as multidisciplinary, rather than interdisciplinary, teams. As a result, each member contributes uniquely to a patient's cardiac program, but all members do not have equal status in decision-making processes. Decisions may not be arrived at jointly and may exclude patients' preferences or ignore their lifestyles. The nurse coordinator who is able to work effectively with each team member to ensure continuity and integrated planning is a key to success.

CHANGING REHABILITATION SCENE

As changes in the health system reduce hospital length of stay, rehabilitation nurses in facilities and community settings continue to work with patients who are more acutely ill and who have more complex health problems than in the past. Similarly these same patients have fewer days to accomplish rehabilitation goals in a facility before they move on to outpatient or community settings. Rehabilitation nurses are called on to function as case managers and consultants to community programs and to assist with preventing patients from reentering hospitals.

In this reperfusion era, early triage and treatment of persons with acute coronary syndromes changes the immediate course of an acute MI and alters long-term prognosis. Early reperfusion via thrombolytic agents or PTCA decreases the size of infarction and improves regional and global left ventricular function. Cardiac rehabilitation has an increasingly important role as secondary prevention has now become the focus for this patient group.

Cardiac rehabilitation is one of several emerging rehabilitation nursing specialties that deals with patients and settings where increased acuity raises the potential for cardiac and other life-threatening emergencies. Preparation in rehabilitation facilities requires written procedures and equipment to respond to patients' needs. Nurses must be knowledgeable about managing cardiopulmonary emergencies for patients and implementing any advance directives. As a result, nurses may decide to review critical care and medical-surgical content with current clinical guidelines for practice and to learn how to operate equipment or perform procedures associated with these specialty practices.

DEEP VENOUS THROMBOSIS

There is a relatively high incidence of deep venous thrombosis (DVT) in persons with acute MI and CHF. Despite preventive measures, a large number of patients still suffer DVT and its complications during hospitalization and rehabilitation.

Thrombophlebitis refers to an inflamed vein as a result of thrombus formation. Phlebothrombosis is probably the same entity but does not exhibit a marked inflammatory component. DVT refers to either thrombophlebitis or phlebothrombosis in the deep venous system of the legs. The most important consequences of DVT are pulmonary embolism and the syndrome of chronic venous insufficiency. DVT accounts for as many as 800,000 new patients per year (Tierney, McPhee, & Papadakis, 2006). To minimize patient morbidity and mortality, prevention, early diagnosis, and treatment of DVT is paramount.

Factors Associated With DVT

The triad associated with DVT was described in 1846 by Virchow as (1) stasis of blood, (2) increased blood coagulability, and (3) vessel wall injury. One or a combination of these factors may produce the formation of a thrombus. Bed rest and immobilization are associated with decreased blood flow and venous pooling in the lower extremities, increasing the risk of DVT. Persons immobilized by hip fracture, joint replacement, or spinal cord injury are especially at risk for DVT. The risk of DVT is increased in situations of impaired cardiac function and decreased cardiac output. Older persons have a higher incidence compared to younger persons, probably because disorders that produce venous stasis occur more frequently in older persons. Hypercoagulability, a homeostatic mechanism, is designed to increase clot formation, and any conditions that increase the concentration or activation of clotting factors increase the risk of DVT. The loss of body fluids associated with hemoconcentration causes the clotting factors to become more concentrated. Deficiencies in certain plasma proteins that normally inhibit thrombus formation, such as antithrombin III, protein C, and protein S, predispose to DVT. Any conditions that increase the levels of fibrinogen, prothrombin, and other coagulation factors increase the risk of DVT.

Women in the postpartum state are at increased risk. The use of oral contraceptives appears to increase coagulability and predispose to DVT. DVT has been associated with certain cancers. Although the reason for this is largely unknown, it is thought that substances that promote blood coagulation may be released from tissues because of the cancerous growth. Introduction of intravenous catheters traumatizes vessels and increases the risk of DVT. A thrombosis risk factor assessment tool is given in Figure 33-1, and a venous thromboembolism prophylaxis guideline for hospitalized patients is provided in Figure 33-2.

Anatomy and Pathophysiology

A thrombus develops as a result of slowed blood flow in the venous bloodstream and is associated with platelet aggregation.

Each Risk Factor Represents 1 Point
• Age 41-60 years
• Minor surgery planned
• History of prior major surgery (<1 month)
• Varicose veins
• History of inflammatory bowel disease
• Swollen legs (current)
• Obesity (body mass index >25)
• Acute myocardial infarction
• Congestive heart failure (<1 month)
• Sepsis (<1 month)
• Serious lung disease including pneumonia (<1 month)
• Abnormal pulmonary function (chronic obstructive pulmonary disease)
• Medical patient currently at bed rest
• Other risk factors _____

Each Risk Factor Represents 2 Points
• Age 60-74 years
• Arthroscopic surgery
• Malignancy (present or previous)
• Major surgery (>45 minutes)
• Laparoscopic surgery (>45 minutes)
• Patient confined to bed (>72 hours)
• Immobilizing plaster cast (<1 month)
• Central venous access

Each Risk Factor Represents 3 Points
• Age over 75 years
• History of deep vein thrombosis/ pulmonary embolism
• Family history of thrombosis*
• Positive factor V Leiden
• Positive prothrombin 20210A
• Elevated serum homocysteine
• Positive lupus anticoagulant
• Elevated anticardiolipin antibodies
• Heparin-induced thrombocytopenia (HIT)
• Other congenital or acquired thrombophilia Type _____
* Most frequently missed risk factor

Each Risk Factor Represents 5 Points
• Elective major lower extremity arthroplasty
• Hip, pelvis, or leg fracture (<1 month)
• Stroke (<1 month)
• Multiple trauma (<1 month)
• Acute spinal cord injury (paralysis) (<1 month)

For Women Only (Each Represents 1 Point)
• Oral contraceptives or hormone replacement therapy
• Pregnancy or postpartum (<1 month)
• History of unexplained stillborn infant, recurrent spontaneous abortion (≥3), premature birth with toxemia or growth-restricted infant

Total Risk Factor Score _____

Total Risk Factor Score	**Incidence of DVT**	**Risk Level**	**Prophylaxis Regime**
0-1	<10%	Low Risk	No specific measures; early ambulation
2	10-20%	Moderate Risk	ES, IPC, LDUH (5000U BID) or LWMH (<3400U)
3-4	20-40%	High Risk	IPC, LDUH (5000U BID) or LWMH (<3400U)
5 or more	40-80% 1-5% mortality	Highest Risk	Pharmacological: LDUH, LWMH (>3400U)*, Warfarin*, or FXaI* alone or in combination with ES or IPC (*used for major orthopedic surgery)

Legend for scoring: ES—elastic stockings; IPC—Intermittent Pneumatic Compression; LDUH—Low Dose Unfractionated Heparin; LMWH—Low Molecular Weight Heparin; FXa I—Factor X Inhibitor From Caprini, J. A. (2005). Thrombosis risk factor assessment as a guide to quality patient care. *Disease Monograph, 51,* 70-78.
COPD, Chronic obstructive pulmonary disease; *BMI,* body mass index; *SVT,; DVT,* deep venous thrombosis; *PE,* pulmonary embolism.

Figure 33-1 Thrombosis risk factor assessment. (Courtesy Joseph A. Caprini, MD, MS, FACS, RVT, Northwestern University, Chicago, IL.)

The thrombus organizes from its outer margins centrally. In some veins the entire thrombus becomes organized with complete and permanent occlusion of the lumen. If the thrombus is large, involution usually occurs by a process of partial fibrosis and partial lysis, which is probably the result of the action of naturally occurring fibrinolysins in the blood. The center may disappear, but the periphery organizes into a fibrous ring, or in other instances bands of fibrous tissue extend across the lumen of the vein dividing it into many small lumina. The result is some restoration of function of the vein, but there is partial obstruction of the lumen by the remaining fibrous tissue and a decrease in circular diameter.

There are varying degrees of inflammatory reaction, depending on the different layers of the vein involved. The accumulation of inflammatory cells, leukocytes, lymphocytes, and fibroblasts cause congestion of the capillaries in and around the venous walls. The amount of obstruction to venous blood flow is directly related to the size and location of the involved vein. Collateral circulation compensates through superficial veins, and this may also be true in obstruction of the saphenous vein of the leg. Because of the numerous anastomoses that exist, collateral channels may become evident even after obstruction of the superior or inferior vena cava. When thrombosis occurs in the iliofemoral or axillary veins, there is only partial collateral circulation, causing increased venous pressure in the veins. The result is distention of all veins, venules, and capillaries, which causes intense congestion and impedes normal reabsorption of fluids and electrolytes. Progressive edema and pain in the affected limb results.

Assessment

Signs and symptoms of DVT develop acutely and usually persist for 1 to 3 weeks. Acute thrombophlebitis in small or medium veins rarely produces systemic reaction, whereas involvement of the larger vessels may cause the temperature to rise as high as 102° F (39° C). The most common signs of DVT are related to the inflammatory process and include pain, swelling, and deep muscle tenderness. Accompanying signs may be fever, malaise, and an elevated white blood count as well as sedimentation rate. The site of the thrombus formation is somewhat determined by the location of the physical findings (Figure 33-3). The most common sites of DVT are in the venous sinuses in the soleus muscle, the posterior tibial veins, and the peroneal veins. Swelling of the foot and ankle is usually present, although it may be slight or absent. Calf pain and tenderness are common complaints. Femoral vein thrombosis produces pain and tenderness in the distal thigh and popliteal area. The most profound signs are produced when there are thrombi in iliofemoral veins. There is swelling, pain, and tenderness of the entire extremity. DVT in the calf veins may produce pain with active dorsiflexion of the foot (Homans' sign).

Because of the risk of pulmonary embolism, the need for early detection and treatment of DVT is paramount. Diagnostic aids that assist with the diagnosis of DVT include the D-dimer test, duplex ultrasonography, gadolinium-enhanced magnetic resonance venography, and rarely ascending contrast venography (Tierney et al., 2006).

Nursing Diagnosis

Nursing diagnoses appropriate when DVT exists include (1) ineffective tissue perfusion: peripheral, (2) anxiety, and (3) ineffective therapeutic regimen management.

Therapeutic goals in the presence of DVT are to arrest the thrombosis, dissolve existing clots, prevent clot migration, and provide supportive care. With DVT in large veins another goal may be to remove the thrombus. Insertion of a vena cava filter may be used in patients who are at high risk but cannot tolerate anticoagulation.

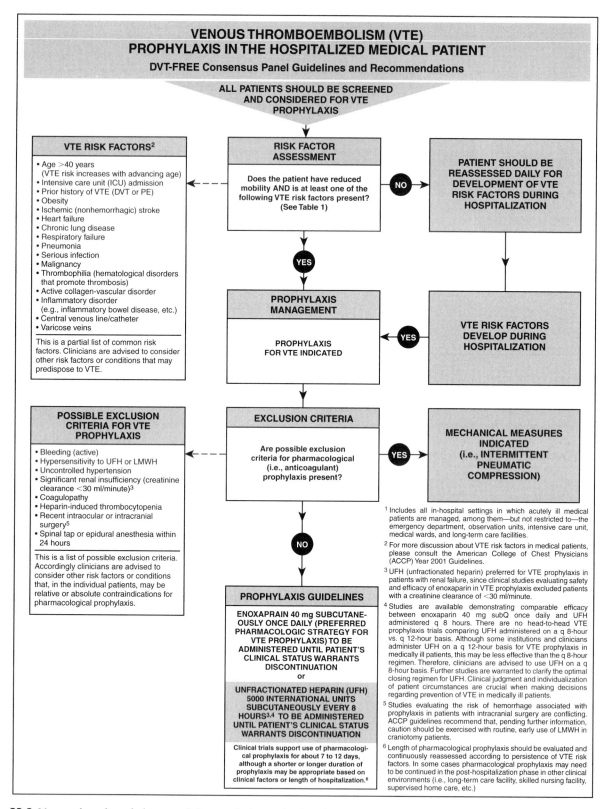

Figure 33-2 Venous thromboembolism prophylaxis in the hospitalized medical patient. (From Bosker, G., & Poponick, J. [2002]. The current challenge of venous thrombosis (VTE) in the hospitalized patient. *Emergency Medicine Reports, 23*(16), 191. Courtesy American Health Consultants, Pearl River, NY. Available at http://www.thrombosis.com/T.htm.)

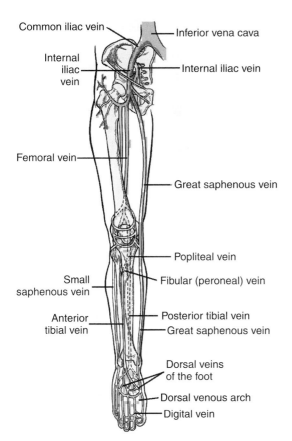

Figure 33-3 Major veins of the lower extremity (anterior view). (From Thibodeau, G. A., & Patton, K. T. [2007]. *Anatomy & physiology* [6th ed.]. St. Louis, MO: Mosby.)

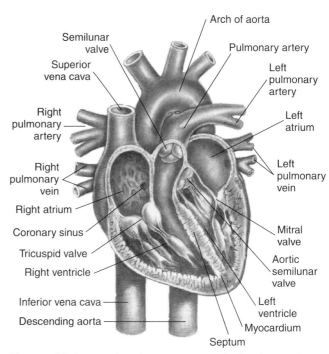

Figure 33-4 Frontal schematic view of the heart. (From Thompson, J. M., McFarland, G. K., Hirsch, J. E., & Tucker, S. M. [2002]. *Mosby's clinical nursing* [5th ed.]. St. Louis, MO: Mosby.)

Intervention

The Nursing Interventions Classification (NIC) interventions related to DVT are embolus precautions, anxiety reduction, and possibly pain management related to affected extremity. Elevation, antiembolism stockings, passive and active range of motion, position change, early mobility, and administration of anticoagulant and pain medications are the appropriate nursing interventions.

CORONARY ARTERY CIRCULATION

Coronary Artery Perfusion

The following anatomical and physiological review describes coronary artery perfusion—impairments are common factors in many cardiac disorders—and contains information that influences nursing assessment and rehabilitation interventions.

The epicardial section of the coronary arteries lies on the surface of the heart. Perforator vessels enter the myocardium, delivering blood to the endocardial and subendocardial areas of the myocardium during diastole. The subendocardial area is the last area of the heart muscle fed by the coronary arteries. This explains why in an MI the damage spreads from the endocardial area outward to the epicardial area.

Three special factors affecting coronary artery perfusion are (1) cardiac cycle, (2) heart rate, and (3) diastolic intraventricular pressure. These factors must be considered while making all nursing assessments related to the coronary artery perfusion. In systole the ventricular wall tension greatly limits blood flow through the coronary perforator arteries. Most coronary circulation occurs during ventricular diastole, while the ventricular walls are "relaxing," which allows a significant reduction in ventricular muscle tension. The significant anatomical parts of the heart are illustrated in Figure 33-4; distribution of the coronary arteries throughout the heart and great vessels is illustrated in Figure 33-5.

The left anterior descending (LAD) artery of the left coronary artery supplies the septum and the anterior portion of the heart, the major portion of the left ventricle. The circumflex artery supplies the lateral portion of the heart, the lesser portion of the left ventricle. The right coronary artery (RCA) supplies the inferior portion of the heart, which includes parts of the right atrium and right ventricle, the sinoatrial node in 55% of persons, and the atrioventricular (AV) node in 90% of persons. The left atrium is supplied by branches arising from the LAD.

Altered Coronary Artery Perfusion

Since 1994 the term acute coronary syndromes (ACS) has been used to refer to patients with ischemic chest pain. ACS represents a continuum of similar disease processes. The continuum is stable angina, unstable angina, non–Q-wave infarction, and Q-wave infarction.

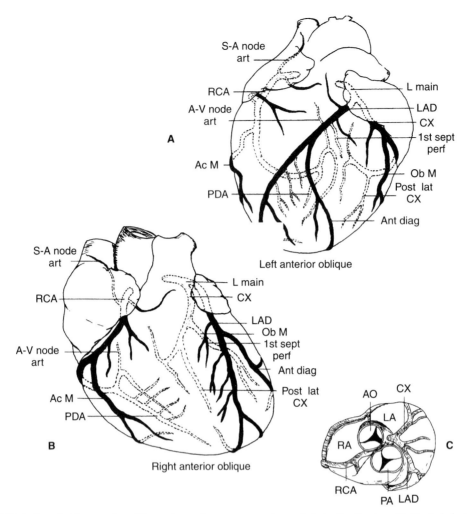

Figure 33-5 **A** and **B,** Left and right anterior oblique views of coronary arteries and their distribution. **C,** Cephalad view of coronary artery distribution in relation to the great vessels. (From Thibodeau, G. A., & Patton, K. T. (2003). *Anatomy & physiology* [5th ed.]. St. Louis, MO: Mosby.) *Ac M,* acute marginal; *Ant,* anterior; *AO,* aorta; *art,* artery; *A-V,* atrioventricular; *CX,* circumflex; *diag,* diagonal; *L,* left; *LA,* left atrium; *LAD,* left anterior descending; *lat,* lateral; *Ob M,* obtuse marginal; *PA,* pulmonary artery; *PDA,* posterior descending artery; *perf,* perforator; *Post,* posterior; *RA,* right atrium; *RCA,* right coronary artery; *S-A,* Sinoatrial; *sept,* septal.

Heart rate is a crucial factor in patients with a coronary syndrome. *Heart rate dictates the length of diastolic perfusion time for coronary arteries.* As the heart rate increases, the diastolic filling time shortens. A patient with stable angina has a threshold heart rate in which diastolic filling time shortens to a point where adequate coronary artery perfusion cannot perfuse stenotic arteries. Rest thwarts anginal episodes. Rest enables the heart rate to slow, and slowed heart rate lengthens the diastolic filling time of the coronary arteries, thereby increasing perfusion. Beta-blockers are an important adjunctive therapy to control heart rate and increase coronary perfusion to the cardiac muscle.

Conditions associated with higher circulating blood volume, such as CHF, may cause myocardial ischemia and anginal symptoms when blood flow to subendocardial areas is reduced. Diastolic intraventricular pressure alters perfusion of blood through the perforator arteries. A high diastolic interventricular pressure reduces the blood flow to the subendocardial area.

Sublingual nitroglycerine or other nitrates relieve anginal symptoms by causing blood to pool in the extremities, which in turn decreases blood return to the heart (preload) and reduces intraventricular diastolic pressure, thereby increasing perfusion.

Stable angina indicates an unchanging atherosclerotic process in the coronary perfusion. Precipitation and relief of anginal symptoms are predictable. In contrast, unstable angina or preinfarction angina suggests an active, dynamic atherosclerotic progression. Symptoms of unstable angina become unpredictable, appear with less exertion, occur more frequently, and tend not to be relieved as readily as with stable angina.

Various symptoms, including angina, are associated with myocardial ischemia. With atherosclerosis, fixed stenotic lesions develop in the coronary arteries. A lesion that occludes 60% or more of an artery can produce myocardial ischemia and anginal symptoms, which often are precipitated by exertion or emotional (dis)stress, accompanied by increased heart rate.

Thus rest is a key intervention once again. At times ischemia of the left ventricle may precipitate transient congestive heart disease. Symptoms of CHF include dyspnea and paroxysmal nocturnal dyspnea. Elderly patients who develop congestive heart disease classically become fatigued, gain weight resulting from edema, and develop cough with dyspnea. A rise in heart rate also occurs in CHF, which decreases coronary perfusion and further aggravates the situation.

Occlusion of the LAD causes an acute anterior wall infarction. These infarctions have a variety of more specific labels depending on the site of occlusion. The higher the occlusion is in the LAD, the more extensive the anterior wall damage and the more extensive the left ventricular pump problem. Persons with LAD occlusions are always at risk for CHF. Conduction problems (e.g., third-degree heart block) have a poor prognosis because of the extent of muscle loss. Occlusion of the circumflex artery is associated with less risk for pump problems.

Occlusion of the RCA produces an acute inferior wall infarction. Inferior MIs are often associated with conduction disorders (frequently temporary) because of disruption of blood supply to the AV node. Right ventricular cardiogenic shock occurs in massive right ventricular infarctions and is often associated with complete heart block. Cardiogenic shock from a right ventricular failure requires definite diagnosis because the therapeutic management is quite different from left ventricular failure.

A CARDIAC REHABILITATION/ SECONDARY PREVENTION PROGRAM

The core components of cardiac rehabilitation/secondary prevention programs are patient assessment, nutritional counseling, lipid management, hypertension management, smoking cessation, weight management, diabetes management, psychosocial management, physical activity counseling, and exercise training. A cardiac rehabilitation program begins within a few days after the patient has had an MI, coronary angioplasty, CABG surgery, heart transplant, or other cardiovascular surgery. For patients with stable angina or CHF, cardiac rehabilitation begins at any point where the patient is considered free of acute symptoms.

Phases of Cardiac Rehabilitation Management

Cardiac rehabilitation is a continuous process that commonly is categorized according to phases. Although in the past phases have been numbered 1 through 4 traditionally, many programs now use the terms *inpatient* and *outpatient* to designate phases. The American Association of Cardiovascular and Pulmonary Rehabilitation (AACVPR) guidelines (2004) identify three phases—inpatient (beginning during hospitalization), followed by a supervised ambulatory outpatient program lasting up to 8 weeks, and continuing as a lifetime maintenance stage at a community facility or at home. Some patients require transitional care in a subacute facility or at home. The continuum of care has become more process oriented than structure oriented with reduced service-delivery interventions over time.

Inpatient Cardiac Rehabilitation

The guideline for cardiac rehabilitation within the inpatient and transitional settings is as follows:

> Following a documented physician referral, patients hospitalized for an event or procedure associated with CAD, valvular disease or cardiac muscle dysfunction should be provided with a program of cardiac rehabilitation consisting of (1) early assessment and mobilization, identification and information regarding cardiovascular disease risk factors and self-care; and (2) a comprehensive discharge-planning session that includes a discussion of follow-up options for transitional care, home programming, and formal outpatient cardiac rehabilitation (AACVPR, 2004, p. 32).

Inpatient cardiac rehabilitation entails a program designed to limit physical and psychological consequences of the acute cardiac illness for the patient who is still hospitalized. The average length of stay is 3 to 4 days, possibly shorter for persons with percutaneous transluminal angioplasty or uncomplicated MI, and up to 2 weeks with persons who have complicated MI and other CHD pathological processes. The major components are risk assessment, early ambulation and physical activity, and education of patients and families. Progressive activity is often integrated into clinical pathways or other protocol formats and performed by unit staff to ensure more timely and more aggressive delivery of rehabilitation. Education is focused on predischarge priorities (survival teaching) such as recognition of signs and symptoms, do's and don'ts for home, and medication instruction. Posthospital follow-up is arranged as part of discharge planning. Patients not ready for discharge home may require transitional care, whereas healthier patients may be referred to start outpatient programs within 1 or 2 weeks after the event. To fulfill the secondary prevention mission of cardiac rehabilitation, the provision of risk factor intervention programs, education, counseling, and exercise training is mandatory. Comprehensive risk reduction education is paramount during cardiac rehabilitation.

Patient and Family Assessment. Assessment guidelines for inpatient cardiac rehabilitation are as follows:

1. The patient's personal goals for rehabilitation should be assessed for readiness to learn and readiness for activity in order to facilitate compliance and postevent adjustment. As appropriate, goals should be developed for such areas as physical function, return to work, risk factor reduction, psychological well-being, and family and social adjustment.
2. Before activity begins, a cardiac rehabilitation staff member with appropriate skills and competencies should perform a baseline physical assessment. This assessment should include, but not be limited to, listening to heart and lungs sounds, palpating peripheral pulses, evaluating gross musculoskeletal strength and flexibility, and assessing the patient's self-care capability. Results of the assessment should be documented along with baseline heart rate,

blood pressure and cardiac rhythm strip (AACVPR, 2004, pp. 35-36).

To begin cardiac rehabilitation, the patient must be considered stable, that is, (1) no new/recurrent chest pain in the past 8 hours, (2) creatine kinase (CK) and/or troponin levels are not rising, (3) no new signs of uncompensated failure (dyspnea at rest with bibasilar rales), and (4) no new significant abnormal rhythm or electrocardiogram (ECG) changes in past 8 hours. Patients are considered for activity progression when activity response include (1) an adequate heart rate, (2) adequate systolic blood pressure rise to within 10 to 40 mm Hg from rest, (3) no new rhythm or ST changes on telemetry rhythm strips, and (4) no cardiac symptoms such as palpitations, dyspnea, excess fatigue, or chest pain. An additional guideline stresses the importance of a smoking-cessation intervention in the initial phase of cardiac rehabilitation and reads as follows: "the smoking status of each hospitalized cardiac patient must be identified. Educational and behavioral interventions should help patients through the period when they are not smoking in the hospital, assess their readiness to continue smoking cessation after discharge, and provide advice on how to maintain smoking cessation if patients are ready to do so" (AACVPR, 2004, p. 38).

Patients and families are empowered to participate as members of the team when they receive information that is individualized to their needs as soon as possible after hospitalization and throughout the program. A nursing assessment of stressors and coping ability is initiated for both patient and family, with referral for mental health counseling as needed. Patient and family members may have misconceptions or misunderstandings about the disease trajectory or the benefits from participating in a cardiac rehabilitation program. For instance, some may believe that bypass surgery is a curative procedure that expunges cardiac risk. Health beliefs have been found to be important factors influencing a patient's decision and ultimate participation in a cardiac rehabilitation program. Assessment questions related to pertinent learner characteristics are presented in Table 33-1.

Nursing Diagnoses and Therapeutic Goals During Inpatient Cardiac Rehabilitation. For patients who have uncomplicated cardiac disease, MI, or who have received angioplasty, the relevant NANDA International (2007) (NANDA-I) diagnostic categories are risk for activity intolerance, anxiety, and deficient knowledge. Inpatient goals for these patients are early risk assessment and early ambulation so they can be discharged promptly to outpatient rehabilitation care and reenter the community.

Some patients have survived sudden cardiac death or have severe cardiac conditions such as CHF, serious ventricular arrhythmias or complex dysrhythmias, left ventricular dysfunction, myocardial ischemia, or certain specific ECG changes with exercise. Diagnostic categories for these persons may include activity intolerance, decreased cardiac output, and ineffective tissue perfusion. Inpatient goals are risk reduction via intensive monitoring, early diagnosis and treatment of

TABLE 33-1 Education-Related Variables and Assessment Questions

Variable	Questions
Existing knowledge base	What do the patient and family already know? What illness-related experiences have the patient and family had?
Readiness to learn (motivation)	What priority does the patient and family place on learning? What questions or comments are being raised? What factors may be impeding motivation (denial, anger, depression)?
Learning needs	Do the patient and family state these needs specifically? Do nurse, patient, and family agree on needs and on the resulting plan?
Client and family goals	What goals, if any, do the patient and family have in relation to illness, lifestyle changes, or therapeutic regimens?
Client and family energy for learning	Are symptoms present that must be taken into account? Can teaching strategies be geared to the energy level?
Presence of support systems	Will others be learning with the patient and family? Do learning needs of patent and family coincide with those of other support persons?
Time for learning	How much time is available? Can a "time line" be designed with the patient and family?
Potential for understanding	What factors will influence understanding of the content (educational level, language, presence of sensory dysfunction, amount of anesthetic, medications that depress central nervous system, anxiety level)? What resources are available that will promote understanding?

From Jillings, C. R. (1988). *Cardiac rehabilitation nursing.* Rockville, MD: Aspen. Copyright 1988 by Aspen. Reprinted by permission.

problems and complications, conditioning or reconditioning through mobilization (physical activity and exercise), and reentry into the community.

Therapeutic Plan and Interventions. When patients have uncomplicated disease, some Nursing Interventions Classification (NIC) interventions are cardiac care and cardiac care: rehabilitation, teaching: disease process, teaching: prescribed diet, teaching: prescribed activity/exercise, anticipatory guidance, anxiety reduction, teaching: individual, and teaching: prescribed medication. Patients with more severe cardiac problems may fall into several NIC interventions, including cardiac precautions, cardiac care: acute, dysrhythmia management, shock management: cardiac, and hemodynamic regulation. These patients receive intensive monitoring using electrocardiographic telemetry in order to detect problems immediately during activity and exercise. Referral to appropriate members of the cardiac rehabilitation team begins inpatient rehabilitation.

An important goal in rehabilitation, as well as in acute and chronic care, is prevention of DVT. Risk assessment and implementation of a DVT prophylaxis plan accomplish this (see Figures 33-1 and 33-2).

Exercise Component. The exercise component is a foundational piece of cardiac rehabilitation. A major physiological effect of exercise training is improved functional capacity resulting from peripheral effects with reduced fatigue, dyspnea, angina, or related symptoms. Overall musculoskeletal condition and sense of well-being improves. Limited left ventricular function improvement has been found (Goodman et al., 1999). Exercise training has produced improvement in exercise tolerance in both men and women of every age-group, including those older than 75 years. Exercise training also results in improvement of symptoms, including decreased angina, decreased symptoms of heart failure, and improvement in clinical measures of ischemia.

Low to moderate intensity strength training soon after an infarction is effective and may actually have lower complication rates than aerobic exercise. Strength training does not increase peak oxygen consumption or reduce myocardial oxygen demand. Combined training improves aerobic and muscle fitness. The increased basal metabolic rate helps with obesity. Increased insulin sensitivity decreases blood glucose levels and cholesterol.

Regular physical activity is known to protect against the progression of many acquired chronic diseases or development of others and assists in maintaining functional abilities. Low-intensity exercises, 3 times a week for 30 minutes plus warm-up and cool-down time, have been found effective in improving functional capacity and endurance during the maintenance and follow-up phase of cardiac rehabilitation. Initially, more frequent exercise may be needed.

Progressive physical activity is supervised and performed in a gradual sequence of steps to increase a patient's work demand as a means to counter deconditioning, as well as to prevent DVT or pulmonary emboli. Activities and exercise often improve a patient's sense of well-being and control, reduce confusion and depression, and stimulate outlook. Thus within the first 1 to 2 days, patients without medical complications are encouraged to perform grooming and self-care activities, get out of bed for toileting when this requires walking short distances, and perform range-of-motion (ROM) exercises.

Throughout the day a patient takes several short walks after which the nurse monitors blood pressure, heart rate, and ECG readings for signs of changes that would indicate a need for reduction of activities. Principles of energy conservation are important considerations as ROM exercises progress from passive to active; eventually 1- to 2-pound weights can be used as resistance. Soon thereafter, warm-up and stretching activities or mild calisthenics are added to ambulation or treadmill work. Patients who will encounter stairs at home or work practice climbing and descending stairs.

Education Component. Education in inpatient rehabilitation includes the following:

- Empowerment for patient and family as team members, such as answering questions and concerns, determining learning style and needs, and introducing them to the disease trajectory and anticipated interventions
- Disease- or condition-specific content such as anatomy and physiology, medical procedures and tests, purposes of monitoring equipment, cardiac precautions, wound care/precautions, self-care of chest pain, and access to emergency services
- Specific guidelines or instructions such as activity types and levels, including lifting/pushing and weight limitations for lifting, specific exercises, prescribed and OTC medication actions and side effects, diet, tobacco use, activities of daily living, and rest
- Preparatory information such as return to work, stress reduction, sexual activity, risk factor and lifestyle modifications, and follow-up care
- Ongoing monitoring of patient's status

During inpatient cardiac rehabilitation, ongoing monitoring of patient's status includes vital signs, cardiovascular status, respiratory status, fluid balance, and pertinent laboratory values. The patient is monitored for dysrhythmias, signs and symptoms of decreased cardiac output, and pacemaker function if appropriate.

Early Outpatient

The guideline for medical evaluation and exercise testing before entry into an outpatient cardiac rehabilitation program is as follows:

> To establish a safe and effective program of comprehensive CV risk reduction and rehabilitation, each patient should undergo a careful medical evaluation and exercise test before participating in an outpatient cardiac rehabilitation program. The specific components of the medical examination should include a medical history, physical examination and resting ECG. The exercise test should be repeated any time that symptoms or clinical changes warrant as well as in the follow-up assessment of exercise training outcome (AACVPR, 2004, p. 70).

The exercise test uses treadmill equipment with recording monitors and with controls to vary the speed and elevation of the exercise surface as the patient "walks" to evaluate exercise tolerance. A treadmill exercise testing protocol should be selected appropriate to the patient's weight and fitness level. The most frequently used treadmill protocols are the Bruce, the modified Bruce, and the Naughton. Exercise treadmill testing may be symptom limited or submaximal. The goal of submaximal testing is to exercise the patient enough to achieve 70% of maximum predicted rate for the patient's age. There are also minimum requirements for measures assessed during exercise testing (see AACVPR, 2004, p. 76).

Predischarge treadmill testing is used to assess risk stratification and determine a home program and activity or work capacity, as well as to minimize a patient's anxiety about activity. Repeated testing at certain intervals helps in determining whether the exercise prescription needs to be altered. For instance, a patient's health status, medications, or symptoms may change. Repeated exercise testing at intervals may occur as necessary but is recommended at 6 months and 1 year after the initial testing.

Other modalities for exercise testing include exercise nuclear imaging, exercise echocardiography, and pharmacological stress testing. A 6-minute walk test is being used more frequently for low-functioning cardiac patients who are not candidates for treadmill testing. Stationary cycling and arm crank ergometry have been utilized for patients with physical limitations such as limb loss or paralysis. The arm crank enables patients with lower body paralysis or paresis, such as with paraplegia, to be tested provided they have sufficient upper body strength and function. A variety of modified or adapted equipment and devices have been used in exercise testing of persons with disabilities. Generally these consist of modified bicycles to suit patients' abilities such as a supine model or arm- and leg-powered model, or equipment attached to existing wheelchairs that connects the equipment to cycles or similar circular modifications. With modifications that rely on the parts of the body with functional abilities to supply crank or cycle power, the exercise workload should not overtax some parts of the body while achieving necessary cardiovascular levels (American College of Sports Medicine [ACSM], 1998; Wenger et al., 1995).

Following medical evaluation and exercise testing, early outpatient cardiac rehabilitation starts 1 to 2 weeks after the event; the average length of stay is 6 to 8 weeks depending upon each patient's level of risk and access to additional resources outside of the formal cardiac rehabilitation program. Emphasis is on secondary prevention of CHD through risk reduction via focused interventions, education, counseling, and exercise. Self-learning and self-monitoring is promoted among all patients. Program variations are used to facilitate patient inclusion, such as elderly persons or those who have undergone transplant, heart failure, or vascular disease. Today there is increased collaboration with primary care health care providers to facilitate secondary prevention. Alternative settings or delivery systems are in use or being explored for patients unable to participate on-site. Some of these include home-based cardiac rehabilitation and exercise with transtelephonic monitoring and surveillance. Guidelines for the structure of the secondary prevention programing are as follows:

1. All patients should be assessed for the presence and extent of modifiable CVD risk factors, including smoking, hypertension, abnormal lipid profile, diabetes, obesity, psychosocial dysfunction, and inactivity.

2. Depending on their medical history and physiological and psychological status, the majority of patients should be able

to begin aggressive secondary prevention and cardiac rehabilitation while still in the hospital. Appropriate pharmacological therapy, including beta-blocker therapy, aspirin, and angiotensin-converting enzyme (ACE) inhibitors, should also begin during hospitalization. Exercise training should begin within 1 to 3 weeks of discharge from the hospital. Most patients, including those with uncomplicated percutaneous transluminal coronary angioplasty (PTCA)/ stent, can and should begin within 1 week of hospital discharge.

3. Outcomes should include the complete cessation of smoking, improved lipid profiles, controlled hypertension, recognition and treatment of psychological dysfunction, and improved nutrition and physical activity habits (AACVPR, 2004, p 55).

During the outpatient phase, patients and families experience the greatest adjustment. They are vulnerable to experiencing a great deal of anxiety about the type and amounts of activities, developing fears and depressions, misinterpreting instructions about medications or regimens, and encountering problems with instituting lifestyle changes such as preparing diets, stopping smoking, and managing stressors.

Assessment. At the time of entrance into the outpatient cardiac program, the AACVPR guideline (2004) states that all patients should undergo (or have undergone) the following screening and assessments: current medical history (medical or surgical profile (or both), including complications, comorbidities, and other pertinent medical history); physical examination (cardiopulmonary systems assessment and musculoskeletal assessment, particularly upper and lower extremities and lower back); resting 12-lead ECG; current medications, including dose and frequency; CVD risk profile including (1) identification of age and gender and menopausal status if female, (2) use of tobacco products, (3) history of hypertension, (4) lipid profile including total cholesterol, high-density lipoprotein (HDL), low-density lipoprotein (LDL), and triglycerides (before event or more than 6 to 8 weeks after event), (5) nutritional status, especially dietary fat, saturated fat, cholesterol, and calories, (6) body composition analysis (weight, height, body mass index [BMI], waist-to-hip ratio, relative body fatness, waist circumference), (7) fasting blood glucose or hemoglobin A_{1c} and history of diabetes, (8) physical activity status, (9) level of anger and hostility, (10) psychosocial history, particularly evidence of depression, and (11) family history (AACVPR, 2004, p. 58).

In addition, a second guideline states: "All cardiac patients entering exercise rehabilitation should be stratified according to risk for the occurrence of cardiac events during exercise" (AACVPR, 2004, p 62). Risk stratification serves as the basis for individualizing prescription of exercise training and assessing the extent of supervision required. Medical evaluation, exercise treadmill testing, and nuclear scanning are means of evaluating risk for progression of atherosclerosis and risk for adverse cardiac events during prescribed exercise training. Risk stratification is based on clinical assessment of functional capacity, myocardial ischemia, ventricular dysfunction, and arrhythmias (Table 33-2). Patients perform a supervised and monitored treadmill exercise test. Test results are correlated with other factors to form an individualized risk stratification—high, low, or moderate—that is used in the exercise prescription and long-term treatment plan.

Psychosocial Assessment. Many patients recover from a cardiovascular event only to succumb to depression, anxiety, and other behaviors that prevent them from resuming family and social relationships or returning to a satisfactory and productive life. As survival rates from cardiac events have increased, attention to issues surrounding a patient's quality

of life have become more common. Neuropsychological functioning has been examined to determine how this might affect cardiac rehabilitation patients. Patients with moderate to severe depression have been found to be twice as likely to die in the 2 years after a severe cardiac event, apparently because depressed patients have an increased tendency to clot (Shaw, 2000). Upon enrollment in the cardiac rehabilitation program the patient should be assessed for depression using a valid questionnaire. Referral to a mental health professional may be indicated.

Dramatic improvement in depression, energy level, and exercise capacity has been found when patients enroll in cardiac

---

TABLE 33-2 Stratification of Risk for Cardiac Events During Exercise Participation

Risk Level	
Low	**Characteristics of patients at lowest risk for exercise participation (all characteristics listed must be present to remain at lowest risk)**
	Absence of complex ventricular arrhythmias during exercise testing and recovery
	Absence of angina or other significant symptoms (e.g., unusual shortness of breath, light-headedness, or dizziness, during exercise testing and recovery)
	Presence of normal hemodynamics during exercise testing and recovery (i.e., appropriate increases and decreases in heart rate and systolic blood pressure with increasing workloads and recovery)
	Functional capacity ≥7 METs
	Non-exercise testing findings:
	Rest ejection fraction ≥50%
	Uncomplicated MI or revascularization procedure
	Absence of complicated ventricular arrhythmias at rest
	Absence of CHF
	Absence of signs or symptoms of postevent/postprocedure ischemia
	Absence of clinical depression
Intermediate	**Characteristics of patients at moderate risk for exercise participation (any one or combination of these findings places a patient at moderate risk)**
	Presence of angina or other significant symptoms (e.g., unusual shortness of breath, light-headedness, or dizziness occurring only at high levels of exertion [>.7 METs])
	Mild to moderate level of silent ischemia during exercise testing or recovery (ST-segment depression <2 mm from baseline)
	Functional capacity <5 METs
	Non-exercise testing findings:
	Rest ejection fraction = 40%-49%
High	**Characteristics of patients at high risk for exercise participation (any one or combination of these findings places a patient at high risk)**
	Presence of complex ventricular arrhythmias during exercise testing or recovery
	Presence of angina or other significant symptoms (e.g., unusual shortness of breath, light-headedness, or dizziness at low levels of exertion [<5 METs] or during recovery)
	High level of silent ischemia (ST-segment depression ≥2mm from baseline) during exercise testing or recovery
	Presence of abnormal hemodynamics with exercise testing (i.e., chronotropic incompetence or flat or decreasing systolic BP with increasing workloads) or recovery (i.e., severe postexercise hypotension)
	Non-exercising testing findings:
	Rest ejection fraction >40%
	History of cardiac arrest, or sudden death
	Complex dysrhythmias at rest
	Complicated MI or revascularization procedure
	Presence of CHF
	Presence of signs and symptoms of postevent/postprocedure ischemia
	Presence of clinical depression

From Williams, M. A. (2001). Exercise testing in cardiac rehabilitation: Exercise prescription and beyond. *Cardiology Clinics, 19,* 415-431.
BP, Blood pressure; *CHF,* congestive heart failure; *MET,* metabolic equivalent; *MI,* myocardial infarction.

rehabilitation programs. Because social isolation has been found to have a negative impact on prognosis, participation in cardiac rehabilitation has been found to improve social adjustment and functioning. Women have better social outcomes. Training in behavior modification, stress management, and relaxation techniques is effective in lowering levels of self-reported emotional distress and modifying negative affective behaviors. Wenger et al. (1995) concluded "education, counseling, and/or psychosocial interventions, either alone or as a component of multifactorial cardiac rehabilitation, result in improved psychological well-being and are recommended to complement the psychosocial benefits of exercise training" (p. 122).

Quality of life and self-esteem, along with adherence to self-care, medication, and exercise regimens, may be deciding factors in a patient's continued participation in a cardiac rehabilitation program. Concepts such as quality of life are not easy to measure or evaluate. Tools recommended by AACVPR (2004) for assessing quality of life are listed in Box 33-2.

Patients may have difficulty maintaining self-esteem as they face changes in their lifestyle and roles. Depression and anxiety are heightened when a patient is unable to return to former activities, including work. In a downward spiral, the patient assumes a sick role, learns helplessness, and becomes fearful of impending cardiac emergencies—even sudden death. Family members may respond by overly protecting the person or by labeling the patient as being overly concerned or having a "cardiac psychosis."

Some patients respond with rebellious behaviors to regain a sense of control or conversely with avoidance and denial by resorting to addictive behaviors, compulsions, and substance abuse. Patients may develop symptoms of illness secondary to depression such as vague discomfort or pains in the chest, headache, restlessness, insomnia, fatigue, feelings of panic, or altered concentration and memory. A comprehensive cardiac rehabilitation program provides for a patient's psychosocial needs, as well as for physical training. Patients may feel as if they have "given up" control over many areas of their lives and find lifestyle preferences a solace. Change requires energy and commitment, which may be emotionally or psychologically overwhelming for them. The nurse carefully monitors depressed patients because depression has been associated with poorer outcomes and premature termination from cardiac rehabilitation.

Each patient and family needs to receive guidance and coaching to cope with the potential psychosocial problems that commonly occur after a cardiac event and often provoke stressful responses. As a group, patients and families predictably ask questions about similar concerns (Box 33-3). Rehabilitation nurses who are aware of these commonly expressed concerns are able to provide anticipatory guidance about specific responses and work through coping responses that enable patients and families to resist or eliminate stressors.

The nurse and other team members are educating patients and families who are coping at different levels and using various coping behaviors. Educational materials are more effective when they meet individual needs. Readability of all educational materials can be tested in order to meet the needs of specific populations. When selecting educational materials, assess the patient and family concerning the following:
- Diagnosis and health status
- Education and socioeconomic background
- Interest in material and mode of presentation
- Availability of computers, Internet access, CDs and DVDs or other devices
- Cultural or religious preferences
- Literacy level, primary language

BOX 33-2 Tools for Assessing Quality of Life

General Well-Being and Quality of Life
- Dartmouth Primary Care Cooperative (COOP) Information
- Medical Outcomes Study SF-36 (Short Form 36) Health Status Questionnaire
- Sickness Impact Profile
- Nottingham Health Profile
- Quality of Well-Being Index

Psychological Status and Well-Being
- Profile of Mood States
- Beck Depression Inventory
- Center for Epidemiologic Studies Depression Inventory (CES-D)
- Spielberger State-Trait Anxiety Inventory

From American Association of Cardiovascular and Pulmonary Rehabilitation. *Guidelines for cardiac rehabilitation and secondary prevention programs* [4th ed., p. 185]. Champaign, IL: Human Kinetics.

BOX 33-3 Commonly Expressed Concerns After a Cardiac Event

What Can Be Expected From a Patient Regarding
- Emotions
- Symptoms
- Medication side effects
- Response to exercise or activity

When Can a Patient Resume
- Sexual activity
- Driving a car
- Recreational activities or sports
- Work-related activities
- Housework or laundry

How Does a Patient
- Manage stress effectively
- Exercise safely
- Know when to call a physician or emergency responder
- Eat properly
- Meet financial needs
- Modify lifestyle to control risk factors

Data from Karem, C. (1989). *A practical guide to cardiac rehabilitation.* Philadelphia: Aspen.

- Visual, auditory, or other sensory impairments
- Functional abilities
- Age or developmental factors

Millions of persons in the United States are unable to comprehend materials written above the sixth-grade reading level; many are functionally illiterate or speak a primary language other than English. Elderly persons, who account for a large percent of the population, also have a 30% to 40% rate of illiteracy. In addition, many elderly persons require large print, which is visualized better against a contrasting color. For example, dark letters printed on yellow, light blue, or white paper are easier for them to read.

Educational resources are becoming more sophisticated and readily available. For example, educational materials may include anatomical views of coronary arteries showing blockages of the coronary arteries after the angiograms or pictures that illustrate surgical procedures or complementary product guides from companies that manufacture prosthetic valves and pacemakers. A number of major organizations, such as the American Heart Association and private vendor or manufacturing companies, have available educational materials, charts, videocassette tapes, handout materials, interactive computer programs, and anatomical models. Also, many websites are available. Preview any prepackaged or "canned" educational materials to individualize the content to meet patient goals, match program philosophy, and ensure information is current and accurate.

Although patients and family members clearly benefit from a variety of educational materials, materials are selected based on the assessment of their learning needs and styles. As a rule families prefer simple and illustrated materials that provide complete and informative explanations over highly technical data, unless they request otherwise. The nurse controls the temptation to overload them with materials they will *never* use.

Nursing Diagnoses and Therapeutic Goals. Many of the relevant NANDA-I diagnostic categories for inpatient cardiac rehabilitation continue to apply. Additional diagnostic categories may be risk-prone health behavior, ineffective health maintenance, and sexual dysfunction.

The early outpatient goals are to (1) control symptoms, (2) improve functional abilities, (3) improve exercise tolerance, and (4) modify cardiac risk factors. The key lifestyle changes recommended for patients in a cardiac rehabilitation program are the same as those proposed as preventive measures for others:

- Weight management (BMI less than 25 kg/m²)
- Lipid Management National Cholesterol Education Program (NCEP guidelines) to improve LDL/HDL ratio; utilizing low-fat, low-cholesterol diet and may include medications
- Complete cessation of smoking and exposure to second-hand smoke
- Reduction or elimination of alcohol intake
- Incorporation of stress management and effective coping strategies
- Physical activity according to a prescribed exercise program

- Blood pressure control
- Diabetes management

Emerging risk factors include elevated homocysteine levels above 15 mmol/L and elevated C-reactive protein markers.

Therapeutic Plan and Interventions. In addition to cardiac care, cardiac care: rehabilitation, anticipatory guidance, anxiety reduction, teaching: prescribed diet, teaching: prescribed activity/exercise, and teaching: disease process, the NIC classifications in early outpatient cardiac rehabilitation include risk identification, role enhancement, coping enhancement teaching: sexuality, health education and health care information exchange. Lifestyle education joins exercise as a foundational component.

Addressing Patient/Family Learning Needs. Patients and families need to be informed and knowledgeable for effective decision making and problem solving about lifestyle choices, behaviors, and specific interventions. Patients are taught to understand their risk factors and learn about those lifestyle habits or preferences that may help modify or reduce their coronary risk level. Lifestyle changes are one of the few areas over which a patient has direct control. Because lifestyle behaviors are embedded in everyday activities and patterns, as well as having cultural or emotional values, they are difficult to change in the short term and even more difficult to change on a long-term basis.

Education is a key function in cardiac rehabilitation programs and a crucial factor in a patient's long-term outcome, but the "window of opportunity" to provide education may be extremely short. The site and format for an educational program can be adapted to meet the available space and group size. For instance, one-on-one interactions, group classes, discussion groups, peer or support groups, and other configurations are conducted in person, via video, closed circuit television, and chat rooms via the Internet.

Many programs offer a series of educational sessions conducted by the members of the cardiac team. As far as possible, scheduling for educational sessions should be modified so both families and patients are able to attend all sessions. Many programs are offered in the evening or on Saturday mornings. The content of the program provides information about the cardiac event, treatments and procedures, lifestyle activities, exercise prescriptions, and medical alerts. Time for participants to raise concerns and ask questions is exceedingly important. As a result, patients and families often are able to provide assistance to one another by passing along information or sharing solutions to otherwise troublesome problems, which is an empowering activity.

Although an educational program necessarily contains standardized content and information, the nurse assesses each patient and family to identify learner variables that will influence their perspective on learning, identify any barriers to learning, and determine the type and mode most appropriate to be used for this patient's educational materials (Table 33-3).

Exercise Prescription. The exercise component of cardiac rehabilitation is individualized for each patient as a means of

TABLE 33-3 Assessment of Learner Variables in Cardiac Rehabilitation

Variables	Assessment Area
Individual	Demographics Developmental stage Education Prior illness experience
Sociocultural	Culture/ethnicity Beliefs about condition Social construction or meaning
Illness related	Status of illness Stage of intervention Anticipated outcome Physical limitations Social limitations Diagnostic activities
Situational	Patient/family system Extended family/significant others Social network or support system
Cardiac status	Specific symptoms and impact Diagnostics and treatment Therapeutic regimens: diet, exercise, medications Illness trajectory

From Jillings, C. R. (1988). *Cardiac rehabilitation nursing.* Rockville, MD: Aspen. Copyright 1988 by Aspen. Reprinted by permission.

BOX 33-4 Adverse Responses to Inpatient Exercise Leading to Exercise Discontinuation

- Diastolic BP ≥110 mm Hg
- Decrease in systolic BP >10 mm Hg
- Significant ventricular or atrial arrhythmias
- Second- or third-degree heart block
- Signs/symptoms of exercise intolerance, including angina pectoris, marked dyspnea, and electrocardiogram changes suggestive of ischemia

From American Association of Cardiovascular and Pulmonary Rehabilitation. (2004). *Guidelines for cardiac rehabilitation and secondary prevention programs* [4th ed., p. 36]. Champaign, IL: Human Kinetics. *BP,* Blood pressure.

reaching cardiovascular conditioning goals. This is in effect an exercise prescription. Data collection begins with the patient's complete medical history, current health status, medication profile, lifestyle data, and level of fitness based on multiple results from exercise testing including workload, heart rate, and blood pressure, and any signs of dysrhythmia or ischemia. The prescription is a written program or "dosage" for exercise that describes the type or mode of exercise; how often it is to be performed; and the duration, intensity, and rate of progression.

Intensity describes the level of demand at which an activity is performed and is tailored to each patient's status. Patients are monitored closely for signs or symptoms of myocardial ischemia or ventricular dysrhythmias or various other criteria (Box 33-4) for termination of the exercise session. Patients should be familiar with the various scales used during exercise sessions. The most commonly used scale is the Borg scale for rating perceived exertion (AACVPR, 2004, p. 80). Other ratings include angina, claudication, and dyspnea scales. The mode of activity describes how the exercise employs the large muscle groups in sustained and rhythmic activity, most commonly walking. Other appropriate modes include cycling, jogging, rowing, arm ergometry, and aquatic exercises. Duration of exercise refers simply to the length of time an activity is to be performed. When upper extremities are exercised, care is taken related to intensity so that blood pressure is not increased. Patients are taught to avoid the Valsalva maneuver when performing upper extremity exercises and when lifting weights. Learning yoga breathing techniques helps to prevent patients from holding their breath. Initially exercises are

performed at low intensity and should not produce angina, sore muscles, or undue fatigue.

Related to weight training, the American Congress of Rehabilitation Medicine and the American Academy of Physical Medicine and Rehabilitation published the recommendation of DeGroot, Quinn, Kertzer, Vroman, and Olney (1998) that stable cardiac patients on a circuit weight-training program start with initial load between 40% and 60% 1-RM (one repetition maximum) and at least 60 seconds of rest between exercise.

The exercise prescription ensures that the exercise session is both beneficial and safe. Age-related target heart rates are not used as guides for cardiac programs. Guidelines for the exercise prescription are derived from research results and are usually written by an exercise physiologist, who understands the principles and physiology of exercise (ACSM, 1998). Each component of the exercise session is modified further by a patient's prognosis of risk (risk stratification factor), which is used to identify patients who may be a higher risk for developing complications during an exercise session. Other guidelines contain information about patient selection for exercise and contraindications for exercise. Remember that current guidelines are not completely predictive of complications during supervised activity (Paul-Labrador, Vongvanich, & Merz, 1999).

Metabolic Equivalent Method. Exercise and activity requirements are described using the metabolic equivalent (MET) method. One MET is equivalent to the amount of oxygen an individual requires while standing at rest, or 3.5 ml of O_2/kg/min (Woods, Froelicher, & Motzer, 2000). Increased expenditure of energy levels results in multiplication of MET values—that is, a 2-MET activity uses oxygen at twice the rate of a 1-MET resting activity, or an 8-MET activity uses oxygen at 8 times the resting rate.

The MET method is easy to understand and can be related to both occupational and leisure activities. For example, a patient may have ischemic ECG changes at a level of 6 METs on a graded exercise test. Therefore this patient's instructions should direct him or her to perform activities that are at or below the level of 5 METs. Patients often do not estimate the actual energy requirements—METs—for daily activities or leisurely pursuits. Women routinely have been found to underestimate the energy requirements needed to complete household tasks and thus often work at higher MET levels than recommended soon after a cardiac event.

Exercise Regimen. The exercise session or activity program consists of warm-up, conditioning/exercise, and cool down (Woods et al., 2000). The purpose of a warm-up is to prepare muscles and joints for the pending activity, which is exercise. This requires between 5 and 15 minutes of stretching activities and ROM exercises, by which time the resting metabolic rate (1 MET) has increased to a level necessary for beginning the conditioning segment of the session.

The composition of the conditioning activity is guided by the individualized exercise prescription for frequency, intensity, mode, and duration of exercise, which is approximately 20 to 30 minutes. Although frequency may be set at several times daily, exercises sessions for outpatients generally are set for 3 to 5 times a week. Little benefit has been found to be derived from exercise more frequent than 5 times weekly. Persons with diabetes mellitus may need to exercise daily related to maintaining their insulin sensitivity, however. The 5- to 10-minute cool-down segment of the session is extremely important. This cool-down time allows the heart rate to gradually return to normal and prevents venous pooling, which can precipitate hypotension and other cardiac complications.

Ideal climates for exercise are those with less than 65% humidity and temperatures between 40° and 75° F. Exercising under ideal conditions is not always feasible but certainly is preferable for patients who have cardiac conditions. Extremes of heat and humidity are major concerns to health; whenever the humidity exceeds 65%, the metabolic rate required for activities is increased. Excessive heat results in vasodilation, which reduces blood return to the heart, decreases the blood pressure, and elevates the heart rate. Heat stress may occur in hot air or hot water temperatures and may result in the vasodilatation cycle when a patient is using alcohol or nitrates.

Patients may choose to modify the environment or alter their exercise time. For example, in hot, humid climates as found in the South, patients may exercise outdoors in the cooler morning or late evenings; during the day they would use an air-conditioned or environmentally controlled indoor space. On the other hand, cold temperatures also increase peripheral resistance and thus raise the workload of the heart. Patients should consider the fabric and type of clothing worn for exercise so it is appropriate for the weather conditions. For example, covering the mouth and nose with a scarf is effective in prevention of cold-induced bronchospasms. Polypropylene/cool-max fabric wicks away moisture (especially important for persons with diabetes mellitus). No matter the conditions, the patient should be encouraged to drink water before, during, and after each exercise session to prevent dehydration.

The early outpatient phase is the period within which patients experience the highest cardiac mortality rates after hospitalization. Frequent contact, monitoring, and support are essential to assist patients in judging their behaviors and activities and for determining when they have medical complications or emergencies. Many patients return home at low risk and can be monitored effectively by nurses from community-based cardiac rehabilitation programs. A number of models to serve low-risk patients who live in geographically distant areas or who do not have cardiac rehabilitation programs nearby exist. Strategies for promoting success in early outpatient cardiac rehabilitation include the following:

- Provide referrals to community agencies or self-help groups for smoking cessation, weight loss or control, or spousal support meetings.
- Provide referrals for professional assistance such as psychosocial or mental health professionals, nutrition counseling or computerized dietary analysis, or professional assistance with comorbid conditions such as diabetes mellitus.
- Provide resources to assist with stress reduction and management when appropriate.
- Encourage accessible activities and events within tolerance levels to promote socialization.
- Generate written health contracts with assigned responsibilities for accomplishing mutually agreed-upon goals.
- Use logs, checklists, calendars, and other record-keeping aids to encourage patients to perform tasks and steps for meeting goals.
- Assess and intervene with the entire family system and any significant others, not only the patient.
- Ensure programs, groups, and referrals are culturally and religiously relevant and sensitive.

Special Patient Populations and Exercise. Several subgroups of patients require special considerations when planning exercise testing and formulating exercise prescriptions. Elderly persons have more frequent complications that involve deconditioning and may lead to functional limitations and responses that result in ineffective coping. These patients may require a longer time to achieve training goals; they may benefit from learning and practicing energy conservation measures, using low-impact exercises (especially walking or swimming), having longer warm-up periods, modifying or abstaining from exercise in undesirable climatic conditions, and attending to primary health needs.

Patients who have one or more chronic or disabling conditions in addition to cardiac disease require special exercise considerations that take into account requirements of each specific condition and the combined requirements of all the conditions. For example, increased exercise is most likely to alter the MET needs and carbohydrate metabolism for a patient with diabetes mellitus, creating a change in insulin or caloric balance. Patients with lower body impairments need to strengthen the upper body to achieve cardiovascular fitness. Likewise, adjustments are required for patients with respiratory disorders, arthritic conditions, chronic fatigue syndrome, or those who have had a stroke and patients who have been recipients of a pacemaker or a heart transplant.

Modified exercise routines or adapted equipment are needed for those who have altered or impaired function and sensation resulting from spinal cord injury or amputation or who have hemiplegia. However, cardiac rehabilitation teams must use care not to focus only on cardiac management of the disability for these latter patients without attention to the patient's one or more chronic conditions and primary care needs.

Rehabilitation nurses examine program plans to meet cardiac goals to ensure these do not interfere with other constraints or needs a patient may have due to comorbidity. This entails a holistic assessment with provisions to prevent further complications or disabilities in facilities or community settings.

Pertinent issues include safety in the home, primary care and health maintenance, pain management, medication regimens that may become complex or costly, rest and energy conservation, recreation and activities, social network, nutritional requirements, religious or cultural dietary preferences, and use of health systems or products from sources other than the cardiac rehabilitation program.

Teaching Techniques. For each patient and family member, it is important to use educational techniques that educate both hemispheres of the brain. The left hemisphere is the analytic side of the brain, which deals with factual information delivered in a language format. To illustrate, the left hemisphere of the brain is learning when a person makes statements such as, "Tell me about . . ." or "Explain to me . . ." or "I don't understand. . . ." Written materials are examples of tools for left-brain education. In contrast, the right hemisphere is the visual-spatial side of the brain, which prefers to deal with models, drawings, figures, and pictures. The right hemisphere of the brain is learning when a person makes statements such as, "Show me . . ." or "Let me see it. . . ." Diagrams and drawings are methods for educating persons with right-brain learning.

Calendars and other data management tools are inexpensive, portable, and easy to use and interpret. They are useful for recording appointments, class times, reminders for follow-up such as with laboratory test results, and other scheduling matters. The same calendar functions as an activity log. Data records can be maintained to show a profile of a patient's changes in weight, daily glucose levels, vital signs or blood pressure, as-needed medication use, occurrence of symptoms, exercise levels, diet changes, or similar events. When these logs are analyzed to show patterns of behavior, the results become a powerful teaching tool created by the patient.

Maintenance and Follow-Up

Maintenance and follow-up begins within 2 to 3 months of the cardiac event. Cardiac rehabilitation continues long term at the hospital or clinic site, at home, or at a community exercise facility under the direction of rehabilitation staff as well as the patient's self direction. The maintenance and follow-up phase of cardiac rehabilitation is lifelong. Because these patients are now more clinically stable and knowledgeable about their activity limits, professional supervision is tapered. Activities and exercises are more aggressive. Organized educational programs

designed to maintain participation and accomplish lifestyle changes become more important. Access to continuing education is through hospital or community health classes and video/Internet programs. Rehabilitation staff monitor compliance with lifestyle changes through regularly scheduled follow-up via one or all of the following: on-site checkups, telephone calls, e-mail contacts, and mailed surveys.

Assessment. Many patients who have participated in cardiac rehabilitation programs eventually are able to return to work. Older persons are less likely to return to work than those who are in primary wage-earning years unless there are preexisting medical reasons. Although work and working have high value in the United States, patients and employers may have a sense of fear or confusion about an employee's health status after a cardiovascular incident. As with other behavioral questions, sorting out the complex variables in determining whether a patient actually returns to work is not an exact science. Assessment of an individual patient's ability to return to work and the capacity for a safe expeditious return to the workforce is conducted by the entire cardiac rehabilitation team, including the patient's physician.

Return to Work. Physical, psychosocial, and medical factors as well as age, access to work, financial situation, and family support are all factors in a patient's return to work. Examples of questions a patient, family, and employer ask include the following:

- Is the person medically stable and able to return to work?
- How soon can work be resumed and at what level of function?
- Are other comparable, less strenuous positions available?
- Can the same job functions be performed?
- Are there any types of barriers?
- Are physical structure or equipment modifications necessary?
- How does the environment need to be altered?
- Does the person have disability coverage or other financial support?
- Do the patient and company want the patient to return to work?

The cardiac rehabilitation team is prepared to work with a patient and family to assess the readiness to return to work and the conditions for doing so. Initially patients complete a treadmill test to identify and calculate the MET level at which they are able to function safely without encountering problems. Some patients are able to improve their MET score after exercise training for cardiovascular fitness. It is important for patients to have a realistic evaluation of the ability to perform work and other activities so they do not overextend themselves on the job or restrict themselves needlessly. The patient's view of self in the sick role or with learned helplessness is an indicator for a psychosocial assessment, which may reveal a need for counseling before work is attempted.

Nursing Diagnoses and Therapeutic Goals. The additional nursing diagnostic categories for maintenance and

BOX 33-5 Electronic Resources and Support Group Information

Heartmates
PO Box 16202
Minneapolis, MN 55416
http://www.heartmates.com/cardiac.html

Heart Information Network (information resource)
Center for Cardiovascular Education, Inc.
New Providence, NJ
http://www.heartinfo.org

Krames Communication
780 Township Line Road
Yardley, PA 19067
800-333-3032 (6 AM to 5 PM Pacific time)
http://www.krames.com

Prichett and Hull Associates, Inc. (information resource)
3440 Oak Cliff Road NE, Suite 110
Atlanta, GA 30340-3079
800-241-4925
http://www.p-h.com

BOX 33-6 Cardiac Rehabilitation Reference Organizations

The American College of Cardiology
Heart House
9111 Old Georgetown Road
Bethesda, MD 20814-1699
800-253-4636
http://www.acc.org/index.htm

American Association of Cardiovascular and Pulmonary Rehabilitation
401 W. Michigan Street
Suite 2200
Chicago, IL 60611
http://www.aacvpr.org

American College of Sports Medicine
401 W. Michigan Street
Indianapolis, IN 46202-3233
http://www.acsm.org

American Heart Association
7272 Greenville Avenue
Dallas, TX 75231-4596
http://www.americanheart.org

American Nurses Credentialing Center
8515 Georgia Avenue
Suite 400
Silver Spring, MD 20910-3492
http://www.nursingworld.org/ancc

follow-up may be ineffective coping, complicated grieving, noncompliance, ineffective role performance, and social isolation. The therapeutic goals are to integrate lifestyle changes and eventually to accomplish lifelong lifestyle changes, reconstruct one's life in context of health status, and reintegrate into the community. By 6 months after the event, patients and families have begun to recognize that lifestyle changes, self-monitoring, and exercise are lifelong goals. At the same time they have been able to reconstruct their lives within the parameters of the patient's condition and abilities. For some patients this means few changes beyond eliminating detrimental health habits and adhering to exercising; others encounter major adjustments and complications; some have great difficulties or fail.

Therapeutic Plans and Interventions. Cardiac rehabilitation, support group, support system enhancement, emotional support, coping enhancement, counseling, anxiety reduction, role enhancement, and family integrity promotion are NIC interventions during maintenance and follow-up. These interventions are addressed in the following paragraphs specific to cardiac rehabilitation.

Support Systems. Services that are enjoyable, accessible, and acceptable for a patient are more likely to be used. Support groups and social activities for patients and families may promote attendance. Social networks and social support are two factors that have been found to be valid predictors of outcome after MI. Networking among patients and family members is one way to provide needed psychological support throughout all stages of illness and rehabilitation. Involvement of all family members is imperative because family members benefit from networking and sharing experiences whether the patient is in a critical care unit or any of the other stages of recovery.

Support Groups. Support groups may be organized or informal; many become very creative, but they exist to meet the needs of persons who participate in them. For example, separate groups may be organized for spouses, children and parents, or patients to present issues or address specific concerns of the group. Some programs organize groups according to diagnostic criteria such as persons with pacemakers, those with congestive heart failure, persons who receive medical treatment, or those who have surgical interventions.

Electronic support groups are flourishing among patients and families who have personal computers with modem, communications software, and Internet access (Box 33-5). Personal computers offer a new form of networking that can extend locally, nationally, or even internationally. Advantages of electronic support groups include the following:

1. Twenty-four-hour access is available.
2. The system can be used from home or facility.
3. Patients choose topics to read and to which to respond.
4. Patients and family are ensured privacy, anonymity, and control.
5. A hard copy of all transactions can be printed.
6. Professional personnel are able to exchange information and obtain interactive consultations (Box 33-6).

Work Hardening Program. Work hardening is a general term as well as the title for a program that has specific characteristics and goals to determine whether a patient returns to work, or under what auspices. The work hardening program may range from 2 to 8 hours per day. It consists of simulated work-related tasks that may become progressively difficult until the patient is able (or unable) to perform the functional tasks as he or she would be required to do on the job. These tasks are performed under supervision of a trained therapist and in a structured environment.

In some work hardening programs, a patient and team member conduct a detailed workplace assessment, documenting activities that would occur during a typical day. They note details of the work style, such as whether a patient is sitting at a computer terminal versus climbing or lifting versus standing in an assembly line. The workplace environment and availability of services, such as food choices in the cafeteria and location and accessibility of lavatories, are inspected; the patient's commute to work and means of transportation during regular commuting hours are assessed; and the number of stressful situations and the degree to which the patient identifies stressors are noted. The workplace load is calculated in METs, which are compared with the patient's exercise test MET level. The MET level, health status, and exercise prescription are important determinants of the patient's ability to return to work.

Other common components of a work hardening program include functional activities; cardiovascular conditioning; education about proper use of body mechanics to prevent overtaxing, strain, or injury; and a variety of techniques for managing job-related and personal stressors.

Home-Based or Unsupervised Exercise Programs. Patients who are unable to attend or access medically supervised exercise classes may be candidates for home exercise training according to a specific exercise prescription. Under certain conditions patients may be eligible for partial reimbursement for intermittent community health nursing services, therapies, and medical supplies. A large number of community-based providers offer a wide array of health care services for patients with varying payment options. However, patients and families need to be educated to choose services that ensure a complete assessment followed by ongoing coordination, continuity, and communication with the cardiac rehabilitation program.

Modern technology has made home exercise programs more practical by improving communications between a patient and the cardiac rehabilitation center. With the availability of telephone, fax, e-mail, web-based Internet sites, CDs, DVDs; Internet and phone links to health providers, and other electronic telecommunication, patients who would otherwise be without services can access a cardiac rehabilitation team. The nurse as coordinator, educator, advocate, and assessor-evaluator is a key link in communication.

Patients and family members need to be able to demonstrate their knowledge about the individualized exercise prescription, precautions including environmental conditions,

signs and symptoms to be reported to the cardiac rehabilitation team, and criteria for terminating exercise. Emergency telephone numbers should be entered into cellular phones or programed into speed-dial systems. Emergency response or electronic emergency systems are available in many communities. As additional precautions, patients may have emergency medical information devices or wear medical alert bracelets and carry diagnosis and treatment cards. Those who have implanted cardiac pacemakers or implanted cardioverter defibrillators should have special information regarding their status and care readily available.

Patients and families need to make arrangements with the primary physician and members of the cardiac rehabilitation team concerning content of any advance directives or do-not-resuscitate orders. The patient's situation, preferences, and special needs should be known to members of the local emergency response units, the pharmacist, vendors who supply equipment or goods such as oxygen and backup supplies for electricity or heat, and other similar services or personnel.

EVALUATION

Evaluation is a necessary component of a cardiac rehabilitation program to (1) assess the effectiveness in providing patient care, (2) maintain accreditation, (3) seek reimbursement, and (4) use the information to guide quality improvement strategies. Likewise, evaluation is part of the nursing process. Both process and outcome evaluations are appropriate for all phases of the cardiac rehabilitation program.

Process Evaluation

Process evaluation provides a means to judge and document the rehabilitation process, including the activities and behaviors of all team members. The cardiac rehabilitation program can be compared to the published program standards and the published standard competencies for professionals in cardiac rehabilitation. Appropriate standards of care also provide a means to conduct a process evaluation and document all team members' actions.

Outcome Evaluation

Outcome evaluation provides a means to judge and document the effectiveness of the cardiac rehabilitation program. Health and functioning are key outcomes of cardiac rehabilitation. The American Association of Cardiovascular and Pulmonary Rehabilitation Outcomes Committee adopted Green's health education framework (Green, Kreuter, Deeds, & Partridge, 1980) as a model to examine the outcome dimensions of cardiac rehabilitation using the dimensions of health, clinical, and behavioral domains (Pashkow et al., 1995). The AACVPR (2004, p. 184) has since added a new domain to provide measurement options for assessing other aspects of program effectiveness related to patient satisfaction and financial and economic considerations.

These measurements include the patient's perception of physical improvement, satisfaction with risk factor alteration,

TABLE 33-4 Potential Nursing Outcomes Classification (NOC) for Cardiac Rehabilitation

Inpatient Rehabilitation	Early Outpatient Rehabilitation	Maintenance and Follow-Up
Activity tolerance	Activity tolerance	Adherence behavior
	Adherence behavior	Acceptance: health status
Ambulation	Ambulation	
Anxiety level	Anxiety self-control	Psychosocial adjustment: life change
Cardiac pump effectiveness		
Circulation status		
Blood coagulation		
		Compliance behavior
		Coping
	Depression self-control	Depression self-control
Endurance		
Family participation in professional care		
Fluid balance		
		Grief resolution
Cardiac disease management	Cardiac disease management	Cardiac disease self-management
Knowledge: illness care	Knowledge: prescribed activity	
	Health seeking behavior	Health seeking behavior
Medication response		
Rest	Energy conservation	Energy conservation
		Quality of life
Risk control: cardiovascular health	Risk control: cardiovascular health	Risk control: cardiovascular health
		Role performance
Self-care ADL	Self-care status: instrumental ADLs	
		Self-direction of care
		Support group
		Social support
	Symptom control	
Tissue perfusion: cardiac		
Tissue perfusion: peripheral		
		Personal well-being

Data from Moorhead, S., Johnson, M., & Maas, M. (2004) *Nursing Outcomes Classification (NOC)* (3rd ed.). St. Louis, MO: Mosby. *ADLs*, Activities of daily living.

psychosocial adjustments in interpersonal roles, and potential for returning to work at a level commensurate with the patient's skills. An elderly patient's outcome measures may include achievement of functional independence and prevention of premature disability (Singh, Schocken, Williams, & Stamey, 2004).

Cardiac rehabilitation improves subsequent prognosis (Brown, Taylor, Noorani, Stone, & Skidmore, 2003; Jolliffe et al, 2001; Taylor et al., 2004). The 2002 Cochrane review of the effects of exercise-based rehabilitation for patients with coronary heart disease reported a 27% reduction in all-cause mortality for exercise-only cardiac rehabilitation and a slightly less reduction for comprehensive cardiac rehabilitation. Total cardiac mortality was reduced by 31% and 26%, respectively, for each group (Jolliffe et al., 2001). Kodis et al. (2001) and Lavie and Milani (2000) found traditional cardiac rehabilitation improved functional capacity. Verill et al. (2001) found improved quality of life.

Biological factors such as fat distribution, body mass index, and body shape are being studied to determine their impact on cardiac rehabilitation outcomes.

The Nursing Outcomes Classification (NOC) outcomes appropriate to cardiac rehabilitation during one or more of the phases are in Table 33-4.

The most important outcome measurement related to DVT is to decrease the incidence of DVT, thereby decreasing the incidence of pulmonary emboli. The NOC outcomes that are appropriate for DVT are tissue perfusion: peripheral and knowledge: treatment regimen.

IMPLICATIONS

The future of cardiac rehabilitation programs includes offering more individualized services to a greater variety of patients and families regardless of their geographical location. The needs of an aging population and noninsured population in an era of shrinking hospital stays and reimbursement issues are accompanied by social changes in work patterns and lifestyles, electronic technology, and a growing body of research knowledge. Patients with chronic CHF need to be further incorporated into cardiac rehabilitation programs. Reconditioning strategies need to be explored; for example, low-frequency electrical stimulation of quadriceps and calf muscles has been found to increase exercise capacity without increase in cardiac output (Maillefert et al., 1998). Besides weight training, additional strategies such as tai chi chuan, yoga, stress management, and relaxation strategies need to be studied for their possible contribution to cardiac rehabilitation. Findings from research of highly structured and uniform aspects of cardiac rehabilitation programs need to be translated into programs that are available to all patients who have experienced a cardiac event and their families, not only those who are geographically or financially available. Prevention, education for self-care, and lifestyle modification are key components for improved outcomes.

Case Study

Mrs. Doe, a 68-year-old widow, suffered an acute anterior MI complicated by CHF. At discharge from hospitalization she had an ejection fraction of 30%, no signs or symptoms of CHF, no murmur or gallop, and no crackles. She lives 100 miles from the nearest "formal" cardiac rehabilitation program in a rural area with two pets. Her children live out of state. She described her neighbors as "helpful whenever I call."

A treadmill test before hospital discharge documented her tolerance of 1 to 2 METs. Mrs. Doe had been very active with yard and garden work before her MI. Her risk factors for atherosclerosis include total cholesterol level 220 mg/dl (high) and HDL 40 mg/dl (low). She does not use tobacco but has had heavy tobacco smoke exposure until 1.5 years ago. She has type 2 diabetes mellitus and mild rheumatoid arthritis for which she takes Motrin 600 mg qid with Prilosec 20 mg daily. She had a hysterectomy with oophorectomy 10 years ago and is not on estrogen replacement therapy. Mrs. Doe's nursing diagnoses, NIC interventions, and NOC outcomes are presented in Table 33-6.

At Discharge From Inpatient Hospitalization

Because 80% of patients experiencing an acute MI return to pre-infarction activity level, education, activities, and follow-up were designed to facilitate this return to "normal" lifestyle.

Home health care referral was arranged to provide continued education, continued assessment, and on-site follow-up. The home health care agency had a formal program for post-MI and CHF patients using specialty nurses and additional professionals such as physical therapists, dietitians, and social workers. The home health care nurse needed to confer with appropriate cardiac rehabilitation personnel regarding an increase in exercise or activity plan.

MI teaching included definition, cause, healing process, rationale for activity/exercise limitations and recommendations, signs and symptoms to report, and awareness of preinfarctional anginal symptoms.

CHF teaching included definition; cause; factors that lower/raise risk of reoccurrence; signs and symptoms to report; rationale of no-added-salt diet; rationale regarding patient continuing daily weights and reporting cumulative weight gain of 2 pounds to the home health care nurse, physician, or cardiac rehabilitation personnel; daily weight rules (approximate same time, same amount of clothing, no weights on carpeted floor, and use only on set scale [home health care personnel should use patient's scales also]); and importance of early symptom awareness and reporting.

Mrs. Doe was taught what emotions, symptoms, medication side effects, and response to exercise and activity to expect, as well as what to report and to whom.

TABLE 33-5 Nursing Diagnoses, Interventions, and Outcomes Applicable to Mrs. Doe
NIC/NOC

Nursing Diagnosis	Nursing Interventions	Nursing Outcomes: Inpatient Through Maintenance/Follow-Up	
Activity intolerance	Teaching: prescribed activity/exercise	Rest Activity tolerance Ambulation Self-care ADL	Energy conservation/quality of life Activity tolerance/endurance Knowledge: prescribed activity Self-care IADL Adherence behaviors/acceptance: health status/self-direction of care
Decreased cardiac output	Cardiac precautions (inpatient only)	Fluid balance	Same
Ineffective tissue perfusion	Cardiac care: acute (inpatient only) Cardiac care Cardiac care: rehabilitation	Cardiac pump effectiveness Tissue perfusion: cardiac	Same Same
Deficient knowledge	Teaching: disease process Teaching: prescribed diet Teaching: prescribed medications Anticipatory guidance	Knowledge: Illness care Compliance behavior Medication response Coping	
Ineffective health maintenance	Risk identification Health education Health care information exchange	Risk control: cardiovascular health	Health seeking behavior Personal well-being

Data from Moorhead, S., Johnson, M., & Maas, M. (Eds.). (2004). *Nursing outcomes classification (NOC)* (3rd ed.). St. Louis, MO: Mosby; Dochterman, J. M., & Bulechek, G. M. (2004). *Nursing interventions classification (NIC)* (4th ed.). St. Louis, MO: Mosby; and NANDA International. (2007). *NANDA-I nursing diagnoses: Definitions & classification 2007-2008*. Philadelphia: Author.

Case Study—cont'd

The home health care nurse guided Mrs. Doe as to resuming work, sex, driving, recreation (e.g., gardening, club activities), and housework. Together they reviewed which MET activities were permitted and projected when additional activities may be added to the established schedule.

Mrs. Doe was helped to learn how to exercise and eat properly and safely, manage stress, and control risk factors—lower LDL level to below 70 mg/dl, raise HDL level to above 50 mg/dl, and lower triglycerides to below 200 mg/dl; maintain type 2 diabetes mellitus status under strict control, fasting blood sugar (FBS) level between 80 and 110 mg/dl or HbA_{1c} less than 7.0%; maintain blood pressure below 130/85 mm Hg; and maintain BMI below 25 kg/m².

Mrs. Doe learned when to call her physician, her home health care nurse, or the cardiac rehabilitation personnel. Clear lines of communication were put in place for all parties involved by the home health care nurse.

Specific information on which activities were allowed and which were not were provided. The type of exercise was adjusted to Mrs. Doe's life and routines of daily living. She learned what symptoms indicated she should terminate an activity or exercise. She used the rule of thumb that 30 minutes after an activity or exercise she should feel good. If she was tired after 30 minutes, she probably had overdone. She learned not to push the speed of an activity or exercise too fast. Gradually increasing the time of an exercise or activity was preferred before increasing the speed of work.

CRITICAL THINKING

1. Persons with inflammatory arthritis (i.e., rheumatoid arthritis [RA] and systemic lupus erythematosus [SLE]) are at high risk for heart disease. Inflammation in rheumatic disease is a predictor of cardiovascular disease. With the evidence linking inflammation to diseased blood vessels, it is now thought that the inflammation in RA and SLE accelerates the process of atherosclerosis. What needs to be taken into consideration in the management of Mrs. Doe's RA that will promote cardiovascular health, and what may negatively impact her cardiovascular health?

2. What are Mrs. Doe's cardiac risk factors, and what measures should be introduced to lower or control these risk factors?

3. Complete a risk assessment scale for DVT using the tool given in this chapter for the case study patient presented in Chapter 24.

REFERENCES

American Association of Cardiovascular and Pulmonary Rehabilitation. (2004). *Guidelines for cardiac rehabilitation and secondary prevention programs* (4th ed.). Champaign, IL: Human Kinetics.

American College of Sports Medicine. (1998). *Guidelines for exercise testing and prescription* (5th ed.). Baltimore: Williams & Wilkins.

American Heart Association. (2002). *Heart facts 2002: All Americans: Cardiovascular diseases still no.1.* Available from http://www.amhrt.org.

America Heart Association. (2005). *Heart disease and stroke statistics—2005 update.* Dallas, Texas: American Heart Association. Available from http://www.amhrt.org.

Blackburn, G. C., Foody, J. M., Sprecher, D. L., Park, E., Appenson-Hansen, C., & Pashkow, F. J. (2000). Cardiac rehabilitation participation patterns in a large tertiary center: Evidence for selection bias. *Journal of Cardiopulmonary Rehabilitation, 20,* 189-195.

Brown, A., Taylor, R., Noorani, H., Stone, J., & Skidmore, B. (2003). *Exercise-based cardiac rehabilitation programs for coronary artery disease: A systematic clinical and economic review* (Technology Report No. 34). Ottawa, Ontario, Canada: Canadian Coordinating Office for Health Technology Assessment.

Bunker, S., & Goble, A. (2003). Cardiac rehabilitation: Underreferral and underutilization. *Medical Journal of Australia, 179,* 332-333.

DeGroot, D. W., Quinn, T. J., Kertzer, R., Vroman, N. B., & Olney, W. B. (1998). Lactic acid accumulation in cardiac patients performing circuit weight training: Implications for exercise prescription. *Archives of Physical Medicine & Rehabilitation, 79,* 838-841.

Goodman, J. M., Pallandi, D. V., Reading, J. R., Plyley, M. J., Liu, P. P., & Kavanah. T. (1999). Central and peripheral adaptations after 12 weeks of exercise training in post-coronary artery surgery patients. *Journal of Cardiopulmonary Rehabilitation, 19,* 144-150.

Grace, S. L., Abbey, S., Shnek, Z., Irvine, J., Franche, R. L., & Stewart, D. (2002). Cardiac rehabilitation II: Referral and participation. *General Hospital Psychiatry, 24,* 127-134.

Grace, S. L., Evindar, A., Abramson, B., & Stewart, D. (2004). Physician management preferences for cardiac patients: Factors affecting referral to cardiac rehabilitation. *Canadian Journal of Cardiology, 20,* 1101-1107.

Grace, S. L., Evindar, A., Kung, T., Scholey, P., & Stewart, D. (2004). Automatic referral to cardiac rehabilitation. *Medical Care, 42,* 661-669.

Green, L., Kreuter, M., Deeds, S., & Partridge, K. (1980). *Health education planning: A diagnostic approach.* Palo Alto, CA: Mayfield.

Jolliffe, J. A., Rees, K., Taylor, R. S., Thompson, D., Oldridge, N., & Ebrahim, S. (2001). Exercise-based rehabilitation for coronary heart disease. *Cochrane Database Systematic Reviews.* 1:CD001800. The Cochrane Library, Hoboken, NJ: John Wiley & Sons.

Kodis, S., Smith, K. M., Arthur, H. M., Daniels, C., Suskin, N., & McKelvie, R. S. (2001). Changes in exercise capacity and lipids after clinic versus home based aerobic training in coronary artery bypass graft surgery patients. *Journal of Cardiopulmonary Rehabilitation, 21,* 31-36.

Lavie, C. J., & Milani, R. V. (2000). Disparate effects of improving aerobic exercise capacity and quality of life after cardiac rehabilitation in young and elderly coronary patients. *Journal of Cardiopulmonary Rehabilitation, 20,* 235-240.

Maillefert, J. F., Eicher, J. C., Walker, P., Dulieu, V., Rouhier-Narcer, I., Branly, F., et al. (1998). *Journal of Cardiopulmonary Rehabilitation, 18,* 277-282.

Missik, E. (2001). Women and cardiac rehabilitation: Accessibility issues and policy recommendations. *Rehabilitation Nursing, 21,* 141-147.

Mitoff, P. R., Wesolowski, M., Abramson, B. L., & Grace, S. L. (2005). Patient-provider communication regarding referral to cardiac rehabilitation. *Rehabilitation Nursing, 30,* 140-146.

NANDA International. (2007). *NANDA-I nursing diagnoses: Definitions & classification 2007-2008.* Philadelphia: Author.

Pashkow, P., Ades, P. A., Emery, C. F., Feid, D. J., Miller, N. A., Peske, G., et al. (1995). Outcome measurement in cardiac and pulmonary rehabilitation by the AACVPR Outcomes Committee. *Journal of Cardiopulmonary Rehabilitation, 15,* 394-405.

Paul-Labrador, M., Vongvanich, P., & Merz, C. N. B. (1999). Risk stratification for exercise training in cardiac patients: Do the proposed guidelines work? *Journal of Cardiopulmonary Rehabilitation, 19,* 118-125.

Plach, S. K. (2002). Women and cardiac rehabilitation after heart surgery: Patterns of referral and adherence. *Rehabilitation Nursing, 27,* 104-109.

Shaw, G. (2000). *For depressed heart patients rehab can be a lifesaver.* Available from http://healthwatch.medscape.com/medscape/p/G_library/article.asp?RecID-2062527channel-11.

Singh, V. N., Schocken, D. D., Williams, K., & Stamey, R. (2004). *Cardiac rehabilitation.* Available from http://www.medicine.com/pmr/topic180.htm.

Stiller, J. J., & Holt, M. M. (2004). Factors influencing referral of cardiac patients for cardiac rehabilitation. *Rehabilitation Nursing, 29*(1), 18-23.

Taylor, R. S., Brown, A., Ebrahim, S., Joliffe, J. A., Noorami, H., Rees, K. et al. (2004). Exercise-based rehabilitation for patients with coronary artery disease: Systematic review and meta-analysis of randomized controlled trials. *American Journal of Medicine, 116,* 682-692.

Tierney, L. M., Jr., McPhee, S. J., & Papadakis, M. A. (2006). *Current medical diagnosis and treatment.* New York: Lange.

Verill, D., Barton, C., Beasley, W., Brennan, M., Lippard, M., & King, C. (2001). Quality of life measures and gender comparisons. *Journal of Cardiopulmonary Rehabilitation, 21,* 37-46.

Wenger, N. K., Froelicher E. S., Smith L. K., Ades, P. A., Berra, K., Blumenthal, J. A., et al. (1995, October). *Cardiac rehabilitation* (Clinical Practice Guidelines No. 17, AHCPR Publication No. 96-0672). Rockville, MD: U.S. Department of Health and Human Services, Public Health Service, Agency for Health Care Policy and Research and the National Heart, Lung, and Blood Institute.

Woods, S. L., Froelicher, E. S. S., & Motzer, S. U. (2000). *Cardiac nursing* (4th ed.). Philadelphia: J. B. Lippincott.

SUGGESTED READINGS

Balady, G. T., Fletcher, B. J., Froehicher, E. S., Hartley, L. H., Krauss, R. M., Oberman, A., et al. (1994). Cardiac rehabilitation: A statement for healthcare professionals from the American Heart Association. *Circulation, 90,* 1601-1610.

Mosca, L., Manson, J. E., Sutherland, S. E., Langer, R. D., Manolio, T., & Barrett-Conner, E. (1997). Cardiovascular disease in women: A statement for health care professionals from the American Heart Association. *Circulation, 96,* 2468-2482.

National Heart, Lung and Blood Institute. (1998, September). Clinical guidelines on identification, evaluation, and treatment of overweight and obesity in adults. Available from http://www.nhlbt.nih.gov/guidelines/obesity/ob_home.htm.

34

Rehabilitation Following Burn Injury

Patricia L. McCollom, MS, RN, CRRN, CDMS, CCM, CLC

It has been estimated that 1 million people experience a burn injury every year in the United States. Of these, 40,000 persons are admitted to hospitals and more than 4,000 die as a direct result of the injury (Burn Incidence and Treatment in U.S., 2007). Half of those with burns will have injuries severe enough to restrict daily activities in the home, school, or workplace, and burn injuries are a major reason for high medical and treatment costs. Rehabilitation is a critical component of recovery and community reintegration.

Though statistics are significant, review of data reveals declines in the national incidence of burn injury in the past two decades. This decline is in direct relation to prevention and a focus upon burn injury treatment. In addition, during this time period regional burn centers have been developed, smoke detectors are widely used, burn prevention education has expanded, occupational safety has been increased, and consumer product information has been emphasized. The decrease in burn incidence also reflects societal changes, such as a decrease in smoking, changes in cooking practices, and reduced industrial employment (Brown, Helm, & Weed, 2005).

This chapter provides information about burn injuries, treatment, and rehabilitation nursing interventions and outcomes. Although intensive care is necessary for acute burn injury care, it is the rehabilitation philosophy that facilitates return to function, coping with body image change, and dealing with long-term health issues.

INCIDENCE

Children ages 2 to 4 years and young adults ages 15 to 25 years are the age-groups with greater numbers of injuries from burns. Burn injuries rank second only to motor vehicle accidents as a cause of death during childhood.

Elderly persons experience high mortality and morbidity from burns (http://www.burnsurvivor.com/burn_statistics January2006). Older persons may not detect danger when preexisting problems such as altered or impaired judgment, decreased coordination and tactile sensation, or impaired vision or smell inhibit awareness.

Seventy percent of burns result from thermal injury. Thermal injury may be dry heat (flame) or moist heat (hot liquid). Thermal injury results in marked changes in the vascular and metabolic responses of the body, resulting in increased risk for infection, due to loss of skin integrity and postburn immunosuppression. Burns may also be caused by chemicals, electric current, or radiation. Scald injuries are the most frequent type of burn; however, flame injuries are more serious. Electrical and radiation burns may appear less severe on the skin surface but may affect underlying organs with damage that may not be known for days after injury. The direct cost of treating burn injuries is more than $1 billion per year. Indirect costs, including resulting disability, are several billion dollars annually (http://www.burnsurvivor.com/burn_statisticsJanuary2006).

PATHOPHYSIOLOGY

Burns are currently described in the clinical context as partial thickness and full thickness. This terminology more accurately describes the burn, indicating depth and severity of tissue injury (Figure 34-1).

Partial-thickness burns result in destruction of varying depths of the epidermis (outer layer of skin) to the dermis (middle layer of skin). The depth of tissue injury is described as superficial (involving only the epidermis) or deep partial thickness (involving the entire epidermis into the dermis). Partial-thickness burns are painful because nerve endings are injured and exposed. However, because epithelial cells are not destroyed, partial-thickness burns will heal. Blistering indicates deep partial-thickness burns. Blisters may increase in size, resulting from collection of tissue fluid. Dryness and itching are common during healing. The cause of this is

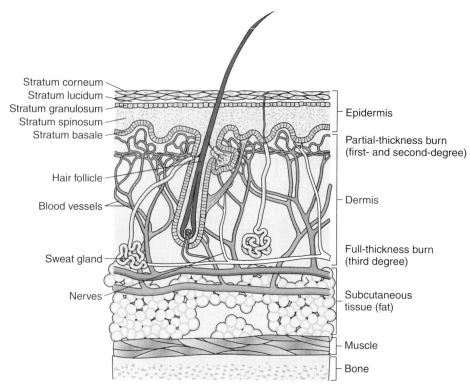

Figure 34-1 Levels of human skin involved in burns. (From Phipps, W. J., Sands, J. K., & Marek, J. F. [1999]. *Medical-surgical nursing: Concepts and clinical practice* [6th ed.]. St. Louis, MO: Mosby.)

increased vascularization, reduction of secretions, and decreased perspiration.

Full-thickness burns result in destruction of the epidermis and the dermis and possible damage to the subcutaneous tissue, muscle, and bone. Nerve endings are destroyed. The wounds become covered by eschar, a dark, thickened substance composed of denatured protein. Surface dehydration causes the eschar to form. Full-thickness burns require skin grafting because epithelial cells are destroyed.

Normal skin function is diminished as a result of burns. There is a loss of protective covering, escape of body fluids, lack of temperature control, loss of sweat and sebaceous glands, and loss of sensory receptors. The severity of these complex changes will determine local response or systemic response.

A major burn injury, despite the cause, is one of the most critical forms of trauma that an individual can endure (Wood et al., 2005). The initial physiological response to partial- and/or full-thickness burn injury is capillary vasoconstriction. Soon after, vasodilation occurs and plasma is released to the injury site. Within 24 hours increased clotting may occur, which will decrease or eliminate blood flow. Without proper blood supply, further cellular death will occur. Because of this dynamic process, the exact depth of a burn injury may not be apparent for 3 to 5 days. During this process massive fluid loss from open wounds and evaporation will occur, resulting in heat loss and elevated metabolism. Furthermore, when

skin integrity is compromised, the body is no longer protected from bacteria and local sepsis will occur rapidly as bacteria enter the wound. If the infection is not monitored closely and treated carefully, tissue will be destroyed. The depth of burn injury may deepen as a partial-thickness burn converts to full thickness. Life-threatening systemic involvement also may occur.

Burn shock may occur as a result of hypovolemia. As fluid escapes to surrounding tissue, edema progresses. Edema progresses until fluid impairs range of motion (ROM) and blood flow to other tissues. Cellular death, damage to peripheral nerves, and sensory and/or motor loss may occur. The respiratory system is affected either by facial/neck edema following burn injury or by hyperventilation and increased oxygen consumption from smoke inhalation, possibly requiring emergent intubation. Other systemic effects involve the gastrointestinal and renal systems. Because of the hemodynamic changes that occur with postburn crises, renal insufficiency as well as gastric dilation and gastrointestinal ileus are concerns. In addition, a suppressed immune system creates an ongoing risk of infection.

Wound Healing

In partial-thickness burns the epidermal cells lining the hair follicles and sweat glands remain intact. Healing occurs as these cells migrate from the wound margin and join any small intact pieces of epithelium to form new epithelium, which will cover the burn wound in 14 to 21 days, depending on the depth of the injury. This newly formed epithelium is extremely delicate and must be shielded until it is capable of performing temperature regulation functions and protecting the body from infection.

Deeper full-thickness burns heal with a different process, which begins with phagocytosis by white blood cells to clear the wound area of debris and bacteria. Fibroblasts secrete collagen at the same time as marginal epithelial cells migrate from the wound periphery and injured venule buds for capillary networks to restore circulation. This process creates granulation tissue that is reddened, highly vascular, warm to touch, and hypersensitive.

Phases of Injury and Goals

The three phases of burn care are the emergent or resuscitative phase, the acute phase, and the rehabilitative phase.

The emergent stage involves critical care, often instituted in the emergency department or on site, at the place of the injury. Goals for this period are to maintain an airway, replace fluids, maintain patient comfort, prevent infection, maintain body temperature, and provide emotional support.

The acute phase encompasses the period from burn injury until the patient is considered stable and until all full-thickness burns are covered with skin. The acute phase focuses upon multisystem stabilization, wound care, infection control, mobility/function, and nutritional support (Box 34-1).

The rehabilitation period focuses upon reentry into the life continuum. Restoration of function and emotional support are the goals of this phase of treatment. Although rehabilitation is an ongoing component of burn care, the process of discharge planning and discharge require rehabilitation nursing interventions to deal with body image change, societal response to the change in appearance resulting from burns, and functional limitations that may affect activities of daily living (ADLs) and work potential. Initial goals set during acute care are directed toward preserving joint mobility strength, endurance, and controlling edema, with some attention to promoting independent self-care and educating patients and families about burn recovery (Weed & Berens, 2005). Rehabilitation goals expand beyond acute care to prevent further disability and complications, such as disfigurement related to scar contracture (Weed & Berens, 2005). The goals of rehabilitation are directed toward minimizing scar contracture formation; increasing flexibility, strength and

---

BOX 34-1 Acute Phase Focus

- Multisystem stabilization
- Wound care
- Infection control
- Mobility/function
- Nutritional support

---

endurance; and promoting independence in normal daily activities (Wood et al., 2005). Long-term goals for patients are to improve physical skills for returning to work or school and for community reintegration.

NURSING PROCESS

Assessment

During initial assessment, information regarding the circumstances surrounding the burn injury must be obtained from the individual or witnesses. Data should include the following:

- How and when the injury occurred
- Duration of contact with the burning agent
- Location when burned
- Presence of explosion
- Age/general health
- Nature of thermal agent

Small children and the elderly have a higher mortality rate (http://www.burnsurvivor.com/burn_statisticsJanuary2006). Concurrent health conditions will affect the individual's ability to withstand the physiological stress of burns.

Objective data will identify the severity of the burn. Burns are classified as major, moderate, or minor, depending upon the size of the burn, the depth, the location, and other complications (Box 34-2).

The "rule of nines" may be used clinically to describe the total body surface area (TBSA) that has been burned. A chart demonstrating anterior and posterior diagrams of the body is divided into areas equal to multiples of 9% (Figure 34-2). The burned areas are typically shaded on the diagrams, allowing the amount of area burned to be calculated. A pediatric chart for the rule of nines exists; however, infants and children will have calculations modified due to their inherent size differences and the depth and location of burns.

Age. The severity of a burn also depends upon the age of the individual. Infants younger than 2 years have a poor response to infection. Older persons with preexisting health conditions may be unable to withstand the physiological stress of the burn injury.

Burn Site. The location on the body is an important consideration in assessment of the patient with burns. A 5% burn to the abdomen of an obese adult female is far different than the same site on a 5-year-old child. Any burn that extends across a joint may cause mobility limitations and require extensive physical therapy. A circumferential burn may cause constrictive contracture, resulting in multiple complications. Any burn causing facial disfigurement results in severe emotional distress, as well as initial concerns about respiratory maintenance, due to structural damage to respiratory anatomy.

Causative Agent. The cause of the burn must be identified because of the direct relationship to treatment and prognosis.

During the rehabilitation phase, ongoing assessment must include the individual's range of motion, complaints of pain and pressure, and response to patient teaching. Special attention must be given to the individual and family responses to body image change. Coping mechanisms must be specified.

Further, the rehabilitation nurse must be prepared to assess the individual's response to positioning, splinting, exercise, and wound care and ability to perform activities of daily living.

Nursing Diagnosis

Nursing diagnosis is defined as a clinical judgment about an individual, family, or community response to actual or potential health problems/life processes that provides the basis for definitive therapy toward achievement of outcomes for which the nurse is accountable (Gordon, 2000).

Determined from analyses of patient data, nursing diagnoses for the person with burns during the rehabilitation period are outlined in Table 34-1.

Expected Outcomes

An expected outcome is defined as a patient state, at a given point in time, reflecting improvement over a state at a prior assessment (Johnson, Maas, & Moorhead, 2004). Outcomes for the burn-injured individual during the rehabilitation phase include the following:

1. Endurance, increased mobility, and increased joint movement
2. Participating in health care decisions; self-direction of care; coping
3. Comfort level
4. Psychosocial adjustment: life changes

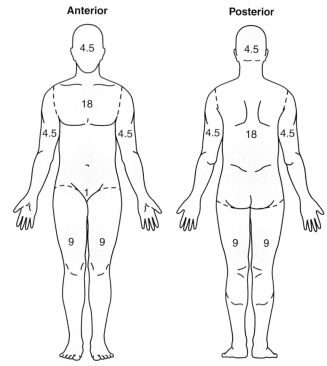

Figure 34-2 Rule of nines. (From Phipps, W. J., Sands, J. K., & Marek, J. F. [1999]. *Medical-surgical nursing: Concepts and clinical practice* [6th ed.]. St. Louis, MO: Mosby.)

BOX 34-2 Burn Classification by Total Body Surface Area Burn Estimate

Minor burn injuries	Less than 15% TBSA in adults (10% in children or elderly persons)
	Less than 2% TBSA full-thickness injury
	Burns in patients with no preexisting disease
Moderate burn injuries	15%-25% TBSA in adults, partial thickness (10%-20% TBSA in children younger than 10 years and adults older than 40 years)
	2%-10% TBSA full thickness
	Burns with no concurrent injury
	Burns in patients with no preexisting disease
Major burn injuries	Partial-thickness injury greater than 25% TBSA (greater than 20% in children younger than 10 years and adults older than 40 years)
	Greater than 10% TBSA, full thickness (children and adults)
	Involvement of face, eyes, ears, hands, feet, or perineum
	Electrical burns
	Burns complicated by inhalation injury or major trauma
	Burns in patients with preexisting disease (diabetes, congestive heart failure, or chronic renal failure)

Modified from Patient Education Program, Burn Unit. (2002). University of Iowa Hospitals and Clinics, Iowa City, IA.
TBSA, Total body surface area.

TABLE 34-1 Nursing Diagnosis During the Rehabilitation Period of Burn Recovery

Nursing Diagnosis	Etiological Factors
Impaired physical mobility	Joint stiffness or contractures; pain discomfort; musculoskeletal impairment
Ineffective health maintenance	Ineffective coping; impairment of support system
Risk for joint contractures	Imposed restrictions by scaring
Chronic pain	Physiological factors and knowledge deficit
Disturbed body image	Non-integration of change in body characteristics
Social isolation	Alteration in physical appearance
Interrupted family processes	Situational transition
Post-trauma syndrome	Injury flashbacks
Imbalanced nutrition requirements	Loss of body fluid

5. Social support
6. Family coping; family functioning
7. Coping; body image acceptance
8. Nutrition

Interventions

Nursing interventions represent those activities that nurses do to assist the individual and/or family with moving toward a desired outcome (McCloskey & Bulechek, 2004).

Interventions Related to Impaired Skin Integrity.

Rehabilitation nursing assessment of the integumentary system goes beyond evaluation of injury sites. By the time the patient has reached the rehabilitative phase, escharotomies, debridements, and grafting procedures have been completed; therefore a patient may enter rehabilitation with a wound that is covered with extremely fragile skin. The goals of wound care during rehabilitative recovery focus on attending to healed areas and donor sites, preventing infection, protecting new skin from further trauma, and preparing skin for compression. Understanding of the physiological alterations of skin resulting from burn injury, along with its impact on lifestyle, underlies all interventions and ongoing management of the individual with burn injury.

Topical agents may be used to prevent infection during the rehabilitation phase. No single topical agent has been demonstrated to be universally effective for burn care. Alternative agents may be used concurrently on different burn sites. The most popular topical agent in use is silver sulfadiazine 1% (Silvadene), a water-based cream effective against gram-positive, gram-negative, and *Candida* organisms. Other agents commonly used include mafenide acetate (Sulfamylon), povidone-iodine, sliver nitrate 5%, and cerium nitrate 1.74%. Over-the-counter topical agents may include bacitracin with polymyxin B and neomycin sulfate.

Persons who have had a burn injury may experience impairments for an extended period following hospitalization. Many of these impairments are difficult to assess and document. For example, heat/cold intolerance, decreased strength and coordination, photosensitivity, or changes in sweating and psychosocial problems may complicate rehabilitation.

A burn injury that extends to the dermis also will destroy hair follicles and sebaceous and sweat glands that arise from this skin layer. Also lost are the abilities for these structures to regenerate. Scar tissue may take up to 2 years to mature; thus the skin is continually changing, healing, and evolving during this posthospitalization phase. As a result, the patient must deal with skin that is thinner, less pliable, drier, more sensitive to temperature changes, and more prone to blistering and itching. Overall preservation of skin integrity is discussed further in Chapter 15.

Dryness. Topical emollients supply external moisture and lubrication to the newly healed skin. Lotions that contain both water (for absorption) and lipid (to retard evaporation) are recommended. In general, it is best to avoid creams, lanolins, and cocoa butter with nonessential or poorly characterized ingredients such as fragrance and exotic plant oils or extracts, which will only mimic adequate lubrication. These nonessential ingredients can cause irritation or contact sensitization. As a supplement a room humidifier may help to reduce epidermal dehydration.

Photosensitivity. Avoiding sunlight exposure for 6 months or longer after a burn injury is recommended to prevent sunburn and permanent hyperpigmentation. Return of melanin pigments to newly healed skin or grafts varies, depending on the extent of injury. Commonsense measures include use of a hat and appropriate clothing, timing of outdoor activities for early morning or late afternoon, and application of sunscreen to newly formed skin. A product with a sun protection factor (SPF) rating of at least 15 should be used when sunlight exposure cannot be avoided. Sunscreens labeled "water resistant" will retain their protective ability for 40 minutes of sweating or swimming, whereas those labeled "waterproof" will retain their effectiveness for up to 80 minutes of activity. New sunscreen products are being developed each season.

Pruritus. Pruritus is a significant problem during the recovery period. If not treated and controlled, the scratching can destroy fragile grafts and healing donor sites. Strategies of daily hygiene, conscientious lubrication, appropriate thermal protection, alternatives to scratching, and antipruritic medications must be incorporated into the patient's lifestyle if successful management is to be achieved. Itching of healing burn areas and new skin can be a severe discomfort. The use of systemic antihistamines in conjunction with topical antipruritic agents may ease some symptoms. An emollient lotion containing menthol (0.25% to 0.5%) and camphor (0.5% to 2%) feels cool to the skin and may provide temporary relief while countering dryness. Refrigerated lotions as cold applications may be soothing for some persons. Topical anesthetics (e.g., pramoxine hydrochloride 1%) are available in ointments, creams, and lotions. Topical benzocaine preparations are not recommended due to potential allergic sensitization.

Interventions Related to Pain Management.

Pain. Severe pain often accompanies partial-thickness burns because of damaged but not destroyed sensory nerve fibers. In contrast, little if any pain is associated with full-thickness injury because nerve endings are in large part destroyed.

Nurses are aware that each patient is the authority on the pain he or she is experiencing. Chapter 23 contains principles for nursing assessment and management of pain and pain relief that apply to patients who have burn injuries. Thus the most valuable nursing intervention with patients who have pain is pain relief through administering prescribed medications (often narcotics), implementing comfort measures, and assisting patients with using alternative techniques. Relaxation techniques of imagery and distraction heighten the effects of analgesia for many patients. These are discussed in more detail in Chapter 23.

Coordinating therapy procedures, anticipating energy requirements for activities, planning for rest periods interspersed with therapies, and promoting time and guidance for self-help strategies contribute to minimizing pain; this in turn allows a patient to participate in ADLs. A patient who is involved in wound care and decision-making processes feels more empowered, thereby enhancing feelings of control related to pain management.

Interventions Related to Impaired Physical Mobility.

Mobility. Assessment of the patient's mobility status is an ongoing process because functional recovery may be a long and laborious process and usually involves interdisciplinary assessments and interventions. Positioning, exercise, compression, and splinting are basic burn rehabilitation treatment procedures. The purpose of these modalities is to prevent loss of function and promote of functional independence.

With advances in splinting and other modalities, most patients can expect to approximate their preinjury level of function. Assistive devices or adapted equipment may be needed to ensure function. Reconstructive surgery may be necessary for a patient to regain function when scar contractures have formed.

Positioning. Proper positioning begins at onset of injury and is evaluated regularly throughout rehabilitation. During the acute phase of injury, proper positioning minimizes edema, provides safe and proper joint alignment, and maintains tendon balance between overstretching and promoting contracture formation. During the rehabilitative phase of recovery the goal is to continue effective positioning to prevent contractures (Helm, Kowalske, & Head, 2005). Because patients are encouraged to become ambulatory as soon as possible, using an assistive device for proper positioning is part of learning upright sitting and standing posture. Whether a patient's wound management dictates total body or partial positioning, various burn injury sites require special attention to prevent complications of pressure necrosis, dependent edema, or flexion contractures. Common factors that may affect positioning are edema, donor sites, graft areas, and respiratory function.

Figure 34-3 illustrates how position devices of cloth rolls, foam wedges, straps, footboards, and slings may be used to assist with proper positioning. Burns involving the head, face, or neck require individualized positioning according to the area burned. Pillows are not recommended because their use may lead to secondary complications, such as neck flexion contractures and pressure to the ears. The supine position,

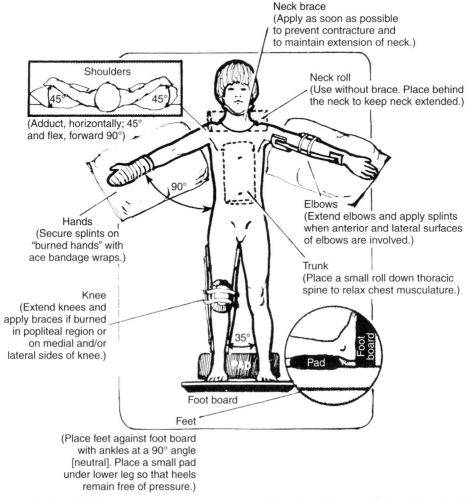

Figure 34-3 Supine positioning of the burn patient to prevent contracture formation. (Courtesy Shriners Burns Institute, Galveston, TX.)

using a small foam pad instead of a pillow, is recommended for severely burned patients. As a general rule, knees, hips, elbows, and interphalangeal joints are placed extended in neutral alignments. Ankles and feet are dorsiflexed at a 90-degree angle, wrists are dorsiflexed at 10 to 20 degrees, and a shoulder is placed in neutral alignment supported in a 90-degree abduction.

Splints are one way to immobilize an area of the body and place it in a position that will preserve or restore function. However, a patient must adhere to a schedule for wearing a splint, practice routine cleaning, and inspect the skin before and on removal of the splint to achieve desired outcomes (Helm, Kowalske, & Head, 2005).

Exercise. Joint function may diminish as a result of bed rest, decreased protein, altered fluid and electrolyte levels, and poor circulation until ultimately contractures occur and heterotopic bone is formed. Full ROM joint exercises for all joints begin early in the wound management process and continue at regular daily intervals. Active and passive exercises may be combined, depending on the patient's capabilities; however, joints are not moved beyond their free range unless prescribed by a physician and directed by a physical therapist.

Successful outcomes of burn injury cannot be achieved when a patient relies solely on the benefits of scheduled therapies. In home and community settings rehabilitation nurses can assist community health nurses and other community resources in intervening with exercise modalities for stretching and increasing ROM that are both creative and cost-effective. In the home, assistive devices such as splints, wedges, pulley systems, slings, shoes, or pillows may be effective in incorporating active and/or passive exercises into daily routines. As part of self-care a patient is expected to follow through with these mobility skills during nontherapy hours, and family members are taught how to assist. A program or system established in the rehabilitation setting will be followed more consistently when it is appropriate and adaptable to the home environment. Ideally a patient will understand, initiate, and incorporate these strategies into everyday routine.

Some patients may find it difficult to adhere to a prescribed exercise program due to pain, diminished endurance, low levels of motivation, other chronic or disabling conditions, or knowledge deficit. The rehabilitation nurse may be instrumental in educating a patient and family about strategic ways to address issues such as anticipating and treating pain before exercise, developing and tolerating wearing schedules of compression garments and splints, coordinating wound management with other treatment regimens, and enduring effective positioning of extremities and trunk. Successful adaptations of these necessary lifestyle changes can be achieved better when patients have incentives for high levels of motivation.

Compression. A primary treatment for prevention and reduction of hypertrophic scarring is compression therapy. After wounds are closed, custom-fitted garments are worn 24 hours every day and are removed only for hygiene and skin care. These garments are worn for as long as 1 to 2 years or until scar tissue matures. Clearly this long-term treatment relies on interdisciplinary teamwork with a fully participating patient and family for successful outcome. Research has demonstrated in some burn centers that flexible dressings provide the same outcome.

Preparation and toughening of the skin to tolerate the custom-fitted garment for such long duration is a primary goal of the interdisciplinary team. Pressure may be applied to burn areas gradually and through various methods. Products such as elastic wraps (ACE bandages), premade tubular elastic garments (Tubigrip), or tailor-made burn garments (Jobst) are designed to apply varying degrees of pressure to the scar tissue. Inserts of foam or silicone may be applied underneath the pressure garment to increase direct pressure to a specific area. The length of time a patient is scheduled to wear a particular pressure application is increased gradually and as tolerated.

Whenever the compression garment or other device is removed, the nurse conducts a complete head-to-toe skin assessment. The nurse specifically pays attention to any pressure areas that may be developing and evaluates skin tolerance to compression treatment. With burn injuries it is not uncommon for blisters to develop on healed areas; these differ from pressure areas. Blisters are evaluated and noted but left intact unless accompanied by signs of infection. Any sign of infection is reported to the physician immediately.

Splinting. Splints are fabricated by an occupational therapist to prevent or correct contractures. As assistive devices they may be used on various parts of the body for support, to promote mobility, and to enable a patient to perform self-care activities. Splinting aids joint positioning and decreases scar contractures and hypertrophy. Splints are necessary to maintain the length of soft tissue joint structures; however, they are used cautiously to avoid prolonged immobilization and fibrosis of soft tissue. Static splints can be used over compression garments to maintain increases in motion that have been achieved with therapeutic exercise. Dynamic splints provide continuous gentle stretch when full motion is not achieved with exercise and activity. Some physicians prefer to use frequent exercise instead of splints (Helm, Kowalske, & Head, 2005).

Nursing interventions with splint treatment include assisting patient and team with initiating and adhering to a tolerable wearing schedule, monitoring skin status, and evaluating the effectiveness of the splint regimen on function and mobility in daily activities. Coordinated interventions with physical and occupational therapy regimens are critical in preventing contractures. Team members, patient, and family must coordinate treatments and devote attention to each phase of the treatment to achieve desired outcomes, which are to preserve function and minimize complications associated with burn injury.

Interventions Related to Ineffective Health Maintenance.

Lifestyle. Assessment of each patient's lifestyle, preferences, and habits as they existed before injury is essential in developing effective and realistic interventions. Patients who learn and practice new strategies to care for their "now new body" will experience improved outcomes. Simple but regular strategies of daily hygiene, vigilant lubrication, avoidance of strong sun exposure and temperature changes, appropriate thermal protection, and antipruritic measures are incorporated as much as possible into lifestyle and preferences. Although these strategies may be intrusive for some, they are necessary for effective long-term skin care management.

Self-Care. Self-initiated programs give patients the psychological benefit of actively participating in their own rehabilitation and promote the habits of a daily routine, which must be conscientiously adhered to after discharge. Active participation in wound care, hygiene, and self-exercise programs are crucial to prevent complications and increase functional ability. The rehabilitation nurse educates patient and family and reinforces modifications for the patient's lifelong lifestyle, not only for the duration of the rehabilitation wound management program.

PSYCHOSOCIAL ADJUSTMENT AND FAMILY INVOLVEMENT

The psychological implications for a patient who has a burn injury are great. Nurses may encounter patients who exhibit a variety of responses and emotional reactions, depending on their phase of recovery. Initially a patient may be delirious as a result of burn shock in combination with medications. Later, depression becomes a major factor as the realization of drastic changes in personal appearance, seemingly endless treatments, and functional implications for the future become more apparent. At some time fear of death is a major concern for many. Other fears commonly expressed by patients are fears of pain, suffering, disfigurement, and prolonged hospitalization and concerns about disruption of lifestyle or survivor guilt.

The nursing goals during these early phases are to decrease pain, to ensure gentle physical care and handling, to answer questions as completely as possible, and to begin to elicit patient and family participation. There is some evidence that children who have burn injuries ultimately may experience less psychological impact than their parents. However, findings from this study do not negate psychosocial adjustment problems for children.

The stress of lifestyle changes and the constant demands of active participation in various preventive procedures can be extremely difficult for many persons. Coupled with body image concerns, functional limitations, adapted lifestyle, and perhaps a changed vocation, the patient reenters society essentially as a changed person with an unfamiliar body. Thus some type of grief response to changed body image usually occurs. These internal changes and adjustments are heightened by the multiple reminders of changes in appearance or ability that a patient will encounter on reentering society. Assertiveness training may help many patients deal with social responses—ranging from avoidance, ridicule, stares, to excessive sympathy—which threaten a patient's self-confidence.

The 1-year-postinjury mark appears to be significant for persons who survive burn injuries. For many, emotional issues are resolved as physical function is restored and most extensive treatment such as compression is completed, and there has been time to adjust to social issues. These factors coincide with scar tissue maturation and improved sensation, which also may be occurring at approximately 1 year. Work and family roles may have been renegotiated by this time.

Family involvement is crucial during both initial and recovery periods. Tremendous sadness or guilt of being a survivor may accompany patients when a loved one was lost as a result of the burn injury event. The family is often the single most important continuing force in a patient's life and the primary resource in redefining identity when the patient reenters the community. Allowing and encouraging regular family visits during all phases of recovery may accomplish the following three goals:

1. Providing a patient opportunity to express emotions and encouraging expression of frustrations and concerns
2. Allowing family members to observe wound healing and adjust to changes in patient's physical appearance and functioning
3. Aiding family in understanding the patient's day-to-day struggles and offering insight into physical and emotional challenges during rehabilitation

The absence of family or a significant other in the ongoing recovery process impedes a patient's motivation and creates further stressors in the discharge process. Depending on the extent of the burn injury and physical functioning, family involvement and support may be a deciding factor in whether a patient returns to live at home or in a skilled care facility.

Sexuality

Although the recovery period following a burn injury may require up to 5 years, a milestone is achieved when a patient is able to look, touch, and care for affected areas. Many times patients have disassociated themselves from the burn areas, perhaps for the first year. Rehabilitation nurses who conduct ongoing assessment will be attuned to a patient's psychological readiness for redefining body image and self-esteem. Sexual functioning becomes a concern as other issues are resolved.

Unpleasant sensations may be due to hypersensitivity of immature scar tissue, irritable feelings from itching, blisters, or changes in heat and cold sensation, which affect normal pleasure response. Often significant others do not know how to deal with sexuality issues. For instance, they may fear causing injury to fragile healing skin sites, may experience frustration with role changes, or in some circumstances may be dealing with their own discomforts resulting from burn injuries incurred during the same event.

If sexual and social adjustment is to be successful, preparation for privacy, time, and supporting patient and family needs for intimacy during all or any phases of recovery is planned. Information regarding sexual potential and emotional adjustment is provided along with specific sexual education on positioning, pleasuring, and alternative methods of sensuality in the reestablishment of intimacy. Questions of fertility may arise secondary to physical injury to genitalia or interruption of organ functioning (e.g., scrotal edema or amenorrhea). Chapter 27 presents a more complete discussion of sexuality and options for persons with chronic or disabling disorders.

Vocational Implications

Various studies show that most people who are employed at the time of their burn injury will return to work. The extent, etiology, and site of burn injury influence a person's return-to-work status. Functional limitations resulting from burn injuries may temporarily or permanently affect the ability to return to work. Related factors include stamina and endurance; tolerance to standing, walking, or sitting; and degree of hand grip and upper extremity strength. A comprehensive medical evaluation by a vocational specialist is required before a patient is cleared to resume occupational roles. Personal fear of reinjury, concern about peer reaction, and an individual's confidence level about resuming a work role may hinder return to work (Vierling, 2005). Vocational issues are a major correlate of long-term psychosocial or emotional problems. When patients hold positive perceptions about how their roles in family, work, social network, and other activities will be resumed, these attitudes indicate strengths toward effective coping and adjustment.

Strength and Resources

All severe burn injuries, regardless of origin, can alter the function of many body systems. Although most systems will recover and resume normal functioning, some processes may be compromised and others will never regenerate. When a patient is able to construct a realistic assessment of these functions, the nurse is able to assess the beginning of psychosocial and emotional recovery, just as wound healing marks the beginning of physical recovery.

Ongoing support from family members and the interdisciplinary team is critical during all phases of institutional care and on community reentry. The rehabilitation nurse functions as advocate, educator, and facilitator to assist patients in realistic appraisal of their status, emphasizing ability rather than limitations or disability. During follow-up appointments, patients need guidance, encouragement, empowerment, and reassurance about emotional adjustments; rehabilitation nurses may use these opportunities to promote effective coping behaviors.

In the community, patients and families benefit from association, awareness, and utilization of community-based services and resources. Examples include hospital- or center-based support groups, peer groups, volunteer or not-for-profit self-help groups established by persons who have themselves survived burn injuries (e.g., Phoenix Foundation or the Knapp Foundation) and national organizations (e.g., American Burn Association).

OUTCOME AND RESTORATIVE NURSING PRACTICE

The transition from patient with a burn injury to a person who survived a burn injury and reentered the community is the ultimate outcome desired following a rehabilitation program. The patient is educated, motivated, and empowered to become the director of his or her own care. The roles of rehabilitation are pivotal to achieving successful outcomes of burn rehabilitation. This is one practice area in the growing field of restorative nursing care. As medical advances continue and health care system changes occur, rehabilitation nurses can anticipate active practice roles in planning, implementing, and evaluating services for patients who require extensive, long-term restorative care for a wide variety of conditions, in addition to those persons with burn injuries.

Case Study

Isabel Dean is a 61-year-old woman who works as a certified nurse aide in a long-term care facility. She has a history of adult-onset diabetes, obesity, and hypertension. Ms. Dean was in the process of preparing a meal and carrying a pot of boiling potatoes to the sink to drain them, when she dropped the pot to the floor. Boiling liquid splashed over both feet and lower legs. She was wearing sport shoes and cotton socks. Emergency medical services transported her to the regional burn center for treatment.

Upon emergency evaluation Ms. Dean was found to have a 10% total body surface area (TBSA) deep partial-thickness burn, circumferential from the toes to midcalf bilaterally. A wound culture was obtained, then wounds were cleansed with sterile water and mild soap. Nonadherent skin was removed. Nursing assessment identified the following:

- *Ms. Dean has been prescribed an oral hypoglycemic and was directed to "avoid sweets." She does not monitor blood glucose levels.*

- *She lives with a significant other in a second-story apartment.*
- *She works over 40 hours per week on the night shift.*
  Objectively, Ms. Dean was assessed as follows:
- *Blood pressure 189/111 mm Hg, respirations 37 breaths per minute, heart rate 109 beats per minute*
- *Lower extremity pulses present per Doppler*
- *Burning, throbbing sensation described in lower extremities*
- *Blood glucose level of 210 mg/dl*
  Nursing diagnoses in this case are as follows:
- *Impaired skin integrity related to thermal injury*
- *Risk for infection related to loss of skin integrity and diabetes*
- *Acute pain related to tissue injury*
- *Impaired physical mobility*
- *Ineffective health maintenance related to burn injury, lack of knowledge of burn process, treatment, and complications*

Continued

Case Study—cont'd

TABLE 34-2 Nursing Interventions and Outcomes Applicable to Ms. Dean NIC/NOC

Nursing Diagnosis	Nursing Outcomes	Nursing Interventions
Impaired skin integrity	Burn sites healed; no complications	Wound care, using strict asepsis Assess wound status with each dressing change Limit ambulation; maintain proper positioning of extremities Administer nutrients and supplements as prescribed Monitor blood glucose levels to maintain control of diabetes
Risk for infection	Infection control	Observe and monitor for signs and symptoms of infection Assess wound status for change in appearance, odor Obtain cultures as indicated Maintain asepsis
Pain related to injury	Pain is managed	Assess pain levels using rating scale Administer analgesics as prescribed Maintain positioning to decrease edema Implement nonpharmacological options for pain control Environmental management: comfort
Impaired physical mobility	Increased endurance and mobility	Assess joint mobility: active and passive Assess patterns of movement and ambulation Maintain positioning Teach regarding activity/exercise Energy management
Ineffective health maintenance	Verbalizes understanding of wound care; performs wound care Identifies necessary care for burn sites Specifies actions to promote health	Assess cognitive and physical abilities to perform wound care Teach patient comfort measures Teach safety/surveillance procedures

Data from Moorhead, S., Johnson, M., & Maas, M. (Eds.). (2004). *Nursing outcomes classification (NOC)* (3rd ed.). St. Louis, MO: Mosby; Dochterman, J. M., & Bulechek, G. M. (2004). *Nursing interventions classification (NIC)* (4th ed.). St. Louis, MO: Mosby; and NANDA International. (2007). *NANDA-I nursing diagnoses: Definitions & classification 2007-2008*. Philadelphia: Author.

CRITICAL THINKING QUESTIONS

1. Considering general principles of psychological care, develop one nursing approach for each of the following issues associated with responses of Isabel Dean to the diagnosis of 10% TBSA deep partial-thickness burns: fear, decreased control, inability to return to work.

2. Discuss the impact of limited mobility upon the potential for rehabilitation in Ms. Dean's case.

3. List the differences in priorities of care for Ms. Dean during the emergent and rehabilitation phases of burn injury.

REFERENCES

American Burn Association. (2007). Burn incidence and treatment in the U.S.: 2007 fact sheet. Available at http://www.ameriburn.org/resources_factsheet.php.

Brown, M., Helm, P., & Weed, R. (2005). Life care planning for the burn patient. In R. Weed (Ed.), *Life care planning and management handbook*. Boca Raton, FL: CRC Press

Gordon, M. (2000). *Manual of nursing diagnosis* (9th ed.). St. Louis, MO: Mosby.

Helm, P., Kowalske, K., & Head, M. (2005). Burn rehabilitation. In DeLisa, J. A., Jr. (Ed.), *Physical medicine & rehabilitation principles and practice*. Philadelphia: Lippincott Williams & Wilkins.

Moorhead, S., Johnson, M., & Maas, M. (2004). *Nursing outcomes classification* (3rd ed.). St. Louis, MO: Mosby.

Dochterman, J., & Bulechek, G. M. (2004). *Nursing interventions classification* (4th ed.). St. Louis, MO: Mosby.

Vierling, L. (2005). Return to work dynamics: A new perspective on the 3 R's. *The Case Manager, 160*(4), 67-69.

Weed, R. O., & Berens, D. E. (2005). Basics of burn injury: Implications for case management and life care planning. Philadelphia: Lippincott Williams & Wilkins.

35

Rehabilitation in Regulatory/Metabolic and Immune System Dysfunction

Deborah J. Konkle-Parker, PhD, FNP
Fleetwood Lostalot, RN, NP, C

Healthy function of the human body relies on regulation to ensure homeostasis and freedom from foreign invasion. Regulation frequently uses negative (or occasionally positive) feedback loops for homeostasis (Figure 35-1). Examples include metabolic/hormonal regulation, temperature regulation, and renal regulation.

Prevention of invasion by bacteria and viruses and subsequent development of disease is accomplished through various mechanisms. The skin is the first line of defense; an intact skin tissue serves to protect the internal environment from harmful organisms that flourish in the external environment. If invasion takes place, however, the body responds by activating the inflammatory process to render these microorganisms incapable of altering homeostasis. If this secondary mechanism fails, the body relies on the complexity of the immune response to neutralize or destroy the invading organisms.

Included in this chapter is a physiological description of the body's regulatory mechanisms related to thermal, metabolic, and endocrine homeostasis. The bulk of this chapter then focuses on the protective mechanisms of the body. Alterations of protective mechanisms are discussed, focusing on human immunodeficiency virus (HIV) disease. Nursing assessment, intervention, and outcomes related to the rehabilitation of individuals with regulation problems are presented. Renal regulation is discussed in Chapter 36.

Common to all of these conditions is the inability of the body to regulate or protect itself, leading to chronic illness and a need for lifelong adaptation. This adaptation necessitates lifestyle changes. Nurses can be instrumental in assisting individuals with chronic diseases with making the necessary changes and living life to the highest level.

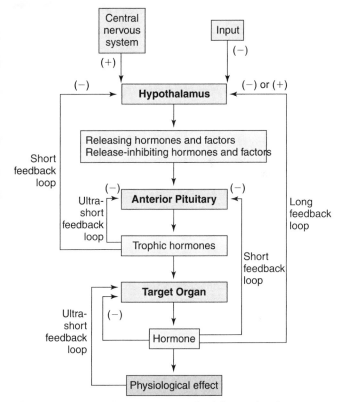

Figure 35-1 Example of negative feedback loop: This shows a general model for release of hormones as directed by the central nervous system or by input from the environment. The hypothalamus is the intermediary organ, providing direction about release of hormones or releasing factors. The releasing glands or target organs then provide feedback to inhibit the continued release of hormones to control hormone and physiological effect to the desired level. (From Phipps, W. J., Sands, J. K., & Marek, J. F. [1999]. *Medical-surgical nursing: Concepts and clinical practice* [6th ed.]. St. Louis, MO: Mosby.)

TEMPERATURE REGULATION

The maintenance of temperature is vital to life. Normal body temperature varies and may range from 96.4° F to 100° F (35.8° C to 37.8° C). For every degree of elevation in body temperature, the demand for oxygen and nutrients increases. Internal body temperature remains relatively constant. Even in altered circumstances, internal defense mechanisms and feedback systems strive to maintain constant body temperature.

Mechanisms of Body Temperature Control

The autonomic nervous system (ANS) controls body temperature, as well as other visceral functions (Guyton & Hall, 2005). The hypothalamus is the body temperature control center. Its function is regulated by neural feedback. Central thermoreceptors in the hypothalamus, spinal cord, abdominal organs, and other central locations, as well as peripheral thermoreceptors in the skin, provide the hypothalamus with information about skin and core temperatures. When temperature is low, the hypothalamus responds by triggering heat production and heat conservation mechanisms. When temperature is high, heat reduction mechanisms are stimulated. Figure 35-2 describes these mechanisms. Heat production and conservation occur with an increase in metabolic rates, vasoconstriction, and increased glycolysis, all mediated by epinephrine. The sympathetic nervous system (SNS) produces an increase in muscle tone,

vasoconstriction, and shivering. Conscious motor functions include voluntary measures to produce heat and conserve heat loss.

High core temperatures stimulate measures of heat loss. Those under control of the autonomic nervous system include sweating to cause heat loss by evaporation, vasodilation and increased respiration to cause greater heat loss through conduction to the cooler outside air, and reductions in muscle tone to decrease heat production.

Elevated Body Temperature

Fever. During fever the body is responding to an altered homeostasis, and the hypothalamus is set at a higher temperature level. The resulting elevated temperature may have a known or an unknown etiology. When the precipitator is an infection, fever may result from the effects of pyrogenic substances secreted by injured cells. The exudate formed contains endogenous or exogenous pyrogens that cause the set point of the hypothalamic thermostat to rise, and within hours the body temperature elevates.

When fever occurs from a disease state, the controlling mechanisms of the hypothalamus fail and temperature continues to rise unless interventions promote heat loss. Neurogenic fever, caused by injury to the anterior hypothalamus, results when the ability to promote heat loss is impaired. This occurs in individuals with severe closed head injuries and basilar skull fractures.

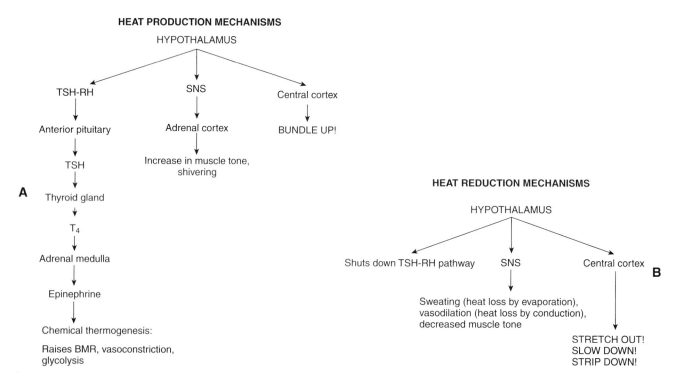

Figure 35-2 Feedback loop involved in temperature regulation. The hypothalamus, having been fed input by peripheral receptors, directs changes in temperature through hormonal pathways, through the sympathetic nervous system, and through the central nervous system. **A,** Heat production mechanisms. **B,** Heat reduction mechanisms.

Patients with spinal cord injury often demonstrate a fever related to the interruption of ANS communication with the hypothalamus during the acute phase after injury. When local reflex activity resumes, the severity of this problem subsides. Other known causes of fever are infections, deep venous thrombosis, tumors, pulmonary embolus, and drug hypersensitivities. Some medications, such as phenothiazines, anticholinergics, diuretics, and certain antihypertensives can interfere with heat loss. In those situations when no clear reason for elevated body temperature is apparent, malignancies or collagen-vascular diseases may be underlying causes.

Specific Conditions Accompanied by Altered Body Temperature

Several pathological states are unique in that they predispose patients to altered ability to maintain normal body temperatures. Examples discussed below are spinal cord injury, head trauma, cerebral vascular accidents, and multiple sclerosis.

Spinal Cord Injury. The disturbed thermoregulatory control in patients with spinal cord injury results from loss of autonomic control over vasomotor activity and the sweating mechanism. See Chapter 14 for further discussion of thermoregulation in spinal cord injury. Patients with complete spinal cord lesions sweat only above the level of the lesion, though those with incomplete lesions can sweat both above and below the level of the lesion. When sweating becomes excessive in persons with lesions above the T6 spinal cord level, autonomic dysreflexia can be suspected (see Chapter 18, Appendix A, for discussion of autonomic dysreflexia). Because controlling body temperature is difficult in patients with high cervical injuries and possible damage to the hypothalamus and brainstem, these patients must be monitored closely. Altered body temperature may be a sign of brainstem or medullary dysfunction. Fever in patients with spinal cord injuries may also be associated with infection, deep venous thrombosis, and emboli.

Head Trauma. Hyperthermia during the acute phase of head trauma is an indicator of damage to the hypothalamus or brainstem and possibly dehydration and infection. When temperature is elevated, metabolic demands grow and more carbon dioxide (CO_2) is released by neural cells into the blood. CO_2 acts as a vasodilator that increases blood volume within the cranial vault thereby increasing intracranial pressure. If the patient already has increased intracranial pressure, hyperthermia leads to further ischemia due to increased intracranial pressure. It is imperative to treat hyperthermia rapidly and effectively in the patient with head trauma. Head trauma is discussed further in Chapter 25.

Cerebrovascular Accidents. Hyperthermia in the acute phase of a cerebrovascular accident (CVA) can result from damage to the brainstem or hypothalamus. Substantial temperature elevations seen in patients with hemorrhagic stroke or subarachnoid hemorrhage may be the result of blood in the cerebrospinal fluid contributing to hypothalamic dysfunction or early aseptic meningitis.

Multiple Sclerosis. Although the reason is unknown, there is increased thermosensitivity in patients with demyelinating disease. Increased core body temperature exacerbates the neurological symptoms of multiple sclerosis (MS). Refer to Chapter 21 for more discussion of MS.

Patient and Family Education

Major goals in the rehabilitation of all patients are to prevent complications and maintain function. Formal and informal education programs are effective for patients to learn about preventing and treating complications and changes in body temperature. Facility-based programs stress ways to prevent infections and fever. Consider that the majority of patients with spinal cord injury readmitted to hospitals are there because of infected pressure sores, urinary tract infections, respiratory tract infections, and generalized septicemia. These patients have impaired sense of hot and cold and must avoid temperature extremes. Patients with cerebrovascular accidents and spinal cord injuries must beware of hot surfaces including stoves, hot water in bathtubs, and overexposure to the sun because they burn severely with short sun exposure. Excessive heat, such as hot baths, can exacerbate symptoms of multiple sclerosis. Prevention strategies are critical to regulating temperature in persons vulnerable to hypothermia or hyperthermia.

ENDOCRINE AND METABOLIC REGULATION

The endocrine system is composed of several glands that secrete hormones to carry out specific metabolic functions. Functions include growth and development, coordinating reproduction, maintaining optimal internal body environment, and initiating adaptive responses when needed (Piano & Huether, 2006).

Hormones operate in a negative or positive feedback system. A negative feedback system turns *off* the release of a chemical substance as it reaches a critical threshold in the blood level, and a positive feedback system turns *on* to release a chemical substance for the same reason. Hormone release occurs either as a response to a change in the cellular environment or as the result of feedback designed to maintain the optimal level of hormone or related substances. In this way, hormone release is influenced not only by levels of the hormones, but also by levels of other chemical factors and by neural control. An example of hormonal regulation is the thyroid hormone negative feedback loop. An example of neural regulation is release of epinephrine from the adrenal medulla in response to stress.

Altered metabolic/endocrine regulation disturbs the internal cellular environment. The result may be persistently altered levels of the actual hormone, as well as the chemical substance the hormone controls. One example of metabolic dysregulation is the process of diabetes mellitus (Huether &

Tomky, 2006). Metabolic regulation frequently requires lifestyle interventions to promote normal functioning. Adequate knowledge of metabolic conditions allows the nurse to positively contribute to overall patient health. To discuss all the aspects of the metabolic syndrome or diabetes mellitus is beyond the scope of this chapter; however, the section following discusses related metabolic/endocrine regulation and rehabilitation issues.

Metabolic Syndrome

The incidence of the metabolic syndrome (MetSyn) has increased to epidemic proportions in recent years. Specific definitions of the MetSyn are debated but generally include hyperglycemia or insulin resistance, hypertension, obesity, and dyslipidemia (Deen, 2004; Eckel, Grundy, & Zimmet, 2005). Acute and chronic treatment of these conditions costs the United States health care system billions of dollars per year in direct and indirect costs. Adequate treatment of these conditions can reduce the immediate and long-term costs and can produce greater quantity and quality of life. The knowledge of definitions, symptoms, and treatment of the MetSyn is important in rehabilitation nursing due to the increasing prevalence and deleterious health effects.

Numerous national and international organizations have provided information to aid in the diagnosis of the MetSyn. The National Cholesterol Education Program Adult Treatment Panel (ATP) III provided the most commonly used diagnostic criteria in the United States (Grundy et al., 2004; Grundy et al., 2005). According to the ATP III, the identification of three of five metabolic indicators leads to the diagnosis of the MetSyn. The indicators include hyperglycemia, elevated blood pressure, dyslipidemia, and abdominal obesity (Box 35-1).

The World Health Organization (WHO), the European Group for the Study of Insulin Resistance (EGIR), the American Association of Clinical Endocrinologists (AACE), and the International Diabetes Foundation (IDF) have also provided diagnostic criteria for the MetSyn. Each grouping of diagnostic criteria includes most of the essential variables. However, the use of numerous definitions has led to some difficulty in adequately reporting the incidence and prevalence of the MetSyn across countries. Reference information for the ATP III, WHO, EGIR, AACE, and IDF is provided in Box 35-2.

The MetSyn as defined by the ATP III is discussed hereafter because it is the most easily integrated into regular clinical practice and most recent recommendations for the U.S. health care system. For ease of understanding the metabolic indicators are discussed as diabetes, hypertension, dyslipidemia, and obesity. However, although the metabolic parameters are discussed individually, they should be viewed as a constellation of conditions, often existing in concert with one another.

Diabetes Mellitus. An estimated 20 million persons in the United States, or about 8% of the population, have diabetes. Prevalence of type 2 diabetes (approximately 90%) is much greater than type 1 diabetes (approximately 10%). Type 1 diabetes is a result of the destruction or defect of the beta cells in the pancreas, usually occurring in childhood, adolescence, or young adulthood. The diagnosis of type 1 diabetes frequently results after the acute development of hyperglycemia and related symptoms (Box 35-3).

Type 2 diabetes is characterized by insulin resistance and obesity and frequently goes undiagnosed. Persons at high risk for type 2 diabetes include those who are overweight or obese. Secondary factors also place overweight or obese persons at higher risk. These factors can include those persons who are in a racial or ethnic minority group, have at risk comorbid conditions (e.g., hypertension, dyslipidemia), a family history of type 2 diabetes, a history of gestational diabetes or birth of a baby weighing more than 9 pounds, or physically inactivity.

An awareness of the diagnostic criteria for diabetes is important. There are three individual avenues to diagnosis of diabetes, each requiring a subsequent comparison level.

BOX 35-1 Clinical Identification of the Metabolic Syndrome

Risk Factor*	Defining Level
Abdominal obesity	Waist circumference
Men	>102 cm (>40 in)
Females	>88 cm (>35 in)
Triglycerides	≥150 mg/dl
HDL cholesterol	
Men	<40 mg/dl
Females	<50 mg/dl
Blood pressure	≥130/≥85 mm Hg
Fasting glucose	≥110 mg/dl

Data from Grundy, S., Cleeman, J., Merz, C., Brewer, H., Clark, L., Hunninghake, D., et al. (2004). Implications of recent clinical trials for the National Cholesterol Education Program Adult Treatment Panel III guidelines. *Circulation, 110*(2), 227-239; and Grundy, S., Cleeman, J., Daniels, S., Donato, K., Eckel, R., Franklin, B., et al. (2005). Diagnosis and management of the metabolic syndrome: An American Heart Association/National Heart, Lung, and Blood Institute scientific statement: Executive summary. *Circulation, 112*, 285-290.
HDL, High-density lipoprotein.
*Identification of three or more factors necessary for diagnosis.

BOX 35-2 Reference Information for Defining the Metabolic Syndrome

National Cholesterol Education Program Adult Treatment Panel (ATP) III: http://www.nhlbi.nih.gov/guidelines/cholesterol/
World Health Organization (WHO): http://www.who.int/en
European Group for the Study of Insulin Resistance (EGIR): http://www.egir.org
American Association of Clinical Endocrinologists (AACE): http://www.aace.com
International Diabetes Foundation (IDF): http://www.idf.org

The diagnostic criteria include (1) the identification of a casual blood glucose level 200 mg/dl or higher with symptoms of hyperglycemia or (2) a fasting blood glucose level 126 mg/dl or higher or (3) a 2-hour postprandial blood glucose level of greater than 140 mg/dl following a 75-g oral glucose tolerance test (American Diabetes Association, 2005).

The goal of diabetes management is euglycemia. Euglycemia is defined as maintaining appropriate preprandial (80 to 120 mg/dl), 2-hour postprandial (less than 140 mg/dl), and bedtime (less than 180 mg/dl) blood glucose levels. Severe alterations in glycemia outside of normal ranges can have both acute and chronic implications. Acute alternations in blood glucose are frequently related to changes in dietary intake, physical activity level, or illness. The hemoglobin A1c (A1c) is the principal method used in assessing overall diabetes control. The A1c is a laboratory test that provides an average blood glucose level of the preceding 2 to 3 months. An A1c of less than 7% is the desired goal. The A1c is used in concert with daily blood glucose levels to determine control.

The nurse and the patient should know signs and symptoms of hypoglycemia and hyperglycemia (see Box 35-3). Self-monitoring of blood glucose level at normal intervals can aid in identifying abnormal blood glucose levels (Weinger, Jacobson, Draelos, Finkelstein, & Simonson, 1995). Acute complications of diabetes include diabetic ketoacidosis or hyperglycemic hyperosmolar syndrome, both characterized by marked hyperglycemia and requiring immediate medical intervention. Chronic complications of diabetes include microvascular (i.e., retinopathy, neuropathy, and nephropathy) and macrovascular (i.e., coronary artery, cerebrovascular, and peripheral vascular disease) complications. The maintenance of euglycemia in diabetes can prevent or reduce the long-term complications associated with diabetes (American Diabetes Association, 2005; Steffes et al., 2005).

If hypoglycemia is noted, glucose or carbohydrate intake can raise blood glucose to acceptable levels. The "rule of 15" is utilized to treat hypoglycemia. If a glucose level of less than 70 mg/dl is noted, 15 g of fast-acting glucose is ingested by the individual, if possible. The blood glucose level is rechecked after 15 minutes. If the blood glucose level is greater than 70 mg/dl, additional ingestion of a complex carbohydrate could be consumed. However, if the blood glucose level remains less than 70 mg/dl, the initial process is repeated until the blood glucose level rises above 70 mg/dl. If a patient is unresponsive or unable to participate in glycemic correction, immediate medical attention is obtained.

Hypertension. An estimated 50 million persons, or approximately 18% of persons in the United States, are hypertensive. Blood pressure levels below 140/90 mm Hg are recommended for persons without risk factors or comorbidities. Box 35-4 provides reference information for the classification of blood pressure levels (National High Blood Pressure Education Program, 2003). For persons with diabetes the goal blood pressure is lowered to less than 130/80 mm Hg (American Diabetes Association, 2005; Whaley-Connell & Sowers, 2005).

Control of blood pressure may require lifestyle modifications including alterations in dietary habits, exercise levels, and possibly weight reduction. Decreasing sodium intake can lower blood pressure levels, and recommendations including the Dietary Approaches to Stop Hypertension (DASH) eating plan could be utilized in appropriate patients (Svetkey et al., 2004). Access to a more detailed review of the DASH diet is provided at the website listed in Box 35-5. Other therapeutic lifestyle changes are discussed later in the chapter because lifestyle interventions with each of the metabolic conditions are similar in scope.

Chronic elevations in blood pressure have harmful effects on numerous body systems and should be avoided. Nurses are aware of orthostatic hypotension, or the rapid lowering of blood pressure when moving into an upright or standing position, for patients who are on antihypertensive therapy. Patients reporting symptoms of vertigo or dizziness upon arising are instructed to remain seated until symptoms resolve. Referral to a health care provider may be required with significant or repeated orthostatic hypotension.

Dyslipidemia. Dyslipidemia has negative correlations with cardiovascular disease. Targets for lipid parameters are based on a risk profile set by the ATP III. All patients do not have

---

BOX 35-3 Signs and Symptoms of Altered Glycemia

Hypoglycemia
- Nervousness
- Fatigue
- Perspiration
- Chills
- Hunger
- Confusion
- Anxiousness
- Irritability
- Dizziness

Hyperglycemia
- Polyuria (frequent urination)
- Polyphagia (frequent hunger)
- Polydipsia (frequent thirst)
- Recurrent infections
- Poor wound healing
- Vision changes
- Fatigue
- Weight loss
- Xerosis
- Impotence

BOX 35-4 Classification of Blood Pressure

Blood Pressure Classification	Systolic Blood Pressure (mm Hg)	Diastolic Blood Pressure (mm Hg)
Normal	<120	and <80
Prehypertension	120-139	or 80-89
Stage 1 hypertension	140-159	or 90-99
Stage 2 hypertension	≥160	or ≥100

From National High Blood Pressure Education Program. (2003). *Report of the Joint National Committee on Prevention, Detection, Evaluation, and Treatment of High Blood Pressure (JNC 7)* (NIH Publication No. 04-5230). Rockville, MD: National Institutes of Health.

the same lipid goals, and each patient is individually assessed to determine appropriate therapeutic interventions.

Risk stratification includes a family history of premature cardiovascular disease (male first-degree relative less than 55 years and less than 65 years in females), high-density lipoprotein (HDL) levels (less than 40 mg/dl), hypertension status (greater than or equal to 140/90 mm Hg or antihypertensive medications), age (greater than or equal to 45 years for males and greater than or equal to 55 years for females), and cigarette smoking. A high-density lipoprotein level of greater than 60 mg/dl is considered a "negative" risk factor, and its presence nullifies one risk factor from the calculation. Each risk factor is given one point, and the total score provides numeric targets for total cholesterol, triglycerides, HDL, and low-density lipoprotein (LDL) levels. If triglyceride levels are greater than or equal to 500 mg/dl, it becomes the primary target because levels in this range place the patient at risk for acute pancreatitis. Otherwise, LDL levels are the primary target. LDL goals include (1) for zero to one risk factors, less than 160 mg/dl; (2) for multiple (two or more) risk factors, less than 130 mg/dl; or (3) previous cardiovascular disease or diabetes, less than 100 mg/dl. However, lower LDL goals (less than 70 mg/dl) may be more appropriate in high-risk patients (Grundy et al., 2004). The Framingham Heart Study cardiovascular risk assessment calculation can also be used to determine risk factors, and a reference is provided at the end of the chapter.

Nurses can recommend therapeutic lifestyle changes to assist with lipid lowering. General recommendations for dietary changes include reducing saturated fat intake (less than 7% of total calories), increasing fiber intake to appropriate levels (20 to 30 g/day), and maintaining a moderate intake of cholesterol (less than 200 mg/day). Weight reduction and increasing physical activity are also recommended for capable patients (Kinney, 2005; Stone, Bilek, & Rosenbaum, 2005). Several medications used in lipid-lowering therapy have notable side effects. HMG-CoA reductase inhibitors (i.e., statins) are frequently used for elevated LDL levels and can cause myopathies in certain patients. Patients experiencing myopathies or other side effects are referred to the appropriate health care provider.

Obesity. It is estimated that over 60% of persons in the United States are overweight or obese. Overweight and obese persons have increased risk for other health conditions, including cardiovascular disease, hypertension, diabetes, sleep apnea, gallbladder disease, arthritis, and certain types of cancer. Weight classifications are established through a body mass index (BMI) calculation: the person's weight in kilograms divided by the square of the person's height in meters. BMI classifications include underweight (less than 18.5), normal (18.5 to 24.9), overweight (25.0 to 29.9), obese class I (30.0 to 34.9), obese class II (35.0 to 39.9), and extreme or obese class III (greater than or equal to 40). Because waist circumference is required for diagnosis of the metabolic syndrome, it is measured with BMI assessments. Patients with a BMI greater than 25.0 and/or a waist circumference of greater than 102 cm (greater than 40 inches) in males or greater than 88 cm (greater than 35 inches) in females require intervention (Allison & Saunders, 2000; Haffner & Taegtmeyer, 2003). Clinical guidelines for the identification, evaluation, and treatment of overweight and obesity can be accessed through the website provided in Box 35-5.

Interventions for overweight or obese patients include weight reduction, increased physical activity, and dietary interventions. A referral to a registered dietitian for counseling and education may be beneficial for the patient. Weight reduction consists of a 1- to 2-pound weight loss per week and is achieved through behavior modifications. Dietary interventions include reduction in caloric intake and evaluation of eating plan. The newly developed U.S. Department of Agriculture food guide pyramid can be individually tailored to each patient, and reference information for the interactive website can be found in Box 35-5. Chapter 16 discusses diet and nourishment in more detail, and alternative measures are found in Chapter 6.

The most cost-effective intervention to increase physical activity is walking. For patients who have been sedentary, walking approximately 10 minutes 2 to 3 times per week is a reasonable initial recommendation. Current recommendations for physical activity are 30 minutes of moderate physical activity 5 times per week. A greater degree or duration of physical activity may be required for significant weight reduction or weight maintenance. However, patients are evaluated to determine if a cardiovascular assessment is need before beginning an exercise program, because many overweight or obese persons frequently have other comorbidities (Bassuk & Manson, 2005; LaMonte, Blair, & Church, 2005). See Chapter 33 for discussion of cardiac rehabilitation.

BOX 35-5 **Additional Resources for Metabolic Disorders**

Dietary Approaches to Stop Hypertension (DASH):
http://www.nhlbi.nih.gov/health/public/heart/hbp/dash/
Framingham Heart Study: http://www.framingham.com/heart/index.htm
Framingham Heart Study/National Cholesterol Education Program Risk Assessment Tool: http://www.nhlbi.nih.gov/guidelines/cholesterol/index.htm
National Heart, Lung, and Blood Institute—Clinical Guidelines on the Identification, Evaluation, and Treatment of Overweight and Obesity in Adults:
http://www.nhlbi.nih.gov/guidelines/obesity/ob_home.htm
United States Department of Agriculture—Food Guide Pyramid:
http://www.mypyramid.gov/

NURSING DIAGNOSIS, INTERVENTIONS, AND OUTCOMES

Due to the considerable interaction among conditions within the MetSyn, nursing diagnosis, interventions, and outcome assessment are frequently interchangeable. The identification

TABLE 35-1 Nursing Diagnoses, Interventions, and Outcomes Applicable to Metabolic Syndrome

Nursing Diagnosis	Nursing Interventions	Nursing Outcomes
Activity intolerance (risk for)	Activity therapy Energy management Exercise promotion	Activity tolerance Endurance Self care
Risk-prone health behavior	Coping enhancement Mutual goal setting	Acceptance: health status Compliance behavior Motivation Health seeking behavior
Decreased cardiac output	Acid-base management Electrolyte management Fluid management Cardiac care	Circulation status Electrolyte and acid/base balance Hydration Tissue perfusion
Caregiver role strain (risk for)	Caregiver support Role enhancement	Caregiver emotional health Caregiver-patient relationship Knowledge: health resources Social support
Ineffective coping	Coping enhancement Decision-making support	Acceptance: health status Impulse self-control
Risk for falls	Fall prevention Medication management	Blood glucose levels Nutritional status
Ineffective health maintenance	Financial resource assistance Health education Teaching: disease process Support system enhancement	Knowledge Health seeking behavior Risk detection Self-direction of care Spiritual health
Risk for infection	Immunization/vaccination management Infection control Nutrition management	Immunization behavior Nutritional status Self care Wound healing
Deficient knowledge	Health education Teaching	Knowledge Knowledge: diabetes management Knowledge: health promotion Diabetes self management
Imbalanced nutrition: more than body requirements	Behavior modification Weight management Weight reduction assistance	Weight control Health beliefs: perceived ability to control
Risk for peripheral neurovascular dysfunction	Peripheral sensation management Exercise therapy Pain management	Risk control Risk detection
Ineffective tissue perfusion: renal	Fluid/electrolyte management Dialysis access maintenance	Circulatory status Fluid balance Kidney function

Data from Moorhead, S., Johnson, M., & Maas, M. (Eds.). (2004). *Nursing outcomes classification (NOC)* (3rd ed.). St. Louis, MO: Mosby; Dochterman, J. M., & Bulechek, G. M. (2004). *Nursing interventions classification (NIC)* (4th ed.). St. Louis, MO: Mosby; and NANDA International. (2007). *NANDA-I nursing diagnoses: Definitions & classification 2007-2008*. Philadelphia: Author.

of normal and abnormal levels for diabetes, blood pressure, lipids, and obesity is vital to goal achievement. There are numerous nursing diagnoses related to the MetSyn. For example, interventions for ineffective coping may require enhancement of coping skills or decision-making support. Desired outcomes of interventions may include health status acceptance or impulse self-control. To present all nursing

diagnosis, interventions, and outcomes related to the MetSyn is beyond the scope of this chapter, but individual examples are presented. Table 35-1 lists several nursing diagnoses related to the MetSyn. Individual patient assessment limits the breadth of perceived diagnoses, and distinct treatment plans are needed for each patient (Dochterman & Bulechek, 2004; Moorhead, Johnson, & Maas, 2004).

Rehabilitation Issues Related to Metabolic Regulation

Health Risks Associated With Metabolic Disorders.

There are numerous microvascular and macrovascular complications related to uncontrolled metabolic disorders. The appropriate knowledge of current standards and recommendations of diabetes, hypertension, dyslipidemia, and obesity allows the nurse to implement or support appropriate nursing diagnoses, interventions, and outcomes necessary to improve or maintain health. Medication adherence, weight reduction, dietary changes, and increased physical activity are individual avenues that promote healthy living and can reduce long-term complications. Acute changes in health related to metabolic disorders can include changes in glycemia, blood pressure, and/or adverse reactions to medical therapy. Regular monitoring of metabolic disorders by the nurse and patient can lead to a reduction in adverse events.

THE IMMUNE RESPONSE

Primary functions of the immune system are defense from invasion by destroying foreign microorganisms, homeostasis by removing worn-out cellular components, and surveillance by perceiving and destroying mutant cells. The immune system protects the body from foreign invaders, whether disease-producing microorganisms or abnormal cells such as cancer. Actually, the immune system is the third and slowest line of defense against such invasion. An intact skin provides the first line of defense. The inflammatory response is next in responding to an invading organism that breeches the barrier formed by the skin.

The inflammatory response consists of cellular components and processes, each with a unique role in maintaining the balance of homeostasis. After annihilating or neutralizing harmful organisms by phagocytosis, the inflammatory process removes the offenders from the site, confines them to limit their effectiveness, stimulates and enhances the immune response, and promotes healing (McCance & Huether, 2006). When this powerful defense is ineffective or fails, the immune system responds.

Immune System

Acting much as a surveillance mechanism, the immune system monitors the internal environment for foreign agents. As a complex system of organs and cells capable of distinguishing self from nonself, it remembers previous invaders and reacts according to needs as they arise. The primary organs of the immune system are the thymus, lymph nodes, spleen, and tonsils. Contributing to the effort of the immune response are lymphoid tissues in nonlymphoid organs and circulating immune cells, such as T cells, B cells, and phagocytes (Mandell, Bennett, & Dolin, 2005).

The lymph system continuously filters the blood. Lymph nodes distributed throughout the body have large clusters in the axillae, groin, thorax, abdomen, and neck. The nodes filter the lymph fluid and foreign materials and are reservoirs for specialized immunological T and B cells.

Antigen and Antigen-Antibody Response

The immune system responds to the invasion of the body by foreign material, called antigens. Some antigens are capable of producing disease, whereas others, although not disease-producing, are recognized as foreign and can elicit an immune response. Although capable of differentiating self from nonself, the immune system cannot differentiate harmful organisms from nonharmful ones.

Immunity is a normal adaptive response that protects the body from disease by resisting and attacking offending organisms. Acquired immunity can be active, developed on exposure to an antigen whereby antibodies are programmed to protect the body from illness with future exposures. These antibodies are specific, often providing lifetime immunity against another attack by the same antigen. Lifetime active immunity may develop from exposure to a specific antigen via inoculation. Passive immunity, on the other hand, is temporary immunity involving the transference of antibodies from one person or from another source to the patient.

Cells of the Immune Response

At least three types of cells are involved in the immune response to foreign material: the T cell, the B cell, and the macrophage. Each cell has a distinct responsibility and contributes to the integrity of the body as a whole. Sets of each cell type contain effector cells capable of attacking and destroying a particular antigen and memory cells that are imprinted with the antigenic code. The memory cells remember and recognize the antigen within minutes of a subsequent exposure (Mandell et al., 2005).

Immune Deficiency

Infection, cancer, and other chronic diseases contribute to a reduced effectiveness of the immune response. Large cancer tumors are able to release antigens into the blood that combine with circulating antibodies to prevent them from attacking tumor cells. Furthermore, tumor cells may possess special blocking factors that coat tumor cells and prevent destruction by killer T cells. This understanding is basic to planning care. In addition, infection with HIV is another major cause for immunodeficiency.

Multiple sclerosis, in which long-term steroid therapy is the mainstay of treatment, and HIV are examples of chronic immunosuppression. In HIV disease there is markedly depressed T-lymphocytes function with reduced numbers of T4 cells, impaired killer T-cell capacity, and increased numbers of suppressor T cells. By selectively invading and infecting T cells, the virus damages the very cell whose function it is to orchestrate the identification and destruction of virus as an antigen (Mandell et al., 2005).

HUMAN IMMUNODEFICIENCY VIRUS

HIV is a retrovirus, carrying genetic information in ribonucleic acid (RNA) rather than in deoxyribonucleic acid (DNA). HIV infects the particular T cell known as the CD4+ cell by binding to it and inserting its RNA into the $CD4_2$ cell. Through the action of reverse transcriptase, HIV is able to reprogram the genetic materials of the infected $CD4_2$ cell. When activated to reproduce, the $CD4_2$ cell produces more HIV, instead of viable and functional $CD4_2$ lymphocytes. The newly produced virus can then infect other $CD4_2$ lymphocytes (Dolin, Masur, & Saag, 2003; Mandell et al., 2005).

Epidemiology

As this chapter is written, new findings are emerging about the epidemiology and etiology of HIV infection and acquired immunodeficiency syndrome (AIDS). HIV infection is a chronic disease manifesting itself in a variety of ways, with AIDS being considered the extreme clinical manifestation. Before the advent of highly active antiretroviral therapy (HAART), the median AIDS-free time was 10 years, with subsets of patients progressing at slower or more rapid rates. Administering potent suppressive therapy has greatly lengthened AIDS-free time and decreased rates of conversion to AIDS and AIDS-related mortality rates (Bartlett & Gallant, 2004).

In states where HIV is a reportable condition, it can be seen that the incidence continues to rise. Reported cases are considered only "the tip of the iceberg" related to actual case rates in the United States and globally. AIDS has increased exponentially because of the lack of accessible treatment and prevention modalities in many developing countries. Anticipated life expectancy has plummeted in these countries from the high number of AIDS deaths. In the United States

incidence has been greater in homosexual and bisexual men, though the rate is increasing in the heterosexual community, particularly in the Southeast. In Africa, South America, and the Caribbean sexual transmission occurs more often between men and women. In Asia and Eastern Europe transmission through intravenous (IV) drug use is also highly prevalent. Other groups of people at significant risk for developing AIDS include sexual partners of high-risk individuals and children born to high-risk parents because AIDS is transmitted through blood and blood products or sexual intercourse (Mandell et al., 2005).

HIV Disease Progression

Rehabilitation nurses may encounter patients in any one of the four stages of HIV disease (Figure 35-3). The first stage is the acute infection period, during which there is viral transmission, primary HIV infection, and seroconversion. After the virus is transmitted, symptomatic primary infection occurs in approximately 80% to 90% of individuals (Bartlett & Gallant, 2004), followed within 6 months by seroconversion. Until that time a typical HIV antibody test may be negative, although a test for actual viral particles and a p24 antigen is positive. The CD4+ count may be in the normal range (650 to 2500 cells/mm³) and is usually considered to approximate a value of about 1000 cells/mm³. This is a highly infectious period, because the level of HIV virus in body fluids is quite high.

The second stage is asymptomatic infection, when patients may be unaware of their HIV disease but are capable of transmitting the disease to others. Although asymptomatic,

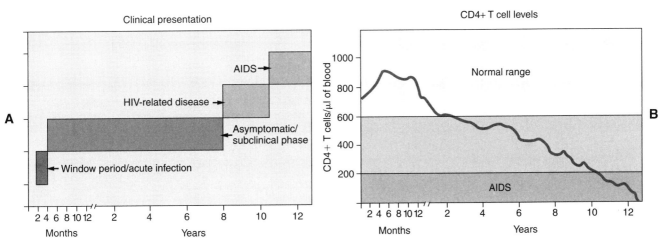

Figure 35-3 Staging of HIV disease. **A**, Typical time frame of progression from HIV infection to AIDS. During the *initial phase* the patient may experience flulike symptoms, characterized by fever, lymphadenopathy, and possibly a rash. Antibodies against HIV are not yet detectable (window period), but viral products, including p24 antigen, viral RNA, and infectious virus may be detectable in the blood a few weeks after infection. During the *second phase* of infection the patient is generally asymptomatic. Viral replication is active during this phase, antibodies are detectable in the blood, and CD4+ T cell levels are generally decreasing at rates relative to the amount of virus present (viral load). During the *third phase*, the patient becomes symptomatic, exhibiting constitutional symptoms and few opportunistic infections. The viral load generally continues to increase and CD4+ T cell levels continue to drop. During the *fourth*, and last, *phase* the patient has been diagnosed with AIDS with a CD4+ T cell count of less than 200, or opportunistic infections or malignancies. **B**, CD4+ changes during advancement from human immunodeficiency virus 1 (HIV-1) infection to acquired immunodeficiency syndrome (AIDS). (From Huether, S. E., & McCance, K. L., [2004]. *Understanding pathophysiology* [3rd ed.]. St. Louis, MO: Mosby.)

the virus is not latent but is actively replicating and destroying CD4+ cells. Individuals may have a variety of mild complaints, such as persistent generalized lymphadenopathy (PGL), fatigue, or various dermatological complaints (e.g., seborrheic dermatitis, psoriasis, pruritic folliculitis). At this point the CD4+ count usually ranges from 500 to 750 cells/mm³ (Dolin et al., 2003).

The symptomatic stage begins with PGL, weight loss, fatigue, and a multitude of worsening dermatological, musculoskeletal, or gastrointestinal complaints. Fevers or night sweats, weight loss, fatigue, and diarrhea are common. The CD4+ count ranges from 200 to 500 cells/mm³ with first symptoms, with wide variation. This stage extends into the AIDS stage, when opportunistic infections and malignancies may develop as a result of immune system dysfunction.

The fourth stage, AIDS, is a clinical diagnosis assigned to individuals who have opportunistic infections or unusual malignancies or those with CD4+ counts below the threshold of 200 cells/mm³, which is evidence of inadequate immune response against disease. This stage evolves with ongoing pathological changes that involve multiple body systems. The end or terminal stage of AIDS presents significant challenges to manage repeated opportunistic infections while preserving the patient's self-care and independence. The nurse's role in coordinating the complex interventions and needs for care becomes more difficult.

Clinical Manifestations of HIV Disease and Related Opportunistic Infection

Clinical manifestations of AIDS are frequently the result of opportunistic infections (OIs) preying on an impaired immune system (Figure 35-4). Early in the disease process, OIs are uncommon and may include tuberculosis or candidiasis. Tuberculosis is a reactivation of latent, encapsulated tuberculosis that flourishes because the immune system is unable to control a formerly inactive bacillus. It can become problematic in many stages of HIV disease, with the CD4+ count usually at less than 350 to 400 cells/mm³.

Candidiasis, a candidial infection of mucous membranes, especially in the oral cavity or the vaginal canal, is a common early clinical feature of HIV infection. Oral candidiasis, or thrush, is a marker of HIV disease progression. Thrush is visualized as white plaques on the buccal mucosa, tongue, and throat that can be removed when scraped with a tongue blade (Mandell & Mildvan, 2001).

Other opportunistic infections seen later in the course of HIV disease include *Pneumocystis carinii* pneumonia (PCP), cytomegalovirus (CMV), toxoplasmosis, and *Mycobacterium avium* complex (MAC). These tend to occur when the CD4+ count is under 200 cells/mm³ for PCP and under 50 for CMV, toxoplasmosis, and MAC. PCP is a pneumonia that appears less acute than bacterial pneumonia but causes significant progressive shortness of breath, weight loss, fatigue, and fevers. CMV frequently affects the retina, starting with blurry vision and leading to blindness. Toxoplasmosis, an infection in the central nervous system (CNS), produces headache, seizure, fever, and confusion. MAC is a systemic mycobacterial infection manifested by fever, drenching sweats, weight loss, wasting, fatigue, diarrhea, and abdominal pain. Anogenital herpes simplex (HSV) occurs with decreasing immune function and appears as persistent,

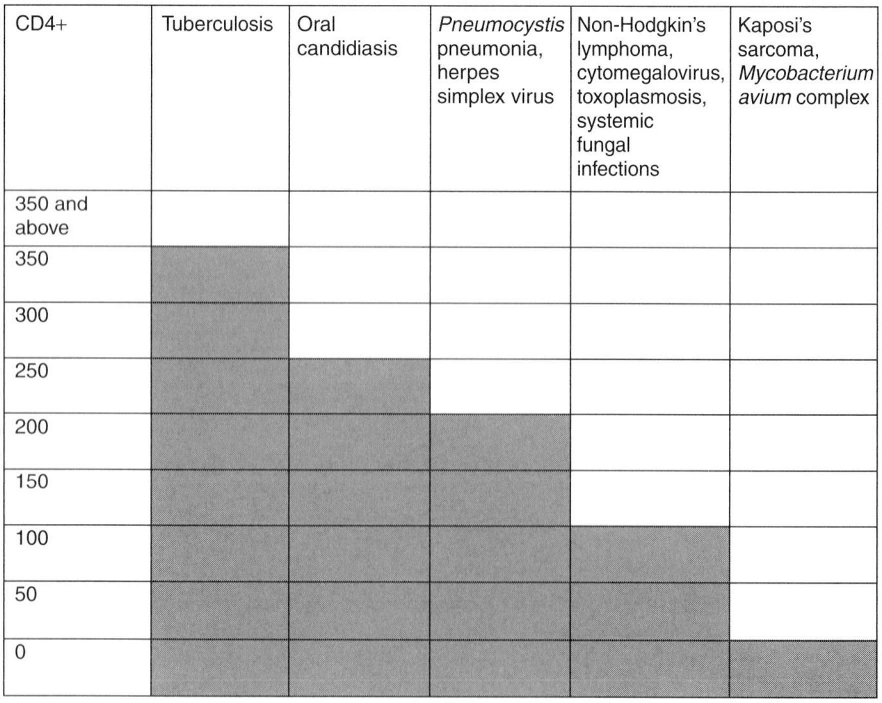

CD4+	Tuberculosis	Oral candidiasis	*Pneumocystis* pneumonia, herpes simplex virus	Non-Hodgkin's lymphoma, cytomegalovirus, toxoplasmosis, systemic fungal infections	Kaposi's sarcoma, *Mycobacterium avium* complex
350 and above					
350	■				
300	■				
250	■	■			
200	■	■	■		
150	■	■	■	■	
100	■	■	■	■	
50	■	■	■	■	
0	■	■	■	■	■

Figure 35-4 Risk of opportunistic infections related to CD4+ count: As immune function worsens, the risk of opportunistic infections increases.

chronic ulcerations over the penis, vulva, or buttocks (Mandell & Mildvan, 2001).

Neoplasias can appear; for example, Kaposi's sarcoma (KS) presents with purplish, hemorrhagic patches, plaques, and nodules (Mandell et al., 2005). In addition, lymphomas can occur as can cervical cancer. Figure 35-4 illustrates the relationship of opportunistic infections with stages of HIV disease.

Physical Systems Affected by HIV

Patients with HIV face a number of infections that affect every organ system. Effects in the nervous system and the gastrointestinal system are especially common.

Nervous System Disorders.
Advancing AIDS involves diffuse and focal central nervous system disorders as well as peripheral neuropathies. People diagnosed with AIDS dementia complex (ADC) may exhibit signs of cognitive, behavioral, and motor disturbances, and each can have a variety of early and late symptoms. A significant number of people with AIDS eventually develop a degree of cognitive, motor, or emotional impairment that can respond favorably to counseling and/or medications. In addition, antiviral medications that cross the blood-brain barrier, such as zidovudine, may decrease symptoms. Later manifestations of central neurological involvement include severe memory loss, speech disturbances, and abnormal reflexes and tone. Gait disturbances from an associated myelopathy may occur, as well as bowel and bladder deficits, strokes, and visual impairment (Price, 2003).

Peripheral nervous system involvement may manifest in four distinct clinical patterns of neuropathy: distal sensorimotor polyneuropathy, inflammatory demyelinating polyneuropathy, mononeuropathy multiplex, and progressive polyradiculopathy (Price, 2003). Outcomes may relate to progressive disease or side effects of medication. Viruses such as varicella-zoster also may cause neuropathies. With neuromuscular complications, lower extremity wasting eventually extends to the upper extremities with proximal muscle weakness and tenderness. Sensory polyneuropathy is a painful paresthesia of the soles of the feet thought to result from HIV infection of the neurons. Although these peripheral neuropathies can be extremely debilitating, few interventions alleviate the pain and distress effectively.

Gastrointestinal Disorders.
The gastrointestinal system is highly vulnerable to the many pathogens capable of invading the immunocompromised patient. This creates some of the most frustrating problems for both the patient and the nurse. The physiological sequelae of HIV in the gastrointestinal tract are an important cause of morbidity and mortality. The pathophysiology of intestinal infection is not understood; however, two mechanisms have been postulated. The first is reduced intestinal immunity, resulting in chronic opportunistic infections that cause altered intestinal functioning. The second is that HIV itself affects the intestinal mucosa and causes malfunctioning. Extensive diarrhea can be seen in

people infected with HIV; this may be caused by bacterial overgrowth, decreased mucosal immune function, and abnormal neural and endocrine function of the intestines (Monkemuller & Wilcox, 2003).

Nutritional Status in HIV Disease.
Compromised nutritional status exacerbates the complicated clinical picture presented by AIDS. Painful oral and esophageal inflammations can cause difficulty with swallowing. Complex drug regimens with adverse interactions and stress of chronicity contribute to persistent anorexia. Diarrhea, malabsorption, and weight loss frustrate efforts to achieve or maintain adequate nutrition. Nurses have an important challenge to assess and implement appropriate interventions to improve the nutritional status of their patients and to understand the relationship among nutrition, HIV infection, and the immune system.

Progressive weight loss is a clinical sentinel symptom resulting from reduced intake, malabsorption, hormone abnormalities, or metabolic abnormalities. Malnutrition with weight loss may adversely affect the function of the immune system and further impair the person's ability to avoid or recover from repeated infections and to manage stressors. Need for nutritional support in HIV arises in early asymptomatic stages and continues during the stage of AIDS. People with asymptomatic HIV benefit from a balanced diet with protein and nutrients. As the disease progresses, progressive involuntary weight loss commonly ensues with reduced food intake, malabsorption, and altered metabolism. These can be exacerbated by anorexia, nausea, infection, chronic diarrhea, malabsorption, and poor food availability. A nurse can refer patients for dietary counseling and home health care services to provide symptom relief and prevent further weight loss. A nutritional assessment includes the following factors:
- Anthropometrics: height, weight, body mass index
- Biochemical tests: albumin, lipids, liver enzymes, renal panel, hemoglobin
- Clinical examination identifying opportunistic infections
- Dietary history
- Economic and social factors

A cohesive team approach is imperative in planning comprehensive care with patients and families. Goals are to maintain body mass and promote self-concept.

Fatigue and Energy Problems Related to HIV Disease.
Although fatigue is common among people with HIV/AIDS, its etiology is unknown. A generalized malaise and loss of motivation unrelated to activity and sleep patterns, generalized fatigue may relate to specific muscle fatigue. Initial complaints are of tiredness, but it persists as a prominent, unexplained symptom. The many physical and psychosocial conditions experienced by immunocompromised people may have profound negative effects on functional level and quality of life. Fatigue has an economic impact as the overriding symptom that leads people with HIV infection to discontinue employment. Unable to work, they lose health

insurance in most instances and turn to public funds throughout the prolonged, slowly progressive deterioration of their illness (Remien, Satriano, & Berkman, 1999).

HIV ACROSS THE LIFE SPAN

Pediatric HIV

Until June 1991 children infected during the perinatal period accounted for 91% of HIV cases up to 13 years of age. Since that time children and adolescents infected as a result of high-risk sexual behaviors account for the majority of the children infected with HIV. Infection with HIV in children with hemophilia has declined since the blood supplies began being tested routinely for HIV (National Center for Health Statistics, National Vital Statistics Reports, March 7, 2005).

Epidemiology. In the United States the number of HIV-infected infants born each year has been reduced to approximately 150 (Centers for Disease Control and Prevention, 2005a). Internationally the number is vastly larger, with 90% of pediatrics cases occurring in developing countries. For example, in sub-Saharan Africa approximately 1,000 infants are born daily with HIV infection (Steele, 2001). In 1994 a landmark multicenter clinical trial showed the use of zidovudine (AZT) taken by the mother reduced perinatal HIV infection from about 30% to about 8% of all births to HIV-positive mothers. The drug is given to the mother during pregnancy, labor, and delivery and to the neonate for 6 weeks. High cost and poor distribution infrastructure have been barriers to making AZT available in developing countries where increased prevalence and incidence of HIV affects women of childbearing age. The Joint United Nations Programme on HIV/AIDS (UNAIDS) has made some impact on this, though the funding is not sufficient to lower the rate of HIV-infected infants to that seen in developed countries. Clinical trials have shown the effectiveness of short-term treatment with low-cost alternative antiviral medications, though they are less effective than the gold standard.

Pregnant HIV-infected women must be identified and offered treatment to halt perinatal transmission of HIV disease. In many cultures identification leads to ostracism, and without finances and infrastructure for treatment of the mother, as well as preventive interventions for the baby, outcomes are limited.

Pediatric Clinical Manifestations. At least two thirds of children who contract HIV disease from their mothers are believed to do so during labor and delivery. Those infants with a positive HIV test at birth are believed to have contracted the disease in utero, whereas those who are HIV negative at birth but seroconvert at a later time (2 to 4 weeks after birth) are believed to have contracted the disease during labor and delivery (Steele, 2001). Children with in utero infection tend to have a more rapid disease course and fare less well. Failure to thrive, recurrent diarrhea, lymphadenopathy, and hepatosplenomegaly are constitutional symptoms that may go unrecognized early in the disease. Oral candidiasis

and diaper dermatitis, chronic nasal discharge, and recurrent otitis media unresponsive to the usual therapies may occur. Frequent bacterial infections are a common complication of HIV disease in children. The progression of the disease may cause damage and dysfunction to one or multiple organs including the central nervous system, heart, lungs, and gastrointestinal systems. Encephalopathy may occur as shown by delays in developmental milestones, impaired cognition and expressive language, spastic paraparesis, ataxia, and hyperirritability (Wong et al., 2000).

Rehabilitation. Rehabilitation efforts are directed to minimizing the deficits caused by the progressive neurological problems. Emphasis is on the maintenance of existing cognitive skills and facilitating developmental achievement with infant stimulation and speech-language therapy. Antiviral treatment lessens the viral load and allows for immune reconstitution. Treatment with triple antiviral treatment is recommended in children as in adults, but dosing, pharmacokinetics, and side effects must be monitored carefully (Steele, 2001).

Referral for physical and occupational therapy assists children with compensating for motor deficits. Rehabilitation programs also address problems and issues generated by the environment of perinatally infected children who are frequently from socially and economically disadvantaged families. Referrals to social services and home health care nurses, as well as community resources, are highly appropriate to incorporate into the rehabilitation plan (Steele, 2001).

Adult Chronic Disease

Psychosocial Challenges. Psychosocial problems are among the most common difficulties associated with HIV disease in the adult population. Dealing with the stigma of AIDS, experiencing loneliness, thinking about death, and needing to make lifestyle changes, coupled with changes in the existing self-concept result in changes in body image and self-esteem. The experience of loneliness and the increased need for social support offers a serious challenge to patients and their caregivers. Isolation may be self-induced because of apathy or changes in personal appearance or due to the stigma associated with this diagnosis. Disclosure to family and friends is an additional psychological strain. Other psychosocial concerns include maintaining sexual integrity, maintaining independent function for activities of daily living, and spiritual distress. Young adults face the risk in parenting a child of infecting the partner and child.

A goal is to promote optimal levels of independent functioning in the community within the limitations imposed by this chronic disease. Educating the patient and caregivers about the nature of the disease and necessary lifestyle changes includes importance of adhering to the plan of care and making changes in sexual and/or drug use practices.

Elderly and HIV

In the United States 1% of men and 2% of women older than age 65 years have AIDS. Because birth control is not an issue for that generation, the use of condoms for protection is less common. HIV is more difficult to treat and has a faster course in the elderly, perhaps owing to underlying deficiencies in the immune system (Linsk, 2000). Antiviral medicines are less tested in the elderly, so pharmacokinetics are less clear. The stigma associated with the disease may mean fear and social isolation. Research is needed regarding HIV disease and aging.

NURSING INTERVENTIONS RELATED TO IMMUNODEFICIENCY

Nurses are integrally involved in protecting a patient with immunodeficiency (Risi & Tomascak, 1998). The nurse has multiple tasks in primary prevention of infection in those with a number of conditions causing immunodeficiency:

* Identify risk factors from the history, such as recent travel, medications that may affect the immune system, drug use, and sexual activity.
* Educate patients to have invasive procedures such as venous access devices or dental work completed and chronic conditions of the skin, scalp, or nail beds treated before starting immunosuppressive therapy.
* Keep immunizations updated to help augment the immune system.
* Reduce neutropenia by administering granulocyte colony-stimulating factor and granulocyte-macrophage colony-stimulating factor.
* Educate patients, family, and significant others about the high risk for infection, and teach the skills for infection control with such basics as cleaning foods thoroughly and cooking meat well. Pets can pose special risks for infectious disease. Emphasize careful hand washing repeatedly. With chronic immunosuppressive conditions, long-term behavior change prevents infection (Risi & Tomascak, 1998).

Nursing Assessment

Patients with HIV or AIDS can present a variety of conditions, from early asymptomatic HIV to advanced AIDS with multiple, complicated problems or multiple system failure. AIDS care requires knowledge in infection control, neurology, oncology, psychiatry, and pediatrics among other areas. Early in the disease, nurses educate patients about interventions and assist them with coping effectively. With advanced AIDS and malnourished patients hospitalized for recurring infection, debilitation, febrile illness, and pain, nursing roles are more intensive. Box 35-6 lists assessment parameters.

History of Present Illness. A history includes risk factors for transmission of HIV and date of diagnosis, as well as data about previous illnesses, treatments, or chronic illness. Transmission history allows for preventive interventions to reduce future spread of HIV and to offer strategies to cope effectively with denial and morbidity. The medication history is connected to past OI history because many OIs are chronic and maintenance medications control infections. Medication history is also imperative for designing a fully suppressive

regimen of HIV medications. Assessment of weight allows understanding of the current wasting status. A nonpurposeful loss of 10% of normal body weight indicates wasting regardless of current weight.

Diagnostic Tests

Laboratory tests specific for HIV are useful for disease staging and treatment decisions. Patients need to understand the tests and their significance. Specific diagnostic tests are the enzyme-linked immunosorbent assay (ELISA) and the Western blot to confirm HIV infection. The major test for staging the disease is the CD4+ count (T-cell count), which indicates the competence of the immune system and shows the extent of destruction of CD4+ cells by the HIV virus. Another key test is the HIV viral load by HIV RNA polymerase chain reaction (PCR) or by branched chain DNA (bDNA), which reports the virulence of infection. Quantitative viral load predicts clinical progression or survival and frequently determines treatment efficacy. Other laboratory tests include genotyping or phenotyping of the infecting HIV virus to reveal mutations that confer resistance to antiviral medications.

HIV itself and the medications used to treat HIV have been shown to cause insulin resistance and hyperlipidemia in some people. Because of the high rate of metabolic disease found in this population, regular monitoring of levels of blood glucose and lipids is also important.

Systems Review

A multiple systems review assists in determining the extent of damage in this all-encompassing disease. Assess the following systems in particular:

BOX 35-6 Nursing Assessment

History
* Risk factors, date of diagnosis, coping, history of opportunistic infections, history of concomitant illnesses, medication history, normal weight before illness
* Laboratory tests specific to diagnosis

Systems Review
* Neurological
* Integumentary
* Gastrointestinal
* Musculoskeletal
* Constitutional symptoms
* Psychiatric, focusing on presence of depression, inability to cope

Physical Assessment
* Functional limitations
* Current opportunistic infections, wasting

Psychosocial Assessment
* Assess readiness to change lifestyle: adherence to medications, sexuality, substance abuse
* Family acceptance, coping, social support

- Neurological—extent of cognitive deficit or peripheral neuropathy
- Integumentary—rashes or lesions
- Gastrointestinal—diarrhea or other malabsorption or appetite problems, nutritional deficit, oral or esophageal candidiasis
- Musculoskeletal—weakness, inability to perform activities of daily living
- Constitutional symptoms—fevers, night sweats, lymphadenopathy, generalized weakness or fatigue, wasting, and pain
- Psychiatric—depression or inability to cope

Physical Assessment

A full physical assessment is important to identify current opportunistic infections with particular focus on the following:

- Cardiorespiratory system for tuberculosis, PCP, and other respiratory illnesses
- Integumentary system for HSV, KS, subcutaneous fungal infections, and other OIs
- Gastrointestinal system, including the oral mucosa, for oral or esophageal candidiasis, KS, MAC, CMV, and other malabsorption problems
- Neurological system, including visual changes, for CMV retinitis, HIV encephalopathy, toxoplasmosis, cryptococcal meningitis, ADC, peripheral neuropathy, or other peripheral or CNS problems
- Musculoskeletal system for HIV wasting, HIV-related myopathies

- Lymphatic system for lymphomas or HIV-related lymphadenopathy

Psychosocial Assessment

Adaptation to HIV disease as a chronic, rather than terminal, disease is critical to successful living. Assess the patient's adjustment, specifically adherence to treatment and modification of sexual lifestyle or drug use. Treatment for HIV disease is complex and must be consistent to prevent resistant mutations of the HIV virus. Treatment involves a minimum of three HIV medications as well as others to control or prevent OIs and those needed to manage metabolic complications

Nurses have influence in the primarily young adult population where privacy about a stigmatizing illness is paramount. Assessment tools for lifestyle change include the Transtheoretical Model of Change, Health Belief Model, screening tools for depression, and for drug and alcohol misuse. Nonjudgmental questioning is important in assessing coping and adaptation to HIV disease because many barriers make adherence to medication regimens and lifestyle changes difficult. Sample questions in Table 35-2 foster frank discussions and interventions based on the Transtheoretical Model of Change. Questions concerning the source of HIV and beliefs about the efficacy of medicines or other therapy reflect the Health Belief Model. The CAGE questionnaire (Table 35-3) is an example of a drug/alcohol assessment tool. There are multiple depression scales (e.g., Zung, Beck, Prime-MD)

TABLE 35-2 Assessment of Medication Adherence

Assessment	Rationale
"I know that it is hard for a lot of people taking medicines every day. What are *your* particular difficulties with them?"	Establish "cons" to adherent taking of medicines. Gives the patient permission to admit to nonadherence, which establishes honesty and acceptance in your relationship. Cons to the behavior generally diminish with time when actively engaging in the behavior.
"Because it is difficult for you to take your medicines every day, why are you taking them? What are the benefits to you in taking your medicines?"	Establish the "pros" to adherent taking of medicines, to increase the individual's investment in the behavior. Pros generally increase as the individual knows more about the purpose and becomes more committed to medicine-taking behavior.
"A lot of people have trouble taking their medicines every day, or sometimes they even stop them completely. There are a lot of medicines, and a lot of people find that very hard to get used to. Side effects can also be a problem. Do you take your medicines regularly every day?"	
If no . . .	Accept individual's concerns/difficulties with the medicines as rational explanations that are appropriate for discussion. Give feedback about health status. Establish personalized pros and cons, and educate/reinforce about consequences of not taking medicines.
If not now but is thinking about It . . .	Encourage expression of negative emotions about taking medicines. Give feedback about health status. Establish personalized pros and cons, and educate/reinforce about consequences of not taking medicines.
If yes, I have recently started . . .	Discuss actual or perceived barriers to regular medicine-taking: access problems, forgetfulness, side effects and present options for addressing those barriers. Support self-efficacy: provide encouragement and feedback. Plan for disruptions in schedule, and for relapses in the future in order to limit the length of time of the relapse.

From Konkle-Parker, D. J. (2001). A motivational intervention to improve adherence to treatment of chronic disease. *Journal of the American Academy of Nurse Practitioners, 13*(2), 66-67.

that are also important in assessing the factors involved with coping with a diagnosis of HIV as well as its treatment.

Social support is critical with any chronic condition that requires lifestyle change. Assessing how well the patient, family, and others understand the disease, accept changes, and use effective coping strategies helps to reveal both spoken and unspoken needs that the nurse may be able to help them meet.

Nursing Diagnoses

Nursing diagnoses with a psychosocial component include the following: risk for ineffective therapeutic regimen management as seen by poor adherence to medications or other lifestyle change; hopelessness; ineffective sexuality pattern; ineffective coping; and disabled family coping (Gordon, 2000). Other diagnoses are related to compromised immune status and opportunistic infections. These include risk for infection related to immune deficiency leading to opportunistic infections; imbalanced nutrition: less than body requirements related to AIDS wasting; diarrhea, related to HIV or to medication therapy; fatigue; chronic pain; and

risk for cognitive impairment (Gordon, 2000). Table 35-4 lists nursing diagnoses with their corresponding interventions and outcomes.

Nursing Goals

The nursing care plan depends greatly on the disease status and extent of disability. The nurse working with those hospitalized for an acute condition concentrates on acute nursing goals for physiological conditions with underlying psychosocial goals. Home health care nurses may consider setting long-term goals with patients toward acceptance and treatment.

Community Health Goals. Community health settings may include care for the community related to HIV prevention and provision of community services to those infected with HIV. Goals in community health include regular health care for continued viral suppression, health maintenance, and case management. The nurse is critical in case management to assess holistic health needs. Ensuring access and removing barriers to care take many forms. Finances or

TABLE 35-3 CAGE Alcohol Screening Questionnaire

Question	Response	
1. Have you ever felt you should *C*ut down on your drinking?	Yes	No
2. Have people *A*nnoyed you by criticizing your drinking?	Yes	No
3. Have you ever felt bad or *G*uilty about your drinking?	Yes	No
4. Have you ever taken a drink first thing in the morning to steady your nerves or get rid of a hangover? (*E*ye-opener)	Yes	No

From Ewing, J. A. (1984). Detecting alcoholism: The CAGE questionnaire. *Journal of the American Medical Association, 252,* 1905-1907. Scoring: Two or more positive answers suggest that the existence of alcohol-related problems is very probable, currently or in the past.

TABLE 35-4 Nursing Diagnoses, Interventions, and Outcomes Applicable to HIV/AIDS   **NIC/NOC**

Nursing Diagnosis	*Nursing Interventions*	*Nursing Outcomes*
Ineffective therapeutic regimen management	Health education	Adherence behavior Knowledge: treatment regimen
Hopelessness	Emotional support	Hope
Ineffective coping	Coping enhancement	Acceptance: health status
Risk for infection	Teaching: disease process, medication management	Treatment behavior
Imbalanced nutrition: less than body requirements	Nutrition management Oral health restoration	Nutritional status Weight: body mass
Diarrhea (related to HIV or to medication therapy)	Diarrhea management	Symptom control
Fatigue	Energy management	Quality of life Endurance
Chronic pain	Pain management	Pain control
Disturbed thought processes	Dementia management Family support	Decision making

Data from Moorhead, S., Johnson, M., & Maas, M. (Eds.). (2004). *Nursing outcomes classification (NOC)* (3rd ed.). St. Louis, MO: Mosby; Dochterman, J. M., & Bulechek, G. M. (2004). *Nursing interventions classification (NIC)* (4th ed.). St. Louis, MO: Mosby; and NANDA International. (2007). *NANDA-I nursing diagnoses: Definitions & classification 2007-2008.* Philadelphia: Author.

transportation may affect access to health care or medications. Situations at home may create problems with adherence. Further education may be needed about HIV or treatments. Isolation may call for connecting with support groups.

Goals in home health care, restricted to those who are homebound and need skilled nursing care, center around physical problems associated with AIDS. Goals include administering intravenous medications as treatment or for maintenance for OIs, enhancing optimal independence, and holistic case management for the individual.

Acute Care Goals. Goals in the hospital include resolving acute OIs, initiating education about maintenance therapy, and ensuring case management. Effective discharge planning ensures that long-term goals are addressed.

Regardless of the setting, partnership with the patient is essential in making permanent adaptation to the disease process and effective health care management, including prevention of further complications. Case management involving referrals to resources is critical to maintaining health. Many communities have local AIDS service organizations and support groups. Table 35-5 contains a list of national resources for those with HIV and AIDS. Sites on the World Wide Web are shown in Table 35-6.

Hospice goals are for those with advanced AIDS when antiviral treatment is no longer effective or patients choose not to participate. The goals include comfort with pain management, control of diarrhea, pacing activities to reduce fatigue, and family support.

Apart from the specific treatments to combat OIs and malignancies, no effective cure exists for AIDS. Treatment goals are to preserve and enhance the immune system; although some approaches are symptomatic, others are highly experimental. The mortality rate for individuals with documented AIDS, at one time 95% at 2 years, has improved dramatically, but the rate and extent of change remain unclear.

NURSING INTERVENTIONS SPECIFIC TO HIV DISEASE

Rehabilitation interventions for HIV occur throughout all levels of prevention. Primary prevention of infection with HIV is to reduce the risks of HIV transmission, secondary prevention is for early screening and diagnosis before extensive immune compromise, and tertiary prevention is for reducing severity of disability. HIV care ranges from care for asymptomatic patients, to adaptation to the disease, to hospice for advanced AIDS.

Primary Prevention

Healthy People 2010 goals pertain to prevention of HIV in the community, as well as reduction of those who advance from HIV to AIDS. Improved medication treatment has not brought a cure or preventive vaccine; thus education about reducing risks remains the best means to contain the epidemic in the United States. Preventive behaviors include ceasing IV drug use, maintaining monogamous sexual relationships, and eliminating vertical transmission from mother to baby. Behaviors to reduce risk include drug use without needle sharing, cleaning needles with bleach, and condom use.

HIV is transmitted during sexual contact, by sharing IV needles or drug paraphernalia, with exposure to infected blood, blood products, or body fluids, and from mother to newborn perinatally. The Centers for Disease Control and Prevention (CDC) developed standard precautions for all professionals to consider blood and body fluids of all patients as potentially infectious for HIV, hepatitis B virus, and other blood-borne pathogens. Standard precautions prevent parenteral, mucous membrane, and nonintact skin exposure to patients' blood as well as other body fluids containing visible blood. Standard precautions also prevent exposure to semen, vaginal secretions, and body tissues as well as cerebrospinal, synovial, pleural, peritoneal, pericardial, and amniotic fluids. These precautions do not apply to feces, nasal secretions, sputum, sweat, tears, urine, and vomit unless they contain visible blood. Standard precautions are not optional; apply them consistently. Nurses must know the standards mandated by the Occupational Safety and Health Administration and organizational policies regarding blood-borne pathogens, as well as environmental or special precautions required during invasive procedures.

Secondary Prevention

Early screening identifies people with HIV before clinical symptoms and the onset of AIDS. State departments of health mandates to control transmission and for secondary prevention

TABLE 35-5 National Resources for Patients With HIV

Resource	Contact Information	Content
National AIDS Hotline	800-342-2437	Hotline for information, counseling
Centers for Disease Control and Prevention	800-458-5231	Publications, epidemiology
National Association of People With AIDS	202-898-0414	Advocacy information, treatment information
AIDS Treatment Data Network	800-734-7104	Record of research data
HIV-AIDS Treatment Information Service	800-HIV-0440	Treatment information
Project Inform	800-822-7422	Linking with HIV services
National Clinical Trials Hotline	800-TRIALS-A	Listing of AIDS clinical trials

should be included in every community health plan. A recent CDC (2006) guideline recommends that all patients in all medical settings should be screened for HIV regardless of risk behavior. The CDC (2005b) reports that in 2005 24% to 27% of those infected with HIV in the United States were unaware of the disease and that there are 40,000 new infections annually (http://www.cdc.gov/hiv/topics/testing/resources). They estimate that those who are unaware of their HIV status account for more than half of the new infections each year. In addition, studies show that those who become aware of their HIV disease generally reduce their risky behavior. For this reason a reduction in the number of people who are unaware of their disease may have an impact on slowing the epidemic.

Tertiary Prevention

Tertiary prevention is to prevent the onset of AIDS and significant morbidity and mortality. For those with HIV, nursing goals have three levels. *Short-term goals* for disease control are medication treatment, suppressing viral replication, and preventing OIs. *Long-term goals* are to control the disease, provide regular health care, and plan for lifestyle changes and adherence. *Lifelong planning* includes patients' recognition of future complications and back-to-work issues, preparing advance directives, and facilitation of a second chance at life or hospice care. Multiple and complex interventions differ with patient needs and situation and with disease progression.

Physiological Interventions

Physiological interventions are to control disease progression, symptoms, and OIs. With *late-stage AIDS*, OIs occur alongside diarrhea, fever, weight loss, and skin breakdown. Monitor and replace electrolytes and fluid volume, use diet and medications for diarrhea and fever, and attend to restoring oral health. Nutrition may be compromised if candidiasis or

TABLE 35-6 Active Websites for Information About HIV Disease and AIDS

Web Address	Subject Matter
http://hopkins-aids.edu	Johns Hopkins AIDS service—professional education
http://hiv.medscape.com	Current medical professional information. Requires registration
http://hivinsite.ucsf.edu	Medical information, prevention and public education, epidemiology, social issues, links to other sites
http://hivatis.org	HIV/AIDS Treatment Information Service—treatment guidelines, clinical trial information
http://thebody.com	The Body: An AIDS and HIV information resource—public and patient-oriented information
http://www.amfar.org	American Foundation for AIDS Research—data derived from AIDS research

mouth sores reduce intake. As more becomes known of long-term side effects of HIV treatment and HIV disease, nurses can expect to manage hyperlipidemia and hyperglycemia alongside HIV disease (Dochterman & Bulechek, 2004).

Hurley and Ungvarski (1994) surveyed home health care requirements of people with HIV/AIDS. They found the most common physiological symptoms were dyspnea, weakness, fatigue and lethargy, pain, and ataxia. Memory deficit, depression, anxiety, impaired judgment, substance abuse, and insomnia occurred most frequently. Needs were assistance with cleaning the home, preparing meals, doing laundry, and shopping.

AIDS-related dementia requires assessment of the type and extent of cognitive deficits. Patients, families, and others need education about this condition. Use written materials, visual cues, and assistive equipment to boost poor memory or concentration. These patients need reminders to adhere to treatment. Medication management of OIs and HIV disease helps combat the *fatigue* that becomes part of the condition. Interventions include counseling about nutrition, reducing pace of activities and environmental stimuli, adequate rest, and adjustment to life changes (Dochterman & Bulechek, 2004). Control of *chronic pain*, usually peripheral neuropathy associated with HIV disease or with medication therapy, is essential to quality of life. Interventions include assessing and monitoring pain and identifying sources of exacerbation using both alternative and complementary or pharmacological interventions (Dochterman & Bulechek, 2004). Chapter 23 discusses pain management in more detail.

Psychosocial Intervention

Active listening as patients express denial, anger, and depression regarding the diagnosis assists patients with working through their feelings. Encouragement to express feelings with full acceptance of the person is a nursing intervention they may not receive from anyone else in their lives; it may help them adjust and form strategies to cope effectively. Patients adjust better if they can assess realistically the impact of the disease, and have facts about their diagnosis, treatment, and prognosis. Other interventions are to promote decision making and encourage spiritual resources. When patients and their families agree to support one another, patients experience less isolation and fewer concerns that a caregiver will be available when needed (Dochterman & Bulechek, 2004).

Medical Treatment

Currently approved antiretroviral drugs are in Chapter 7, though this list changes rapidly with additions of new drugs. Nucleoside reverse transcriptase inhibitors (NRTIs) are the oldest class of antiretroviral drugs, used alone until 1995, when a new class, protease inhibitors (PIs), emerged with improved suppressive power. Another class—nonnucleoside reverse transcriptase inhibitors (NNRTIs)—inhibit the reverse transcriptase enzyme in a slightly different pathway. Figure 35-5 illustrates the drug actions in the HIV trajectory. Drug combinations, such as two NRTIs and one PI or NNRTI, create potent suppression of viral replication. Several new drugs and classes, including nucleotide reverse transcriptase inhibitors and fusion inhibitors have been approved, and others have entered the Food and Drug Administration (FDA) approval process.

Several lipid abnormalities have been noted among those with HIV disease. Medical therapy for HIV disease can contribute to developing risk factors for metabolic disease. Negative medication side effects, including adipose redistribution, can lead to an increase in visceral adipose tissue and abdominal girth and a decrease in adipose distribution in the extremities and face. These factors predispose patients to insulin resistance and diabetes. Medications used for HIV can also cause abnormalities in lipid metabolites. Specific therapies for HIV, including protease inhibitors and nucleoside reverse transcriptase inhibitors, may negatively alter lipid parameters. Triglycerides may be severely altered to the point of changing HIV therapy to decrease the patient's risk for pancreatitis. However, it appears that medical management and HIV disease each contribute to the development of insulin resistance and lipid abnormalities (Grinspoon & Carr, 2005).

Interventions During the Terminal Phase of AIDS

Eventually in the trajectory of the disease, physiological and emotional problems accompanying AIDS affect an individual's ability to function independently. Continuing rehabilitation appropriately supports caregivers that may become depressed. AIDS networks and groups help in support and information. Nurses should help caregivers make informed decisions about care options as the patient enters the terminal phase.

Stages of HIV reproduction

1. HIV enters a CD4+ cell.
2. HIV is a retrovirus, meaning that its genetic information is stored on single-stranded RNA instead of the double-stranded DNA found in most organisms. To replicate, HIV uses an enzyme known as reverse transcriptase to convert its RNA into DNA.
3. HIV DNA enters the nucleus of the CD4+ cell and inserts itself into the cell's DNA. HIV DNA then instructs the cell to make many copies of the original virus.
4. New virus particles are assembled and leave the cell, ready to infect other CD4+ cells.

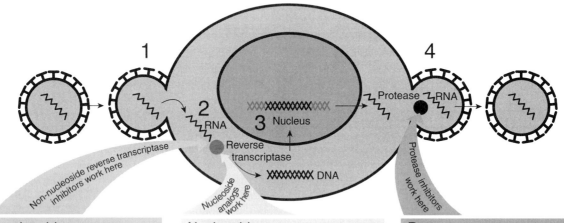

Non-nucleoside reverse transcriptase inhibitors

The newest class of antiretroviral agents, non-nucleoside reverse transcriptase inhibitors (NNRTIs) stop HIV production by binding directly onto reverse transcriptase and preventing the conversion of RNA to DNA. These drugs are called "non-nucleoside" inhibitors because even though they work at the same stage as nucleoside analogs, they act in a completely different way.
VIRAMUNE (nevirapine)
Rescriptor (delavirdine mesylate)
Sustiva (efavirenz)

Nucleoside analogs

The first effective class of antiretroviral drugs was the nucleoside analogs. They act by incorporating themselves into the DNA of the virus, thereby stopping the building process. The resulting DNA is incomplete and cannot create new virus.
Ziagen (abacavir sulfate)
Retrovir (zidovudine; also known as ZDV or AZT)
Epivir (lamivudine; also known as 3TC)
Videx (didanosine; also known as ddI)
Hivid (zalcitabine; also known as ddC)
Zerit (stavudine; also known as d4T)
Combivir (lamivudine/zidovudine)

Protease inhibitors

Protease inhibitors work at the last stage of the virus reproduction cycle. They prevent HIV from being successfully assembled and released from the infected CD4+ cell.
Invirase (saquinavir mesylate)
Crixivan (indinavir)
Norvir (ritonavir)
Viracept (nelfinavir mesylate)
Fortovase (saquinavir)

Note: This information is provided for background only.

Figure 35-5 Areas of impact of antiretroviral medications. A combination of medications that affect different processes in HIV replication can suppress replication to a greater degree. Thus nucleoside or nonnucleoside reverse transcriptase inhibitors are combined with protease inhibitors to effectively inhibit the process of transcription of RNA to DNA and to inhibit the process of combining proteins together to form the basis of a replicated HIV virus. (Courtesy Roxane Laboratories, Inc., Columbus, OH.)

Hospice is an appropriate option for comfort without active curative measures or invasive or diagnostic procedures. An array of services based on a holistic health care philosophy, hospice provides the dying person and family with comfort, autonomy, and emotional and physical support. An interdisciplinary team supports the nurse, who coordinates and supervises all hospice services 7 days a week, 24 hours a day from a hospital or in the home setting or other community programs. Chapter 36 discusses hospice care for patients with end-stage renal disease.

OUTCOMES

Nursing outcomes for patients with HIV disease include physiological and psychosocial outcomes that vary according to the stage of disease and the patient's stage of life. Rehabilitation nurses evaluate the entire range of outcomes to ensure holistic care.

Clinical Endpoints

A high CD4+ count, an undetectable viral load, improved or lack of symptoms, and no OIs indicate physiological control of HIV disease progression. With wasting, outcomes include improved nutrition and weight, especially with more lean body mass that may help resolve diarrhea or mucosa and skin integrity problems (Moorhead et al., 2004).

With fatigue, improved outcomes include endurance in performing activities of daily living and instrumental activities of daily living, rested appearance, and interest in activities as opposed to exhaustion and lethargy. Pain control may reduce impairments in concentration, mobility, and self-care. Cognitive impairment occurs in up to 75% of those with HIV disease and AIDS. Outcomes include early identification and treatment of cognitive deficits and adapting the environment to compensate for permanent deficits. Support systems and interventions are added to maximize cognition as deficits are known (Moorhead et al., 2004).

Adequate nutrition is evidenced by weight and body mass index. Fatigue and activity intolerance and physical changes, such as thinner extremities with increased abdominal girth, are cautions that may indicate complications of HIV disease or complications of medical treatment.

Psychosocial Outcomes

Psychosocial outcomes for long-term adjustment to HIV disease are similar to those with other life-threatening chronic illnesses. Education to minimize complications and facilitate coping, as well as to prevent transmission, is appropriate in the short-term. Outcomes evaluate the patient's ability to describe how to prevent transmission of HIV to others, to avoid contracting OIs, and to demonstrate understanding about *non*transmission to avoid self-imposed isolation. Patients demonstrate learning about the disease when they are able to describe the medication regimen and side effects, sources for medications, and purposes of continual monitoring of CD4+ counts and viral loads. Those who engage in active

partnership with health professionals usually understand the importance of adherence to the regimen (Moorhead et al., 2004). Patients also need to know what signs or symptoms are concerns for medical attention.

Outcomes of adequate coping vary with comfort, pain level, level of independence, support system, and coping strategies. Denial and substance abuse are nonproductive (Moorhead et al., 2004). Functional coping includes acceptance of changes in lifestyle, body image, and spiritual meaning to life. Social stigma is a difficult issue because patients are isolated and feel active persecution in some communities. Although the community is less changeable, interventions involving active listening, support groups, and environmental changes may help patients accept their reality and cope with the loss of relationships. Certainly some patients lose friends and partners to the disease, creating further isolation and loss. Education to prevent transmission, such as protected sexual intercourse and other ways to establish intimacy between partners, can help acceptance.

Outcomes Related to Stage of Disease

Outcomes in early HIV disease differ from advanced AIDS, where the focus is on short-term symptom relief, OI management, and optimal function. Those resistant to antiviral medications no longer obtain an undetectable suppressive response. Patients with advanced disease who have started on new antiviral medications may begin with a short-term focus but find their immune system reconstituted. Instead of terminal planning, they may need to change their outlook by envisioning a longer life. With early HIV disease, patients focus on long-term adaptation to chronic illness by accepting the disease and the resulting changes in life as the highest priority. Refer to Chapter 22 for a more complete discussion about coping and family caregivers.

Outcomes Related to Life Stage

Children. Children infected with HIV need to live as normal a life as possible. Early identification of developmental difficulties with appropriate interventions involves assistance by the school. Families choose whether to inform the school: issues to consider include the likelihood of stigma and discrimination by the school and other students. This fear should be balanced against the benefit of a school nurse, who can provide medication during the day and would understand absences resulting from sickness or treatments and could facilitate acceptance by children and teachers. Medication therapy for children is complex, perhaps more so than for adults. Parents are responsible for young children's adhering to a regimen that can be a burden with frequent dosing and unpleasant medications the child does not like. Active problem solving around these difficulties assists in adherence and supports parents in managing their responsibilities.

Adolescents. Issues important for adolescents involve their desire for peer group acceptance, their need to accept self, and their tendency for taking risks. Outcomes for adolescents are to express self-acceptance, belong to an accepting peer group, and limit risky behaviors, as well as to adhere to the medical regimen. The composition and orientation of peer and support groups directs behaviors in this population.

Adults. For adults psychosocial issues are acceptance of a chronic illness, the resulting altered body image and lifestyle, and the complexities involved in having children. At a time when they envision a career path and intimate partnerships, young adults with AIDS must accept their chronic illness and challenges related to work. This is especially difficult for those who were once disabled but who now can return to work because of the effectiveness of new medications. This psychosocial conflict has been called the "Lazarus phenomenon." Many who prepared to die (before HAART), must now plan how to reconsider life and all the accompanying stressors. For example, Medicaid may deny previously available benefits if disability is no longer an issue, and entering the job market without skills or work history can be difficult. Nurse case managers are instrumental in helping patients resolve these issues and referring them for appropriate resources.

Elderly. Those who are elderly and infected with HIV need to address isolation problems. The prevalence of chronic conditions makes adherence less of an issue. However, elders with HIV tend to self-imposed isolation, fear discrimination and ostracism, and fear loss of age-mates from all causes.

Evaluation of Care With HIV Disease

Clinical Endpoints. Laboratory values and clinical health status, such as undetectable viral loads and rising or stable CD4+ counts, indicate fully suppressed viral replication. Even in a situation of rising viral loads, a patient's health status may remain very good for several years, especially if immune function remains stable. In this situation, however, medication changes may be essential to maintain immune function.

Process Outcomes. Evaluation of nursing care includes process outcomes, as well as clinical endpoints. Satisfaction with care encourages patients to seek health care regularly, an important outcome for any chronic illness. Nurse case managers ensure patients have full access to services for their needs, including housing, transportation, or assistance related to isolation or financial hardship. Access to services is necessary for patients to take medications, keep diets, or visit primary care providers. Patients who express improved quality and satisfaction in their lives and who maintain health reflect effective nursing care.

Evaluation Techniques. Ongoing review and evaluation of interdisciplinary care is a means for continual improvement. Laboratory values and missed appointments are indicators readily available to evaluate clinical care and access to care. More complex evaluation includes periodic surveys for satisfaction with care, to assess quality of life, or to identify

barriers to the therapeutic regimen. Chapter 9 discusses quality improvement in detail.

Implications of Current Trends in Treatment of HIV Disease

Escalating health care costs continue as an economic issue. Initiatives that emphasize community-based care to enhance functional ability in people with AIDS will become more common. No longer an acute/terminal disease, chronic AIDS affects all bodily systems. Musculoskeletal and neurological problems benefit from rehabilitation. Rehabilitation nurses and their teams will have central roles in enhancing the quality of life for individuals with AIDS, in minimizing their functional dependence, and in lowering health care costs (Remien et al., 1999). As more people with AIDS are retained in community settings throughout the trajectory of their illness, it becomes imperative for nurses to develop rehabilitation expertise to address the myriad needs presented by these patients. Chapter 12 explains more about community-based rehabilitation.

Access to Care Issues. Society is clamoring for a solution to the AIDS crisis and issues related to funding for the most efficacious treatment and ultimately for a cure. Although expensive, adequate outpatient treatment is cost-effective provided it occurs before conversion to AIDS and is less costly than hospitalization for OIs.

Low income and lack of insurance have been barriers to outpatient treatment in HIV disease, as well as for other chronic illnesses. In 1990 the Ryan White CARE Act became a federal law. The act was named for the boy who gained national attention when denied schooling in his hometown after officials discovered he had acquired AIDS through blood transfusions for hemophilia. Before he died, Ryan became a spokesperson for those discriminated against for HIV disease. The federal program mandates the following.
- Improving quality and availability of care for those with financial barriers
- Improving access to medical care
- Providing early intervention services
- Providing antiretroviral medications and medicines to treat or prevent opportunistic infections
- Providing education for health care providers on treatment of HIV disease

Unfortunately, because of budget shortfalls, adequate funding for these laudable goals is not always available. As of this writing, several states have waiting lists for antiretroviral medications for people with no insurance.

Political-Economic Issues. Other political-economic issues relate to the definitions of disability and Medicaid coverage. Each state provides Medicaid for their designated populations, but definitions of disability vary and in some states patients must have a diagnosis of AIDS and a history of at least two OIs or major limitations to receive benefits. Thus health care and medications are available for those with advanced disease, but health care is not available to prevent progression to this stage. Recent initiatives in several states allow those with *potential* for catastrophic illness to receive Medicaid, rather than waiting for the disabling effects of the catastrophic illness. This change, authorized by federal legal moves, potentially would include many chronic diseases, such as cancer, diabetes, or congestive heart failure, in addition to HIV disease. The initiatives will be monitored for cost-effective outcomes of providing expensive outpatient health care against the hope to decrease costs from hospitalizations and loss of work.

Those declared disabled because of the severity of their AIDS symptoms, but who now can work because of successful adequate antiretroviral treatments, were mentioned earlier. They face potential loss of disability payments and Medicare or Medicaid; however, even with a full-time job providing health insurance, they find most insurance policies do not pay for "preexisting conditions." Patients have a lapse in coverage at best and uncertainty of benefits. Nurses can assist patients with information and resources for correct understanding of the issues. Some nurses may choose political action.

Global Health Issues. The HIV/AIDS epidemic is raging unchecked in parts of the developing world, particularly in Africa and Asia. Rehabilitation in developing countries includes symptom control and prevention of transmission because expensive antiretroviral medications are not options for many individuals. Transmission from mother to baby is a serious concern because a large percentage of childbearing populations is infected with HIV and funds for medications to prevent perinatal transmission are insufficient. Economic and cultural demands for breast-feeding may infect infants who avoided HIV in utero and at birth. Increasing populations of HIV-infected children further strain resources of poor regions of the world. In the next decade the number of children becoming orphans because of AIDS will increase dramatically, and a large segment of the workforce will be dead or dying from AIDS. This dire future for developing countries is a preview of the grim realities in the world.

In order to address this profound global health threat, the United Nations has developed UNAIDS, which is the main advocate for accelerated, comprehensive, and coordinated global action on the epidemic. The mission of UNAIDS is to lead, strengthen, and support an expanded response to HIV and AIDS that includes preventing transmission of HIV, providing care and support to those already living with the virus, reducing the vulnerability of individuals and communities to HIV, and alleviating the impact of the epidemic.

In response to this, U.S. President George W. Bush provided funding for UNAIDS through a program called the President's Emergency Plan for AIDS Relief (PEPFAR) to provide antiretroviral medications for 14 severely affected nations: Botswana, Cote d'Ivoire, Ethiopia, Guyana, Haiti, Kenya, Mozambique, Namibia, Nigeria, Rwanda, South Africa, Tanzania, Uganda, and Zambia. In addition, other developed nations provided the funding to attempt to meet the UNAIDS goal of 3 million people on HAART by 2005 through the use of generic antiretroviral medication combinations that are made available only to these countries. Although this goal of "3 by 5" was not met, the will to create the goal has been an important start to stabilizing the health and political situations in these countries.

Continued Need for Knowledge of HIV Disease. Information about HIV disease and its medical treatment is changing with multiple implications for practice, research, administration, and professional education. The research agenda about HIV and its treatment and prevention is very active, causing rapid changes in guidelines. Education updates about medications, clinical guidelines, and behavioral aspects can be a focus of therapeutic partnerships between patient and professional.

Clearly, rehabilitation nurses need support for continuing education so they are prepared to meet the needs of these patients. Education should include content about providing emotional support for patients and providers in a field where loss of life is still all too common. Selected websites with updated information are listed in Table 35-6.

Ethical Issues. Our existing knowledge base provides an adequate foundation for designing delivery strategies and for planning interventions to meet the complex physiological and psychosocial needs of the person with HIV/AIDS. Professional nurses are responsible for keeping fully informed of changes in the epidemiology of and treatment approaches for this disease and to modify their care accordingly. Nurses have challenges to define critical pathways and initiate case management approaches that will direct holistic yet cost-effective care for patients. Ethical dilemmas continue about disclosure and confidentiality with HIV disease. As patient advocates, nurses must be diligent in their efforts to respect the patient's rights. Chapter 3 discusses ethical issues in rehabilitation in more detail.

Case Study

Lisa Meyer, a 38-year-old woman, was admitted to the hospital with a blood glucose level of 602 mg/dl after coming to the emergency department one night having had fevers and malaise for 2 days. She said that she had been diagnosed with diabetes 10 years ago, but 6 years ago, when she had her first child, she stopped taking her medicines or monitoring her diet. Now a single mother with two small children, ages 2 and 6, she felt that she simply could not cope with all that life had given her. Because of her continued high fevers and profuse night sweats, she was tested for HIV and was identified as positive for HIV antibodies.

After being discharged from the hospital, Ms. Meyer had a renewed interest in monitoring her blood glucose levels. She was instructed by the nurse educator to check her blood glucose level twice daily, before breakfast and before dinner. Along with checking blood glucose levels, she began a walking program with her neighbor. After 3 consecutive days of walking 30 minutes per session, she began to have "weird" feelings, and her vision was somewhat blurred. She referenced her hospital discharge notes and found the sheet discussing hypoglycemia. She immediately checked her blood glucose level, which was 68 mg/dl. In accordance with her discharge notes, she ate three glucose tablets totaling 15 g of carbohydrates. After 15 minutes, Ms. Meyer again checked her blood glucose level, which was now 90 mg/dl.

Ms. Meyer began to attend the infectious disease clinic for care of her HIV disease, and blood was drawn to stage her disease. Her CD4+ count was 260 cells/mm³, showing that she had significant damage to her immune system but was not yet in the stage of AIDS. Her HIV RNA viral load was 58,268. At the recommendation of her nurse practitioner, Ms. Meyer began treatment for her HIV disease, after coming to the realization that this would be critical in her desire to continue to live to take care of her children and further her education. Her initial treatment was stavudine 40 mg BID, lamivudine 150 mg BID, and efavirenz 600 mg at bedtime. She developed the habit of taking her insulin along with her medications every morning and again in the afternoon, thus controlling both her HIV disease and her diabetes. After approximately 3 months, she began to complain of numbness in her feet and tingling in her hands. This progressed to the point where the numbness was accompanied by tenderness in her feet, so that she could not wear her shoes. Because of her diabetes, her care providers were not sure if this was caused by her past history of uncontrolled blood glucose levels or related to her HIV disease or the treatment of her HIV. Stavudine was changed to abacavir 300 mg BID, and medications were added to relieve the neuropathy pain. She began to inspect her feet daily for possible unfelt skin breakdown and to take extra care to protect the numb extremities as well as to control her blood glucose levels. Within 2 months after the change of HIV

medications, her neuropathic pain had resolved, and she was able to go back to work.

Within 6 months, her viral load was undetectable and her CD4+ count had risen to 340 cells/mm³. The nurse instructed her that the medications only controlled her disease and did not cure it and that the viral load would increase markedly if she stopped her medications. This increase in viral load would resume damaging her immune system and could cause resistance to her medications. Because of this education, she continued to take her medications regularly every day.

While watching television one afternoon, she heard an advertisement for a lipid-lowering medication, encouraging patients to know their cholesterol levels. She was taking a lipid-lowering medication but did not know her cholesterol levels. She had an appointment with a nurse educator the following day and decided to ask about her cholesterol. The nurse informed her that her latest cholesterol panel was abnormal, and her LDL cholesterol was 168 mg/dl. She then asked, "What is normal?" The nurse informed the patient that all persons with diabetes or those with a history of heart disease are automatically placed in the high-risk group. Based on the latest guidelines, her LDL should be less than 100 mg/dl. However, even lower LDL levels may be more beneficial. Ms. Meyer felt encouraged to take her cholesterol-lowering medication on a daily basis and to participate in therapeutic lifestyle changes, if able.

One year after hospitalization, Ms. Meyer has an HgbA$_{1C}$ of 6.5%, a CD4+ count of 420 cells/mm³, and an HIV RNA viral load of less than 50. Through continued medical care for both diabetes and HIV, she came to the realization that she could live a normal life with both these disease states, as long as she continued in treatment for both. She feels very good, although she continues to worry about her weight, which has not decreased to the extent she would like. She has a job at the day care center that cares for her youngest child and has begun a new romantic relationship. In the last 2 weeks her daily glucose readings have varied widely due to changes in her eating habits, although this friend walks with her several days a week. She hopes to get married and have more children.

CRITICAL THINKING

1. In what ways can you encourage self-monitoring of blood glucose levels and self-management of diabetes?
2. How can you as a rehabilitation nurse assist this patient in disclosing her HIV to this new romantic partner?
3. There are risks and benefits when an HIV-infected woman becomes pregnant, especially when the father is not HIV infected. What are those risks, and how can you counsel her and help her to arrive at plans to minimize the risks?

REFERENCES

Allison, D., & Saunders, S. (2000). Obesity in North America: An overview. *Clinics of North America, 84*(2), 305-332.

American Diabetes Association. (2005). Clinical practice recommendations. *Diabetes Care, 28*(1), 1-79.

Bartlett, J. G., & Gallant, J. E. (2004). *Medical management of HIV infection.* Baltimore: Johns Hopkins University, Department of Infectious Diseases.

Bassuk, S., & Manson, J. (2005). Invited review: Epidemiological evidence for the role of physical activity in reducing risk of type 2 diabetes and cardiovascular disease. *Journal of Applied Physiology, 99*, 1193-1204.

Boss, B. J. (2006). Alterations of neurologic function. In K. L. McCance & S. E. Huether (Eds.), *Pathophysiology: The biologic basis for disease in adults and children* (5th ed., pp. 547-603). St. Louis, MO: Mosby.

Centers for Disease Control and Prevention. (2005a). HIV/AIDS surveillance report 2005. Available at http://www.CDC.gov.

Centers for Disease Control and Prevention. (2005b, March 7). *National vital statistics reports.* From the Centers for Disease Control and Prevention National Center for Health Statistics, National Vital Statistics System.

Centers for Disease Control and Prevention. (2006, September 22). Revised recommendations for HIV testing of adults, adolescents, and pregnant women in health-care settings. *MMWR. Morbidity and Mortality Weekly Report, 55*(RR14), 1-17.

Deen, D. (2004). Metabolic syndrome: Time for action. *American Family Physician, 69*(12), 2875-2882.

Dochterman, J. M., & Bulechek, G. M. (2004). *Nursing interventions classification (NIC)* (4th ed.). St. Louis, MO: Mosby.

Dolin, R., Masur, H., & Saag, M. S. (2003). *AIDS therapy* (2nd ed.). Philadelphia: Churchill Livingstone.

Eckel, R., Grundy, R., & Zimmet, P. (2005). The metabolic syndrome. *Lancet, 365*(9468), 1415-1428.

Ewing, J. A. (1984). Detecting alcoholism: The CAGE questionnaire. *Journal of the American Medical Association, 252*, 1905-1907.

Gordon, M. (2000). *Manual of nursing diagnosis* (9th ed.). St. Louis, MO: Mosby.

Grinspoon, S., & Carr, A. (2005). Cardiovascular risk and body-fat abnormalities in HIV-infected adults. *New England Journal of Medicine, 352*(1), 48-62.

Grundy, S., Cleeman, J., Merz, C., Brewer, H., Clark, L., Hunninghake, D., et al. (2004). Implications of recent clinical trials for the National Cholesterol Education Program Adult Treatment Panel III guidelines. *Circulation, 110*(2), 227-239.

Grundy, S., Cleeman, J., Daniels, S., Donato, K., Eckel, R., Franklin, B., et al. (2005). Diagnosis and management of the metabolic syndrome: An American Heart Association/National Heart, Lung, and Blood Institute scientific statement: Executive summary. *Circulation, 112*, 285-290.

Guyton, A., & Hall, J. (2005). *Textbook of medical physiology* (11th ed.). Philadelphia: W. B. Saunders.

Haffner, S., & Taegtmeyer, H. (2003). Epidemic obesity and the metabolic syndrome. *Circulation, 108*, 1541-1545.

Huether, S. E., & Tomky, D. (2006). Alterations of hormonal regulation. In K. L. McCance & S. E. Huether (Eds.), *Pathophysiology: The biologic basis for disease in adults and children.* (5th ed., pp. 683-734). St. Louis, MO: Mosby.

Hurley, P., & Ungvarski, P. (1994). Home healthcare needs of adults living with HIV disease/AIDS in New York City. *Journal of Association of Nurses in AIDS Care, 5*, 33-40.

Kinney, J. (2005). Challenges to rebuilding the US food pyramid. *Current Opinion in Clinical Nutrition & Metabolic Care, 8*(1), 1-7.

LaMonte, M., Blair, S., & Church, T. (2005). Physical activity and diabetes prevention. *Journal of Applied Physiology, 99*, 1205-1213.

Linsk, N. (2000). HIV Among older adults: Age-specific issues in prevention and treatment. *The AIDS Reader, 10*(7):430-440.

Mandell, G. L., Bennett, J. E., & Dolin, R. (Eds.). (2005). *Principles and practice of infectious diseases* (6th ed.). Philadelphia: Elsevier Churchill Livingstone.

Mandell, T. G. L., & Mildvan, D. (2001). *Atlas of AIDS.* Philadelphia: Current Medicine, Inc.

McCance, K. L., & Huether, S. E. (2006). *Pathophysiology: The biologic basis for disease in adults and children* (5th ed.). St. Louis, MO: Mosby.

McCloskey, J. C., & Bulechek, G. M. (Eds.). (2000). *Nursing interventions classifications (NIC)* (3rd ed.). St. Louis, MO: Mosby.

Monkemuller, K. E., & Wilcox, C. M. (2003) *Diseases of the esophagus, stomach, and bowel.* In R. Dolin, H. Masur, & M. S. Saag (Eds.), *AIDS therapy* (2nd ed.). Philadelphia: Churchill Livingstone.

Moorhead, S., Johnson, M., & Maas, M. (Eds.). (2004). *Nursing outcomes classification (NOC)* (3rd ed.). St. Louis, MO: Mosby.

National High Blood Pressure Education Program. (2003). *Report of the Joint National Committee on Prevention, Detection, Evaluation, and Treatment of High Blood Pressure (JNC 7)* (NIH Publication No. 04-5230). Bethesda, MD: National Institutes of Health.

Piano, M. R., & Huether, S. E. (2006). Mechanisms of hormonal regulation. In K. L. McCance & S. E. Huether (Eds.), *Pathophysiology: The biologic basis for disease in adults and children* (5th ed., pp. 655-734). St. Louis, MO: Mosby.

Price, R. W. (2003). Neurologic disease. In R. Dolin, H. Masur, & M. S. Saag (Eds.), *AIDS therapy* (pp. 737-757). New York: Churchill Livingstone.

Remien, R. H., Satriano, J., & Berkman, A. (1999). Acquired immune deficiency syndrome and human immunodeficiency virus. In M. G. Eisenberg, R. L. Glueckauf, & H. H. Zaretsky (Eds.), *Medical aspects of disability* (pp. 53-67). New York: Springer.

Risi, G. F., & Tomascak, V. (1998). Prevention of infection in the immunocompromised host. *American Journal of infection Control, 26*, 594-603.

Steele, R. W. (2001). *2001 American Academy of Pediatrics National Conference and Exhibition: Pediatric infectious disease highlights.* MedScape Pediatrics. Available from http://www.medscape.com/viewarticle/415038_1.

Steffes, M., Cleary, P., Goldstein, D., Little, R., Wiedmeyer, H., Rohlfing, C., et al. (2005). Hemoglobin A1c measurements over nearly two decades: Sustaining comparable values throughout the Diabetes Control and Complications Trial and the Epidemiology of Diabetes Interventions and Complications study. *Clinical Chemistry, 51*(4), 753-758.

Stone, N., Bilek, S., & Rosenbaum, S. (2005). Recent National Cholesterol Education Program Adult Treatment Panel III update: Adjustments and options. *American Journal of Cardiology, 96*(4A), 53E-59E.

Svetkey, L., Simons-Morton, D., Proschan, M., Sacks, F., Conlin, P., Harsha, D., et al. (2004). Effect of the Dietary Approaches to Stop Hypertension diet and reduced sodium intake on blood pressure control. *Journal of Clinical Hypertension, 6*(7), 373-381.

Weinger, K., Jacobson, A., Draelos, M., Finkelstein, D., & Simonson, D. (1995). Blood glucose estimation and symptoms during hyperglycemia and hypoglycemia in patients with insulin-dependent diabetes mellitus. *American Journal of Medicine, 98*(1), 22-31.

Whaley-Connell, A., & Sowers, J. (2005). Hypertension management in type 2 diabetes mellitus: Recommendations of the Joint National Committee VII. *Endocrinology & Metabolism Clinics of North America, 34*(1), 63-75.

Wong, D. L., Hockenberry-Eaton, M., Wilson, D., Winkelstein, M. L., Ahmann, E., & DiVito-Thomas, P. A. (2000). *Whaley & Wong's nursing care of infants and children* (6th ed.). St. Louis, MO: Mosby.

36

Renal Rehabilitation

Christy A. Price Rabetroy, MSN, RN, NP

Acute renal failure is the abrupt decline of normal renal function, usually within a period of 3 days to 3 weeks. The primary causes are obstruction, exposure to nephrotoxic drugs, and ischemia after prolonged hypotension, leading to acute tubular necrosis (ATN). Elderly persons who undergo extensive cardiac and vascular surgeries and critically ill patients with multiple system failure are representative of most individuals affected by acute renal failure. Some individuals survive their acute renal insult, only to suffer chronic kidney disease (CKD) because of the injury resulting to kidney function. Humans lose 1 ml/min of glomerular filtration rate (GFR) for every year after age 40 (Mathers, 1998). Along with the natural aging process, concurrent events or conditions, such as surgeries, infections, hemorrhage, cardiomyopathy, hypertension, and diabetes mellitus, directly influence or compromise renal function in the acutely ill and elderly.

CKD often has an insidious onset over 3 months to 20 years or results from complications of acute renal failure that is unresolved within 3 months. Over 20 million people in the United States have CKD, which is now classified in five stages. When referring to a patient's health status, CKD stages 1 to 5 is the current terminology, which is outlined in Table 36-1. However, when referring to the Medicare program for funding for dialysis and kidney transplantation, end-stage renal disease (ESRD) remains the correct terminology. ESRD, or CKD stage 5, means cessation of normal renal function to a level at which the patient cannot sustain life without dialysis or kidney transplantation. In the United States the primary causes of ESRD in 2004 were diabetes mellitus (53%), hypertension (28%), and glomerulonephritis (10%) (U.S. Renal Data System [USRDS], 2005). Patients with diabetes and hypertension account for the majority of persons with ESRD; however, this condition is associated with other diseases, including polycystic kidney disease, secondary vasculitis, hereditary nephritis, drug-induced nephropathy, and pyelonephritis.

Patients have potential for multiple metabolic disturbances, such as electrolyte imbalances, fluid imbalance, bone disease, anemia, uremia, risk for infections, risk for bleeding, skin disorders, altered glycemic control, and hypertension.

In addition, persons with ESRD are confronted with significant dietary restrictions, extensive medication regimens, individualized dialysis prescriptions, frequent comorbid conditions, and procedural complications from their dialysis treatments and/or renal transplantation. The nursing interventions are covered under the Nursing Interventions Classification (NIC), although specific interventions necessary for the renal patient may be modified from the NIC (Dochterman & Bulechek, 2004).

REHABILITATION OF THE PATIENT WITH ESRD

Successful rehabilitation of patients with ESRD has long been recognized as one of the failures of the Medicare ESRD program. Passage of PL92-603 in 1972 assured persons who are eligible for Medicare coverage of renal dialysis and transplantation regardless of age. At that time about 10,000 persons with ESRD were receiving dialysis treatment in the United States, and estimates were that roughly 70% of these individuals would receive kidney transplants and most would to return to gainful employment (Evans, Blagg, & Bryan, 1981; Iglehart, 1993). These objectives have never been realized,

TABLE 36-1 Classification of Stages of Chronic Kidney Disease

Stage	Creatinine Clearance	Intervention
1	>90 ml/min	Monitor
2	60-89 ml/min	Blood pressure control, monitor urine for protein
3	30-59 ml/min	Refer to a nephrologist
4	15-29 ml/min	Anemia management, blood pressure control, prepare for dialysis or kidney transplant
5	<10-15 ml/min	Initiate dialysis

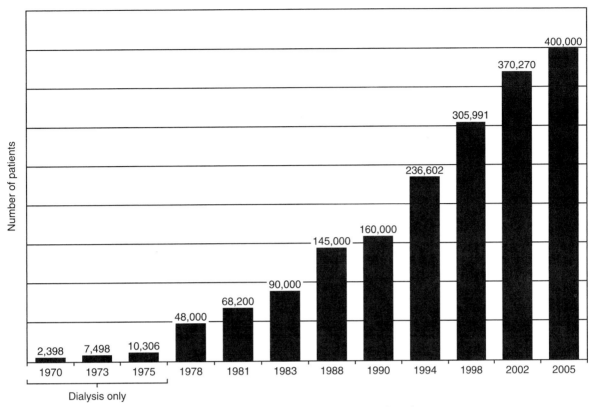

Figure 36-1 The combination of dialysis and renal transplant has allowed more patients to survive.

primarily because the providers shifted the focus of dialysis and transplantation to technology and pharmaceutical advances. The biochemical and physiological concerns overshadowed patients' psychosocial and emotional concerns; financial and scientific agendas arbitraged patients' longevity and took precedence over their quality of life. Figure 36-1 shows the growth in the number of patients with ESRD from 1970 to 2003 (Burten & Hirshman, 1976; Maxwell & Sapolsky, 1987; USRDS, 2005). In the early years of dialysis nearly 75% of patients were treated with home dialysis. The philosophy was to emphasize independence, self-care, and rehabilitation for age-appropriate tasks.

The most controversial issues in ESRD treatment today are selection of individuals for chronic renal replacement therapy and identification of those to be withdrawn from therapy. Who decides when the burden of disease and necessary treatment outweigh benefits (McCormick, 1993)? In the 1960s, patient selection committees decided who would be offered dialysis. Often referred to as "death committees," their selection criteria are listed in Box 36-1 (Alexander, 1962; Fox & Swazey, 1974; Price, 1992). By 1972, exclusionary criteria were eliminated, granting universal access to services so that merely the discovery of ESRD ensures treatment, regardless of defined benefit to the patient. A lack of appropriate evaluation of patients created an inequity in Medicare funding; that is to say, chronic kidney care for 0.05% of those eligible

for Medicare engulfs nearly 6.7% of the entire Medicare budget, amounting to a covered amount of approximately $72,450 per person per year for dialysis only (USRDS, 2005). Because Medicare pays 80% of expenses, remaining funds are obtained from Medicaid, private insurance, or self-payment. As the largest financier of dialysis services, Medicare allocates more than $18 billion annually to care for 93% of patients in the United States with ESRD (USRDS, 2005). In 1999 a work group with physicians specializing in nephrology, nurses, social workers, patients, ethicists, federal government employees, and primary and critical care physicians met to develop a clinical guideline: Shared Decision Making for the Appropriate Initiation and Withdrawal of Dialysis for Patients With ARF and ESRD ("RPA/ASN Guidelines," 2000). The group proposed nine recommendations for consideration of appropriate dialysis therapy and/or withdrawal. The goals of the guideline are to promote shared decision making between professionals and patients and to promote sound ethical and medical decision making in light of the person's condition.

COMPREHENSIVE CARE OF THE PATIENT WITH ESRD

Care of patients with renal failure requires the specialty knowledge and practice skills of multiple professionals. Every person with this condition has, at a minimum, a primary care

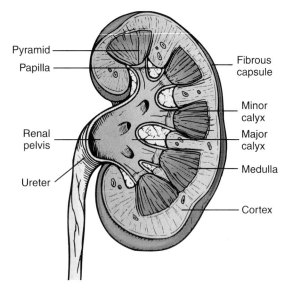

Figure 36-2 Frontal section of the kidney. (From Phipps, W. J., Sands, J. K., & Marek, J. F. [1999]. *Medical-surgical nursing: Concepts and clinical practice* [6th ed.]. St. Louis, MO: Mosby.)

provider, nephrologist, nephrology nurse, social worker, and renal dietitian involved in the care. A nephrology nurse practitioner greatly enhances the care and outcomes for these patients by addressing comprehensive care for their health care needs. The nurse practitioner often coordinates necessary health care services with the patient's primary care provider. Unfortunately, most dialysis centers no longer provide the services of a rehabilitation counselor. Apart from hospitalization, in which acutely ill persons have numerous providers, patients with CKD need varying levels and kinds of services and providers at certain periods in the course of their illness. Many patients with CKD lead very active, productive lives and are fully engaged in family and community activities, whereas other patients require occasional home health care, physical or occupational therapy, or other rehabilitative services.

At one time, when the average age of patients with renal disease was 42 years, rehabilitation often included returning the patient to gainful employment. With a current average age of 64 years for new patients with renal disease, rehabilitation goals have shifted to having patients with ESRD achieve age-appropriate developmental tasks that are comparable with those of their age-matched peers in the general population. Patients who are debilitated or deconditioned need extended and extensive community services. However, whether these services are provided is regulated by insurance or other reimbursement sources, rather than patient needs. For some, rehabilitation consists of referral to specific community services for transportation, grocery and pharmacy delivery, and information about opportunities for peer interaction or socialization. Finally, hospice or end-of-life care is available to those who decide to forgo or withdraw dialysis therapy. Hospice or other professionals specializing in terminal care must be involved to ensure death with dignity in the environment or place that is the patient's choice.

OVERVIEW OF RENAL ANATOMY

Macroanatomy

Most humans (more than 90%) have two kidneys at birth. Because one kidney is sufficient for proper physiological functioning, a person may not discover until later in life that he or she has only one kidney. The gross anatomy is not complex; the kidneys sit retroperitoneal and between T12 and L3. An adult kidney weighs about 300 g, is 10 to 13 cm long, and 5 to 7 cm wide. Kidneys have one or more renal arteries and veins that receive blood from the heart and return it back into the vascular circulation. The kidneys are perfused with approximately 25% of the cardiac output, or 1 to 2 L/min, processed at the glomerulus. A single ureter delivers urine to the bladder at a rate of $1\frac{1}{2}$ to 2 L/24 hours. The kidney is surrounded by a protective cover, or *fibrous capsule*. Figures 36-2 and 36-3 illustrate the gross anatomy of the kidney and components of the urinary system.

Microanatomy

The microanatomy of the kidney is very complex in structure and function. The kidney is separated into the outer cortical region and the inner medullary region. Within the cortex and juxtamedullary section, each kidney has nearly one million nephrons, or functional units. Each nephron is comprised of a glomerulus; Bowman's capsule; proximal convoluted tubule; loop of Henle; distal convoluted tubule; collecting duct; and a peritubular capillary system, or vasa recta. Figure 36-4 depicts the microscopic renal anatomy.

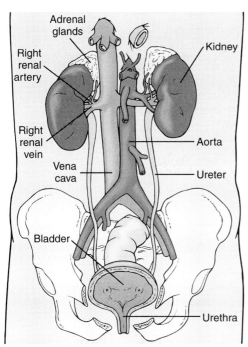

Figure 36-3 Organs and structures of the urinary system. (From Lewis, S. L., Collier, I. C., Heitkemper, M. M., & Dirksen, S. R. [2000]. *Medical-surgical nursing: Assessment and management of clinical problems* [5th ed.]. St. Louis, MO: Mosby.)

OVERVIEW OF RENAL PHYSIOLOGY

Functionally the kidneys are responsible for maintaining the body's internal milieu or homeostasis, acid-base balance, electrolytes and fluid balance, removal of toxins or waste products, and production or regulation of certain hormones or biochemical factors (Lancaster, 2001). To achieve the balance and precision of maintaining physiology, the processes controlled by the kidneys must occur without interruption. As outlined in Table 36-2, each segment of the nephron performs a special task toward normal kidney function.

Glomerulus

The renal processes begin at the glomerulus, where an ultrafiltrate of whole blood is created. Formed cells and protein are absent in ultrafiltrate, and this ultrafiltrate is isotonic with plasma, which helps explain why hematuria and proteinuria are abnormal (Whelan & Whelan, 1999). Creatinine is freely filtered at the glomerulus across the Bowman's capsule and not appreciably reabsorbed or secreted in the remainder of the tubule system. This process makes creatinine clearance the gold standard for assessing kidney function or GFR. Normal GFR for adults is 100 to 125 ml/min for males and 85% of this amount for females, or 85 to 110 ml/min. Recalling that kidney function begins to decline at age 40 years, it is extremely important to consider overall health status in estimates of kidney function.

The Cockcroft and Gault formula is commonly used to estimate creatinine clearance (Zawada, 1994) and to classify the stage of CKD (see Table 36-1):

$$\text{Creatinine clearance} = (140 - \text{Age in years}) \times \text{Weight in kilograms} \div 72 \times \text{Serum creatinine}$$

A comparison formula for estimating creatinine clearance is the Modification of Diet in Renal Disease (MDRD) which is becoming the standard calculation used by many laboratories (Poggio, Wang, Greene, Van Lente, & Hall, 2005).

A systemic infection, radiographic procedure, prolonged hypotension, or aggressive surgical intervention may add insult and further dysfunction to an already deteriorating kidney. Equally important is the protein-binding status of drugs (e.g., heparin, warfarin, antibiotics, and digoxin) that should not be filtered at the glomerulus. Therefore drug monitoring for therapeutic levels is essential for anyone with kidney dysfunction. The natural aging process and its relationship to kidney function and drug metabolism must also be factored into interventions and pharmacological management. Some medications need to be dose adjusted for creatinine clearance of less than 30 ml/min or less than 10 ml/min. Every medication must be checked for renal clearance before ordering or administrating.

Similar to all solid organs, the kidney depends on sufficient pressure to function. It has an amazing ability to autoregulate effectively within mean arterial blood pressures between 80 and 180 mm Hg. The afferent and efferent arterioles are capable of dilating or constricting as necessary to accommodate high or low pressures. However, autoregulation stops at a systolic blood pressure of about 70 mm Hg or mean arterial pressure of 60 mm Hg. This phenomenon explains the damage incurred to kidney function when patients remain in a state of prolonged hypotension. Damage may begin if hypoperfusion states exist beyond 30 minutes.

Proximal Convoluted Tubule

The processing of the ultrafiltrate begins immediately in the proximal tubule. The body essentially takes back the electrolytes and nutrients necessary to maintain the proper internal milieu. Namely, sodium, potassium, urea, bicarbonate, glucose, phosphates, and amino acids are reabsorbed in sufficient quantity into the peritubular system for return to the general circulation. The reabsorption of bicarbonate is the primary renal component that contributes to proper acid-base balance of the body. The pulmonary system contributes by regulating the carbon dioxide content of blood. Together they maintain proper blood pH between 7.35 and 7.45. The kidneys also process the ammonia ion and titratable acids to contribute to proper acid-base balance.

If the transmembrane potential, or necessary amount of a particular factor, is exceeded, then the excessive amount remains in the filtrate and is eliminated in the urine. This phenomenon can be seen in a person with diabetes whose blood glucose level is elevated or in a person under stress after surgery with glucose found in the urine (if the serum glucose

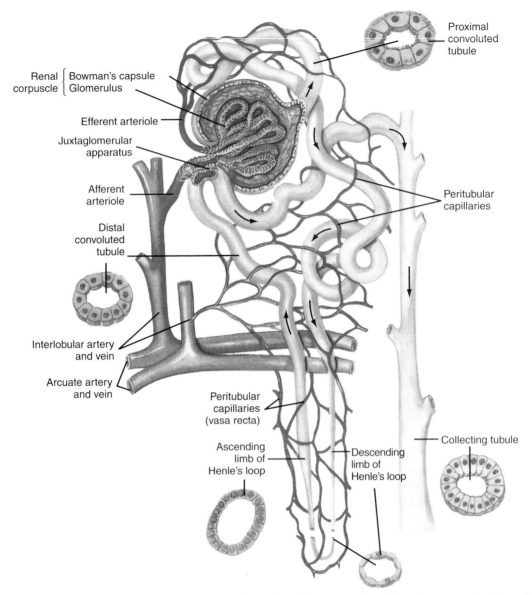

Figure 36-4 The nephron is the basic functional unit of the kidney. This illustration of a single nephron unit also shows the surrounding peritubular blood vessels. (From Thibodeau, G. A., & Patton, K. T. [1999]. *Anatomy & physiology* [4th ed.]. St. Louis, MO: Mosby.)

level exceeds 180 mg/ml, the transmembrane potential for glucose has been reached).

Loop of Henle

The loop of Henle is primarily responsible for the processing of sodium, chloride, and water. Through a complex system of countercurrent multipliers, an exchange mechanism, and a sodium chloride pump, the kidney concentrates and dilutes urine. The thin descending loop is permeable to water, concentrating the filtrate as water moves out into the peritubular capillary system, or vasa recta. The thick ascending loop is impermeable to water, having a diluting effect when sodium and chloride move out as the filtrate moves along the loop up to the distal convoluted tubule.

TABLE 36-2 Description of Functions of the Nephron by Segments

Segment of Nephron	Functions
Glomerulus	Creates an ultrafiltrate of plasma (formed cells that are protein free)
Proximal tubule	Reabsorbs two thirds of filtered Na^+, Cl^-, and H_2O Reabsorbs HCO_3^-, glucose, K^+, PO_4, proteins, uric acid, amino acids Secretes H^+, NH_4^+, organic acids, and bases
Loop of Henle	Reabsorbs NaCl
Distal tubule	Reabsorbs Na^+, Cl^-, and H_2O Secretes H^+, K^+, and NH_4^+
Collecting duct	Reabsorbs Na^+, Cl^-, and H_2O Secretes H^+, K^+, and NH_4^+

Distal Convoluted Tubule

The distal convoluted tubule receives this hypo-osmotic, very dilute urine from the loop of Henle. A major function of this segment of the nephron is to reabsorb the water and sodium depending on current physiological needs. The distal tubule operates in part under the influence of renin and aldosterone. Renin stimulates the liver and lungs to produce angiotensin I and angiotensin II, respectively. Angiotensin, a very potent vasoconstrictor, elevates blood pressure. Renin also stimulates the secretion of aldosterone from the adrenal medulla, allowing the kidneys to hold on to sodium in exchange for potassium.

The initial section of the distal tubule has a region of very specialized cells called the *juxtaglomerular apparatus*, or *macula densa* (see Figure 36-4). The macula densa borders a segment of the afferent arteriole that eventually receives the blood from the renal artery. The afferent arteriole pushes against the macula densa only when the circulatory volume and pressure of the blood inside the arteriole are high. The volume reflects the hydration status; hypervolemia results in a high pressure, and hypovolemia results in a low pressure. High pressure and volume are interpreted as a need to relieve the volume, and therefore the macula densa does not secrete renin and the adrenal glands do not secrete aldosterone. Alternatively, in a low-pressure state the macula densa secretes renin, leading to secretion of angiotensin and aldosterone. The distal tubule responds by reabsorbing sodium and water. This mechanism operates consistently and assists the body in maintaining a normal circulatory volume and blood pressure. This is the same mechanism of action exerted by a class of drugs prescribed for hypertension—angiotensin-converting enzyme (ACE) inhibitors and angiotensin receptor blockers (ARBs). On the other hand, some patients take potassium-sparing diuretics, such as spironolactone, amiloride, and triamterene, to prevent the excessive loss of potassium in the distal tubule. In early stages of CKD, furosemide or hydrochlorothiazide may be acceptable.

Collecting Duct

The distal tubule and collecting duct are the sites of action of antidiuretic hormone (ADH). As its name implies, ADH triggers removal of water in this final segment of the nephron. ADH is secreted by the posterior pituitary gland in response to osmotic receptors in the carotid bodies and right atrium of the heart. The collecting duct of the nephron operates under the influence of ADH to assist in maintaining normal blood volume and osmolarity. Caffeine, alcohol, and cold temperature inhibit ADH secretion, explaining the increased need to urinate.

Secretion, another important process, takes place throughout the nephron but mainly in the distal tubule. Secretion is a process whereby the body removes, or eliminates, unnecessary or unneeded elements, such as potassium, antibiotics, acids, phosphates, and a small amount of creatinine. It transfers electrolytes, drugs, ammonia, and other elements from the peritubular capillary system into the tubule to be excreted in the urine.

Hormone Production

The kidneys, particularly the nephrons and peritubular capillary system, act to maintain the harmony and balance in the body. When homeostasis is disrupted, life cannot be sustained apart from pharmacological, nutritional, and renal replacement therapy supports. The kidneys also are a site of action and responsible for production of proteins and the hormones erythropoietin and prostaglandins. Erythropoietin stimulates the bone marrow to produce red blood cells; without this stimulus individuals eventually become severely anemic. Prostaglandins play a role in blood pressure control and filtration at the glomerulus.

FACTORS ASSOCIATED WITH FUNCTIONAL HEALTH STATUS

Epidemiology of Renal Disease

CKD may present as a single system or a multiorgan failure disease; in either case, all aspects of life are affected. Not only are patients subject to restrictions or barriers to their lifestyle, they have many questions and fears. This population of patients has had sufficient exposure to dialysis therapy and transplantation to dread lifelong reliance on machines, dietary restrictions, frequent infections and comorbidities, repeated hospitalizations, and constant confrontation with the high mortality associated with ESRD. Once dialysis begins, life expectancy shortens significantly, averaging less than 8 years for patients older than 40 (RPA/ASN, 2000). Mortality rates vary with age at onset, ethnicity, and renal diagnosis and range from less than 2 years to 18 years after the onset of dialysis. When an individual decides to stop or withdraw from dialysis voluntarily, life expectancy ranges from a few days to 2 to 3 weeks.

Approximately 70% of those with ESRD on dialysis have a comorbid diagnosis of diabetes mellitus and/or hypertension, both of which are known to place undue stress on the body and its functions. Similarly, too many adults and children are overweight and lead sedentary lives. The alarming rate of adolescent onset of type 2 diabetes mellitus may significantly increase the growth of CKD patients in the future. These conditions eventually may damage the kidneys, although they could be managed through lifestyle changes. In 2003 the incidence of patients with ESRD in the United States, 338 per million population, and the prevalence of patients, 1,496 per million population (USRDS, 2005), continued to rise but could be curtailed under the recommendations of *Healthy People 2000* and *Healthy People 2010*. In particular, *Healthy People 2010* identifies chronic kidney disease as a target area because of the psychosocial impact and the clinical and financial resources involved in treatment.

Ethnic Variables

Chronic renal disease is found across all groups—socioeconomic, ethnic, and cultural. Whether related to genetics, access to adequate health care, nutrition, education, or other factors, African Americans have a high incidence of hypertension. African Americans, followed by Native Americans, have a greater incidence of chronic renal disease and diabetes mellitus than do white, Asian, or Pacific Island peoples (USRDS, 2005). Age increases the likelihood of ESRD; it is uncommon in individuals younger than 18 years. Use of illegal and/or certain legal drugs, such as nonsteroidal antiinflammatory drugs (NSAIDs), are implicated as a cause in the United States.

NURSING PROCESS

Nursing Assessment

The nursing assessment begins with the initial history and physical examination for gathering objective and subjective data. The complete history includes chief complaint, present medical illnesses, past medical history, family history, social history, medications, allergies, lifestyle activities, and a review of systems. Collect data in light of the patient's renal function (e.g., CKD stage 1 to 5). The patient's renal function dictates nursing interventions and planning for total health care needs.

When obtaining the history, the nurse pays particular attention to and documents risk factors for kidney dysfunction, such as hypertension, obesity, diabetes, smoking, prescription and nonprescription drug history, and hereditary diseases. Excessive intake of NSAIDs can have a negative effect on function of both normal and compromised kidneys. Care should be taken to document use of herbal medicines or dietary supplements. Questions about predisposing factors, concurrent illnesses, lifestyle practices, and environmental stimuli that have the potential for worsening the renal dysfunction or complicating the treatment modality need to be addressed. For the acutely ill person, include data about recent surgeries, infections, hemorrhage, or prolonged illness.

Physical Examination

In addition to conducting a comprehensive physical examination, the nurse assesses for conditions and nursing diagnoses that relate to chronic renal disease (Lancaster, 2001). Assessment components specifically related to CKD and potential findings and nursing diagnoses are presented in Table 36-3.

Nursing Diagnoses

The potential medical and nursing diagnoses related to patients with CKD are numerous because of the complex nature of kidney dysfunction, the etiology of the individual's disease, the secondarily involved organ systems, and the need for aggressive dialytic and/or transplant therapies. Patients are at risk for hyperkalemia and hypokalemia, hypercalcemia and hypocalcemia, azotemia, anemia, chronic cough, fluid overload, peripheral edema, pulmonary edema, dehydration, systemic and local infections, malnutrition, cerebral atrophy, muscle atrophy, cardiomyopathy, left ventricular hypertrophy, congestive heart failure, bleeding and clotting abnormalities, peripheral neuropathy, bone disease, diarrhea, fatigue, sexual dysfunction, sleep disturbances, and pain. Patients may have difficulty with coping effectively; fear and anxiety; mild to severe depression; dealing with anger, loss of independence, social isolation, reliance on intricate life-sustaining technology; family role changes; and decreased life expectancy. Palliative and end-of-life care are essential for those who decide to forgo or withdraw from dialysis.

The rehabilitation nurse is unlikely to find every problem in this huge spectrum of potential nursing and medical diagnoses in a patient. However, the key to appropriate care of patients with CKD is using the nursing process completely so that potential problems and unusual situations are discovered and interventions are timely and therapeutic. The goal for every patient must be safe, effective therapy in a supportive, partially compensatory or fully compensatory approach that is individualized to his or her specific needs or death with dignity on the patient's own terms. These goals are congruent with the Nursing Outcomes Classification (NOC) expectations (Moorhead, Johnson, & Maas, 2004).

Nursing Interventions for the Patient Receiving Hemodialysis

About 87% of patients with ESRD in the United States use in-center hemodialysis (HD) as their chronic renal replacement therapy (USRDS, 2005). Although fewer than 1% of patients use HD at home compared with nearly 70% in the 1970s, home HD (HHD) is once again becoming a popular therapy. Approximately 13% of patients are maintained on home peritoneal dialysis (PD). The rehabilitation nurse coordinates patient therapies with the dialysis center treatment schedule. The NIC interventions may need to be adapted for individualized treatment.

Schedules

Information about the location of the dialysis center, hours of operation, and telephone and pager numbers for the physicians, nurse practitioners, nephrology nurses, social worker, and renal dietitian should be posted. The routine treatment schedule is 3 to 4 hours of HD on alternate days, 3 times per week. This means that the patient is away from home for 5 to 6 hours each treatment day; children are not scheduled during normal school hours.

Planning for care at home or in a rehabilitation center should not be done immediately before or after a patient's HD treatment because the patient is the most biochemically imbalanced before dialysis and generally physically fatigued after dialysis. Patients receiving HD rarely feel completely well, partially because of the accumulation of uremic toxins resulting from their kidneys' inability to function normally, which includes the processing of fluid, electrolytes, and toxins 24 hours per day. Furthermore, patients who are noncompliant with the total HD regimen (i.e., including diet modifications and a medication regimen) have more health-related problems with higher morbidity and mortality.

Treatment

Hemodialysis is a very aggressive life maintenance therapy that processes a patient's total blood volume many times through

TABLE 36-3 Physical Assessment Finding for a Patient With Renal Disease

System	Finding	Rationale
Neurological	Dizziness, light-headedness	Uremia, hypotension, anemia
	Slow thought processes	Uremia, anemia, cerebral atrophy
	Decreased sensation	Peripheral neuropathy
Cardiac	Hypertension/hypotension	Fluid overload or dehydration
		Noncompliance with medication regimen
		Cardiomyopathy, CHF
	Irregular pulse	Hyperkalemia/hypokalemia, hypocalcemia
	S_3, rub	Fluid overload, uremic pericarditis
Pulmonary	Cough, congestion,	CHF, fluid overload, side effect of medications
	Decreased oxygenation	Fluid overload, pulmonary edema
	Decreased breath sounds	Rales, rhonchi, crackles
	Cyanosis, decreased capillary refill	Anemia
Gastrointestinal	Diarrhea	Uremia, dietary factors
	Constipation	Side effect of medications
	Epigastric pain/discomfort	Uremia, peritoneal fluid pressure
	Impaired gastric mobility	Side effect of diabetes
	Nausea/vomiting	Uremia, inadequate dialysis
	Occult blood in stool	Uremia, heparin dosing for HD or PD
Skin	Dryness, scaling	Dehydration, uremia
	Ulcerations	Hyperphosphatemia
	Erythema, induration	Hematoma over vascular access
	Erythema, drainage	HD or PD catheter site infection
	No bruit or thrill	Clotted vascular access
	Pruritus	Uremia, hyperphosphoremia
	Ecchymosis	Heparin dosing, hematoma
Musculoskeletal	Decreased DTRs	Hypokalemia
	Muscle weakness	Hyperkalemia/hypokalemia
	Muscle atrophy	Malnutrition
	Fatigue/poor endurance	Anemia
Reproductive	Decreased sexual function	Anemia, uremia
	Decreased libido	Anemia, depression
	Irregular menses	Uremia, hormone imbalance

NOTE: Patients may have same or similar findings with different etiological factors.
CHF, Congestive heart failure; *DTRs*, deep tendon reflexes; *HD*, hemodialysis; *PD*, peritoneal dialysis; S_3, third heart sound.

an artificial kidney. Figure 36-5 demonstrates the components of an HD system; Figure 36-6 shows a hemodialysis machine. The HD process restores fluid balance; normalizes electrolytes; and removes uremic toxins through a complex system of pumps, pressures, concentration gradients, blood flow rates, dialysate flow rates, and ultrafiltration. Although HD maintains life, it falls far short as a facsimile of native renal function. Each month the dialysis prescription changes according to laboratory analyses of a comprehensive metabolic profile, complete blood count, and dialysis adequacy. Iron indices are obtained every 3 months, and aluminum and parathyroid hormone levels are measured semiannually.

Vascular Access

Each patient has vascular access for the blood to process through the HD system. Figure 36-7 shows a native arteriovenous fistula (AVF) and a synthetic arteriovenous graft (AVG).

These blood accesses are placed in the lower or upper arm, usually in the nondominant arm, or in the thigh area. An AVF generally requires 2 to 3 months of maturation before successful cannulation can be achieved, whereas an AVG does not require time for development so cannulation can be attempted after 2 to 3 weeks. Should problems occur or a clot form in the access, the other arm or leg remains an option. Unfortunately, most accesses do not last the lifetime of the patient, especially grafts that last less than 2 years; a native fistula lasts longer. Home health care must include daily cleansing of the extremity, auscultating the bruit, feeling for the thrill, and observing for signs and symptoms of infection. The patient cannot wear tight clothing or jewelry. The vascular access extremity is not used for measuring blood pressures, drawing blood, or placing an intravenous catheter. Figure 36-8 shows a patient on HHD who has self-cannulated his AVF.

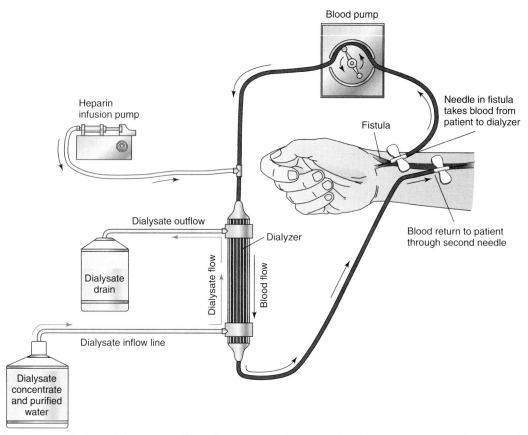

Figure 36-5 Components of a hemodialysis system. (From Lewis, S. L., Collier, I. C., Heitkemper, M. M., & Dirksen, S. R. [2000]. Medical-surgical nursing: Assessment and management of clinical problems [5th ed.]. St. Louis, MO: Mosby.)

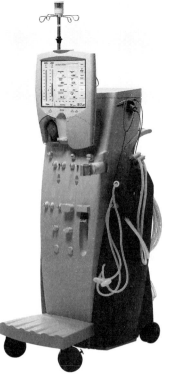

Figure 36-6 Hemodialysis machine. (Courtesy Baxter Healthcare Corp, Deerfield, IL.)

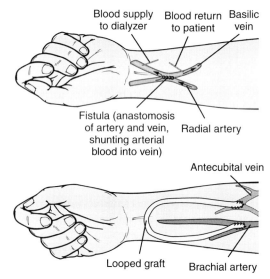

Figure 36-7 Methods of vascular access for hemodialysis. **A**, Internal arteriovenous fistula. **B**, Looped graft in forearm. (From Lewis, S. L., Collier, I. C., Heitkemper, M. M., & Dirksen, S. R. [2000]. *Medical-surgical nursing: Assessment and management of clinical problems* [5th ed.]. St. Louis, MO: Mosby.)

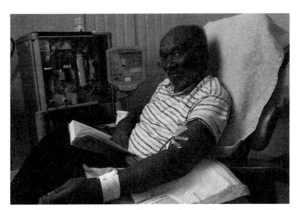

Figure 36-8 Patient receiving hemodialysis in his home. (Courtesy Aksys Limited, Libertyville, IL.)

The bruit on a vascular access is the sound created as the blood is redirected from the high-pressure artery to a low-pressure vein; it sounds like a passing train. The thrill is the sensation created by the blood being redirected from an arterial inlet through a thin-walled vein or synthetic graft to a venous outlet; it has a vibrating feeling. If either the bruit or thrill is not evident, suspect a thrombosed vascular access. The patient family or nurse must telephone the vascular surgeon, the nephrologist, nephrology nurse practitioner, or dialysis unit staff member. An access can undergo thrombolysis through interventional radiology or surgery if the procedure is attempted within 24 to 48 hours of clot formation in an AVF and less than 2 weeks in an AVG. When the vascular access appears infected or the patient has signs and symptoms of systemic infection, evaluate the vascular access and initiate antibiotic therapy. Accessing a dialysis catheter or cannulation of a fistula or graft is an opening into the circulatory system that is at high risk for infection. Sterile technique and proper flushing are essential to prevent local infection or bacteremia.

Figure 36-9 illustrates the positioning of intrajugular and subclavian catheters that often are the only vascular access patients may have in place when their circulatory systems are unable to support an AVF or AVG.

Diet

Renal dietary restrictions are essential with ESRD. Although composition varies with nutritional status, age, and diagnosis, the dietary intake is limited in protein, potassium, sodium, glucose, phosphorus, and fluid intake. A renal dietitian performs a thorough dietary history and helps the patient plan meals. A rule of thumb is 1 to 1.5 g/kg of protein, 2 to 3 g of sodium, 60 to 90 mEq of potassium, and 600 to 800 mg of phosphorus per day. Fluid restriction is 1000 to 1200 ml plus urine output. Fluid restrictions may vary depending on the individual's energy-expending activities, insensible losses, and seasonal or environmental temperatures. During a home assessment the nurse learns the patient's food habits and preferences and ascertains his or her understanding of the

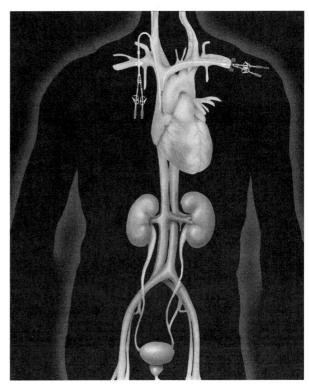

Figure 36-9 Intrajugular and subclavian hemodialysis catheters. (Courtesy Bard Access Systems, Salt Lake City, UT.)

renal diet. Education in light of the patient's beliefs and values may assist him or her to adhere to dietary restrictions (Lancaster, 2001; Wilson, 1995). Written guides for the renal diet, special renal diet recipe books, and fast food or other restaurant listings for food content are convenient aids to ease the meal selection process. Patients who do not adhere to the diet are at risk for hyperkalemia, hyperphosphatemia, fluid overload, bone disease, worsening hypertension, hyperparathyroidism, skin problems, and death. The goal is for patients to make lifestyle choices that are conducive to a healthy life and help prevent complications resulting from noncompliance.

Medications

With ESRD, patients can expect a host of medications to control their disease process. For instance, patients take vitamins, iron supplements, antihypertensive agents, insulin, phosphate binders, calcium carbonate, antidepressants, and potentially many other medications. Children may take human growth hormone to promote near-normal stature. Individualized insulin or oral hypoglycemic agent regimens are prescribed for diabetes but must be changed at the stage of renal replacement therapy to accommodate for the increased insulin resistance that coincides with advancing renal dysfunction. Patients with diabetes mellitus may need less insulin or oral hypoglycemic agents as their renal failure advances, but with a standard 200 mg/dl concentration of glucose in dialysate fluid, they can experience more fluctuations in the blood glucose level between days on and off dialysis treatment.

Thus home blood glucose testing becomes an increasingly important measure for the patient with diabetes and ESRD.

Hypertension control waxes and wanes with HD treatments; blood pressure may be elevated before dialysis, then low afterwards. Blood pressure management is very individualized, and not all patients need pharmaceutical interventions. All classes of drugs have a place in the armamentarium of treatment for hypertension. Antihypertensive drugs have no set regimen; however, they often are not given before HD to prevent hypotension during therapy.

What is critical is a regimen that works for the person, and most patients benefit from supportive counseling to maintain compliance with their medication regimens and dietary and fluid restrictions. Lobley (2001) describes a multidisciplinary approach shown to be effective in achieving the desired outcome of reasonably well-controlled hypertension. As with many approaches to preventive or restorative health care, the emphasis is on patient education.

Phosphate binders, calcium carbonate, calcium acetate, lanthanum carbonate, and sevelamer are prescribed with meals to promote the binding of dietary phosphorous and elimination in the stool. If calcium carbonate is used as a calcium supplement, it is ingested between meals. Water-soluble vitamins are taken after hemodialysis. Prolonged imbalance of calcium and phosphorous results in elevated parathyroid hormone levels and eventually bone disease. Most patients are prescribed a vitamin D analog to promote control of parathyroid hormone and foster proper bone metabolism. Patients must avoid foods and medications containing magnesium and aluminum because these elements are excreted via the kidney. Patient education includes information about medications that interact and food-medication combinations.

Activity

Patients with ESRD do not produce sufficient erythropoietin and are anemic. Introduced in 1987, epoetin alpha has benefited patients by stimulating the production of red blood cells. Epoetin alpha is administered either intravenously (IV) or subcutaneously (Sub-Q) during the dialysis treatment. Data from a monthly complete blood count are used to regulate the dose. For the epoetin alpha to be more effective, IV iron preparation may be administered during dialysis therapy to replete lost iron stores (Bowe & Ammel, 2005). Under the Medicare ESRD program in accordance with the Dialysis Outcomes Quality Initiatives (DOQI), the goal for administration of epoetin alpha is to maintain the patient's hematocrit level between 33% and 36% ("Clinical Practice Guidelines for Hemodialysis Adequacy," 1997; "Clinical Practice Guidelines for Vascular Access," 1997). Thus patients with ESRD remain anemic with the inherent side effects of fatigue, shortness of breath, dyspnea on exertion, and poor exercise tolerance, although regular exercise within limitations is extremely important in rehabilitation of these patients (Colangelo, Stillman, Kessler-Fogil, & Kessler-Hartnett, 1997; Karmiel, 1996; Pianta & Kutner, 1999; Sabath, 1999).

The deconditioned state of patients with ESRD has renewed interest in mild to moderate regular exercise, a multidisciplinary approach, physical therapy, and encouraging children to participate in all school activities and organized sports (Schrag, Campbell, Ewert, Hartley, Niemann, & Ross, 1999; Solomon, 1999). Sexual dysfunction, either related to decreased libido or impotence secondary to uremia and anemia, is a major inhibitor to involvement and maintenance in relationships.

In rehabilitation nursing the assessment includes the patient's ability to participate in regular exercise, sexuality concerns, and lifestyle behaviors. Interventions must cover all areas of activity.

Psychosocial/Emotional

Patients with ESRD receiving HD as their chronic renal replacement therapy often struggle to cope effectively with their disease and technology; denial and depression are prominent. Children have developmental, growth, and maturation issues that can result in maladaptive behaviors. Rehabilitation nurses are prepared to meet patients along their continuum of adaptation and recommend strategies to improve outcomes.

NURSING INTERVENTIONS FOR THE PATIENT RECEIVING PERITONEAL DIALYSIS

Although home PD continues to be an option for patients with ESRD, only 13% receive this therapy. The procedures and equipment for two standard clinical practices, continuous ambulatory peritoneal dialysis (CAPD) and continuous cycling peritoneal dialysis (CCPD), are illustrated in Figure 36-10, A and B. PD is a self-care treatment. The patient connects tubing to a peritoneal catheter that is surgically implanted in the peritoneal cavity (Figure 36-11). The semipermeable peritoneal membrane exchanges fluid, electrolytes, and toxins via the concentration gradient between the patient's vascular supply and the dialysate solution. Fluid, potassium, phosphorus, amino acids, glucose, and other substances are exchanged and eliminated from the body. PD may not be an option for patients with impaired sight or manual dexterity or who have had extensive abdominal surgeries with residual scar tissue.

Schedules

CAPD involves manual performance of three to five exchange procedures, which allows for draining filling, and dwelling peritoneal fluid over a 24-hour period. The same procedures are performed in CCPD with the use of a peritoneal dialysis machine, usually during a time when the patient is sleeping. Either way, peritoneal effluent is disposed of every day. Ideally, children use CAPD or CCPD to avert pain associated with vascular access cannulation, to improve nutrition, and to encourage their involvement in age-appropriate activities. PD procedures can be performed in the home, school,

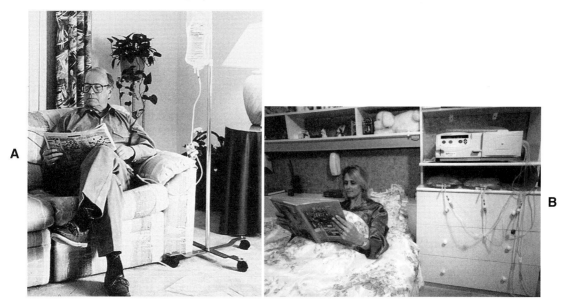

Figure 36-10 A, Ambulatory patient using Y-set peritoneal dialysis system for an exchange. B, Continuous cycling peritoneal dialysis (CCPD). (Photos courtesy Baxter Healthcare Corp, Deerfield, IL.)

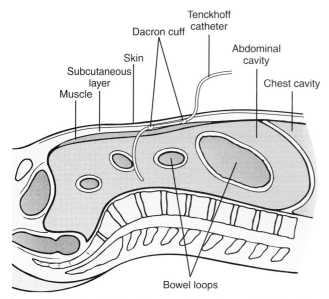

Figure 36-11 Tenckhoff catheter used in peritoneal dialysis. (From Lewis, S. L., Collier, I. C., Heitkemper, M. M., & Dirksen, S. R. [2000]. *Medical-surgical nursing: Assessment and management of clinical problems* [5th ed.]. St. Louis, MO: Mosby.)

or office daily and generally can accommodate the patient's schedule, preferences, and needs.

Patient Training

The renal rehabilitation team evaluates the patient and situation for opportunities to promote shared decision making. The nephrology nurse and social worker make home visits to identify barriers to successful management of home therapy. Structurally the patient needs a separate area or room to perform CAPD or a table at bed height for the cycler machine for CCPD. Most patients and family quickly grasp essential points, but learning the principles and techniques and troubleshooting for complications requires 3 to 5 days of training. With experience they become proficient. Various pedagogical devices such as charts, videos, demonstrations, and written materials positively influence the outcomes (Szczepanik, 1995). Rehabilitation nurses who learn the techniques themselves improve their understanding of the therapy and better assist patients.

The patient being treated with CAPD performs daily exchanges with 1500 to 3000 ml of peritoneal solution using strict sterile technique; each exchanges takes about 30 to 45 minutes. The fill volume, prescribed by the nephrologist or nephrology nurse practitioner, requires 10 to 15 minutes to complete. The drain time also varies, generally 30 to 45 minutes, and the dwell period ranges from 4 to 6 hours and overnight. For ease in remembering, the prescribed schedule is before breakfast, lunch, dinner, and retiring for the evening. For CCPD, every evening the patient sets up the cycler machine using strict sterile technique and then in the morning disconnects the machine at completion of therapy, again with sterile technique. Parameters for drain time, fill volume and time, and dwell time are programmed into the machine.

Diet

Patients using CAPD or CCPD have fewer dietary restrictions than patients using HD because PD is performed daily.

Patients learn how to assess their weight and fluid status daily and how to choose 1.5%, 2.5%, or 4.25% dextrose peritoneal solution to control fluid removal. The higher the dextrose in the solution, the greater the osmotic gradient and therefore the more fluid removed from the intravascular and interstitial spaces. A newer PD solution called Icodextran is a maltose-based solution that particularly helps diabetic patients in controlling their blood glucose levels. However, Icodextran may be used only once a day. Because fluid removal occurs daily, most of what is consumed is removed within 24 hours. Little fluid accumulates when the correct plan for exchanges is followed and the peritoneal membrane operates properly, and because urea, creatinine, potassium, and sodium are removed daily, there is little chance of their building in the blood. However, more albumin is lost in the peritoneal effluent than in HD, so patients must increase their protein intake. In general, patients receiving PD feel better and have a better nutritional status than patients receiving HD, provided the patients receiving PD follow procedures and the prescribed regimen. Monthly laboratory analyses of the comprehensive metabolic panel and complete blood count direct the dialysis prescription. Increased potassium may be needed to prevent hypokalemia.

Medications

Patients receiving PD often use the same medications prescribed to patients with HD but in lower doses. Again, because PD is performed every day, blood pressure management may be remarkably improved, and the antihypertension regimens can be simplified. Supplements such as vitamins, iron, or calcium are routinely prescribed. Phosphate binders must be consumed with meals.

Patients with diabetes who are receiving PD must incorporate a new regimen for insulin or oral agents because the peritoneal solutions have a heavy dextrose content that adds calories to the diet. Usually the insulin requirements increase, or insulin may be needed to control hyperglycemia. Once patients recognize their unique requirements, management becomes routine. One advantage for persons with ESRD using PD is their ability to add regular insulin to the peritoneal solution, thereby avoiding insulin injections 2 to 4 times a day. Home health care nurses need to learn techniques for adding medication into the peritoneal solution should a patient require this.

Patients at home self-administer epoetin alpha subcutaneously 1 to 3 times a week much like an insulin injection. When diet is improved and less blood lost, these patients do not require the medication. Monthly complete blood counts are used to regulate epoetin alpha.

Infection Risks

Patients receiving PD are taught proper techniques for care and cleaning of the catheter exit site and to observe for erythema, drainage, tenderness, leaking, or bleeding. They have responsibility for monitoring for infection or complications and notifying the clinic to obtain cultures and oral antibiotics. Antibiotic ointment, usually mupirocin, or povidone-iodine may be applied around the exit site with daily dressing changes. A more serious risk is peritonitis should an infectious agent gain entry into the peritoneal cavity during an exchange or when the catheter becomes disconnected. Patients learn to monitor for cloudy effluent, abdominal pain, fever, and chills. If peritonitis is apparent, they save the first cloudy bag of effluent, then perform two or three rapid flushes for 30 to 60 minutes. Depending on facility protocols, some patients inject antibiotics into the next exchange solution. The first cloudy bag is submitted for cultures and cell count. Generally patients are not hospitalized, and home health care nurses are instrumental in assisting these often frightened and uncomfortable persons. Intraperitoneal antibiotics are continued for 10 to 14 days.

Activity

Patients with ESRD who are using CAPD or CCPD are extremely independent and proficient in self-care. Because they have no activity restrictions, they play sports and function as energy permits. Often those receiving HD report more sexual inactivity than patients receiving PD. Some dialysis centers discourage swimming, soaking in a hot tub, or bathing in a bathtub; all discourage football. As the equipment, catheters, and training have improved, many centers set special precautions such as showering and changing the exit site dressing immediately after participating in these activities. Some recommend enclosing the end of the catheter in a plastic bag for protection; others modify colostomy bags around the site and end of the catheter. These techniques may be helpful to home health care nurses who plan to assist patients with physical therapy or bathing.

Psychosocial/Emotional

Home self-care is superior to HD in fostering independence because patients can adapt their daily activities around their need for dialysis. Most studies suggest or confirm that patients performing home self-care have a more positive outlook on life and therefore more effective coping with the disease and chronic renal replacement therapy. Patients tend to remain fully involved in age-appropriate activities and to less often reverse roles or interfere with family norms. However, those receiving PD are at risk for fatigue with their chronic treatment and need support, education, and counseling, as well as encouragement and reinforcement of their self-care agency.

NURSING INTERVENTIONS FOR THE PATIENT WITH A RENAL TRANSPLANT

Patients with kidney transplant constitute 25% of the ESRD population, or 95,347 patients in 2003 (USRDS, 2005). Renal transplantation is the treatment of choice for children. In the past, eligibility ended at 60 years; however, some transplant centers perform renal transplants for patients 72 years old or in older patients with excellent health. Kidney donations from cadavers have leveled at about 9000 per year, but more donations are arriving and being accepted from living persons who are relatives and nonbiological or emotionally related donors. There has also been an increase in Good Samaritan donors, or anonymous live donors. The system of organ distribution is problematic, and policy is in a state of flux in the United States. Discussion is ongoing about the most efficient, practical, and fair way to distribute organs for transplantation. Medical rationing of health care does exist when solid organs are involved. Approximately 65,000 persons in the United States await a kidney transplant, and more than 80,000 wait for some solid organ transplant.

Typical patients who receive a kidney transplant are fully involved in age-appropriate activities and require little extra assistance—a scene that may change as more people survive longer with a kidney transplant. These persons manage their immunosuppressive medications and other health care needs and have no dietary restrictions. The only concern is avoiding activities that put the patient at risk for any blunt trauma to the abdomen, the donor kidney site (Figure 36-12). Patients are discouraged from activities such as horseback or motorcycle riding and playing contact sports.

Recipients live with an ever-present awareness of potential organ rejection. The signs and symptoms are similar to those experienced by anyone advancing toward ESRD and renal replacement therapy. Patients also must remain alert to their increased risk for opportunistic infections secondary to immunosuppression management; less obviously, they have increased risk for malignancy after years of immunosuppressive therapy.

NURSING OUTCOMES AND GOALS FOR RENAL PATIENTS

The complex nature of ESRD and renal replacement therapies requires partnership between the patient and family, the nephrology providers, and when appropriate, the rehabilitation nurses (Kutner, 1998). As noted earlier, the greatest flaw in the ESRD program in the United States is the lack of planning for successful rehabilitation of a growing population of patients. When the program began, the patient's social worth, gainful employment, and contribution as a member of society were factors in the decision process for future care. Rehabilitation with return to independence and active community participation set treatment goals. When the federal government passed PL92-603, ensuring dialysis or kidney transplant, the nephrology community rejoiced at being relieved of the rationing of a then scarce resource. The anticipation in the early 1970s was sound medical assessment and evaluation to ensure the appropriate initiation and withdrawal of renal replacement therapies. Although rehabilitation remained a concern, funds were directed to enhance opportunities for patients to meet expected outcomes. Within a few years, after it became evident that the idealistic goals would not be met, funding became less abundant. Rehabilitation nurses and counselors were eliminated. Nephrology nurses

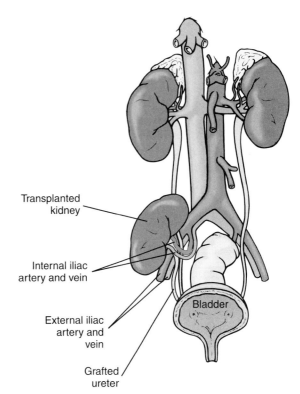

Figure 36-12 Surgical placement of transplanted kidney. (From Lewis, S. L., Collier, I. C., Heitkemper, M. M., & Dirksen, S. R. [2000]. *Medical-surgical nursing: Assessment and management of clinical problems* [5th ed.]. St. Louis, MO: Mosby.)

have largely been replaced with unlicensed assistive personnel who function as dialysis technicians. Many nephrologists retired or left the field, and fewer new physicians select nephrology as a career path. Finally, the patients with ESRD are older, sicker, more dependent, and often less involved in age-appropriate activities. Lately, there has been a renewed interest in and programs directed at patient outcomes from groups like the National Kidney Foundation and the American Association of Kidney Patients.

In summary, outcomes for the patient with renal disease are within biochemical, cognitive, and affective domains. Biochemical goals are to remain in complete fluid, electrolytes, and acid-base balance. Essentially the body's internal milieu is maintained within the limits of established norms for all plasma and tissue components. Cognitively patients must comprehend the disease process, prescribed regimen, potential complications of the disease and/or dialytic therapy, and health promotion and resources. Affective goals are to develop effective coping skills and therapy adherence, family normalization, and personal quality of life. When the disease process and treatment result in a highly compromised quality of life, the patient and family goals shift to palliative care and a comfortable death with dignity. Patients, families, and providers must participate in a coordinated effort toward individualized goals for unique needs of the person.

The success in achieving these expected outcomes rests on the following three steps:

1. Establish practices of appropriate initiation and withdrawal of dialysis based on weighing benefits versus burdens to the patient and family.
2. Reinstitute appropriate levels of funding and professional manpower (i.e., primary care physicians, nephrologists, nephrology nurse practitioners, nephrology nurses, renal dietitians, social workers, and rehabilitation and home health care nurses).
3. Enhance efforts to promote patients' self-care and independence with their full participation in shared decision making and health care planning. Patients with ESRD must identify resources in the community and develop a network and system for support. Rehabilitation nurse advocates can address these issues and facilitate partnership between the local community and the family.

Case Study

For several years Mr. Stone, 57, has been dialyzed in the evenings at a chronic patient clinic. He was employed as an accountant for a large corporation, so he would drive to the clinic after working an 8- to 10-hour day. Although dialyzing in the evening allowed him time to relax, read the newspaper, or watch television, it was extremely fatiguing for him to drive home after receiving his treatments. In addition, his diet suffered, because he would pick up a fast-food meal on his way to the clinic. His body stature of 6 feet 4 inches and 180 pounds precluded him from being a good candidate for peritoneal dialysis. The routine thrice weekly hemodialysis treatments were minimally adequate to meet his physiological needs, anemia control, calcium and phosphorus balance, and removal of uremic toxins. However, his nurse practitioner and nephrologists clearly realized there would be a clinical benefit to his receiving more frequent dialysis. Years earlier he had done well with a kidney transplant, but eventually it failed. After several months of encouragement, he finally agreed to transfer to a local home hemodialysis (HHD) training program for self-care training.

During a 6-week HHD training program Mr. Stone learned to set up his machine, troubleshoot various machine alarm situations, cannulate his arteriovenous fistula, document his medical record, safely terminate his treatment, and clean and disinfect his machine at the end of treatment. With assistance from his wife, he was a successful graduate of the HHD program. The home health care nurses and biomedical technician arranged for a few water, electrical, and plumbing adjustments in his home, plus they organized a place in his home for him to have HHD. Sterile supplies were delivered to his home monthly. He thoroughly enjoyed and benefited from more time with his family and decreased fatigue and stress related to driving home after dialysis late in the evening. With the comfort of home cooking, his diet has improved. After a couple of weeks of home support from nurses he is once again independent, and he has been able to continue his full-time career. Table 36-4 provides NIC and NOC information for Mr. Stone.

Mr. Stone has been on HHD for over 4 years. With the flexibility of HHD he generally dialyzes 4 or 5 times per week for varying lengths of treatment. His blood pressure, fluid status, anemia, bone disease, and emotional status are within normal limits without the necessity of expensive medication regimens. The quality of time spent with his family has enriched their relationships, and his wife is not only his marriage partner, but also his dialysis partner. He has not been hospitalized for several years. However, he has required periodic assistance from home health care nurses for glucose monitoring, treatment of skin infections, and a fractured tibia secondary to a fall on ice. He is a model patient who has demonstrated successful rehabilitation, despite the inherent problems related to CKD.

CRITICAL THINKING QUESTIONS

1. Mr. Stone has been asked to represent his company at a national sales meeting for a week. His wife will be joining him. What considerations can the rehabilitation nurse assist him with in arranging for his planned trip, because he will be taking his dialysis machine with him?
2. Mr. Stone's wife, and dialysis partner, is planning a visit to their daughter's house to help her care for the grandchildren for a week. Mr. Stone is unable to go this time because of his work, but he will need a dialysis partner to continue his home treatment. Is there a way for the rehabilitation nurse to coordinate his home health care for the week?
3. The winter has been rough, and Mr. Stone fell on the ice and sustained a closed fracture of his left tibia. How can the rehabilitation nurse assist with his home treatment?
4. Mr. Stone was fortunate, and he received a kidney transplant. He is now home doing well, but there is always the possibility of needing dialysis again in the future. What home considerations should be made for safe storage of his dialysis supplies for a few months, and how can the rehabilitation nurse assist him with his transplant medication regimen?

Case Study—cont'd

TABLE 36-4 Nursing Interventions and Outcomes Applicable to Mr. Stone (CKD) NIC/NOC

Nursing Interventions	*Nursing Outcomes*
Acid-base management: metabolic acidosis	Electrolyte and acid/base balance
Electrolyte management	
Electrolyte management: hyperkalemia	
Electrolyte management: hyperphosphatemia	
Fluid/electrolyte management	
Fluid management	Fluid balance
Dialysis access maintenance	Hemodialysis access
Hemodialysis therapy	Kidney function
	Patient satisfaction: physical care
	Activity tolerance
Environmental management: home preparation	Patient satisfaction: physical environment
Environmental management	Family physical environment
Home maintenance assistance	
Nutritional management	Nutritional status
Nutritional counseling	Nutritional status: energy
	Nutritional status: nutrient intake
Health care information exchange	Knowledge: health resources
Health education	Knowledge: health promotion
Anticipatory guidance	
Learning facilitation	
Decision making	Decision making
Family integrity promotion	Family normalization
Family support	
Self care assistance	Self care status

REFERENCES

Alexander, S. (1962). They decide who lives, who dies. *Life Magazine, 9*, 102-125.

Bowe, D., & Ammel, D. (2005). Using CQI strategies to improve and simplify IV iron and anemia management: A dialysis facility's experience. *Nephrology Nursing Journal, 32*(4), 535-543.

Burton, B., & Hirshman, G. (1976). Demographic analysis: End stage renal disease and its treatment in the United States. *Journal of Dialysis, 1*(2), 47-51.

Clinical practice guidelines for hemodialysis adequacy and peritoneal adequacy. (1997). *American Journal of Kidney Diseases, 30*(3 Suppl. 2), S15-S66.

Clinical practice guidelines for vascular access and anemia of chronic renal failure. (1997). *American Journal of Kidney Diseases, 30*(4 Suppl. 3), S150-S191.

Colangelo, R., Stillman, M., Kessler-Fogil, D., & Kessler-Hartnett, D. (1997). *Rehabilitation Nursing, 22*(6), 288-292, 302.

Dochterman, J. M., & Bulechek, G. M. (2004). *Nursing interventions classification (NIC)* (4th ed.). St. Louis, MO: Mosby.

Evans, R., Blagg, C., & Bryan, F. (1981). Implications for health care policy. *Journal of the American Medical Association, 245*(5), 487-492.

Fox, R., & Swazey, J. (1974). *The courage to fail: A social view of organ transplantation and dialysis.* Chicago: University of Chicago Press.

Gordon, M. (2000). *Manual of nursing diagnosis* (9th ed.). St. Louis, MO: Mosby.

Iglehart, J. (1993). Health policy report: The end stage renal disease program. *New England Journal of Medicine, 328*(5), 366-371.

Karmiel, J. (1996). The easy bike program: An exercise during dialysis program. *Topics in Clinical Nutrition, 12*(1), 74-78.

Kutner, N. (1998). Rehabilitation of the renal patient. In J. Parker (Ed.), *Contemporary nephrology nursing* (pp. 405-431). Pitman, NJ: AJ Jannetti.

Lancaster, L. (2001). *ANNA core curriculum for nephrology nursing* (4th ed.). Pitman, NJ: AJ Jannetti.

Lobley, L. (2001). Using nursing diagnosis to achieve desired outcomes for hemodialysis clients. *Advances in Renal Replacement Therapy, 4*(2), 112-124.

Mathers, T. (1998). The geriatric patient. In J. Parker (Ed.), *Contemporary nephrology nursing* (pp. 481-513). Pitman, NJ: AJ Jannetti.

Maxwell, J., & Sapolsky, H. (1987, June). The first DRG: Lessons from the end stage renal disease program for the prospective payment system. *Contemporary Dialysis & Nephrology*, 26-34.

McCormick, T. (1993). Ethical issues in caring for patients wit renal failure. *American Nephrology Nurses Association Journal, 20*(5), 549-555.

Moorhead, S., Johnson, M., & Maas, M. (Eds.). (2004). *Nursing outcomes classification (NOC)* (3rd ed.). St. Louis, MO: Mosby.

Pianta, T., & Kutner, N. (1999). Improving physical functioning in the elderly dialysis patient: Relevance of physical therapy. *American Nephrology Nurses Association Journal, 26*(1), 11-14.

Poggio, E., Wang, X., Greene, T., Van Lente, F., & Hall, P. (2005). Performance of the Modification of Diet in Renal Disease and Cockcroft-Gault equations in the estimation of GFR in health and in chronic kidney disease. *Journal of the American Society of Nephrology, 16*, 459-466.

Price, C. (1992, February). Is it time again for patient selection criteria? *Nephrology News & Issues*, 18-20.

RPA/ASN guidelines aimed at helping nephrologists make difficult decisions on initiation, withdrawing dialysis therapy. (2000, January). *Nephrology News & Issues*, 14-16.

Sabath, R. (1999). Exercise evaluation of children with end stage renal disease. *Advances in Renal Replacement Therapy, 6*(2), 189-194.

Schrag, W., Campbell, M., Ewert, J., Hartley, S., Niemann, J., & Ross, D. (1999). Multidisciplinary team renal rehabilitation: Interventions and outcomes. *Advances in Renal Replacement Therapy, 6*(3), 282-288.

Shared decision-making in the appropriate initiation of and withdrawal from dialysis, clinical practice guideline. (2000). Washington, DC: Renal Physicians Association and American Society of Nephrology.

Solomon, D. (1999). Focus on rehabilitation: Teamwork that works. *Advances in Renal Replacement Therapy, 6*(3), 278-281.

Szczepanik, M. (1995). Assessment and selection considerations: ESRD patient materials and media. *Advances in Renal Replacement Therapy, 2*(3), 207-216.

U.S. Renal Data System. (2005). *2003 Annual data report.* Available from www.cms.hhs.gov/esrd.

Whelan, C., & Whelan, W. (1999, September/October). The management of hematuria and proteinuria in the adult primary care setting. *The American Journal for Nurse Practitioners,* 29-34.

Wilson, B. (1995). Promoting compliance: The patient-provider partnership. *Advances in Renal Replacement Therapy, 2*(3), 199-206.

Zawada, E. (1994). Indications for dialysis. In J. Daugirdas & T. Ing (Eds.), *Handbook of dialysis* (2nd ed., pp. 3-9). Boston: Little, Brown.

37

Cancer Rehabilitation

Patricia L. McCollom, MS, RN, CRRN, CDMS, CCM, CLC

Cancer is a group of diseases characterized by uncontrolled growth and spread of abnormal cells. The causes may be external, such as tobacco, chemicals, or radiation, or internal, such as hormones, inherited gene mutations, or immune conditions (American Cancer Society, 2007).

Cancer is the second most common cause of death in the United States, and an estimated 9.8 million persons have or have had the disease (American Cancer Society, 2005). The number of survivors increases annually because of advances in patient education, early detection, and new treatment and technology. Cancer is now considered a chronic condition, with associated functional, physical, emotional, and spiritual sequelae. The Association of Rehabilitation Nurses (ARN) and the Oncology Nurses Society (ONS) collaborated to develop the following statement published in February 2000 and revised in 2003 without change.

> The sequelae of cancer are best addressed through a comprehensive oncology rehabilitation program. The focus of the program must be collaborative and interdisciplinary, whether based in acute, sub-acute or home health care.
>
> It is the position of ARN and ONS that:
> - Oncology rehabilitation is part of quality cancer care, which is a right of all citizens.
> - Oncology rehabilitation is an option for all patients at any stage of cancer.
> - Oncology rehabilitation incorporates the individual with cancer and the family as fully informed partners and decision makers.
> - Oncology rehabilitation includes timely access to and reimbursement for a coordinated, comprehensive interdisciplinary approach.
> - Oncology rehabilitation is coordinated and delivered by competent rehabilitative cancer care providers.
> - Accountability and coordination of quality oncology rehabilitation care are best accomplished by registered nurses who have been educated and certified in oncology or rehabilitation specialties.

Collaboration by these professional organizations represents a foundation for advancement of rehabilitation care for patients with cancer.

CANCER TREATMENT BASICS

Surgical intervention in cancer treatment is designed to resect the tumor tissue from the space-occupying area. Tumor control surgery options include prophylactic procedures to remove tissue or organs susceptible to malignancy, breast conservation surgery for breast cancer, and highly complex surgical procedures for pancreatic, bowel, or brain cancer, including palliative procedures.

Adjuvant therapy such as chemotherapy or hormonal therapy has been demonstrated to improve longevity and quality of life for cancer patients. Using breast cancer as an example, tamoxifen has been used with promise. In one trial conducted by the National Surgical Adjuvant Breast and Bowel Project (NSABP), in a 5-year follow-up, women treated with chemotherapy and tamoxifen demonstrated a 91% disease-free survival and a 96% overall survival. Another new hormonal manipulation therapy is known as aromatase inhibitors. In initial 2005-2006 trials this family of drugs shows improved survival with fewer side effects.

Radiation is cancer treatment that uses ionizing radiation to deposit energy that injures or destroys cells in the area treated. Radiation damages normal cells as well; however, they are able to regenerate. Radiotherapy may be used to treat solid tumors or diseases of the blood-forming and lymphatic systems. Other treatments showing promise for cancer are angiogenesis inhibitors, immune-modulating drugs, targeted therapies, lasers, photodynamic therapy, cryotherapy, radiofrequency ablation, and vaccines.

CANCER AND REHABILITATION

With the prevalence of newly diagnosed and existing patients with cancer, it is apparent that rehabilitation interventions will play an increasing role in cancer care. The outcomes of rehabilitation/restorative care in cancer treatment are the following:

1. *Quality of life:* Improved clinical outcomes related to body image enhancement, bowel/bladder management, emotional support, family support, health education, mutual goal setting, pain management, self-care, and elimination.

2. *Service:* Improved process outcomes resulting in increased patient/family satisfaction, provider satisfaction, and payer understanding of the treatment plan.

3. *Cost management:* Improved functional abilities and perceived control by the patient results in decreased inpatient stays and improved response to treatment.

ISSUES IN CANCER TREATMENT

Medical treatment for cancer is continually changing as a result of research, clinical trials, and new discoveries. Recent research has contributed to outpatient chemotherapy, supportive therapy to address many symptoms, especially nausea and fatigue, and potential cures for various types of cancer.

Clinical Trials

Clinical trials represent research in which patients participate in the clinical evaluation of methods to prevent, diagnose, and treat cancer. Clinical trials are important in establishing safe levels of drugs for humans, determining whether a treatment influences a particular disease or symptom, and comparing current standards of care with new protocols to improve patient outcomes. Clinical trials represent the current methodology for monitoring and comparing treatment protocols for cancer care and treatment. It is through clinical trials that objective evaluations of new treatment can be completed. Institutions participating in clinical trials must adhere to rigid guidelines established by the Food and Drug Administration (FDA) and the Office of Protection from Research Risk (OPRR). Further, all clinical trials must be approved and maintain standards as established by institutional review boards. Patients are closely monitored, and reports of patient responses are submitted to the FDA for evaluation of safety and treatment efficacy.

Screening trials examine options for early diagnosis for cancer. Prevention trials research new approaches, such as diet, supplements, vitamins, or other medication, with the aim of lowering the risk of development of specific types of cancer (National Cancer Institute, 2003).

Treatment trials actually test new drugs, surgical intervention, or radiation therapy. Quality-of-life trials study methods to improve comfort and quality of life for cancer patients (Canadian Cancer Society, 2005).

Reimbursement

The goal of oncology care is to provide timely, appropriate, and cost-effective treatment and care to patients diagnosed with cancer (ARN, 2003). In the world of changing health care paradigms, the rules for reimbursement under managed care may represent a major issue in cancer treatment.

Communication with payers to approve cancer treatment becomes a critical component of achieving the oncology care goals. Barriers to effective communication may be identified in two sectors. First, oncology providers often have limited knowledge of the types of health plans and their legal impact on care. The providers may have little understanding of the

plan's contractual financial agreements or requirements and may have difficulty articulating the treatment plan to the payer. Conversely, the payer may have little clinical knowledge about the needs and treatment of patients with cancer. The payer also may have difficulty translating the language of cancer care into the language of managed care.

Recommendations for resolution of reimbursement issues for cancer care by providers are as follows:

- Obtain preauthorization for care as outlined in the treatment plan by submitting requests in writing, outlining expected outcomes.
- Supply a rationale for treatment, specifying objective information to support requested procedures and protocols. Evidence-based practice guidelines are valuable tools in developing a rationale for treatment.
- Provide a detailed treatment plan.
- Know the payer's appeal process after denial of authorization.

Reimbursement conflicts are a direct result of external efforts to control patient care costs. Approval/denial issues are at the heart of growing litigation in health care. Improved communication, promoting collaboration, may be the single tool for resolution of these issues.

GOALS FOR CANCER REHABILITATION

Treatment goals for cancer rehabilitation are collaboration, communication, coordination of care, patient education, consistency of information across the continuum, and support for the patient/family unit. Rehabilitation philosophy promotes these treatment goals. Cancer survivors must deal with disability and functional impairment just as general rehabilitation patients do (Beck, 2003).

Psychosocial support is one outcome of the treatment goals. Research of the literature demonstrates that cancer care results in decreased physiological, psychological, and social functioning, which develops into severe distress for the patient and caregivers. Treatment plans for patients with cancer must address these issues, from a rehabilitation perspective, to achieve outcomes of increased function and positive health change.

It is interesting to note that both specialty nursing practices of oncology and rehabilitation identified "energy management" as a core intervention. Rehabilitation nurses noted the need for body image enhancement and specified many interventions directed at patient empowerment. Because of these interventions, as identified by practitioners, nursing activities in this chapter will focus upon fatigue and body image enhancement. The principles of rehabilitation nursing, described throughout this text and directed toward patient empowerment, should be applied in care delivery for patients with cancer.

FATIGUE

The feeling cannot even be described! It is as if all of life is in slow motion—no even worse—still frames, connected to one another and going on around me, not a part of me. Sounds are processed in syllables, not words. And, oh the effort to even move across the room. . . . I would have chemotherapy on Fridays. Saturday the slowness would begin and by the afternoon, sleep was my only refuge. I would sleep, often without turning for hours. Some weeks I would sleep until Tuesday mornings, only getting out of bed to go to the bathroom—and of course to drink the gallons of fluid to help wash the poison from my soul.

These are the words of a breast cancer patient sharing the response she had to chemotherapy. Fatigue is defined as "an overwhelming sustained sense of exhaustion and decreased capacity for physical and mental work at usual levels" (Johnson et al., 2001). Fatigue is one of the most prevalent complications for patients with cancer and frequently influences quality of life and outcomes of treatment. Although the etiology of fatigue is not understood, multiple variables contribute to fatigue in patients with cancer. Both chemotherapy and radiation therapy are known to contribute to fatigue. Medications prescribed to treat various symptoms, such as pain or nausea, may have the side effect of fatigue. Physiological factors include anemia, metabolic disturbances, and nutritional deficits. The patient with cancer may be experiencing depression, lack of sleep, fear, and stress. As these factors combine, the human body responds with a retreat to a state of rest. Cancer rehabilitation can be a component of management of fatigue because it assists the patient with altering activities of daily living through use of energy conservation (Beck, 2003).

Assessment of Fatigue

In order to specify appropriate nursing interventions, a comprehensive nursing assessment must be completed. Understanding of the cancer diagnosis and treatment plan is critical for the nurse as a basis for assessment of fatigue.

Nursing assessment of fatigue must rely on the patient's self-report. It is important to ask the patient his or her definition of fatigue. Words such as exhaustion, lethargy, tiredness, or lack of energy are most frequently used to describe fatigue. Symptoms may vary, and each patient's perception of fatigue is unique.

When the presence of fatigue has been stated by the patient, an in-depth approach to gather information is needed. Questions must be directed to determining the onset, duration, and patterns of fatigue. The nurse must inquire regarding methods used to alleviate fatigue or factors that exacerbate the fatigue experience.

Because fatigue has a major impact upon quality of life, assessment includes gathering information about how the fatigue is affecting physical, emotional, and mental well-being. Questions may include the following:
- Do you have problems remembering?
- Are you able to complete projects start to finish?
- Are you involved in social situations?
- Do you feel sad or depressed?

To assess the physiological impact of fatigue, note anemia and hemoglobin and hematocrit levels. Review laboratory studies for metabolic changes and the chemotherapy or

BOX 37-1   Nursing Diagnosis: Fatigue

Nursing Interventions	Nursing Outcomes
Sleep enhancement	Hours of sleep documented
	Sleep patterns identified
	Sleep quality identified
	Sleep routine specified
	Feelings of rejuvenation after sleep
	Wakeful at appropriate times
	Energy maintained at consistent levels
Counseling/emotional support	Fear control
	Depression control
	Health beliefs clarified
	Uses relaxation techniques
	Remains productive
	Maintains a sense of purpose
Energy management	Performance of usual routine
	Rested appearance
	Concentration
	Exhaustion not present
	Lethargy not present
	Libido

Modified from Moorhead, S., Johnson, M., & Maas, M. (2004). *Nursing outcomes classification* (3rd ed.). St. Louis, MO: Mosby.

radiation treatment plan. Nutritional status may be assessed by monitoring weight and recording intake. The following are questions for the patient to assist in determining physiological impact:
- Are you able to participate in your usual daily activities?
- Describe your exercise program.
- How do you think fatigue is affecting your life?
- Describe your daily food intake.

Assessment of fatigue is imperative in order to define interventions to manage fatigue. Management of fatigue promotes the patient's ability to participate in the completion of healing and treatment.

Interventions for Fatigue

Once assessment is complete, specific interventions can be identified to assist the individual with managing fatigue. Interventions should address sleep and rest, depression, anxiety, and inactivity. Physiological interventions should address anemia, nutrition, infection, and pain (Box 37-1).

Fatigue associated with cancer may be seen before, during, and after treatment. Patients, in follow-up after treatment, report ongoing fatigue for months or longer. Rehabilitation nurses involved in providing care must be aware of this response to develop appropriate plans to assist survivors and promote quality of life.

BODY IMAGE

At first I could deal with the loss of my breast. But my hair . . . that was my dignity! For the year I was bald, I cried every time I looked into the mirror. After a while, there were no more tears . . . (words of a cancer patient)

One of a human's earliest self-states to evolve is that of the body image concept. This concept involves the individual's perception of his or her physique, body symmetry, boundaries of the body, agility, and the aesthetics of the total appearance. Our sense of body image is acquired from verbal and nonverbal input from the environment. Any change in the perception of one's body image results in significant impact on emotional health.

Assessment of Disturbed Body Image

Individuals with the diagnosis of cancer may have a change in appearance or loss or limits of a body part. The result could be negative feelings or perceptions about the changes, which may impact response to treatment and quality of life.

Nurses again must rely upon self-report from the patient. Nurses must be alert to the patient's verbalizations regarding the change in body structure or feelings of fear of rejection or the reaction of others. Patients may repeat negative responses to body changes or dwell on past appearance.

During assessment the following questions may provide data to formulate a nursing diagnosis of *disturbed body image:*

* What do you see as the changes in your body?
* Are there lifestyle changes you are experiencing since your diagnosis?
* Do you continue your usual social activities?

Other cues the rehabilitation nurse may note include the patient's body language. Is the body part hidden or overexposed? Does the patient touch or decline to look at the changed body part?

Management of response to body image change is critical to promoting quality of life and preventing long-term emotional complications for the patient. It is through assessment of response to body image change that a clear plan for interventions may be identified.

Interventions for Disturbed Body Image

Body image enhancement is defined as improving a patient's conscious and unconscious perceptions and attitudes toward his or her body (McCloskey, Dochterman & Butechek, 2004). In dealing with implementation of interventions the nurse may function as a counselor to promote effective coping behaviors and to assist the patient/family with constructing a positive attitude toward treatment and ongoing requirements for care. Box 37-2 identifies nursing interventions and correlating outcomes.

It may require months or years for a patient to become adjusted to an altered body image and for associated problems to resolve. Support groups for patients, family members, and friends are active in most community settings and can be an important adjunct in implementing interventions to promote positive outcomes.

BOX 37-2 Nursing Interventions and Outcomes for Disturbed

Nursing Interventions	Nursing Outcomes
Body image enhancement	Indicators: • Positive perception of own appearance and body functions • Congruence between body perception and reality • Description of affected body part • Willingness to touch affected body part • Satisfaction with body appearance • Satisfaction with body function • Adjustment to change in appearance • Willingness to use strategies to enhance appearance and function

Modified from Gordon, M. (2000). *Manual of nursing diagnosis* (9th ed.). St. Louis, MO: Mosby.

SUMMARY

With improved outcomes for individuals with cancer, this medical diagnosis has now been identified as a chronic and/or disabling condition. Furthermore, an individual with a disability may have a dual diagnosis of a cancer. Patients who are expected to improve following diagnosis and treatment for cancer may require therapeutic and preventative interventions, adaptive equipment, or assistive devices common in rehabilitation settings. Patients seeking oncology rehabilitation include those with breast or bone reconstruction, grafts, amputations, surgical removal of muscle or tissues, sectioning or removal of functional parts, altered sensory function, or chronic pain.

Oncology rehabilitation may be preventative, restorative, supportive, or palliative. Patients with cancer have clear need for the rehabilitation process, which addresses a health-oriented approach to promote maximum functioning. In dealing with oncology in rehabilitation the nurse and other team members, patient, and family constitute a sociocultural, psychoemotional, holistically interactive unit dedicated to identifying and mobilizing a patient's internal and external coping resources. Rehabilitation outcomes improve when a patient has an active support system and professional support for appropriate referrals and care. Box 37-3 lists contact information for some of the leading cancer support organizations in the world.

BOX 37-3 Nurse/Patient Resources

American Association for Cancer Education (AACE)
P.O. Box 601
Snellville, GA 30278-0601
http://rpci.med.buffalo.edu/departments/education/aace2.html

American Cancer Society
1599 Clifton Road NE
Atlanta, GA 30329
404-320-3333
http://www.cancer.org

American Institute of Cancer Research
1759 R Street NW
Washington, DC 20009
202-328-7744; 800-843-8114
Fax: 202-328-7226
http://www.aicr.org

American Society of Clinical Oncology (ASCO)
435 North Michigan Avenue, Suite 1717
Chicago, IL 60611
312-644-0828

Association of Community Cancer Centers (ACCC)
11600 Nebel Street, Suite 201
Rockville, MD 20852
301-984-9496

Canadian Cancer Society
10 Alcorn Avenue, Suite 200
Toronto, Canada M4V 1E4
Canada
416-961-7223
http://www.cancer.ca

Cancer Archives
http://cure.medinfo.org/lists/cancer/index.html

Cancer Care, Inc.
1180 Avenue of the Americas
New York, NY 10036
800-813-HOPE

Cancer Federation, Inc.
21250 Box Spring Road
Morena Valley, CA 92388
714-682-7989

Cancer Guide
http://cancerguide.org/

Cancer Hotline
800-525-3777; 800-638-6070 (Alaska); 800-636-5700
   (District of Columbia)
808-524-1234 (Hawaii, call collect)

Cancer Information Service (CIS)
NIH Building 32, Room 10A 24
Bethesda, MD 20892
1-800-4-CANCER; 1-800-638-6070 (Alaska)
808-524-1234 (Hawaii; in Oahu, dial direct; call collect from
   neighboring islands)

Cancer News on the Net
http://www.cancernews.com

International Society of Nurses in Cancer Care
Mulberry House, The Royal Marsden Hospital
Fulham Road
London SW3 6JJ
England
071-252-8171, ext. 2123

International Union Against Cancer
3 rue du Conseil General
1205 Geneva
Switzerland
http://www.uicc.ch/

Memorial Sloan-Kettering Cancer Center
1275 York Avenue
New York, NY 10021
212-639-2000
http://www.mskcc.org/

**National Cancer Institute—International Cancer
   Information Center**
(CancerNet and CancerFax)
Building 82, Room 123
Bethesda, MD 20892
800-4-CANCER; 301-496-4907
Fax: 301-402-0212
http://www.nci.nih.gov/

National Coalition for Cancer Survivorship (NCCS)
1010 Wayne Avenue, 5th Floor
Silver Spring, MD 20910
301-650-8868; 301-565-9670

National Foundation for Cancer Research
7315 Wisconsin Avenue, Suite 500-W
Bethesda, MD 20814
301-654-1250
Fax: 301-654-5824

OncoLink (cancer information site)
http://www.oncolink.upenn.edu

Oncology Nursing Society
501 Holiday Drive
Pittsburgh, PA 15220
412-921-7373
http://www.ons.org

Society of Gynecologic Oncologists
401 N. Michigan Avenue
Chicago, IL 60611
312-644-6610
http://www.sgo.org/

Case Study

Pamela Martin is a 61-year-old woman who was diagnosed with breast cancer in 1996. She underwent a modified radical mastectomy and a 6-month protocol of chemotherapy followed by 5 years of tamoxifen (Nolvadex). In 2004 she was diagnosed with breast cancer recurrence to the bones. She was prescribed letrozole (Femara) 2.5 mg daily and zoledronic acid (Zometa) 4 g IV monthly.

Ms. Martin began experiencing right hip pain during the summer of 2004. Thinking she was merely feeling effects of aging, she was devastated to learn of recurrence. As a self-employed consultant, her diagnosis impacted every facet of her life. Major symptoms were pain, impaired mobility, and sleep disturbance.

CRITICAL THINKING QUESTIONS

1. What are the potential side effects of medications that will have an impact on this woman's quality of life?
2. What are rehabilitation nursing interventions to address these side effects?
3. How will Ms. Martin's anxiety regarding recurrence affect the treatment plan?
4. What patient education information is critical to a long-term positive outcome in this case?
5. What referrals would be appropriate?

REFERENCES

American Cancer Society. (2005). *Cancer facts and figures, 2007.* Retrieved January 09, 2006, from http://www.cancer.org.

Association of Rehabilitation Nurses. (2003). *Position on rehabilitation of people with cancer.* Glenview, IL.

Beck, L. (2003). Cancer rehabilitation: Does it make a difference? *Rehabilitation Nursing, 28*(2), 42-47.

Canadian Cancer Society. (2005). *Definition of quality of life trials.* Retrieved January 09, 2006, from http://www.cancer.ca/ccs/internet/standard/0,3182,3172_372029_168816178_langId-en,00.

Gordon, M. (2000). *Manual of nursing diagnosis* (9th ed.). St. Louis, MO: Mosby.

Johnson, M., Bulechek, G., McCloskey, J., Dochterman, J., Maas, M., & Moorhead, S. (2001). *Nursing diagnosis, outcomes, and interventions NANDA, NOC, NIC linkages.* St. Louis, MO: Mosby.

National Cancer Institute. (2003). *Clinical trials.* Retrieved January 09, 2006, from http://www.cancer.gov/clinicaltrials.

North American Nursing Diagnosis Association. (2005). *Nursing Diagnosis: Definitions and classification (2005-2006).* Philadelphia, PA: Author.

Page numbers followed by b indicate boxes; f, figures; t, tables.

Joints
    assessing ROM of, 217-218
    contractures of. *See* Contractures, joint
    glenohumeral subluxation of, 402
    movements of, 393t
    principles for protecting, 414b
    in rheumatoid arthritis, 405f
    after spinal cord injury, 251
    structure and function of, 205, 392
    in therapeutic exercise, 221
Journal writing
    as complementary therapy, 78
    in coping process, 454
    in spiritual care, 601, 604
Judgement, impaired, 526
Juvenile rheumatoid arthritis (JRA), 395-396, 395t

K

Kaposi's sarcoma, 716f, 717
Katz rating scales, 217
Kegel exercises, 222, 355, 357, 357b
Keller, Helen, 485
Kennedy, Eunice, 34, 625
Kessler, Henry, 4
Kessler Rehabilitation Institute, 9
Kidney, 732-735, 732f, 733f
Kidney dialysis. *See* Renal dialysis.
Kidney disease. *See* Chronic kidney disease (CKD).
Kidney transplantation
    about, 742-743
    access to, 730-731, 731b
Kinesic therapy, 204
Kinesics of communication, 505
Kinesiology, 214t
Kinesthesia perception, 219
Kinesthetic learners, 64
Kinetic therapy, 272
King's Open Systems Framework and Theory of Goal
        Attainment, 17, 17f
Klein-Bell Scale, 217
Knee jerk reflex, 212, 218t
Knee-ankle-foot orthoses (KAFOs), 225t, 231
Knees, deformities of, 403, 404f
Knowledge deficit
    in cardiac rehabilitation, 682, 694t
    in communication deficits, 514t
    cultural competence on, 85t
    in HIV/AIDS prevention, 727
    in impaired nutritional status, 284
    in metabolic syndrome, 713t
    in neuromuscular disorders, 444t
    on sexual health, 570t, 579-580, 583
    on skin care, 270t
    on stroke process, 175t
Kohlberg's theory of moral development, 35

L

Laboratory data
    to assess skin integrity, 264
    for diabetes, 711
    for HIV/AIDS, 717
    for musculoskeletal disorders, 405-406
    in pulmonary rehabilitation, 311
    for wound infection, 274
Lactose intolerance, 378
Lambert, Jonathan, 484
Lane, Sir Arbuthnot, 369

Language
    development of, 499, 500t
    effective, 499
    high-level skills in, 507-510
    prosodia in, 504
Language barriers
    affecting learning process, 65
    in cardiac rehabilitation, 687
    FIM sheet on, 136f
    in reporting health status, 71
    supportive behaviors for, 516b, 518b
Language disorders
    in children, 503-504, 512
    developmental disability and, 618, 619
    terminology/definitions for, 501-502
    types of, 502-503
Language dysfunction, 501
Laryngeal hypophonia, 510
Larynx, 285-286, 287
Laser therapy, low-level, 80
Lateral positions, 223-224, 224f
Laughter, 78, 603
Lavage irrigation, pulsed, 276
Laws. *See* Legislation on rehabilitation; Regulations on
        rehabilitation.
Laxatives
    abuse/overuse of, 378, 386-387
    in bowel training program, 381, 382, 388
    dependency on, 379
    history of use of, 369
    types of, listed, 106-107t
"Lazarus phenomenon," 726
Lead poisoning. *See* Environmental factors.
Leadership, nursing, 125-127
Learning activities, 66, 66t
Learning process
    in cardiac rehabilitation, 687, 688t
    in patient education, 62-67
Learning readiness/style, 63-64
Learning theories, 59-61, 61b
Leave policies, 34
Leg cramps, nocturnal, 556
Legal issues in rehabilitation
    advocacy role and, 34
    in case management, 197
    case study on, 42-43b
    in conflict resolution, 37b
    in developmental disabilities, 625-626
    in nursing process, 40, 42-43
    in rehabilitation nursing, 38, 39-40
Legislation on rehabilitation, 39-40
    across life span, 7-9
    for developmentally disabled, 610-611, 623-624
    history/evolution of, 3, 5
    limits of, 184
    regarding special education, 643
    summaries of, 40b, 41b
    universal design in, 201
Leininger's Culture Care Theory, 19-20, 82-83
Leisure. *See* Recreational activities.
Length of stay (LOS)
    and community-based rehabilitation, 181
    in fiscal management, 130
    and patient safety, 162
Leprosy, 493
Leukotriene modifiers, 101-102t
Libido. *See* Sexual response.